Fourth Edition

Fundamentals for Sleep Professionals

Fundamentals for Sleep Professionals

Cynthia D. Mattice, MS, RPSGT, FAAST
Clinical Support Ambassador
Advanced Sleep Management
Frisco, Texas

Rita J. Brooks, MEd, REEG/EPT, RPSGT, FAAST
Director of Diagnostic Services
Capital Health System
Trenton, New Jersey

Teofilo L. Lee-Chiong, MD
Professor of Medicine
National Jewish Health
Denver, Colorado
Professor of Medicine
University of Colorado Denver
Aurora, Colorado
Chief Medical Liaison
Philips SRC
Murrysville, Pennsylvania

Wolters Kluwer
Philadelphia • Baltimore • New York • London
Buenos Aires • Hong Kong • Sydney • Tokyo

AAST | THE COMMUNITY FOR SLEEP-CARE PROFESSIONALS

Acquisitions Editor: James Sherman
Senior Development Editor: Ariel S. Winter
Editorial Coordinator: Varshaanaa SM
Marketing Manager: Kirsten Watrud
Production Project Manager: Kirstin Johnson
Manager, Graphic Arts & Design: Stephen Druding
Manufacturing Coordinator: Lisa Bowling
Prepress Vendor: S4Carlisle Publishing Services

Fourth edition

9 8 7 6 5 4 3 2 1

Printed in Mexico

Library of Congress Cataloging-in-Publication Data

ISBN-13: 978-1-975260-73-6

Library of Congress Control Number: 2026931268

shop.lww.com

QUADM0426

Preface

Imagine discovering this textbook for the first time a century from now—well worn, with its creased edges and pages filled with highlights and annotations, evident testaments of the countless occasions it had been read over the years. Or perhaps the book remains pristine, having never fulfilled the role it was intended for by the owner who acquired it.

A few thoughts immediately come to mind. What was the purpose of the authors and editors when they created this compendium? It was, after all, published during the first quarter of the 21st century, when the internet and artificial intelligence had already established themselves as vital sources of expertise and, regrettably, misinformation. Was it hubris, ignorance, or shortsightedness that led them to believe they could capture the fundamental concepts of the field of sleep health care in a single collection? Did the authors and editors seriously consider the pitfalls as well as the dangers of such an assumption? You wonder how much of the materials would have stood the test of time and remained relevant a year, a decade, or a century hence. Finally, you ask yourself if there were unintended negative consequences of such an endeavor—that by promoting best practices based on evidence or consensus, they had fossilized the discipline into standardized policies and procedures that failed to address the unique needs, resources, experiences, and expectations of the diverse patients and communities that they served.

As you kept reading, you start to identify several of the themes that must have guided the authors and editors in their work. You discern that there was a firm belief in interconnectedness—that each person's actions, decisions, plans, and behavior have an impact both on another individual and on the global human society. There was also an appreciation of the multiplicity of solutions to health-related questions that were enabled by ongoing advances in science, technology, and advocacy, and a commitment to knowledge creation and lifelong learning. These aspirations demanded continuous internal and external dialogues by sleep health care professionals.

You may, then, recognize the true intent of the authors and editors, that is, they merely wished to ensure that these conversations continue. They wrote *to* future generations of sleep health care professionals by sharing their achievements, limitations, hopes, and anxieties. They wrote *about* the future of sleep health care by reestablishing its foundations in the principles of patient respect and autonomy, equitable access to care, and environmental sustainability and healing. And lastly, they wrote *for* the future of sleep health care by reaffirming their responsibilities in enhancing the well-being of all human beings and of the planet.

We hope that the future you, in reading this book, might consider that the authors and editors have achieved their goal.

Cynthia D. Mattice
Rita J. Brooks
Teofilo L. Lee-Chiong

Acknowledgments and Dedication

The editors extend appreciation and thanks to all the authors who contributed chapters to this edition and the associate editors who dedicated significant time to review and edit many of the chapters, namely, Chad Eiken, Elizabeth Y. Wiesemann, and Carlos Teixeira.

We also thank Ariel S. Winter, senior development editor at Wolters Kluwer, and the AAST Board of Directors for their untiring assistance and counsel throughout the process.

Finally, this textbook would not have been possible without the support of the following individuals—it is to them that we dedicate this fourth edition of *Fundamentals for Sleep Professionals:*

Ed Mattice, Keely Mattice, Lucy Gordon and Elly Gordon, Marc Brooks, Kiersten Brooks, Riley Brooks, Dolores Grace Zamudio, and Zoe Lee-Chiong.

Cynthia D. Mattice
Rita J. Brooks
Teofilo L. Lee-Chiong

Contributors

Fayçal Abdenbi, PhD
Scientific & Medical Affairs Liaison
Sleep & Respiratory Care
Philips
Suresnes, France

Lacey Adams, Associate of Arts, RPSGT, CCH
Clinical Solutions Specialist
Customer Success
EnsoData
Hoover, Alabama

Kevin Adley, RPSGT, CCSH
Regional Sales Manager
ZOLL Itamar
Glenview, Illinois

Debbie Akers, AS, RRT, RPSGT, FAAST
Polysomnographic Technologist
Scoring
Advanced Sleep Management
Virginia Beach, Virginia

Kevin Asp, CRT, RPSGT, FAAST
President
Sleep
SomnoSure
Richmond, Texas

Jon W. Atkinson, BS, RPSGT, FAAST
Sleep Technologist
Scoring
Advanced Sleep Management, Ohio Sleep Consulting and Recording Services
Lancaster, Ohio

Matthew J. Balog, DrPH, MBA, CCSH, RPSGT
Pediatric Clinical Sleep Educator
Pediatric Sleep Medicine
Advocate Children's Hospital
Park Ridge, Illinois

Angelica Benitez, BSc, RPSGT
Clinical Education Manager
Business Development
BMC Medical
Cali, Colombia

Lisa M. Bond, RPSGT, RST, FASST
Director of Scoring Services
Scoring
Advanced Sleep Management, LLC
Bryan, Texas

Rita J. Brooks, MEd, REEG/EPT, RPSGT, FAAST
Director of Diagnostic Services
Capital Health System
Trenton, New Jersey

Paul R. Carney, MD, FAES
Professor, Neurology and Pediatrics
Director, Pediatric Neurology and Epilepsy
Department of Neurology
University of North Carolina
Chapel Hill, North Carolina

Dottie Covey-Elleby, BS, RPSGT
Department Chair
Polysomnography
Fayetteville Technical Community College
Fayetteville, North Carolina

Rui M. de Sousa, BSc, RPSGT, FAAST, RST
Polysomnographic Technologist
Neurophysiology
Sunnybrook Health Sciences Centre
Toronto, Ontario, Canada

Tripat Deep Singh, MBBS, MD, RPSGT, RST, CCSH
Director
Sleep Medicine
Academy of Sleep Wake Science
Patiala, Punjab, India

Pamela DeYoung, BA, RPSGT
Clinical Research Supervisor II
Pulmonary Critical Care and Sleep Medicine
University of California San Diego
San Diego, California

Aleshia L. Dorst, RPSGT
Sleep Tech II
Sleep Lab
National Jewish Health Hospital
Denver, Colorado

Iain Duncan, BSc, MSc
Deputy Lead Sleep Physiologist
Sleep Disorders Centre
Queen Victoria Hospital, NHS Trust
East Grinstead, West Sussex, United Kingdom

Chad Eiken, MBA, RPSGT, CSSH
Director of Clinical Programs
ZOLL Itamar Medical
Minneapolis, Minnesota

Todd Eiken, RPSGT, FAAST
Vice President of Product Development
Dymedix Diagnostics, Inc.
Shoreview, Minnesota

J. Emerson Kerr III, BS, MBA, RRT, FAAST, RPSGT
Vice President
Market Development and Strategic Partnerships North America
Nox Medical
Alpharetta, Georgia

Lisa M. Endee, MPH, RT, RRT-SDS, RPSGT, FAARC
Clinical Associate Professor
Department of Respiratory Care
School of Health Professions
SHP Drowsy Driving Prevention Program
American Association for Sleep Technologists (AAST) Board of Directors
Long Island Regional Director, New York State Society for Respiratory Care (NYSSRC)
Chair, Education and Research Committee, NYSSRC
Co-Chair, Membership Committee, NYSSRC
Stony Brook University
Stony Brook, New York

George P. Evans, RPSGT, BS
Manager
Capital Health Center for Sleep Medicine
Hamilton, New Jersey

Laree J. Fordyce, MS, RPSGT, RST, CCSH, FAAST, ESRS
Somnologist-Technologist
Clinical Sleep Educator
Sleep Medicine
Calgary, Alberta, Canada

Rachel Fordyce, BAS, RPSGT, CCSH, RST, Technologist-Somnologist (ESRS)
Sleep Technologist
Calgary, Alberta

Michael Furgason, RPSGT, RST, CCSH, FAAST
Manager
Sleep Disorders Center
Cleveland Clinic Martin
Palm City, Florida

James D. Geyer, MD, FAASM
Professor, Director Sleep Medicine, Medical Director of Behavioral Sleep Medicine
College of Community Health Sciences
The University of Alabama
Tuscaloosa, Alabama

Kelly W. Gladden, RRT, RPSGT, CCSH
Sleep Navigator
Sleep Center
Wellstar Health System
Roswell, Georgia

Kathryn Hansen, BS, CPC, CPMA
Executive Director
Society of Behavioral Sleep Medicine
Lexington, Kentucky

Monica M. Henderson, RN, RPSGT
Sleep Clinic Program Manager
UMC-Neurology and Sleep Medicine, College of Community Sciences
The University of Alabama
Tuscaloosa, Alabama

Daniel L. Herold, RPSGT, FAAST
Technology and Information Specialist
Centers For Sleep Medicine
Mayo clinic
Rochester, Minnesota

Richard Johannes Herstein, MD, MHA, MBA, BA
Founder and Clinical Director
Sleep Medicine
Stuart Sleep
Stuart, Florida

Auburne Hutchins, RPSGT, MHA, PhD
Director
Sleep Medicine
Texas Children's Hospital
Houston, Texas

Byron Jamerson, RPSGT, RST, CCSH, FAAST
US Clinical Manager
Sales Support
Nox Medical
Chattanooga, Tennessee

Danieliza Juniis-Johnson, MSE, LPN, RPSGT, RST
Clinical Coordinator
Sleep Center
Medbridge Healthcare
Valhalla, New York

Nila J. Kappely, RRT, RRT-SDS, RPSGT, CCSH, RPFT
Associate in Applied Science in Respiratory Care
Sleep Tech III & Sleep Educator
Mercy Sleep Center
Mercy Hospital Oklahoma City
Oklahoma City, Oklahoma

Amy Korn-Reavis, MBA, RRT, RPSGT, CCSH, FAAST
Scorer
Sleep Lab
Nemours Hospital
Lake Nona, Florida

Laura A. Linley, CRT, RPSGT
EVP Operations
Advanced Sleep Management LLC
Dallas, Texas

Su Jeong Linstrom, RPSGT, RST, BS
Clinical Manager of the Sleep Program
Children's Hospital Colorado
Aurora, Colorado

Darius Loghmanee, MD, FAAP, FAASM, DABIM
Advocate Children's Hospital
Park Ridge, Illinois

Elise A. Maher, BS, MA
Clinical Operations Manager
System Sleep Testing Centers
University Hospitals
Cleveland, Ohio

Gerald George Mannikarote, MBBS, MBA
Vice President
Executive Leadership
Medigy
Fort Worth, Texas

Jayme R. Matchinski, JD
Chief Legal Officer
Dedicated Sleep, LLC
Chicago, Illinois

Cynthia D. Mattice, MS, RPSGT, FAAST
Clinical Support Ambassador
Scoring Department
Advanced Sleep Management
Norman, Oklahoma

Laura McFarland, BS, RRT-SOS, RPSGT
Polysomnographic Technologist
Pulmonology and Sleep
Allina Health
Minneapolis, Minnesota

Robert Miller, RPSGT
Senior Vice President of Commercial Strategy
Daybreak
Rockwell, North Carolina

Amanda Moore, RPSGT, AAS Polysomnography, BS
Program Director/Instructor
Polysomnography and Neurodiagnostic Technology
Alvin College
Alvin, Texas

Jessica Moore, BS, RPSGT
Account Executive
Sales
EnsoData
Charles Town, West Virginia

Angela P. Neal, RPSGT
Sleep Technologist
Mercy Sleep Center
Oklahoma City, Oklahoma

Tiffany Nealy, MD
Sleep Medicine Fellow Physician
Sleep Medicine
Macon & Joan Brock Virginia Health Sciences at Old Dominion University
Norfolk, Virginia

Keir Morrison Noe, RPSGT, RST, CCSH
Sleep Navigator
Sleep Services Admin
WellStar Healthcare
Austell, GA

Jennifer Parr-Christmas, CRT, RPSGT
DCH Sleep Center
Northport, Alabama

Regina Patrick, BA, RPSGT, RST
Freelance Medical Writer/Editor
Toledo, Ohio

Kevin Postol, DDS
Owner
Gateway Center for Sleep Apnea and TMJ Therapy
Twin Oaks, Missouri

Andrea Ramberg, MS, CCSH, RPSGT
Clinical Solutions Director
Customer Success
EnsoData
Harvard, Illinois

James A. Rehill, MBA, RPSGT
Cardiopulmonary
Legacy Mount Hood Medical Center
Gresham, Oregon

Jorge Rey, CCSH, RPSGT
Regional Sales Director
Huxley Medical
Baytown, Texas

Kimi Clark Rodahaffer, AAS, RPSGT, CCSH, FAAST
Senior Clinical Solutions Specialist
Customer Success
EnsoData
Denver, North Carolina

Jeremy James Roy, BS, CCSH, RPSGT
Director of Scoring and Physician Education
Clinical Services
Persante Healthcare, Inc
Mt. Laurel, New Jersey

Jordan E. Rusk, BS, RPSGT, CCSH, Pediatric Sleep Certificate
Program Director and Full Time Faculty
Polysomnography
Lone Star College- Kingwood
Kingwood, Texas

Christina Saulys, BA, RPSGT, ACRP-PM, FAAST
Vice President, Project Solutions
Clinilabs
Eatontown, New Jersey

Katherine M. Sharkey, MD, PhD
Professor
Psychiatry and Behavioral Medicine and Internal Medicine
Wake Forest University School of Medicine
Winston-Salem, North Carolina

Joshua Eric Shore, RPSGT, CSE
Clinical Sleep Specialist
Home Sleep Testing Division
ZOLL Itamar
St. Louis, Missouri

Johnathan Simpson, RPSGT
Operations Coordinator
Sleep
Northwestern Medicine
Chicago, Illinois

Patrick Sorenson, MA, RPSGT
Research Associate
Sleep and Neurodevelopment Services
The National Institute of Mental Health
Bethesda, Maryland

Christopher K. Speigner, BS, RPSGT, CCSH
Regional Sales Manager – Central US
NOX Medical, LLC
Waxahachie, Texas

Shanna Steven, RPSGT, R.EEGT
Lead Technologist
Sleep Lab
Kalispell, Montana

Stephen Tarnoczy, BSRT, RRT , RRT-SDS, RRT-NPS, RPSGT, CCSH , FAAST
Respiratory Therapist/PSG Technologist
Oklahoma City, Oklahoma

Carlos Teixeira, BSc, EST
International Sleep Disorder Specialist
Assistant Professor EEG and Sleep
Instituto Politécnico de Saúde do Norte
Escola Superior de Saúde do Vale do Ave (ESSVA)
Vila Nova de Famalicão, Portugal

Jatin Tekchandani, MSBME, R. EEG T., RPSGT
Chief Elevator Operator
Intellimedics International
Kingwood, Texas

Melinda O. Trimble, RPSGT
Retired
Protem, Missouri

Kimberly A. Trotter, MA, RPSGT, FAAST
Manager
Sleep Lab
UCSF Benioff Children's Hospital
Oakland, California

Robert N. Turner, RPSGT
MS Community Counseling
Clinical Supervisor
Sleep Disorders Center
HCA HealthONE Rose Medical Center
Denver, Colorado

Matthew Uhles, MS, RPSGT, RST
Chief Operating Officer
Clayton Sleep Institute/Saint Louis University
Kirkwood, Missouri

Edwin M. Valladares, MS, RPSGT
Adjunct Professor in Biomedical Engineering & Healthcare Administration
Oral Roberts University
College of Science and Engineering and College of Health Sciences
Tulsa, Oklahoma

Sarah Wahhab, RPSGT
Director, Clinical Outreach
Sleep Services
Advanced Sleep Management
Melissa, Texas

Kristina Weaver, RPSGT
Executive Director Population Health and Care Transitions
Population Health and Sleep Center
Parrish Healthcare
Titusville, Florida

Jill West, BA, RPSGT, CCSH
Sleep Clinical Specialist
Department of Education
Cadwell Industries, Inc
Ogden, Utah

Chad Whittlef, BSc, PgCert
Senior Sleep Physiologist
Sleep Disorders Centre
Guy's & St Thomas' Hospital
London, United Kingdom

Robyn V. Woidtke, MSN Ed, RN, CCSH, RPSGT, FAAST
Principal
RVW Clinical Consulting
Castro Valley, California

David F. Wolfe, MSEd, RRT-SDS, RPSGT, FAAST
Educator
Education and Professional Development
Crouse Health
Syracuse, New York

Associate Editors

Chad Eiken, MBA, RPSGT, CSSH
Director of Clinical Programs
ZOLL Itamar Medical
Minneapolis, Minnesota

Carlos Teixeira, BSc, EST
International Sleep Disorder Specialist
Assistant Professor EEG and Sleep
Instituto Politécnico de Saúde do Norte
Escola Superior de Saúde do Vale do Ave (ESSVA)

Elizabeth Y. Wiesemann, MA, RPSGT, CCSH
Supervisor
NYU Sleep Disorders Center
Garden City, New York
Adjunct Instructor
Hudson Valley Community College
Troy, New York

Contents

Appendices and Glossary are available online as a supplement.

Introduction

The Continuing Evolution of Sleep Medicine

JON W. ATKINSON, RITA J. BROOKS, CYNTHIA D. MATTICE, TRIPAT DEEP SINGH, KEVIN POSTOL, J. EMERSON KERR III, AND LAREE J. FORDYCE

As the field of sleep medicine has evolved, so too has the role of the sleep professional—adapting to meet the changing needs of physicians, fellow clinicians, and, most importantly, patients. While technology has brought greater automation, the need for hands-on, compassionate care remains vital. At the heart of this care is a belief we hold firmly: people take care of people. Within this ecosystem, the expertise of the sleep professional is essential.

Sleep professionals serve not only as skilled technicians but also as key patient educators. Their work is grounded in technical proficiency, clinical standards, and a deep understanding of sleep science and patient care. *Fundamentals for Sleep Professionals*, published by Lippincott in collaboration with the American Association of Sleep Technologists (AAST), was created to support this vital role with clarity, depth, and purpose.

Originally released in 2007, the original textbook, *Fundamentals of Sleep Technology*, was developed through a close partnership between AAST, editorial team, and Lippincott Williams & Wilkins. The goal was to offer sleep professionals a trusted resource that could serve both as an introduction to the field and a reliable reference in daily practice.

For students entering the profession, it represents the standard of care. For those preparing for certification and registry, it provides critical exam support. And for experienced professionals, it remains a go-to guide for continuous learning and clinical excellence. Drawing on the insights of respected clinicians, educators, and leaders in the field, the textbook delivers a comprehensive overview of sleep physiology, disorders, diagnostics, and treatment. Case studies, review questions, and evidence-based guidelines throughout the text give readers the tools to connect theory to real-world application.

Over the course of our careers, we have seen sleep technology grow from a niche discipline to a vital component of modern health care. With this growth comes the need for a new generation of technologists—professionals who are not only technically skilled, but also clinically insightful, curious, and engaged. *Fundamentals for Sleep Professionals* is an indispensable resource in shaping these future leaders. Whether you are preparing for board exams, onboarding new staff, or revisiting core concepts, we invite you to use this textbook not only as a manual, but as a reflection of the high standards, passion, and purpose that define our profession.

Sleep technology has evolved rapidly in the last 50 years. Polysomnography (PSG) has transitioned from analog to digital machines, positive airway pressure (PAP) therapy was identified as a treatment for obstructive sleep apnea (OSA), and various advanced forms of PAP therapy and interfaces were introduced to treat sleep-disordered breathing (SDB). In the last decade with advancements in mobile phone technology, mobile apps and wearables are now marketed to monitor our health including sleep. The first professional bodies involved in the development of sleep medicine and sleep technology were established in the United States and Europe. In the past 20 years, additional professional bodies have formed, including in many countries, that are performing important work in the development of sleep medicine and technology. The development of sleep science, sleep medicine, and sleep technology has been codependent on advances in both recording and treatment technology.

Despite all the advances in sleep technology, the technologist must still possess a good working understanding of the basics of polysomnographic technology, including amplifiers, filters, sensitivities, expected frequency ranges of physiologic parameters, and troubleshooting. Today's acquisition technologist has high-quality snore sensors, pressure transducers, thermocouples and thermistors, respiratory effort sensors, and pulse oximeters as well as various types of electrocardiogram (EKG) and electroencephalogram (EEG) electrodes with many sleep centers using single use EEG electrodes. There are multiple vendors supplying these sensors as well as a variety of preparation materials and supplies needed to perform sleep studies.

Sleep medicine and technology and, for that matter, medicine in general, is in a constant state of flux; the future is certainly difficult to predict. Given the past and recent developments on multiple fronts, technology will continue to improve. Industry is in constant search of the "ultimate" PAP interface, with smaller and quieter flow generators and more potential "bells and whistles" to establish a better control of the marketplace. Computer equipment will improve with higher quality amplifiers, higher resolution monitors, faster processors to handle more information, and larger, cheaper storage devices. Software will become increasingly user-friendly.

Opportunities for technologists to specialize will become more abundant. The growth of sleep medicine will continue as patient volumes increase. Technology will continue to make sleep medicine more accessible across the world and will assist physicians and sleep professionals to improve the sleep of our patients. As the sleep medicine and technology fields continue to grow globally, we can anticipate better diagnostics and treatments for our patients throughout the world.

EVOLVING ROLES OF SLEEP PROFESSIONALS

Industry growth has provided opportunities for sales, marketing, and installation and training positions. Industry will continue to expand, and new technology will continue to develop with a continuing need for sleep technology professionals to fill multiple roles.

As the growth in sleep testing facilities continues, opportunities for traveling technologists and training consultants will be created. There are positions for sleep professional educators at community colleges and in stand-alone training programs. We are indeed no longer merely denizens of the night. We have become a diverse group of individuals with varying interests who have one thing in common: a passion for sleep. It is that passion that keeps sleep professionals involved in sleep medicine and technology whatever the capacity.

CMS reimbursement for portable, unattended polysomnography and actigraphy has led to significant growth in home sleep testing. Actigraphy is a very useful tool particularly for diagnosis and treatment of insomnia and circadian rhythm disorders.

SLEEP TECHNOLOGY: A GLOBAL PERSPECTIVE

The first professional bodies involved in the development of sleep medicine and sleep technology were established in the United States and Europe. In the past 20 years, additional professional bodies have formed including in many countries that are performing important work in the development of sleep medicine and technology.

MECHANISMS OF SLEEP AND WAKEFULNESS

Hans Berger, a German psychiatrist, discovered electroencephalography (EEG) in 1929 (1), which later led to the study of sleep states in humans and the discovery of rapid eye movement (REM) sleep (2). Newer techniques like genetic approaches, gene therapy, optogenetics, and chemogenetics and clustered regularly interspaced short palindromic repeats (CRISPR)-Cas now allow researchers to understand the finer details of sleep-wake regulation and are also assisting to better understand the causes and treatments of sleep disorders.

The genetic approach has improved understanding of two sleep disorders: narcolepsy and advanced sleep phase syndrome. Emmanuel Mignot found mutation in hypocretin receptor 2 inch canine narcolepsy using forward genetics, and Masashi Yanagisawa's group found narcoleptic symptoms in orexin knockout mouse (3). In advanced sleep phase syndrome, forward genetics revealed that individuals with this disorder have a mutation in the *hPer2* gene (4), and reverse genetics established that mice with this mutation also demonstrated a shorter period of sleep-activity cycle (5).

TECHNOLOGY AND SLEEP DIAGNOSTICS

Computer-Assisted Sleep Scoring and Interscorer Reliability

Manual scoring of sleep and associated events has been the standard worldwide, and interscorer reliability (ISR) is an important issue in quality control. The American Academy of Sleep Medicine (AASM) frequently revises the scoring manual, the latest manual, Version 3, being released in 2023.

Younes et al have highlighted that inattention errors and bias contribute little to interscorer variability (6); rather, the difference is due to equivocal epochs that can be assigned one or two sleep stages by trained technologists (6). They indicate digital information regarding key sleep staging variables (spindles, delta wave duration, and objective sleep depth) is needed to reduce scoring variability and that better training or refining the scoring rules is not going to improve ISR (6). Younes et al showed that providing digital information regarding key sleep staging variables (spindles, delta wave duration, and objective sleep depth) improved ISR (6). Younes et al also showed that manual scoring of NREM sleep stages is highly variable and unreliable among experienced sleep professionals (7). Technologists varied widely in scoring N1 and N3 sleep stages (7). The AASM also reported the lowest agreement in scoring of N1 and N3 sleep among different scorers globally in their ISR program (7). They suggested the use of automated analysis of slow-wave activity as a potential solution (7). Several computer-assisted sleep scoring systems have been validated against human scoring, which has not only improved interscorer variability but also shortened the time required to score one sleep study considerably. Recently, researchers in Singapore developed a real-time automatic sleep staging system that can be cloud based, allowing multiple users to perform real-time sleep staging at the same time (8). This system can score an entire night's sleep recording with an accuracy on par with expert human scorers but much faster (5 seconds compared with 30-60 minutes).

It requires considerable practice and knowledge to learn manual sleep staging. There are very few technologists trained in manual scoring of sleep stages in developing countries, which is a limiting factor in starting more sleep labs in these countries. Computer-assisted sleep scoring systems make scoring simple and may be very useful in extending the reach of sleep facilities to patients in developing countries.

Consumer Sleep Technologies

Consumer sleep technologies (CSTs) have become very popular within our society for self-monitoring sleep. They are primarily used for sleep induction, wake induction, self-guided sleep assessment, entertainment, social connection, information sharing, and sleep education. The primary delivery platforms for CSTs are:

- Mobile device platforms,
- Wearable platforms,
- Embedded platforms,
- Desktop or website platforms, and
- Accessory appliance platforms.

The manufacturers of these technologies update them at a rapid pace, and the medical community cannot keep up. By the time any study is published validating the technology, a new version of the technology has already been released.

A recent study reported that only 32.9% of sleep apps contained information supporting their claims, 15.8% included clinical input, and 13.2% contained links to sleep literature. Also, apps contained information on how sleep is affected by alcohol or drugs (23.7%), food, daily activities, and stress (13.2%). However, no guidelines or validation of data generated by CSTs shows how sleep is affected by different disease states and how to use the data to manage different disease states long term.

Technology is becoming an integral part of human lives. Whether we like it or not, patients will come to the clinic asking us to interpret the data from these devices. Instead of throwing the data away in light of no evidence, we should take a look at the data to see whether it makes any sense clinically. These technologies are at least engaging consumers and making them self-aware and interested in their own health.

Home Sleep Apnea Testing

Prevalence of OSA has increased in the US population and in recent years, there is a trend toward increased Home Sleep Apnea Testing (HSAT) use because the number of patients has increased and PSG being an expensive test is a big burden on public health systems. In Western societies where PSG and PAP treatments are reimbursed, economic analysis has found HSAT to be a more cost-effective test compared to PSG.

OSA in the Asian population is not different from that in Western societies. However, in most Asian countries (except Japan) where PSG and PAP treatments are not reimbursed by the public health system or private insurance companies, the high costs of PSG and PAP treatments impede the diagnostic and treatment process. The number of trained professionals in the field of sleep medicine and sleep technology is few in developing countries. Given the high burden of SDB in the Asian population, the high cost of PSG which is not reimbursed by public health systems or private insurance companies, and few trained professionals, there is a need for a simple, low-cost, and reliable test to diagnose patients with SDB in developing countries. HSAT and computer-assisted sleep scoring may play an important role in developing countries to extend services of sleep diagnostics to patients with SDB.

AASM guidelines for diagnostic testing of OSA in adult patients (9) recommend HSAT for diagnosing uncomplicated adult OSA patients with increased risk of moderate-to-severe OSA. If a single HSAT is negative, inconclusive, or technically inadequate, a PSG can be performed for the diagnosis of OSA. HSAT should not be used for the diagnosis of OSA in patients with significant cardiorespiratory disease, potential respiratory muscle weakness because of neuromuscular condition, awake hypoventilation or suspicion of sleep-related hypoventilation, chronic opioid medication use, and history of stroke or severe insomnia (9).

A large proportion of patients may be eligible for HSAT in developing countries where PSG and PAP therapies are not reimbursed. In selected OSA patients without comorbidities, HSAT followed by auto-PAP (APAP) treatment is as effective as a PSG–continuous positive airway pressure (CPAP) titration strategy and may be beneficial to many patients in developing countries. However, HSAT is not free of limitations. Some HSAT devices do not record body position, which makes it difficult to study positional OSA and recommend positional therapy. Most HSAT devices do not record sleep, but only total recording time (TRT). As a result, AHI may be underestimated with HSAT.

The AASM provides detailed guidelines for HSAT in the scoring manual, highlighting technical requirements and reporting parameters including scoring rules for respiratory events (3).

The AASM scoring manual defines the respiratory event index (3) as the number of apneas plus the number of hypopneas divided by monitoring time (not TST). Monitoring time is defined as TRT minus time patient was awake as assessed by asking the patient, upright body position, regularity of respiration, or actigraphy minus the time of artifact (3). This gives a close approximation to TST and a more reliable estimation of AHI.

Because HSAT does not record sleep and hence arousals cannot be scored, it may lead to underscoring of hypopneas that are not associated with desaturation but are associated with arousal. This limitation can be overcome by choosing an HSAT device that records sleep.

Central apneas are another challenge for this technology because snoring generally does not occur in patients with central apnea.

Global Sleep Medicine and Technology

In Europe, the European Sleep Research Society (ESRS) and other local sleep societies are leading the way in the development of sleep medicine and technology.

The World Sleep Society was formed in 2016 with the merger of the World Association of Sleep Medicine (WASM) and the World Sleep Federation (WSF). The official society website is www.worldsleepsociety.org. The society has four different types of individual membership options including full, regular, student, and technician memberships.

The journal *Sleep Medicine* is the official society journal. The society conducts World Sleep Day in the month of March every year. Recognition for those performing research and working in sleep medicine includes awards in different areas of sleep medicine and sleep research.

The World Sleep Congress is held every 2 years in one of the member countries across the globe.

SUMMARY

There have been many new developments in sleep diagnostics and technology, and new ways of doing things are emerging rapidly. Computer technology is rapidly becoming integrated in the practices of sleep medicine and technology. Telemedicine, HSAT, and computer-assisted technologies along with consumer devices that track sleep are mainstream practices today. Technology is making sleep medicine more accessible across the world and assisting physicians and sleep professionals to improve the sleep of our patients. These practices are growing rapidly, and many are being developed and utilized successfully across the globe where the cost of care for patients with sleep disorders has been prohibitive in the past. As the sleep medicine and technology fields continue to grow globally, we can anticipate better diagnostics and treatments for our patients throughout the world.

MAJOR TRENDS THAT WILL LIKELY IMPACT THE FIELD OF SLEEP HEALTH CARE: A DENTIST'S PERSPECTIVE

With an estimated 54 million Americans suffering from OSA (10)—and Healthy Sleep 2030 continuing to report that there is little to no detectable change in the proportion of adults with sleep apnea symptoms who are getting evaluated by a health care provider (11), wearables, artificial intelligence (AI) and other technologies have emerged and provide a significant opportunity to increase people's awareness of poor sleep. It will be up to the sleep community to ensure we have the infrastructure in place to discuss sleep health with our patients, help them easily navigate diagnosis and offer personalized treatment to ensure that patients are properly managed.

Precision medicine has been increasingly prioritized by both researchers and clinicians. It is certain that the trend of offering patients personalized treatment options for OSA will continue to evolve and impact the field for the better. As treatments for OSA continue to emerge and research supports their efficacy, patients will have more flexibility with treatment options (12). Given that most current treatments require patients to decide each night whether they are going to manage their OSA, it is imperative that patients choose a therapy they can tolerate. Oral appliance therapy provides a proven, effective option for patients who cannot tolerate PAP, are not interested or do not qualify for a surgical procedure, or do not want to take medication regularly. In the recent CHOICE trial, after 1 month of oral appliance therapy (OAT) and CPAP, patients were able to choose their therapy, alternating between the therapies as they wished. During the crossover phase, adherence was higher for OAT than CPAP. During the observation phase, most of the patients (55%) chose to use both therapies and of those who alternated therapies, 83% were highly adherent to therapy (13). This study reinforces the importance of patient autonomy in deciding which therapy to use for OSA—patients want more of a say in their treatment and will demand that health care providers listen to their needs.

Alongside this, advances in research and AI will help to better identify responders to the various OSA therapies, better informing the treatment options discussed with each patient. As larger sets of genomic, phenotypic, and demographic data are assessed, health care professionals will be able to more easily identify patients who are likely to respond to specific OSA therapies. This will allow us to provide personalized treatments that are more effective and have fewer adverse effects in a more time effective manner.

Another trend impacting the field of sleep health care is patients demanding convenience. Across the board, there is a significant workforce shortage in sleep medicine. Patients will continue to demand more accessible ways to be diagnosed and treated. There are not enough sleep physicians, qualified dentists (14), sleep professionals, behavioral sleep specialists, and other trained health care providers to ensure patients, regardless of their geographic location, have convenient access to screening, diagnosis, treatment, and appropriate managed care. Telehealth offers some remedy for this situation. The AASM recently released a position statement advocating for permanent access to telehealth for sleep medicine, citing that telehealth appointments have increased access to care for many patients (15).

This is the ideal time for interdisciplinary collaboration to provide effective, targeted therapy to patients. Embracing technological advances and expansion of providers is key. It is important that all sleep health care providers come together to ensure our models of care focus on delivering optimal patient care in a manner that is convenient, utilizes the most appropriate sleep health care provider, and delivers optimal patient care.

Sleep health care has always been an interdisciplinary field. In regard to OSA, a growing interest in the impact of sleep on overall quality of life and health, technological advances, and an increase in the treatment options offered by different providers, there is a great opportunity to expand treatment to the millions who need it, but doing so requires a balance of exploring areas where training of health care providers can increase access to care while recognizing the limitations of their training and expertise. Working in a collaborative, interdisciplinary fashion will ensure more patients get screened, diagnosed, and effectively treated with as few complications as possible.

REFERENCES

1. Dement W. History of sleep physiology and medicine. In: Kryger M, Roth T, Dement W, eds. *Principles and Practice of Sleep Medicine*. 4th ed. Elsevier; 2005.
2. Berger H. Hans Berger on the electroencephalogram of man: the fourteen original reports on the human electroencephalogram. *NervKrankh*. 1929;87:527.
3. Troester MM, Quan SF, Berry RB, et al; American Academy of Sleep Medicine. *The AASM Manual for the Scoring of Sleep and Associated Events: Rules, Terminology and Technical Specifications*. Version 3. American Academy of Sleep Medicine; 2023.
4. Vogel G. Studies in the psychophysiology of dreams, III: the dream of narcolepsy. *Arch Gen Psychiatr*. 1960;3: 421-428.
5. Rechtschaffen A, Wolpert E, Dement W, et al. Nocturnal sleep of narcoleptics. *Electroencephalogr Clin Neurophysiol*. 1963;15:599-609.
6. Younes M, Hanly PJ. Minimizing interrater variability in staging sleep by use of computer-derived features. *J Clin Sleep Med*. 2016;12(10):1347-1356.
7. Younes M, Raneri J, Hanly P. Staging sleep in polysomnograms: analysis of inter-scorer variability. *J Clin Sleep Med*. 2016;12(6):885-894.
8. Patanaik A, Ong JL, Gooley JJ, Ancoli-Israel S, Chee MWL. An end-to-end framework for real-time automatic sleep stage classification. *Sleep*. 2018;41(5): zsy041. doi:10.1093/sleep/zsy041
9. Kapur VK, Auckley DH, Chowdhuri S, et al. Clinical practice guideline for diagnostic testing for adult obstructive sleep apnea: an American Academy of Sleep Medicine clinical practice guideline. *J Clin Sleep Med*. 2017;13(3):479-504.
10. Benjafield AV, Ayas NT, Eastwood PR, et al. Estimation of the global prevalence and burden of obstructive sleep apnoea: a literature-based analysis. *Lancet Respir Med*. 2019;7(8):687-698.
11. U.S. Department of Health and Human Services. Healthy People 2030: sleep. Accessed May 6, 2025. https://odphp.health.gov/healthypeople/objectives-and-data/browse-objectives/sleep
12. Stewart GM, Tong BK, Cistulli PA. Precision medicine approaches in obstructive sleep apnoea: the role of dentist-sleep physician partnerships. *Aust Dent J*. 2024;69 suppl 1(suppl 1):S21-S30.
13. Hamoda MM, Huynh N, Ayas NT, et al. Continuous positive airway pressure and mandibular advancement splints: the CHOICE multicentre, open-label randomised clinical trial. *Eur Respir J*. 2025; 65(4):2401100.
14. Levine M, Cantwell M, Postol K, Schwartz D. Dental sleep medicine standards for screening, treating, and management of sleep-related breathing disorders in adults using oral appliance therapy. *J Dent Sleep Med*. 2025;12(2).
15. Vohra KP, Johnson KG, Dalal A, et al. Recommendations for permanent sleep telehealth: an American Academy of Sleep Medicine position statement. *J Clin Sleep Med*. 2025;21(2):401-404.

SECTION I
Anatomy and Physiology

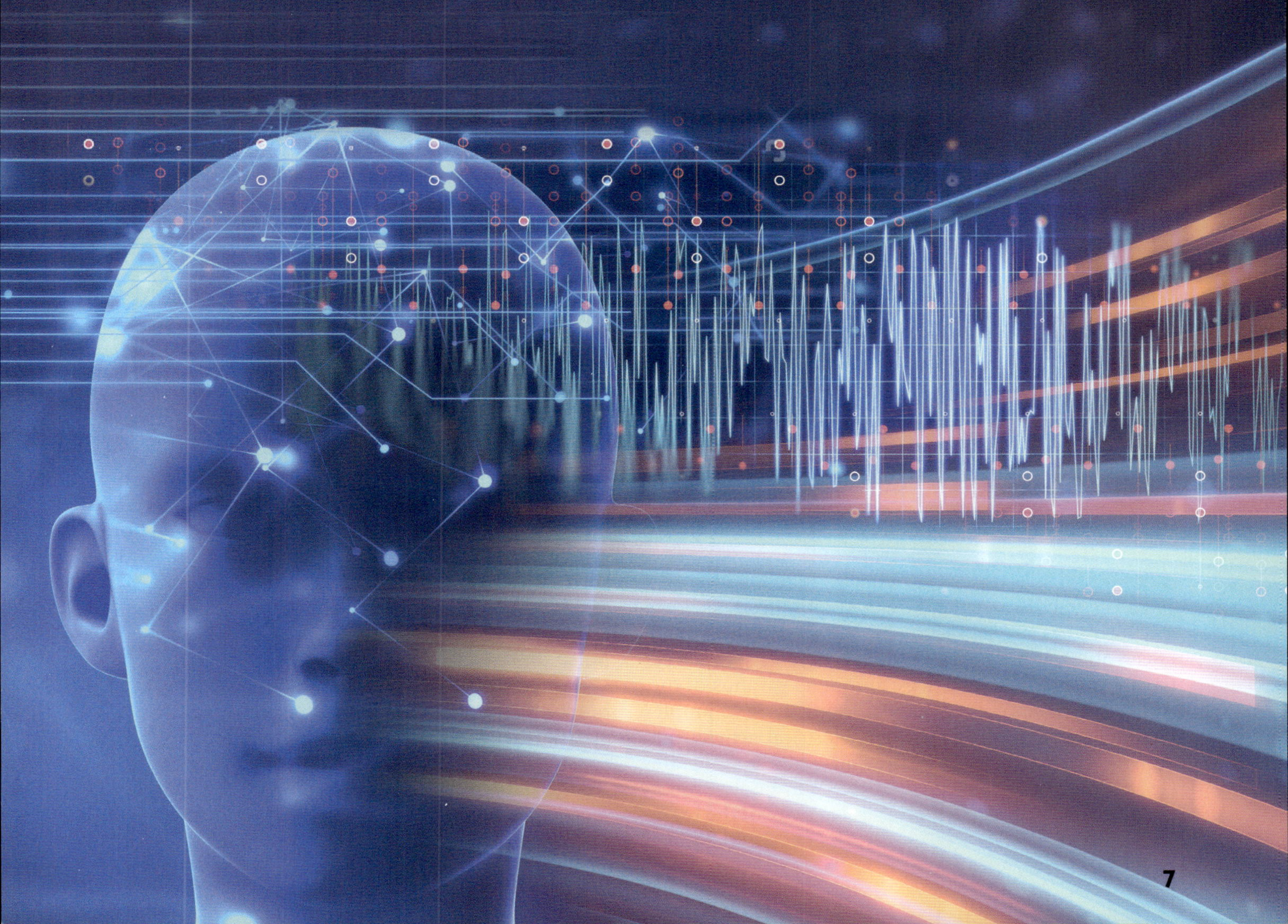

Chapter 1
The Biologic, Anatomic, and Physiologic Aspects of the Biopotentials of Sleep

REGINA PATRICK

KEY CONCEPTS/LEARNING OBJECTIVES

The key chapter concepts include describing the basic anatomy of the eye, brain, heart, and respiratory system; the biopotentials of the heart, muscles, skin, and eyes; how individual cells generate electrical potentials; how surface electrodes attached to the skin record the electrical potentials associated with many cells rather than individual cells; and skin anatomy and the principles of recording biopotentials using surface electrodes.

KEY TERMS

Biopotential
Electroencephalogram
Electromyogram
Electrooculogram
Neuron
Neurotransmitter
Reticular formation
Suprachiasmatic nucleus

A polysomnograph (PSG) is a device that measures the electrical activity generated by the brain, heart, skeletal muscles, and eyes. The activity is extremely small, but a PSG is able to record this activity through sensors placed on the scalp, chest, chin, legs, and outer canthus of the eyes. The sensors relay the electrical activity to amplifiers that increase the signal. The electrical activity can then be viewed in a visual form on a polysomnogram (ie, the recording produced by a PSG). On a polysomnogram, the recording of the electrical activity of the brain is called an electroencephalogram (EEG); the electrical activity of the heart, an electrocardiogram (ECG); the electrical activity of the muscles, an electromyogram (EMG); and the electrical activity of the eyes, an electrooculogram (EOG). A polysomnogram also presents information on respiratory activity, which is transmitted by respiratory sensors that detect airflow and air pressure changes through the nose and mouth and by sensors that detect mechanical activity created by respiratory movements of the chest and the abdomen. The signals from these sensors are transformed into an electrical signal, amplified, and viewed on the respiratory channels of a polysomnogram.

The first portion of this chapter describes how biopotentials are generated and briefly describes the biopotentials of the heart, brain, muscle, integumentary (ie, skin) cells, and eye. The second portion of this chapter gives a basic description of the anatomy of the brain, heart, and respiratory system with an emphasis on their physiologic relation to sleep.

BIOPOTENTIALS

In living organisms, a biopotential is an electrical activity that results from chemical processes (ie, biochemical processes). In living cells, biopotentials result from the movement of ions (ie, electrically charged atoms or molecules) across a cell's membrane. The fluid within a cell (ie, intracellular fluid or cytoplasm) contains ions such as sodium (Na^+), potassium (K^+), chloride (Cl^-), and calcium (Ca^{2+}). The fluid that surrounds a cell is called "extracellular fluid"; it contains these same ions but at different concentrations.

The relative difference in the net charge between the intracellular and extracellular fluid of a cell creates an electrical potential across the cell's membrane. Potential (from Latin *potentia*, meaning "power") refers to the work needed to move ions across a cell's membrane. A cell's baseline electrical potential—that is, when it is not transmitting a signal—is called its "resting potential" or "membrane polarization." A decrease in a cell's electrical potential (ie, a decrease in the electrical difference across the cell membrane) is called "depolarization." An increase in a cell's electrical potential (ie, an increase in the electrical difference across the cell membrane) is called "hyperpolarization."

Depolarization and hyperpolarization occur through the movement of ions across a cell's membrane. Depolarization can occur if an excess of positively charged ions from the extracellular fluid enters the intracellular fluid or if an excess of negatively charged ions from the intracellular fluid enters the extracellular fluid. Thus, depolarization results in the intracellular fluid becoming more positive. Hyperpolarization can occur if an excess of negatively charged ions from the extracellular fluid enters the intracellular fluid or if an excess of positively charged ions from the intracellular fluid enters the extracellular fluid. Thus, hyperpolarization results in the intracellular fluid becoming more negative.

A cell's potential is usually expressed by the electrical charge, usually in millivolts (mV), of its intracellular fluid with respect to the fluid outside the cell. A cell's potential is expressed as a positive value (eg, +55 mV) when the electrical charge of the intracellular fluid is more positive than that of the extracellular fluid, and a cell's potential is expressed as a negative value (eg, −55 mV) when the electrical charge of the intracellular fluid is more negative than that of the extracellular fluid.

Ions move across a cell's membrane through ion channels, which are proteins interspersed on the surface of a cell's membrane. The molecular structure of the proteins that make up an ion channel is arranged in a way that gives the ion channel a unique "shape." This shape allows only certain ions to flow into or out of a cell. A change in the shape of an ion channel changes how it functions. For example, a small change in an ion channel's shape may allow a sudden increase or decrease in the rate at which certain ions flow through the ion channel. In the process, the electrical potential between intracellular and extracellular fluids changes and a cell may become depolarized or hyperpolarized.

After the process of depolarization or hyperpolarization begins, ion channels quickly work to restore the resting potential. Restoration of the resting potential is called "repolarization." However, as one area of a cell's membrane undergoes repolarization, the process of depolarization (or hyperpolarization) continues along the length of the cell's membrane like a wave. Newly depolarized (or hyperpolarized) areas quickly undergo repolarization as the wave of depolarization (or hyperpolarization) continues along the cell's membrane. Depolarization typically enhances the propagation of a signal from cell to cell, whereas hyperpolarization typically inhibits the transmission of signals from cell to cell (Figure 1-1).

Nerve cells (ie, neurons), muscle cells, and heart cells are unable to transmit an impulse until the electrical potential decreases (ie, depolarizes) to a certain level. The point at which an impulse becomes possible is called the "threshold potential." The electrical potential that exists when a cell is transmitting an impulse is called its "action potential."

Biopotentials measured on the surface of the body are extremely small—one-millionth or one-thousandth of a volt (microvolt [μV] or millivolt [mV], respectively). The following sections briefly describe the biopotentials that occur in the heart, brain, muscles, and skin.

Cardiac Biopotentials

Biopotential changes in the heart are involved in the rhythmicity of heart contractions. The sinoatrial (SA) node is the pacemaker of the heart. It is in the right atrium, which is one of two upper chambers of the heart. (The plural of atrium is "atria.") The resting potential of the SA node cells is −90 mV. Certain ion channels in the cells of the SA node allow a continuous outflow of K^+ and inflow of Na^+ ions, which causes the cell's intracellular environment to become more positive (ie, the cells depolarize). When the cells depolarize to their threshold potential at approximately −60 mV, calcium ion channels suddenly open, which allows the sudden influx of Ca^{2+} ions into the cells, further enhancing the depolarization process. An impulse results and spreads quickly throughout the heart's left and right atria. The impulse spreads so quickly that the atrial myocytes (ie, heart muscle cells) contract in synchrony. After the atrial contraction, the atria repolarize. Meanwhile, the wave of depolarization spreads

+ + + + + + + + + (Extracellular fluid)	– – – – – – – – + + + + ++ + + + + ++ + + + + ++ + ++ ++ + + + + +++ ++
(Cell membrane)	Point of stimulation >
– – – – – – – – – (Intracellular fluid)	+ + + + + + + + – This depolarization travels down the membrane as ion channels restore polarization across both sides of a cell's membrane > > > > > >

Figure 1-1 Net electrical charges across a cell membrane during depolarization.

downward toward the atrioventricular (AV) node, which is another set of pacemaker cells. The AV node is at the bottom of the right atrium and just above the right ventricle. The AV node acts as a relay point between the atria and ventricles. The resting potential of the AV node cells is −60 mV. Once these cells become depolarized, they relay the signal to the bundle of His (also called the AV bundle), which is a group of specialized muscle fibers that travel down the ventricular septum and then divide into the right and left bundle branches within the septum. The right and left bundle branches each further divide into Purkinje fibers, which spread throughout the ventricular walls. Depolarization of the bundle of His causes the ventricles to contract in synchrony. One heart contraction takes approximately 0.8 seconds.

Brain Biopotentials

The brain is made up of billions of neurons. A brain wave represents the collective activity of biopotential changes occurring among the neurons. A neuron has a central portion (ie, the cell body) and extensions branching from the cell body. A neuron may have one or more short extensions (ie, dendrites) and a single long extension (ie, axon) branching from the cell body. Dendrites receive impulses and transmit them through the cell body; an axon carries the impulse away from the cell body. A neuron's resting potential ranges between −60 and −70 mV; its threshold potential is approximately −55 mV. When a neuron reaches its action potential, an impulse travels down the neuron's axon to the axon's terminal. At the terminal, the axon releases neurotransmitters such as serotonin, acetylcholine, and glutamic acid. When a neurotransmitter exits the axonal terminal, it enters a small space between the neuron's axonal terminal and the dendrite of an adjacent neuron. This space is called the "synaptic cleft." The average distance between cells in the synaptic cleft is approximately 20 to 30 nm. (A nanometer is one-billionth of a meter.) The neurotransmitter travels across the synaptic cleft and attaches to a receptor on the surface of an adjacent neuron's dendrites or cell body. Once the neurotransmitter is attached to the receptor, it can depolarize the neuron and cause the neuron to reach its action potential. In this way, electrical impulses are transmitted from neuron to neuron.

Muscle Biopotentials

A muscle contraction begins when a stimulus triggers an action potential within a neuron that innervates the muscle. The action potential travels down the neuron's axon toward the axonal terminal. At the terminal, neurotransmitters are released into the neuromuscular junction (ie, the synapse between the axon of a neuron and a muscle fiber). The neurotransmitter travels across the neuromuscular junction to attach to receptors on the muscle fiber. The resting potential of skeletal muscle is −95 mV, and the threshold potential is −50 mV. Once the neurotransmitter attaches to the receptors on the muscle fiber, Na^+ ions flood into the muscle fiber. The muscle fiber depolarizes until it reaches its action potential. The action potential quickly spreads to other muscle fibers and results in a muscle contraction.

Integumentary (Skin) Biopotentials

The outermost layer of the skin (ie, epidermis) consists of dead cells, which do not have electrical activity. However, two layers beneath the epidermis—the dermis and, below it, the hypodermis—have electrical activity (Figure 1-2). In polysomnography, the biopotentials of the skin (ie, dermis and hypodermis) are not measured. However, oil, sweat, and dead skin cells on the surface of the skin can create a barrier between the skin's surface and an electrode. This electrical barrier is called "resistance." Resistance can interfere with the recording of EEG, EMG, and ECG signals.

The metal of the electrode and the conductive electrode paste used in electrodes can retain some of the electrical charge recorded from the body. This storage is called "capacitance." The combination of capacitance and resistance is called "impedance." Excessive impedance can hinder the recording of a signal received by an electrode and affect the quality of a recording. An impedance meter is an instrument used to measure the impedance formed between an electrode and the surface of the skin. In polysomnography, impedance is measured in kilo-ohms (ie, 1,000 ohms; often denoted as "kΩ"). Properly cleaned skin should ideally have a reading of 5 kΩ or less (1).

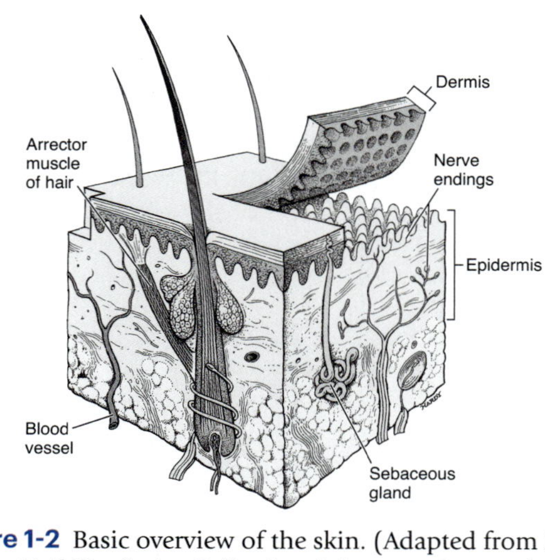

Figure 1-2 Basic overview of the skin. (Adapted from Neil O. Hardy, Neil Hardy Art Collection, Westport, Connecticut.)

Eye Biopotentials

The eye is a fluid-filled, globe-shaped organ. A round, clear, convex membrane—the cornea—extends slightly outward from the front of the eye. A circular, colored membrane—the iris—is visible though the cornea and gives a person's eye its color. The iris opens and contracts in response to low and high light intensity, respectively. Light enters the eye through an open circular center (ie, the pupil) in the iris. A transparent biconvex lens, situated behind the iris, focuses light onto the retina, a membrane that lines much of the inner surface of the eye (Figure 1-3).

The process of vision begins in the retina, following the refraction (ie, bending) of light, which occurs when light passes from air into the denser materials of the cornea, aqueous humor, and lens. Refraction helps focus light onto the retina. Through chemical reactions triggered by light (ie, photochemical reaction), visual cells in the retina (eg, cones, rods) transform light energy into a neurologic impulse that is transmitted from the retina, through the optic nerve, to the visual center of the brain where it is interpreted.

The electrical potential of the retina's visual cells before undergoing a photochemical reaction (ie, the retina's resting potential) is approximately −30 to −40 mV. When a particle of light (ie, a photon) strikes the rods and cones, ion channels on the surface of these cells change their shape. The shape change prevents positively charged sodium and potassium ions from entering the cells while allowing positively charged calcium ions to exit the cells. These two actions cause the intracellular environment of the rods and cones to become more negatively charged (ie, hyperpolarized). Hyperpolarization of the rods and cones can approach −80 mV.

Epithelial cells that line the outer surface of the cornea secrete positively charged ions such as sodium (Na^+) and potassium (K^+) into the cornea and excrete negatively charged ions out of the cornea. This process creates a potential of approximately +30 to +40 mV across the membrane of the cornea. Owing to the positive charge of the cornea and the negative charge of the retina, an electrical potential exists between the front and the back of the eye. This potential is called the "corneoretinal potential."

An EOG records changes that occur in the corneoretinal potential with eye movement. In polysomnography, two electrodes are used to record an EOG. Both electrodes are placed on the outer canthus (ie, eye socket ridge), with one electrode placed above the midline of the outer canthus and the other placed below the midline of the outer canthus. (The right electrode is typically placed above the midline and the left electrode is placed below the midline [Figure 1-4].)

As the eyes move in tandem (ie, conjugate eye movements), one electrode will be closer to the cornea, whereas the other will be closer to the retina. Hence, one electrode will record a positive impulse (recorded as a downward deflection), whereas the other electrode will record a negative impulse (recorded as an upward deflection) as the eyes move around (Figure 1-5).

Therefore, placing one electrode above the midline and the other below the midline on the outer canthus

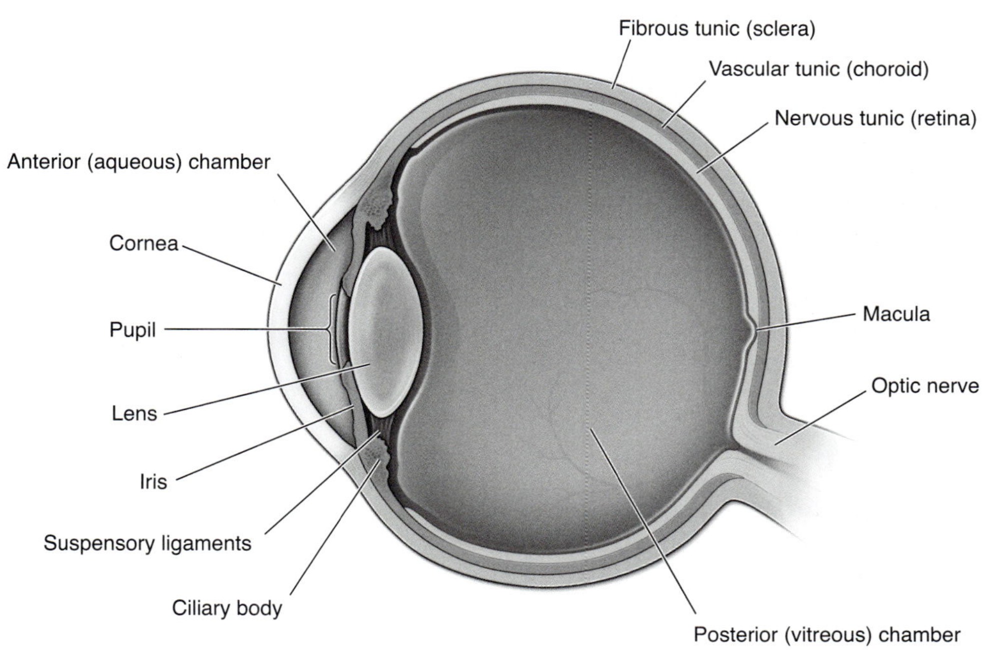

Figure 1-3 Basic eye anatomy. (Reprinted with permission from Detton AJ. *Grant's Dissector*. 16th ed. Wolters Kluwer; 2016. Figure 7-57.)

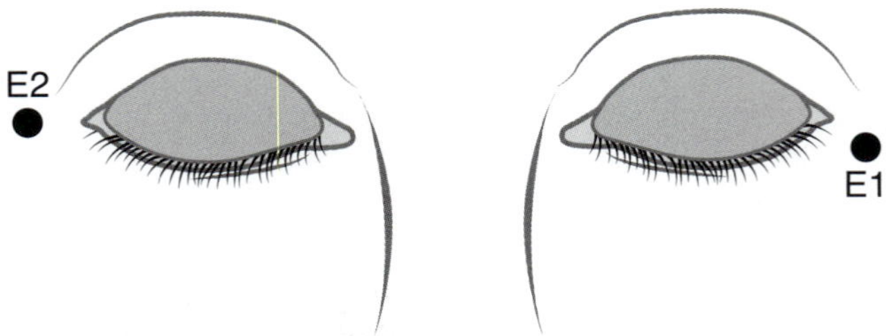

Figure 1-4 Electrode placement on the outer canthus.

is important. If both electrodes are placed in the same horizontal plane, vertical eye movements would be recorded as moving conjunctively (ie, both EOG channels deflect in the same direction, or "in phase") rather than disjunctively (ie, both EOG channels deflect in opposite directions, or "out of phase").

ANATOMY AND PHYSIOLOGY OF THE BRAIN

The brain consists of the cerebrum (which consists of the left and right hemispheres), the midbrain, the brainstem (ie, the stalk-like portion of the brain that connects the cerebral hemispheres with the spinal cord; the brainstem contains the midbrain, pons, and medulla), and the cerebellum (which has two hemispheres and extends from the back of the brainstem). Several brain structures involved in sleep and wakefulness are in the brainstem (eg, locus coeruleus, reticular formation, raphe nuclei) or near the base of the brain (eg, thalamus, suprachiasmatic nucleus [SCN], hypothalamus, and the pineal gland). These structures have the following roles in sleep.

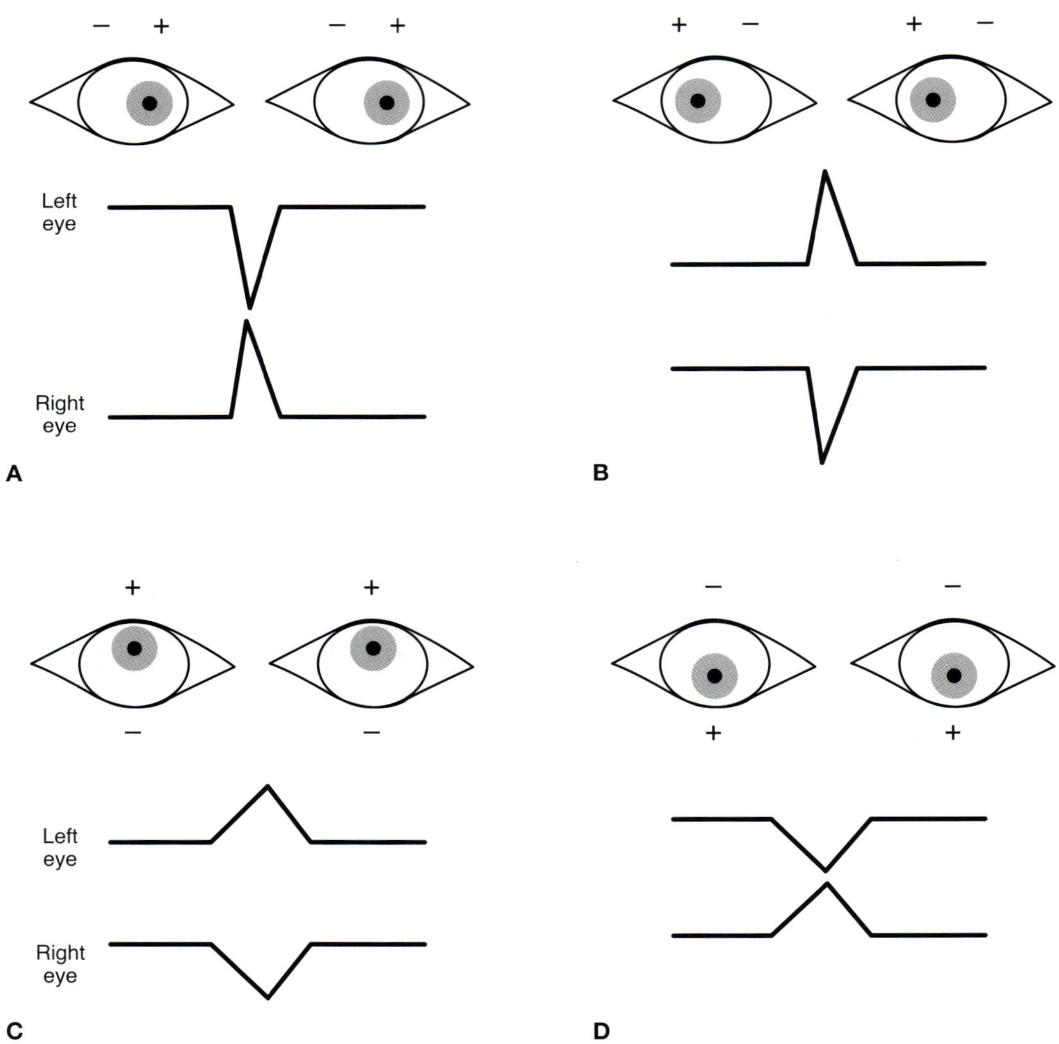

Figure 1-5 Positive and negative changes of the eyes and the left eye and right eye signals on the electrooculogram with eye movements. A: Eyes looking left. B: Eyes looking right. C: Eyes looking up. D: Eyes looking down.

Locus Ceruleus

The locus ceruleus (pronounced "LOH-kus suh-ROO-lee-us"), a small, blue-tinged area in the back of the brainstem, is involved in rapid eye movement (REM) sleep and in wakefulness (2,3) (Figure 1-6). The locus ceruleus contains neurons that release or are activated by norepinephrine, serotonin, and choline (ie, norepinephrinergic, serotoninergic, and cholinergic neurons, respectively). These neurons fire quickly during wake, begin to slow their firing with the onset of sleep, continue to slow their firing as sleep deepens, and then nearly stop firing during REM sleep. The locus ceruleus contains "REM-off" cells, a group of neurons that inhibit REM sleep (ie, the action of these cells ends a REM period). The REM-off cells become increasingly active as REM sleep progresses and ultimately hinder the activity of "REM-on" cells (ie, specialized cells that induce the onset of a REM period), which are in the pons and basal forebrain.

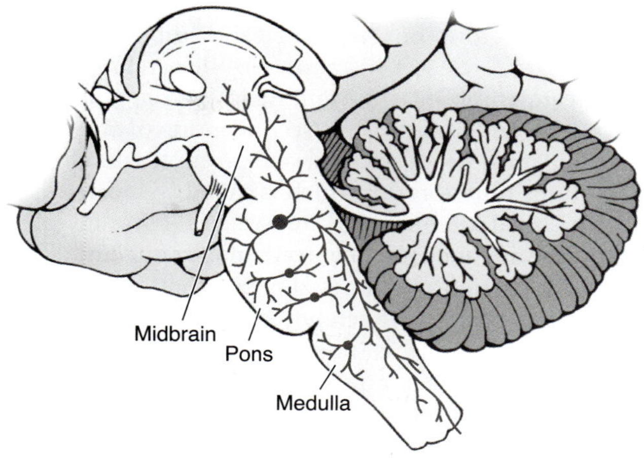

Figure 1-7 Ascending and descending axons in the reticular formation. (Reprinted with permission from Siegel A, Sapru HN. *Essential Neuroscience*. 4th ed. Wolters Kluwer; 2019. Figure 22.6.)

Reticular Formation

The reticular formation consists of diffuse groups of nerve cells that are embedded within a wealth of nerve fibers (Figure 1-7), which gives it a mesh-like appearance when examined using a microscope. (In Latin, *reticulo* means "net.") The reticular formation runs throughout the inner core of the midbrain, pons, and medulla and fills the spaces between major nuclei and nerve tracts in the brainstem.

The alternation between sleep and wake cycles results from the neural interplay between the reticular formation and the cerebral cortex. The thalamus, a structure located just above the brainstem, relays signals between the cerebral cortex and the reticular formation. Increased cerebral activation activates the reticular formation and consequently wakefulness. During sleep, fewer impulses arise from the cerebral cortex; therefore, activation of the reticular formation is decreased.

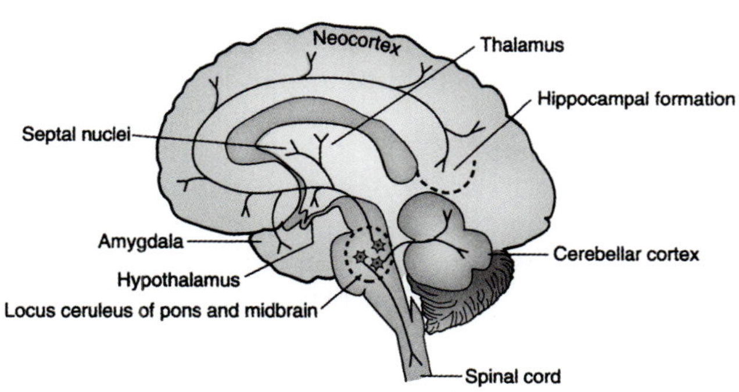

Figure 1-6 Locus ceruleus. (Reprinted with permission from Gould DJ, Brueckner JK, Fix JD. *High-yield Neuroanatomy*. 5th ed. Wolters Kluwer; 2016. Figure 20-4.)

The reticular formation has two components: the ascending reticular formation and the descending reticular formation. Of these two components, the ascending reticular formation (also called the "reticular activating system") is most directly involved in sleep and wake cycles, and it has a role in the overall degree of central nervous system activity. The ascending reticular formation receives sensory signals traveling from the periphery toward the brain; the signals are first relayed to the thalamus. From there, the signals are relayed to the cerebral cortex of the brain. The pathway from the thalamus to the cortex is called the "thalamocortical pathway." Neurons of the thalamocortical pathway release excitatory neurotransmitters, such as glutamate, dopamine, noradrenaline, serotonin, and histamine, to the cerebral cortex. These neurotransmitters are involved in wakefulness.

The descending reticular formation receives information from the hypothalamus and is involved in the degree of activity in the autonomic nervous system (ie, the sympathetic and parasympathetic nervous systems collectively). Activation of the descending reticular formation allows the body to withstand the increase in autonomic nervous activity that occurs with wakefulness. An increase in the heart rate, respiratory rate, and muscle tone activates the descending reticular formation and thereby forms a positive feedback loop (ie, as one factor increases, another factor also increases). The positive feedback loop is controlled by various dampening neural systems in the brain. If it were not dampened, the result would be an extreme arousal state and consequently a seizure.

Another arousal pathway in the brain extends from the reticular formation to the hypothalamus and, finally, to the cerebral cortex. This pathway is called the "reticulo-hypothalamo-cortical pathway." In the hypothalamus, a group of cells, called the "tuberomammillary nucleus," releases histamine to the cerebral cortex. The greatest amount of histamine in the cerebral cortex is synthesized during wake. A second group of cells in the hypothalamus produces the wake-promoting excitatory neurotransmitter orexin, which is called "hypocretin."

The basal forebrain (ie, the base of the frontal lobe) has pathways that are involved in arousal and REM sleep. Acetylcholine-synthesizing neurons in the basal forebrain project to the cerebral cortex. The neurotransmitter acetylcholine is involved in wakefulness and facilitates REM sleep. The highest brain level of acetylcholine is synthesized during wake and REM sleep. The pons also contains a group of cholinergic neurons (ie, REM-on cells) that facilitate REM sleep.

Reticular deactivation leads to sleep. This deactivation results from neuronal activity in the forebrain, pons, medulla, and cerebellum. For example, the basal forebrain contains neurons that synthesize the inhibitory neurotransmitter γ-amino butyric acid (GABA). These neurons project to the cerebral cortex, to the histamine-producing neurons of the tuberomammillary nucleus in the hypothalamus, and to the reticular formation. In these regions, GABA inhibits the activation of the reticular activating system through a negative feedback system (ie, as one factor increases, another factor decreases) and thereby induces sleep.

Raphe Nuclei

The reticular formation contains several groups of cells, collectively called the "raphe nuclei," which consist of the caudal linear nucleus, dorsal raphe nucleus, median raphe nucleus, raphe magnus nucleus, raphe obscurus nucleus, and raphe pallidus nucleus. The raphe nuclei are clustered near the junction that separates the left and right sides of the brainstem. This junction is called the "raphe" (in Greek, *raphe* means "seam"). Nerve fibers that project from the raphe nuclei release the excitatory neurotransmitter serotonin to all parts of the brain, which contributes to wakefulness. During wake, the raphe nuclei neurons fire rapidly. They reduce their firing rate with sleep onset and increasingly reduce firing until nearly becoming quiescent in REM sleep. Exactly what triggers the cells to reduce their firing rate with sleep onset is unknown. A possibility is that other neurons such as GABAergic neurons (ie, neurons that are activated by or synthesize GABA) indirectly or directly regulate the activity of other neurotransmitters involved in sleep.

Thalamus

The thalamic reticular nuclei are embedded within a thin layer of myelinated fibers, called the "internal medullary lamina," in the thalamus. The thalamic reticular nuclei neurons are GABAergic and project from the thalamus to the reticular formation. During slow-wave sleep, the thalamic reticular nuclei neurons rhythmically shift between depolarization and hyperpolarization, which results in the rhythmic bursting pattern of slow waves that occur during slow-wave sleep. The transition from sleep to wake occurs when, through the influence of excitatory neurotransmitters such as glutamate and acetylcholine, the thalamocortical neurons inhibit this rhythmic bursting pattern.

Suprachiasmatic Nuclei, Hypothalamus, and Pineal Gland

SCNs are important in the alternation between sleep and wake cycles. These nuclei are in the anterior hypothalamus. They receive signals through the retinohypothalamic tract, the geniculohypothalamic tract (ie, the pathway between the geniculate bodies [ie, four small round masses just beneath the thalamus] in the upper brainstem and the nearby hypothalamus), and the raphe nuclei.

The retinohypothalamic tract is formed by the axons of retinal ganglion cells, which extend from the retina to the hypothalamus and the SCN. It is important in establishing the circadian rhythmicity of the sleep and wake cycle. The retina, a thin multilayered lining inside the eye, contains two types of light-sensitive visual cells: rods and cones. Rods allow a person to see in dim light settings and to detect motion, whereas cones allow a person to perceive color.

When light strikes the rods and cones, photopigments (eg, the protein rhodopsin) in these cells chemically transform the light energy into an action potential. The signal is relayed from the rods and cones to bipolar cells and finally to the ganglion cell layer in the retina. Fibers extending from the ganglion cells exit from the back of the eye as the optic nerve and project into the lateral geniculate bodies, which are involved in vision. The signals are relayed from the geniculate bodies to the visual center in the occipital lobe.

As mentioned previously, in the retinohypothalamic tract, some fibers from the retinal ganglion cells relay signals from the retina to the SCN in the anterior hypothalamus. The SCN then relays signals to the pineal gland, a pinecone-shaped structure within the groove formed by the juncture of the two halves of the thalamus. Depending on the strength of the signals, the pineal gland increases or decreases its secretion of the sleep-promoting neurotransmitter melatonin. High-intensity light (eg, daylight) decreases the pineal gland's production of melatonin, whereas low-intensity light (eg, nightfall) increases its production of melatonin.

ELECTROENCEPHALOGRAM ACTIVITY OF THE BRAIN DURING SLEEP

Electrodes used for recording EEG signals in polysomnography are too large to detect the activity of a single neuron. The signal recorded from an EEG electrode actually reflects the change in the collective electrical activity of numerous neurons on the surface of the brain beneath the site of the electrode. The change in the collective neuronal activity is called a "brainwave." On the EEG channels of a PSG, brainwaves fluctuate in characteristic ways for each stage of sleep and wake. Brain waves of interest in polysomnography are alpha waves, theta waves, beta waves, spindles, K-complex waveforms, sharp vertex waves, delta waves (ie, slow waves), and sawtooth waves. These waveforms are identified by frequency (ie, the number of waves [cycles] per second, usually expressed in Hertz [Hz]); by peak-to-peak amplitude (representing the signal voltage); and by morphology (ie, shape). Each stage of sleep has unique EEG waveforms.

Wake

During wake, the EEG shows low-amplitude, high-frequency activity. With the eyes closed during relaxed wakefulness, alpha waves (so named because they were the first brain waves discovered) (4) initially appear intermittently among low-amplitude, high-frequency waves and ultimately become the dominant wave. (On opening the eyes, the waves drop out.) Alpha waves have a frequency of 8 to 13 Hz and are most prominent in the occipital region (5) (Figure 1-8).

Stage N1 Sleep

Alpha waves drop out and theta waves appear with the onset of sleep (ie, stage N1). Theta waves have a frequency of 4 to 7 Hz (Figure 1-9) and are the predominant waves of stage N1 sleep (5).

Stage N2 Sleep

A sharp vertex wave is a transient wave that commonly appears during the transition from stage N1 to stage N2 sleep (5). These sporadic waves have a negative (ie, upward)

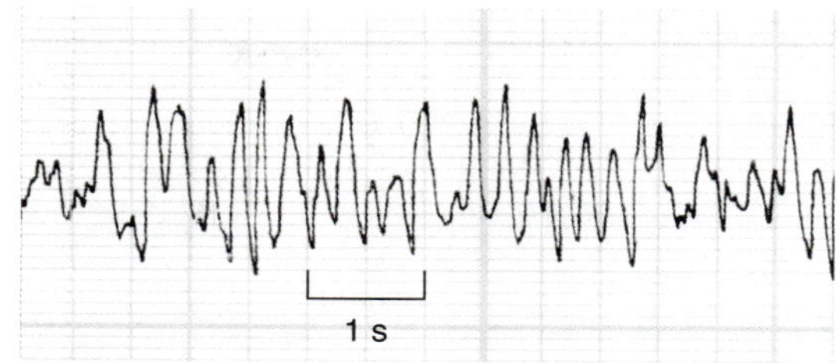

Figure 1-9 Theta waves in stage N1 sleep.

deflection and last less than 0.5 seconds. The amplitude of these waves is maximal in the central channels; however, no amplitude criterion exists for a sharp vertex wave (Figure 1-10).

As sleep progresses from stage N1 sleep to stage N2 sleep, the EEG amplitude remains somewhat low, but short bursts of fast, short-lasting activity begin to appear. These bursts are called "spindles" and are one indicator of the onset of stage N2 sleep (5). Spindles have a frequency of 11 to 16 Hz (more commonly 12-14 Hz) and typically last approximately 0.5 to 1.5 seconds. Their maximal amplitude occurs in the central channels.

A second waveform that can indicate the onset of stage N2 sleep is the K-complex (5). A K-complex is a short-lasting wave that begins with a sharp negative (ie, upward) deflection, followed by a slower positive (ie, downward) component. The duration of a K-complex is 0.5 seconds or longer. The maximal amplitude is usually in the frontal channels (Figure 1-11).

Stage N3 Sleep (Slow-Wave Sleep)

As sleep progresses from stage N2 to slow-wave (ie, stage N3) sleep, high-amplitude waves—slow waves (also called "delta waves")—begin to appear (5). Slow waves have a frequency of 0.5 to 2 Hz and a voltage of 75 μV or greater (Figure 1-12). As N3 sleep progresses, the slow waves become increasingly dominant. They are most readily detected in the frontal channels.

Stage R Sleep (Rapid Eye Movement Sleep)

As sleep progresses from N3 sleep to REM sleep (also called "stage R sleep"), the voltage of the EEG waves

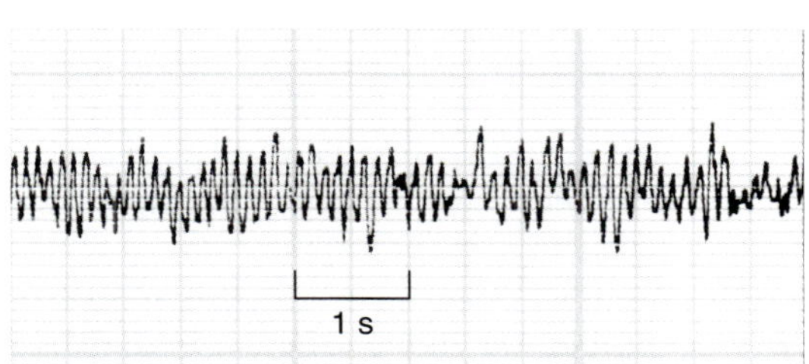

Figure 1-8 Alpha waves in stage N1 sleep.

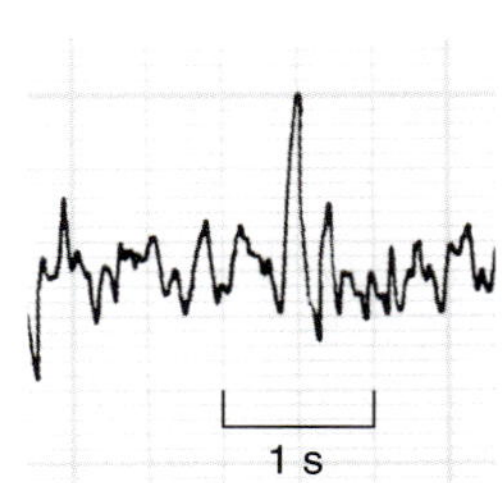

Figure 1-10 Sharp vertex wave in stage N2 sleep.

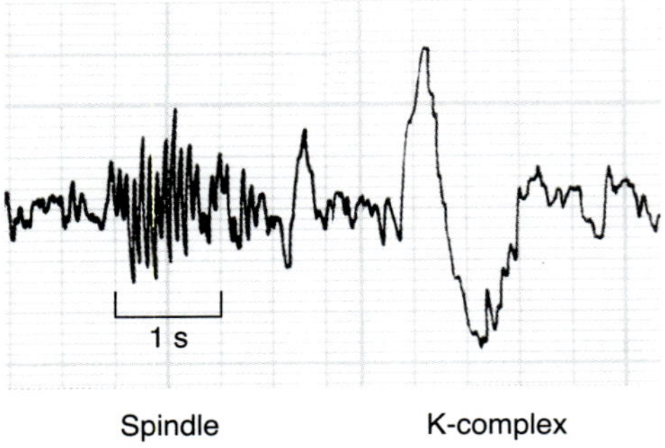

Figure 1-11 K-complex and spindle in stage N2 sleep.

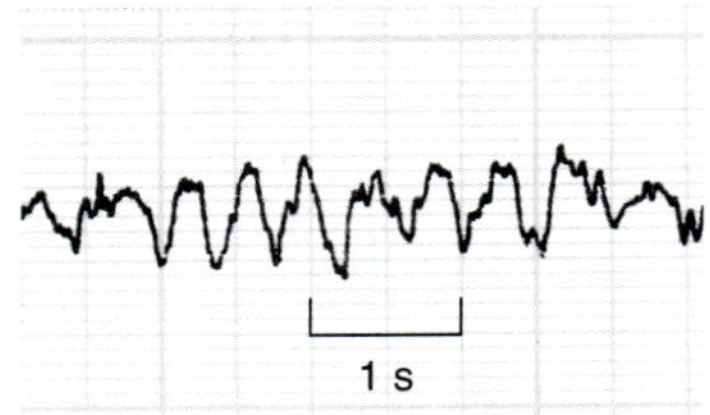

Figure 1-13 Sawtooth waves in rapid eye movement sleep.

dramatically decreases, and the EEG appears very similar to stage N1. However, other channels on the PSG reveal features in this sleep stage that do not occur in N1 sleep. Just before the onset of stage R sleep, the electromyography channel (ie, chin channel) shows the sudden loss of muscle tone, as reflected by a thick line suddenly becoming a thin line on the chin EMG channel. Bursts of waves, called "sawtooth waves," which resemble jagged theta waves, intermittently appear (5). The frequency of sawtooth waves (2-6 Hz) is within the theta frequency range of 4 to 7 Hz (Figure 1-13). The amplitude of sawtooth waves is highest in the central channels. Sawtooth waves often appear just before the onset of conjunctive eye movements (ie, the eyes move in unison; however, the signals of the left and right eye movements deflect in opposite directions on the EOG). The EEG of REM sleep is very similar to that of stage N1 sleep; however, REM sleep is distinguished from stage N1 sleep by non-EEG features such as the lack of muscle tone and the appearance of REMs.

ANATOMY AND PHYSIOLOGY OF THE HEART

The heart is a cone-shaped, four-chambered muscular organ. Its apex points downward and slightly to the left in the chest and its base points upward in the chest. The base of the heart contains two atria and the apex of the heart contains two ventricles. The atria and ventricles make up the four chambers of the heart. The cardiac septum is a muscular wall that splits the heart longitudinally into left and right halves. The atrial septum forms a border between the left and right atria and the ventricular septum forms a border between the left and right ventricles. Valves separate each atrium from its corresponding ventricle. The tricuspid valve separates the right atrium from the right ventricle, and the mitral valve separates the left atrium from the left ventricle.

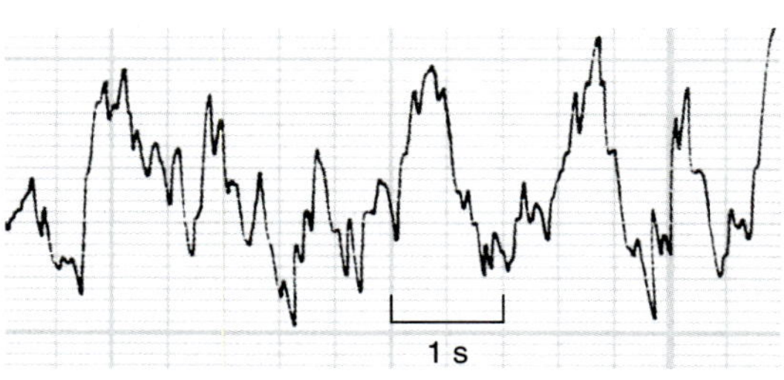

Figure 1-12 Slow waves in slow-wave sleep.

A heartbeat begins with the simultaneous contraction of the atria. When they contract, the tricuspid and mitral valves open to allow blood to flow from each atrium into its corresponding ventricle. After the ventricles are filled, the tricuspid and mitral valves close as the ventricles contract. Ventricular contraction expels the blood into the pulmonary trunk (right ventricle) and into the aorta (left ventricle). The pulmonary trunk takes the blood to the lungs for oxygenation while blood in the aorta travels throughout the body to oxygenate the body's tissues. Blood that is oxygenated in the lungs is returned to the left atrium by the pulmonary vein. Blood that has gone through the body tissues ultimately loses oxygenation and is returned to the right atrium by the inferior and superior venae cavae (singular, vena cava; these veins are the largest in the body). Once the atria are filled, this process begins again.

A heart muscle cell is called a "cardiomyocyte." Cardiomyocytes are short, flat, branching quadrangular cells shaped somewhat like a thick X. The branches of a cardiomyocyte are joined with the branches of another myocyte by dense fibrous bands called "intercalated discs." Gap junctions and desmosomes of one myocyte are juxtaposed with those of another myocyte through the intercalated discs.

A gap junction is a channel that is formed by a hexagon-shaped protein on a cell's membrane. Within the center of the hexagonal protein is a pore (ie, channel) through which ions and proteins and other small molecules can pass from one cell to the next. The distance between the gap junctions of adjacent cells is extremely small, approximately 2 to 3 nm. Such a short distance allows electrical energy to be transmitted quickly from cell to cell, so that an impulse originating in one part of the heart can spread quickly enough to cause the myocytes to beat in synchrony.

Desmosomes are dense circular bodies scattered just beneath and attached to the cell membrane. Thin fibers extend from each desmosome and insert into the desmosome of adjacent myocytes. The thin fibers anchor myocytes tightly together so that myocytes do not come apart during contractions.

An impulse for a heartbeat normally begins in the SA node. The SA node is functionally and histologically a specialized group of cells in the upper right atrium. The SA node cells usually act as the heart's pacemaker. However, under certain conditions, other cells can take over as the heart's pacemaker, which will be discussed later in this section. Pacemaker cells are modified myocytes that do not contract. They instead transmit rhythmic impulses by undergoing a continual process of depolarization and repolarization.

The rhythmic impulses from the SA pacemaker cells induce rhythmic depolarization of the atrial myocytes, resulting in rhythmic atrial contractions. The signals are relayed to the AV node, a group of pacemaker cells located at the bottom of the right atrium. The AV node depolarizes and relays the signals to the bundle of His, which is a group of specialized pacemaker fibers. The bundle of His fibers exit from the AV node and travel downward through the septum (ie, the muscular portion of the ventricular septum). In the upper region of the interventricular septum, the bundle of His breaks into left and right branches. These branches travel down the interventricular septum toward the heart's apex. At the apex, the left bundle branch breaks into many fibers as it spreads itself throughout the muscular wall of the left ventricle, and the right bundle branch similarly spreads itself throughout the muscular wall of the right ventricle. When an impulse passes through the bundle of His, the ventricular myocytes depolarize, which causes the ventricles to contract. A heartbeat (ie, atrial contraction followed by ventricular contraction) normally takes approximately 0.8 seconds.

The AV node cells or the bundle of His fibers can set the heart's rhythm in case disease or injury to the SA node prevents it from transmitting a signal. The AV node or bundle of His fibers can take over as pacemaker because each has its own intrinsic rhythm: the AV node can generate 40 to 60 impulses per minute and the bundle of His fibers can generate 30 to 40 impulses per minute (5). The SA node normally sets the heart's rhythm because it can generate impulses at a rate of 60 to 100 impulses per minute and therefore can override the impulses of the AV node or the bundle of His fibers. If an injury occurs at or near the SA node, the AV node takes over as the heart's pacemaker because it can generate signals more quickly than the bundle of His fibers. If injury affects the SA node and AV node, the His fibers may then take over as the heart's pacemaker (Figure 1-14).

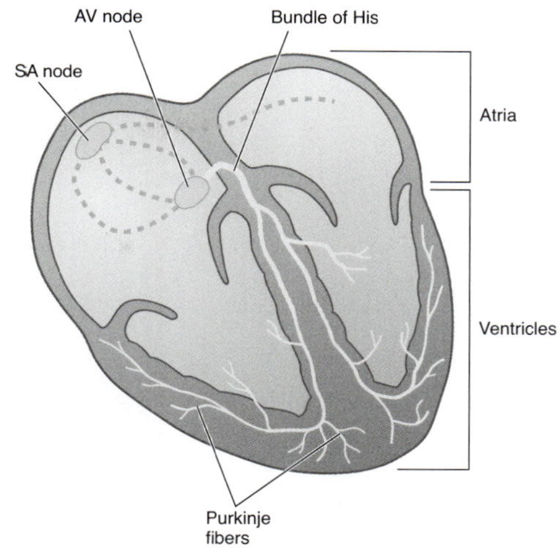

Figure 1-14 The conducting system of the heart. Impulses originating in the sinoatrial (SA) node are transmitted through the atria, to the atrioventricular (AV) node, to the bundle of His, and, through Purkinje fibers, to the ventricles. (Reprinted with permission from Frandsen G, Pennington SS. *Abrams' Clinical Drug Therapy: Rationales for Nursing Practice*. 10th ed. Wolters Kluwer Health/Lippincott Williams & Wilkins; 2014. Figure 25.1.)

Pulmonary and Systemic Circulation

Two separate cardiovascular circuits exist for blood flowing into and out of the heart. The first circuit is the pulmonary circuit. In this circuit, blood flows from the heart to the lungs and back to the heart. The second circuit is the systemic circuit. In this circuit, blood flows from the heart, throughout the body to oxygenate all of the body's cells, and then returns to the heart (Figure 1-15).

The pulmonary circuit begins at the right atrium. Deoxygenated blood from the body's tissues is returned to the right atrium through the venae cavae. The superior vena cava brings deoxygenated blood from the head and neck to the right atrium, and the inferior vena cava brings deoxygenated blood from the rest of the body to the right atrium. When the atria contract, the right atrium pumps the blood through the tricuspid valve into the right ventricle. When the ventricles contract, the right ventricle pumps blood through the pulmonary valve and into the pulmonary trunk. This vessel branches to become the left and right pulmonary arteries, which carry the deoxygenated blood away from the heart and to the lungs. In the lungs, the pulmonary arteries branch and become increasingly smaller as they travel to the alveoli, where the blood within the vessels undergoes gas exchange.

The lungs contain millions of alveoli, sac-like outpouchings that contain air that flows into and out of the lungs with each breath. The outer surface of each alveolus is surrounded by a mass of capillaries consisting of a network of microscopic vessels that connect the

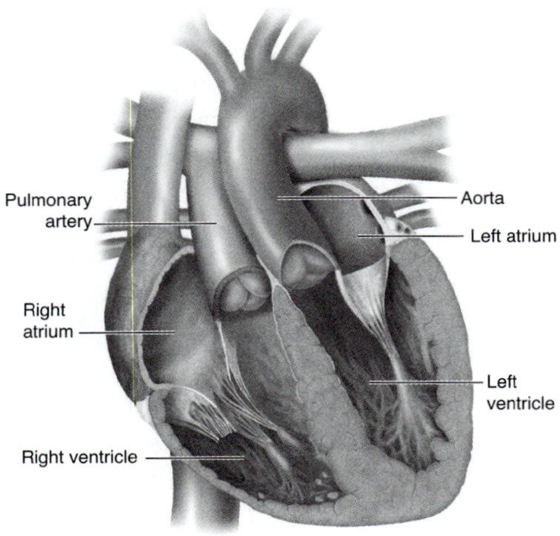

Figure 1-15 Pulmonary blood flow. The pulmonary circuit carries deoxygenated blood from the heart to the lungs (via the pulmonary trunk) for oxygenation and returns oxygenated blood to the heart, whereas the systemic circuit transports oxygenated blood from the heart throughout the body (via the aorta) to nourish cells and returns deoxygenated blood to the heart. (Reprinted with permission from Lee EY. *Pediatric Thoracic Imaging*. Wolters Kluwer; 2019. Figure 4.27.)

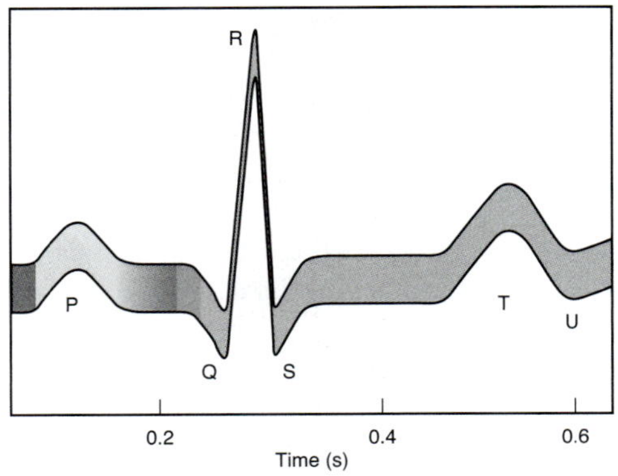

Figure 1-16 The cardiac waveforms: P, QRS, and T waves. (Reprinted with permission from Plowman SA, Smith DL. *Exercise Physiology for Health Fitness and Performance*. 5th ed. Wolters Kluwer; 2017. Figure 11.4B.)

venous system with the arterial system. Oxygen in the alveolar air diffuses through the alveolar wall and enters the surrounding pulmonary capillaries. Hemoglobin molecules in the red blood cells in the capillaries pick up oxygen—thereby oxygenating the blood—whereas carbon dioxide in the blood diffuses from the capillaries across the alveolar membrane into the alveolus. On exhalation, the carbon dioxide is expelled into the external environment. The oxygenated blood flows out of the arterial capillaries and enters the venous capillaries. The oxygenated blood flows through the venous system and returns to the left atrium of the heart via the left and right pulmonary veins.

Once in the left atrium, the blood enters the systemic circuit. When the atria contract, the now oxygenated blood is pushed through the mitral valve and enters the left ventricle. On ventricular contraction, the left ventricle pumps the blood through the aortic valve into the aorta, which is the largest artery in the body. The aorta arches over the heart and then descends through the thorax and abdomen to the lower trunk of the body, where it splits into two main branches that carry blood to the legs. Throughout its descent through the thorax and abdomen, arteries branch off the aorta. Each of these branches becomes increasingly smaller until joining a capillary bed associated with a tissue (eg, tendons, organs such as the liver). At the capillary bed, the oxygenated arterial blood provides oxygen to the body's tissues. As the blood travels from the arterial capillaries to the venous capillaries, the blood ultimately flows into the inferior and superior vena cava, both of which take the blood to the right atrium. On atrial contraction, the right atrium pumps blood into the right ventricle, and blood reenters the pulmonary circuit. Thus, with each heartbeat, some blood is always entering the pulmonary circuit and some blood is entering the systemic circuit.

An artery is a vessel that carries blood away from the heart and a vein is a vessel that carries blood to the heart. Therefore, in the pulmonary system, arteries are blue because the blood is deoxygenated and veins are red because the blood is oxygenated. In the systemic system, the converse is true.

Cardiac Waveforms

In polysomnography, cardiac waveforms of interest on an ECG channel are the P wave, the QRS complex, and the T wave (Figure 1-16). The P wave represents the depolarization (ie, contraction) of the atria. It appears as a small upwardly curved stroke. The P wave is quickly followed by the QRS complex, an angular down-up-down stroke that represents the depolarization of the ventricles. Repolarization of the atria occurs at the same time as the contraction of the ventricles; however, the QRS complex has a larger voltage and therefore is more easily recorded than the waveform for atrial repolarization. The T wave represents the repolarization of the ventricles. Its shape is somewhat similar to the P wave, but it is a little broader.

ANATOMY AND PHYSIOLOGY OF THE RESPIRATORY SYSTEM

Oxygenating the blood is the function of the respiratory system. The respiratory system consists of the upper airway and the lower airway (Figure 1-17). The upper airway consists of the nose and nasal passages, the oral

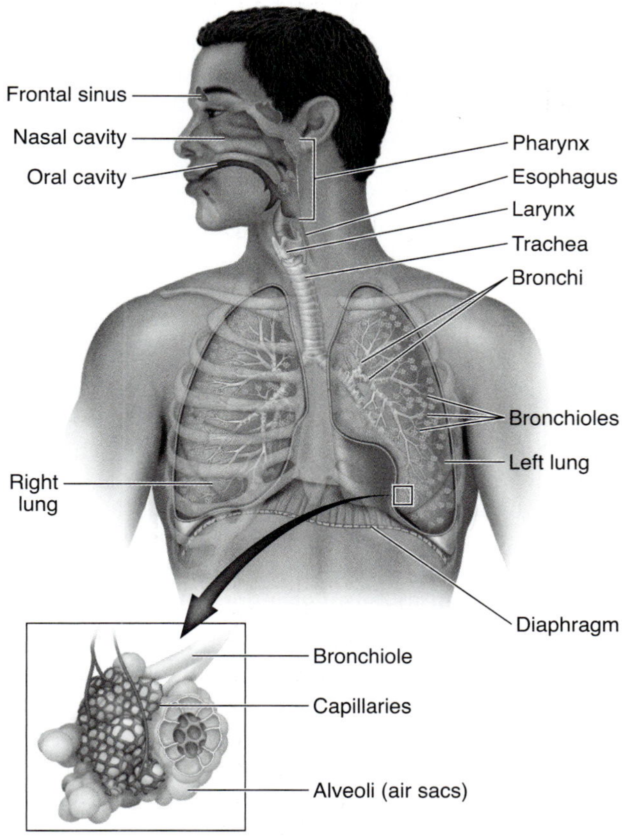

Figure 1-17 The respiratory system. (Reprinted with permission from McConnell TH, Hull KL. *Human Form, Human Function: Essentials of Anatomy & Physiology*. Wolters Kluwer Health/Lippincott Williams & Wilkins; 2011. Figure 13-2.)

cavity (ie, mouth), and the pharynx (ie, throat cavity). The nasal passage and oral cavity open into the pharynx.

The pharynx begins at the back of the nasal cavity and ends at the larynx and is divided into three major regions: the nasopharynx (ie, the region extending from the back of the nasal cavity to the soft palate), the oropharynx (ie, the region extending from the soft palate to above the epiglottis [the cartilaginous membrane that covers the larynx when a person swallows]), and the laryngopharynx (ie, the region extending from below the epiglottis to the larynx). The larynx contains the vocal cords, which expand and contract to control the entrance of air into and out of the lungs when a person is talking or breathing.

The larynx opens into the trachea, a cartilage-ringed, rigid tubular structure (often called the windpipe). The trachea branches into two bronchi (singular, bronchus), which are also ringed by cartilage. As the bronchi descend into the lungs, they become progressively smaller while increasingly losing the protective rings of cartilage. Minute extensions of the bronchi, called "bronchioles," consist of smooth muscle supported by connective tissue. A bronchiole continues to divide until it forms a terminal bronchiole, which ends the air conducting portion of the respiratory system. A terminal bronchiole branches into several respiratory bronchioles, each of which is capped by an alveolar sac. The surface of an alveolar sac contains round outpouchings called alveoli. The surface of each alveolus is covered by capillaries.

Gas exchange—the movement of oxygen into the blood and carbon dioxide out of the blood—occurs on the surface of each alveolus on an alveolar sac. On inhalation, the oxygen in the alveolar air diffuses through the alveolar wall, passes through the wall of surrounding capillaries, and finally enters the capillary blood. Once in the capillary blood, most of the oxygen is picked up by hemoglobin molecules in red blood cells and is ultimately transported throughout the body tissues. Carbon dioxide in the capillary blood diffuses out of the capillaries, passes through the alveolar wall, and enters the alveolar air. On exhalation, the carbon dioxide is expelled from the lungs.

Breathing Control Mechanisms

The rhythmicity of inhalation and exhalation involves the interplay between several nuclei in the brainstem (collectively called the "respiratory center"), the aorta, and the carotid arteries. Nuclei outside the brain are called "peripheral nuclei" and nuclei within the brain are called "central nuclei." Peripheral nuclei that are involved in respiration are the aortic bodies, the carotid body, and baroreceptors in the aorta and carotid arteries. Some central nuclei that are involved in respiration are the apneustic center, pneumotaxic center, ventral respiratory group, and dorsal respiratory group.

Peripheral Nuclei

Aortic bodies lie along the aorta. These bodies are small groups of cells that are especially sensitive to changes in the blood level of oxygen (O_2); they also respond to changes in the blood level of carbon dioxide (CO_2) and changes in the blood concentration of hydrogen ions (ie, pH, a measure of acidity [ie, pH <7] or alkalinity [ie, pH >7]; pH 7 = neutral). The aortic bodies increase their firing rate in response to a low blood O_2 level (ie, hypoxemia); high CO_2 blood level (ie, hypercapnia); or a pH level less than or equal to 7.35, which represents increased blood acidity (ie, acidemia). The increased firing rate of the aortic bodies induced by hypoxemia, hypercapnia, or acidemia results in a person taking deep, fast breaths.

The aortic bodies decrease their firing rate in response to a high blood O_2 level (ie, hyperoxemia), low CO_2 blood level (ie, hypocapnia), or a pH level greater than or equal to 7.45 (ie, alkalemia [increased blood alkalinity]). The decreased firing rate of the aortic bodies, induced by hyperoxemia, hypocapnia, or alkalemia, results in a person breathing in shallow, slow breaths.

The carotid body is a mass of cells lodged within the bifurcation of each carotid artery (Figure 1-18). The left and right carotid arteries extend from the top of the aorta, pass through the neck, and supply oxygenated blood to the neck, face, skull, and brain. At the level of the neck, each carotid artery splits into two branches. The point where a carotid artery splits is called the "carotid bifurcation."

The carotid bodies are sensitive to changes in blood levels of O_2, blood pH, and CO_2. The aortic bodies increase their firing rate in response to hypoxemia, hypercapnia, or acidemia and decrease their firing rate in response to hyperoxemia, hypocapnia, or alkalemia. The carotid and aortic bodies relay signals to the respiratory center, which is in the medulla oblongata and pons in the brain. The respiratory center neurons increase or decrease their firing rate in correlation with the frequency of signals received from the carotid bodies and aortic bodies. The depth and rate of respiration correspondingly increase or decrease.

Baroreceptors (in Greek, *baros* means "pressure") are embedded within the wall of a blood vessel—in particular, the aortic arch and the carotid sinus (ie, a dilated area at the base of the internal carotid artery near the carotid bifurcation)—and respond to changes in the pressure exerted by blood flowing through the vessel. With increasing vascular pressure, baroreceptors increase their firing rate. As a consequence, a person has an increased rate and depth of respiration. The converse occurs when the vascular blood pressure decreases.

Central Nuclei

The respiratory center consists of several nuclei in the medulla and pons. These central nuclei are responsible for different aspects of respiration. Four nuclei that are important in respiration are the ventral respiratory group, the dorsal respiratory group, the apneustic center, and the pneumotaxic center. The term "pontine respiratory group" is often used to describe the pneumotaxic and apneustic centers collectively (Figure 1-19).

The ventral respiratory group and the dorsal respiratory group are in the medulla. The ventral respiratory group neurons become stimulated during strong, active

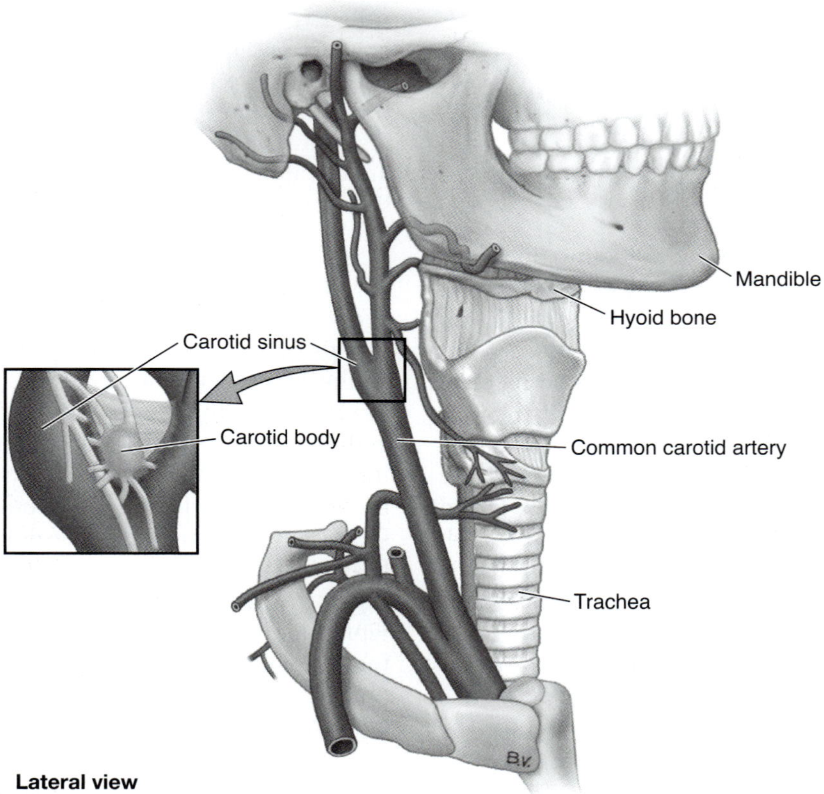

Figure 1-18 The carotid body is an ovoid mass of tissue that lies at the bifurcation of the common carotid artery. It is a chemoreceptor that monitors the level of oxygen in the blood. (Modified with permission from Agur AMR, Dalley AF II. *Grant's Atlas of Anatomy*. 14th ed. Wolters Kluwer; 2017. Figure 8.15C.)

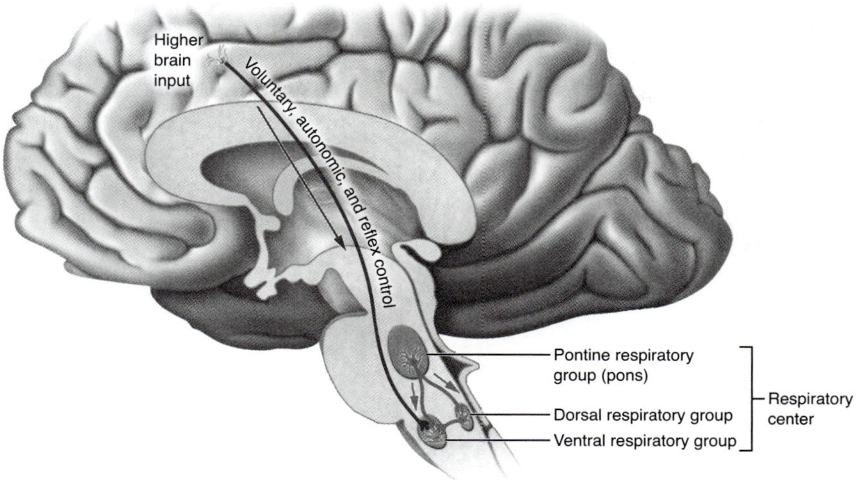

Figure 1-19 Respiratory control centers. The pontine and dorsal respiratory groups send information to the ventral respiratory group, which sets the basic respiratory rhythm by altering motor nerve activity supplying inspiratory muscles. The respiratory center then receives inputs from peripheral and central chemoreceptors and higher brain regions. (Reprinted with permission from McConnell TH, Hull KL. *Human Form, Human Function: Essentials of Anatomy & Physiology*. Wolters Kluwer Health/Lippincott Williams & Wilkins; 2011. Figure 13-15.)

respiration. They are involved in respiratory muscle movement when a person voluntarily controls inspiration and expiration. The ventral and dorsal respiratory group nuclei can modify the activity of other respiratory motor neurons. The ventral respiratory group neurons primarily fire during inhalation and exhalation, particularly during active breathing (eg, during exercise or forced breathing). The dorsal respiratory group neurons primarily fire during inhalation and are more involved in normal, quiet breathing. Both groups work in conjunction with other structures in the brainstem (eg, pontine respiratory group, reticular formation) to regulate the rhythm and rate of breathing.

The pontine respiratory group nuclei consist of the apneustic center and the pneumotaxic center. The apneustic center promotes the inspiratory phase of a breath. The pneumotaxic center rhythmically inhibits the inspirations induced by the apneustic center and thereby sets the stage for the expiratory phase of a breath. The interplay between these four nuclei within the respiratory center makes respiration possible, whether breaths are occurring automatically (ie, involuntarily) or whether a person is voluntarily changing the breathing rate and frequency.

SUMMARY

Sleep professionals must understand how the brain, heart, skeletal muscles, and eyes generate electrical activity. Without understanding why certain settings are used on a channel, a technologist will be unable to recognize artifacts and quickly make corrections when an artifact occurs in a channel. Without understanding how normal physiologic signals are produced, a technologist will be unable to determine when an abnormal physiologic signal is occurring (ie, normal EEG waves vs abnormal EEG waves during a seizure; a normal heart rhythm on an ECG vs heart arrhythmias such as premature ventricular contractions), which can potentially put a patient's life at risk. Without an understanding of how certain factors such as blindness or a skin problem can alter the biochemical generation of signals, a technologist will not adjust electrode placement on a patient or adjust the PSG recording settings to produce a desired signal on the sleep record. Most importantly, by having a clear understanding of the anatomy and the physiology of biopotentials, a technologist will be capable of producing a sleep record with signals that are accurately recorded (eg, with the correct polarity) and channels that are artifact free.

REFERENCES

1. American Association of Sleep Technologists. *AAST Technical Guideline: Standard Polysomnography*. American Association of Sleep Technologists; 2021. Accessed March 14, 2025. https://www.aastweb.org/Portals/0/Docs/Resources/Guidelines/AAST%20PSG%20Guideline%20Final.pdf

2. Mortazavi N, Talwar P, Koshmanova E, et al. REM sleep quality is associated with balanced tonic activity of the locus coeruleus during wakefulness. *J Biomed Sci*. 2025;32:35. doi:10.1186/s12929-025-01127-9
3. Koshmanova E, Berger A, Beckers E, et al. Locus coeruleus activity while awake is associated with REM sleep quality in older individuals. *JCI Insight*. 2023;8:e172008. doi:10.1172/jci.insight.172008
4. Berger H. On the human electrocephalogram. Über das Elektrenkephalogramm des Menschen. *Arch Psychiatr Nervenkr*. 1929;87:527-570. doi:10.1007/BF01797193
5. Berry RB, Wagner MH, Ryals SM. *Fundamentals of Sleep Medicine*. 2nd ed. Elsevier Health Sciences; 2025.

Chapter 2
Regulating Sleep and Waking—Circadian and Homeostasis

DAVID F. WOLFE

KEY CONCEPTS/LEARNING OBJECTIVES

The key concepts for this chapter include describing the ascending reticular activating system's role in maintaining wakefulness, reviewing the brain structures and processes for activating rapid eye movement (REM) and non-REM sleep, and the circadian and homeostatic influences on the regulation of sleep.

KEY TERMS

γ-Aminobutyric acid
Aminergic
Cholinergic
Glutamate
Histaminergic
Hypocretin
Locus ceruleus
Melanin-concentrating hormone
Reticular formation
Tuberomammillary nucleus

Various areas of the brain are responsible for allowing the body to enter different sleep stages, as well as regulate sleep and wake. Neuromediators (within these brain locations) known mainly for having wake-promoting properties include serotonin, norepinephrine, histamine, hypocretins, acetylcholine, dopamine, glutamate, and γ-aminobutyric acid (GABA). Melanin-concentrating hormone and adenosine are known for promoting sleep. GABA can promote both sleep and wake depending on its localization and interaction with other neurotransmitters (1).

CIRCADIAN AND HOMEOSTATIC PROCESSES

Two important processes in regulating sleep and wake are the circadian rhythm and homeostatic sleep drive. The balance of each of these processes helps individuals sleep well, whereas disturbances of each of these systems may cause difficulty sleeping. The homeostatic drive for sleep decreases during sleep and increases during wakefulness, whereas the circadian process diminishes its alerting signal during the night to help promote sleep and increases during the day to promote alertness (2).

Homeostatic Drive

The homeostatic sleep drive increases with sleep debt—the more hours awake, the higher the drive to sleep. Although processes exist that cause continued alertness within an individual with excessive sleep debt, the only way to satisfy the homeostatic drive to sleep is by sleeping. High cognitive workload promotes sleep homeostatic responses by increasing subjective sleepiness and fatigue, but it also delays sleep onset, producing a global sleep homeostatic response by reducing wake after sleep onset (3).

Circadian Rhythm

With its alerting effects, the circadian rhythm opposes the homeostatic drive to sleep. Through specialized retinal photoreceptors containing melanopsin, the suprachiasmatic nucleus (SCN), located in the anterior hypothalamus, receives input from light. The input of light to the SCN inhibits melatonin secretion by the pineal gland (2), producing alertness. When the SCN receives input from low levels of light (dark), melatonin is secreted from the pineal gland, causing a decrease in alertness.

The pineal gland produces melatonin from the amino acid tryptophan. Melatonin is secreted not only into the blood but also into the cerebrospinal fluid. Daytime plasma melatonin concentrations are at least

10-fold lower than nocturnal concentrations (4,5). The secretion of melatonin begins at 3 or 4 months of age, concurrent with sleep consolidation at night. Nighttime melatonin levels then increase rapidly, peaking at 1 to 3 years of age, at which point it begins to decline (6) Melatonin nocturnal serum concentrations decline across puberty (7). Peak nocturnal melatonin concentrations in 70-year-olds decrease to only a quarter or less of what they are in young adults (8).

Ocular light exposure induces a range of neurobehavioral, neuroendocrine, and circadian responses, including melatonin suppression, circadian phase resetting, and enhancement of alertness and performance. These responses are most sensitive to blue (short-wavelength, 450-480 nm) visible light (9). Before bedtime, sleep improves when subjects looked through amber lenses (blocking blue wavelength light) instead of clear lenses (10). Nighttime light exposure acutely suppresses melatonin and increases alertness in a dose-dependent manner. Independent of melatonin suppression, daytime white light exposure has also been shown to increase alertness (9).

Although inherent and set genetically, the circadian system is modifiable. Zeitgebers, meaning "time givers" in German, entrain or align the internal clock, which cycles with a period slightly longer than 24 hours: about 24.2 hours in adults (11) and 24.3 hours in adolescents (12). Although zeitgebers include meals, exercise, and social contact, the most potent stimuli to entrain the circadian phase is bright light (13).

HYPOTHALAMUS

In addition to the SCN, the hypothalamus contains another important system for sleep: the ventrolateral preoptic (VLPO) area. The VLPO and the median preoptic nuclei contain sleep-active neurons. Insomnia and sleep fragmentation are produced by a loss of VLPO neurons (14). Neurons in the VLPO contain GABA and galanin—they are relatively inactive during wake. Most sleep-active neurons in the VLPO are active during nonrapid eye movement (NREM) and REM sleep and are activated by sleep-inducing factors including prostaglandin D2 and adenosine (15). Caffeine is an adenosine antagonist, causing arousal (16).

Hypocretins (1 and 2) are arousal-promoting peptides that are only found in the lateral hypothalamus. The tuberomammillary nucleus (TMN) receives GABAergic inhibitory connections from melanin-concentrating hormone containing neurons and excitatory inputs from hypocretin-containing neurons. The TMN contains histaminergic neurons. The tonic discharge from these neurons induces and maintains wakefulness, while their silence is responsible for slow-wave sleep (1).

LOCUS CERULEUS

Located in the brainstem (pons), the locus coeruleus inhibits the VLPO, leading to wakefulness. In addition, norepinephrine-, choline-, and serotonin-containing neurons, within the locus ceruleus, fire quickly during wake. With the onset of sleep, the neurons fire slower and continue to slow as sleep deepens. During REM sleep, the neurons cease firing (17). The locus ceruleus is involved in inhibiting REM sleep with REM sleep-off neurons. As REM sleep progresses, these cells become increasingly active, eventually obstructing the activity of REM sleep-on neurons found in the pons and basal forebrain (18,19).

BASAL FOREBRAIN

Activation of the basal forebrain leads to acetylcholine release, resulting in wakefulness or REM sleep. Inhibition of acetylcholine release in the basal forebrain, by adenosine, leads to slow-wave sleep (17). Major cholinergic output of the central nervous system occurs in the basal forebrain (20). Other important neurotransmitters in the basal forebrain, involved in promoting sleep and wake, include GABA, glutamate, and vesicular glutamate transporter 3 (1).

RAPHE NUCLEI

The raphe nuclei are located in the reticular formation of the brainstem. Through thalamus, serotonin-containing neurons of the raphe nuclei promote the emergence of slow-wave cortical activity (21). Similar to the locus ceruleus, raphe nuclei cells are most active and variable during waking, particularly in response to novel stimuli. Also similar to the locus ceruleus, these cells do not fire in REM sleep (17) because of the decrease in aminergic system activity (serotonin-containing raphe neurons and norepinephrine-containing locus ceruleus) (19) and fire relatively slowly during slow-wave sleep (17).

ASCENDING RETICULAR ACTIVATING SYSTEM

The ascending reticular activating system (ARAS) comprises several neuronal circuits, traveling through the thalamus, connecting the brainstem (reticular formation) to the cerebral cortex. The ARAS also includes the hypothalamus and basal forebrain and consists of dorsal and ventral pathways. Both pathways are involved in cortical activation (20), causing neurons in the ARAS to fire at a higher rate during wakefulness. Because of external stimuli, the ARAS provides an inhibitory influence by reducing afferent (sensory neurons) activity during sleep. In other words, during sleep, fewer impulses arise from the cerebral cortex and decrease ARAS activation.

The ARAS is also involved in REM sleep. Interaction of brainstem aminergic, cholinergic, and GABAergic neurons controls the activity of glutamatergic reticular formation neurons. This leads to REM sleep, resulting in REMs, muscle atonia, cortical activation, and dreaming (20).

THALAMUS

Located just above the brainstem is the thalamus. Within the thalamus is the thalamic reticular nuclei, which contain GABAergic neurons that project from the thalamus to the reticular formation. The rhythmic bursting pattern of slow waves seen during slow-wave sleep is caused by the thalamic reticular nuclei neurons rhythmically shifting between depolarization and hyperpolarization (18). The thalamocortical neurons inhibit this rhythmic bursting pattern through the influence of excitatory neurotransmitters, such as acetylcholine and glutamate, causing the transition from sleep to wake (18,19).

CONCLUSION

The reticular formation is the primary generator of wakefulness. As the circadian rhythm and homeostatic sleep drive balance to achieve sleep and wakefulness, the hypothalamus, brainstem, basal forebrain, and thalamus assist in sleep–wake balance and maintaining REM and NREM sleep.

REFERENCES

1. Falup-Pecurariu C, Diaconu S, Tint D, Falup-Pecurariu O. Neurobiology of sleep (review). *Exp Ther Med*. 2021;21(3):272.
2. Malkani R, Zee PC. Basic circadian rhythms and circadian sleep disorders. In: Chokroverty S, Thomas RJ, eds. *Atlas of Sleep Medicine*. 2nd ed. Elsevier; 2014:119.
3. Goel N, Abe T, Braun ME, et al. Cognitive workload and sleep restriction interact to influence sleep homeostatic responses. *Sleep*. 2014;37(11):1745.
4. Lynch HJ, Wurtman RJ, Moskowitz MA, et al. Daily rhythm in human urinary melatonin. *Science*. 1975; 187(4172):169.
5. Lynch HJ, Jimerson DC, Ozaki Y, et al. Entrainment of rhythmic melatonin secretion in man to a 12-hour phase shift in the light/dark cycle. *Life Sci*. 1978; 23(15):1557.
6. Kennaway DJ, Stamp GE, Goble FC. Development of melatonin production in infants and the impact of prematurity. *J Clin Endocrinol Metab*. 1992;75:367.
7. Waldhauser F, Weiszenbacher G, Frisch H, et al. Fall in nocturnal serum melatonin during prepuberty and pubescence. *Lancet*. 1984;1:362.
8. Waldhauser F, Lynch HJ, Wurtman RJ. Melatonin in human body fluids: clinical significance. In: Reiter RJ, ed. *The Pineal Gland (Comprehensive Endocrinology)*. Raven Press; 1984:345.
9. Rahman SA, Flynn-Evans EE, Aeschbach D, et al. Diurnal spectral sensitivity of the acute alerting effects of light. *Sleep*. 2014;37(2):271-281.
10. Shechter A, Kim EW, St-Onge MP, et al. Blocking nocturnal blue light for insomnia: a randomized controlled trial. *J Psychiatr Res*. 2018;96:196.
11. Czeisler CA, Duffy JF, Shanahan TL, et al. Stability, precision, and near-24-hour period of the human circadian pacemaker. *Science*. 1999;284:2177.
12. Carskadon MA, Labyak SE, Acebo C, et al. Intrinsic circadian period of adolescent humans measured in conditions of forced desynchrony. *Neurosci Lett*. 1999;260:129.
13. Dunlap JC, Loros JL, DeCoursey PJ. *Chronobiology: Biological Timekeeping*. Oxford University Press; 2004.
14. Fuller PM, Zee PC, Buxton OM. Sleep mechanisms. In: Kryger M, Avidan A, Berry R, eds. *Atlas of Clinical Sleep Medicine*. 2nd ed. Elsevier; 2014.
15. Berry RB. Neurobiology of sleep. In: Berry RB, ed. *Fundamentals of Sleep Medicine*. Elsevier; 2012:91-100.
16. McGinty D, Szymusiak R. Sleep-promoting mechanisms in mammals. In: Kryger MH, Roth T, Dement WC, eds. *Principles and Practice of Sleep Medicine*. 4th ed. Elsevier; 2005:179.
17. Garcia-Rill E. Mechanisms of sleep and wakefulness. In: Lee-Chiong TL Jr, Sateia MJ, Carskadon MA, eds. *Sleep Medicine*. Hanley & Belfus; 2002:33.
18. Patrick R. The biologic, anatomic, and physiologic aspects of the biopotentials of sleep. In: Mattice C, Brooks R, Lee-Chiong T, eds. *Fundamentals of Sleep Technology*. 3rd ed. Wolters Kluwer; 2020:36.
19. Reinoso-Suarez F, de Andres I, Rodrigo-Angulo M, et al. Brain structures and mechanisms involved in the generation of REM sleep. *Sleep Med Rev*. 2001; 5(1):63-77.
20. Brown RE, Basheer R, McKenna JT, et al. Control of sleep and wakefulness. *Physiol Rev*. 2012;92(3): 1087-1094.
21. Culebras A. Normal sleep. In: Lee-Chiong TL Jr, Sateia MJ, Carskadon MA, eds. *Sleep Medicine*. Hanley & Belfus; 2002:1094.

Chapter 3
Sleep Deprivation

LISA M. BOND AND CYNTHIA D. MATTICE

KEY CONCEPTS/LEARNING OBJECTIVES

The key concepts for this chapter include a review of the recommended sleep requirements for all age groups, the adverse effects of sleep deprivation, differentiation between acute total sleep deprivation and chronic partial sleep deprivation, and methods employed in the diagnosis of sleep deprivation. The clinical features of insufficient sleep syndrome and countermeasures available to combat sleep deprivation associated with shift work are also reviewed.

KEY TERMS

Armodafinil
Bright light
Caffeine
Melatonin
Modafinil
Shift work
Sleep deprivation
Sleep duration
Sleep fragmentation

Sleep technologists are in a unique position both to evaluate and to experience the consequences of sleep deprivation. Because most sleep disorders evaluated by polysomnography (PSG) are the result of qualitative or quantitative disturbances in sleep, the technologist is at the front line of the evaluation. In addition, most sleep recordings are made during the patient's usual sleep hours, requiring sleep technologists to work during the evening and night. Often, the shift is 10 to 12 hours in length though the workweek is often limited to three nights per week. As shift workers, technologists are likely to experience sleep deprivation and will need to have a working knowledge of the consequences and countermeasures available. A recent advertisement representing a training program for sleep technologists indicated that candidates would need to "remain awake, alert, and maintain good interpersonal skills throughout the night as well as demonstrate the ability to get proper sleep during the day." The challenges for the sleep technologist are significant.

NORMAL SLEEP REQUIREMENTS

Sleep requirements differ among individuals and within different age groups. In recognition of this, in 2015, the National Sleep Foundation (NSF) updated what is considered normal sleep requirements for various age groups (1). The NSF also broke down recommendations for sleep for adults into three categories rather than just one for all adult ages and created new age grouping for younger adults ages 18 to 25, adults ages 26 to 64, and older adults ages 65 and above. The scientifically grounded guidelines were developed based on a rigorous, systematic review of scientific literature on sleep duration, health, performance, and safety. The different age categories now have recommended sleep amounts, what may be appropriate, and what is not recommended.

It is no longer sufficient to simply say an adult should get 8 hours of sleep each night. Sleep technologists need to be aware of how much sleep is recommended for each age group. Even with sufficient sleep time, sleep quality is still important to enable best function. The best indicator of sufficient good-quality sleep is waking up feeling refreshed, alert, and performing at a peak level during wake time.

In 2016, the American Academy of Sleep Medicine (AASM) developed a consensus statement on the recommended amount of sleep for pediatric populations that indicates that infants aged 4 to 12 months should sleep 12 to 16 hours per 24 hours, including naps. At 1 to 2 years of age, the recommendation is 11 to 14 hours per 24 hours including naps. The recommendation for children 3 to 5 years of age is 10 to 13 hours per 24 hours, including naps. By the age of 6, most children no longer nap, and the recommended amount of sleep for children between 6 and 12 years of age is 9 to 12 hours per 24 hours. The recommendation for teenagers 13 to 18 years of age is 8 to 10 hours of sleep per 24 hours (2).

DEFINITION OF SLEEP DEPRIVATION

Sleep deprivation in an individual can be caused by insufficient duration of sleep (quantitative sleep deprivation), a fragmented or interrupted sleep period (qualitative sleep deprivation), or a combination of both factors. Sleep deprivation can be either chronic or acute. The subjective assessment of the quality of sleep is based on the amount of sleep, continuity of sleep, and depth of the sleep. See Table 3-1 for the NSF's sleep duration recommendations (1).

Acute sleep deprivation refers to no sleep or a reduction in the usual total sleep time, typically lasting 1 or 2 days (3,4). Chronic sleep insufficiency (also called sleep restriction) exists when an individual routinely sleeps less than the amount required for optimal functioning.

PREVALENCE OF SLEEP DEPRIVATION

The prevalence of sleep deprivation in the industrialized world appears to be on the rise. In June 2023, the Centers for Disease Control and Prevention's (CDC) Preventing Chronic Disease section published a research brief reporting that more than a third of Americans were not getting enough sleep on a regular basis. The major consequences of chronic sleep deprivation are fatigue, excessive daytime sleepiness, clumsiness, weight changes, and adversely affected cognitive function. Consequences can also include motor vehicle or industrial accidents, negative socioeconomic and public health outcomes, reduced academic and job performance, and a reduced sense of well-being. Sleep researchers have long reported that sleep deprivation can affect your physical health and emotional well-being. In a world that is increasingly changing into a "global community," the encroaching demands on the sleep-wake cycle of an individual pose a significant dilemma.

Historically, major industrial disasters, such as those at Chernobyl nuclear power plant in 1986, Three Mile Island nuclear power plant in 1979, Bhopal toxic gas leak in 1984, the Texas City BP oil refinery explosion in 2005, and the Colgan air crash in 2009, and serious accidents, such as those involving the Space Shuttle Challenger in 1986, the Exxon Valdez oil spill in 1989, American Airlines Flight 1420 crash in 1999, and train derailment in Bronx, NY, in 2013, have been attributed to errors in judgment caused at least in part by sleepiness in the workplace.

The US National Highway Traffic Safety Administration (NHTSA) reports 100,000 car crashes caused by drowsy driving each year, resulting in an estimated 1,500 deaths per year. People who are sleep deprived have nearly 3 times the risk for type 2 diabetes than non–sleep-deprived individuals and have an increased risk for high blood pressure and a 48% increased chance of developing heart disease. Getting less than 5 hours of sleep nightly puts an individual at a 50% higher risk

Table 3-1 National Sleep Foundation's Sleep Duration Recommendations

Age	Recommended (hours)	May Be Appropriate (hours)	Not Recommended (hours)
Newborns 0-3 mo	14-17	11-13 18-19	<11 >19
Infants 4-11 mo	12-15	10-11 16-18	<10 >18
Toddlers 1-2 y	11-14	9-10 15-16	<9 >16
Preschoolers 3-5 y	10-13	8-9 14	<8 >14
School-age children 6-13 y	9-11	7-8 12	<7 >12
Teenagers 14-17 y	8-10	7 11	<7 >11
Young adults 18-25 y	7-9	6 10-11	<6 >11
Adults 26-64 y	7-9	6 10	<6 >10
Older adults ≥65 y	7-8	5-6 9	<5 >9

Reprinted from Hirshkowitz M, Whiton K, Albert SM, et al. National Sleep Foundation's sleep time duration recommendations: methodology and results summary. *Sleep Health*. 2015;1(1):40-43. Copyright © 2015 National Sleep Foundation. With permission.

of obesity as there is an increase in the hunger hormone ghrelin and a decrease in the appetite-control hormone leptin.

The NSF celebrates Sleep Awareness Week in March every year to emphasize the connection between sleep and our overall health. During this week, the NSF releases the results of their survey of Americans regarding the state of the nation's sleep health.

TYPES OF SLEEP DEPRIVATION

Acute, Chronic, and Total Sleep Deprivation

Acute sleep deprivation refers to no sleep or a reduction in the usual total sleep time, usually lasting 1 or 2 days. Chronic sleep insufficiency or deprivation (also called sleep restriction) exists when an individual routinely sleeps less than the amount required for optimal functioning. Chronic sleep restriction has been shown to cause similar deficient cognitive performance as two nights of total sleep deprivation (TSD), meaning that even moderate sleep restriction can seriously impair the functioning of healthy adults.

A study published in 2024 examined the effect of TSD on the brain. TSD was noted to increase or blunt autonomic nervous system and cortisol responses to stress. It appears that TSD may modify the nature of physiologic responses to daily challenges, influencing health outcomes. From studies done in 1894 on puppies, 1898 on dogs, different rat studies (5,6), and in 1896 on humans (7), as well as from individuals who have prion disease, referred to as fatal familial insomnia, we have learned that prolonged sleep loss leads to a range of psychological problems and death.

Accumulating research in both animals and humans has demonstrated profound behavioral and physiologic consequences from sleep deprivation. Animal sleep deprivation studies have suggested that sleep is critically important for survival and is probably vitally important in thermoregulation, energy balance, and immune function. Totally sleep-deprived rats show a characteristic picture of weight loss, skin lesions, and ultimately death after 11 to 22 days of TSD. As they deteriorate, the animals exhibit marked increases in energy expenditure, an increase in heart rate, large increases in food intake, rises in plasma norepinephrine, and declines in plasma thyroxine. It is theorized that the increased energy expenditure is an attempt to maintain body temperature despite excessive heat loss during sleep deprivation. Available studies in humans suggest a far less profound physiologic response to sleep deprivation over periods of up to 11 days.

Studies of sleep deprivation in humans suffer from certain methodologic limitations. It is unethical to deprive human subjects of sleep to the point of producing medical consequences. Motivations of both experimenter and subject can have a large impact on results, particularly on data related to behavior and mood.

Despite these methodologic limitations, numerous studies of human sleep deprivation have been published. The most obvious consequence of acute sleep loss is excessive sleepiness. The impact of TSD can reduce the latency of sleep onset on the Multiple Sleep Latency Test (MSLT), which is taken into account in the AASM practice parameter that recommends 6 hours of sleep time prior to the performance of the MSLT. Various studies have addressed the impact of sleep deprivation on subjective and objective measures of sleepiness, as well as psychomotor vigilance, performance, memory tasks, and mood. This will be described later in this chapter. Technologists should keep in mind that characteristics of each individual, such as age, may affect the severity of sleep loss consequence and ability to recover.

Recovery From Total Sleep Deprivation

The sleep technologist will be asked, and will need to know, if sleep loss can be recovered. Early studies suggested that only a small fraction (10%-20%) of the total sleep time lost during deprivation is recoverable. However, those studies allowed ad-lib time in bed, and an individual's motivation to get out of bed resulted in an underestimation of the true recovery. In a study that enforced a 24-hour time in bed following sleep deprivation, subjects recovered 72% and 42% of the total sleep lost during the 24- and 48-hour periods, respectively, of deprivation (6).

For sleep recovery, the hours slept and the intensity of the sleep are important. Some of the most refreshing sleep occurs during deep sleep. Although such sleep's true effects are still being studied, it is generally considered a restorative period for the brain. Sleeping more hours allows the brain more time in this rejuvenating period (7).

Chronic and Partial Sleep Deprivation

More common than acute TSD is chronic partial sleep deprivation, which may accumulate over several days. This type of sleep restriction occurs in everyday life in those who voluntarily restrict their sleep time or during travel across time zones. For example, when a person with a usual nocturnal sleep need of 8 hours gets only 7, a 1-hour "sleep deficit" or "sleep debt" is created. If this pattern is sustained over 1 week, the "sleep debt" is roughly equivalent to a full night of total sleep loss. Despite the frequent occurrence of this type of chronic partial sleep deprivation in the population, it is not readily recognizable.

Several experimental studies have looked closely at this issue. In evaluating partial sleep restriction over a

2-week period, it has been shown that chronic restriction of sleep to 6 hours or less per night produced cognitive performance deficits equivalent to up to two nights of TSD. Equally important, subjects in the study were largely unaware of the increasing cognitive deficits. In a related study from the same group, impairment from sleep loss was significantly different among individuals and stable within individuals, suggesting that an individual's vulnerability to sleep loss was an inherent trait.

Chronic sleep restriction is also associated with a higher overall mortality rate. In fact, both short and long sleep durations are associated with an increase in mortality from cardiovascular disease as well as total mortality (7). A large-scale prospective study of Japanese men and women aged 40 to 79 years confirmed that, compared with 7 hours of sleep, short sleep duration of 4 hours or less was associated with a 2-fold increase in mortality from coronary heart disease for women and a 1.5-fold increase in mortality from noncardiovascular disease/noncancer and a 1.3-fold increase in total mortality for both men and women. Clearly, optimal sleep duration is a key factor in overall health (8,9).

DIAGNOSING QUANTITATIVE SLEEP DEPRIVATION

The *International Classification of Sleep Disorders*, 3rd edition, lists insufficient sleep syndrome (ISS), also known as behaviorally induced ISS, insufficient nocturnal sleep, chronic sleep deprivation, and sleep restriction, under Central Disorders of Hypersomnolence (10). This sleep disorder is extrinsic—it originates from causes outside of the body. Diagnostic criteria consist of daily need to sleep, or lapses into sleep, during the day (for children there is a complaint of behavioral abnormalities attributed to sleepiness).

The sleep time, obtained via personal history, sleep logs, or actigraphy, is shorter than expected for the age group. The patient curtails sleep by an alarm clock or wakening by others and generally sleeps longer on weekends and vacations. The curtailing of sleep is present most days for at least 3 months. Extending the total sleep time resolves symptoms of sleepiness. The symptoms are also not better explained by another untreated sleep disorder, medication effects, or a medical, neurologic, or mental disorder. Actigraphy is commonly used with sleep diaries for 2 to 3 weeks to help document the patient's time in bed, sleep latency, total sleep time, and sleep efficiency. PSG and MSLT are not required to establish this diagnosis. Rather, a therapeutic trial of longer sleep episodes is used, and if the longer sleep durations lead to resolution of the symptoms, this is sufficient to diagnose ISS.

If PSG is performed, it would reveal reduced sleep latency and a greater than 90% sleep efficiency, reflecting the need for more sleep. It is also common to see slow-wave sleep (SWS) rebound (10) at the expense of other non–rapid eye movement (NREM) stages. An MSLT would show excessive sleepiness with N1 seen in most naps and a short sleep onset. It is often common to see N2 in 80% of the MSLT naps, and sleep-onset rapid eye movement periods (SOREMPs) can occur. As the MSLT can have two SOREMPs and a short sleep latency, ISS can be confused with narcolepsy along with other disorders of hypersomnolence. This confusion can be heightened by the growing epidemic of ISS among adolescents and young adults. It is therefore important that a clear and accurate sleep history of normal sleep amounts be obtained.

SELECTIVE SLEEP DEPRIVATION AND RECOVERY

Rapid Eye Movement Sleep Deprivation

Animal experiments have shown that selective rapid eye movement (REM) sleep deprivation leads to increased motor activity and aggression as well as reduced pain thresholds, memory impairment for recently acquired tasks, and a decrease in the seizure threshold. Selective deprivation studies in humans suggest that this leads to increasingly shorter REM sleep latencies. A REM rebound, or temporary increases in REM sleep activity, may also be observed. Short REM sleep latencies and REM rebound suggest that REM pressure exists; if so, it is postulated to be related to the composition of prior sleep rather than prior wakefulness. Through unknown mechanisms, selective REM deprivation actually enhances alertness in experimental human subjects.

Slow-Wave Sleep Deprivation

In human experimental studies, it was found to be more difficult to deprive a person of stage N3, or SWS, than REM sleep. Subjects required 5 to 7 times as many arousals to deprive them of stage N3 sleep than to deprive them of REM sleep during each night of selective sleep deprivation. Daytime performance after selective stage N3 and REM sleep deprivation conditions in humans has also been tested, yet decrements were not found after as many as seven nights of either stage N3 or REM sleep deprivation. It is clear from the available research that the major predictor of performance during these sleep loss paradigms was the total amount of time spent asleep, regardless of sleep stage parameters.

However, even though the deprivation of SWS may not objectively affect daytime performance, SWS deprivation appears to result in meaningful changes in daytime pain levels and the sensation of fatigue. In a study of healthy subjects, both REM sleep and SWS interruption decreased mechanical pain thresholds. An increase in pain thresholds followed recovery sleep. Similar studies in middle-aged women without musculoskeletal complaints showed that three nights of selective SWS deprivation decreased pain thresholds. The subjects also reported generalized discomfort, fatigue, and reduced vigor. The qualitative changes of alpha wave intrusion into SWS have been associated with chronic syndromes (eg, fibromyalgia), but critical reviews by numerous investigators have failed to show a direct connection between the alpha-delta electroencephalography (EEG) sleep pattern and pain complaints among patients with chronic pain.

SLEEP FRAGMENTATION

Sleep fragmentation is best described as the interruption of sleep with frequent, brief arousals characterized by increases in EEG frequency or bursts of alpha activity and, occasionally, transient increases in skeletal muscle tone. These arousals generally last 3 to 15 seconds, usually do not result in prolonged wakefulness, and may not alter the sleep stage scoring of a standard 30-second epoch on a polysomnogram. Many times, the sleep technologist will be able to identify the arousing condition or stimulus (apneas, leg movements, and pain), and other times, no arousing stimulus will be identifiable.

Several studies have shown that sleep fragmentation without overall sleep loss per se is associated with reduced daytime function, similar to that seen from acute sleep deprivation and TSD. This phenomenon has been evaluated by simulating the sleep-disrupting effects of apnea with performance of a standardized awakening after each minute of sleep for two consecutive nights in normal adults. Following this experimental sleep disruption, subjects were significantly sleepier than they were at their baseline. The level of impairment was similar to that seen after periods of total sleep loss of 40 to 64 hours.

ADVERSE EFFECTS OF SLEEP DEPRIVATION

The adverse effects of sleep deprivation on human function are wide ranging and include excessive sleepiness; alterations in immune, cardiovascular, and hemodynamic changes; and alterations in hormone production. Not getting enough sleep, and enough good-quality sleep, has been shown to increase the risk of or exacerbate high blood pressure, heart disease, obesity, diabetes, anxiety, depression, irritability that can damage relationships, and profoundly affect the ability to think clearly and react quickly as well as form memories. Being sleep deprived can be very dangerous. Testing has shown that the hand-eye coordination of individuals driving while sleep deprived was just as bad as, if not worse than, that of drunk drivers. Being sleep deprived magnifies the effect of alcohol on the sleep-deprived body beyond what is seen in a normal rested individual. Most of these issues are beyond the scope and purpose of this review, but some of the behavioral changes described earlier in this chapter deserve elaboration.

Every sleep technologist should know and recognize the basic signs of sleep deprivation, which include irritability and moodiness, reduced ability to cope and deal with stress, lack of motivation, difficulty concentrating, memory problems, impaired motor skills, drowsiness when driving, feeling sluggish in the afternoon, needing a nap to get through the day, difficulty getting out of bed in the morning, relying on the snooze button, weight gain, frequent colds, and infections.

Daytime Sleepiness

Daytime sleepiness is the feeling of being drowsy and sluggish most days to the extent that it can interfere with work, school, or relationships. It is not the same as fatigue, which is characterized as low energy. It is also not depression, where there is a reduced desire to perform normal activities, even those that are enjoyable. Though this is not a disorder, it is a serious symptom and the one most people list as a chief complaint for why they are seeking help in a sleep clinic. Daytime sleepiness can be measured subjectively by use of the Stanford Sleepiness Scale (SSS) or the more commonly used Epworth Sleepiness Scale (ESS). However, for an objective measurement, one would need to perform the MSLT after an adequate overnight PSG test.

A result of greater than 10 in the ESS is considered significant and requires further medical assessment (11). Sleep questionnaires have also been developed for both pediatric patients and adolescents with variations on the questions. For example, "sitting and watching TV" would be changed to "sitting, watching TV or a video." "Sitting in a classroom at school during the morning" may be substituted for "sitting inactive in a public place (theater, movie, meeting, etc.)."

The two-process model described by Borbély (12) best answers the question: Why do we feel sleepy? The homeostatic sleep drive is driven by the amount of prior wakefulness. It is physiologic, linear, and cumulative. The "sleep load" or sleep need increases as an individual becomes progressively sleepier with each passing hour. Superimposed is a second process, the circadian rhythm, driven by the "biologic clock" and influenced by the time of the day. A reduction in circadian alertness leads to increased sleepiness that occurs roughly at the same time each day. These two processes interact with each other—the circadian rhythm influences how sleepy a sleep-deprived individual feels. After a night without sleep, one may be fairly alert at 10 AM, because the circadian increase in alertness counteracts the accumulated physiologic sleep need, but in the afternoon, biologic and physiologic influences may combine to create an intense need for sleep. The most vulnerable times to feel sleepy appear to be between 5 and 8 AM and 2 and 4 PM (independent of a lunch-time meal), and the most likely times to feel alert seem to be between 10 AM and 12 noon and again in the evening. Mary Carskadon, PhD, has summarized the concept nicely: "Regardless of how many hours you've been awake, the most sleepy time occurs as the circadian 'night' is ending; the least sleepy time occurs at the end of the circadian day."

Cognitive Functioning, Memory, and Mood Disturbance

Various studies have addressed the impact of sleep deprivation on subjective and objective measures of sleepiness, as well as psychomotor vigilance, performance, memory tasks, and mood. Impairment of immediate recall for elements placed in short-term memory is a classic finding in sleep deprivation experiments. The pattern of memory deficits shows some functional similarities to adult aging and alcohol intoxication.

Degradation of nonexecutive components of cognition, such as information intake, that accounted for the overall impairment in subjects' performance on cognitive tasks also occurs. A study on the effects of sleep deprivation published in the journal *Sleep* in 2010 appeared to show that the sleep-deprived brain is capable of processing information, but this information may be distorted before it can be processed. Individuals who are sleep deprived, such as emergency responders, police officers, military personnel, and medical personnel, who often have little opportunity for adequate sleep, risk their ability to make sound decisions in safety-critical environments.

A meta-analysis of available data suggested that mood is more affected by sleep deprivation than either cognitive or motor performance. Despite the possibility of self-reporting errors, it is likely that sleep deprivation has a negative effect on mood. For example, the therapeutic effects of sleep deprivation on endogenous depression have long been recognized. Because depression can be associated with a decrease of functional serotonergic neurotransmission, afflicted patients may exhibit significant mood improvement after one night of sleep deprivation even though they may complain of sleep loss. This antidepressant effect is likely related to the enhancement of central serotoninergic neurotransmission, similar to that described for antidepressants such as selective serotonin reuptake inhibitors. When selective REM sleep deprivation was employed in patients with endogenous depression, mood improved and was associated with improvement in the abnormal temporal distribution of REM sleep.

Dietary Changes and Increases in Obesity

The CDC reports that during the 2-year period of August 2021 to August 2023, 40.3% of the US adult population age 20 and up were obese. There are several factors including sleep deprivation that influence this growing problem of obesity. Studies have demonstrated an association between insufficient sleep and an increased appetite. Individuals with adequate amount of sleep are more likely to make healthy food choices. Conversely, sleep deprivation promotes overeating and inactivity, with the increase in caloric consumption derived from less healthy choices such as snack foods. Studies have demonstrated that sleep curtailment leads to decreased leptin and elevated ghrelin, agents that provide feedback to hypothalamic regulatory centers that control food intake. The changes reported would likely lead to increased food consumption and weight gain. Chronic or partial sleep loss may increase the risk of obesity and diabetes by affecting glucose regulation and increasing insulin resistance. During experimentally induced sleep loss, healthy individuals showed decreased insulin sensitivity without adequate compensation in beta-cell function, resulting in an impaired glucose tolerance and increased diabetes risk. It has been reported that school-age children (4-10 years of age) with more variable sleep schedules and shorter sleep durations were at higher health risk for altered insulin levels and adverse metabolic outcomes leading to obesity. Weight gain from sleep deprivation has also been shown to result from a dysregulation of the neuroendocrine control of appetite, leading to excessive food intake and decreased energy expenditure.

Effects on Pain Thresholds and Increases in Spontaneous Pain

Improving sleep quantity and quality is important in the treatment of patients with chronic pain disorders. Studies performed on female patients at Johns Hopkins University School of Medicine have shown that sleep-deprived individuals have a decrease or absence of SWS, which can be a risk factor for the exacerbation of chronic pain ranging from tension headaches to fibromyalgia (13). These findings support the need for aggressive treatment of insomnia and other sleep quality issues as an adjunct to other modalities directed at treating chronic pain.

Motor Vehicle Accidents

The American Automobile Association (AAA) Foundation for Traffic Safety reports that between 2017 and 2021, 17.6% of all fatal crashes involved a drowsy driver. In a study done by the AAA, drowsiness was assessed using a validated measure of the percentage of time that an individual's eyes are closed. Using this measure, drowsiness was identified in 8.8% to 9.5% of all crashes reviewed and 10.6% to 10.8% of crashes that resulted in significant property damage, airbag deployment, or injury (14). Studies have shown that fatigue-related crashes are more common for truck drivers with irregular schedules (67%) than those with regular schedules (38%). The challenges that face us are predicting performance and vehicular safety on the basis of driver fatigue. Previous studies have shown that the most important crash predictor is the duration of the driver's most recent sleep period. In the future, artificial intelligence will be used to develop an analytic approach to predict fatigue and drowsiness and the effect on reducing vigilance and the impact on reaction time.

In a review of vehicle accidents specifically attributed to driver "fatigue," a prominent 24-hour pattern was identified, showing a major peak at 3 AM and a minor peak at 3 PM. This bimodal pattern closely mirrors the known circadian propensity to sleep (2-7 AM and 2-5 PM) seen in human studies of healthy, noncomplaining individuals.

Studies have also affirmed that sleep-deprived drivers are just as dangerous as drunk drivers. Subjects who drove after being awake for 17 to 19 hours performed worse than those with a blood alcohol level of 0.05%. Twenty to 25 hours of wakefulness produced performance decrements equivalent to those observed at a blood alcohol concentration of 0.10%, a level deemed unsafe and unacceptable when working or driving. Driving while drowsy is considered a risk to others' personal safety by 8 out of 10 people. In addition, 9.7% of drivers report they have fallen asleep or nodded off during the past year, even though 30% report that they continue to drive in spite of being tired and having a difficult time keeping their eyes open.

INTERVENTIONS TO COMBAT SLEEP DEPRIVATION IN SHIFT WORKERS

Sleep technologists may suffer from shift work disorder because of the nature of the field. Most people sleep at night, and most technologists work at night, monitoring, recording, and intervening with treatment for many sleep disorders. Sleep technologists are intimately familiar with shift work and are in a unique position to help others that need to deal with a 24-hour society. The traditional 9-AM-to-5-PM day shift has been replaced in many industries with evening shifts, night shifts, and rotating shifts.

According to the NSF, roughly 15% of our full-time labor force is working in shifts. In the 2008 NSF poll, 63% of shift workers (vs 89% of nonshift workers) reported that their jobs allowed them to get enough sleep. Though not all shift workers suffer from shift work disorder, about 10% of those working rotating shifts are believed to have a shift disorder of some type, and roughly 25% to 30% of any type of shift worker do suffer from symptoms such as excessive sleepiness and insomnia regularly.

The diagnostic criteria for shift work disorder in the *International Classification of Sleep Disorders*, 3rd edition, lists the following requirements to diagnose shift work disorder:

1. Insomnia or excessive sleepiness paired with a reduction of total sleep time that is associated with a recurring work schedule that overlaps the usual sleep times
2. The symptoms must have been present for, and the patient must have been working in shift for, at least 3 months.
3. A disrupted sleep-and-wake pattern demonstrated by a sleep log or actigraphy monitoring over a minimum of 14 days that includes both work and free days
4. There is no other current sleep disorder; medical, neurologic, or mental disorder; medication use; poor sleep hygiene; or substance use that can explain the symptoms.

Several strategies have been developed to address the impairments associated with shift work.

Education

In 1999, the US Department of Transportation targeted shift workers and teens in a new program implemented to combat the problem that fatigue and sleepiness present for highway safety. An NHTSA program provided materials and guidance for employers, shift workers, and shift workers' families. NHTSA administrator Ricardo Martinez stated, "Shift workers cannot be expected to adapt to society's schedules. Society must adapt to these workers' schedules." The NHTSA continues to combat drowsy driving. Information is available at the NHTSA's website at https://www.nhtsa.gov/risky-driving/drowsy-driving. Several preventive strategies have been suggested to minimize the effect of sleep deprivation on shift workers. The effective use of days off to catch up on sleep is critical. However, studies of medical residents working the night float shift (rotating night shift) revealed that they slept less even though they had ample opportunity to sleep during the day after each night shift. Furthermore, they had decreased vigor and increased fatigue during the night float shift, and their fatigue scores correlated significantly with omission errors during the night float rotations but not during daytime rotations.

Sleep loss is cumulative; it is important to begin a new work schedule without an existing sleep debt. This generally requires two nights of unrestricted sleep, as it is not possible to stock up in anticipation of sleep debt in the future. Exercise also has a role in helping to cope with shift work. Moderate exercise is preferred to intensive training. For day shifts, exercise is best timed after the shift. For night shifts, exercise should be timed before an evening nap.

The following recommendations may help individuals (including sleep technologists) who are coping with shift work. Remember that there is no substitute for getting adequate sleep.

1. Limit continuous performance schedules to 12 to 16 hours.
2. Schedule adequate time off duty to protect sleep and sanity.
3. Know the times of greatest impairment and maximum alertness.
4. Avoid driving between 2 and 9 AM.
5. Recognize behavioral changes as an indication of dangerous levels of fatigue.
6. Provide performance backups during times of impairment.
7. Avoid alcohol.
8. Realize that there is no substitute for sleep.

Work Environment

It is important when working evening or night shifts that the workplace be bright and cool to support alertness and productivity on the job. Bright light does not need to be constant, even 20 to 30 minutes can help shift workers to be more alert. If possible, schedule the work that requires the most concentration and skill when workers are in their most alert state. The drowsiest time for night shift workers is roughly 3 to 5 AM. Workers should avoid working more than a few consecutive nights and, if possible, schedule at least 2 days off after working a night shift rotation.

Dealing With Rotating Shifts

Some jobs require working rotating shifts, which is possibly the most physically demanding adjustment for shift workers. Still there are things that can be done to make even rotating shifts easier to handle. A clockwise rotation is much easier to adapt to than a counterclockwise rotation. This is a more natural change for the body. A pattern of day shift to evening shift to night shift to day shift would be the preferred pattern to follow. Rotating every 2 to 3 days is also easier on you physically than rotating every 5 to 7 days or randomly rotating even when following the clockwise pattern. Rotating shift workers should also begin to adjust before their shift change if possible. Delaying sleep by an hour or two before the day of the change can also make the change a bit easier.

Sleep Schedule

Shift workers should maintain consistent bedtimes and rise times, including nights off work. Delaying sleep by an hour or two to allow some daytime activities that cannot be avoided can be appropriate. However, flipping completely back to days and then back to nights is not healthy or advised. Doing so can make it more difficult to return to work and function optimally and to sleep again during the daytime when needed.

Bright Light

Evidence supports a role for appropriately timed bright-light exposure. It has been demonstrated that there is improvement in nocturnal alertness and daytime sleep in night shift workers who were exposed to bright light in their workplace followed by attenuating morning light (using dark sunglasses) on the way home from work. Light boxes, which produce 10,000 lux, once large and cumbersome, now can be easily purchased and are small and more compact. Working with a sleep specialist can help determine the best time and the appropriate amount of time for bright-light sessions for maximum effectiveness. Sessions are normally between 15 and 30 minutes in length. Light boxes are familiar devices to most sleep technologists in that they are aware of light therapy for treating circadian rhythm disorders and seasonal affective disorder. However, light therapy can also be used to help with managing working the night shift.

Blue Light

It has been shown that low-intensity blue light exposure can promote alertness during prolonged nighttime performance testing. Low-intensity blue light exposure may be a valuable option to be applied in situations where bright-light therapy may not be appropriate, such as in certain occupational settings. Testing on daytime workers has demonstrated subjective improvement in alertness, performance, and even fatigue when working under blue-enriched white lights instead of standard white lighting. However, it should be noted that the blue light emitted by electronic devices can also affect individuals and delay sleep onset. Shift workers, like all workers, should be attentive to turning off and discontinuing the use of such devices before sleep.

Eating Habits

Eating healthy is important for shift workers, regardless of shift, though it may be difficult. The best practices for night shift workers include having a lunch-like meal upon awakening to energize for your "day." Early in the shift, a small dinner meal or snack is appropriate. Later in the shift, small healthy snacks every couple of hours can help to maintain alertness and energy. At the end of the shift, a small breakfast is best to improve daytime sleep.

Meals should be balanced between proteins, low-glycemic-index foods, fruits and vegetables, and carbohydrates. Eat for energy and avoid junk foods that cause sluggishness. Preplanning meals and snacks ahead of time is also a best practice and assists with wiser choices. To achieve better eating habits, bring your own food to work. Most to-go foods and vending machine foods are high in salt, fat, and sugars, and the temptation to upsize is high. Drink plenty of water and stay away from soft drinks because even the diet versions are unhealthy.

Napping

Napping is an effective strategy for those who suffer sleep deprivation as the result of shift work or prolonged work schedules. It is important to take advantage of the circadian rhythm and normal periods of sleepiness. Night shift workers who took a 90-minute-to-2-hour nap before their shift were able to prevent sleepiness. Later naps produced deeper sleep, but workers awakened with grogginess because of sleep inertia. When time will not allow a 90-minute-to-2-hour nap, the nap timing should be limited to 45 minutes to avoid entering SWS. Even a 20-minute nap at work on the night shift between 1 and 3 AM can improve performance on the first night shift but not the second.

Exercise

Exercise triggers an increase in body temperature and improves alertness. Shift workers that engage in brief bouts of aerobic exercise experience less sleepiness and more alertness during their shift.

Sleep Aids

The temptation to use a sleeping pill to fall asleep during the day is high and many over-the-counter sleep aids are available. However, they cannot reset the circadian clock; not even the prescription sleep aids can do that. Many sleep aids also become less and less effective over time. Antihistamines are a common ingredient in over-the-counter items that people use as sleep aids, but the side effect of drowsiness when awake can be severe. This could lead to drowsy driving or difficulty being alert while working.

Sleep Hygiene

The practice of following basic sleep hygiene is important. Blackout curtains to darken rooms, and the use of "white noise" to help block daytime sounds is even more important for shift workers. Schedule repairs and deliveries outside of scheduled sleep hours as much as possible. Silence phones and consider setting up an alternate contact for an emergency during sleep hours. Protect sleep time and maintain good sleep habits to improve functioning during a night shift.

Stimulants

Caffeine

The alerting effect of caffeine has been recognized for centuries. Caffeine-containing beverages and over-the-counter tablets help individuals ameliorate the impact of both voluntary and involuntary sleep deprivation. In general, its effects last 3 to 5 hours yet may last for 10 or more hours in caffeine-sensitive individuals. The alerting effect is dependent on habitual use, body mass index, and previous food intake. Strategies for caffeine use have been developed for workers and call for avoidance when already alert (eg, the beginning of a daytime shift or just after a nap). Caffeine is best ingested 1 hour before the expected time of decreased alertness, which on the night shift would probably be between 3 and 5 AM. Consumption should be stopped at least 3 hours ahead of the planned bedtime. Users of caffeine need to be aware of the potential side effects, such as diuresis (dehydration), anxiety, irritability, tremulousness, and insomnia. It has been suggested that in drivers, the combined use of caffeine and a nap may counteract sleepiness. Knowing that the effect of caffeine is usually delayed by 30 minutes after ingestion, drivers who employed the use of caffeine followed by a short nap incurred the benefits of both.

Modafinil

Medications should not be the first line of treatment for shift workers. Modafinil, a unique wake-promoting agent, is approved for use in treating sleepiness associated with shift work. This drug was originally developed for the treatment of narcolepsy. It is generally well tolerated and associated with few side effects; it is relatively long acting and does not usually cause peripheral sympathetic stimulation. Studies have suggested a lower misuse and dependency potential when compared with older stimulant drugs. Modafinil has been shown to attenuate physiologic sleepiness and neurobehavioral deficits that occur during the hours of a typical night shift. In a study exploring the efficacy of modafinil prophylactically given for maintaining the performance of aviators in simulators despite 40 hours (2 days and 1 night) of continued wakefulness, the drug showed some promise, but nausea, vertigo, and dizziness were common. When compared with D-amphetamine, modafinil had comparable beneficial effects on mood, fatigue, and cognitive performance with fewer side effects. When compared with 600 mg of caffeine in normal adults following 40 continuous hours of wakefulness, both drugs improved performance and vigilance equally. In a randomized, placebo-controlled study, improvements in alertness and performance were found with 200 mg of modafinil in measures of sleep latency, clinical impression rating, sustained-attention performance, and patient-estimated sleepiness. However, the benefits were small, and in those treated, high levels of sleepiness and impaired performance persisted at night.

Many sleep technologists, like other night workers, suffer from shift work sleep disorder (SWSD), which is caused by an inability of some shift workers to adapt to the major misalignment between their work and rest schedules. The US Modafinil Study Group reported that the effect of modafinil taken 30 minutes before the night shift in patients with excessive sleepiness was the result of SWSD. Modafinil significantly improved functioning and quality of life and at the same time did not show adverse effects on intended sleep. The drug was well tolerated and did not lead to meaningful changes in safety parameters when compared with placebo.

Armodafinil

Armodafinil is another oral wakefulness-promoting agent used in the treatment of narcolepsy, SWSD, and residual daytime sleepiness complaints in patients with obstructive sleep apnea treated with continuous positive airway pressure. The Food and Drug Administration–approved dose of armodafinil is 150 to 250 mg taken as a single dose in the morning or 150 mg taken 1 hour before the start of the night shift in patients with SWSD. Armodafinil dose reductions should be considered for patients with severe hepatic impairment or for older patients in whom elimination may be slowed. Unlike modafinil, there is a lower risk of serious rash or hypersensitivity reaction with the use of armodafinil. The incidence and type of psychiatric symptoms associated with armodafinil are expected to be similar to those of modafinil.

Melatonin

Melatonin, a secretory product of the pineal gland, is known to be important in synchronization of circadian rhythms. Exogenous melatonin has been used to treat the symptoms of circadian maladaptation associated with night shift work and jet lag. By taking melatonin before the start of the first four of eight afternoon/evening sleep episodes before night shift (a 7-hour advance of the sleep schedule), subjects were found to have larger phase advances than those who took a placebo (15). However, only a few studies have addressed the impact of melatonin in practical, real-life situations. Cavallo et al (16) gave melatonin or placebo to physicians training in pediatrics during the morning after night shift work and found no improvement in measures of sleep, mood, and five of six measures of attention in the melatonin group when compared with the placebo group. It is safe to say that there is insufficient evidence to recommend melatonin as part of the strategy to combat sleep loss in night shift workers.

SUMMARY

Quantitative and qualitative sleep deprivation is a widespread problem with serious health consequences both for the individual and for society. Sleep technologists are in a unique position to understand sleep deprivation from a "personal" perspective and to employ their knowledge of sleep physiology to advise their patients and improve their own performance.

REFERENCES

1. Hirshkowitz M, Whiton K, Albert SM, et al. National Sleep Foundation's sleep time duration recommendations: methodology and results summary. *Sleep Health*. 2015;1(1):40-43.
2. Paruthi S, Brooks LJ, D'Ambrosio C, et al. Recommended amount of sleep for pediatric populations: a consensus statement of the American Academy of Sleep Medicine. *J Clin Sleep Med*. 2016;12(6):785-786.
3. Cirelli C. Insufficient sleep: definition, epidemiology, and adverse outcomes. *UpToDate*. 2025. Accessed March 19, 2025. https://www.uptodate.com/contents/insufficient-sleep-definition-epidemiology-and-adverse-outcomes
4. Patrick GTW, Gilbert JA. On the effect of loss of sleep. *Psychol Rev*. 1896;3:469-483.
5. Rechtschaffen A, Bergmann BM, Everson CA, et al. Sleep deprivation in the rat: Integration and discussion of the findings. *Sleep*. 1989;25:68-87.
6. Dispersyn G, Sauvet F, Gomez-Merino D, et al. The homeostatic and circadian sleep recovery responses after total sleep deprivation in mice. *J Sleep Res*. 2017;26:531-538. doi:10.1111/jsr.12541
7. Van Dongen HPA, Baynard MD, Maislin G. Systematic interindividual differences in neurobehavioral impairment from sleep loss: evidence of trait like differential vulnerability. *Sleep*. 2004;27:423-433.

8. Ferrie JE, Shipley MJ, Cappuccio FP, et al. A prospective study of change in sleep duration: associations with mortality in the Whitehall II cohort. *Sleep*. 2007;30:1659-1666.
9. Satoyo I, Hiroyasu I, Chigusa D. Association of sleep duration with mortality from cardiovascular disease and other causes for Japanese men and women: the JACC study. *Sleep*. 2009;32(3):259-301.
10. American Academy of Sleep Medicine. *International Classification of Sleep Disorders*. 3rd ed. American Academy of Sleep Medicine; 2014.
11. Johns M. About the ESS. Accessed June 23, 2018. http://epworthsleepinessscale.com/about-the-ess/
12. Borbély AA. A two process model of sleep regulation. *Hum Neurobiol*. 1982;1:195-204.
13. Smith M, Edwards R, McCann U, et al. The effects of sleep deprivation on pain inhibition and spontaneous pain in women. *Sleep*. 2007;30:494-505.
14. Owens JM, Dingus TA, Guo F, et al. Prevalence of drowsy driving crashes: estimates from a large-scale naturalistic driving study. AAA Foundation for Traffic Safety. 2018. https://aaafoundation.org/prevalence-drowsy-driving-crashes-estimates-large-scale-naturalistic-driving-study/
15. Sharkey KM, Eastman CI. Melatonin phase shifts human circadian rhythms in a placebo-controlled simulated night-work study. *Am J Physiol Regul Integr Compr Physiol*. 2002;282:R454-R463.
16. Cavallo A, Ris D, Succop P, et al. Melatonin treatment of pediatric residents for adaptation to night shift work. *Ambul Pediatr*. 2005;5:172-177.

SUGGESTED RESOURCES

AAA—https://aaafoundation.org/

Centers for Disease Control and Prevention—https://www.cdc.gov/pcd/issues/2023/22_0400.htm

National Sleep Foundation—https://www.thensf.org/

Occupational Safety and Health Administration—https://www.osha.gov/worker-fatigue

Chapter 4
Respiratory Anatomy and Physiology

DAVID F. WOLFE

KEY CONCEPTS/LEARNING OBJECTIVES

On completion of this chapter, the reader should be able to:

1. Identify the anatomic name and location of each portion of the respiratory system from the mouth to the blood flowing through the lungs, including the relevant respiratory muscles and their control. Discuss the physics of respiratory gas exchange, the role of oxygen and carbon dioxide concentration gradients, and the thin membranes involved in gas exchange. Describe several aspects of the relationship between ventilation and perfusion of the lungs, including anatomy, gas exchange, and neural/chemical control of ventilation.
2. Describe the general effects of sleep on respiratory and cardiovascular control of ventilation. Describe the differential effects of waking, nonrapid eye movement sleep, and rapid eye movement sleep on ventilation and heart rate. Identify and describe the more common pathologic states associated with breathing control mechanisms, including central apnea/hypopnea, obstructive apnea/hypopnea, treatment-emergent central sleep apnea, Cheyne-Stokes respiration, and periodic breathing.

KEY TERMS

Bicarbonate
Carbonic acid
Carbonic anhydrase
C-fiber receptors
Chemoreceptors
Concentration gradients
Expiratory reserve volume
Functional residual capacity
Inspiratory reserve volume
Intrapleural space
Parietal pleura
Rapidly adapting receptors
Slowly adapting receptors
Visceral pleura

Respiration is, in all animals, a vital process responsible for the delivery of oxygen (O_2) to the tissues to support metabolism and the removal of the metabolic waste gas, carbon dioxide (CO_2). The major mechanisms of this exchange of gases between the external and internal environments are (1) simple passive diffusion along concentration gradients and (2) transport of these gases by the circulatory system. Concentration gradients refer to the difference in the concentration of a gas or liquid across a semipermeable barrier. In very small animals, such as single-celled organisms, gaseous diffusion occurs across their cell membranes, but larger organisms have distances that are too great for passive diffusion. Animals evolved a few very effective solutions, for example, a closed circulatory system and highly vascularized lungs or gills. Lungs (or gills) provide a specialized structure for placing a large amount of circulating body fluid (eg, blood) very close (<1 mm) to a large amount of environmental media (eg, air). Proximity across a permeable membrane that separates different concentrations of O_2 and CO_2 allows rapid movements of both gases down their concentration gradients, normally in opposite directions.

In higher chordate animals, respiratory transfer of CO_2 and O_2 is a two-step, cyclic process. The first step is at the interface between the body tissues (eg, muscle cells, liver cells) and the circulating lung capillary blood. This step is characterized by O_2 movement from blood plasma across the thin separating membrane that makes up the capillary wall and into a metabolizing tissue (eg, muscle or brain). Concurrently, the CO_2 liberated by tissue metabolism diffuses from the metabolizing cells across the tissue capillary membrane and into the circulating blood.

The second step occurs in the lungs between the lungs' airspaces and the circulating blood in very small capillaries within the lungs. Opposite from the tissue part of the cycle, gas movements in the lung are characterized by O_2 movement from the air within the lung into the pulmonary capillary blood, whereas CO_2 moves from the capillary blood into the minute air spaces called "alveoli" within the lung. The next expiration then expels most of the CO_2, and the next inspiration replenishes the O_2 supply. This two-part process is termed "gas exchange." The transfers of metabolic gases are passive processes because both gases are simply moving down their concentration gradients at both the pulmonary and the tissue locations.

Necessary and complementary components of this process are the circulation of blood and ventilation of the lungs. Therefore, the heart and blood vessels are essential components of respiration and are intimately involved in blood gas homeostasis. Breathing control mechanisms exist to control the concentrations of O_2 and CO_2 in the lung air and, subsequently, blood within the lung, which is carried to the tissues to support normal metabolism. In other words, the controls of respiratory movements are based mostly on sensory signals from the brain and body chemoreceptors, sensing O_2 levels, and CO_2/pH levels. These sensory signals come mostly from chemosensitive neurons in the brainstem, especially the medulla, the carotid bodies in the neck, and the aortic bodies on the aortic arch. The carotid and aortic bodies are chemosensitive to O_2 and CO_2/pH. These signals then "feed back" to the brainstem controllers, which then reduce hypercapnia (an excess of CO_2) or hypoxia (a deficiency of O_2 in the airways) by increasing ventilation and cardiac output. This is a classic example of a negative feedback loop used to control some critical physiologic variable. These respiratory actions are well coordinated with the cardiovascular system to achieve effective blood gas homeostasis.

In humans and other mammals, the respiratory drive to ventilate the lungs is mostly performed by neural networks in the brain. In fact, much of the brainstem and significant portions of certain "higher" areas of the brain are devoted to respiratory and cardiovascular control, especially cardiopulmonary coordination. Although purely physical and biochemical factors can and do affect respiration, by far, most mechanisms for maintaining and adjusting pulmonary ventilation are found in the brainstem and spinal cord. As a first step into the mechanisms used to control gas exchange, we review the structural components of the system, because a basic biologic principle is the intricate interdependence between form (anatomy) and function (physiology).

A REVIEW OF RESPIRATORY-RELATED ANATOMY AND PHYSIOLOGY

Any comprehensive discussion of respiratory function requires a review of thoracic, circulatory, and central nervous system (CNS) structure. Respiration and respiratory control encompass many anatomic and physiologic features that interact to meet very specific goals of homeostasis. One excellent example of this interaction is that of the circulatory and respiratory systems. The O_2 content and the CO_2 content within the circulatory system are the focus of the homeostatic controllers of ventilation.

Upper Respiratory Tract

Air drawn into the nasal passages and oral cavity is humidified, filtered, and warmed (in cooler climates) at the beginning of the pathway (Figure 4-1). Humidification of the incoming air is complete, resulting in pulmonary airspaces with 100% water saturation. The inside surfaces of the oral cavity and tongue contribute to water saturation of the incoming breath and also collect particulates from the incoming air, using surface water and turbulent airflow. In addition to humidification, the mucus membranes of the irregularly shaped turbinates within the nasal passages promote turbulence in the airflow, which assists the filtering of particulates. Air turbulence serves to increase filtering efficiency because small particles in the inhaled, turbulent air are more likely to eventually contact a mucus membrane than would particles within a straight streamlined airflow. Nasal hairs also serve to create turbulence in the nasal airflow to maximize the filtering and humidification of the inspired air. These hairs also screen out large particles in the air stream. The captured particles (dust, ash, pollen, skin flakes, etc.) are then swallowed, coughed out, or blown out of the nose by a sneeze. The main utility of this physical process is that the amount of particulate matter going into the lung is minimized.

Just behind the nasal passages and the oral cavity is the pharynx, essentially the upper part of the throat. As suggested by Figure 4-1, nasal and oral air mix here before passing into the larynx; this portion of the upper airway is located between the pharynx and the trachea and contains the vocal cords. The pharynx is a common

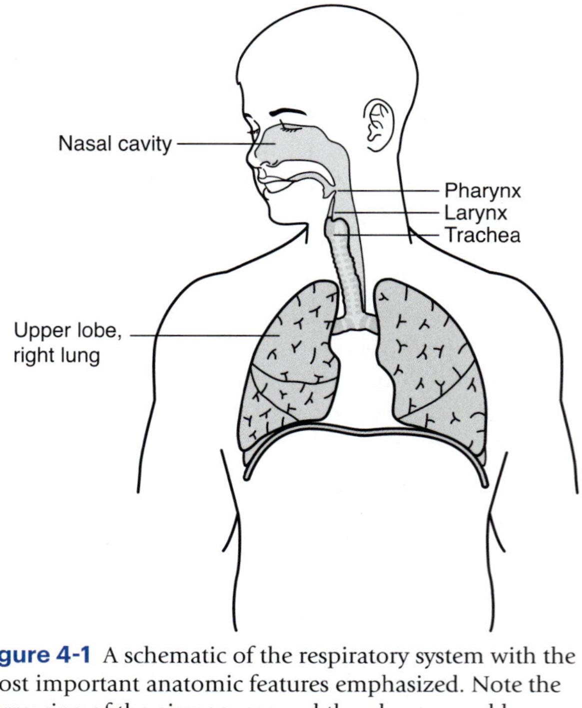

Figure 4-1 A schematic of the respiratory system with the most important anatomic features emphasized. Note the narrowing of the airspace around the pharynx and larynx.

site for airway collapse or partial obstruction, especially during supine sleep. The collapse may lead to a complete occlusion, called an apnea, or a partial collapse allowing some airflow, called a hypopnea. Muscles of the larynx and pharynx respond to sleep like most other skeletal muscles, with a significant decrease in muscle tone and reactivity (1). Most of the upper airway is surrounded by pharyngeal and laryngeal muscles that are important in airway rigidity, airway size, coughing, and speech. A bolus of food or water activates complex laryngeal motor reflexes, which guide the bolus into the esophagus, away from the vocal cords and trachea.

The pharynx and the larynx are the usual sites for obstructive ventilatory events; that is, both structures tend to collapse and occlude the airway. One common scenario is when the back of the tongue relapses onto the posterior walls of the pharynx. The relapse is often caused by insufficient tongue muscle activation during sleep, especially in supine sleep and obesity. This is the classic description of obstructive sleep apnea (OSA), or obstructive hypopnea. The insufficiency is partly related not only to the normal decrease in motor tone during sleep but also to anatomic features, such as the tongue's size and mass and/or micrognathia (small, recessed chin). The most important aspect of obesity in relation to obstructive apnea is when the area under the chin is obese and flaccid, allowing the tissue to sag into the mouth cavity leading to obstructions (2). Obviously, supine sleep significantly exacerbates the obstruction. In that position, the tissue sags toward the back of the throat, increasing the effect of an obstruction in the airway.

Other airway obstructions often occur because of sleep-related relaxation of the pharyngeal and/or laryngeal muscles, allowing negative airway pressure to pull the posterior wall of the airway forward toward the tongue and the front side of the airway. This obstruction usually creates either an apnea or a hypopnea. Airflow through the vocal cords and trachea is low resistance and generally unremarkable. This continuum from the mouth and nares to the superior end of the trachea represents the upper respiratory tract.

Lower Respiratory Tract

The lower respiratory tract begins at the upper end of the trachea (Figure 4-1); this then connects to the pulmonary trunk, which soon branches into the right and left bronchi (Figure 4-2). At the first branching level, the trachea splits into right and left bronchi. The left bronchus branches into two smaller sections, whereas the right bronchus branches into three. The lung tissue supplied by these five bronchi corresponds to the five lobes of the lung: three lobes of the right lung and two lobes of the left lung. Branching continues, ending with the alveoli and the alveolar ducts. These levels are where gas exchange takes place.

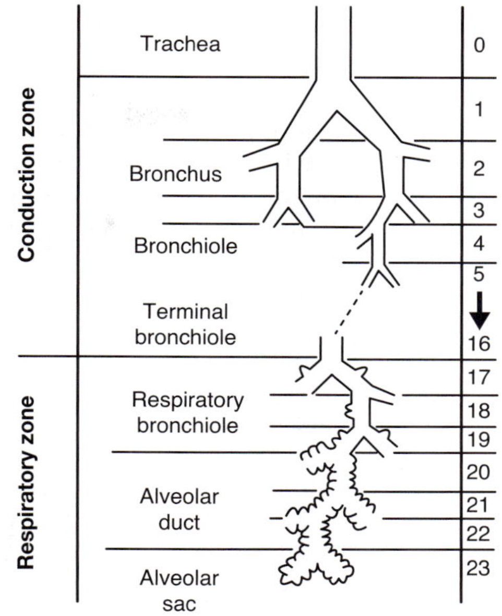

Figure 4-2 This diagram represents the branching of the respiratory conduction system of the lung. There is no real "airflow" after the terminal bronchioles; the distances are so short that diffusion moves the gases. Note that from the trachea to the later branches and terminal bronchioles, total airway volume is increasing as the individual airway size decreases.

The walls of the alveoli are composed of pulmonary epithelial cells and pulmonary capillaries carrying deoxygenated venous blood. There are two important cell types lining the alveolus: type I pneumocytes and type II pneumocytes. Type I cells make up the cell membrane or walls. The less numerous type II cells are the source of a substance called "surfactant," which reduces surface tension on the inner alveolar walls. The reduced (and variable) surface tension stabilizes the alveolus, making collapse less likely (3). The narrow divide (0.5 μm) between air in the alveoli and venous blood in the capillaries greatly facilitates gas exchange across the alveolar membrane with the nearby red blood cells (RBCs).

When a reduced RBC (depleted of O_2) reaches the alveolar membrane, the venous O_2 pressure is approximately 40 mm Hg, and the alveolar air, half a micron away, is about 100 mm Hg. This concentration gradient moves alveolar O_2 easily across the membrane into the blood plasma and then into the RBC. The Po_2 value for the exiting capillary blood, on its way to the left atrium of the heart, is approximately 150 mm Hg. In contrast, the CO_2 pressure is about 45 mm Hg in venous blood and about 40 mm Hg in oxygenated alveoli, a relatively small concentration gradient. In healthy people, the transfer of that 5 mm Hg of CO_2 takes about one-fourth second (similar to the time for RBC oxygenation), well before the RBC exits the pulmonary capillary (~0.75 seconds).

Vascular Anatomy of the Lungs and Heart

It should be clear that the cardiovascular system is intimately involved in breathing control mechanisms. The flow of blood generated by the heart is how O_2 reaches the tissues and how CO_2 gets to the alveoli to be expired. There is a considerable symmetry between the vascular structure and the airway structure in the lower reaches of the lungs. This is necessary to bring the smallest airways and the very small pulmonary capillaries into close contact while maintaining sufficient blood pressure to keep the small vessels open and sufficient airway pressure to keep the most vulnerable airways open.

Venous blood from the body reaches the heart through two large veins: the superior vena cava and the inferior vena cava. The superior vena cava carries blood from the head, arms, and upper torso; the inferior vena cava carries blood from the legs and lower torso. These two large veins converge on the right atrium. During the part of the cycle when the cardiac muscle is relaxed, blood flows through the right atrium via the tricuspid valve and pools in the right ventricle (Figure 4-3). When the ventricle is full, systole (cardiac muscle contraction) begins with contraction of the right atrium, forcing atrial venous blood into the already full ventricle. This stretches the ventricular muscle, raising the ventricular blood volume and pressure. The tricuspid valve between the right atrium and the right ventricle closes just as the right ventricle contracts. Contraction of the right ventricle expels the venous blood, forcing it through the pulmonary valve of the heart into the pulmonary artery and, eventually, the pulmonary capillaries of the alveoli within the lung. For the now-oxygenated blood exiting the alveoli, it is the same process back to the heart. The pulmonary capillaries come together to form very small veins, which merge with others to form a somewhat larger vein, and so on. Finally, this O_2-saturated blood travels the pulmonary vein back to the left atrium of the heart. As with the right side, the left atrium is, essentially, a primer pump to create sufficient intraventricular pressure to stretch the cardiac muscle and maximize the efficiency of the ventricular contraction. The left ventricle then expels its volume of oxygenated, low CO_2 content blood into the arterial circulation (Figure 4-3).

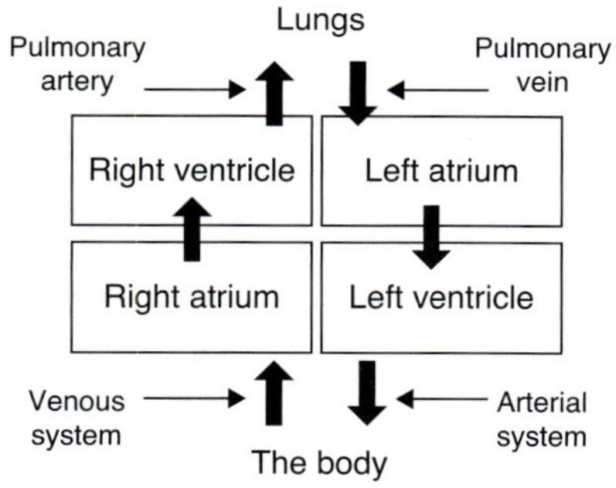

Figure 4-3 A simple schematic of the circulatory cycle within the heart, lungs, and body. Large arrows demonstrate the direction of blood flow in and out of the lungs and heart. Small arrows indicate body anatomy involved: right heart (pulmonary artery and venous system) and left heart (pulmonary vein and arterial system).

The circulatory structure of the cardiopulmonary system is the one place in the body where venous blood is carried in an "artery," because it is exiting the right ventricle but is still deoxygenated and hypercapnic (an excess of CO_2). Similarly to the airway conduction system, the large pulmonary artery coming from the right ventricle enters the lung and branches down to the level of the alveolar ducts and alveoli. Once the venous blood is into the pulmonary capillaries surrounding an alveolus, the CO_2 within that blood flows down its concentration gradient, across the pulmonary membrane, into the alveolar air. At the same time, inspired O_2 moves down its concentration gradient, across the alveolar membrane into the "venous" blood in the pulmonary capillaries, changing it to oxygenated arterial blood.

Thoracic Anatomy and Function

The main muscles of inspiration are the diaphragm and the external intercostals. Both are common skeletal muscles controlled by spinal motor nerves. The diaphragm and the external intercostals act in concert to create negative intrapulmonary pressure, resulting in airflow into the trachea, or inspiration. During an inspiration, ambient air enters the body through the nares, mouth, or both. Then, the air stream passes through the many branches of the airways, eventually reaching the vicinity of many alveoli. Diffusion moves the O_2 the rest of the way into the alveoli and their capillaries.

The air within the pathways from the mouth and nares down to the terminal airways constitutes a significant volume that is not involved in an exchange of O_2 and CO_2. This is because air is in the passageways of the lung, not in the portions involved in gas exchange. This is the "conduction" portion of the respiratory system. The "respiratory" portion of the lungs is composed of the alveoli, alveolar ducts, and respiratory bronchioles. These are the levels at which gas exchange occurs. The airway conduction system is graphically demonstrated in Figure 4-2.

One of the two respiratory "pump" muscles is the diaphragm, necessary for normal ventilation, although many other muscles assist the diaphragm in producing ventilation. Ventilation is the physical consequence of normal cyclic respiratory muscle activity. Diaphragmatic contraction, due to CNS activation, causes the thoracic cavity floor to descend, making the thoracic cavity larger and creating negative pressure to draw in air from the environment, that is, inspiration. The diaphragm has almost no involvement in expiring air from the lungs. The other major inspiratory pump muscles are the external intercostals, which connect adjacent ribs. During inspiration, the external intercostals contract to pull the chest wall outward and upward to increase thoracic cavity size, contributing to the decrease in intrapulmonary pressure and making the chest wall stiffer (less compliant). There are also several sets of secondary, or accessory, inspiratory muscles. Accessory respiratory muscles include those in the abdomen, neck, pharynx, larynx, nose, tongue, and upper chest.

In polysomnography, changes in abdominal and thoracic circumference are usually recorded to assess ventilatory effort. This technique actually measures the displacement because of the external intercostals—diaphragmatic contraction does not increase chest circumference. This is still useful because it provides a relatively easy index of respiration, without complicated and invasive procedures or imaging.

In normal "at-rest" ventilation, expiration is entirely passive. Because during normal breathing no expiratory muscle activity is required, cyclic inspiration is the emphasis of the control system at rest. Of course, active expiration by expiratory muscles is often necessary, such as in exercise, to more quickly expel the breath and allow for appropriately rapid ventilation. The main expiratory muscles are the internal intercostals and abdominal muscles, but others also assist. Expiratory pump muscles act to increase intrathoracic pressure in order to increase intrapulmonary pressure and push air out of the lungs more quickly.

The conducting airways, from the mouth and nose to the lungs, are not involved in gas exchange but are surrounded by both skeletal and smooth muscles that act to control the flow of air to and from the lungs (Figure 4-2). Muscles of the upper respiratory tract are especially relevant in sleep medicine because of their involvement in OSA. The usual site of an obstruction is an area of the upper airway where muscles are relatively flaccid, or abnormally large. Muscles of the pharynx, larynx, and tongue make up this group. These too are skeletal muscles and, like the other accessory respiratory muscles, have functions other than ventilation—for example, swallowing, speech, and movement of the head, neck, or shoulders. Airway muscles are activated in a specific phase of respiration (inspiration or expiration), but they are not responsible for controlling intrathoracic pressures and, therefore, are not respiratory pump muscles.

OSA/hypopnea arises from insufficient compensation by muscular control systems for certain anatomic and postural features or deficiencies, such as the chin and neck obesity described earlier. This insufficiency is often not due to any change in the CNS controllers or blood gas reflexes but simply due to the weight of the tongue (or tonsils) and the lack of physical support while sleeping supine. Sleep is a critical factor in apneas/hypopneas because neural output to all skeletal muscles, except the diaphragm, is reduced during sleep (4). OSA is an excellent illustration of the interaction between structure and function and of the impact of the neurophysiologic state, sleep, on those interactions.

The lungs themselves have no muscles for movement and are not physically attached to the chest wall; instead, an alternate mechanism evolved to couple the lungs to the thoracic wall. The outer surface of the lungs is called the "visceral pleura." The visceral pleura also covers the mediastinum, a midline "structure" between the lungs that includes the trachea, heart, great vessels, thymus, and esophagus. The inside surface of the thoracic cavity is lined by a layer of epithelium called the "parietal pleura." The visceral pleura is held to the parietal pleura by negative intrapleural pressure. It is important to realize that there are no anatomic features that hold the lungs against the inner thoracic walls. This physical coupling of the two pleura, resulting from the negative intrapleural pressure, ensures that the volume of the lungs varies directly with the size of the thoracic cavity. The pleura are mostly impervious to gases, helping maintain the negative pressure. Because there is normally almost no "space" in the "intrapleural space" (2-5 mL), it is often referred to as a "potential space." Negative intrapleural pressure results from elastic recoil of the respiratory muscles and lungs and the surface tension of the aqueous film lining the inner alveolar surface. Elasticity is a structural property of lung tissue. Emphysema reduces elastic recoil through the destruction of alveolar walls and their pulmonary capillaries (5). The resulting enlargement of that airspace represents a greatly reduced surface area for gas exchange.

The term "pneumothorax" is used to convey a loss of negative pressure in the intrapleural space because of an opening to the atmosphere or into the lung. When the negative pressure is lost, the two pleura separate, and air flows into the newly enlarged space. This effectively uncouples the close adhesion between inspiratory chest wall movement and lung expansion, that is, the lung collapses. A pneumothorax may occur spontaneously or as a result of trauma involving an opening in either of the pleura. For example, a stab or gunshot wound that penetrates both pleura can allow air from the atmosphere into the intrapleural space and the lung, removing the negative pressure gradient. This is a medical emergency requiring immediate assistance.

In patients without penetrating trauma of the chest wall, the diagnosis is usually based on the presence of chest pain, increased heart rate, tachypnea, hypoxemia, and shortness of breath. x-rays are also helpful in diagnosing a pneumothorax. Acute pneumothorax is usually treated with a needle aspiration of the intrapleural space and/or a chest tube. Both procedures require hospitalization. Other treatments include supplemental O_2 and positive pressure ventilation. A chronic spontaneous pneumothorax can occur in the lung, often near the apex, and creates a hole in the visceral pleura, allowing lung air to flow into the negative pressure of the intrapleural space.

Innervation of the Respiratory Muscles and Blood Vessels

The diaphragm and external intercostals are driven by specific motor nerves from the spinal cord. The diaphragm is the main controller of ventilatory movements and is driven by the phrenic nerves. The external intercostals are the most relevant to respiratory control mechanisms. The output carried by the phrenic nerve is from the bilateral phrenic areas of the spinal cord gray matter. The spinal phrenic area is, in turn, controlled from specific areas in the brainstem. Neural control is addressed later in this chapter.

In addition to the inspiratory muscles, there are important expiratory muscles as well. The most important expiratory muscles are the internal intercostals and the abdominal muscles. Like the external intercostals, the internal intercostals are driven by nerves that emanate from the full length of the thoracic segment of the spinal cord. Motor nerves to the abdominal muscles derive from the lumbar portion of the spinal cord.

Blood vessel diameter, and subsequently pressure, is actively controlled by the sympathetic nervous system. The main output nuclei controlling cardiovascular sympathetic neurons are located in the brainstem and hypothalamus; these areas are driven by many inputs from several brain areas. The parasympathetic system has no known significant impact on the control of blood pressure. The other major controlling variable is the heart rate. The intrinsic heart rate is derived from the sinoatrial (SA) node, located in the right atrium. This "baseline" rate is normally modulated by many factors but mostly by the sympathetic system and the parasympathetic system. Usually, sympathetic excitation is associated with increased heart rate, enhanced cardiac muscle contractility (force of contraction), increased motor tone throughout the body, and often, an increase in blood pressure. The parasympathetic effects are mostly the opposite of the sympathetic effects.

RESPIRATORY PHYSIOLOGY

Respiratory function is based on the need to acquire O_2 for normal metabolism and to remove the metabolic waste gas, CO_2. A paradox of this physiologic mechanism is that the respiratory system does not try to eliminate *all* of the CO_2 in the lungs. Instead, the neurally mediated respiratory control system actively maintains CO_2 at approximately 40 mm Hg. The respiratory system is an important component of acid-base (pH) balance within the body. Within RBCs, the combination of CO_2 and water (H_2O) into carbonic acid (H_2CO_3) is catalyzed by carbonic anhydrase. Blood plasma does not have this important enzyme. Carbonic acid dissociates to hydrogen (H^+) and bicarbonate ions (HCO_3^-). Maintaining CO_2 at approximately 40 mm Hg results in an O_2 pressure lower than it would be without the high level of CO_2, illustrating the importance of the role played by the respiratory system in acid-base balance. Figure 4-4 shows the effects of various agents on the oxyhemoglobin dissociation curve, including acidity and P_{CO_2}: decreased P_{CO_2} or increased pH shifts the curve to the left, decreasing P_{O_2} for a given hemoglobin (Hb) saturation (increasing the Hb's affinity for O_2). Most relevant to the patient is where they are on the *x*-axis when the controlling factors are expressed (↑P_{CO_2}, ↓pH).

In what follows, there are many descriptions of gradients and concentration differences. Often, it is important to know the quantity of some gas, mixed with other gases and contained within some space (like a lung or the earth's atmosphere). The quantitative measure of that specific gas is the partial pressure (Table 4-1), conventionally in millimeters of mercury (mm Hg). The total of all partial pressures in the earth's atmosphere is the barometric pressure, approximately 760 mm Hg. The partial pressure of O_2 in our atmosphere is 158 mm Hg. Because 158 divided by 760 equals 0.208, the O_2 in our atmosphere is approximately 21%. Almost all the rest is nitrogen, with a partial pressure of 596 mm Hg (78.4%

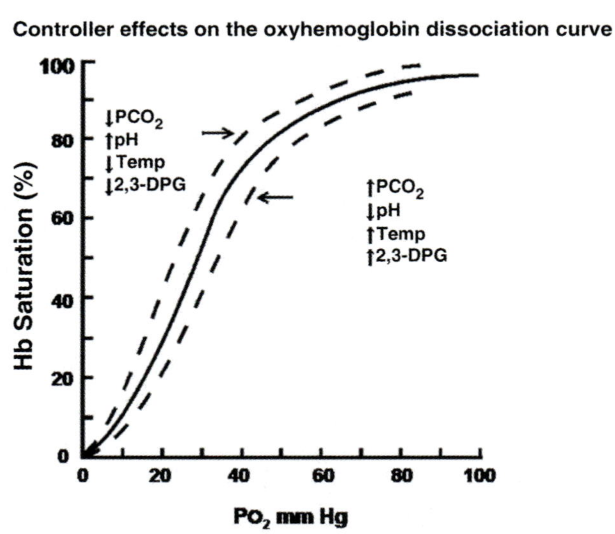

Figure 4-4 The oxyhemoglobin dissociation curve. This graph illustrates that the basic function for hemoglobin (Hb) is the uptake of, or dissociation from, oxygen (O_2) molecules. The broken lines describe the effect of four variables on O_2 release from Hb. These effects are much greater when the patient is on the steep part of the curve. 2,3-DPG, 2,3-diphosphoglycerate.

Table 4-1 Partial Pressures (mm Hg)

Compartment	O_2	CO_2
Atmosphere	158	0.3
Alveolar air	97-100	~40
Pulmonary capillary	100-45	~46
Arterial blood	~100	36-44
Arterial capillary	60-65	~40
Tissues	~40	45-48
Venous blood	40-50	46.0

of barometric pressure). Also, there is usually water in the atmosphere, with some obvious exceptions. A generalized value for the partial pressure of water in the atmosphere is 5.7 mm Hg or 0.008%.

$$P_{baro} = PO_2 + PN_2 + PH_2O = 759.7$$

There is a very small amount of other gases in the atmosphere, such as argon (0.93%) and CO_2 (0.03%). Still more gases are also present in air but at very low concentrations.

The following is an illustrative example of a gradient: if the partial pressure of O_2 in arterial capillary blood is 62 mm Hg and the partial pressure of O_2 in an adjacent metabolizing cell is 35 mm Hg, then the O_2 gradient is 27 mm Hg, from blood to tissue cells. The steeper is the gradient, the greater is the force or speed of gas movement.

Respiratory Volumes and Capacities

There are several "compartments" within the respiratory system: first, the body trunk cavity lined with parietal pleura, then the thoracic cavity, then the lungs themselves within the visceral pleura, the upper airway, the trachea, the conducting portion of the bronchial tree, and, finally, the cavities within alveoli and alveolar ducts. These compartments comprise the pulmonary structure.

It is necessary to know the various volumes and capacities to understand the usual clinical pulmonary function testing (PFT) (Table 4-2). The first example is tidal volume (V_T), the volume of air moved in a single breath, usually in milliliters (mL) or liters (L). V_T multiplied by the respiratory rate (breaths per minute) gives the minute ventilation (liters per minute), an important clinical parameter describing the amount of air moved in 1 minute. Low levels of minute ventilation are a common accessory to apnea of any type. The maximum volume that one can inspire beginning at the end of a normal inspiration is the inspiratory reserve volume (IRV). Similarly, the expiratory reserve volume (ERV) is the volume that can be expired from the end of a normal expiration. This information from the reserve volumes can indicate deficiencies that do not become evident until the patient

Table 4-2 Respiratory Volumes and Capacities

Space/Structure	Volumes (mL)	Capacities (mL)
Tidal volume (V_T)	500	
Inspiratory reserve volume (IRV)	3,000	
Expiratory reserve volume (ERV)	1,100	
Residual volume (RV)	1,300	
Total lung capacity	IRV + V_T + ERV + RV	5,900
Vital capacity	IRV + V_T + ERV	4,600
Function residual capacity	ERV + RV	2,400
Inspiratory capacity	V_T + IRV	3,500
Physiologic dead space	155	
Anatomic dead space	150	
Intrapleural space	2-5	

All values approximate.

tries to exercise. Exertion requires extra energy and O_2 and the removal of excess CO_2 created by the increase in metabolism with exertion. This need to restore normal or optimal concentrations requires ventilation to increase and move into the IRV and likely the ERV as well. Different pathologies affect different volumes in different ways and can be quite valuable in diagnosis.

Measures of various volumes within the respiratory system are very important in diagnosing disease or injury in the lungs (Figure 4-5; Table 4-2); examples include pulmonary fibrosis, asthma, and chronic obstructive pulmonary disease (COPD). Knowledge of these pressures, volumes, and capacities is essential in PFT.

Almost all the lung volumes can be measured by a device called a "spirometer," a clinical instrument for measuring ventilatory movements in terms of relative volume changes. The spirometer measures and records the changes in the volume of inhaled or exhaled air continuously across ongoing respiratory cycles. A change in spirometer volume is equal to the amount of air expired (or inspired) by the patient. Performing several ventilatory maneuvers allows assessment of specific volumes using spirometry, which is very useful in the diagnosis of several obstructive diseases, for example, asthma and COPD.

The volume in the lung remaining at the end of a normal expiration is the functional residual capacity (FRC). The FRC is composed of the ERV and the residual volume

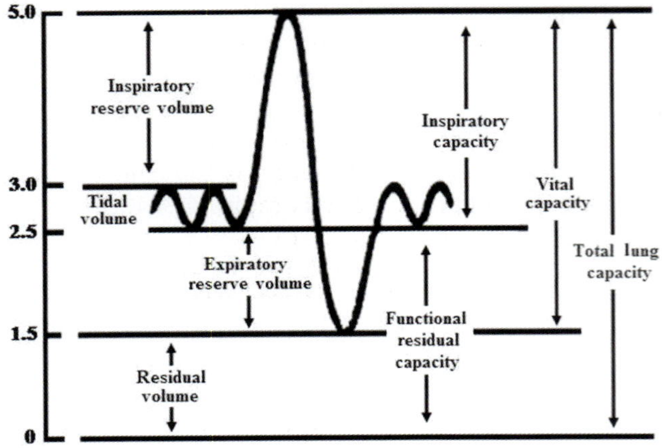

Figure 4-5 The various lung volumes and capacities as defined by a spirometry trace. These volumes are measured using specific breathing maneuvers while attached to a spirometer. *y*-axis is in liters (L).

(RV): FRC = ERV + RV. RV is the volume of air remaining after a maximum expiration. RV cannot be quantified by spirometry, but it can be estimated or quantified by other more extensive, and sometimes invasive, tests.

In another spirometric test, the patient is asked for a maximal inspiration, followed by a maximal expiration; the difference (range) between the peak and trough volumes defines vital capacity (VC). VC is the combination of V_T, ERV, and IRV: VC = V_T + ERV + IRV. In many texts, the VC is referred to as the forced VC, which refers to the use of maximum force on both inspiration and expiration. As may be clear by now, a capacity is the sum of two or more volumes. Total lung capacity (TLC) is the sum of VC (V_T + IRV + ERV) and RV.

RV is the only volume that cannot be measured by spirometry. This derivation is problematic because one of the limits of the RV range is zero (0). FRC also cannot be derived by spirometry because FRC contains RV, along with ERV. Spirometry measures volumes as differences between two definable limits or landmarks, such as ERV derived from the volume at the end of a maximal expiration *relative to* the lung volume at the end of a normal expiration. RV cannot be measured by spirometry because absolute values are needed, not relative values. Therefore, other procedures must be used to measure an absolute value such as RV. Because RV cannot be directly measured (quantitatively), TLC cannot be derived from spirometry as that would require absolute values for RV.

RV is one portion of the lung that does not directly participate in normal gas exchange. In this area, lacking sufficient ventilation, diffusion distances are large and inefficient. This volume is not adequately replenished with atmospheric air, and removal of CO_2 is slow. Therefore, in RV, O_2 levels are low (hypoxia) and CO_2 accumulates (hypercapnia).

Anatomic and Physiologic Dead Space

"Dead space" refers to those areas within the lung that are not participating in gas exchange. These are volumes of great importance because they represent the useless ventilation of an area that has little or no blood flow. Dead space is inevitable in a complex structure like the lung, but changes in dead space usually indicate a pathologic process or event. Essentially, increased dead space represents inefficiency in ventilation. There are two important types of dead space: anatomic and physiologic.

Most of the anatomic dead space is represented by the volume of the conducting airways: nares, pharynx, larynx, trachea, bronchi, bronchioles, and terminal bronchioles. Their membranes are thick and fibrous, resulting in rigidity; effective gas exchange is practically impossible in those tissues. Anatomic dead space (in milliliters) is roughly equal to a person's weight in pounds (6,7).

Another type of dead space is physiologic dead space. This represents areas that could engage in gas exchange but do not for some reason, for example, insufficient pulmonary blood flow (*Q*) to some portion of the lung to maintain normal gas exchange. Dead space reduces gas exchange and can lower O_2 levels in the arterial system.

Circulatory abnormalities can also create shunting. This refers to the absence of ventilation through some area in the lung, while perfusion of that area continues. One hallmark of shunt is an increase in the difference between the PO_2 in the alveolus (PAO_2) and PaO_2 (partial pressure of O_2 in the arterial blood); normally, this difference is due to a drop in PaO_2 rather than an increase in PAO_2. The normal difference is small (<5 mm Hg). A larger difference normally results from a reduced PaO_2 and indicates incomplete oxygenation of the arterial blood.

The magnitude of the shunt can be expressed by the shunt fraction, which expresses the percentage of blood in the cardiac output that is not ventilated. Intrapulmonary shunting (low ventilation with normal right heart output) can be a major cause of hypoxemia in pulmonary edema and pneumonia.

The application of supplemental O_2 to a patient will either increase the PaO_2 or have no significant effect. If the patient shows an increased level of arterial O_2 in response to supplemental O_2, they probably have a ventilation/perfusion mismatch; if the patient has nearly the same PaO_2 with supplemental O_2, the problem is likely a shunt.

Measuring the PAO_2 for comparison with the PaO_2 is problematic regarding access to small groups of alveoli, which are microscopic blind sacs. A good estimate for the partial pressure of alveolar O_2 can be derived with the alveolar gas equation:

$$P_AO_2 = FIO_2(P_{atm} - PH_2O) - PaCO_2 / R$$

The uppercase *P* represents partial pressure, "A" denotes alveolar, "a" denotes arterial, FI is fraction inspired (normally 0.21), P_{atm} indicates atmospheric (barometric) pressure (usually near 760 mm Hg), and R signifies the respiratory quotient, which is the ratio between the O_2 consumed and the CO_2 produced. The normal value for R is 0.8 but varies from approximately 0.6 to 1.1, usually because of dietary differences. For example, a diet high in carbohydrates may result in a higher respiratory quotient.

Lastly, a blood clot (embolus) in a pulmonary arteriole in the wall of ventilated alveoli creates physiologic dead space because perfusion is reduced in that area. The RV also contributes to physiologic dead space. However, most physiologic dead space results from low blood flow, creating an inequality between ventilation and perfusion. A rough average for normal anatomic dead space is 150 mL, and physiologic dead space is about 155 mL, for a total of approximately 305 mL in a normally functioning respiratory system. Refer to Table 4-3 for normal values for several of the most relevant respiratory variables.

Gas Exchange and Transport

Gas exchange refers to the movements of O_2 and CO_2 between the atmosphere and the metabolizing cells of the body. Respiratory gas exchange occurs in two different areas of the body. One is the membrane between alveolar air spaces and the deoxygenated, CO_2-laden blood entering the pulmonary capillaries, that is, alveolar capillaries. This particular exchange includes the movement of CO_2 from the blood into the alveolar air spaces and O_2 moving from the air spaces into the pulmonary/alveolar capillary blood. Although it takes an RBC about 0.75 seconds to traverse a typical pulmonary capillary, it takes only 0.25 seconds for about 95% of the blood to be oxygenated (6). Note that the equilibration point is only one-third of the way through the capillary. This is another example of "built-in" extra capacity to increase the rate of blood flow and ventilation. The second area for gas exchange is between the arterial capillaries and the metabolizing tissues, for example, muscle cells, liver cells, or neurons. In this exchange, the gas movements are reversed. Here, O_2 in the blood diffuses into the tissues to support metabolism, whereas CO_2 moves from the tissue into the local venous capillaries. In both locations, the movements of both respiratory gases are driven by their respective concentration (or partial pressure) gradients.

There is another important factor at work that greatly increases the O_2-carrying capacity of the blood but, at the same time, has little effect on the PO_2 gradient between the blood and the tissues. That factor is Hb, a complex molecule with a proteinaceous part (a globin molecule) and an iron-dependent pigment molecule with four heme groups attached (heme is an organic molecule containing nitrogen). Each heme group contains an atom of ferrous iron (Fe^{2+}), and each Fe^{2+} atom can carry one molecule of O_2. Hence, one Hb molecule can carry up to four O_2 molecules. The globin molecule actively controls the affinity of the iron atoms for O_2 and plays a major role in gas exchange between Hb and the tissues and efficient oxidation in the lungs.

The O_2–Hb Dissociation Curve

The complex relationship between HbO_2 (percent saturation) and plasma PO_2 (mm Hg) is commonly illustrated with the O_2–Hb dissociation curve (Figure 4-4). The most obvious feature of this curve is the sigmoid (S-shaped) nature of the relationship. This shape is a direct result of particular properties of the Hb molecule, especially that once the first heme is oxidized, there is an increase in O_2 affinity of the three remaining hemes. Stated differently, the shape of the curve represents a facilitation of the *release* of O_2 when exposed to the low

Table 4-3 Normative Values

Term	Parameter	Value	Other
Partial pressure O_2	PO_2	100 mm Hg	Value—lung, arterial blood
Tidal volume	V_T	400 mL	Normal value
Minute ventilation	Vdot	6 L/min	Normal value
Breath frequency	*f*	10 breaths/min	Normal value
Minute circulation	Qdot	100 mL/min	Value—bronchial circulation/flow
Barometric pressure	*B*	760 mm Hg	Atmospheric press, sea level
Dead space	*D*	~150 mL	
Arterial O_2	PO_{2a}	95 mm Hg	
Venous O_2	PO_{2v}	40 mm Hg	Also for "mixed" venous
O_2 concentration in air/inhaled	FIO_2	0.2094	Inhaled air is 21% O_2
CO_2 concentration/exhaled	$FECO_2$	0.045	Exhaled air is 4.5% CO_2

O_2 levels characteristic of metabolizing tissues (↓PO_2, <60 mm Hg) and, conversely, the quick, efficient capture of O_2 when exposed to ventilated alveolar air (↑PO_2, >60-70 mm Hg). The flat portion of the curve at the top of the graph represents a weak effect of PO_2 on percent Hb saturation in that area of the curve when both PO_2 and HbO_2 are high. In that upper area, Hb-bound O_2 is relatively unaffected by modest falls in PO_2, which can happen when there are lung regions that are underventilated or underperfused. In spite of the fall in PO_2, the blood maintains a lower, but still adequate, O_2 storage. While sitting (or during mild exercise in fit people), most of the O_2 needs of the body are supplied by dissolved O_2 and a small amount of Hb-bound O_2. Dissolved O_2 must fall approximately 40 mm Hg (40%) for a fall in Hb saturation of only 7% to 10%. Because most O_2 is carried by Hb, not dissolved, O_2 content (= HbO_2 + PO_2) is mostly preserved. However, once the inflection of the curve is reached, a much smaller further drop in PO_2 is accompanied by a rapid, large drop in saturation (and O_2 content), that is, the steep portion of the curve. These unique properties of Hb provide considerable extra capacity for effective gas exchange. The sheer volume of HbO_2 in the blood provides a ready source of O_2 to maintain metabolism and appropriate gas concentration gradients, even during intense exercise.

One example of biophysical factors modulating the O_2 affinity of Hb, the Bohr effect, describes the effects of local acidity (H^+) on affinity between heme and O_2 (Figure 4-4). As PCO_2 rises (eg, during exercise), the amount of coupling of CO_2 with water ($H_2O + CO_2$) also rises, creating more of the intermediate form H_2CO_3 (carbonic acid). Carbonic acid quickly dissociates into hydrogen ions (H^+) and bicarbonate ions (HCO_3^-). Bicarbonate ions are essential in acid-base homeostasis, in that bicarbonate ions are the main base (opposite of acid) within that regulatory system. The release of hydrogen ions lowers the pH, which reduces the affinity of heme for O_2. In other words, if during exercise the H^+ concentration goes up (lower pH), the heme groups tend to release their O_2 molecules to maintain the exercise. This is referred to as the Bohr effect, which occurs in the metabolizing tissues (↑PCO_2, ↓pH, ↓PO_2) and increases O_2 availability to counteract the acidosis. Other factors modulating heme affinity for O_2 include temperature and concentrations of CO_2, adenosine triphosphate, and phosphate. Increases in muscle temperature, for example, tend to release O_2 from Hb.

It is noteworthy that the mechanism for the fine control of O_2 delivery to the tissues is largely accounted for by the interaction between many metabolic factors (PO_2, temperature, pH, PCO_2, etc), all shifting the basic controller, the slope, and/or shape of the oxyhemoglobin dissociation curve, to the left or right (Figure 4-4). Using the single factor of acidity may illustrate the impact of moderate changes in pH on Hb saturation and O_2 content. With PO_2 at 45 mm Hg and a normal pH of 7.4, the Hb saturation is approximately 80%; however, at the same PO_2, but with a more acidic pH of 7.2, Hb saturation is approximately 70%. Therefore, an acidosis of 7.2 leads to a considerable loss of Hb saturation and O_2 content of the blood. Under the same conditions, but with an alkalosis (pH 7.6), the percentage of Hb that is saturated is 85% to 90%, a 5- to 10-point increase from the normal condition. The degree of change is smaller in alkalosis than in acidosis because of the very small slope of the upper part of the dissociation curve. Other important variables such as increased temperature and increased levels of inorganic phosphate in the body shift the oxyhemoglobin dissociation curve to the right, as with acidosis. Generally, an increase in metabolism is associated with a shift of the curve to the right, favoring O_2 release to maintain activity and oxygenation.

CO_2 Storage and Transfer

Practically all of the CO_2 in the body is generated by tissue metabolism. About 10% of the CO_2 is in the plasma and 90% within the RBC. However, only about 5% of total CO_2 in the blood is dissolved, and another 5% reacts within the plasma, which alters the form of the CO_2. For example, a noncatalyzed reaction with water incorporates the CO_2 into a bicarbonate ion, but very slowly (3). The presence of carbonic anhydrase within the RBC catalyzes the reaction, creating large amounts of bicarbonate ions; this is the reason for the large difference in the percentage of CO_2 between plasma and within the RBC. In fact, the majority of the CO_2 in the body is held in bicarbonate ions—HCO_3—not as CO_2. Some of the hydrogen ions liberated by the carbonic acid bind to Hb, triggering O_2 release from the Hb molecule into the RBC plasma and, then, into the blood.

Ventilation-Perfusion Ratios ($\dot{V}_A/\dot{Q}$)

A common occurrence in the normal lung is the temporary partial collapse of small areas of alveoli and alveolar ducts, which reduces the effectiveness of gas exchange. Most of these underventilated alveoli are still perfused with deoxygenated pulmonary capillary blood. This condition significantly reduces gas exchange in that area, whereas in other areas of the lung, gas exchange is normal or even elevated. The ventilation-perfusion ratio ($\dot{V}_A/\dot{Q}$) of this local area of partly or completely collapsed alveoli will fall substantially because the local alveolar collapse represents a decrease in the numerator, $\dot{V}_A$, whereas $\dot{Q}$ is relatively unchanged. The O_2 content of the arterial blood, as it leaves the lung, is diluted by the low or absent contribution from the fully or partially collapsed areas. Normal healthy people at rest have some small amount of collapsed alveoli and dilution ($\leq$4%) but can still be fully functional, that is, these small few collapsed areas have little impact on the normal values of Po_2, O_2 content, or Pco_2. The unchanged pulmonary arterial blood (still hypoxic and hypercapnic) then mixes with and dilutes the plasma gas concentrations, altering the O_2 and CO_2 stores. The result is a small decrease in the whole-body average arterial O_2 level (6).

When an abnormally low amount of ventilation occurs (hypopnea or apnea), $\dot{V}_A$ is reduced. This is commonly because of increased amounts of alveolar collapse, while Q remains normal, and the $\dot{V}_A/\dot{Q}$ falls. The airway blockage also leads to changes in the gas concentrations of the unventilated alveoli; there, gas concentrations become equal to those of venous blood. Alveolar O_2 falls from a Po_2 of 100 to 40 mm Hg, and alveolar Pco_2 increases from 40 to 45 mm Hg (7).

A somewhat different result is seen when the lungs are ventilated normally but underperfused in some areas, again effectively reducing or preventing gas exchange within that area. In this case, alveolar O_2 levels can go up as the blood flow drops, increasing the $\dot{V}_A/\dot{Q}$ above 1. This is because O_2 is not being absorbed from the alveoli because of the underperfusion. However, the increase in Po_2 has little effect on total body O_2 content. Pco_2 is essentially zero when $\dot{V}_A/\dot{Q}$ is high.

Another way of describing this two-way $\dot{V}_A/\dot{Q}$ pathology is that a low (<1) $\dot{V}_A/\dot{Q}$ is associated with a respiratory pathology (collapsed alveoli), whereas a high $\dot{V}_A/\dot{Q}$ is normally associated with a cardiovascular problem. Usually, the problem is a full or partial blockage of pulmonary capillaries or of the upstream arteries that feed the pulmonary capillaries. Deficiencies in either $\dot{V}_A$ or pulmonary blood flow are referred to as a "$\dot{V}_A/\dot{Q}$ mismatch."

Disease or injury may adversely affect cardiac output or lung surface area and consequently decrease blood flow through the lung. Moderately low blood flow does not usually result in significant hypoxia because of the extra unused capacity for gas exchange. If it takes 0.6 seconds (more than twice the normal requirement of 0.25 seconds) to accomplish adequate gas exchange, it is still accomplished. This rapid equilibration is due mostly to the thinness of the alveolar membrane (<0.5 mm), but the substantial concentration gradient for O_2 (95% arterial to 40% venous) also contributes to rapid O_2 movement.

Because the normal $\dot{V}_A$ in humans is approximately 5,250 mL/min and the normal cardiac output (Q) is 5,000 to 6,000 mL/min, the normal $\dot{V}_A/\dot{Q}$ ratio is approximately 1. If an obstructive problem arises upstream from the pulmonary capillaries, effectively occluding blood flow into the alveoli, then the alveolar gases soon become equal to inspired gas (Po_2 = 150 mm Hg; Pco_2 = 0 mm Hg) but are not absorbed into the blood. In this case, supplemental O_2 can help increase mean arterial O_2. However, if a total blockage occurs in the airways, then the alveolar gas concentrations mimic those of the "venous" blood arriving through the pulmonary arteries. With the airway blockage, supplemental O_2 has little effect on arterial saturation mainly because a greater supply of O_2 does not matter if the O_2 is not absorbed. In a situation where blood flow is compromised and $\dot{V}_A$ is normal or higher, the $\dot{V}_A/\dot{Q}$ is large (>1) because $\dot{Q}$ is low. Similarly, when blood flow is normal but ventilation is significantly reduced, the $\dot{V}_A/\dot{Q}$ is small in magnitude (<1). Hypoxia is one of several factors that causes pulmonary arterial vasoconstriction in the lungs. In patients with cardiopulmonary disease, hypoxemia is usually caused by $\dot{V}_A/\dot{Q}$ mismatch.

From the clinical perspective, an important distinction must be made for the effects of gravity on blood and lung tissue. The effect of gravity varies somewhat between upright and reclining; upright posture results in a greater effect on the blood, which is massive compared with the nearly weightless air. When upright, gas and blood stratify between the base of the lung and the apex but in different directions. In that posture, blood pressure is higher in the base of the lung than in the apex, while air stratifies in the opposite direction. Volume is one parameter affected by gravity, such that the base of the lung contains more volume than the apex. Also, at the base of the lung, Pco_2 and O_2 content is higher than at the apex. Nearer to the apex, $\dot{V}_A/\dot{Q}$ and Po_2 are larger than values at the base. It is important to acknowledge that the posture of a patient under examination has an impact on several aspects of cardiopulmonary function and must be taken into account during a clinical measurement. Likewise, it is clear that alveolar function in one region of the lung is not equal to the function in another area.

Work of Breathing

The work of breathing is a relevant topic owing to the high levels of exertion and muscle activity that accompany many respiratory pathologies, such as emphysema and OSA. Of course, normal respiration also incurs work. The "work" is muscular work used in inspiration and often in expiration too. Most of the muscular work is overcoming elasticity of the lungs and thorax, and part of that elasticity results from the natural tendency of alveoli to collapse from surface tension, even with surfactant. Another important component of the work of breathing is overcoming airway resistance, especially during high airflow rates, as with exercise. The type of airflow is an important factor in airway resistance. A laminar flow incurs less airway (or vascular) resistance than a turbulent flow. A third source of work of breathing is related to moving inelastic structures such as the liver and stomach, which is particularly an issue in obese patients. The proportions of the overall work of breathing are overcoming elasticity—65%, airway resistance—28%, and displacement of organs and tissues—7% (3).

NEURAL CONTROL OF VENTILATION

The nervous system is essential for the act of breathing and is responsible for the signals transmitted by nerves to the respiratory muscles. The neural signals also modulate respiratory sensitivity to CO_2 and O_2, which is especially relevant during sleep when the incoming neural signals are reduced in strength. Many neural structures participate in the control of respiration; a few have already been mentioned. Most of the areas responsible for the control of normal breathing are in the medulla, pons, and cerebellum.

Respiratory Rhythm Generation

The basic respiratory rhythm is created and controlled by the CNS. The phrenic nerve output to the diaphragm comes from cervical spinal nuclei called the "phrenic nucleus" (C3-C5). The medulla is that portion of the brain just "above" (rostral to) the spinal cord. The basic, at-rest, respiratory rhythm is created by a network of neurons in the medulla that fire mostly together, resulting in sustained (~1-3 seconds) muscle contractions of the diaphragm and external intercostals, followed by the loss of inspiratory muscle activity, and relaxation of the respiratory muscles. Expiration occurs passively when at rest, as stretched muscles and lungs shorten (elastic recoil), pushing out the breath (8).

Central sleep apnea is caused by a lack of respiratory drive from the brainstem and phrenic nucleus. Most likely, this event is caused by insufficient neural activity in the respiratory rhythm generator within the medulla. This lack of respiratory drive occurs only in sleep, suggesting that the central pattern generator, in some relatively rare individuals, requires greater brainstem arousal to allow normal function. Common treatments for central sleep apnea are respiratory stimulants such as theophylline and related compounds; caffeine is used in some central apnea cases.

Many influences converge in the nucleus of the tractus solitarius (NTS), also known as the solitary tract, and nearby structures that not only control respiration but also affect the autonomic system (heart rate, arterial pressure, cardiac force, etc.). In fact, there is quite a bit of spatial and physiologic overlap between the respiratory and autonomic controllers. These other autonomic influences modulating respiration come from all levels of the nervous system but most importantly, from the pons (just above the medulla), hypothalamus, and cerebellum (3).

Neurally mediated coordination between the cardiovascular and respiratory control systems serves to appropriately match respiratory airflow and blood flow through the lungs. The main controlling influences on the phrenic nucleus are the respiratory pattern generator (in the brainstem), P_{CO_2}/pH, and P_{O_2}. The brain's response to increased CO_2 is more robust than the response to hypoxia. The neural control system uses these many incoming sensory signals concerning P_{CO_2}/pH, hypoxia, stretch, blood pressure, temperature, and so on to determine how *much* gas exchange is needed. The required change in ventilation requires alterations in the activity of the muscles controlling ventilation and, thus, of those controlling the respiratory gas pressure gradients. These mechanisms of blood gas maintenance are extremely rapid and efficient in healthy people.

NERVOUS SYSTEM ANATOMY AND FUNCTION

The two most relevant CNS areas for respiration are the medulla and the pons (Figure 4-6). There are two main areas within the medulla that drive respiratory muscles: the dorsal respiratory group, which is mostly inspiratory, and the ventral respiratory group (VRG), which is related to both inspiration and expiration. Many other brainstem and higher CNS areas modulate those two outputs to "fine-tune" respiration. The pons is also an important source of the effects of rapid eye movement (REM) sleep on respiration in which respiratory variability increases in both amplitude and frequency.

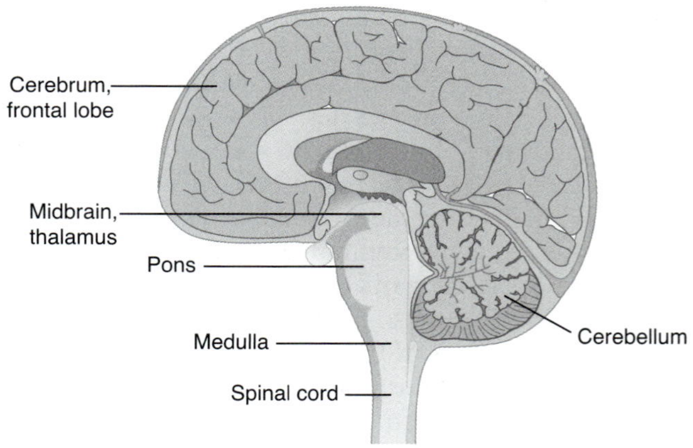

Figure 4-6 The major anatomic regions of the brain. Respiratory and most cardiovascular control is centered in the medulla and pons and assisted by the fastigial nucleus of the cerebellum and the hypothalamus.

There are an unknown number of chemosensory areas that monitor the amount of O_2, CO_2, and acidity in the blood, but the most well-known group of brain chemoreceptors lies on the ventral surface of the medulla. This group of medullary neurons makes up the classical central chemoreceptors. Central chemoreceptors seem to provide the major drive to the basic respiratory rhythm; that is, without some CO_2 sensory stimulation in this area, respiration tends to slow or stop. This is an important reason why the respiratory control system does not completely eliminate CO_2, because CO_2 is essential to the acid-base balance of the body and, likely, the centrally mediated drive to breathe. Central chemoreceptors are the main sensors for CO_2, but they also respond to acidic pH and low Po_2.

There are two sets of peripheral chemoreceptors that are similar to the central chemoreceptors but not identical. These sensors are called "peripheral" because they reside outside the CNS. One set of peripheral chemoreceptors is in the carotid bodies, which are located at the bifurcation of the common carotid arteries in the neck. The other set is located in the aortic arch of the upper chest. Most of the monitoring of O_2 in the blood is performed by the peripheral chemoreceptors. It is now known that several other brain sites are also chemoreceptive to CO_2 (9), but their relative contribution to respiration is largely unknown.

The carotid bodies' sensory nerve fibers make up a part of the carotid sinus nerve and also carry information on arterial blood pressure. Those arterial pressure sensors, called "baroreceptors," are in the carotid sinus, adjacent to the carotid bodies. Chemoreceptor information from the aortic arch conducts baroreceptor information. Both sets of peripheral chemoreceptors (and their associated baroreceptors) send their sensory information back to the NTS. The NTS is the first target for many important peripheral sensory inputs from the respiratory and cardiovascular systems, such as oxygenation, CO_2, arterial blood pressure, lung stretch, pulmonary irritant receptors, and others.

Practically all of the secondary respiratory muscles, for example, shoulder muscles, chest muscles, and abdominals, are also controlled by brainstem cell groups, especially the VRG, but these muscles are also controlled by more conventional motor systems located outside of the brainstem. An important point concerning neuromuscular control of ventilation is that many of those muscle actions must also accommodate the other nonventilatory functions of the respiratory system, such as swallowing, talking, postural control, defecation, vomiting, and locomotion.

One of the more important brainstem controllers is the NTS, which processes sensory signals from both respiratory and cardiovascular systems, although mostly in different subregions (10). The medulla is also the major source of sympathetic (autonomic) drive to constrict the blood vessels of skeletal muscles, the kidneys, and other viscera and to participate in the control of the heart rate. In fact, it is possible that the chemoreceptors and the sympathetic neurons of the ventral medulla are one and the same. The extensive anatomic overlap between respiratory and cardiovascular control is just one reflection of the complex functional coupling of the two systems. For example, increased blood flow through exercising muscles, mediated in part by the medulla, is necessary to carry the additional CO_2 away from the tissues, modulating the CO_2 concentration gradient between the intracellular environment and the blood plasma. Respiratory insufficiency, leading to low oxygenation (hypoxia), causes increased sympathetic activity that leads to higher heart rate and blood pressure. These changes in sympathetic activity compensate for the low O_2 levels by increasing the delivery rate of blood. Therefore, respiration and cardiovascular control are fundamentally linked by common goals of cardiopulmonary homeostasis.

Innervation of the Respiratory Muscles

The intercostal muscles (both external and internal) and other thoracic and abdominal muscles also receive innervation from spinal motor neurons in the ventral parts of the lower cervical and thoracic spinal cord. These spinal motor neurons receive input from many of the same medullary cell groups that project to the phrenic nucleus (10,11). Other accessory respiratory muscles, such as those in the upper airway (pharynx, larynx, and tongue), are innervated by cranial motor nerves such as the facial (VII), the glossopharyngeal (IX), and the hypoglossal (XII) nerves. Although the primary function of the upper airway muscles is to maintain an open airway during inspiration, a secondary function is the regulation of the rate of expiratory airflow using constriction and relaxation of the airway. The change from nasal breathing to mouth breathing (and vice versa) is also controlled by upper airway muscles (pharyngeal). Although many of these ventilatory muscles are driven by the same medullary cell groups, they often have maximal activity during a selective portion of the inspiratory (or expiratory) phase, such as late inspiration or early expiration. Different timing of accessory muscle activations in both inspiration and expiration are important control features that serve to reduce the work of breathing and maximize gas exchange. In addition, as respiratory activation is intensified by large blood gas disturbances, the degree of accessory muscle participation increases.

Although skeletal muscles make up the main functional component of ventilation, smooth muscle is used in the tracheal and bronchial airways for constriction or relaxation. The parasympathetic branch of the autonomic nervous system innervates these muscles. Although this aspect of respiratory control is mediated by autonomic (parasympathetic) structures, it is incorrect to refer to respiratory control as an "autonomic" system; it is a somatomotor system (albeit a very specialized one) just as the control of chewing or walking is a somatomotor system. The parasympathetic innervation of the airways is mainly from the vagus nerve and uses acetylcholine to constrict the airways; therefore, anticholinergic drugs can be used for airway muscle relaxation, for example, in asthma (12).

Basic Respiratory Pattern Generation

The source of the cyclical alternation of inspiration and expiration is a long-running controversy in various branches of the biomedical community. The arguments fall into two major groups: the pacemaker hypothesis and the network hypothesis (10). However, there is little controversy that the basic respiratory rhythm is generated in the medulla, regardless of how it is generated. The basic respiratory rhythm produced by either scenario is then modified and controlled by reflexes and other influences to match ventilation to changing physiologic needs, such as exercise and sleep.

The pacemaker hypothesis states that there exists a group (or groups) of medullary neurons that independently create the basic respiratory rhythm, similar to the pacemaker cells in the SA node of the heart. A group of pacemaker neurons does seem to exist in the ventrolateral part of the medulla, very near to a major output path to the phrenic nucleus (in the VRG), but it is doubtful that these neurons are solely responsible for normal respiration (10).

The network hypothesis states that the basic respiratory rhythm arises from a complex interplay between various types of inspiratory and expiratory neurons. These cell types are, once again, localized to the medulla but distributed over several nuclei (5,10,13). In rather simplistic terms, neurons that depolarize preferentially in the early part of the inspiratory phase inhibit all other cell types but have decreasing influence over the course of the inspiration. This network concept has somewhat greater acceptance than the pure pacemaker hypothesis, although there are medullary neurons (surgically isolated) that cyclically activate inspiratory or expiratory muscles, constituting a pacemaker. However, it is unclear whether this greatly reduced ventilation can be sustained for long periods and increased metabolism. The basic oscillation between inspiratory and postinspiratory cells likely requires stimulation from outside the respiratory pattern–generating network; that external stimulation may come from central chemoreceptors (10).

Because this chapter addresses the control of breathing, this brief introduction to rhythm generation is useful even though rhythm generation is not well understood; it provides some physiologic separation between the centralized, respiratory pattern generator and the multitude of respiratory-related reflexes that adjust that basic respiratory rhythm. This diversity of controlling influences is a reflection of the necessity to coordinate many different physiologic and behavioral demands on the respiratory system. Although most of the reflexes act on various brainstem respiratory neuronal groups, some act more directly on the phrenic nucleus and the other spinal areas controlling the intercostals and other accessory respiratory muscles (14).

Chemical (Blood Gas) Control of Ventilation

The primary function of the respiratory control system is regulation of the partial pressures of CO_2 and O_2 in arterial blood and plasma. This is accomplished by sensory signals from the various chemoreceptors and is the main driver of respiration. This sensory information is used by the brain to adjust ventilation to bring the gas concentrations back to their respective "set points." In most scenarios, the peripheral chemoreceptors respond to blood gas disturbances more quickly than the central chemoreceptors, allowing very rapid responses to transient changes. Those set points for CO_2 and O_2 vary with sleep and disease states and are reflected in their arterial concentrations. For example, part of the reason that respiration during non-REM sleep is slower and deeper is a reduced sensitivity of chemoreceptors to CO_2.

It is important to remember that pH is also a variable controlled by the respiratory system, especially CO_2 control. The level of CO_2 has a direct effect on pH because CO_2 and H_2O naturally combine to form carbonic acid, which dissociates into H^+ and bicarbonate (HCO_3^-). Carbonic anhydrase is an important catalyst (enzyme) in the reactions of CO_2 and water but only within RBCs (not plasma). Bicarbonate and certain proteins are important buffers for acidity in the plasma and cerebrospinal fluid (CSF). The main problem with high CO_2 levels in the blood is its influence on the production of H^+ ions in the body. Acidity must be tightly controlled because small deviations (~0.2 pH units) can adversely affect many different biochemical and physiologic processes, and extremes of pH can be toxic.

Increases in P_{CO_2} (or decreases in P_{O_2}) activate the chemoreceptors, which then directly influence the medullary respiratory networks to increase V_T (the volume of a single breath) and, likely, respiratory frequency as well. There are varying degrees of relative change in the two parameters depending on the particular disturbance and physiologic context. In mild exertion, it is common to have the augmentation of V_T but not frequency. The increase in ventilation leads to an enhanced excretion of CO_2, which leads to a decreased stimulation of the chemoreceptors—another classic example of a negative feedback loop. The changes in blood gases that elicit alterations in respiration are so small, and the effectiveness of the chemical control of respiration is so great, that during mild-to-moderate exercise almost no differences can be detected in arterial P_{CO_2}.

Because the classical chemoreceptors lie on or just beneath the surface of the medulla, they respond to pH/P_{CO_2} disturbances in CSF, not the blood. However, CSF levels of respiratory gases depend on the arterial plasma levels. Therefore, CSF is an important intermediary between the blood and the central chemoreceptors. The normal value of arterial pH is approximately 7.4, whereas the usual pH of CSF is about 7.32.

These blood gas sensory stimuli also influence cardiovascular reflexes, with hypoxia, hypercapnia (high P_{CO_2}), or acidity being generally sympathetically activating. Hypoxia, hypercapnia, and/or a pH of less than 7.3 initiate sympathetic reflexes to increase heart rate, cardiac output, and often blood pressure. The dual action of chemoreceptors in blood gas homeostasis is another reflection of the coupling between respiratory and cardiovascular control systems and the requirements of efficient gas exchange. An increase in ventilation would be ineffective without a corresponding increase in blood perfusion of the lungs and tissues.

Imagine a possible real-life occurrence—you are about to miss your bus to campus. You cognitively recognize the need to hurry, so you begin to run. Muscles throughout your body increase activity for locomotion and balance. The increased muscular activity requires greater metabolism, which consumes more O_2 and produces more CO_2. These changes are reflected by your falling concentrations of O_2 and rising concentration of CO_2, altering the concentration gradients that existed before you began to run. That is, more O_2 diffuses from the blood to the tissues because tissue O_2 levels are lowered (because of increased consumption), which then increases the concentration gradient from arterial blood to the tissue. CO_2 diffuses from the working tissues into the blood, raising your P_{CO_2} and lowering pH.

These changes in blood gases are sensed by the various chemoreceptors in contact with the arterial blood and CSF, which then activate respiration through neuronal networks. Just as importantly, this sudden bout of exercise requires that blood flow through the lungs be increased to make best use of the increased ventilation and exchange of gases; therefore, cardiac output must be increased. This is accomplished by increasing your heart rate and making adjustments to the strength of each beat, which are, in part, mediated by neural systems. Blood pressure may or may not change depending on the type of exercise and other factors. In addition to increased activation of the phrenic nucleus, the expiratory muscles are activated by medullary respiratory networks (recall that during rest, expiration is passive, ie, not driven by muscular contraction) and the participation of accessory inspiratory muscles is increased, as is necessary for rapid respiratory rates. This increase in ventilation then enhances the expiration of CO_2 and the delivery of O_2, which offsets the changes caused by the dash for the bus. Homeostasis is maintained, and you just make the bus—a little acidic maybe, but your knowledge of respiratory control assures you that as soon as your chemoreceptors detect the correction, your breathlessness will subside.

Other Respiratory Reflexes

Several respiratory reflexes act to protect the respiratory system (eg, cough, antioverinflation). At least three broad classes of sensory receptors are involved in these protective reflexes: slowly adapting receptors, rapidly adapting receptors, and C-fiber nerve endings. There is some degree of overlap in the function of the reflexes mediated by these three classes of receptors, all of which reside in the lungs and airways and practically all of which use the vagus nerve to transmit their information back to the brainstem.

Slowly adapting receptors are mainly stretch receptors residing in the smooth muscle of the conducting airways, which mediate the Hering-Breuer inflation reflex. This most well known of the respiratory protective reflexes acts to restrict overinflation of the lung. An important role for this reflex in neonates and infants is widely accepted; however, another role for the reflex in adults during exercise seems likely. Bronchoconstriction and, possibly, lung deflation below normal expiratory volume also activate these receptors.

The second major type of pulmonary receptor is the rapidly adapting type, which is also referred to as irritant receptors and which can initiate many different responses, such as cough, rapid breathing (tachypnea), breath holding, and/or airway constriction. Several activators for the rapidly adapting receptors exist, including hyperinflation and deflation, but unlike the slowly adapting receptors, which are mechanoreceptors, the rapidly adapting type is also quite sensitive to several different noxious chemicals—hence the name "irritant receptors." Examples of chemical stimulants of these receptors are ammonia, cigarette smoke, edema, distilled water, and sulfur dioxide, but other stimulants also exist. In addition, irritant receptors may be involved in asthma "attacks" in which certain asthma mediators stimulate airway irritant receptors that are pathologically hypersensitive, initiating a strong airway constrictor reflex involving increased vagal parasympathetic activity (12). Other factors, both neural and nonneural, are also involved in asthma.

C-fiber endings are the most numerous of the pulmonary receptors and are stimulated by both mechanical and chemical stimuli. The activating stimuli and the resulting respiratory reflexes of these receptors are very similar to those for rapidly adapting irritant receptors. There are two classes of C-fiber receptors based mainly on where they are found—pulmonary and bronchial. Activation of pulmonary C-fiber receptors usually evokes apnea, bradycardia, hypotension, and bronchoconstriction. Activation of the bronchial receptors elicits rapid shallow breathing, bronchoconstriction, and increased secretion of mucus onto the surface of the airways. Both classes of C-fiber receptors (and rapidly adapting receptors) can cause cough.

Cardiovascular reflexes also affect respiration. One example is the effect of changes in blood pressure on respiration. Increases in blood pressure are sensed by the baroreceptors in the carotid sinus and the aortic arch, which then increase their firing rates. These sensory signals are passed to the NTS, which distributes the information to various brain sites, where the signal causes a reduction in sympathetic drive to the blood vessels and returns blood pressure to "normal" levels. The respiratory component of the baroreflex involves a reduction in ventilation during hypertension and a small increase during low blood pressure (hypotension) (8). This is the classic baroreceptor reflex (or baroreflex).

SLEEP AND RESPIRATION

Sleep is a very important modulator of respiration and cardiovascular function. Part of that effect is caused by the general reduction in muscle tone characteristic of sleep. Another effect on breathing is that during sleep, energy needs are considerably lower than during waking and especially so for active waking. A reduced need for energy and O_2 is representative of the behavioral aspect of sleep, that is, reduced metabolism.

Effects of Normal Sleep on Respiratory Control

Sleep affects respiration in several ways. Most notable is the reduction in respiratory rate during non-REM sleep compared with waking. In addition, respiratory variability is lowest in non-REM sleep. Generally, the deeper stages of non-REM sleep (ie, N3, slow-wave sleep) are associated with slower, deeper, and less variable breathing than non-REM sleep stages N1 and N2. Heart rate and heart rate variability are also lowest in non-REM sleep. Respiration during REM sleep is more like waking than during non-REM sleep in terms of rate, depth, and variability.

The sensitivity of the respiratory system to CO_2 is affected by the sleep-wake state. CO_2 sensitivity is highest during waking and lowest during quiet, non-REM sleep, with REM sleep having intermediate sensitivity (9). A difference in sensitivity means that for a given increase in P_{CO_2}, the respiratory response is greater in waking than in non-REM sleep. This is a large part of the reason respiration is slower during non-REM sleep (especially N3, slow-wave sleep) than waking or REM sleep. Concentrations of CO_2 in the blood are slightly higher during non-REM sleep. The abrupt decrease in P_{CO_2} sensitivity at sleep onset while the "waking" P_{CO_2} level persists (for a few dozen seconds) may be a mechanism of sleep-onset central apneas (15,16).

Compared with non-REM sleep, REM sleep is associated with respiratory frequency increases, smaller V_T, and greater variability. A significant portion of that greater variability is caused by changes in respiratory pattern (eg, tachypnea) associated with periods of REMs. In addition, the reduction in muscle tone during non-REM sleep and the loss of accessory respiratory muscle activity in REM sleep are factors in sleep-related respiratory patterns and variability.

Arousal as a Respiratory Drive

Waking respiratory frequencies are higher and more variable than either type of sleep. These state-related differences are a result of the higher metabolic needs during waking and activity and of the neural-stimulating action of arousal or wakefulness (13) on respiratory control systems, cardiovascular systems, and other brain networks. In other words, the major effect of sleep on respiration may be the removal of the stimulating effect of waking.

Respiration is affected by sleep and arousal in another way that has even more clinical significance—that of a sleep-related decrease in the basal level of skeletal muscular activity. Compared with waking, non-REM sleep is characterized by a reduction in muscle tone throughout the body; in REM sleep, muscle activity is at its lowest. In fact, a scoring criterion for REM sleep is muscular paralysis, as reflected by a nearly flat electromyographic signal during polysomnography (17). The diaphragm is the only skeletal muscle not inhibited by sleep (or at least not *as* inhibited). The large decline in tonic muscle activation includes the accessory respiratory muscles; consequently, the rhythmic drive to assist in ventilation is reduced during non-REM sleep and practically disappears in REM sleep.

Sleep-Disordered Breathing

There are many kinds of sleep-disordered breathing, including not only the common obstructive and central apnea/hypopnea but also Cheyne-Stokes respiration/periodic breathing and treatment-emergent central sleep apnea. Loss of muscular tone in the upper airways during supine sleep is the major factor in OSA. OSA is easily the most common type of apnea, partly because of the increase in the incidence of obesity. During an obstruction, the airway muscles are unable to maintain an open airway because of the loss of the wakefulness stimulus, usually in conjunction with supine sleeping, obesity, airway narrowing, muscular disease, and/or abnormal craniofacial structure. The reduction in muscle tone during non-REM sleep can lead to airway turbulence, airway narrowing, or complete occlusion.

Central apnea is the lack of respiratory drive to the diaphragm and the subsequent lack of airflow. The mechanisms for this are uncertain, but in healthy adults, many central apneas are likely because of a short-lasting drop in P_{CO_2} during sleep that can happen after a sigh or hyperventilation (18). The occasional central apnea is not pathologic. On the contrary, those patients with clinically significant central apnea or hypopnea are more difficult to treat compared with those with obstructive symptoms. A relative lack of arousal stimuli to the central pattern generator is the usual way a central apnea is initiated.

Cheyne-Stokes respiration is characterized by a period of central apnea/hypopnea, followed by gradually increasing ventilation, usually to hyperventilation, then gradually decreasing back to apnea/hypopnea. The entire cycle takes 30 to 90 seconds and can reflect slow chemoreceptor responses or impaired circulatory function associated with heart failure. These symptoms are suggestive of a neurologic problem, usually in association with congestive heart failure (CHF).

Treatment-emergent central sleep apnea is seen in a relatively small subset of OSA patients when positive airway pressure is applied. Central apneas emerge during the titration portion of a polysomnographic recording. In these patients, the resolution of their obstructive and mixed events seems to lead to a greater propensity for central apneas. Continuous positive airway pressure may be contraindicated for these patients. The common therapy for treatment-emergent central sleep apnea is the use of adaptive servo-ventilation (ASV). Note that warnings have been posted by equipment manufacturers and the American Academy of Sleep Medicine suggesting that ASV should not be used in patients with CHF with an ejection fraction of less than 45% because of the risk of mortality (19). ASV devices respond to arrhythmic ventilatory movement, usually central and obstructive apneas, with appropriate pressure support and disengage when the respiratory pattern stabilizes. Much research is directed at processes of treatment-emergent central sleep apnea and, subsequently, more effective treatments.

SUMMARY

The primary function of the respiratory system is to maintain blood gases (O_2 and CO_2) and pH at optimal levels. O_2 and CO_2 move down their respective concentration gradients between the blood and the cells and then again between the blood and air within the alveoli of the lungs. Rhythmic ventilation by respiratory muscles exchanges the air in the lungs with fresh air to remove the CO_2 and replenish O_2. These blood gases must be tightly controlled to allow sufficient metabolism and vigorous activity.

CNS networks are not only centered in the medulla and spinal cord but are also affected by neural systems in other brain areas. The respiratory rhythm of inspiration and expiration is generated in the medulla, most likely by several different neuronal types, although a single type may form the basis of the inspiratory phase. This basic rhythm is powerfully affected by sensory signals concerning the level of CO_2 and O_2 in the blood and the CSF. There are two categories of chemoreceptors: the central chemoreceptors, mainly near the surface of the rostral part of the ventrolateral medulla, and peripheral chemoreceptors, which are in the carotid bodies and aortic arch. These sensory signals are used to adjust ventilation to compensate for a change in blood gases, returning them to their optimal levels.

The diaphragm is the main respiratory muscle, and therefore output from the medulla is directed mainly at the phrenic nucleus of the spinal cord that innervates the diaphragm. However, accessory respiratory muscles play an essential role in ventilation, especially during physical activity. These accessory muscles are powerfully affected by sleep and the sleeping body position (reclining), which can contribute to pathologic processes and conditions. Sleep and arousal are powerful modulators of respiratory and cardiovascular function to the extent that arousal and wakefulness are significant activating factors for both systems and are notably absent during sleep.

REFERENCES

1. Ayappa I, Rapoport DM. The upper airway in sleep: physiology of the pharynx. *Sleep Med Rev*. 2003;7(1):9-33.
2. Victor L. Obstructive sleep apnea. https://pubmed.ncbi.nlm.nih.gov/10593319/
3. Lambertson C. Respiration. In: Mountcastle VB, ed. *Medical Physiology*. 14th ed. Mosby; 1980:1677-1842.
4. Horner RL, Liu X, Gill H, et al. Selected contribution: Effects of sleep-wake state on the genioglossus vs. diaphragm muscle responses to CO_2 in rats. *J Appl Physiol*. 2002;92(2):878-887.
5. West JB. *Pulmonary Pathophysiology: The Essentials*. 2nd ed. Williams & Wilkins; 1982:61-64.
6. West JB. Pulmonary gas exchange. In: Brobeck J, ed. *Best and Taylor's Physiological Basis of Medical Practice*. 10th ed. Williams & Wilkins; 1979.

7. Schwartzstein RM, Parker MJ. The gas exchanger: matching ventilation and perfusion. In: *Respiratory Physiology: A Clinical Approach*. Lippincott, Williams & Wilkins; 2006.
8. West JB. *Respiratory Physiology: The Essentials*. 3rd ed. Williams & Wilkins; 1985.
9. Nattie EE. Central chemosensitivity, sleep, and wakefulness. *Respir Physiol*. 2001;129(1-2):257-268.
10. Feldman JL, McCrimmon DR. Neural control of breathing. In: Squire LE, Bloom FE, McConnell SK, et al, eds. *Fundamental Neuro-Science*. 2nd ed. Academic Press; 2003:967-990.
11. West JB. Control of breathing. In: Brobeck J, ed. *Best & Taylor's Physiological Basis of Medical Practice*. 10th ed. Williams & Wilkins; 1979.
12. de Jongste JC, Longejan RC, Kerrebijn KF. Control of airway caliber by autonomic nerves in asthma and in chronic obstructive pulmonary disease. *Am Rev Respir Dis*. 1991;143(6):1421-1426.
13. Richter DW. Generation and maintenance of the respiratory rhythm. *J Exp Biol*. 1982;100:93-107.
14. Mack SO, Kc P, Wu M, et al. Paraventricular oxytocin neurons are involved in neural control of breathing. *J Appl Physiol*. 2002;92(2):826-834.
15. Horner RL, Rivera MP, Kozar LF, et al. The ventilatory response to arousal from sleep is not fully explained by differences in CO_2 levels between sleep and wakefulness. *J Physiol*. 2001;534(pt 3):881-890.
16. Nakayama H, Smith CA, Rodman JR, et al. Effect of ventilatory drive on carbon dioxide sensitivity below eupnea during sleep. *Am J Respir Crit Care Med*. 2002; 165:1251-1260.
17. Rechtschaffen A, Kales A, eds. *A Manual of Standardized Terminology, Techniques and Scoring System for Sleep Stages of Human Subjects*. UCLA Brain Information Service/Brain Research Institute; 1968.
18. Dempsey JA, Smith CA, Harms CA, et al. Sleep-induced breathing instability. *Sleep*. 1996;19(3): 236-247.
19. Aurora RN, Bista SR, Casey KR, et al. Updated adaptive servo-ventilation recommendations for the 2012 AASM guideline: "The treatment of central sleep apnea syndromes in adults: practice parameters with an evidence-based literature review and meta-analyses". *J Clin Sleep Med*. 2016;12(5):757-761. doi:10.5664/jcsm.5812

Chapter 5
Oxygen and Gas Exchange in the Body

STEPHEN TARNOCZY

KEY CONCEPTS/LEARNING OBJECTIVES

The key concepts for this chapter include a review of the exchange of gases within the body as well as the outside environment, methods for oxygen delivery to the tissues throughout the body; the relationship between oxygen and hemoglobin and factors that alter their relationship; how disease may impact oxygen diffusion, transport, and/or delivery; the types of hypoxia, hypoxemia, and ischemia; and how supplemental oxygen affects the healthy and compromised patient.

KEY TERMS

Alveoli
Anemia
Anemic hypoxia
Circulatory hypoxia
External respiration
Hemoglobin
Hypoxemia
Internal respiration
Ischemia
Ventilation

The human organism is a magnificent and complex balance of systems that work in tandem to maintain our balance of systems or homeostasis—all equally important but none as influential as the exchange of gases at the cellular level or respiration.

RESPIRATION VERSUS VENTILATION

A very important concept surrounding this topic of discussion is the distinction between respiration and ventilation, which are two very different processes. Ventilation is defined as "the process of moving gas (usually air) in and out of the lungs" (1). This is completely independent of respiration, where the exchange of gas actually occurs either in the lungs (external respiration) or at the level of the tissues inside the body (internal respiration). These two very important areas will be addressed, but only respiration will be covered in this chapter. The mechanism of ventilation (moving air in and out of the lungs) will be covered in another forum. It is important to realize that ventilating a patient does not ensure that respiration is actually taking place and vice versa. Rather than dwelling on these two distinctions, let us examine the forces and laws that govern the miracle of respiration.

External Respiration

The exchange of gas between the body and the outside environment is referred to as "external respiration." The process of external respiration takes place between the lungs and the atmospheric air we breathe. This takes place in the tiny spherical sacs of the lungs, called "alveoli," and the blood supply carried in by very tiny blood vessels in the lungs, called the "pulmonary capillaries." Collectively, we refer to the conjoining of these two systems as the "alveolar-capillary membrane" (ACM). The process of gas exchange at this level is one of physics and pure diffusion, the movement of gas from an area of high concentration to an area of low concentration, until the two areas are equilibrated or equal. As we take air in or inhale air (inhalation), we are bringing in a gas (air) that comprises primarily nitrogen (N_2) and 20.9% oxygen (O_2). The amount of oxygen in the inspired air, or the fraction of inspired oxygen (FIO_2), is greater inside the alveoli than the amount of oxygen contained in the pulmonary capillaries. Utilizing the gradient of diffusion and movement of gas from a high to a low concentration, oxygen leaves the alveoli, crosses the ACM, and enters the red blood cell (RBC). As oxygen moves in, carbon dioxide (CO_2) is simultaneously moving out. Again, under the laws of diffusion, the amount of CO_2 inside the RBC is significantly higher than the amount of CO_2 inside the alveoli, and CO_2 diffuses from the RBC into the alveoli to be excreted or expired during exhalation. Under normal conditions, this takes place very quickly at the level of the ACM, usually in about 0.25 seconds. The amount of contact time that the average RBC has with the ACM is about 0.75 seconds.

Internal Respiration

After the exchange of gas in the lungs, oxygenated blood returns to the heart to be distributed throughout the body through the left ventricle, arteries, and the body's systemic circulation. The blood travels the arterial circulation to be distributed throughout the body and to its many organ systems. As the RBCs make their way through the smaller blood vessels, they eventually reach the arterial capillaries of the body. These capillaries are the end point of a network of blood vessels that feed the entire body with nutrients, electrolytes, and oxygen. At the capillary level, much as in the capillaries of the lungs, the RBC comes into contact with the capillary wall and the adjoining tissues.

Under normal circumstances, internal or cellular respiration utilizes oxygen to create energy, with the waste product primarily being CO_2 through the aerobic pathway of the Krebs cycle. At the tissue level, the amount of oxygen inside the RBC is greater than the amount outside the RBC in the tissues, and O_2 moves out of the RBC and into the tissues. Again, simultaneous exchange of CO_2 is taking place as CO_2 leaves the tissues and moves into the plasma and RBC for return to the lungs and elimination; then the process starts all over again. The concentration of CO_2 is greater in the tissues compared with the RBC, so CO_2 leaves the tissues and diffuses out into the plasma and RBC. The transport of both CO_2 and O_2 within the body is a bit more complex than described here, but it sets the foundation for further discussion.

ATMOSPHERIC GAS AND PARTIAL PRESSURES OF OXYGEN

Depending on where you live, the atmosphere of the air you breathe exerts a pressure that is equal to about 760 mm Hg, 1 atm, or 14.7 pounds per square inch (psi). At higher altitudes above sea level, that pressure gradually begins to decrease. As you go below the sea level, the opposite occurs, and the pressure actually increases by 760 mm Hg, 1 atm, or 14.7 psi for every 33 ft you are below the water's surface! The concentration of gas or the amount of oxygen in room air of 21% never changes, but rather the pressure that it is under in the atmosphere changes, causing the gas to behave differently. Take a balloon and blow it up. You have a balance of air pressures that keep the balloon inflated. You have air inside the balloon exerting a force outward in all directions against the inside wall. You have air in the atmosphere exerting pressure on the balloon at 760 mm Hg. *Keeping all other variables constant,* if you were to take the balloon and submerge it in a pool of water, the balloon would shrink in size. Elevating the same balloon several thousand feet will cause it to expand. The gas in the balloon never went anywhere, but the environmental pressure on the outside of the balloon changed! Now notice the phrase *keeping all other variables constant* because that is very important when you are dealing with any gas and demonstrating its physical properties.

Regardless of the units of measure used, the atmospheric pressure (760 mm Hg) is a combination of all the gases in room air. Because room air is made up primarily of nitrogen and oxygen, these two gases make up the greatest percentage of the atmospheric pressure of 760 mm Hg. For example, room air is 21% oxygen and 79% nitrogen. There are additional "trace" gases or elements also present in extremely small amounts, but the air we breathe is primarily nitrogen and oxygen. Of the 760 mm Hg pressure exerted by the atmosphere, 160 mm Hg pressure is exerted by oxygen, and 600 mm Hg pressure is exerted by nitrogen. Because air does not comprise 100% pure gas but rather is a mixture of these two elements, we refer to the pressures exerted by nitrogen and oxygen as *partial pressures.* Adding these two pressures together, we get the 760 mm Hg of total pressure exerted by our atmosphere on an average day. This calculation is known as Dalton's law of partial pressure: *The partial pressure of a gas is equal to the concentration of that gas (expressed as a decimal) × the atmospheric pressure (760 mm Hg in our example).*

Therefore,

$$\left.\begin{matrix}\text{The partial pressure of}\\ \text{of nitrogen }(PN_2)\end{matrix}\right\}\begin{matrix}=0.79\times 760\text{ mm Hg}\\ =600\text{ mm Hg}\end{matrix}$$

$$\left.\begin{matrix}\text{The partial pressure of}\\ \text{oxygen }(PO_2)\end{matrix}\right\}\begin{matrix}=0.21\times 760\text{ mm Hg}\\ =160\text{ mm Hg}\end{matrix}$$

$$\text{Total atmospheric pressure}\left.\right\}\begin{matrix}=PN_2(600)+PO_2(160)\\ =760\text{ mm Hg}\end{matrix}$$

The change in atmospheric pressure at higher elevations requires hikers or climbers attempting summit assaults on Everest to bring canisters of oxygen to facilitate their climb. As you reach altitudes of 1 mile or greater, the air becomes "thinner" or, better phrased, the atmospheric pressure significantly decreases as you rise in altitude.

Let us calculate partial pressures of these gases at 30,000 ft elevation where atmospheric pressure is about 250 mm Hg:

$$\left.\begin{matrix}\text{The partial pressure of}\\ \text{nitrogen }(PN_2)\end{matrix}\right\}\begin{matrix}=0.79\times 250\text{ mm Hg}\\ =197.5\text{ mm Hg}\end{matrix}$$

$$\left.\begin{matrix}\text{The partial pressure of}\\ \text{oxygen }(PO_2)\end{matrix}\right\}\begin{matrix}=0.21\times 250\text{ mmHg}\\ =52.5\text{ mm Hg}\end{matrix}$$

$$\left.\begin{matrix}\text{Total atmospheric pressure}\\ \text{at 30,000 ft}\end{matrix}\right\}\begin{matrix}=PN_2\ 197.5+PO_2(52.5)\\ =250\text{ mm Hg}\end{matrix}$$

Notice that the concentration of gases or the composition of air did not change but that the partial pressures of both gases dropped markedly compared with a sea-level pressure of 760 mm Hg. The PO_2 dropped by more than one-third! This is why there are emergency oxygen masks in airline cabins; if the internal pressure suddenly drops, supplemental oxygen is required because the surrounding air at 30,000 ft contains insufficient oxygen.

This is also why patients with abnormally low levels of oxygen in their blood (hypoxemia) are treated by giving them supplemental oxygen to breathe through a mask or oxygen cannula. Although we are not changing atmospheric pressure by administering oxygen, we are changing the concentration of oxygen that the patient inspires, or, more correctly, we are increasing the patient's FIO_2.

So, to complete our sample calculations, let us calculate the partial pressure of these gases while climbing our mountain, breathing extra oxygen from a tank, estimating that we have increased the FIO_2 from 0.21 of room air to 0.40 by putting our oxygen masks on . . .

$$\left.\begin{array}{r}\text{The partial pressure of}\\ \text{of nitrogen } (PN_2)\end{array}\right\}\begin{array}{l}=0.60\times 250 \text{ mm Hg}\\ =150 \text{ mm Hg}\end{array}$$

$$\left.\begin{array}{r}\text{The partial pressure of}\\ \text{oxygen } (PO_2)\end{array}\right\}\begin{array}{l}=0.40\times 250 \text{ mm Hg}\\ =100 \text{ mm Hg}\end{array}$$

$$\left.\begin{array}{r}\text{Total atmospheric pressure}\\ \text{at 30,000 on } O_2\end{array}\right\}\begin{array}{l}=PN_2(150)+\\ =PO_2(100)=250 \text{ mm Hg}\end{array}$$

Using a higher FIO_2 with supplemental oxygen, we were able to correct for the lower partial pressure of oxygen at the higher altitude. We will utilize similar strategies to treat patients with lower than normal blood oxygen levels (hypoxemia).

DIFFUSION OF RESPIRATORY GASES ACROSS THE ALVEOLAR-CAPILLARY MEMBRANE

When gas (room air) enters the body through inhalation, it makes its way through the conducting airways of the respiratory system and eventually to the level of the alveolus. Only gas that comes into contact with the alveolus has the potential to participate in gas exchange. The word potential is used because there are a variety of factors that must exist in order for the transfer of gases or external respiration to occur. The presence of disease, as well as the equally important role of pulmonary capillary perfusion, determines how well gases diffuse or exchange across the alveolar-capillary junction.

There are multiple factors associated with the diffusion process, any one of which can fail or become impaired, leading to impaired gas exchange and resulting in harm to the patient. We will analyze the anatomy first and then specifically talk about CO_2 and O_2 exchange in the alveoli.

The alveoli are small sac-like structures attached to the terminal bronchioles that are recognized as the last branching or division of the tracheobronchial tree. Starting with the trachea, the airways branch off into 23 divisions until they split into the terminal bronchioles. Air is brought in and out of the chest as a result of changing pressures in the thorax, but gas movement at this level is through Brownian movement of pure diffusion from an area of high concentration to an area of low concentration. This pressure gradient or drive can be altered or accelerated depending on the general health of the structural system and the presence of either pulmonary or cardiovascular disease (2).

Each alveolus is wrapped in a net of capillaries that surround the spherical lung unit to provide blood supply and enable gas exchange. As oxygen moves out of the alveolus, it crosses a series of thin yet significant layers of tissue on its journey out of the alveolus, moves across the alveolar cell wall, through the capillary membrane wall, into the blood plasma, across the membrane wall of the RBC, and finally adheres to the hemoglobin (Hgb) molecule in the RBC. Depending on the overall health of the individual, this process may occur unhindered, or there may be significant barriers at the tissue level that impede the diffusion of oxygen. All these structures and tissues can be diseased, scarred, or underperfused, which will make gas exchange significantly less efficient. The end result is lower oxygen content in the arterial circulation and, potentially, a simultaneous increase in carbon dioxide in the bloodstream when damage becomes severe.

A similar process of diffusion occurs at the tissue level of the arterial capillaries. When an RBC comes into contact with tissue that is in need of O_2, the drive or diffusion gradient causes the relatively higher concentration of O_2 to move out of the RBC and across the barriers and diffuse into the cellular tissue that is in need of oxygen. However, if not enough oxygen was efficiently exchanged at the alveoli, there will be insufficient oxygen available when the RBC arrives at the tissue level, resulting in hypoxemia.

Patients with a history of pulmonary disease such as emphysema or fibrosis can suffer from a variety of conditions that alter the normal diffusion process. Changes in the alveoli and eventual destruction of lung function because of smoking or by scar tissue formed as the lungs tried to repair themselves from previous disease resulting in fibrosis produces varying degrees of damage from unnoticeable to extremely debilitating. It is sometimes very difficult for the clinician to determine through physical examination and history the extent of damage and the potential challenges the patient may present in the sleep center. Key indicators for potential ACM damage are a history of smoking, occupational health exposure, or any type of pulmonary fibrosis, to name a few. The definitive test to evaluate ACM function is pulmonary function testing with arterial blood gases.

Pulmonary function testing is used to determine a patient's baseline status and level of damage. The results of this testing in the patient record are an invaluable tool in assessing patients with significant pulmonary disease that we sometimes see in the sleep center.

Gas exchange, as previously stated, is just as much a function of ventilation as of perfusion. The circulatory system is the delivery pathway back and forth to where respiration can occur. The first component of gas exchange is getting the RBC to the lungs and exchanging gases across a healthy ACM. The second component is the delivery system and getting the RBC to the tissue level where it is needed and perfusing the areas where gas exchange needs to occur. When these two systems become unbalanced, significant impairment of gas exchange and/or delivery of oxygen or elimination of CO_2 can result. The body has a unique system that accommodates these potential challenges that lead us to discuss the relationship between Hgb and oxygen.

OXYGEN-HEMOGLOBINDISSOCIATION CURVE

The relationship between oxygen and Hgb of the RBC is a complex one; however, it is quite simple to understand. Oxygen and Hgb, just like two magnets, have an attraction to each other. The closer the magnets, the stronger the attraction, and the opposite is true as you spread the magnets farther away. There are a few conditions that can make oxygen more or less attractive to Hgb. Temperature, blood pH, and CO_2 levels of the blood can all affect the attraction or *affinity* of oxygen and Hgb. Factors that make oxygen more attractive to Hgb are decreased CO_2, decreased temperature, and increased pH. These factors result in oxygen binding more readily at the lungs and staying bound to the RBC more strongly at the tissue level. Factors that make oxygen less attractive to Hgb include increased CO_2, increased temperature, and decreased pH. With these factors in place, oxygen binds at the alveolar level less readily and is freed up at the tissue level much more easily. So, what does this mean?

Under normal circumstances in healthy individuals, there is really no significant alteration in gas exchange related to these differences in affinity. There is a problem, however, in individuals who do not have normal oxygen levels. The oxygen-Hgb relationship curve is not linear but rather S-shaped with a rapid downward slope in the middle of the curve. In patients who have less than normal blood oxygen levels because of cardiopulmonary disease, these shifts in affinity can be most detrimental. In the real world of health care, a majority of patients who are sick will have an increased temperature and an increased CO_2 level, which often results in a decreased pH. As you recall, these factors make oxygen slightly less attractive to Hgb, and the uptake at the ACM level may not be ideal, resulting in a less than normal oxygen level in the blood. This is our patient with chronic obstructive pulmonary disease, emphysema, and cardiopulmonary disease who has such significant impairment of gas exchange that they fall in the middle of the S-shaped oxyhemoglobin dissociation curve, and any slight shift or movement on that curve (affinity) can have huge consequences on the amount of oxygen available at the tissue level. So, how do we compensate?

Fortunately, the body's rate of oxygen consumption is not all or nothing, and there is a great deal of oxygen in reserve. As each Hgb molecule can hold up to four oxygen molecules, there is a tremendous carrying capacity evident. If we assume that the arterial Hgb sites are all bound with oxygen, yielding a 100% oxygen saturation, at the tissue level when oxygen is released, generally only one oxygen molecule unbinds from Hgb, leaving the other three oxygen molecules intact. The remaining three of the four Hgb molecules with bound oxygen yield an oxygen saturation equal to 75% as the RBC returns in the venous circulation back to the heart. This also clearly demonstrates that the body consumes only about 25% of the oxygen available under normal conditions. This leaves a tremendous amount of oxygen available in reserves if needed. As an individual increases their demand for oxygen, the body is normally able to accommodate without issue. Again, the difficulty arises for those individuals who have less than normal arterial Hgb saturation, to start with, leaving their oxygen reserves severely compromised to the point where the slightest increase in demand for oxygen can tax them to the point of respiratory insufficiency.

HYPOXEMIA/HYPOXIA/ISCHEMIA

The terms hypoxemia and hypoxia are, unfortunately, used interchangeably quite often, yet they mean very distinctly different things. Although both of these terms relate to lower than normal oxygen levels, hypoxemia is specifically a lower than normal oxygen level in the blood, whereas hypoxia is lower than normal oxygen level in the tissues, which leads to ischemia. Theoretically, it is possible to have one without the other, and their clinical significance varies and therefore warrants discussion.

Hypoxemia is usually related to the integrity and efficiency of gas exchange at the ACM. If not enough oxygen diffuses across in the lungs, then the RBC will not pick up sufficient oxygen to saturate the Hgb in the arterial circulation (generally 97% or greater). Hypoxia occurs when there is not enough oxygen present at the level of the tissues, resulting in ischemia; there are several different causes and types of hypoxia.

This is where the nomenclature starts to get a bit tricky. Review the definition of hypoxemia; if there are low oxygen levels to start with at the level of gas exchange in the lungs, then it makes sense that there will be lower than normal oxygen available to the tissues. Therefore, hypoxia, caused by hypoxemia, is referred to as *hypoxic hypoxia*. Another type of hypoxia is caused by insufficient RBCs in the blood (anemia). When there are an insufficient number of Hgb molecules to accept oxygen, there will not be enough oxygen delivered to the tissues. This is referred to as *anemic hypoxia*.

Remember that oxygen delivery is reliant just as much on the circulatory system to transport the RBC as it is on the gas exchange that occurs in the lungs; if the body has vascular damage or underperfusion of the tissues, it is called *circulatory hypoxia*. In circulatory hypoxia, the arterial oxygen content may be completely normal, but there is a problem with the delivery system, and the oxygen-rich blood cannot reach the site where gas exchange occurs because of a fault in the circulatory system.

The last and rarer form of hypoxia is caused by any condition that interferes with or impedes the body's ability to use oxygen normally. The example often used is cyanide poisoning resulting in *histotoxic hypoxia*.

Correcting Hypoxemia

In the sleep center environment, frequent desaturation events related to sleep-disordered breathing (SDB) are a nightly occurrence. Pressurization of the upper airway using continuous positive airway pressure (CPAP), bilevel, or adaptive servoventilation can benefit the alveolar exchange mechanism by enabling the alveoli to remain distended and participate in gas exchange. Often, pressurization alone can maintain a patient's oxygen level within a normal range. Occasionally, in the presence of severe SDB or in concert with pulmonary disease, the need to increase FIO_2 may arise and necessitate the adjunct of supplemental oxygen.

Assuming that the patient has no preexisting cardiopulmonary conditions, the primary cause of hypoxemia is the interruption of gas exchange in the lung and does not usually involve damage to the airway control mechanism. Logically, this should be corrected by resolving the upper airway obstruction, and normal oxygen levels in the blood should resume. These otherwise healthy patients may suffer from normal alveolar hypoventilation changes associated with the resumption of restored physiologic sleep. This can sometimes result in borderline hypoxemia that responds in the sleep lab with an additional 1- to 2-cm H_2O increase in baseline CPAP. Occasionally, increasing the FIO_2 may be necessary to address persistent hypoxemia in the absence of breathing-related events. Implementation of supplemental oxygen should be initiated following department protocols and parameters as established by the center medical director.

SUMMARY

The exchange of gases with the atmosphere as well as within the body occurs utilizing well-defined processes in the field of biochemistry and within the laws of physics. If these normal processes are disturbed or interrupted, then the consequence of altered gas exchange mechanisms may occur. By understanding the laws that govern these processes, it is possible to apply concepts that we use in the sleep center to create mechanisms to correct this disturbance. The challenge is that sometimes we get only a few brief hours of diagnostic and therapeutic time to evaluate and treat individuals in a single night. A good understanding of the normal gas exchange process allows the technologist to apply that knowledge to understanding how the body responds to an alteration in that normal mechanism and take corrective action in an effort to restore normal physiologic function.

REFERENCES

1. Wilkins RL, Stoller JK, Kacmarek RM. *Egan's Fundamentals of Respiratory Care*. 12th ed. Mosby; 2021.
2. West JB. *Pulmonary Pathophysiology*. 7th ed. Lippincott Williams & Wilkins; 2008.

SUGGESTED READINGS

Des Jardins T. *Cardiopulmonary Anatomy & Physiology*. 4th ed. Delmar; 2008.

Des Jardins T, Burton GG. *Clinical Manifestations and Assessment of Respiratory Disease*. 6th ed. Mosby; 2011.

Chapter 6
Cardiac Anatomy and Physiology

LISA M. ENDEE

KEY CONCEPTS/LEARNING OBJECTIVES

The key concepts for this chapter include describing the components of the cardiovascular system and the functional anatomy of the heart, discussing the cardiac conduction system, the generation and transmission of an impulse along its path, and its relationship to the cardiac cycle, describing the basic concepts of cardiac electrophysiology and how ion channels facilitate the transmission of an impulse through action potentials, identifying the main components of the electrocardiogram (ECG) waveform, including normal morphologies and measures of a normal sinus rhythm, and understanding the importance of the ECG in monitoring patient safety in the sleep lab.

KEY TERMS

Action potential
Afterload
Cardiac cycle
Conduction system
Depolarization
Diastole
Preload
Repolarization
Systole
Transmission of impulses

FUNCTIONAL ANATOMY OF THE CARDIOVASCULAR SYSTEM

An essential part of a full-night polysomnogram is the electrocardiogram (ECG). The ECG is a graphic illustration of the electrical activity of the heart and is crucial to monitoring a patient's cardiovascular status. Knowledge of basic cardiac anatomy and electrophysiology will assist the reader to achieve a better understanding of the ECG and its components.

Heart Anatomy

The heart is a four-chambered muscular organ that lies in the thorax, posterior to the sternum and intercostal cartilages. It sits on the superior surface of the diaphragm and is the largest organ in the mediastinum, weighing approximately 2 g/lb of ideal body weight. The wall of the heart is composed of three layers. The most superficial of these layers is the epicardium. The epicardium contains an outer fibrous connective tissue and an inner serous pericardium. The space between these layers, the pericardial sac, contains about 25 mL of fluid that acts to reduce friction of the beating heart. Just underneath the pericardium is the muscular middle layer of the heart, the myocardium, which, in addition to its contractile properties, has the capacity to conduct electrical impulses to its cells. The endocardium, a sheet of endothelium resting on a thin layer of connective tissue, is the innermost layer of the heart and extends outward to include the valves of the heart.

The four chambers of the heart are the right and left atria, superiorly, and the right and left ventricles, inferiorly. The two sides of the heart are divided internally by the interventricular septum. Atrioventricular (AV) valves are made up of leaflets of connective tissue connected to fibrous cords called chordae tendineae. They connect to muscular projections (papillary muscles) from the inner surface of the heart wall. The AV valves sit between the atria and the ventricles and function to prevent backward blood flow. Specifically, the tricuspid valve contains three leaflets and lies between the right atrium and the right ventricle. The mitral or bicuspid valve contains two leaflets and sits between the left atrium and the left ventricle. The two semilunar valves are made up of leaflets attached to a fibrous ring of endothelium: The pulmonic semilunar valve lies between the right ventricle and the pulmonary trunk, whereas the aortic semilunar valve sits between the left ventricle and the aorta (Figure 6-1).

The right atrium is the receiving chamber for deoxygenated blood returning from systemic circulation and is fed by the superior vena cava, inferior vena cava, and coronary sinus. Deoxygenated blood enters the right atrium and flows through the tricuspid valve into the right ventricle. The right ventricle pumps the blood through the pulmonic semilunar valve and into

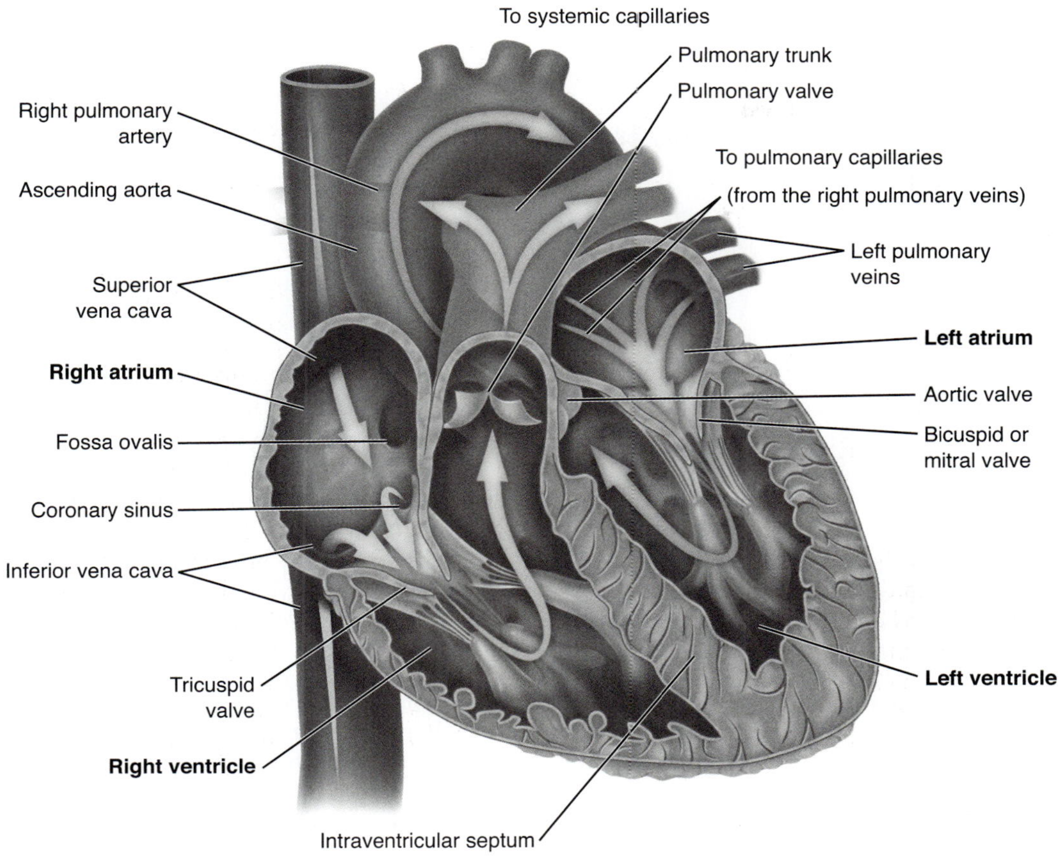

Figure 6-1 Anatomic view of cardiac blood flow. (Reprinted with permission from Archer P, Nelson LA. *Applied Anatomy & Physiology for Manual Therapists*. Wolters Kluwer Health/Lippincott Williams & Wilkins; 2013. Figure 10.8A.)

the lungs for oxygenation. Once oxygenated, the blood then returns to the left atrium of the heart. Here, it passes through the mitral valve into the left ventricle. With each beat of the heart, the left ventricle pumps this oxygen-rich blood through the aortic valve into the aorta and out to the body, where it delivers oxygen to the tissues.

Coronary Circulation

The heart itself is nourished with a rich blood supply by coronary arteries extending over the surface of the epicardium. The right and left coronary arteries arise from the base of the aorta, just above the aortic valve, and surround the heart like a crown. The left coronary artery passes posterior to the pulmonary trunk and then divides into two branches. The left anterior descending (LAD) artery runs anterior and downward toward the apex of the heart. This artery is also referred to as the left anterior interventricular artery. In its path, the LAD artery branches to supply oxygen to the free wall of the right and left ventricles, anterior papillary muscle, anterior two-thirds of the septum, and much of the conduction tissue, namely, the bundle of His and right and left bundle branches. The other branch, the circumflex artery, encircles the heart, following the groove between the left atrium and the ventricle (coronary sulcus), and runs posteriorly to supply oxygen to the left atrium and the posterior and lateral portions of the left ventricle. In approximately 45% of people, the circumflex branch also supplies blood to the sinoatrial (SA) node. The right coronary artery (RCA) travels in the coronary sulcus between the right atrium and the right ventricle on the anterior surface of the heart. At the top of the ventricular septum posteriorly, the RCA becomes the right posterior descending artery (posterior interventricular artery), which runs parallel to the ventricular septum. Finally, at the inferior border of the heart, the artery branches off to become the marginal artery. In its path, the RCA and its branches supply oxygen to most of the right atrium, including the SA node and AV nodes, the right ventricle, and part of the bundle of His (Figure 6-2).

The coronary veins return deoxygenated blood from the heart wall into the right atrium. Specifically, the great (anterior), middle (posterior), and small (inferior) cardiac veins drain into the coronary sinus, located in

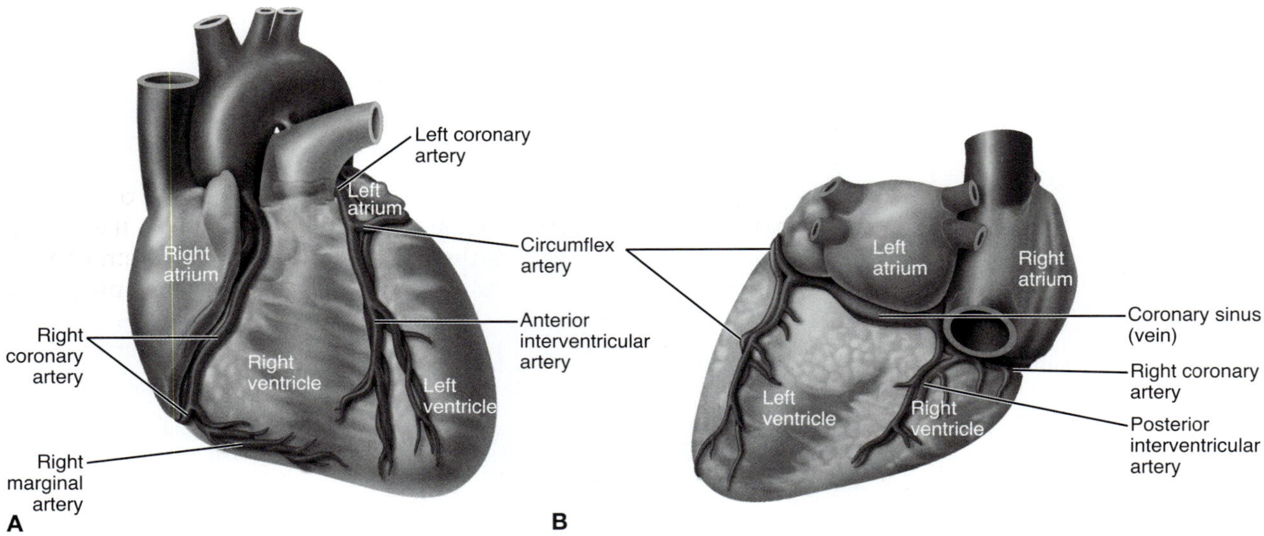

Figure 6-2 Coronary circulation. The coronary circulation, anterior (A) and posterior (B) views. Blood is supplied to the heart muscle via the coronary vessels. The major vessels of the coronary circulatory loop are shown here. (Reprinted with permission from Nath J. *Stedman's Medical Terminology*. 2nd ed. Wolters Kluwer; 2017. Figure 10.5.)

the posterior coronary sulcus. Coronary artery anatomy can vary significantly among people. The anatomic distribution often has no physiologic implications in the normal healthy heart.

Conduction System

The conducting system of the heart includes the SA node, the AV node, the bundle of His, right and left bundle branches, and the Purkinje fibers. This specialized network of cells making up the conduction system is the cardiac muscle cells modified for spontaneous excitation and rapid conduction of an action potential. The primary pacemaker of the heart, the SA node, is located in the posterior wall of the right atrium near the opening to the superior vena cava. All of the cells in the conducting system have automaticity, that is, the ability of self-excitation. However, those in the SA node fire spontaneously at a faster rate than the others, at a frequency between 60 and 100 bpm.

Once an impulse is generated at the SA node, the action potential spreads quickly through the cardiac muscle cells and internodal pathways of the right atrium and left atria (Bachmann bundle), causing simultaneous depolarization and contraction. At the same time, the impulse is conducted through the conduction pathway to the AV node located in the interatrial septum. Because the AV node is the only connection of impulse between the atria and the ventricles, the action potential slows here, causing a slight delay (approximately 0.10 seconds) and allowing time for atrial kick and ventricular filling. This delay in conduction at the AV node also has the protective function of preventing excessive impulse rates from entering the ventricles. Consequently, the AV node can also serve as a backup pacemaker with a rate between 40 and 60 should the SA node fail to initiate an impulse. Thus, the AV node has a significant role in preserving cardiac function.

The action potential continues along the conduction pathway to the AV bundle (bundle of His), a fibrous projection of cells, which enters the interventricular septum and divides into right and left bundle branches. The right and left bundle branches then project endocardial nerve branches (Purkinje fibers), which turn superiorly into the ventricular walls, extending into the myocardium and the inner surfaces of the ventricles. Once an electrical impulse enters the bundle of His, the conduction through the bundle branches and Purkinje fibers is extremely fast, about 1 to 4 m/s! This rapid conduction of the impulse to the apex of the heart allows simultaneous depolarization of both ventricles, with a wave of contraction traveling superiorly, effectively pumping blood up and out through the great vessels (Figure 6-3).

Innervation

Cardiac muscle fibers generate spontaneous contractions that are coordinated into a functional heartbeat by the electrical conduction mechanisms inherent in the heart itself. However, the activity of the heart is also influenced by inputs from the nervous system.

The heart receives two opposing neural inputs belonging to the autonomic nervous system. Both send motor neurons to certain cardiac muscle cells. One input comes from the cells of the parasympathetic nervous system, whose synaptic terminals in the heart release the neurotransmitter acetylcholine. The effect of acetylcholine is to decrease the rate of depolarization during the

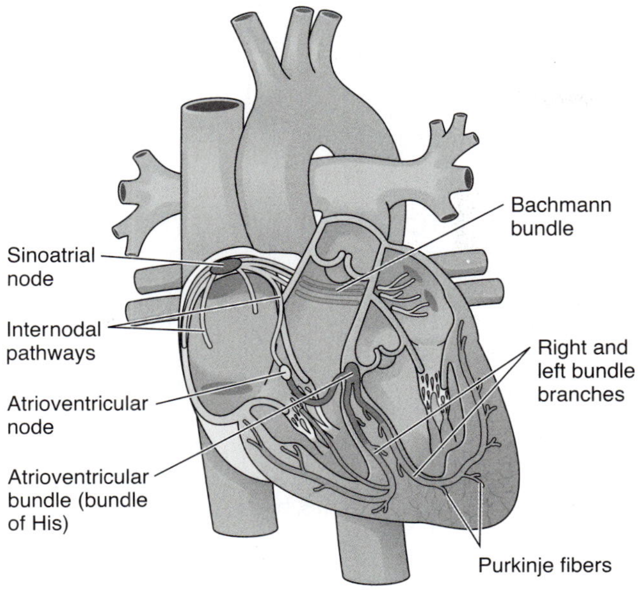

Figure 6-3 Conduction pathway of the heart. (Reprinted with permission from Plowman SA, Smith DL. *Exercise Physiology for Health Fitness and Performance*. 5th ed. Wolters Kluwer; 2017. Figure 11.4A.)

pacemaker potential of the SA node. This has the effect of increasing the interval between successive action potentials, thereby decreasing the rate at which the pacemaker drives the rate of the heartbeat.

The second neural input to the heart comes from cells of the sympathetic nervous system, whose synaptic terminals release the neurotransmitter norepinephrine. Activation of this input increases the heart rate. This effect is also mediated through the pacemaker potential, which depolarizes more rapidly after the activation of the sympathetic input. Both factors accentuate the depolarizing trend during the pacemaker potential.

Cardiac Muscle

A cardiac muscle cell is made up of contractile units known as sarcomeres. Within the sarcomere are long thread-like structures called myofibrils. Myofibrils are made up of two types of contractile proteins, or myofilaments, called actin and myosin. Cross-bridges that project from myosin fibers link themselves to the thinner actin filaments, giving the muscle cell a striated appearance. When cardiac muscle cells receive an electrical impulse, the actin filaments slide over myosin filaments, shortening the sarcomere. The shortening of adjacent sarcomeres effectively shortens the entire muscle cell.

The plasma membranes of adjacent myocardial cells form a structure known as intercalated discs. These junctions contain desmosomes, which join adjacent cells, and gap junctions, which allow electrical signals to pass directly from cell to cell. This complex network of electrically linked cells, through which an impulse can travel quickly, sets the environment for the simultaneous contraction of many cells. This is crucial for the heart to pump efficiently.

Cardiac Cycle

The cardiac cycle describes the sequence of events that occur within the heart with each heartbeat. It is described in terms of the mechanical events of the atria and ventricles (contraction or relaxation) and the pressure and volume changes as blood flows through the vessels and chambers. The cardiac cycle can also be correlated to the electrical activity occurring through the conduction system and the ECG, which will be discussed later in the chapter. One cardiac cycle is one beat of the heart and lasts approximately 0.8 seconds during a normal resting adult heart rate. The cardiac cycle can be divided into two phases: systole, the contractile phase, and diastole, the filling or relaxation phase.

The diastolic phase is normally about 500 ms, or two-thirds of the cardiac cycle. It begins with the relaxation of the ventricles following systole. As the ventricular myocardium relaxes, the pressure within the ventricle declines. When the pressure falls below that of the atria, the AV valves open as a result of the pressure differential. When these valves open, blood that has entered the right atrium (from the vena cava) and left atrium (from the pulmonary veins) passively flows into the ventricles. This portion of diastole is called the ventricular filling phase, where about 75% of the blood volume enters the ventricles passively. At the end of this phase, the SA node initiates an impulse, and atrial depolarization occurs. The contraction of the atria, also called atrial kick, forces the remaining blood from the atria into the ventricles. Atrial kick contributes about 20% to 30% of the total ventricular end-diastolic volume.

Ventricular systole is approximately one-third of the cardiac cycle. It begins with the depolarization of the ventricles, which initiates ventricular myocardial contraction, causing pressure to rise within the ventricles. When the pressure inside the ventricles exceeds that of the atria, the AV valves close. At this point, with both the AV and the semilunar valves closed and the volume of blood inside constant, the continued contraction of the myocardium causes a rise in pressure within the ventricles. This phase is known as *isovolumetric contraction*.

When the pressure in the left ventricle reaches about 80 mm Hg and the right ventricle about 8 mm Hg, the semilunar valves open, because these pressures exceed those of the aorta and pulmonary artery, respectively. At this point, the cardiac cycle enters the rapid ejection phase. With the semilunar valves open, contraction of the myocardium rapidly forces blood out of the ventricles into the great vessels. The aorta receives oxygenated blood from the left ventricle to be circulated throughout the body, whereas the pulmonary artery receives deoxygenated blood from the right ventricle to participate in gas exchange in the lungs.

As the blood flow out of the ventricles slows and the myocardium relaxes, intraventricular pressure declines. When the pressure falls below that of the great vessels, the semilunar valves close. This marks the end of systole. With both valves closed, the ventricles enter a phase of *isovolumetric relaxation*; pressure within the ventricles declines until it falls below that of the atria, the AV valves open, and the cycle repeats.

Regulation of Cardiac Activity

Both intrinsic and extrinsic factors are responsible for the regulation of cardiac activity. Extrinsic regulation of cardiovascular activity involves, most notably, the autonomic nervous system. The role of sympathetic and parasympathetic nerve pathways has been discussed previously. Pharmacologic influences have also become incredibly specific in the extrinsic regulation of cardiovascular activity; however, they are too numerous and beyond the scope of this chapter. Our discussion will focus instead on the intrinsic mechanisms involved in the regulation of cardiac activity.

Cardiac output is the amount of blood pumped by one ventricle and is measured in liters per minute. It is a product of heart rate (beats per minute) and stroke volume (liters per beat). Stroke volume, in turn, is dependent on several different factors, including preload, afterload, and contractility. Preload of the heart describes the stretch on the ventricular myocardium prior to contraction. The Frank-Starling model describes the recoil properties of an elastic object. Specifically, the greater the stretch on an elastic object up to the outer limit of normal, the greater the recoil. In this case, a greater stretch on the ventricular myocardium will result in a greater force of contraction. Because the ventricular myocardium is stretched by the amount of blood that exists in the ventricle prior to contraction, an increased venous return will produce greater tension on the myocardial wall, resulting in a greater force of contraction and stroke volume.

Afterload describes the resistance against which the heart must pump blood, known as the systemic vascular resistance. Thus, changes in vascular tone will affect stroke volume and, ultimately, cardiac output. For example, increased systemic vascular resistance in the form of arterial vasoconstriction results in a greater afterload and will cause a decrease in the strength, velocity, and/or duration of ventricular contraction. Valvular and other cardiac diseases can impact preload, afterload, and/or contractility, ultimately resulting in diminished stroke volumes and cardiac output.

Normal cardiac output for a healthy young adult is approximately 5 to 6 L/min. By increasing stroke volume and/or heart rate, the heart can increase its cardiac output up to 25 L/min. This portrays the heart's ability to intrinsically adjust its pumping capacity to alterations in venous return. In addition, the heart matches the outputs of the two ventricles to keep a balance of the systemic and pulmonary circuits.

THE SYSTEMIC VASCULAR SYSTEM

The systemic vascular system is an intricate network of passages that delivers oxygen-rich blood to needy cells of the body. Oxygenated blood, originating in the heart, is pumped out of the aorta and channeled into arteries, arterioles, and capillaries, where major organ systems such as the heart, brain, and organs are nourished. Veins, in turn, carry deoxygenated blood, high in carbon dioxide, from the tissues back to the heart, where it is channeled into the pulmonary vascular system to reclaim its oxygen supply and dispose of waste products. Oxygen-rich blood then reenters the heart, and the endless loop of circulating blood continues. Blood flow within the vascular system is maintained by pressure gradients between different blood vessels. Specifically, the mean aortic blood pressure is normally about 90 mm Hg, whereas the mean central venous pressure, measured at the vena cava, is normally close to 0 mm Hg. Changes in vascular resistance, or resistance to flow, within different organ systems or tissues, control the distribution of blood according to the need. For example, tissues with increased metabolic demand will signal nervous system inputs to decrease blood vessel tone. This results in vasodilatation, making blood more available to the starved tissue.

Systemic arterial blood pressure is the pressure exerted by blood against the walls of a blood vessel per unit area. It is normally measured at the brachial artery by a sphygmomanometer (blood pressure cuff), which temporarily occludes blood flow and measures the pressure at which blood flow returns to the artery. Arterial blood pressure consists of a higher systolic pressure, which represents the contraction of the ventricles and outflow of blood, and a lower diastolic component, which corresponds to the relaxation of the ventricles. Normal adult systemic arterial blood pressure is approximately 120/80 mm Hg.

The cardiovascular system is extremely efficient in maintaining an adequate and effective blood pressure to drive blood throughout the entire body despite changes in body position or fluid volume. In addition, it has the intrinsic ability to adjust blood pressure to local tissue oxygen requirements and metabolic demands. Specialized sensory neurons such as baroreceptors and chemoreceptors, found within the walls of the arteries and specific areas of the heart, sense changes in volume and blood chemistry. Feedback loops involving the cardiovascular regulatory center found in the medulla oblongata of the brain respond with appropriate adjustments to variables such as heart rate, vascular tone, and cardiac output.

CARDIAC ELECTROPHYSIOLOGY

Membrane Potentials

The plasma membrane, the outside casing holding the cell intact, is made up of a phospholipid cell layer with ion channels that allow for selective permeability. At any one time, there is an electrical voltage difference across the plasma membrane (the membrane potential) caused by unequal distribution of ions on each side. The potential directly influences the movement of charged particles (positive and negative ions) across the cell membrane. Electrical energy stored in the membrane potential is tapped to generate signals that can be passed from one cell to another. The common molecules that exist in the body are water and simple inorganic molecules. Fluids in the body can be divided into one of two parts. They can be part of either the extracellular fluid (ECF) or the intracellular fluid (ICF). The barrier between these two compartments is the plasma membrane of the cell. The ECF is high in both sodium, a positively charged ion, and chloride, a negatively charged ion, but low in potassium, whereas the ICF is low in sodium and chloride, but high in potassium. This difference is maintained and regulated by the ion channels residing in the plasma membrane, which acts as a selective permeable barrier permitting some substances to cross while excluding others. Major organic cellular anions inside the cell, such as protein, are the cell's biochemical machinery, and the plasma membrane is impermeable to this special group of molecules.

Ion Channels and Gates

An electrical voltage difference exists between the inside and the outside of the cell, the inside being more negative than the outside. The difference is measured in millivolts (mV) and is referred to as the membrane potential of the cell. The membrane is permeable only to some ions. Ion channels are the routes that ions travel to gain access into the cell. These channels exhibit ion selectivity, which allows some inorganic ions to pass through but not others. These channels are designed to permit entry only to certain permeating ions of appropriate size and charge. This enables the cell to limit their rate of passage. However, these ion channels are gated and not always open. The gates open only for a brief period and are then closed again. In most cases, the gates open in response to specific stimuli. There are different ways in which these channels are gated and different types of stimulation that cause them to open. One of the main types of stimuli is caused by an intracellular mediator, referred to as an ion-gated channel (Table 6-1).

Action Potentials

Action potentials are defined as rapid, transient electrical excitations of the cell's membrane. Action potentials are simply impulses that allow for long-distance signaling within a system. Action potentials within the cardiomyocytes can last for several hundred milliseconds, with a timed sequence of permeability changes. The sequence consists of a rapid depolarizing phase, a long-lasting plateau phase, and a concluding repolarizing phase (Figure 6-4).

The action potential of a cardiomyocyte begins from a resting membrane potential that approximates −90 μV. The initial depolarization phase of the cardiac action potential is prompted by the opening of the voltage-gated sodium channels. This action allows a rapid influx of positively charged sodium ions across the membrane. This causes the inside of the cell to very quickly become more positive, increasing the overall voltage (membrane potential), and driving a rapid depolarization of the cell.

During the plateau phase, the sodium channels close and the voltage-gated potassium channels open. As a result, there is a movement of positively charged potassium ions out of the cell, reducing the voltage slightly. However, soon after, the calcium ion channels open, resulting in a slow movement of positively

Table 6-1 Summary of Ionic Channels of Cardiac Muscle Membrane

Principal Ion	Response to Depolarization	Speed of Response	Inactivation	Function
Na^+	Opens	Fast	Fast, but incomplete	Initial depolarization
K^+	Closes	Fast	None	Maintains plateau
K^+	Opens	Slow	Little	Repolarization
K^+	Opens because of Ca^+ influx	Slow	Closes as internal Ca^+ falls	Repolarization
Ca^+	Opens	Slow	Slow	Maintains plateau and prolongs contraction

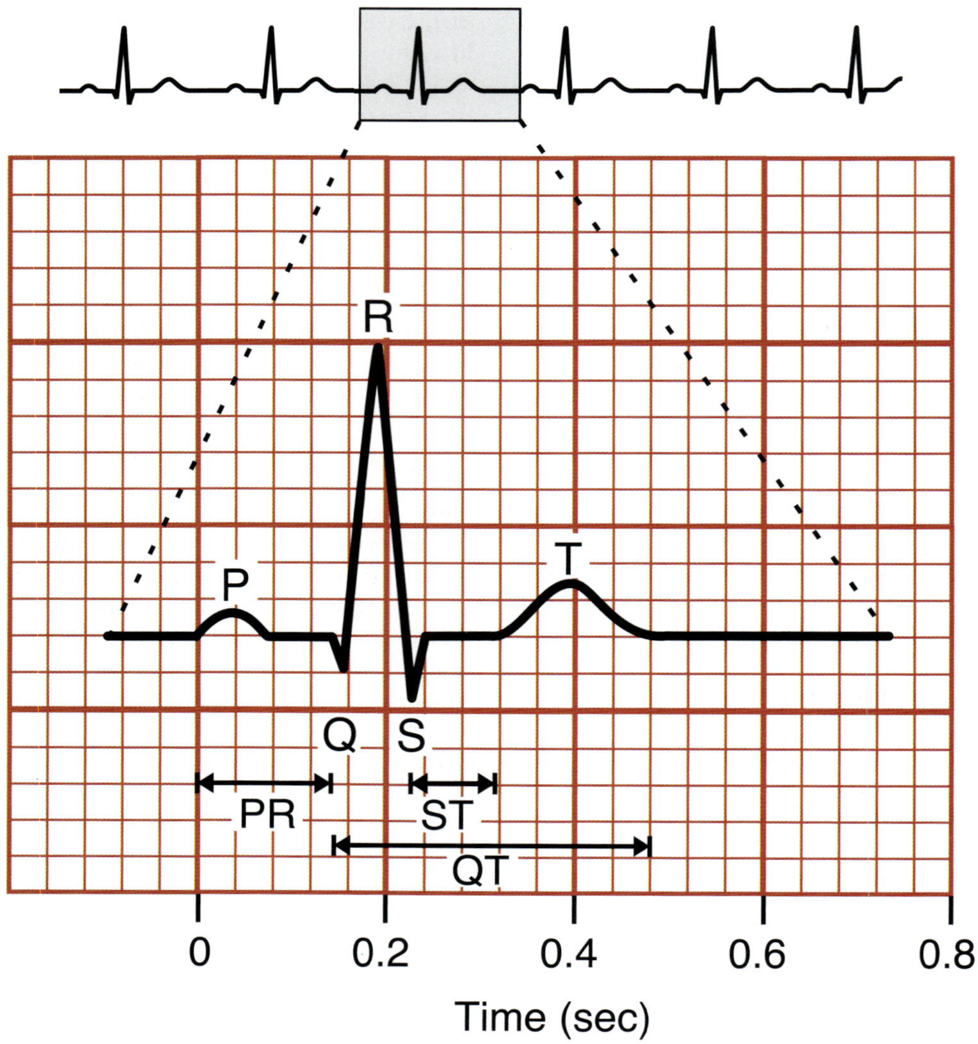

Figure 6-4 A cardiac action potential portraying a rapid depolarizing phase, a long-lasting plateau phase, and a concluding repolarizing phase.

charged calcium ions into the cell. This concurrent influx of calcium ions and efflux of potassium ion results in a voltage plateau. In cardiac muscle fibers, the contraction is maintained by the influx of calcium ions across the plasma membrane during the plateau phase of the cardiac action potential. This voltage plateau is unique to cardiac muscle fibers, allowing additional time at the higher membrane potential so that the chambers can fully contract and pump blood out.

In the final phase, the calcium ion channels close, while potassium continues to move out of the cell via the open voltage-gated potassium channels. As a result, the inside of the cell becomes more negative, and the membrane potential approaches resting potential of -90 μV. This phase is associated with repolarization and relaxation of the heart.

The duration of the contraction in cardiac muscle is controlled by the duration of the action potential, specifically during the plateau phase. This provides an important mechanism by which the pumping action of the heart can be regulated. Medications such as calcium channel blockers, for example, prevent calcium from entering the heart and arteries. Since calcium is responsible for the sustained and strong contraction seen in the plateau phase, these medications promote relaxation of the blood vessels, slowing of the heart rate, and reduction in the force of contraction.

Transmission of Impulses

To effectively pump blood, there must be a coordinated contraction of all of the individual muscle fibers making up the walls of the heart. When an action potential is generated in a cardiac muscle fiber, it causes action potentials in their surrounding neighbors. This type of excitation spreads rapidly through all the muscle fibers of the heart chamber, ensuring that all the muscle fibers within that chamber contract in a coordinated fashion.

At the ends of each cardiac cell, the plasma membranes of neighboring cells come into close contact at the intercalated discs. The contact at this point is sufficiently close to enable the electrical current flowing inside of one fiber to cross directly into the interior of the next fiber. This electrical current will pass through the point of least resistance. This low-resistance path from one cell to another becomes possible through gap junctions. These structures directly connect the interiors on the joined cells, so ions can pass directly through the gap junctions from one cell to another.

When electrical current passes from cell to another, as in cardiac muscle, those cells are considered to be electrically coupled. If two cells are coupled through gap junctions, a response to the injected current occurs in both cells because the ions carrying the current inside of the cell can pass directly through the gap junction. This electrical coupling among cardiac muscle fibers explains how coordinated contraction occurs in all of the fibers of a chamber.

Within the electrical membrane potential of a spontaneously beating cardiac cell lie a series of spontaneous action potentials. After each action potential, the potential falls back to its normal negative resting value and then begins to depolarize slowly. This slow depolarization is called a pacemaker potential and is caused by spontaneous changes in ionic permeability within the membrane.

THE ELECTROCARDIOGRAM

The ECG records the electrical activity of the heart as a waveform and is accomplished by placing various electrodes on the chest, arms, and legs to detect and amplify voltage activity. Consider the function of the ECG recording as a voltmeter that records the differences in electrical voltages (potentials) generated by depolarization of heart muscle. The ECG provides information about the heart rate, rhythm, and electrical conduction.

Electrode Placement

Electrode placement for an ECG can range from a simple 2-lead placement to a full 12-lead comprehensive setup, which provides the ability to view the heart's electrical activity from different angles and planes. A lead is a record of electrical activity between two electrodes. Each lead records the average current flow at a specific time during the cardiac cycle in a particular portion of the heart. There are three types of leads: limb, augmented, and precordial (chest) leads. Each lead has both a positive and a negative electrode that senses the magnitude and direction of the electrical forces caused by the spread of waves of both the depolarization and repolarization throughout the myocardium.

The position of the positive electrode on the body determines the portion of the heart that is seen by each of the leads. If the wave of depolarization (electrical impulse) moves toward the positive electrode, the waveform recorded on the ECG graph paper will appear upright, relaying a positive deflection (1). If the wave of depolarization moves toward the negative electrode, the waveform recorded will be inverted, appearing downward or as a negative deflection. A biphasic waveform, which is both partly positive and partly negative, is recorded when the wave of depolarization moves perpendicularly to the positive electrode.

The recommended ECG placement for a standard polysomnogram is a single modified Lead II, which is derived from two electrodes, one placed below the right clavicle at the midclavicular line and the other on the left lower torso, midaxillary, in the sixth or seventh intercostal space. Alternative placement is a single modified Lead I, which is derived from two electrodes, one placed below the right clavicle at the midclavicular line and the other placed below the left clavicle at the midclavicular line. Additional leads may be placed if clinically indicated. A 3-lead placement may be utilized, as it provides a backup channel for re-referencing if one should become displaced during the course of the testing (1).

Normal Electrocardiogram Rhythm

A normal sinus rhythm, reflected in the ECG, includes the appearance of a P, QRS, and T wave during one cardiac cycle. The P wave represents atrial depolarization (contraction). This waveform is normally 0.08 to 0.12 seconds in duration. and the amplitude should be less than 3mm. The QRS wave represents ventricular depolarization (contraction) and should measure between 0.06 and 0.10 seconds. Atrial repolarization occurs simultaneously with ventricular contraction; thus, there is no visual representation on the tracing. The PR interval is measured from the beginning of the P wave to the beginning of the QRS complex, with normal values between 0.12 and 0.20 seconds. The last positive waveform is the T wave, which represents ventricular repolarization. The interval between the end of the QRS and the beginning of the T wave (ST interval) should normally rest at electrical baseline. Finally, the QT interval is measured from the beginning of the QRS complex to the end of the T wave, is normally less than or equal to 0.44 seconds, and varies with the heart rate (Figure 6-5).

Normal heart rates for adults range from 60 to 100 beats per minute. This will be reflected and determined in the ECG tracing by the number of QRS

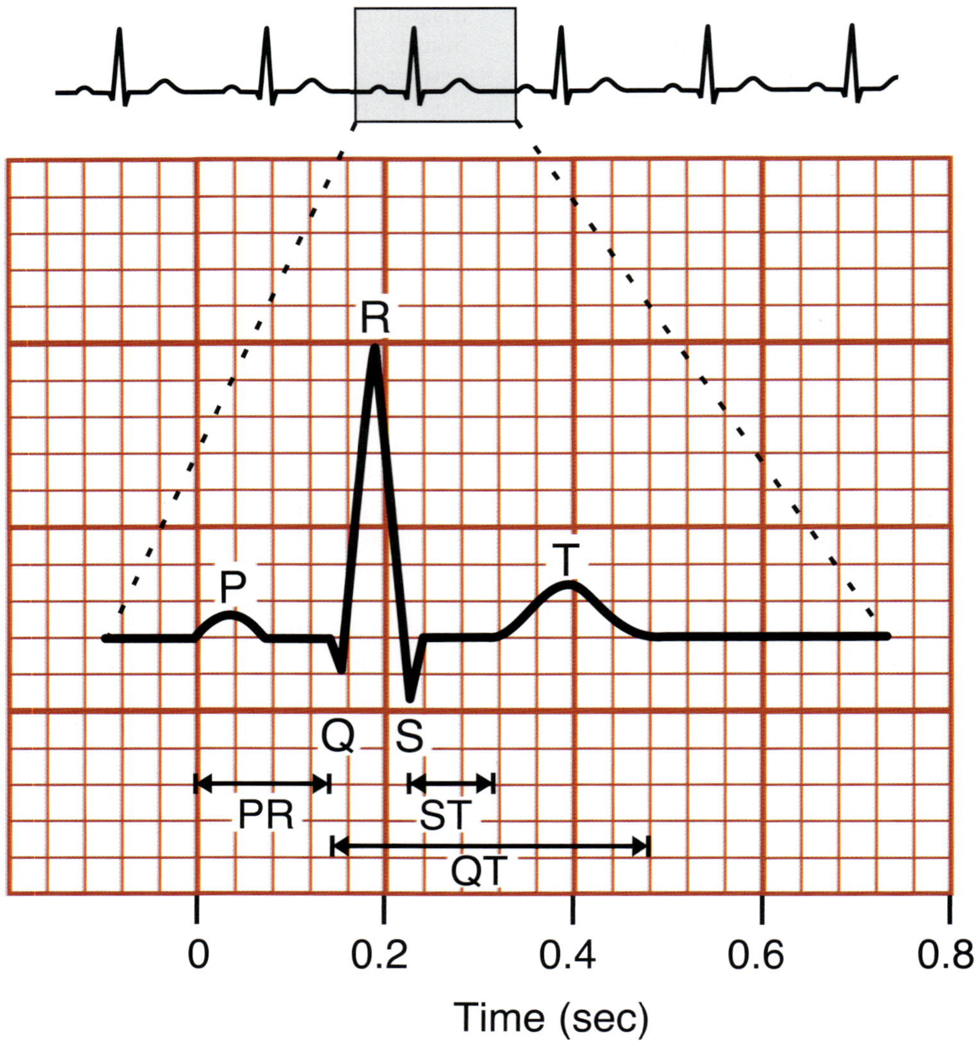

Figure 6-5 Normal electrocardiography tracing showing a normal sinus rhythm. Shown are the P, QRS, T, and U waves, which represent electrical activity in different parts of the heart. Intervals measure from one wave to the next; segments are smaller components of the tracing.

complexes per minute. In a normal sinus rhythm, the P, QRS, and T waves should all appear in correct sequence with normal values for all measures.

Respiration may alter the heart rate and rhythm. For example, it is common to see sinus arrhythmia, especially in children. This benign condition is caused by the pressure fluctuation within the thorax that occurs during normal breathing. Specifically, during inhalation, when thoracic pressure is more negative, you may see a heart rate deceleration, whereas cardiac acceleration may be noted during exhalation.

Electrocardiogram Patterns Commonly Seen in Sleep

A typical sleep study includes an ECG channel for the purpose of monitoring a patient's cardiac status throughout the testing. Many of the parameters that define a sleep disorder can cause changes in the cardiac rate and rhythm. Therefore, it is important that the sleep technologist be able to recognize abnormal cardiac rhythms. Apnea and hypopnea episodes, typical of obstructive sleep apnea (OSA), are often followed by arousals and/or hypoxemia (low oxygen saturation). Further, frequent arousals during sleep commonly result in changes in heart rate. Bradycardia (heart rate <50 bpm) may be noted during an apneic/hypoxic episode, whereas tachycardia (heart rate >90 bpm) or rate acceleration may accompany the arousal that follows. If the patient has severe OSA, this pattern may be observed throughout the night. Repeated episodes of apnea and hypopnea with oxygen desaturation may also be associated with premature atrial contractions or other atrial dysrhythmias such as atrial fibrillation or atrial flutter. Supraventricular tachycardia is an example of a supraventricular dysrhythmia that may be noted and is characterized by a fast, narrow complex rhythm that begins and ends very abruptly. Lastly, the sleep technologist may encounter patients who have other comorbidities, such as underlying cardiac disease. In this case, ventricular dysrhythmias, such as premature ventricular contractions and bigeminy, or conduction abnormalities, may be noted. For this reason, it is important that the sleep technologist carefully review the patient's past medical and cardiopulmonary history as well as current medications before the patient arrives. This can better prepare the technologist for what to expect while monitoring the patient.

Besides obtaining quality sleep study, the most important role of the sleep technologist is to maintain patient safety. Sleep technologists must be certified in basic life support, be familiar with emergency protocols, and participate in annual emergency protocol drills. By monitoring the cardiac rate and rhythm, they will be prepared to recognize changing and deteriorating rhythms and know when it becomes necessary to call for help. For a more detailed discussion of cardiac arrhythmias, refer to Chapter 37.

CONCLUSION

This section has provided a brief overview of the normal cardiac anatomy and electrophysiology, including the specialized functions and mechanics of the cardiac muscle, the cardiac cycle, the electrical impulse conduction pathways, and the way in which this relates to the entire cardiovascular system. Patients undergoing sleep studies may exhibit any number of cardiac dysrhythmias. Sleep technologists must be prepared to recognize and identify these rhythms and, when necessary, act appropriately. A strong understanding of the anatomy and electrophysiology of the heart can better prepare them for this task and greatly improve patient safety.

REFERENCES

1. Amerman EC. *Human Anatomy and Physiology*. 2nd ed. Pearson; 2018.

SUGGESTED READINGS

AAST. Fundamentals of EKG: Module 1: Cardiac anatomy and physiology. Online Educational Training. https://learn.aastweb.org/products/fundamentals-of-ekg

Jensen B, Boukens B. *The Cardiac Conduction System: Evolution, Development, and Therapeutic Potential*. 1st ed. Academic Press; 2025.

Pappano AJ, Wier WG. *Cardiovascular Physiology*. 11th ed. Elsevier Enhanced Digital Version; 2019.

Chapter 7
General Human Physiology for the Sleep Technologist

REGINA PATRICK

KEY CONCEPTS/LEARNING OBJECTIVES

The key concepts for this chapter include a basic understanding of human anatomy and physiology, unique functions of the endocrine system, the renal system, the digestive system, the immune system, the genitourinary system, the musculoskeletal system, metabolism, and thermoregulation in humans, and how dysfunction in these systems can impact sleep as well as why certain sleep disorders are associated with dysfunction in one or more of these systems.

KEY TERMS

Digestive system
Electrolyte
Endocrine system
Genitourinary system
Immune system
Metabolism
Musculoskeletal system
pH
Renal system
Thermoregulation

The brain is the primary organ that controls sleep and wake. However, the function of many other body systems can impact sleep. This chapter will discuss the basic functions of the endocrine, renal, digestive, immune, genitourinary, and musculoskeletal systems; metabolism; and thermoregulation. This chapter will also discuss sleep disorders that are associated with dysfunctions in these systems.

THE ENDOCRINE SYSTEM

The endocrine system consists of several glands that secrete hormones that affect different organs (ie, target organs). The glands release their hormones directly into the bloodstream or into lymph (ie, a transparent yellow liquid that flows through lymphatic vessels). Once the hormone travels to a target organ, it may affect the metabolism or function of the target organ. The hypothalamus, pituitary, pineal gland, thyroid, parathyroid glands, adrenal glands, gonads, and pancreas are a few organs that make up the endocrine system (Figure 7-1).

Overview of Endocrine Hormone Classification

Three types of hormones produced in the endocrine system are steroid hormones, protein hormones (also called "peptide hormones"), and amine hormones. Steroid hormones are synthesized from cholesterol and secreted by the adrenal cortex, testes, and ovaries. Examples of steroid hormones are cortisol, aldosterone, testosterone, and estrogen. Protein hormones consist of amino acids that are bound together with peptide bonds. In a peptide bond, the amine group ($-NH_2$) of one amino acid binds with the carboxyl group ($-COOH$) of another amino acid. Most hormones in the body are protein hormones. Insulin and calcitonin are examples of protein hormones. Amine hormones contain amino acids, but the acids do not form peptide bonds. Melatonin, thyroxine, and epinephrine are examples of amine hormones.

The release of many hormones is controlled by a negative feedback system. In such a system, when one substance reaches a certain level, it inhibits the release of another. For example, when the blood glucose level is high, the release of insulin inhibits the release of glucagon; when the blood glucose level is low, the release of glucagon inhibits the release of insulin. A negative feedback loop helps maintain proper levels of other substances (in this case, glucose) and proper functioning of the body. See Table 7-1 for a synopsis of the endocrine hormones and their main functions.

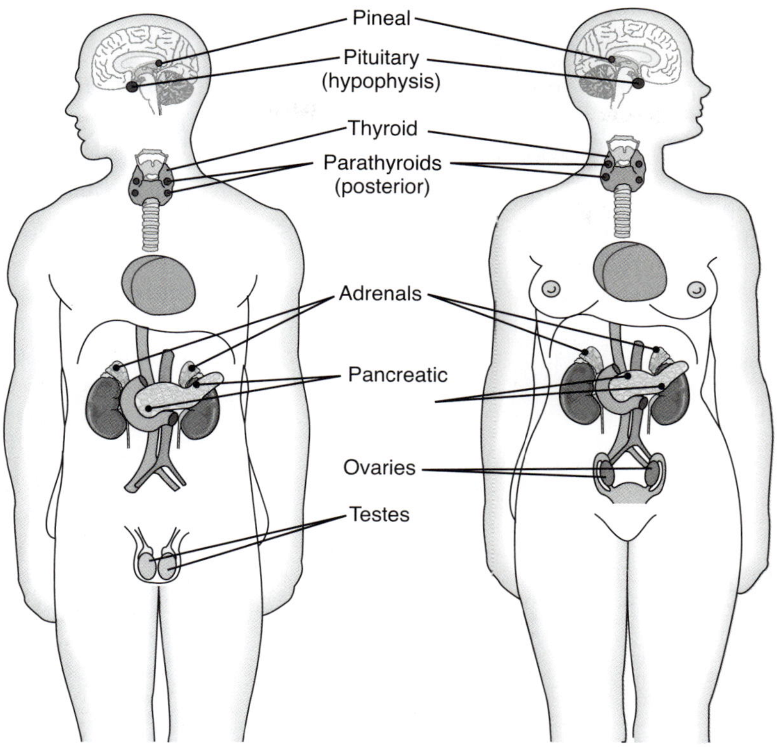

Figure 7-1 The endocrine system is composed of glands with the primary function of hormone secretion. (Reprinted with permission from Taylor JJ, Cohen BJ. *Memmler's Structure and Function of the Human Body*. 10th ed. Wolters Kluwer Health/Lippincott Williams & Wilkins; 2013. Figure 11-2.)

Table 7-1 The Source and Main Action of Various Endocrine Hormones

Source Organ	Endocrine Hormone	Target Organ	Action of the Hormone
Adrenal gland			
Medulla (inner core)	Epinephrine[a]	Blood vessels, liver, lungs, brain	Involved in the "fight-or-flight" response in times of stress (eg, increases blood pressure by increasing the strength and rate of heart contractions and vasoconstriction) Assists in the breakdown of glycogen to glucose in the liver to provide energy during times of stress Bronchodilation Acts as a neurotransmitter in the brain (eg, activates the reticular formation in the brain)
	Norepinephrine[a]	Blood vessels, heart	Increases heart rate and vasoconstriction in response to hypotension (ie, low blood pressure)
Cortex (outer portion)			
Inner layer	Sex hormones: testosterone, estrogen	Reproductive organs	Involved in the development of sex characteristics
Middle layer	Glucocorticoids: cortisol	Immune cells, liver, kidney	Involved in the metabolism of carbohydrates, protein, and fat Promotes diuresis Reduces inflammatory processes

(continued)

Table 7-1 The Source and Main Action of Various Endocrine Hormones (*continued*)

Source Organ	Endocrine Hormone	Target Organ	Action of the Hormone
Outer layer	Mineralocorticoids: Aldosterone	Kidney	Promotes water retention Regulates the concentration of electrolytes (eg, sodium, potassium)
Gonads			
Ovaries (women)	Estrogen	Female genitalia (eg, uterus)	Involved in menstruation, the development of female reproductive organs and secondary sex characteristics (eg, pubic hair)
Testes (men)	Testosterone	Male reproductive organs	Involved in the development of male reproductive organs and secondary sex characteristics (eg, pubic hair, facial hair), spermatozoa formation, muscle growth
Heart			
Atrial wall	Atrial natriuretic peptide	Kidney	Stimulates the excretion of sodium and water by inhibiting the reabsorption of water and sodium in nephrons, which reduces blood volume and blood pressure Reduces the levels of renin, aldosterone, and antidiuretic hormone
Hypothalamus			
Anterior hypothalamus	Corticotropin-releasing hormone	Anterior pituitary	Stimulates the anterior pituitary to release adrenocorticotropic hormone (ACTH)
	Dopamine	Brain, kidneys, adrenal gland, anterior pituitary	Involved in the transmission of signals from neuron to neuron in the brain; in sleep, mood, and motor function; and in the regulation of blood flow in the kidneys Acts as a precursor to norepinephrine Inhibits the release of prolactin (a hormone involved in lactation) by the anterior pituitary
	Growth hormone-releasing hormone	Anterior pituitary	Stimulates the anterior pituitary to release growth hormone
	Somatostatin	Anterior pituitary	Inhibits the anterior pituitary production of growth hormone
	Thyrotropin-releasing hormone	Anterior pituitary	Stimulates the anterior pituitary to produce thyroid-stimulating hormone
Posterior hypothalamus	Antidiuretic hormone	Posterior pituitary	Stored in the posterior pituitary
Pancreas			
Islets of Langerhans			
Alpha cells	Glucagon	Liver, fat tissue	Stimulates the conversion of glycogen into glucose, which is then released into the bloodstream, when blood glucose levels are low
Beta cells	Insulin	Liver, muscles, many other body cells	Promotes the removal of glucose from the blood into cells (thereby reducing blood glucose levels) when blood glucose levels are high Involved in protein and glycogen synthesis Involved in the conversion of glucose to glycogen in the liver
Parathyroid gland	Parathyroid hormone (also called parathormone)	Intestine, kidneys, and skeletal system	Involved in the utilization of calcium and phosphate in the body

Table 7-1 The Source and Main Action of Various Endocrine Hormones (*continued*)

Source Organ	Endocrine Hormone	Target Organ	Action of the Hormone
Pineal gland	Melatonin	Suprachiasmatic nuclei	Promotes sleep and is involved in the circadian rhythm
Pituitary gland			
Anterior pituitary	Adrenocorticotropic hormone (ACTH)	Adrenal cortex	Stimulates the adrenal cortex to increase its secretion of hormones such as cortisol
	Gonadotropic hormones: follicle-stimulating hormone, luteinizing hormone	Ovaries, testes	Promotes estrogen and testosterone production, involved in menstrual cycle, stimulates spermatozoa formation
	Thyroid-stimulating hormone	Thyroid	Stimulates the release of thyroid hormones
Posterior pituitary	Antidiuretic hormone (also called "vasopressin")	Kidney, smooth muscles of arterioles	Stimulates the resorption of water from urine into the blood, which reduces urine output Increases the constriction of blood vessels
Thyroid	Calcitonin	Skeletal bones	Inhibits the breakdown of bone
	Thyroxine (also called T_4) and tri-iodothyronine (also called T_3)	All cells	Stimulate energy metabolism in cells

[a]Epinephrine and norepinephrine are commonly called adrenaline and noradrenaline, respectively.

ENDOCRINE ORGANS

Hypothalamus

The hypothalamus is a structure that lies at the base of the brain. The optic tract and optic chiasm (the point at which fibers of the left and right optic nerves cross to the opposite side of the brain) form part of the hypothalamus. The hypothalamus also contains various nuclei (ie, groups of cells having a specialized function) that are involved in water balance, maintaining body temperature (ie, thermoregulation), sleep, and food intake. Extending by a stalk from the hypothalamus is the pituitary, a gland that contains an anterior lobe and a posterior lobe. The anterior hypothalamus (ie, front portion of the hypothalamus) produces various hormones that are transported into the anterior pituitary through special blood capillary network; on arriving at the anterior pituitary, the posterior hypothalamic hormones stimulate the release of or inhibit the production and release of anterior pituitary hormones. In the posterior hypothalamus (ie, the back portion of the hypothalamus), the axons of neurosecretory cells (ie, neurons or nerve-like cells that secrete substances that act on another structure) extend from the posterior hypothalamus into the posterior pituitary. These neurosecretory cells synthesize hormones in the posterior hypothalamus; the hormones are then transported to the terminals of the axons in the posterior pituitary, where they are stored and then released when necessary.

Pituitary Gland

The pituitary gland, which is located below the hypothalamus, extends from the hypothalamus by a stalk and consists of two distinct parts: a front portion (ie, the anterior pituitary) and a rear portion (ie, the posterior pituitary). The anterior pituitary receives various releasing and inhibiting hormones from the hypothalamus. As their name implies, these hormones cause the anterior pituitary to release hormones (eg, growth hormone-releasing hormone stimulates the anterior pituitary to release growth hormone) or inhibit their production and release of hormones (eg, somatostatin inhibits the anterior pituitary's production of growth hormone). The posterior pituitary gland acts as a reservoir for various hypothalamic hormones such as antidiuretic hormone and releases them into the bloodstream when needed. The anterior pituitary histologically consists of the endocrine tissue, whereas the posterior pituitary histologically has the structure of nerve tissue.

Pineal Gland

The pineal gland is a small, flattened, cone-shaped gland in the upper rear brainstem. It receives sensory information from the optic nerves such as the level of light. It produces several hormones, the most important of which is the sleep-promoting hormone melatonin.

Thyroid

The thyroid is a butterfly-shaped gland that lies in front of the lower portion of the throat, just above the trachea. It secretes and stores various thyroid hormones (eg, thyroxine [T_4], triiodothyronine [T_3], and calcitonin). Thyroxine and triiodothyronine are involved in regulating a person's metabolic rate, and calcitonin is involved in maintaining proper calcium levels in the body.

Parathyroid Glands

The parathyroid glands are four small glands on the posterior surface of the thyroid. The parathyroid glands produce parathyroid hormone (also called "parathormone"), which has a role in the regulation of calcium and phosphate levels in the body.

Adrenal Gland

The adrenal gland is a small organ that lies on the top of the kidney. It consists of an inner core (ie, the medulla) and an outer portion (ie, cortex) that covers the medulla. The medulla secretes epinephrine and norepinephrine, which are released to prepare the body for the "flight or fight" response in times of stress. The adrenal cortex has three layers, each of which secretes different hormones. The cortex's outermost layer secretes mineralocorticoids. These chemicals maintain the level of mineral salts (eg, sodium chloride) in the body. The main mineralocorticoid produced by the adrenal cortex is aldosterone. The middle layer of the cortex produces glucocorticoids. These chemicals are involved in maintaining the blood glucose level and maintaining blood pressure. The main glucocorticoid produced by the adrenal cortex is cortisol. The innermost level of the cortex secretes small amounts of sex hormones (eg, testosterone and estrogen).

Gonads

The gonads are organs that produce the reproductive cells. The gonads in men are the testes, which produce spermatozoa; the gonads in women are the ovaries, which produce ova (ie, egg cells). The testes produce the sex hormone testosterone, and the ovaries produce estrogen. These hormones are involved in reproductive behavior, fertility, and the development of secondary sex characteristics (eg, facial hair in men).

Pancreas

The pancreas is an oblong gland situated behind the stomach. The surface of the pancreas contains microscopic groups of specialized cells, scattered like islands among the pancreatic cells. These cells are called the "islets (or islands) of Langerhans." Two types of cells exist within each islet of Langerhans—alpha and beta cells. The alpha cells secrete the hormone glucagon, which converts the liver starch glycogen into glucose when blood glucose levels are low; the beta cells secrete insulin, which reduces the blood glucose level when glucose levels are too high. Insulin and glucagon are antagonistic in their actions.

Endocrine Function and Sleep Disorders

The secretion of endocrine hormones normally increases and decreases with circadian rhythmicity. For example, the production of melatonin normally increases in the evening (thereby promoting sleep) and decreases in the morning (thereby promoting wakefulness). Factors such as night shift work, blindness, or dysfunction of certain hypothalamic cells can disrupt the rhythmic production of endocrine hormones. This disruption can lead to sleep and wake cycles that occur at undesired times (eg, advanced or delayed sleep phase) or lead to the destruction of the cyclicity of a person's sleep and wake cycles (eg, non-24-hour sleep-wake rhythm disorder [formerly called "circadian rhythm sleep-wake disorder—free-running rhythm" (1)]). As a result, a person may struggle with sleep problems such as insomnia or excessive daytime sleepiness (EDS).

The production of melatonin is influenced by a person's exposure to light. In the normal eye, light stimulates the retina, which relays signals through the optic nerves. The signals ultimately reach the pineal gland, which produces melatonin. The greater the amount of light, the greater the number of signals reaching the pineal gland and the less the amount of melatonin it produces. As dark progresses through the evening, melatonin production increases and ultimately induces sleep. Night shift work, working frequently changing shifts, and blindness can alter a person's exposure to light and disrupt the production of melatonin and lead to sleep problems.

Night Shift Work/Frequently Changing Shifts

A person who works third shift typically works all night in a lighted setting and drives home in the bright light of morning. Both of these factors reduce the production of melatonin. Once the person arrives home, they may have difficulty going to sleep at a desired time because of the reduced melatonin level. Once a person falls asleep, the delayed sleep onset can shorten the person's sleep time and result in struggles with sleepiness when the person is awake during a work shift.

A shift worker can take steps to shift the time at which the greatest amount of melatonin production occurs. Reducing daytime exposure to light can help shift the melatonin production to daytime hours and thereby promote sleep during the day. For example, after working a shift, the worker could drive home with dark sunglasses on and use room-darkening shades in the bedroom. However, the ability to reset and maintain a consistent rhythm of melatonin production may not be possible if shift changes are frequent (eg, every week).

Blindness

Some blind people—especially people who have no light perception—have a non-24-hour sleep-wake rhythm. In a person with a non-24-hour sleep-wake rhythm disorder, the sleep-wake phases move forward every day rather than remaining stable at the same time every day. For example, the person may fall asleep at 8:00 PM one night, fall asleep the next night at 9:00 PM, fall asleep the following night at 10:00 PM, and so forth. When trying to follow a normal sleep-wake schedule, people with a non-24-hour rhythm may experience a period of struggling with excessive sleepiness, a period of "normal" sleep, and a period of insomnia (ie, difficulty initiating or maintaining sleep). This disruption in sleep patterns occurs because the unstable sleep-wake cycles shift in and out of phase with the societal norm.

Dysfunction of Hypothalamic Cells

In a 1999 dog study, scientists reported that a mutation in the hypocretin (also called "orexin") receptor 2 gene was responsible for narcolepsy (2). Hypocretin is an excitatory neurotransmitter. Later research on humans revealed that hypothalamic cells that produce the wake-promoting excitatory neuropeptide orexin are inexplicably and irreversibly destroyed in some people with narcolepsy (3). The primary symptom of narcolepsy is EDS. This symptom may be accompanied by cataplexy (ie, the sudden, temporary loss of skeletal muscle tone), hypnagogic or hypnopompic hallucinations (ie, realistic dream imagery occurring with sleep onset or on awakening, respectively), and paralysis on awakening from sleep or on going to sleep (ie, sleep paralysis). The latter three symptoms may be the result of the muscle atonia and dream imagery features of rapid eye movement (REM) sleep intruding into wake. In recent years, scientists have noted another symptom in people with narcolepsy: disrupted nighttime sleep (4), characterized by frequent arousals that occur for no apparent reason such as obstructive sleep apnea. The arousals may reflect a dysfunction in the neural control of sleep and wake.

Orexin-producing neurons project from the hypothalamus into brainstem areas such as the locus ceruleus, raphe nuclei, and reticular formation. These areas are involved in various aspects of REM sleep and wakefulness. Therefore, the destruction of orexin-producing hypothalamic cells may be involved in the improper manifestation of REM sleep features in wake, sleep disruption, and sleepiness in narcolepsy.

THE RENAL SYSTEM

The renal system consists of the kidneys, ureters, and urinary bladder (Figure 7-2). The urinary system maintains blood volume, removes waste, regulates blood pressure, and is involved in maintaining pH balance in the blood.

The kidney is a bean-shaped organ that is approximately the size of a fist. The ureter is a fibromuscular tubular structure that descends from the kidney to the urinary bladder. It transports urine (an amber fluid that is a waste product) from the kidney to the urinary bladder. The urinary bladder is a musculomembranous sac in the front portion of the pelvis. It receives urine and voids it to the exterior of the body through the urethra (a membranous canal).

Each kidney contains millions of nephrons (Figure 7-3), which are the structural component of the kidney. Each nephron contains a glomerulus (a ball-like cluster of capillaries), a proximal convoluted tubule and distal convoluted tubule, and a collecting tubule. Afferent arterioles (ie, microscopic arteries) bring blood from the renal artery into the glomerulus. A hollow-walled structure, called Bowman capsule, surrounds each glomerulus. (To use an analogy, imagine a fist that is pushed into a balloon so that the balloon surrounds the fist: the fist represents the glomerulus and the balloon, Bowman capsule.) Some blood plasma exits from the glomerular capillaries and enters the hollow wall of the surrounding Bowman capsule. The remaining blood flows out of the glomerulus through the efferent arteriole. The efferent arteriole branches to form a capillary

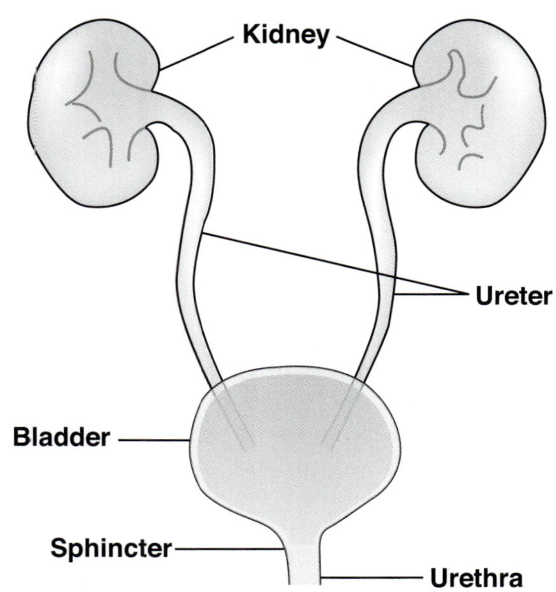

Figure 7-2 The renal system. (National Institute of Diabetes and Digestive and Kidney Diseases, National Institutes of Health, Bethesda, Maryland.)

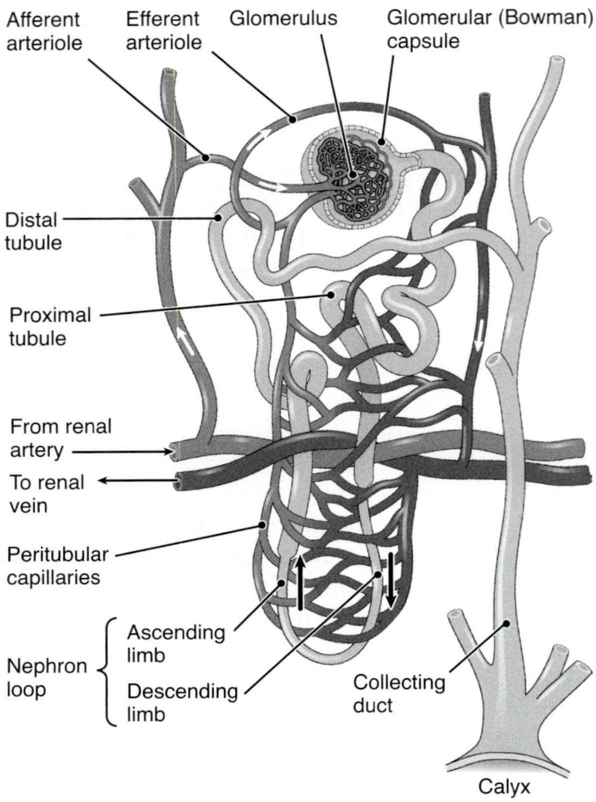

Figure 7-3 A nephron and its blood supply. The nephron regulates the proportions of water, waste, and other materials in urine based on to the body's constantly changing needs. A nephron consists of a glomerular capsule, convoluted tubules, the nephron loop (also called the loop of Henle), and a collecting duct. Blood filtration occurs through the glomerulus in the glomerular capsule. Materials that enter the nephron can be returned to the blood through the surrounding peritubular capillaries. (Reprinted with permission from Knight L. *Medical Terminology: An Illustrated Guide Canadian Edition*. 2nd ed. Wolters Kluwer Health/Lippincott Williams & Wilkins; 2013. Figure 13.3.)

network, called the "peritubular capillaries," that surrounds a nephron's tubules. The peritubular capillaries drain blood into veins that ultimately feed into the renal vein. The renal vein takes blood away from the kidney.

The blood plasma in the hollow wall of Bowman capsule empties into the proximal convoluted tubule. This fluid is called the "glomerular filtrate." Once the glomerular filtrate is in the proximal convoluted tubule, ions such as sodium and chloride, glucose, and amino acids exit from the glomerular filtrate and enter the surrounding perivascular capillaries, and thereby reenter the bloodstream. This process is called "reabsorption." Through reabsorption, most nutrients and approximately 65% of salt and water in the glomerular filtrate in the proximal tubule are returned to the blood. Electrolytes, which are positively or negatively charged molecules or atoms such as sodium (Na^+), potassium (K^+), bicarbonate (HCO_3^-), and calcium (Ca^{2+}), are also reabsorbed from the glomerular filtrate. Some nitrogen-containing compounds (eg, urea), ions, salts, and water are not reabsorbed from the glomerular filtrate and are excreted as waste.

The glomerular filtrate next passes through the loop of Henle, which has a descending arm and an ascending arm. The glomerular filtrate becomes increasingly concentrated as it flows down the descending arm and then up the ascending arm of the loop of Henle. The glomerular filtrate then travels to the distal convoluted tubule. In the distal convoluted tubule, salt and water continue to be reabsorbed into the bloodstream. As the filtrate passes through the loop of Henle, chemical compounds such as uric acid, creatinine, ammonia, hydrogen ions, and drugs (eg, penicillin) exit from the perivascular capillaries and enter the glomerular filtrate. In this way, these compounds are removed from the blood. By the time the glomerular filtrate passes through the distal convoluted tubule, it is urine. The urine drips into the collecting duct and descends through the collecting duct to the renal pelvis, which joins the ureter. The ureter transports the urine into the urinary bladder.

Renal Control of Electrolyte Balance

The kidneys maintain the balance of electrolytes in the body. Electrolytes are ingested with foods and are lost through perspiration and feces. Some important electrolytes are Na^+, K^+, Ca^{2+}, HCO_3^-, phosphate (PO_4^{3-}), and chloride (Cl^-). The amount of electrolytes taken into the body must equal the amount lost by the body. Losing a greater amount of electrolytes than what is consumed can set the stage for heart arrhythmias, muscle cramps, and other problems.

The steroid hormone aldosterone, which is produced and released by the adrenal gland, regulates sodium and potassium levels in the body. Aldosterone is released when the blood sodium level is low. It acts on the tubules to increase sodium reabsorption into the blood. When the blood potassium level is high, aldosterone causes potassium ions to be excreted into the glomerular filtrate and exit the body through urine. Potassium is usually excreted in the form of potassium salts such as potassium chloride (KCl).

Other hormones can impact the kidney's regulation of electrolytes. For example, the distal tubules are sensitive to the actions of parathyroid hormone (ie, parathormone) and calcitonin. Parathyroid hormone causes calcium to be reabsorbed from the distal tubules into the blood and thereby raises the blood calcium level. Calcitonin decreases the reabsorption of calcium, phosphate, and sodium ions from the distal tubules and thereby allows these electrolytes to be excreted in the urine.

Atrial natriuretic peptide (a protein) has the opposite action of aldosterone. Atrial natriuretic peptide is secreted from the heart's atrial wall in response to increased intravascular volume or stretching of the atria beyond the normal dimension. It stimulates the kidney tubules to excrete sodium into the urine (ie, natriuresis), which causes more water to enter the urine. Natriuresis reduces fluid volume in body tissues and blood pressure.

Renal Control of Acid-Base Balance

The kidneys also regulate the acid-base balance (ie, pH, the concentration of hydrogen ions [H^+]) of body fluids. An improper acid-base balance can result in problems such as sleep-disordered breathing, excessive sleepiness, coma, and death.

In a solution, acids release hydrogen ions (thereby increasing the hydrogen concentration of the solution), and bases remove hydrogen ions (thereby decreasing the hydrogen concentration of the solution). The concentration of hydrogen ions is expressed by pH. A fluid with a pH of 7 is neutral, a fluid with a pH less than 7 is acidic, and a fluid with a pH greater than 7 is basic (ie, alkaline).

The pH of many body fluids is normally maintained within a narrow range. For example, the normal pH of arterial blood ranges between 7.35 and 7.45. A person experiences acidosis (ie, too acidic) if the arterial blood pH is less than 7.35 and experiences alkalosis (ie, too alkaline) if the arterial blood pH is greater than 7.45. The narrow pH range in the blood and the other body fluids is maintained by various buffers.

A buffer is a solution containing two or more chemical compounds that prevent drastic changes in pH when an acid or a base enters a system (eg, the bloodstream). A buffer usually contains a weak acid and its corresponding salt. The salt of an acid is formed when one or more of the hydrogen atoms in the acid have been replaced by other molecules. An example of a buffer is carbonic acid (H_2CO_3) and its salt sodium bicarbonate ($NaHCO_3$).

A buffer helps the kidneys regulate the acid-base balance. For example, lactic acid, a waste product of muscle metabolism, easily dissociates in solution. In a solution such as blood, lactic acid dissociates into lactate ($C_3H_5O_3^-$) and hydrogen (H^+) ions. The negatively charged lactate ions interact with the sodium ions from the sodium bicarbonate molecules to form sodium lactate. The remaining hydrogen ions from the lactic acid bind with the bicarbonate ions from the sodium bicarbonate molecule to form carbonic acid. Carbonic acid is a weak acid and therefore does not increase the acidity of the fluid drastically. In this way, the pH is buffered against the greater increase in acidity that would have been caused by lactic acid.

When the blood is too acidic, hydrogen ions are transported into the lumen of the tubules, enter the glomerular filtrate, and are ultimately excreted in urine. The bicarbonate ions are transported out of the glomerular filtrate and into the perivascular vessels surrounding the nephrons. These actions reduce the acidity of the blood.

When the blood is too alkaline, fewer hydrogen ions are excreted into the urine. Bicarbonate ions (which act as a base) are not easily reabsorbed into the blood from the tubules; therefore, they remain in the glomerular filtrate and are excreted in the urine. These actions increase the acidity of the blood.

Circadian Rhythmicity and Kidney Function

Kidney function (eg, filtration, urine production, salt and water balance) normally varies according to a circadian (ie, 24-hour) rhythm. For example, the glomerular filtration rate is normally at its highest during the day (peaking at approximately 2-3 PM) and falls to its minimum in the middle of the night; sodium excretion and urine production are highest during the day and fall to their minimum at night; and urine is more dilute in the day and more concentrated at night.

What remains unclear is the extent to which circadian rhythmicity in kidney function is influenced by external factors or is intrinsic to kidneys (ie, internally driven, regardless of external factors such as the environmental light level). Some research indicates that this fluctuation is driven by light and dark phases (5). For example, the excretion of urine is increased in the day (ie, light phase) and decreased at night (ie, dark phase). However, some research indicates that circadian rhythmicity in kidney function is intrinsic (6). In animals that are bred to lack certain genes that control the circadian rhythm, the circadian variation in kidney function is abolished, even when the animals are exposed to consistent light/dark cycles (6).

Circadian Rhythmicity of Normal Kidney Function

The interrelation between renin (a protein and enzyme), angiotensin (a hormone), and aldosterone (a mineralocorticoid) helps maintain proper sodium balance, fluid volume, and blood pressure. When blood flow in the kidneys decreases, the kidneys release renin, which is involved in the production of the powerful vasoconstrictor angiotensin II. Angiotensin II also stimulates the production of aldosterone, which promotes sodium and water retention and thereby raises blood pressure. The production of renin decreases once blood pressure is sufficiently raised. The levels of renin, angiotensin II, and aldosterone are generally higher in the morning and lower in the afternoon and evening. However, the production of these and other substances varies with sleep stages. Other substances include cortisol (a glucocorticoid involved in diuresis [increased urine excretion] and natriuresis [sodium excretion in urine]), and atrial natriuretic peptide lowers blood pressure by reducing renin, angiotensin II, and aldosterone levels.

During sleep, the production of hormones involved in kidney function fluctuates with the sleep state. The secretion of renin increases during non-REM sleep and decreases during REM sleep. Aldosterone increases and decreases in correlation with renin production during sleep. However, aldosterone and cortisol levels quickly increase dramatically when a person awakens from sleep. This sudden rise in aldosterone and cortisol levels may be related to the activation of the hypothalamus-pituitary-adrenal (HPA) axis with wake. The HPA axis is involved in the interplay between hormones produced by the hypothalamus, pituitary, and adrenal cortex. For example, the hypothalamus produces corticotrophin-releasing hormone, which causes the anterior pituitary to release adrenocorticotropic hormone, which then induces the release of aldosterone from the adrenal glands. Thus, aldosterone production may be influenced by changes in renin production during non-REM and REM sleep but may be under the influence of cortisol during wake. By contrast, cortisol production appears to be weakly linked with REM sleep and non-REM sleep (7).

Impaired Kidney Function and Sleep Disorders

Kidney failure (ie, the inability of the kidneys to excrete metabolites or to retain electrolytes at normal physiologic levels in the blood) can occur because of decreased blood supply to the kidneys, damage to the kidney tissues, or obstruction to the outflow of urine. Kidney failure can be acute (ie, sudden onset) or chronic. Acute kidney failure, if diagnosed quickly, can often be reversed with medical treatment. Acute kidney failure can progress to end-stage renal disease, uremic syndrome (ie, kidney failure comprising a group of symptoms such as a metallic taste in the mouth, the formation of a layer of uric acid crystals on the surface of the skin [ie, uremic frost], muscular twitching, pain, hypertension, mental confusion, and edema), and death. Poorly controlled diabetes, high blood pressure, and chronic glomerulonephritis (ie, inflammation of the glomeruli) are some common causes of chronic kidney failure. Impaired kidney function or kidney failure can cause the blood to become too acidic or too alkaline and negatively impact sleep. People with impaired kidney function or kidney failure can experience sleep-disordered breathing, insomnia, alterations in the circadian rhythm, restless legs syndrome (RLS), and EDS (8).

Sleep-Disordered Breathing

Central Apnea and Cheyne-Stokes Breathing

Neurons in the respiratory center in the brain are sensitive to pH changes in the blood. Therefore, blood pH is involved in the rhythmicity of breathing and in the depth of breathing. Acidosis normally induces increased firing of the respiratory center neurons and causes a person to take deep, fast breaths. Alkalosis normally induces decreased firing of the respiratory center neurons and causes a person to take shallow, slow breaths. However, a chronic state of acidosis or alkalosis, which may occur with impaired kidney function or chronic kidney failure, can alter the respiratory center's response to acidosis and alkalosis.

Improper responses to pH can set the stage for the manifestation of central sleep apnea (ie, the cessation in the respiratory drive, resulting in a lack of respiratory effort) and Cheyne-Stokes respiration (ie, a rhythmic breathing pattern characterized by a gradual increase in the depth and rate of breathing, followed by a gradual decrease in both, often progressing to a central apnea before the cycle repeats). Frequent arousals resulting from these respiratory events during the night can result in EDS, fatigue, difficulty concentrating, and other symptoms associated with insufficient sleep.

Obstructive Sleep Apnea

Obstructive sleep apnea (OSA) is the cessation in breathing (ie, apnea; from the Greek *apnoia*, meaning "no breath") caused by upper airway tissues (eg, fat tissue, tonsils, adenoids) blocking the upper airway during sleep. With airflow impeded, the blood oxygen level falls. However, a person continues to make respiratory movements. Once the blood oxygen falls below a certain level, an arousal occurs, and a person awakens briefly (usually for a few seconds) to take some deep breaths, which restores the oxygen level. Once the oxygen level is restored, the person promptly resumes sleep. Many episodes of apnea can occur during a sleep period. A person who has five or more episodes of apnea per hour may be diagnosed with OSA. Owing to the arousals from sleep, a person may struggle with symptoms such as EDS, impaired cognition, and diminished daytime functioning.

OSA is very common among people with end-stage renal disease. Exactly why OSA is so prevalent in patients with end-stage renal disease is unclear. A possibility is a phenomenon called "rostral fluid shift." During the day when a person is awake and mobile, fluid volume is greater in the lower extremities because of gravity. However, when a person lies horizontally in bed, fluid shifts from the legs toward the neck (ie, fluid moves rostrally [toward the oronasal region]). Excess fluid accumulation in the upper airway tissues can swell these tissues and contribute to upper airway narrowing and blockage and thereby lead to OSA.

Insomnia

Insomnia is difficulty in initiating or maintaining sleep. It is usually secondary to (ie, the result of) another problem. In people with end-stage renal disease, insomnia may occur because of the physical stress of managing their disease (eg, the timing of the hemodialysis session), long-term dialysis treatment, and pain.

For unclear reasons, people whose hemodialysis sessions are scheduled for early morning appear to have a greater problem with insomnia compared with people whose sessions are scheduled for the afternoon (9). A possible explanation for this phenomenon is that patients with the early morning session may become conditioned to waking up early. By contrast, patients whose sessions are scheduled in the afternoon are often tired and sleepy after hemodialysis, which may enhance their sleep; thus, they report fewer problems with insomnia.

Patients undergoing long-term hemodialysis and older patients receiving hemodialysis have greater problems with insomnia, compared with younger patients receiving hemodialysis. With aging or long-term dialysis treatment, symptoms associated with chronic dialysis treatment (eg, itchiness, bone pain) can delay the onset of sleep at a desired time or disrupt sleep. The effect of concurrent diseases such as cardiovascular disease (eg, heart failure with Cheyne-Stokes breathing) and neurologic disease (eg, RLS) can also contribute to insomnia in patients on long-term dialysis treatment.

Pain or discomfort due to changes in bone structure, muscle cramps, abdominal pain, etc., can delay the onset of sleep at a desired time. Pain may be so intense that it awakens a person and causes difficulty going back to sleep. High levels of parathyroid hormone can contribute to bone pain. Parathyroid hormone causes the release of calcium from the bone into the blood and other fluids. Excess levels of the hormone weaken the bone structure (ie, osteoporosis), and thereby result in bone pain, fractures, and tenderness, and affect other organs such as the kidneys (eg, kidney stones), the muscles (eg, weakness, tremors, cramps), and the gastrointestinal system (eg, abdominal pain, nausea, vomiting).

Alteration in the Circadian Rhythm

The level of the sleep-promoting hormone melatonin is normally highest during the night and lowest during the day. The nocturnal production of melatonin is lower in people with chronic kidney disease than in healthy individuals. In addition, the circadian rhythmicity of melatonin production is abolished in some people who are on hemodialysis (10). This reduced production may contribute to problems with initiating or maintaining sleep. Why the melatonin concentration is lower in hemodialyzed patients is unclear.

Restless Legs Syndrome

Symptoms of RLS begin to manifest in the evening shortly before bedtime as a person sits or lies relaxed. Unpleasant sensations in the calves or legs cause a person to irresistibly move the legs to relieve the sensations (eg, walking, rubbing them against bed sheets). The relief is short lived, and a person has to repeatedly go through efforts to relieve the sensations. These efforts at relief can delay the onset of sleep. The sensations usually stop just as a person is falling asleep. However, if the person awakens during the night, the symptoms can recur, and a person will go through the same efforts to relieve them, thereby delaying sleep. In healthy individuals without kidney disease, RLS and periodic limb movement have been associated with low levels of iron in the brain (11,12). Iron is involved in the production of the hormone dopamine (which has a role in motor function). However, some people with RLS have normal levels of iron. Therefore, the relationship between iron and RLS is unclear. In people undergoing hemodialysis, RLS may be related to increased levels of urea, creatinine, or other nitrogen-containing substances. Excess levels of these substances may contribute to central and peripheral nerve damage and thereby contribute to symptoms of RLS.

Excessive Daytime Sleepiness

EDS, like insomnia, is usually secondary to other problems in people with chronic kidney disease or kidney failure. EDS can be caused by uremia (ie, high blood levels of nitrogen-containing substances such as ammonia), disrupted sleep because of RLS or periodic limb movement disorder (ie, a disorder in which the foot or leg rhythmically contracts intermittently during sleep and can induce arousals from sleep), or sleep apnea. Neurologic changes such as uremic encephalopathy (ie, brain disorder caused by uremia); low levels of the amino acid tyrosine, which is involved in dopamine production; the release of inflammatory cytokines during dialysis; high diurnal levels of melatonin; and a change in the circadian rhythmicity of body temperature may lead to problems with sleepiness at unwanted times. Addressing these factors can help alleviate EDS. For example, switching to nocturnal hemodialysis treatment—a slower, longer hemodialysis treatment that takes place at night while a person sleeps—can remove toxic substances from the blood on a more frequent basis, compared with the conventional three times weekly hemodialysis treatment, and thereby reduce the impact of toxic substances on the brain and other body tissues.

THE DIGESTIVE SYSTEM

The digestive system begins at the mouth and ends at the anus (Figure 7-4). The digestive system consists of the gastrointestinal tract and several accessory organs. The mouth, esophagus, stomach, and the small and large intestines make up the gastrointestinal tract. The salivary glands, liver, gallbladder, and pancreas are accessory organs that support the function of the digestive tract. Two major functions of the digestive system are (1) to break down large food molecules (eg, starch, proteins, lipids) into small molecules (eg, glucose, amino acids, or fatty acids) and (2) to absorb small molecules into the bloodstream. Once in the bloodstream, these substances can be absorbed and used by the body's tissues.

Digestion and Absorption

Digestion begins when food is taken into the mouth and ground down (ie, chewed) by the teeth. In the process of chewing, the salivary glands secrete fluids such as mucus that lubricate the food and enzymes such as amylase that break down starches into sugars. Once the food is chewed sufficiently, it is swallowed, and the mass of food (ie, a bolus) begins to travel down the esophagus. Rhythmic muscular contractions (ie, peristalsis) push the bolus downward toward the stomach. At the lower portion of the esophagus, the bolus passes through the lower esophageal sphincter (LES, which is just above the diaphragm) and the cardiac sphincter (which is below the diaphragm). Once the bolus has passed through the cardiac sphincter, it enters the stomach.

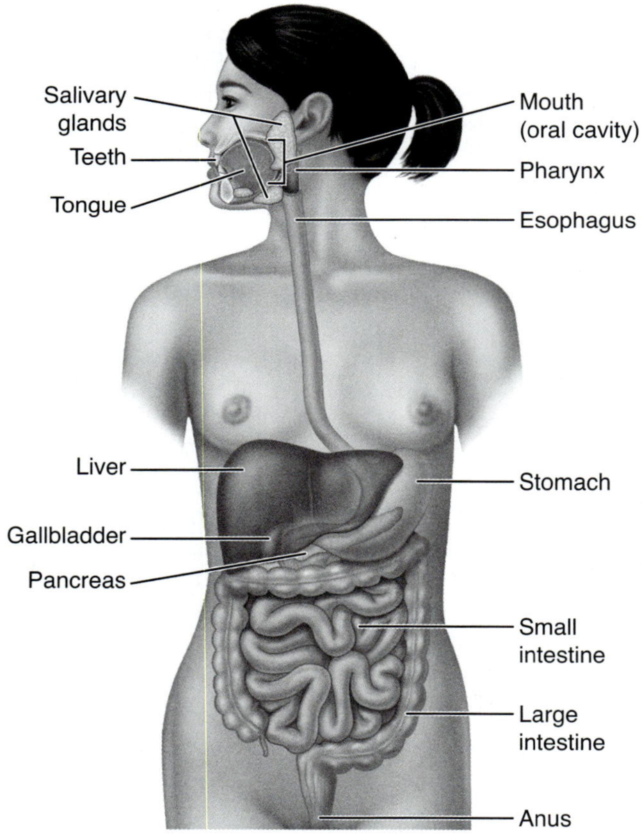

Figure 7-4 The digestive system extends from the mouth to the anus. Accessory organs secrete various substances (eg, saliva, bile, and pancreatic juice) into the digestive tract. (Reprinted with permission from Cohen BJ, Hull K. *Memmler's The Human Body in Health and Disease*. 13th ed. Wolters Kluwer; 2015. Figure 19.1.)

In the stomach, the bolus is subjected to the physical churning actions of the muscular layers of the stomach and to the chemical actions of gastric juice, which is secreted by gastric glands and contains strong protein-digesting enzymes, mucus, and hydrochloric acid. These processes change the bolus into a soup-like liquid called "chyme." The chyme is pushed in spurts from the stomach into the duodenum, the first portion of the small intestine. Most digestion takes place in the duodenum.

The duodenum contains several glands: the crypts of Lieberkühn, which release enzymes that further break down chyme; Brunner glands, which secrete mucus to protect the intestinal lining from acid; and Paneth cells, which release peptides and enzymes that maintain healthy gut bacteria and defend the intestinal system against pathogens. Pancreatic juice is released into the duodenum from the pancreas via the pancreatic duct, whereas bile is produced by the liver, stored in the gallbladder, and released into the duodenum via the bile duct. Pancreatic juice contains bicarbonate ions, protein-digesting enzymes (ie, peptidases), and other enzymes (eg, trypsin). Bile is a golden brown to green-yellow alkaline fluid that contains various chemicals such as electrolytes, cholesterol, and bile salts. Bile is synthesized in the liver but is stored in and released by the gallbladder. The pancreas releases pancreatic juice through the pancreatic duct. The gallbladder squeezes bile through the cystic duct. It then flows through the common bile duct, which merges with the pancreatic duct just before inserting into the duodenum. Bile helps break down large fat globules into small globules. The small fat globules are further broken down by enzymes, a process called "emulsification." Brunner glands in the duodenum produce mucus, which helps neutralize the acidity of chyme.

Chyme next passes through the jejunum and finally through the last portion of the small intestine, the ileum. The jejunum and ileum contain villi and microvilli. The villi are finger-like projections that extend from the inner surface of the jejunum and ileum. The microvilli are finger-like projections that extend from each epithelial (ie, surface) cell of a villus. Within each villus is a network of capillaries and lymph vessels (called "lacteals"). The products of protein, carbohydrate, and nucleic acid digestion are actively transported or diffuse out of the chyme and into the blood vessels within a villus, whereas the products of fat digestion enter the lacteals. The villi also absorb water from chyme as it passes through the jejunum and ileum. Chyme consequently becomes an increasingly concentrated semisolid liquid.

From the ileum, the semisolid liquid (now called "feces" or "stool") enters the first portion of the large intestine, a large sac-like structure called the "cecum" (pronounced "SEE-kum"). The large intestines do not have villi or microvilli, and no chemical digestion occurs in these intestines. However, the large intestines reabsorb some water and ions. These intestines contain bacteria that break down the undigested material in the stool. This bacterial action results in the release of nutrients and the synthesis of vitamins (eg, vitamin K and certain B vitamins) that then enter the bloodstream from the large intestines.

After passing through the cecum, the stool travels up the ascending colon (which is on the right side of the abdomen), then travels horizontally through the transverse colon (which is just beneath the liver, gallbladder, and stomach), and, finally, travels down the descending colon (which is on the left side of the abdomen). At the level of the pelvis, the colon makes an S-like curve (ie, the sigmoid colon) and becomes the rectum. The rectum terminates in the anal canal. At the end of the anal canal is a sphincter called the "anal sphincter." By the time the stool has reached the anus, much of its water has been reabsorbed and it has been compacted into a firm mass that primarily contains undigested material (eg, fiber), bacteria, and other material. The release of stool through the anus is called "defecation."

Neural and Hormonal Mechanisms of Digestion

In recent years, three hormones—leptin, orexin (also called hypocretin), and ghrelin (pronounced "GRELL-in")—have been investigated to clarify their roles in digestion and sleep. Each of these hormones has neurotransmitter and hormonal properties. Some of the effects these hormones have on digestion are described in the following paragraphs.

Leptin is produced by many body tissues, but especially by fat tissue. Leptin receptors exist in the brain, in fat, and in other tissues. Insulin regulates leptin production, and cross-talk between insulin and leptin receptors has been observed in the brain (13).

In the hypothalamus, leptin inhibits the actions of orexin-secreting cells (14). Hence, an antagonistic interplay exists between orexin (which promotes appetite and food intake) and leptin (which reduces appetite). This interplay may be involved in weight control.

Orexin is produced within the hypothalamus by a group of specialized neurons (ie, orexinergic neurons). Orexin stimulates glucose uptake and the formation of fat tissue. It may temporarily regulate energy utilization. The orexin level rises immediately before eating (ie, when glucose levels are low) and falls immediately after food has been ingested.

Ghrelin increases appetite and promotes food intake. It is produced and secreted primarily by the stomach and, to a lesser extent, by the hypothalamus. The vagus nerve, which contains ghrelin receptors, relays signals from stomach-derived ghrelin to the brain. An increased level of glucose inhibits the production of orexin, whereas prolonged fasting can increase the ghrelin level.

Digestive Function and Sleep Disorders

A digestive disorder that affects sleep is gastroesophageal reflux disorder (GERD). In GERD, gastric juices flow backward (ie, reflux) from the stomach, through the LES, and into the esophagus during sleep. Gastric juices are very acidic; therefore, if reflux occurs frequently, esophageal tissues can become irritated or destroyed.

GERD occurs when the LES is weak or when excessive pressure is exerted on the stomach that the LES cannot withstand. In some people, decreased LES pressure and, consequently, gastric reflux can be promoted by the ingestion of certain foods (eg, orange juice and chocolate), substances (eg, alcohol and nicotine), or drugs (eg, atropine, diazepam, and calcium channel blockers). Any factor that increases the intra-abdominal pressure—including OSA—can also lower the LES pressure and contribute to GERD.

Symptoms of GERD can occur either during wake or during sleep. The most common symptom of GERD is heartburn (ie, a sense of warmth or pain felt behind the breastbone that may travel up toward the neck). The heartburn may be severe enough to mimic angina (ie, spasmodic thoracic pain that may radiate to the arms and be associated with a sense of suffocation). Other GERD symptoms are pain on swallowing, difficulty swallowing (irritation from gastric juices may induce stricture at the level of the LES because of esophageal spasm or esophagitis, which would then hinder the passage of food through the esophagus), and regurgitation during sleep. When GERD occurs during sleep, a person will complain of having episodes of abrupt awakenings with coughing, choking, or a mouth full of saliva. These actions can interfere with a person's sleep and result in symptoms of insufficient sleep (eg, EDS).

Leptin is involved in decreasing appetite. In animal studies, the administration of leptin induces weight loss and decreases appetite (15). However, some people have a higher than normal leptin level but are obese. For example, people with OSA tend to be obese and have higher than normal leptin levels. The resistance of leptin receptors to the effects of leptin may explain this finding. However, research is continuing toward clarifying the association between leptin resistance and obesity.

THE IMMUNE SYSTEM

The immune system helps the body resist harmful substances and microorganisms through the actions of immune cells or through chemical means. Immunity involving the actions of immune cells is called "cell-mediated immunity." Immunity involving chemical factors is called "antibody-mediated immunity."

The process of immunity begins after a foreign microorganism or substance enters the body. Macrophages, a type of white blood cell, engulf, consume, and digest the offending microorganism. Pieces of the microorganism's proteins (ie, antigens) are preserved and displayed on the surface of the macrophage. The macrophage moves toward lymph vessels, which convey the cell to lymphoid tissues (eg, lymph nodes). In a lymph node, the macrophage encounters a helper T-lymphocyte, which is a type of immune cell. The foreign proteins on the surface of the macrophage interact with receptors on the surface of the helper T-lymphocyte. This interaction causes the helper T-lymphocyte to produce various proteins called "lymphokines." Depending on the type of lymphokine produced, one of two types of immune cells becomes stimulated: T-lymphocytes or B-lymphocytes. If T-lymphocytes are stimulated, the immune response is cell-mediated immunity. If B-lymphocytes are stimulated, the immune response is antibody-mediated immunity.

Cell-Mediated Immunity

In cell-mediated immunity, an immune cell directly interacts with a microorganism or foreign molecule. T-helper cells release cytokines that stimulate the multiplication of cytotoxic T-lymphocytes, which search for cells displaying the foreign antigen. On finding a cell with the antigen, the cytotoxic cell attacks and destroys the foreign cell. To prevent this immune response from destroying normal tissue, another type of lymphocyte, called a "suppressor T-lymphocyte," inhibits the activity of the cytotoxic T-lymphocyte as an increasing number of antigen-containing foreign cells are destroyed.

Antibody-Mediated Immunity

In antibody-mediated immunity, a macrophage (which ingests a foreign cell and displays the foreign cell's antigen on its surface) encounters different types of B-lymphocytes in lymphoid tissue. It ultimately encounters a B-lymphocyte that has the specific antibody to its antigen. An antibody is a large protein that is also called an immunoglobulin (Ig). The presence of an antigen induces the synthesis of an antibody. An antibody is the chemical complement to an antigen, so that it alone can chemically react with the antigen. A helper T-lymphocyte binds with a B-lymphocyte and a T-lymphocyte. Only when this complex is formed does the B-lymphocyte begin to multiply and produce sister cells that are programmed to produce the antibody. B-lymphocytes produce antigen-specific antibody molecules at a fast rate. Within hours, many B-lymphocytes are transformed into plasma cells, which only produce the antibody.

Five types of antibodies are immunoglobulin G (IgG), immunoglobulin M (IgM), immunoglobulin A (IgA), immunoglobulin D (IgD), and immunoglobulin E (IgE). IgG is the most common; it confers resistance to disease. IgM is the first antibody to appear when an infection occurs. IgA interacts with microorganisms at the body surface and along other tracts that are open to the environment (eg, respiratory tract). IgD acts as a receptor site on the B-lymphocyte. IgE is produced during allergic reactions.

Cell-mediated immunity is involved in the delayed allergic response, whereas antibody-mediated immunity is involved in the immediate allergic response. An immediate allergic response (also called "type I allergic response") manifests minutes after exposure to an allergen (ie, an antigen). A delayed allergic response, also called "type IV allergic response," manifests 12 to 48 hours after exposure to an antigen. In the immediate allergic response, symptoms can appear within minutes because antibodies produced by B cells can quickly enter the blood and travel to the site of an antigen. Symptoms of cell-mediated immunity take longer to manifest because it takes longer for T cells to multiply and then travel to the site of the antigen. Whether a person undergoes an immediate or delayed response is determined by which immune cells—B cells or T cells—are most active.

Immune Function and Sleep Disorders

Neurons that control sleep interact closely with the immune system. This phenomenon is evidenced, for example, when a person has an infectious disease such as the flu and feels sleepy. During the infection, the production of certain immune factors such as cytokines induces sleep. Two sleep disorders that may involve a dysfunctional immune response are narcolepsy and Kleine-Levin syndrome. Both disorders involve hypersomnia (ie., the excessive need for sleep or excessive sleepiness when awake).

Narcolepsy

Several factors support the involvement of the immune system in narcolepsy. Some people with narcolepsy report that their symptoms began after an infection. A high percentage of people with narcolepsy have the *HLA-DQB1*0602* gene, which belongs to a class of genes (HLA-DQB1) that is associated with other immune disorders. As stated earlier in this chapter, hypocretin-producing hypothalamic cells in people with narcolepsy are inexplicably destroyed, a possible result of autoimmune destruction.

Kleine-Levin Syndrome

Kleine-Levin syndrome consists of several symptoms, the foremost of which is hypersomnia. A person with Kleine-Levin syndrome experiences hypersomnia lasting 16 to 20 hours per day that occurs one or more times per year, with the hypersomnia phase ranging from 2 days to 4 weeks at a time. The hypersomnia is not secondary to another factor such as a mental disorder (eg, depression), the physiologic effects of a substance (eg, a drug of misuse or medication), or a medical condition (eg, a metabolic disorder). In addition to the hypersomnia, one or more of the following symptoms will be present:

- The person is rousable during the episode, but when awake, the person has abnormal cognition or mood (eg, confusion and lethargy).
- The person has excessive, compulsive eating.
- The person has abnormal behavior (eg, irritability and aggression).
- The person is hypersexual and exhibits inappropriate sexual behavior (eg, masturbating in public and making unwanted sexual advances).

After the episode of hypersomnia, the person's alertness, cognition, and behavior return to normal. The person may not remember what occurred during the episode. Nearly one-half of people with Kleine-Levin syndrome report having had an infection, such as COVID-19, days before the onset of symptoms (16).

THE GENITOURINARY SYSTEM

The genitourinary system consists of the ureters, the urinary bladder, and the urethra (Figure 7-2). A ureter is a long tube extending from each kidney that carries urine from the kidney to the urinary bladder. The urinary bladder expels urine through the urethra, a tube that extends from the base of the urinary bladder.

In men and women, the sphincter muscle of the urethra lies slightly below the neck of the bladder (ie, where the urethra extends from the bladder). It encircles the urethra and compresses it to keep urine in the bladder. Another muscle, called the "sphincter muscle of the urinary bladder," is a circular layer of fibers that surrounds the opening of the urethra at the level of the bladder.

As the bladder fills, stretch receptors in the urinary bladder become stimulated. As a result, the receptors induce a reflexive contraction of the bladder and relaxation of the urethral and urinary bladder sphincter muscles. This action allows urine to be voided from the bladder.

Genitourinary Function and Sleep Disorders

Genitourinary phenomena that may occur during sleep are enuresis, nocturia, and erectile dysfunction. The first two phenomena can disrupt sleep. The third phenomenon does not disrupt sleep, but its manifestation during sleep can be related to other problems.

Enuresis

A person is normally able to sense when the bladder needs voiding. The uncontrolled voiding of urine (ie, urinary incontinence) can occur for various reasons such as neurologic disorders (eg, stroke), enlarged prostate (in men), and urinary tract infection. In some people, uncontrolled voiding occurs only during sleep. Urinary incontinence that occurs only during sleep is called "enuresis" (ie, bed-wetting).

Enuresis typically occurs in children (especially boys) who are past the age that urinary control during the night is normally achieved. However, enuresis can occur in adults. In children, enuresis tends to occur during slow-wave sleep. Why enuresis tends to occur in this stage is unclear.

A factor that may contribute to enuresis in children is OSA. Enuresis may be induced by the excessive intra-abdominal pressures that occur during a child's efforts to breathe. The excessive pressure may be strong enough to induce relaxation of the urethral sphincter muscle, which then results in enuresis. Other factors that can contribute to enuresis are urinary tract infection, urinary tract obstruction, and psychological stress.

Nocturia

A person with nocturia awakens one or more times during the night to urinate. Nocturia can result from a disruption in the normal circadian rhythm in urine concentration. Urine is normally less concentrated in the daytime and more concentrated in the night. The circadian rhythmicity in the production of antidiuretic hormone, which reduces the excretion of urine, contributes to this variation. Antidiuretic hormone levels are normally higher at night (thereby reducing urine volume, which allows a person to sleep through the night) and lower during the day when a person is active and consuming fluids and needs to excrete more urine. Nocturia can also result from a medication effect (eg, diuretics); overactive bladder; kidney or lower urinary tract disorders; or cardiovascular, endocrine, or metabolic disorders.

Erectile Dysfunction (Impotence)

During the night, men normally have an erection during each REM sleep period. (The erection is unrelated to the dream content.) During wake, erectile dysfunction (ie, inability to achieve or maintain an erection) can occur because of psychological factors. People with erectile dysfunction due to psychological factors can have normal REM sleep-related erections. Therefore, the lack of an erection during an REM sleep period indicates that physiologic, rather than psychological, factors are responsible. Some physiologic factors that can contribute to erectile dysfunction are vascular disease, type II diabetes, and spinal cord lesion. Erectile dysfunction can also be an adverse drug effect. For example, some antihypertension drugs block α-adrenergic receptors on nerves that are involved in an erection, thereby contribute to erectile dysfunction. Newer antihypertension drugs are able to reduce blood pressure by acting on β-adrenergic receptors while allowing the α-adrenergic receptors to remain functional. This action allows a man to have an erection while allowing the antihypertension drug to exert its blood pressure–lowering effect. Other drugs associated with erectile dysfunction are selective serotonin-reuptake inhibitors (eg, fluoxetine, sertraline, and paroxetine); cholesterol-lowering drugs (eg, atorvastatin, simvastatin, and rosuvastatin); antidepressant drugs such as selective serotonin-reuptake inhibitors (eg, fluoxetine, sertraline, and paroxetine); tricyclic antidepressants (eg, amitriptyline and nortriptyline); and monoamine oxidase inhibitors (eg, phenelzine); opioids (eg, morphine, oxycodone, and hydrocodone); and antianxiety medications such as benzodiazepines (eg, diazepam, lorazepam, and alprazolam).

THE MUSCULOSKELETAL SYSTEM

A skeletal muscle is an organ that originates from and inserts into some part of the skeleton. For example, the anterior tibialis muscle, which can be felt on the outer side of the shin bone (ie, tibia), originates from the upper lateral surface of the tibia and inserts onto the first metatarsal bone (located beneath the base of the big toe) and onto the medial cuneiform bone (located within the instep). The contraction of a skeletal muscle causes the skeleton to move. For example, contraction of the anterior tibialis muscle flexes the foot. Muscle movement induced by contractions can be voluntary (eg, skeletal muscles) or involuntary (eg, muscles of the intestines, bladder, and blood vessels).

Skeletal muscle is often called "striated muscle" because of its striped appearance (Figure 7-5). A muscle is in actuality a bundle of muscle fibers. Each muscle fiber contains 4 to 20 rod-like filaments (ie, myofibrils). A myofibril is approximately 1 to 2 μm in diameter and 100 μm in length. Each myofibril consists of shorter disk-like units called "sarcomeres." Sarcomeres are stacked end to end (somewhat like a stack of checkers) to create the myofibrils. Sarcomeres give a muscle fiber its striped appearance.

A sarcomere is composed of two types of filaments: thin and thick filaments. A black line (Z line) exists where the thin filaments of one sarcomere interweave with the thin filaments of an adjacent sarcomere. Thick filaments overlap thin filaments in the center of the sarcomere, resulting in another darkened area called the "A band." A thin darkened region, the H zone, exists within the very center of the A band. The A band consists of only thick filaments. The lightest portion of the

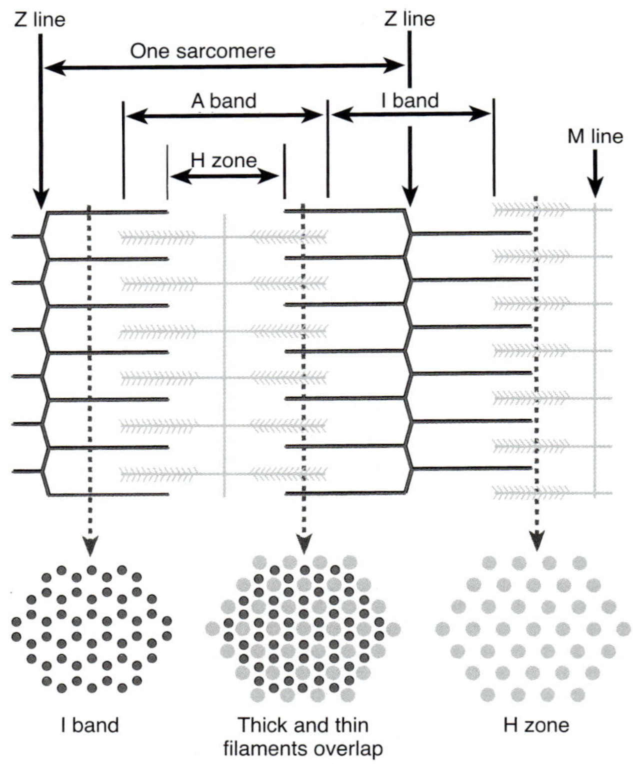

Figure 7-5 Molecular organization of the sarcomere. The arrangement of the elements in a sarcomere viewed longitudinally and as cross-sections through selected regions of the sarcomere. The myofilaments overlap at different parts of the sarcomere. (Reprinted with permission from Rhoades RA, Bell DR. *Medical Physiology: Principles for Clinical Medicine*. 5th ed. Wolters Kluwer; 2018. Figure 8.2.)

sarcomere is the I band, which exists between the edge of the Z line and the outer edge of the A band.

A muscle contraction begins when a stimulus triggers an action potential within a neuron that innervates a muscle fiber. The action potential travels down the axon of the neuron. When the action potential reaches the axon's terminal, neurotransmitters are released from the terminal into the neuromuscular junction (NMJ), which is the synapse between the axons of a neuron and a muscle fiber. The neurotransmitters travel across the NMJ to attach to receptors on a muscle fiber.

At this point, contraction of a muscle occurs through the following process. Once a neurotransmitter attaches to a muscle receptor, sodium ions flood into the muscle fiber, thereby reducing its electrical potential (ie, depolarizing it). The action potential then travels through the muscle fiber and ultimately spreads to other muscle fibers.

The resting potential of skeletal muscle is −95 mV, and the threshold potential is −50 mV. When a muscle fiber contracts, the thin filaments of sarcomeres are drawn close together. The thick filaments remain in place in the center of the sarcomere as the thin filaments slide over them. The thick filaments may provide the energy to the thin filaments for contraction. However, scientists are continuing to investigate this possibility.

Musculoskeletal Function and Sleep Disorders

Problems with the musculoskeletal system can interfere with sleep. Some musculoskeletal problems that may affect sleep are fibromyalgia, arthritis, thoracic deformities, and neuromuscular disorders.

Fibromyalgia

Fibromyalgia is a chronic pain syndrome involving fatigue, morning stiffness, widespread muscle pain, cognitive problems, and poor sleep quality. No pathology such as inflammation or degenerative changes have been detected that can explain the symptoms of fibromyalgia.

Diagnosing fibromyalgia and treating it can be problematic. It has many symptoms in common with other disorders. For example, hypocalcemia (ie, low blood calcium level) and low vitamin D level can result in muscle soreness and tenderness, hypothyroidism can result in fatigue, and infections such as Lyme disease and arthritis can result in pain that is similar to fibromyalgia. These disorders can be easily diagnosed through testing, whereas no definitive test exists for fibromyalgia. Adding to the difficulty in diagnosing fibromyalgia, people with fibromyalgia may also have nonpain complaints such as gastrointestinal problems (eg, irritable bowel-like symptoms and nausea), mood disorders (eg, depression), and sleep disturbances (eg, insomnia and RLS). People with fibromyalgia tend to have alpha-delta sleep, which manifests on an electroencephalogram (EEG) as alpha waves superimposed on the delta waves of slow-wave sleep. This pattern indicates that the person is awake and asleep at the same time. People with the abnormal EEG pattern of alpha-delta sleep—even individuals without a diagnosis of fibromyalgia—complain of feeling unrested.

Arthritis

Arthritis is inflammation of the joints. It can occur as a result of an infection (eg, rheumatic fever), noninfectious degenerative processes (eg, osteoarthritis), or genetic factors (eg, ankylosing spondylitis). A person with arthritis has pain, stiffness, and/or swelling of the joints. The pain may be most noticeable in the morning or after sitting or lying in one position for a long time. Arthritis may affect the small joints of the hands or feet or larger joints such as the hip and spine. People with arthritis may complain of being unable to go to sleep at a desired time because of joint pain or inability to remain asleep because the pain awakens them.

Thoracic Deformities

A thoracic deformity can result from a deformity in the alignment of the spine, a ribcage deformity, or both. A thoracic deformity can impede normal respiratory movements and consequently impact sleep. Examples of thoracic deformities are kyphosis and scoliosis, and examples of ribcage deformities are pectus excavatum (commonly called "funnel chest") and pectus carinatum (commonly called "pigeon chest").

Kyphosis and Scoliosis

Kyphosis and scoliosis both involve a deformity in the alignment of the spine. In kyphosis, the spine curves in an anteroposterior direction at the level of the thorax or thoracolumbar region or sacrum, giving the back an excessively rounded appearance. Kyphosis is commonly called a "hunchback." In scoliosis, the spine curves at the level of the thorax, lumbar region, or thoracolumbar region in a lateral direction (ie, to the left or right), giving an S-like curve to the spine. In some people with scoliosis, the spine twists on its axis in addition to having the lateral curvature. Scoliosis often occurs in association with kyphosis and lordosis (ie, an anterior curvature of the spine in the lumbar region, often called a "swayback").

The spinal curvature in kyphosis and scoliosis can result from collapse of the vertebrae because of disease (eg, arthritis and osteoporosis), deformity of the vertebrae, genetic factors, compression fractures of the vertebrae, and disk degeneration. Backache or back pain can be associated with kyphosis and scoliosis and may impact the onset of sleep or the maintenance of sleep.

Kyphosis and scoliosis can impair a person's ability to expand the chest wall and thereby reduce lung capacity. Reduced lung capacity may lead to hypoventilation (ie, insufficient airflow in and out of the lungs) and consequently chronic hypoxemia (ie, low blood oxygen level) and hypercapnia (ie, excessive blood carbon dioxide level). Prolonged hypoventilation can disrupt the normal physiologic responses to improper levels of oxygen and carbon dioxide. The result can be sleep-related breathing disorders such as hypopnea (ie, shallow breathing), central sleep apnea (ie, cessation in breathing due to the lack of the respiratory drive), and OSA (ie, cessation of breathing due to upper airway blockage).

In some cases of kyphosis and scoliosis, the curvature of the spine may be severe enough to compress and damage the spinal cord, which may then result in spastic paraplegia (ie, spasticity [stiffness] and paralysis of the lower portion of the body from the point of injury downward). This injury may negatively affect the movement of the respiratory muscles and contribute to hypoventilation or sleep-related breathing disorders.

Ribcage Deformity

Pectus excavatum and pectus carinatum both result from a deformity of the ribcage and sternum (ie, breastbone). In pectus excavatum (from Latin meaning "excavated chest"), the sternum appears sunken. In pectus carinatum (from Latin meaning "keel chest"), the chest is narrow but protrudes abnormally in the front, reminiscent of the shape of a ship's keel. Depending on the severity of the deformity, pectus excavatum and pectus carinatum may restrict lung movement, thereby affecting lung function (eg, hypoxemia), and may cause pain. These factors may then disrupt sleep.

Neuromuscular Disorders

Neuromuscular disorders such as multiple sclerosis, postpolio syndrome, and quadriplegia (ie, paralysis affecting all four limbs) affect the transmission of neurologic signals involved in muscular movement. When impaired neurologic signals affect the muscles of respiration (eg, diaphragm, intercostal muscles), respiratory movements can be altered and make ventilating the lungs difficult. Chronic insufficient respiratory movements may lead to hypoventilation and improper blood levels of oxygen and carbon dioxide and induce dysfunction in the sensitivity of receptors that detect oxygen and carbon dioxide levels. People with neuromuscular disorders may consequently develop respiratory failure (ie, persistent abnormally low level of oxygen or abnormally high level of carbon dioxide) and sleep-related breathing disorders such as hypopnea and OSA. Severe oxygen desaturations and hypercapnia can occur, especially during REM sleep. In people with neuromuscular disease, low nocturnal levels of oxygen may contribute to nocturnal or morning headache, and disrupted sleep may contribute to daytime sleepiness.

METABOLISM

Metabolism is the sum of all physical and chemical processes in a living organism that maintain its various physiologic activities (eg, respiration) and provide energy. Metabolism can be affected by a person's nutrition: the consumption of foods containing the proper amounts of carbohydrates, fats, proteins, vitamins, and minerals. Improper amounts of these substances can result in malnutrition.

The liver has important roles in metabolism. For example, the liver secretes bile, which breaks fat molecules into smaller molecules; it synthesizes and releases into the bloodstream protein molecules such as albumin; and it stores minerals such as iron and certain vitamins such as vitamins A, D, and K.

The pancreas also has an important role in metabolism. It synthesizes insulin and glucagon. The opposing effects of these hormones normally maintain proper blood glucose levels.

Metabolism consists of two components: catabolism (ie, the breakdown of large molecules into smaller molecules) and anabolism (ie, the buildup of large molecules from smaller molecules). Catabolism releases energy, whereas anabolism requires energy. Carbohydrates, fats, proteins, vitamins, and minerals undergo metabolism in the following ways.

Carbohydrate Metabolism

Carbohydrates are molecules that are composed only of carbon, hydrogen, and oxygen atoms. A carbohydrate can be simple sugars such as glucose, fructose, galactose, or a starch (ie, a complex molecule composed of several sugar molecules). During digestion, simple sugars are absorbed from the small intestines and enter the bloodstream. The bloodstream transports the sugars through the hepatic portal vein into the liver. The sugars are converted into glucose. The glucose is then available for use by other body tissues.

The body's cells take carbohydrates into their cytoplasm (ie, the fluid surrounding a cell's nucleus). In the cytoplasm, carbohydrate molecules are broken down and release carbon dioxide and water as waste products.

Insulin facilitates the transfer of glucose through a cell's membrane (ie, it facilitates the uptake of glucose into the cell). This uptake removes glucose from the blood. If insulin is produced in insufficient amounts or if insulin receptors on the surface of a cell cannot respond to the effects of insulin correctly (ie, insulin resistance), glucose cannot enter the cell. The result is excess amounts of glucose remaining in the blood, a condition called "diabetes mellitus" (ie, diabetes type II).

In liver cells and in muscle cells, an excess amount of glucose is stored as glycogen, which is a large, branched molecule consisting of several glucose molecules joined together. The process of creating glycogen from glucose is called "glycogenesis." When the glucose level is low, liver cells break down glycogen into its glucose components. The breakdown of glycogen into glucose is called "glycolysis." If the available sources of glucose are depleted (eg, during starvation), glucose can be synthesized from noncarbohydrate sources such as fatty acids, amino acids, and glycerol. Fatty acids are a group of organic (ie, carbon-containing) molecules that are a constituent of fat. Amino acids are molecules that are the basic components of proteins. Amino acids are joined together in a unique sequence to form a specific protein. Glycerol is a sugar alcohol that is a constituent of many lipids (ie, fat and fat-like substances).

Fat Metabolism

In the process of digestion, fat molecules are broken down into fatty acids and glycerol. Three fatty acid molecules bind with a glycerol molecule to form a triglyceride molecule. Enzymes in the liver break down a triglyceride molecule into its glycerol and fatty acid components. However, some triglycerides are stored in fat tissue. A fatty acid must be bound with a blood plasma protein such as albumin to allow it to enter a cell.

Before a lipid (eg, cholesterol) can travel through the blood to a cell, it must be bound with a protein to form a lipoprotein. Lipoproteins are classed by their density (the greater the amount of protein, the denser the molecule). Three classes of lipoproteins are very low-density lipoprotein (VLDL), low-density lipoprotein (LDL), and high-density lipoprotein (HDL). Two other classes of lipoproteins are chylomicron (also called "ultra low-density lipoprotein"), which consist of 85% triglyceride, 13% lipid, and 2% protein and are less dense than the VLDL, and intermediate lipoproteins, which consist of approximately 24% to 30% triglyceride, 8% to 10% cholesterol, and 10% to 12% protein and have a density between that of VLDL and LDL.

A VLDL particle consists of approximately 60% triglyceride, 15% cholesterol, and 10% protein; an LDL particle consists of approximately 50% triglyceride, 50% cholesterol, and 25% protein, and an HDL particle consists of approximately 5% triglyceride, 20% cholesterol, and 50% protein. Lipoproteins transport cholesterol to the liver. The liver then breaks down lipoproteins into their lipid and protein constituents. LDL is often called "bad cholesterol" because of its high percentage of cholesterol. HDL is often called "good cholesterol" because of its lower percentage of cholesterol. In addition, LDL carries cholesterol from the liver to cells throughout the body (including the cells of blood vessels), whereas HDL carries cholesterol away from the body's cells to the liver for elimination. These actions contribute to the "bad" and "good" qualities of LDL and HDL, respectively.

The breakdown of fat occurs in the cytoplasm of cells. Once glycerol is separated from fatty acid molecules, glucose may be synthesized from the glycerol, depending on the body's needs. Mitochondria in a cell's cytoplasm break down fatty acids for energy.

A by-product of fat metabolism is the formation of ketone bodies, which comprise three organic molecules: acetone, β-hydroxybutyric acid, and acetoacetic acid. Ketone bodies can be used for energy when glucose levels are depleted. An excessive amount of ketone bodies in body tissues and fluids is a condition called "ketosis." Ketosis causes the body to become acidic. If left untreated, ketosis can lead to coma and death. Ketosis can occur in diabetics because the reduced level of insulin or insulin resistance results in an insufficient amount of glucose molecules entering the body's cells, although an excessive amount of glucose remains in the blood. The body senses a starvation state and begins to form glucose from fat tissue. During the process, ketone bodies are produced as a waste product. As a result of the excessive level of ketone bodies, a person may have a fruity smell to their body and breath. Other situations that can set the stage for ketosis are starvation (eg, anorexia nervosa) and a high-fat, low-protein diet.

The anabolism of fat (ie, fat storage) normally occurs if there is too much glucose in the blood. In this situation, glucose is converted to fatty acids. In the liver, the fatty acids are used to form triglycerides.

Protein Metabolism

In the gastrointestinal tract, protein molecules are broken down into amino acids. From the intestines, the amino acids are transported to the liver. In the liver, the amino acids may be reassembled into proteins or released into the bloodstream to be transported to other cells. In the cells, the amino acids are linked in specific sequences to form specific proteins. Some amino acids are used for energy. An amino acid may be essential (ie, it must be obtained from the diet) or nonessential (ie, it can be synthesized in the body, even if there is no dietary source).

Vitamin Metabolism

Vitamins generally act as coenzymes. They bind with a protein molecule to form an active enzyme. The active enzyme takes part in vital metabolic processes such as fatty acid production and energy expenditure. A vitamin can be fat or water soluble. A fat-soluble vitamin is absorbed with dietary fats. Vitamins A, D, E, and K are fat soluble. They are not normally excreted in the urine but instead are stored in the fat tissue in the body. Taking fat-soluble vitamins in excess can be toxic. A water-soluble vitamin is absorbed with water from the gastrointestinal tract. All B vitamins and vitamin C are water soluble. These vitamins are excreted in the urine and must be replaced daily through the diet. The vitamins have the following roles in metabolism.

Fat-Soluble Vitamins

Vitamin A is important for many biologic activities affected by metabolism such as bone growth, reproduction, immune response, and proper functioning of the retina. Vitamin D affects the utilization of calcium, which has a role in enzymatic processes involved in metabolism. Vitamin E is important in the formation of red blood cells, which carry oxygen to the body's tissues. Oxygen is then used in various metabolic processes. Vitamin K is needed for the production of some B vitamins.

Water-Soluble Vitamins

The B vitamins consist of several molecules. Some of the more commonly known B vitamins are vitamin B_1 (ie, thiamine), B_2 (ie, riboflavin), B_3 (ie, niacin), B_5 (ie, pantothenic acid), B_6 (ie, pyridoxine), B_{12} (ie, cyanocobalamin), biotin, and folic acid. Vitamins B_1, B_2, and B_3 are involved in energy expenditure at the cellular level. Vitamin B_5 aids the actions of enzymes that are involved in fat and carbohydrate metabolism. Vitamin B_6 aids the actions of enzymes that break down amino acids (eg, the degradation of tryptophan), is involved in the conversion of glycogen to glucose, and is involved in fat metabolism. Vitamin B_{12} is required for the synthesis of proteins. Biotin is involved in the degradation of amino acids and in the metabolism of fatty acids. Folic acid is involved in the breakdown of amino acids and energy expenditure in cells.

Vitamin C (also called "ascorbic acid") is needed for certain enzymes to function optimally. It improves the absorption of iron, a metallic element that has a role in energy expenditure in the cells and in the transport of oxygen to cells.

Mineral Metabolism

Inorganic elements (ie, minerals) are needed for various metabolic processes. Minerals are involved in a variety of physiologic processes, such as enhancing the activity of various enzymes and contributing to maintaining osmotic pressure in body fluids. Some minerals that are involved in metabolism are calcium, sodium, potassium, phosphorus, magnesium, iodine, sulfur, copper, cobalt, manganese, and zinc. These minerals have the following effects on metabolic processes.

Calcium and phosphorus have a role in many enzymatic processes involved in metabolism. Sodium and potassium have a role in protein synthesis, maintaining water balance in body tissues, and transporting molecules such as glucose across a cell membrane. Magnesium is a component of many enzymes involved in metabolism and is involved in the creation of energy in cells. Iodine is necessary for the formation of thyroid hormones (eg, thyroxine and triiodothyronine) that regulate the metabolic rate of all cells. Sulfur is used in the production of several amino acids and is a constituent of some vitamins such as thiamine, which is involved in carbohydrate metabolism. Copper is a constituent of many proteins and enzymes involved in metabolism. Cobalt is a constituent of vitamin B_{12}, which is needed for the synthesis of various proteins. Manganese activates a number of enzymes that are involved in metabolism. Zinc is a constituent of several enzymes involved with metabolism and has a role in protein synthesis.

Metabolism and Sleep Disorders

Faulty metabolism of carbohydrates, fats, proteins, minerals, and vitamins can negatively affect sleep. Two sleep disorders that may result from impaired metabolism are metabolic syndrome and RLS.

Metabolic Syndrome

Metabolic syndrome is a cluster of symptoms that reflect impaired metabolism. A person with metabolic syndrome has the following features: (1) fasting hyperglycemia (ie, excess blood sugar level) resulting from diabetes mellitus type II or from impaired glucose tolerance and/or insulin resistance; (2) high blood pressure; (3) overweight with abdominal obesity (ie, fat deposits primarily around the waist); (4) dyslipidemia (ie, improper levels of fat and fat-like substances in the blood) with a decreased HDL cholesterol level and an elevated triglyceride level. Obesity can increase the amount of fat tissue in the upper airway; therefore, a person with metabolic syndrome may be at greater risk of having sleep-disordered breathing, in particular OSA. Owing to frequent sleep disordered breathing–related arousals from sleep, people with metabolic syndrome who have OSA may struggle with sleepiness, inattentiveness, and other symptoms of insufficient sleep. In some people with metabolic syndrome, OSA may make it more difficult to control glucose levels and high blood pressure.

Restless Legs Syndrome

In a person with RLS, uncomfortable sensations in the legs begin in the evening soon before bedtime. For some people, the uncomfortable sensations affect the legs and the arms. To relieve such sensations, the person feels compelled to move the legs by walking, by rubbing them against the bed sheets, by stretching, or by other actions. The relief is short-lived, and a person must repeat the actions frequently to obtain relief. These efforts at relief can delay a person going to sleep at the desired time. The sensations drop out soon before or just at the onset of sleep. If a person awakens during the night, the same sensations may recur and thus delay the onset of sleep. A person with RLS may struggle with EDS because of disturbed sleep at night.

Why RLS occurs is unclear. For some people, the cause appears to be related to low levels of iron or improper utilization of iron (11,12). However, some people with RLS have normal iron levels. Iron-containing dopamine (D_2) receptors exist on the basal ganglia neurons. The basal ganglia are a collection of nuclei at the base of the brain. Some of these nuclei are involved in movement. Insufficient amounts of iron or the impaired metabolism of iron may therefore be involved in the uncomfortable sensations and irresistible urge to move the legs. Scientists continue to investigate the role of iron in RLS.

THERMOREGULATION

Thermoregulation is the maintenance of heat within a certain range. The maintenance of the body temperature between 97 °F (36.1 °C) and 100 °F (37.7 °C) is an example of thermoregulation. The maintenance of the body temperature results from the combination of heat production and heat loss. Heat production in the body is primarily a consequence of metabolism—much energy is released as food is broken down into molecules. Other factors such as muscle movement can produce heat in the body.

Four factors that can result in heat loss are radiation, evaporation, conduction, and convection. In radiation, heat is lost from the body in infrared waves to the external environment; in evaporation, heat-retaining water in sweat and exhaled air vaporizes, thereby drawing heat away from the body; in conduction, heat is directly transferred from the body through contact with an external object such as water or air; and in convection, atoms and molecules in contact with the body absorb heat from the body (ie, through conduction), but move away from the body, only to be replaced by more atoms and molecules that similarly absorb heat from the body. (Wind or water currents can enhance the process of convection.)

The hypothalamus is responsible for thermoregulation in the body. Certain neurons within the hypothalamus function as a thermostat. When the body temperature falls below a certain point (ie, the set point), blood flow to internal organs increases, whereas blood flow to extremities decreases. These actions conserve heat in the core of the body. When the body temperature rises above the set point, the opposite process occurs.

Temperature-sensing receptors in the skin (ie, peripheral thermal receptors) relay signals to temperature-sensing receptors in the hypothalamus (ie, central thermal receptors). Central thermal receptors in the hypothalamus are sensitive to temperature changes in the blood. The peripheral thermal receptors form a negative feedback loop with the central thermal receptors in the hypothalamus to maintain body temperature.

If the central thermal receptors sense that the blood is too hot, blood flow to the extremities increases, whereas blood flow to the internal organs decreases. At the skin, radiation, evaporation, conduction, and convection occur and reduce the temperature of the blood. The cooled blood then travels to the inner organs, thereby cooling them.

Fever-inducing chemicals, called "pyrogens" (from the Greek *pyro-* meaning "fire" and *gen-* meaning "to produce"), induce the hypothalamus to reset the set point to a higher level. As a result, a person with a fever will feel cold and the body will make efforts to conserve or produce body heat (eg, vasoconstriction of skin vessels and shivering). When the fever is over, other chemicals (eg, prostaglandins) act on the hypothalamus to reduce the set point. As a consequence, a person will feel hot, and the body will make efforts to reduce the body heat (eg, sweating and vasodilation of skin vessels).

Thermoregulation During Sleep

A person's core body temperature cycles in correlation with the sleep-wake rhythm. Core body temperature decreases during the sleep phase and increases during the wake phase. During sleep, thermoregulatory responses differ, depending on the sleep stage. As a consequence, when a person is exposed to an excessively cold or hot environment during sleep, responses such as shivering to increase body temperature or sweating to decrease body temperature are altered. For example, sensitivity to a hot or cold environment is reduced in REM sleep, compared with non-REM sleep and wakefulness. In a cold environment, shivering occurs during sleep stages N1 and N2 but not during slow-wave sleep or REM sleep, and sweating is increased in slow-wave sleep compared with other sleep stages, whereas the onset of sweating is delayed in REM sleep.

Such alterations in thermoregulation during sleep can affect sleep architecture when a person is exposed to an excessively hot or cold environmental temperature. For example, the duration of REM sleep and, to a lesser extent, slow-wave sleep decreases because a person awakens more easily when a room is excessively hot or cold.

With sleep onset, skin vessels vasodilate, which cools the blood. The cooled blood ultimately travels to the organs in the body, which lowers the core body temperature and further promotes sleep. Some scientists, therefore, believe that skin temperature rather than core body temperature may promote sleep. In addition, brain temperature decreases during slow-wave sleep but increases during REM sleep. To what extent brain temperature contributes to the thermosensitivity of the body during sleep is unclear.

Thermoregulation and Sleep Disorders

Shift Work/Frequently Changing Shifts

A person's core body temperature rises and falls according to a circadian rhythm, rising to its highest point during the evening from approximately 4:00 to 6:00 PM and falling to its lowest point during the night at approximately 4:00 AM. Attempting to sleep when the core body temperature is at its highest can lead to difficulty initiating and maintaining sleep (ie, insomnia), and attempting to remain awake when the body temperature is at its lowest may be difficult. Many physiologic processes such as melatonin secretion easily change their rhythms (ie, become entrained) to a new schedule somewhat quickly; however, the rhythmicity of core body temperature is not as easily entrained. When shifting to a new schedule, the core body temperature is one of the last biologic rhythms to become entrained (17). Because it takes a long time for body temperature to become entrained, one-third of shift workers may continue to struggle with sleepiness or insomnia at undesired times—even though the worker is carefully avoiding excessive exposure to daylight and maintaining a regular sleep-wake schedule.

Hot Flash

Some menopausal women experience the consequences of a sudden, temporary fluctuation in temperature control, commonly called a "hot flash." A hot flash is a heat dissipation response that begins with a sudden sense of warmth that is associated with sweating on the face, neck, and chest and peripheral vasodilation (eg, the face may become suddenly red). The sense of warmth is followed soon after by a sense of extreme cold that may be associated with shivering. A hot flash can occur during wake or during sleep (in which case a woman may awaken with her bedsheets drenched in sweat).

Hot flashes are often reported by menopausal women, leading to the common belief that they are related to low levels of estrogen. However, hot flashes can also occur in other stages of a woman's life (eg, during breastfeeding) when estrogen levels are still elevated. Some research also indicates that estrogen levels do not differ between symptomatic and asymptomatic menopausal women.

A logical assumption is that hot flashes are triggered by a sudden downward resetting of the hypothalamic set point because a woman's core body temperature does not increase during the episode. Hence, a woman would feel warm, although the environmental temperature does not change. Evidence obtained using telemetry pills (ie, an ingestible sensor that internally monitors physiologic phenomenon such as core body temperature) indicates that a small or no elevation in the core body temperature occurs immediately before or during a hot flash (18) and that the thermoneutral zone (ie, the range in which sweating, peripheral vasodilation, and shivering do not occur) is virtually nonexistent in symptomatic women. By contrast, the thermoneutral zone exists in asymptomatic women. The small temperature elevation occurring within a reduced thermoneutral zone may trigger a hot flash. Animal studies suggest that increased central sympathetic activation reduces the thermoneutral zone. Research has revealed that central sympathetic activation is elevated in women who have hot flashes.

Hot flashes can occur anytime. When experienced at night, they may disrupt sleep. Some women who have hot flashes during sleep awaken cold and with drenched sheets. These consequences can interrupt sleep—especially if she needs to change bedsheets after an episode or if she has several episodes during the night.

SUMMARY

Problems with sleep and wake are not limited to a dysfunction in the brain. As this chapter discussed, many factors in the function of the endocrine, renal, digestive, immune, genitourinary, and musculoskeletal systems, as well as metabolism and thermoregulation, can contribute to impaired sleep or wakefulness by impacting brain function or by other means.

REFERENCES

1. Berry RB, Wagner MH, Ryals SM. *Fundamentals of Sleep Medicine*. 2nd ed. Elsevier Health Sciences; 2025.
2. Lin L, Faraco J, Li R, et al. The sleep disorder canine narcolepsy is caused by a mutation in the hypocretin (orexin) receptor 2 gene. *Cell*. 1999;98:365-376. doi:10.1016/s0092-8674(00)81965-0
3. Thannickal TC, Moore RY, Nienhuis R, et al. Reduced number of hypocretin neurons in human narcolepsy. *Neuron*. 2000;27:469-474. doi:10.1016/s0896-6273(00)00058-1
4. Maski K, Mignot E, Plazzi G, Dauvilliers Y. Disrupted nighttime sleep and sleep instability in narcolepsy. *J Clin Sleep Med*. 2022;18:289-304. doi:10.5664/jcsm.9638

5. Zhang J, Qiu L, Liu Z, et al. Circadian light/dark cycle reversal exacerbates the progression of chronic kidney disease in mice. *J Pineal Res*. 2024;76:e12964. doi:10.1111/jpi.12964
6. Ansermet C, Centeno G, Nikolaeva S, Maillard MP, Pradervand S, Firsov D. The intrinsic circadian clock in podocytes controls glomerular filtration rate. *Sci Rep*. 2019;9:16089.
7. Johnston JG, Pollock DM. Circadian regulation of renal function. *Free Radic Biol Med*. 2018;119:93-107. doi:10.1016/j.freeradbiomed.2018.01.018
8. Ezzat H, Mohab A. Prevalence of sleep disorders among ESRD patients. *Ren Fail*. 2015;37:1013-1019.
9. Hariharan N, Chkhikvadze L, Mateshvili A, et al. Association of sleep problems with dialysis shifts in patients undergoing hemodialysis in Tbilisi, Georgia. *Cureus*. 2024;16:e63733. doi:10.7759/cureus.63733
10. Russcher M. *Circadian Rhythm Disturbances in End-stage Renal Disease*. Thesis. Vrije Universiteit Amsterdam; 2015. Accessed March 14, 2025. https://research.vu.nl/files/42141322/preliminary%20matter.pdf
11. Li J, Moore Ht, Lin L, et al. Association of low ferritin with PLM in the Wisconsin Sleep Cohort. *Sleep Med*. 2015;16:1413-1418. doi:10.1016/j.sleep.2015.05.015
12. Manconi M, Garcia-Borreguero D, Schormair B, et al. Restless legs syndrome. *Nat Rev Dis Primers*. 2021;7:80. doi:10.1038/s41572-021-00311-z
13. Boucsein A, Kamstra K, Tups A. Central signalling cross-talk between insulin and leptin in glucose and energy homeostasis. *J Neuroendocrinol*. 2021;33:e12944.
14. Goforth PB, Leinninger GM, Patterson CM, Satin LS, Myers MG Jr. Leptin acts via lateral hypothalamic area neurotensin neurons to inhibit orexin neurons by multiple gaba-independent mechanisms. *J Neurosci*. 2014;34:11405-11415.
15. Ge TT, Yao XX, Zhao FL, et al. Role of leptin in the regulation of food intake in fasted mice. *J Cell Mol Med*. 2020;24:4524-4532. doi:10.1111/jcmm.15110
16. Nasrullah A, Javed A, Ashraf O, Malik K. Possible role of COVID-19 in the relapse of Klein-Levin syndrome. *Respir Med Case Rep*. 2021;33:101445. doi:10.1016/j.rmcr.2021.101445
17. Reddy S, Reddy V, Sharma S. Physiology, circadian rhythm. In: *StatPearls* [Internet]. StatPearls Publishing; 2025. Updated May 1, 2023. Accessed March 14, 2025. https://www.ncbi.nlm.nih.gov/books/NBK519507
18. Bailey TG, Cable NT, Aziz N, et al. Exercise training reduces the acute physiological severity of post-menopausal hot flushes. *J Physiol*. 2016;594:657-667. doi:10.1113/JP271456

Chapter 8
Sleep Across the Life Cycle

NILA J. KAPPELY AND ANGELA P. NEAL

KEY CONCEPTS/LEARNING OBJECTIVES

The key concepts for this chapter include defining sleep, the characteristic aspects of normal sleep in different age groups, and the recommended amount of sleep for people from birth to old age.

KEY TERMS

Chronologic age
Conceptional age
Gestational age
Hypnogram
Phase advance
Phase delay
Sleep architecture
Sleep consolidation
Sleep cycle
Sleep regulation

Sleep is a vital component of health. Along with proper nutrition and physical activity, good sleep provides a foundation for physical and emotional wellness. For sleep to be "healthy," it needs to be of sufficient duration and timing, and without abnormalities or disturbances (1). Sleep technologists must be well versed in the nature of human sleep across the lifespan. This knowledge allows technologists to compare the sleep and sleep habits of patients studied to what is expected for their age group. Sleep health education is an important component of the sleep technologist's core job responsibilities. The role of the sleep technologist is expanding with a new focus on patient education and therapy management. Technologists with specific education and a certification in clinical sleep health are assuming a larger role in providing sleep hygiene and disease-specific education for patients with sleep disorders and assisting in the management of their therapies. Caring for patients at all levels includes a discussion of basic sleep health. Questions relating to sleep needs and basic sleep hygiene practices are routinely discussed in sleep centers, often during polysomnography hookup procedures. Every patient interaction is an opportunity for sleep technologists to enhance patient knowledge regarding the importance of sleep.

SLEEP CHARACTERISTICS

Sleep is a state of being unaware of and unresponsive to the outside world that is immediately reversible (2). Resting with eyes closed in a recumbent position in darkness may look like sleep, but there is no disconnection from the surroundings. Likewise, coma or a state of unconsciousness is not sleep. A person in a coma may be disconnected from the outside world as if asleep but cannot be immediately awakened. In the sleep center, sleep is identified by observation of a combination of behavioral, physiologic, and electroencephalographic (EEG) features. Sleep in people of all ages is classified into two states: rapid eye movement (REM) and non-REM (NREM) sleep. The rhythmic cycling of REM and NREM patterns, including wake, and the NREM stages of N1, N2, and N3, and REM throughout the course of the sleep period is referred to as sleep architecture. A visual graph of sleep architecture, called a hypnogram, provides an overview of the patient's night of sleep. Figure 8-1 demonstrates the sleep-stage hypnograms of three patients who underwent an in-laboratory polysomnogram. There are physiologic variables and EEG parameters specific to a certain state of sleep and wakefulness. Sleep stages are determined by assessing EEG, electrooculogram and electromyogram activities, and patient observation. The evaluation of these parameters will be discussed in detail in Chapter 76, Adult Sleep Scoring. Sleep is essential for the maintenance of brain and bodily functions in all age groups.

Sleep behaviors demonstrate great variability between individuals, cultures, societies, and geographic regions (3). They are affected by external factors such as parental beliefs, cultural traditions, socioeconomic status, work and school schedules, use of media, and education about sleep hygiene. Nevertheless, extensive sleep research makes it possible to understand and

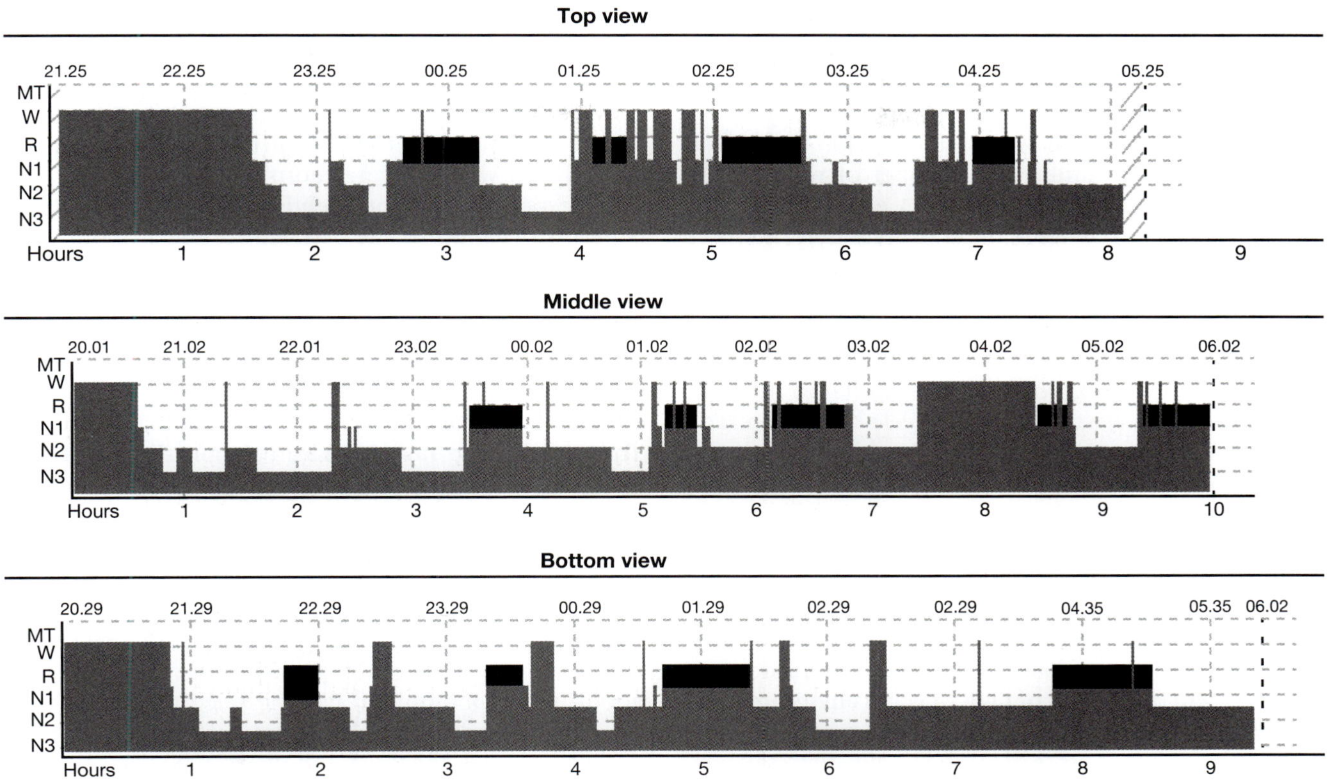

Figure 8-1 Three sleep-stage hypnograms.

predict sleep-wake patterns in different periods of the life cycle (3). The most noticeable age-related developments in sleep and sleep-wake rhythms take place around birth and during the first year of life. They include consolidation of sleep, reductions in the number and duration of naps, and changes in EEG. In the span of infancy through young childhood, sleep is considered particularly essential for development. By age 2, a child has spent about half of their life sleeping (2). Significant changes in sleep occur throughout the lifespan. See Figure 8-2 for the National Sleep Foundation's (NSF) recommended sleep duration requirements (4).

DEVELOPMENT OF SLEEP-WAKE PATTERNS IN INFANTS AND CHILDREN

Newborns: 0 to 3 Months

Full-term infants are those who are born between 39 and less than 41 weeks of gestation (5). The American Academy of Sleep Medicine (AASM) classifies infants as premature if less than 37 weeks' gestation, full-term if 37 to 42 weeks, and postterm if born after 42 weeks' gestation (6). Sleep technologists need to know and document three "ages" of their newborn patients: gestational,

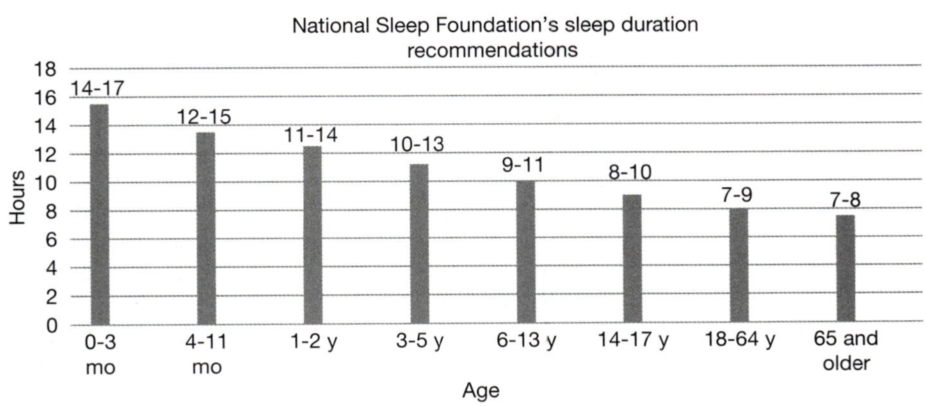

Figure 8-2 Recommended sleep durations.

conceptional, and chronologic. The term "gestational age" (GA) refers to the time from the first day of the mother's last menstrual period to the day of delivery, expressed in weeks. The conceptional age (CA) is the GA plus the number of weeks since birth. The baby's chronologic age is simply the number of weeks since birth. It is necessary to know the CA of newborns and infants in the sleep center in order to accurately interpret the EEG. The EEG characteristics of sleep differ based on conceptional, not chronologic age. A baby born 6 weeks ago is considered 6 weeks of chronologic age, but if born 9 weeks before term, will have a CA of 37 weeks. That infant's sleep patterns would appear similar to those of a newborn who was born at 37 weeks' gestation. For sleep-stage scoring purposes, the AASM identifies a patient from full-term birth to 2 months' chronologic age as newborn. For sleep study scoring purposes, the AASM uses the term neonate for a baby's first 28 days after birth, and infant at age 1 month to 1 year (6).

Full-term newborns sleep approximately 14 to 17 hours per day. Unfortunately for new parents, that sleep occurs in short bouts distributed throughout the day and night, regardless of light or other environmental cues. Bottle-fed babies tend to sleep for approximately 2 to 5 hours at a time versus breastfed babies, who sleep in 1- to 3-hour periods (7). Within the sleep period, sleep cycles occur in which the sleep state alternates between REM and NREM, lasting approximately 50 minutes. Interspersed are periods of wakefulness lasting between less than 1 and 2 hours. Sleep-wake cycles depend not so much on circadian rhythm, which is not fully developed at birth but on hunger and satiety (7) and comfort. An observer can recognize sleep visually, as the eyes remain closed, with noticeable squirming, sucking motions, and small body movements and twitches upon falling asleep. Newborns enter sleep through REM. At this age, approximately half the baby's sleep is REM, and the other half is NREM. Preterm infants have a higher percentage, as much as 80%, of REM sleep. Undisturbed sleep periods are vital to newborn development, and special care should be taken to preserve the natural sleep periods of the newborn. Particular attention should be paid to preterm babies in the neonatal intensive care area. These patients should have as few disruptions to their REM sleep as possible. Studies have shown that undisturbed sleep periods, when compared to unnaturally disturbed sleep periods, improve cognition in later development (8). There is wisdom in the old saying "never wake a sleeping baby," particularly in the first few months of life.

Issues related to sleep in newborns are often in association with congenital abnormalities or prematurity. Airway compromise with resulting hypoxia and hypercapnia may be seen. Sleep studies on patients in the neonatal intensive care unit are not uncommon. Sleep-disordered breathing is seen in this and all other age groups. Sudden infant death syndrome is most likely to occur between birth and 4 months post term. Digestive issues can create sleep-wake problems. Colic and gastroesophageal reflux are seen. Other issues relate to parental expectations of the newborn that are not aligned with their newborn's sleep behaviors. The NSF's expert panel recommends that babies in the 0- to 3-month age group sleep between 14 and 17 hours (4). Babies should sleep in a safe environment, supine, on a firm mattress, and without a pillow (7).

Infants: 4 to 11 Months

As infants develop, their sleep undergoes many changes. The overall sleep needs reduce to approximately 12 to 15 hours, although there is significant variation among infants. Sleep begins to consolidate at night, with longer nighttime sleep periods and shorter day sleeps. Sleep regulation, the infant's ability to self-soothe and fall asleep without assistance, often begins at about 3 months post term (7). Infants and young children with poor sleep regulation can be a source of great stress for parents. At about 3 to 4 months of age, the sleep cycles begin to increase in length, and the infant enters sleep through NREM, although the transition may not be complete until 8 months of age (9). About this time, EEG develops patterns that will be evident in childhood and beyond. These EEG changes allow for categorizing NREM sleep into three separate stages. Stage N1 is the light stage of sleep that usually occurs at sleep onset. This stage lasts only a few minutes before the infant transitions to stage N2. This stage of sleep is identified by the brain waves named K-complexes and sleep spindles. K-complexes generally appear beginning at 5 months post term, and sleep spindles become evident between 4 and 6 weeks post term. The initial cycle of stage N2 generally lasts from 5 to 25 minutes. Stage N3 sleep, also known as slow-wave sleep (SWS) or deep sleep, is identified electrographically by the predominance of high-voltage slow waves, which can first appear anywhere from 2 months post term to 5 months post term. Stage N3 usually lasts about 30 minutes. REM sleep appears in the infant EEG as low-voltage high-frequency waves. REMs occur, as do decreased muscle tone and the grimaces, twitches, and sucking motions previously mentioned. Between birth and age one, there is a reduction in the amount of REM sleep.

By about 6 months of age, infants should be sleeping through the night with longer periods of daytime wakefulness and shorter daytime naps. REM percentage decreases to about 30%. Many healthy infants have given up nighttime feedings at around 6 months of age. Continued nighttime feedings may result more from a learned behavior or parental preference than from hunger. By 1 year of age, overall sleep will likely be reduced by another hour, and naps may decrease from a total of 3 to 4 hours to 1 hour or less. The number of naps needed may be as few as one.

Issues with infants at this age include those associated within the first 3 months postterm, although the likelihood of sudden infant death syndrome is very low at age one. Nighttime awakenings and sleep-related rhythmic movement are also common around age 1. The NSF recommends that infants between 4 and 11 months of age sleep between 12 and 15 hours, including naps, with normal ranges of as few as 10 and as many as 18 hours of sleep (4). The AASM recommends that infants from 4 to 12 months of age sleep 12 to 16 hours for optimum health (1). Good sleep habits, including consistent bedtimes, bedtime routines, and putting the infant to bed drowsy, are important. Special items such as blankets or stuffed animals can help infants self-soothe and develop the ability to fall asleep on their own.

Toddlers: 1 to 2 Years

At this age, total sleep time averages 11 to 14 hours, including one or two naps of approximately 2 to 3 hours. By age 1, babies generally enter sleep via NREM sleep, which continues throughout the lifespan. Toddlers begin to develop signs of morningness or eveningness, in terms of their natural propensity for wakefulness, tiredness, and sleep times. The REM-NREM sleep cycle increases to 60 to 70 minutes. The proportion of REM to NREM sleep decreases to 30% between 1 and 2 years (9). Stage N3 sleep occupies much of NREM. During this stage of development, as parents can attest, sleep restriction or deprivation, even of a very short duration (missed afternoon nap), may create an inability to self-regulate, often resulting in a temper tantrum or inconsolable crying spell. Also at this age, sleep issues associated with moving from co-sleeping to independent sleeping or moving from crib to bed are common. Bedtime routines are important to develop to help with easy transition to sleep. Other issues can include problems with falling asleep, nighttime awakenings, and head-banging. Both the AASM and the NSF recommend a total sleep time of 11 to 14 hours in this age group, including naps, for optimal health (1,4). A range of as little as 10 hours and as much as 18 may be within normal.

Preschoolers: 3 to 5 Years

By ages 3 to 5, children sleep about an hour less than toddlers. Naps are reduced to one by age 3 and most likely eliminated by age 5. REM percentage continues to decline closer to the level of adulthood (20% to 25%), and the sleep cycle increases to 90 minutes. A significant portion of NREM sleep is stage N3, which is associated with a high arousal threshold. It can be difficult to awaken a child from SWS. Disorders of arousal, usually as a result of waking from SWS, include confusional arousals, sleepwalking, and sleep terrors. Other sleep issues that may arise for the first time in this age group are often a result of imagination and inability to distinguish fantasy from reality. Fear of monsters, ghosts, witches, and werewolves can create bedtime resistance and fearful awakenings. Increased language skills allow children to negotiate, stall, and challenge parents regarding bedtime rituals. Other issues at this age include nightmares and bedwetting, in addition to the sleep problems of infants and toddlers. Both the AASM and the NSF expert panels recommend 10 to 13 hours of sleep per 24-hour period, including naps (1,4).

School Age: 6 to 12 Years

In the period from about 5 years to puberty, nighttime sleep is typically a consistent 10 hours per night. With parental oversight, school routines often require early rise times, which is generally not a problem for grade-school-age children. They often wake by themselves and rise early even on nonschool days. Sleep propensity during the day is very low (10). Perhaps the term "sleeps like a baby" should be "sleeps like a grade schooler," because children of this age normally have boundless energy during the day and little trouble going to bed, falling asleep, and staying asleep at night. REM approaches adult proportions, and nearing puberty, stage N3 declines in amount and percentage. Throughout the childhood stage, N3 is prominent in the beginning of the night. Disorders common in the younger age groups also appear in school-age children, although battles over bedtime and requests for nighttime comforting to return to sleep may become less common. Other issues can include insufficient sleep from later bedtimes, sleep disruption from caffeine, and poor sleep hygiene. Restless legs syndrome, periodic limb movement disorder, and narcolepsy can also be seen. The AASM recommends between 9 and 12 hours of sleep, and the NSF recommends 9 to 11 hours for optimal health, with a range of as little as 7 to as much as 12 hours per night (1,4).

Teenagers: 13 to 18 Years

Sleep-wake schedules and total sleep times change dramatically in the teenage years. Around puberty, there is a significant phase delay: a shift in the sleep and wake times caused by circadian rhythm alteration. Where prepubertal children's circadian timing correlates well with early bedtimes and grade school start times, high school students tend to stay up later at night and have difficulty waking for school. This almost 2-hour shift causes a reduction in total sleep time, and increase in sleep debt, which is the difference between what is required to be fully rested and what is achieved. In addition to the biologic propensity to stay up late, many high school students have extracurricular activities, jobs, social lives, virtual lives on social media, and family obligations that make a reasonable bedtime difficult. Most students needing to be at a bus stop at 6 AM will accrue a large sleep debt. Children 13 to 18 years old need about 8 to 10 hours of sleep per night. The sleep debt that builds up during the week, along with staying up extra late on Friday and Saturday nights, often creates very late rise times on Saturday and Sunday. Although the sleep debt may be partially repaid on the weekend, there is difficulty falling asleep on Sunday night. Then the weekly cycle begins again. The student is required to rise early, against their natural tendency, until the weekend. As parents can attest, high school students tend to be sleepy, mopey, groggy, and crabby in the morning, yet have a "second wind" in the late evening, making an early bedtime even more difficult.

Sleep-stage changes occur across adolescence. In addition to a decrease in total sleep time by about an hour, there is a significant decrease in SWS. Sleep efficiency may decrease because it can be difficult to fall asleep at bedtime (prolonged sleep latency). Although total sleep time recommended for optimal health by both the AASM and the NSF is 8 to 10 hours, with a normal range of 7 to 11 hours (1,4), many in this age group get less sleep. A host of issues related to insufficient sleep may occur, including drowsy driving, psychomotor impairment, and behavioral issues such as moodiness, lack of motivation, and poor judgment (7). Sleep disorders that may appear in this age group include delayed sleep-wake phase disorder and insomnia, in addition to the disorders associated with younger children.

SLEEP AND WAKE IN YOUNG AND MIDDLE-AGED ADULTS

Young and middle-aged adults with no sleep problems sleep on average 7 to 9 hours per night. A typical night consists of a fairly short sleep latency, a few minutes of N1, progressing to N2 and N3 sleep, followed by the first REM period about 90 minutes after falling asleep. This ultradian (occurs rhythmically more than once per day) pattern repeats itself every 90 to 110 minutes, with less N3 as the night progresses but longer REM periods. Healthy sleepers will have a sleep efficiency (the percentage of time in bed asleep) of over 90%. REM occupies 20% to 25% of sleep, occurring in four to six discrete episodes (11). As adults reach middle age, their total sleep time decreases by about an hour. The N3 sleep percentage continues to decline throughout adulthood and into old age. Men have a more pronounced decrease in SWS than women. Studies show that both hormones, the phases of the menstrual cycle, and menopause can significantly impact sleep, a topic explored further in Chapter 9, Sleep and Women. Prolonged work hours, stress, and family obligations often lead to self-imposed sleep restriction, resulting in decreased total sleep time. Chronic medical conditions that develop in adulthood may negatively impact sleep. The incidence of many adult sleep disorders increases in this age group. Chronic medical conditions impact the quantity and quality of sleep and the prevalence of sleep disorders, particularly toward middle age. As a person's overall wellness declines, even in the absence of a diagnosed condition, sleep is affected. Insufficient physical activity, obesity, alcohol, marijuana, and cigarette consumption can negatively impact sleep.

Sleep and Aging

Sleep patterns continue to change in older adults. The NSF defines older adults as those 65 and over. A pronounced loss of N3, particularly in men, occurs. By age 70, men have approximately 5.5% N3, whereas women have about 17% N3 sleep (12,13). REM also decreases, but only by 2% to 3% from middle age (12,13). An increase in N1 sleep occurs, as does the incidence of arousals and awakenings from sleep. Sleep efficiency decreases from greater than 90% in early adulthood to about 79% in those over 70 (12,13). The older adults experience increased difficulty with phase shifting. Bedtime and rise times tend to remain fairly constant, but when traveling or changing bedtimes, sleep becomes difficult. Napping is common, which may interfere with nighttime sleep. Phase advancing, causing early bed and rise times, is prevalent. Newspapers are often delivered in over 55 communities by 5 AM to avoid customer complaints. Older adults often spend more hours in bed than needed, reducing sleep efficiency and leading to sleep complaints. Incidence of sleep disorders is high in this population. Insomnia and sleep-related breathing disorders are prevalent, as are restless legs syndrome and periodic limb movement disorder. Common chronic conditions such as heart disease, chronic obstructive pulmonary disease (COPD), diabetes, Alzheimer disease, dementia, attention deficit disorder (ADD), attention-deficit/hyperactivity disorder (ADHD), depression, and generalized anxiety disorder (GAD) negatively impact sleep and contribute to sleep disorders. Medications to treat these conditions may also disturb sleep. Chronic pain causes short sleep durations and fragmented sleep. The NSF recommends 7 to 8 hours of sleep for optimal health for older adults (2).

SUMMARY

Sleep begins in fetal life and changes throughout the lifespan. The first year of life sees many changes, both in the wake and in the sleep patterns of babies. At birth, babies spend the majority of a 24-hour period asleep, in short bouts of sleep interspersed with short periods of wakefulness. As infants age, sleep consolidates, the sleep cycle lengthens, and a clear day-night pattern emerges. Sleep patterns and needs continue to change, particularly in adolescence and throughout teenage years, when intrinsic phase delays often conflict with early school start times. Sleep in the middle-aged, and certainly in the older population, can be of sufficient duration and quality but is often disturbed by underlying chronic conditions and physiologic changes associated with aging.

Patients often ask their sleep technologist about sleep quality and quantity. An understanding of the sleep needs, patterns, and cycles of patients throughout the lifespan prepares technologists to advise patients on their sleep needs and behaviors. The importance of a good night's sleep cannot be overemphasized.

REFERENCES

1. Paruthi S, Brooks LJ, D'Ambrosio C, et al. Recommended amount of sleep for pediatric populations: a consensus statement of the American Academy of Sleep Medicine. *J Clin Sleep Med*. 2016;12(6):785-786.
2. Dement W. *The Promise of Sleep*. Random House; 1999.
3. Jenni OG, Carskadon MA. Sleep behavior and sleep regulation from infancy through adolescence: normative aspects. *Sleep Med Clin*. 2007;2:321-329.
4. Hirshkowitz M, Whiton K, Albert SM, et al. National Sleep Foundation's sleep time duration recommendations: methodology and results summary. *Sleep Health*. 2015;1:40-43.
5. American College of Obstetricians and Gynecologists. Committee opinion no. 579: definition of term pregnancy. *Obstet Gynecol*. 2013;122:1139-1140.
6. Troester MM, Quan SF, Berry RB, et al; for the American Academy of Sleep Medicine. *The AASM Manual for the Scoring of Sleep and Associated Events: Rules, Terminology and Technical Specifications. Version 3*. American Academy of Sleep Medicine; 2023.
7. Mindell J, Owens J. *Pediatric Sleep*. Wolters Kluwer; 2015:9-36.
8. Weisman O, Magori-Cohen R, Louzoun Y, et al. Sleep-wake transitions in premature neonates predict early development. *Pediatrics*. 2011;128:706-714.
9. Sheldon SH, Ferber R, Kryger H. *Principles and Practice of Pediatric Sleep Medicine*. Elsevier; 2005:56.
10. Carskadon MA, Keenan S, Dement WC. Nighttime sleep and daytime sleep tendency in preadolescents. In: Guilleminault C, ed. *Sleep and Its Disorders in Children*. Raven Press; 1987:43-52.
11. Carskadon MA, Dement WC. Monitoring and staging human sleep. In: Kryger MH, Roth T, Dement WC, eds. *Principles and Practice of Sleep Medicine*. 5th ed. Elsevier Saunders; 2011:16.
12. Bliwise DL. Normal aging. In: Kryger MH, Roth T, Dement WC, eds. *Principles and Practice of Sleep Medicine*. 4th ed. Elsevier Saunders; 2005:24-36.
13. Garbarino S. Sleep disorders across the lifespan: a different perspective. *Int J Environ Res Public Health*. 2020;17(23):9025. doi:10.3390/ijerph17239025

Chapter 9
Sleep and Women

ELIZABETH Y. WIESEMANN

KEY CONCEPTS/LEARNING OBJECTIVES

The key concepts for this chapter include identifying key differences between females and males in sleep disorders, recognizing the hormonal impacts on sleep across the female lifespan, understanding sleep disorder treatment responses for females, knowing accommodations to make for female patients in the sleep lab, and recognizing the critical need for further research on women and sleep.

KEY TERMS

Cognitive Behavioral Therapy for Insomnia (CBT-I)
Endometriosis
Estradiol
Gonadotropin-releasing hormone (GnRH)
Insomnia
Luteinizing hormone (LH)
Menopausal hormone therapy (MHT)
Menopause
Perimenopause
Postmenopause
Postpartum
Pregnancy
Progesterone
Puberty

Sleep is a fundamental physiologic process essential for optimal well-being, profoundly affecting physical and mental health, as well as cognitive and brain function (1,2). In contemporary society, the increasing prevalence of sleep disturbances presents significant public health challenges (1). A critical area of focus within sleep medicine is the distinct landscape of women's sleep health, which exhibits notable sex differences in sleep patterns, perceived sleep quality, and the manifestation of sleep disorders compared to men (1,3). These disparities arise from a complex interplay of biologic, physiologic, psychological, and socioecological factors unique to women across their lifespan (4,5).

Despite objective measures such as polysomnography (PSG) or actigraphy often indicating comparable or even superior sleep efficiency, shorter sleep-onset latency, and longer total sleep time in women, there is a consistent and paradoxical trend: women frequently report more subjective sleep complaints and dissatisfaction (3,5).

This discrepancy between objective sleep metrics and subjective experience is not merely a "complaint" but signifies a fundamental difference in how sleep health is perceived and experienced by women. The subjective experience of sleep quality is deeply influenced by a confluence of factors unique to women, including hormonal fluctuations, the presence of chronic pain, psychological states such as anxiety and depression, and the cumulative burden of social and occupational roles (4–6). These factors can lead to a persistent feeling of unrefreshing or inadequate sleep, even when underlying sleep architecture appears within conventional objective parameters.

This divergence between objective findings and subjective reports presents a significant clinical challenge. Overreliance on objective data alone risks overlooking genuine patient distress and failing to identify the multifaceted issues contributing to perceived poor sleep. Such an oversight can lead to delayed or missed diagnoses, particularly for conditions where subjective symptoms are prominent, such as insomnia. Furthermore, a patient's perception of poor sleep can exacerbate psychological distress, creating a negative feedback loop that further impairs overall well-being.

For sleep technologists, understanding this dynamic is paramount. It emphasizes that a woman reporting "poor sleep" warrants thorough investigation, irrespective of initial objective findings. This necessitates a shift toward a comprehensive biopsychosocial assessment model in clinical practice, prioritizing detailed history taking that includes inquiries about perceived sleep quality, daytime functioning, mood, pain, and life stressors. Such an approach empowers technologists to advocate for further specialized investigations or tailored interventions, even when objective data may seem unremarkable.

Before 1993, women were very rarely included in clinical trials in the United States, so much so that in 1977, the U.S. Food and Drug Administration (FDA) created a guideline to exclude women of reproductive age from participating in early stages of clinical research, except for life-threatening conditions. This decision was not reversed until 1993, when the United States Congress passed a law requiring the inclusion of women in National Institutes of Health sponsored clinical trials. In 1994, the United States Federal Drug and Drug Administration established the Office of Women's Health to promote the inclusion of women in clinical trials and advance women's health care. In research conducted by Harvard Medical School, it is shown that as of 2019, women are still substantially underrepresented in clinical trials for major diseases (7). In 2025, the American Academy of Sleep Medicine (AASM) launched a task force aimed at promoting sleep health in women. Their goal is to increase awareness of women's health issues and increase funding opportunities for research focused on including women.

The unique biologic and psychosocial factors affecting women necessitate a gender-specific approach to assessment, diagnosis, and treatment in sleep medicine (2,3). A failure to acknowledge these differences can result in the underdiagnosis, misdiagnosis, and suboptimal management of sleep disorders in women (3,8). This chapter aims to equip sleep technologists with specialized knowledge to more effectively serve female patients, recognizing their unique vulnerabilities and symptom presentations (2,3).

APPROACHES TO ACQUIRING SLEEP STUDIES IN WOMEN

Acquiring accurate sleep study data in women presents unique challenges, often leading to underdiagnosis or delayed treatment, particularly for conditions like obstructive sleep apnea (OSA). A significant disparity exists in PSG referrals, with men being referred twice as often as women (9). This difference is largely attributed to lower awareness of sleep disorders in women, as men are more frequently referred due to abnormal observations by their bed partner (13.3% of men vs 6.9% of women) (9). Traditional screening questionnaires for OSA, which often rely on classic male symptoms like loud snoring and witnessed apneas, are less sensitive in identifying OSA in women due to their atypical symptom presentation (3).

When evaluating women for sleep disorders, clinicians must be aware of these gender-specific differences. Women with OSA often present with nonspecific symptoms such as fatigue, insomnia, mood disturbance, nocturia, and poor sleep quality, rather than overt snoring or excessive daytime sleepiness (3,10). Consequently, a comprehensive clinical history that probes these less obvious symptoms is critical (3).

Polysomnographic data also exhibit gender differences. While men typically show higher total apnea-hypopnea index (AHI) values, women often have a lower total AHI but a higher REM-AHI (apnea-hypopnea index during rapid eye movement sleep) (3,10). Notably, the REM-AHI may not differ significantly between sexes, even when the total AHI is lower in women, highlighting its importance in evaluating OSA severity in female patients (3,10). This suggests that a focus solely on total AHI might underestimate the severity of OSA in women. Furthermore, women generally exhibit better sleep quality parameters during PSG, including higher total sleep time, sleep efficiency, and percentage of REM sleep, even when diagnosed with OSA (10).

Beyond PSG, other methods are valuable for assessing sleep in women. Actigraphy and sleep diaries can provide insights into sleep patterns, movement, and fragmentation in the home environment over extended periods (11). These tools are particularly useful for midlife women who may experience sleep disturbances due to pain or nocturnal vasomotor symptoms (VMS), as they can objectively capture less efficient sleep and self-reported less restful sleep (11). The use of wearable electronics is also increasing, allowing for more representative measurements of sleep in the home environment and enabling women to self-diagnose sleep disorders (4). Higher day-to-day variability in sleep onset and duration has been associated with longer time to achieving pregnancy in women, highlighting the utility of actigraphy in reproductive health contexts.

Ultimately, the approach to acquiring sleep study data in women must be tailored to their unique physiologic and symptomatic profiles. This involves a heightened awareness among clinicians and technologists of atypical presentations, a willingness to utilize a broader range of diagnostic tools, and a focus on interpreting results with a gender-specific lens (2,3).

SEX DIFFERENCES IN SLEEP DISORDERS

Sleep disorders manifest differently between men and women, affecting prevalence and symptom presentation. Recognizing these sex differences is crucial for accurate diagnosis and effective management (Table 9-1).

Insomnia is consistently reported at higher rates in women across the lifespan compared to men (1,3,6,12,13). While objective measures of sleep often show women having better sleep efficiency, shorter sleep-onset latency, and longer total sleep time, women paradoxically report more sleep problems, dissatisfaction, and difficulty maintaining sleep (5,10). This suggests that factors beyond basic sleep architecture contribute to the subjective experience of poor sleep

Table 9-1 Key Sex Differences in Sleep Disorders

Sleep Disorder	Prevalence in Women vs Men	Typical Symptom Presentation in Women	Typical Symptom Presentation in Men
Insomnia	Consistently higher in women across the lifespan (1,3,6,10,12).	Difficulty initiating/maintaining sleep, poor sleep quality, fatigue, mood disturbance, higher presleep arousal, perceived severity (1,5,6,12).	Less frequent, more likely to hold false beliefs about insomnia; cope with poor health behaviors (5).
Obstructive sleep apnea (OSA)	Less common in premenopausal women than men, but prevalence doubles postmenopausally, becoming comparable to men (3)	Fatigue, insomnia, mood disturbance, nocturia, impaired memory, morning headache, reflux, enuresis; less prominent snoring (3,10). Often symptomatic at lower AHI values (3)	Loud snoring, witnessed apneas, excessive daytime sleepiness (9,10)
Restless legs syndrome (RLS)	Slight female predominance (3)	Leg discomfort, urge to move legs, often worse in evening/night, relieved by movement (3)	Leg discomfort, urge to move legs, often worse in evening/night, relieved by movement (3)
REM sleep behavior disorder (RBD)	More common in men (3)	Sleep talking, dream enactment (3)	Acting out dreams, often violent (3)
Central sleep apnea (CSA)	High-loop-gain CSA more common in men (3). OHS with lone hypoventilation more common in women (3)	OHS with lone hypoventilation more common (3)	High-loop-gain CSA (eg, Cheyne-Stokes respiration) more common (3). Stronger ventilatory response to arousal (3)

AHI, apnea-hypopnea index; OHS, obesity hypoventilation syndrome.

quality in women, including higher presleep arousal and a greater perceived severity of their sleep issues (5).

OSA presents a distinct gendered pattern. While OSA is generally more prevalent in men, its prevalence in women doubles after menopause, becoming comparable to that in men (3). This shift is partly attributed to the decline in protective ovarian sex hormones, such as progesterone, which influences upper airway stability and ventilation (3,4). Crucially, women with OSA often present with atypical symptoms that differ from the classic male presentation. They are frequently symptomatic at lower AHI values and report symptoms such as sleep fragmentation, poor sleep quality, insomnia, fatigue, mood disturbances, and nocturia, rather than loud snoring or excessive daytime sleepiness (3,10). This atypical symptom profile contributes to the underdiagnosis of OSA in women (3). Polysomnographic findings also vary; women with OSA may have a lower total AHI and non-REM-AHI compared to men, but their REM-AHI is typically higher and may not differ significantly from that of men (3,10). This highlights the importance of considering REM-AHI in women's OSA evaluation. Women also tend to have a lower collapsibility of the upper airway and a lower arousal threshold compared to men, which can lead to more respiratory-related arousals and symptoms of disturbed sleep (3).

Restless legs syndrome (RLS) shows a slight female predominance, and its prevalence may be linked to fluctuations in dopamine levels (3). In contrast, REM sleep behavior disorder (RBD) and high-loop-gain central sleep apnea (CSA) are more common in men (3). Men also exhibit a stronger ventilatory response to arousal, predisposing them to postarousal central apneas. However, obesity-related hypoventilation syndrome (OHS) with lone hypoventilation (without relevant OSA) is more common in women, and its prevalence increases after menopause (3).

SLEEP ACROSS THE FEMALE LIFESPAN

Sleep patterns and health are dynamically influenced by the distinct physiologic and hormonal changes that occur across a woman's lifespan. Understanding these transitions is crucial for comprehensive sleep care.

ADOLESCENCE

Adolescence represents a pivotal developmental stage marked by the maturation of sleep regulatory systems. However, this biologic maturation frequently conflicts with psychosocial and societal pressures, resulting in insufficient and mistimed sleep for many young individuals. Adolescents typically experience a delayed shift in their intrinsic circadian rhythmic system, pushing their natural alertness and preferred bedtimes later into the evening and night (14). Concurrently, societal demands, particularly early school start times, often necessitate earlier wake-up times on school nights, leading to chronic sleep restriction and irregular sleep schedules, with compensatory longer sleep durations on weekends (14).

Pubertal changes in sleep behavior coincide with a significant decline in deep (slow-wave) sleep and its electroencephalographic (EEG) correlate, delta spectral power (14). This decline commences around ages 11 to 12 years and persists until 16.5 years, notably occurring approximately 1 year earlier in girls than in boys, suggesting a potential role for sex hormones in driving these changes (14). The increase in pulsatile luteinizing hormone (LH) secretion, a key indicator of pubertal onset, is initially restricted to sleep and occurs during or immediately following N3 sleep, indicating that entry into N3 sleep may stimulate gonadotropin-releasing hormone (GnRH) and LH secretion during puberty (14). Research further indicates that girls with OSA who exhibit abnormal sleep architecture may experience relatively delayed thelarche (breast development) compared to girls without OSA, emphasizing the potential impact of poor sleep hygiene on the developing reproductive axis (14). Earlier pubic hair development in girls has been associated with later bedtimes or shorter sleep duration, with adrenal androgens hypothesized to play a role in these maturational sleep changes (14). A systematic review and meta-analysis found a significant inverse association between longer sleep duration and a lower risk of early puberty, an association that may be modified by other factors such as body mass index (15).

This evidence points to a complex, dynamic feedback loop between sleep, hormones, and pubertal development. Adequate, high-quality sleep, particularly deep sleep, appears to be a physiologic prerequisite or facilitator for optimal hormonal signaling during puberty. Conversely, the hormonal shifts of puberty, especially adrenal androgens, seem to inherently influence sleep architecture, such as the observed decline in deep sleep. Disruptions to sleep, including those caused by sleep disorders like OSA, could interfere with this delicate hormonal balance, potentially affecting the timing and progression of pubertal development. The association between longer sleep duration and a lower risk of early puberty suggests a regulatory or protective role of sleep in developmental timing, implying that insufficient sleep might accelerate pubertal onset in some contexts. Thus, chronic sleep disruption or restriction during adolescence could directly interfere with the neuro-reproductive axis, potentially delaying or altering pubertal development. Conversely, the physiologic changes inherent to puberty can inherently alter sleep patterns, making adolescents more vulnerable to sleep phase delays and insufficient sleep. This creates a reinforcing cycle where poor sleep can negatively affect development, and developmental changes can make healthy sleep more challenging.

Clinicians working with adolescent patients must be acutely aware of these intricate developmental and hormonal sensitivities. Beyond assessing for common sleep disorders, they should consider the potential reciprocal impact of sleep on pubertal progression and vice versa. Early identification and intervention for sleep problems in adolescent girls could have significant positive impacts on their long-term reproductive health, mental well-being, and overall physiologic development, extending beyond immediate sleep improvements. This also highlights the need for interdisciplinary collaboration with pediatric endocrinologists and gynecologists.

The accumulated sleep debt and associated daytime sleepiness in adolescents have profound implications for mental health and well-being (13). Sleep deprivation has been shown to increase worry in younger adolescents, indicating an increased vulnerability to elevated anxiety when sleep-deprived (13). Furthermore, short sleep duration and later parent-set bedtimes are associated with higher levels of perceived stress, mood disturbance, suicidal ideation, unhappiness, interpersonal problems, poor perceived health, school absence due to illness, and fatigue in adolescent populations (13).

REPRODUCTIVE YEARS

During the reproductive years, sleep is significantly influenced by the menstrual cycle, with women often reporting better subjective sleep quality during their follicular and ovulatory phases compared to the late luteal and premenstrual phases (4). Progesterone and its metabolites are generally associated with sleep-promoting effects. A steep decline in progesterone, such as that occurring during the late luteal phase, is consistently linked to sleep disruption, increased wakefulness after sleep onset, and brief arousals (4). In contrast, endogenous estrogen levels show no clear or consistent correlation with sleep alterations during the menstrual cycle (4).

Women are generally more susceptible to psychological and sleep difficulties, with insomnia disorder being notably more prevalent in women than men (1,6,9,12). This higher prevalence is attributed to a combination of biologic factors, including hormonal differences and changes across a woman's life, and psychosocial factors, such as anxiety, depression, and stress related to gender role expectations (6).

Endometriosis, a chronic gynecologic disease characterized by ectopic endometrial-like tissue causing chronic pain and infertility, profoundly impacts psychological health, leading to increased stress, fatigue, and mental health disorders (6). Crucially, endometriosis is strongly associated with significant sleep disturbances, including poor sleep quality, excessive daytime sleepiness, and insomnia (6). The high prevalence of sleep difficulties in women with endometriosis is often attributed to the interplay of hormonal fluctuations, mood disorders, and the chronic pain associated with gynecologic dysfunction (6). There is a bidirectional association between sleep health and psychological well-being in women with endometriosis, where pain and anxiety symptoms are also bidirectionally linked (6).

The evidence clearly demonstrates a complex, multifactorial etiology where chronic pain, hormonal dysregulation (inherent to or exacerbated by conditions like endometriosis), and psychological distress (anxiety, depression) do not act in isolation but in a synergistic, perpetuating cycle that severely impairs sleep. The bidirectional association between sleep health and psychological well-being is a key mechanism in this dynamic. The constant presence of pain and the physiologic stress it induces can directly disrupt sleep architecture. This sleep disruption, in turn, can lower pain thresholds, worsen mood disorders, and diminish coping mechanisms, making the individual more vulnerable to the overall burden of their condition. Without addressing the underlying gynecologic condition, the chronic pain, and the psychological distress, sleep interventions alone may be insufficient or only provide temporary relief. Sleep complaints in women of reproductive age, particularly those with chronic pelvic pain or gynecologic conditions, are often deeply rooted in a complex interplay of physical and mental health factors. A thorough medical history, extending beyond typical sleep questions to include menstrual health, pain history, and mental health screening, is crucial. This information aids in identifying potential underlying conditions like endometriosis and advocates for integrated care with gynecologists, pain specialists, and mental health professionals, ensuring a truly holistic approach to patient management.

PREGNANCY AND POSTPARTUM

Pregnancy and the postpartum period are times of profound physiologic and emotional change, consistently associated with frequent sleep disruption (4). As pregnancy progresses, sleep quality worsens and duration shortens, largely due to physiologic factors such as increased nocturnal micturition, gastroesophageal reflux, and musculoskeletal discomfort (4). Pregnancy is also recognized as a risk factor for the development or aggravation of sleep-disordered breathing and RLS (4).

During pregnancy, sleep disruption appears to be more strongly associated with these changing physiologic factors than with absolute changes in estrogen or progesterone levels, which may mask any direct hormonal effects on sleep (4). However, progesterone may offer a protective role against OSA in pregnant women (4). After childbirth, the sharp decrease in progesterone postpartum was not found to be directly related to changes in REM sleep (4).

Poor sleep quality during both pregnancy and the postpartum period is a significant and consistent risk factor for the development of postpartum depression (PPD) and is strongly associated with increased symptoms of depression and anxiety (16,17). Observational studies indicate that high-quality sleep reduces the odds of developing anxiety and lessens the severity of depression and anxiety symptoms in the postpartum period (17). A longitudinal study revealed that less stable maternal sleep, characterized by higher sleep variability, is associated with lower maternal sensitivity during mother-infant interactions. This association was particularly noted among mothers with high levels of social support, highlighting the importance of sleep stability (18).

This finding suggests that for mothers whose basic needs for support are met, the subtle effect of fragmented or unstable sleep on higher order cognitive and emotional functions, such as maternal sensitivity, becomes more apparent and impactful. In environments with strong social support, the lack of sleep stability might be a more direct and unmasked determinant of a mother's capacity for sensitive interactions. Conversely, for mothers with low social support, the overwhelming stressors of their environment might obscure the specific link between sleep stability and sensitivity, or their sleep might be so universally poor that this specific relationship is less discernible.

This highlights that "good sleep" for a new mother is not only about total hours but also about its consistency and restorative quality. Unstable or fragmented sleep, even if total duration is seemingly adequate, can impair a mother's executive functions, emotional regulation, and attentional resources. This impairment directly affects her ability to respond sensitively and consistently to her infant's cues. Social support, while generally protective, might create a context where mothers have the mental and emotional bandwidth to experience and manifest the effects of sleep instability more acutely in their interactions, or it might be that in the presence of support, sleep stability becomes the key limiting factor for optimal maternal functioning. Sleep technologists should expand their assessment of postpartum women beyond just sleep duration and perceived quality to include inquiries about sleep stability and fragmentation.

Furthermore, understanding the patient's social support context is crucial for interpreting sleep complaints and tailoring interventions. Interventions should not only aim for increased sleep quantity but also prioritize strategies that promote more consistent and stable sleep. This also suggests that while social support is vital, it does not negate the direct need for effective sleep interventions to optimize maternal well-being and mother-infant bonding. Systematic reviews and meta-analyses demonstrate that postpartum sleep interventions effectively reduce the severity of depressive symptoms (16,17). These interventions, often nonpharmacologic, represent a potential low-cost, nonpharmacologic strategy for the prevention and treatment of postpartum mental illness (16). Shorter sleep duration in the postpartum period has also been associated with greater postpartum weight retention (17).

MENOPAUSE AND POSTMENOPAUSE

The menopausal transition is a period of heightened vulnerability to sleep difficulties due to significant hormonal shifts, particularly declining estrogen and progesterone levels (4). These hormonal changes are often accompanied by VMS such as hot flashes and night sweats, increased prevalence of mood disorders, and age-related disruptions to circadian rhythm, all of which contribute to sleep disturbances (4,11). The risk of sleep-disordered breathing, especially OSA, also significantly increases after menopause (4). The prevalence of OSA doubles postmenopausally, becoming comparable to that observed in men (9). This increase is partly attributed to the decrease in protective ovarian sex hormones, particularly progesterone, which has sleep-promoting effects and influences upper airway stability (4,9). Declining or low progesterone levels during the menopausal transition are strongly associated with sleep disturbances, including increased arousals and more wake after sleep onset (4). Low estradiol levels are linked to lower sleep efficiency, increased sleep-disordered breathing, and frequent movement arousals (4). Importantly, fluctuations and the rate of change in estrogen levels, rather than just absolute levels, are also associated with sleeping problems (4). Follicle-stimulating hormone (FSH) levels are significantly higher in peri- and postmenopausal women with insomnia and are negatively related to sleep efficiency and increased wake after sleep onset (4).

Women in the menopausal transition and postmenopause are often symptomatic at lower AHI values for OSA and present more frequently with symptoms of sleep fragmentation and poor sleep quality, such as insomnia, nocturia, and fatigue, rather than the classic male symptoms of loud snoring or excessive daytime sleepiness (3,10). This differing presentation can lead to significant underdiagnosis of OSA in this population (9). Nocturnal VMS (hot flashes, night sweats) are direct contributors to restlessness and wakefulness, further complicating sleep assessment (11).

The body of evidence reveals a critical diagnostic challenge: As women age and enter menopause, their risk of OSA increases dramatically, yet their symptom presentation often deviates significantly from the "classic" male phenotype. Their symptoms are more subtle, internal, and easily misattributed to general aging, menopausal symptoms, or primary insomnia. This "silent" or atypical progression means OSA is highly likely to be underdiagnosed in postmenopausal women, especially if clinicians rely on male-centric screening questions or if there is no bed partner to report overt snoring. The increase in REM-AHI in women (9,10) further suggests a specific physiologic manifestation that might be overlooked if only overall AHI is considered. The decline in protective female sex hormones (estrogen and progesterone) directly contributes to increased upper airway collapsibility and altered ventilatory control in menopausal women, leading to a higher incidence and severity of OSA. This physiologic change, combined with a lack of awareness of atypical female symptoms among health care providers, contributes to significant diagnostic delays and undertreatment. Clinicians must be vigilant for these nontraditional presentations of OSA in menopausal and postmenopausal women. Proactive questioning about fatigue, insomnia, mood changes, and nocturia, even in the absence of loud snoring, is essential. This understanding can significantly improve early detection and intervention for OSA in this vulnerable population.

PSYCHOLOGICAL, MENTAL HEALTH, AND LIFESTYLE FACTORS

Women demonstrate an increased susceptibility to both sleep difficulties and mental health issues throughout their lives, commencing in adolescence (13). Insomnia disorder is the most prevalent sleep disorder in the general population, and numerous studies and systematic reviews consistently show it to be more common in women than in men (1,6,9,12,13). This higher prevalence is attributed to a combination of biologic factors, including hormonal differences and their fluctuations across a woman's lifespan, and psychosocial factors, such as anxiety, depression, and stress related to gender role expectations (6).

There is a well-established bidirectional association between sleep health and psychological well-being in women (6,12). For instance, studies indicate that women with insomnia symptoms consistently report higher levels of fatigue, anxiety, and depression, along with a lower perception of quality of life, irrespective of time (12). This connection is particularly evident in the context of chronic pain conditions. Endometriosis, a chronic gynecologic disease characterized by pain and infertility, significantly affects psychological health, leading to heightened stress, fatigue, and various mental health disorders (6). Women with endometriosis report more severe insomnia symptoms and lower psychological well-being compared to controls, with pain and anxiety symptoms also bidirectionally associated (6). The high prevalence of sleep difficulties and insomnia in women with endometriosis is often attributed to the complex interplay of hormonal fluctuations, mood disorders, and the chronic pain stemming from gynecologic dysfunction (6). These findings underscore the importance of assessing and treating sleep difficulties in this population, as it can contribute to a significant improvement in psychological well-being and overall quality of life (6).

Lifestyle factors also play a crucial role in women's sleep health. High levels of perceived stress are associated with shorter sleep durations in adolescents (13). The impact of acute stressful situations, such as the COVID-19 lockdown, on insomnia in women has yielded discordant results across studies, with some indicating increased insomnia in women during the pandemic and others showing no significant sex differences or even a higher prevalence in men in certain age groups (1). However, one study noted that women scored higher on insomnia scales and reported worse total sleep duration, well-being, and daytime sleepiness after COVID-19 infection, suggesting a greater impact of the inflammatory response on women's sleep (1). These findings highlight the need for health care professionals to consider individualized treatment and prevention strategies that account for sex differences in risk factors for insomnia and circadian rhythm disorders (1). Furthermore, beliefs about lifestyle factors causing psychological distress can influence mental health stigma, which is relevant when considering the holistic approach to women's sleep and mental health (7,12).

SOCIAL, ROLE-BASED, AND OCCUPATIONAL CONTRIBUTORS

Sleep health is profoundly influenced by a socioecological framework encompassing individual, interpersonal, and broader social/societal domains (5). Within this framework, gender roles and societal expectations significantly shape women's sleep experiences. Women often report a greater need for sleep and tend to sleep more than men across most life stages, yet this difference is frequently explained by work/family responsibilities and gendered time tradeoffs.

Traditional gender expectations regarding housework and child-rearing contribute to gender differences in sleep duration, with women often bearing a disproportionate share of these responsibilities (5). The demands of child-rearing are associated with increased psychological and behavioral burdens for women, directly affecting their sleep (5). For example, the COVID-19 pandemic highlighted how family responsibilities accounted for gender differences in insomnia among frontline health care workers (5). Co-sleeping with a partner can also influence sleep patterns, with some studies indicating increased sleep fragmentation (arousals after sleep onset) for female partners and others suggesting that living with a partner predicts better sleep health, particularly for women (5). The emotional health of relationships also plays a role, with individuals in higher functioning relationships reporting better sleep outcomes (5).

Occupational stress is another prevalent issue that negatively impacts sleep quality (19). While the association between occupational stress and sleep quality is consistent across various industries, specific gender-related findings exist. In one study involving emergency department health care workers, poor sleep quality and insomnia were common, and the relationship between poor sleep and burnout was significantly stronger in women compared to men (20). The relationship between sleep quality and burnout was affected by both gender and clinical role (20). Another study found that significantly more women than men experienced high job strain, insomnia, and daytime sleepiness among nurses in Italy (19). For these women, the level of social support was significantly and negatively associated with insomnia and daytime sleepiness (19). These findings underscore the importance of person-level factors and the specific occupational context in understanding the sleep-burnout relationship in women. Furthermore, occupational balance, including adequate time for recovery and sleep, is associated with good sleep quality in women (19).

The gender disparity in insomnia is amplified in populations with intersectional identities (5). For instance, female active US military service members and female combat veterans report higher rates of insomnia and utilize more sleep aids than their male counterparts (5). Black, middle-aged women in the United States with higher perceived racism had increased odds of clinically significant insomnia (5). Sexual and gender minority populations are twice as likely to be diagnosed with insomnia as cisgender counterparts (5,7). These findings emphasize the importance of assessing intersectional identity across socioecological domains, as broader societal factors, such as the level of sexual minority support in a given state, can influence sleep outcomes (5).

CLINICAL TREATMENT APPROACHES

Effective clinical management of sleep disorders in women necessitates a gender-specific approach that acknowledges the unique biologic and psychosocial factors influencing their sleep health (2,3). A one-size-fits-all approach, often based on male-centric research, may lead to suboptimal outcomes.

Cognitive Behavioral Therapy for Insomnia (CBT-I) is widely recognized as a first-line nonpharmacologic treatment for insomnia, and its effectiveness is particularly well documented in menopausal women (21). A scoping review evaluating randomized controlled trials found that CBT-I significantly improves sleep quality and reduces insomnia severity in menopausal women (20). This therapy has demonstrated superiority over other interventions such as sleep restriction therapy and sleep hygiene education (21). Importantly, the improvements in sleep quality achieved through CBT-I have been observed to persist for up to 6 months posttreatment, offering a sustainable solution with fewer side effects compared to pharmacologic alternatives (21). However, current research on CBT-I efficacy in menopausal women has predominantly focused on white and well-educated populations, highlighting a need for further study in diverse groups (21).

Pharmacologic treatments for sleep disorders in women require careful consideration due to pharmacokinetic differences between sexes. For instance, zolpidem was the first drug in the United States to have different recommended doses for women versus men, reflecting variations in absorption, metabolism, and excretion rates (5). The FDA has advised dose reductions in women and older adults for many pharmacotherapies due to risks of cognitive and behavioral changes, including driving impairment (5). For postmenopausal women, menopausal hormone therapy (MHT) should be considered as a treatment choice for insomnia, particularly when menopausal symptoms are closely related to sleep disturbances (22). Melatonin and 5HT-based drugs are also preferentially recommended alongside MHT due to their fewer side effects (22). While eszopiclone, zolpidem, and suvorexant have shown short-term improvements in global and sleep outcomes compared to placebo, the comparative effectiveness and long-term efficacy of pharmacotherapies for insomnia are not fully established (5).

Integrative care models, rooted in a biopsychosocial approach, offer promising avenues for treating women with sleep conditions (23). These models emphasize person-centered care, delivered collaboratively by interdisciplinary health teams that may include physicians, psychologists, physiotherapists, and specialists in complementary and alternative medicine (CAM) (23). Such approaches have demonstrated positive results on sleep quality and patterns, offering both physical and psychological benefits for women across different life stages (23). This holistic framework allows for a more comprehensive understanding and management of the complex factors, contributing to women's sleep problems.

WOMEN AND POSITIVE AIR PRESSURE TREATMENT

Women's response to positive air pressure (PAP) treatment is lacking a large body of data. Manufacturers of PAP equipment have made masks for female patients with smaller cushions, frames, and straps to better fit female dimensions. Research released in 2015 by Resmed showed that compared to their standard Automatic Positive Airway Pressure (APAP) algorithm the "for Her" APAP algorithm resulted in less overall flow limitations. Aside from that, there were not statistically significant differences between the standard and "for Her" algorithm (24). There is a need to more thoroughly research women's response to PAP treatment.

A study from 2017 looked at CPAP adherence in 29 women over the age of 45 (25). After 2 years, it was found that approximately half of the participants were still compliant. There was no statistically significant difference between the age or OSA severity of the nonadherent versus the adherent group (25). Interestingly, 66.7% of the married participants lived alone, while 33.3% of the adherent group were married (25). Conversely, 21.4% of nonadherent participants lived alone and 78.6% of the nonadherent participants were married (25). There is some indication from this and other work that partner intimacy can affect adherence. The adherent group had statistically significant worse severity of symptoms of daytime sleepiness independent of AHI (25). This suggests that women with fewer overt symptoms may need more support adhering to CPAP treatment (25). A contrasting study with a sample size of 16 women had no adherent CPAP users among unmarried participants and a 40% adherence rate in the married cohort (26). These contradictory studies highlight the need for more research on women and PAP treatment.

ACCOMMODATIONS IN THE SLEEP LAB

In general, if a patient mentions any accommodation that can be made during the study to facilitate a more comfortable experience, it is best to provide it. Extra accommodations create a much more pleasant experience for the patient and result in a higher quality sleep study due to the patient being less restless and more able to sleep, resulting in better sleep study data with less fragmentation and better sleep maintenance. There are particular accommodations that women may find especially helpful to aid in the best possible sleep during their sleep lab stay.

Giving the patient adequate information prior to the sleep study allows the patient to plan and be mentally prepared for the procedure. Advise women prior to the study that nightgowns are not practical pajamas for a sleep study. It is best to wear two pieces with either shorts and a top or pants and a top due to the wire placement. Nail polish and nail extensions should be removed to make sure the pulse oximeter signals are accurate. Nail polish, especially dark nail polish, and false nails or nail tips will prevent the light from the pulse oximeter from functioning properly. The patient will need to remove any hairpieces glued to the scalp and, if possible, remove any extensions in the hair prior to the sleep study. Make sure the patient is aware that there will be extensive amounts of paste in the hair that require washing with water and shampoo to remove so they can plan hair styling services.

Safety is a concern for most patients and can be of special concern for patients with a traumatic history. Make sure your patient is aware of all safety precautions taken at your facility, such as doors being locked, security patrolling, panic alarms, and other protocols related to safety. This creates an environment of safety, allowing the patient to be more at ease.

For women with religious restrictions or a history of trauma, ensuring that they are cared for by female techs can be extremely helpful. There are women who cannot have a sleep study without the assurance of female-only health care providers. Especially in cases with a history of trauma, anxiety about safety may be so severe that they need a family member, friend, or family member to stay in the lab. In these cases, ensure that the person accompanying the patient is aware they cannot sleep in the bed with the patient, as that will interfere with the acquisition of the study. Most labs do have a chair in the room or one that can be brought in for the support person to sleep. Advise the support person that if they are disruptive to the study, they may be asked to leave. Careful screening of patients can assist in determining the most effective strategy for a patient with a history of trauma.

If independent temperature controls are available in rooms, ensure the patient is comfortable with the temperature of the room upon arrival and just before going to sleep. While any patient can get cold through the night, in general, anecdotally, women have a tendency to request more extra blankets. Make sure that your lab has an ample supply of blankets and, if possible, socks.

During perimenopause and menopause, women can experience hot flashes. Lighter-weight blankets, air conditioning, and fans can assist in combating these. Aside from causing the patient discomfort, night sweats can generate sweat artifact in signals that make the study difficult to score. If you see sweat artifact, it is important to attempt to help the patient cool down.

For pregnant patients, pregnancy or body pillows can aid in comfort. Encourage pregnant patients to bring these pillows from home for their study. Restless leg symptoms can be very prevalent in pregnant populations. Letting the patient know prior to lights out that they can get up and walk around if needed to relieve sensations in the legs can be helpful for any patient trying to sleep with this condition.

Nighttime can be a time of very heavy menstrual flow due to the relaxation of muscles during sleep. This can create a very uncomfortable and embarrassing situation for the patient. Providing access to feminine hygiene products can be very reassuring to patient. If your facility provides these products, make sure the patient is aware of how to access these products. If a patient menstruates on the blankets or sheets, assure them not to worry about it and that you will make sure the linens are laundered properly.

Patients with chronic pelvic pain due to menstruation, endometriosis, and other conditions may need to bring pain medicine to be able to complete the study successfully. Some women find heating pads or hot water bottles to ease pelvic pain. Encourage patients to bring these items or any other items they can use for pain relief to ease these conditions, as the pain associated with these conditions can be very disruptive to sleep.

CONCLUSIONS

The intricate relationship between women's health and sleep is profoundly influenced by a dynamic interplay of hormonal, physiologic, psychological, and socioecological factors across the lifespan. Women consistently report more subjective sleep problems despite sometimes exhibiting objectively better sleep parameters, highlighting the critical importance of a comprehensive biopsychosocial assessment that values the patient's lived experience.

Hormonal fluctuations are central to women's sleep health. During adolescence, sleep patterns are intricately linked to pubertal development, with deep sleep potentially stimulating LH secretion, while sleep disruptions like OSA may delay pubertal milestones. In the reproductive years, menstrual cycle phases, particularly the late luteal phase, are associated with sleep disturbances, and chronic conditions like endometriosis demonstrate a reinforcing cycle of pain, hormonal imbalance, and sleep impairment. Pregnancy and the postpartum period are marked by significant sleep disruption primarily due to physiologic changes; with poor sleep quality strongly linked to postpartum mental health issues and reduced maternal sensitivity. The menopausal transition presents a heightened vulnerability to sleep difficulties, including a doubling of OSA prevalence, driven by declining estrogen and progesterone, and presenting with atypical symptoms often leading to underdiagnosis.

Psychological factors such as anxiety and depression are bidirectionally associated with sleep health in women, and these are often exacerbated by chronic pain and gender role expectations. Social, role-based, and occupational contributors, including family responsibilities, gendered time tradeoffs, and occupational stress, significantly impact women's sleep quality and duration. The sex differences in sleep disorders necessitates a tailored approach, as women often present with different symptoms for common conditions like OSA and insomnia, leading to diagnostic challenges.

These findings underscore the imperative of adopting a gender-specific and holistic approach to patient care. This includes:

- Prioritizing subjective experience: Recognizing that a woman's report of poor sleep is a valid and critical indicator, even if objective measures appear normal.
- Comprehensive history taking: Probing for hormonal status, chronic pain, mental health symptoms, and socio-occupational stressors.
- Awareness of atypical presentations: Being vigilant for nontraditional symptoms of sleep disorders, especially OSA in menopausal women, and considering REM-AHI as a key diagnostic metric.
- Tailored diagnostic approaches: Utilizing a range of sleep study methods, including actigraphy and sleep diaries, to capture the nuances of women's sleep patterns.
- Promoting integrated care: Advocating for multidisciplinary collaboration with gynecologists, endocrinologists, pain specialists, and mental health professionals to address the multifaceted nature of women's sleep health.
- Creating an accommodating environment of care in the sleep lab to ensure the most comfortable experience possible.

Future research must continue to explore sex differences in sleep disorders; investigate the efficacy of interventions in diverse female populations; and deepen the understanding of the complex interplay between sleep, hormones, and socioecological factors throughout a woman's lifespan. By embracing these gender-specific considerations, sleep technologists can become more effective, providing a more optimal sleep diagnostic and treatment experience, empowering women to achieve optimal sleep health and overall well-being.

REFERENCES

1. Pajėdienė E, Urbonavičiūtė V, Ramanauskaitė V, Strazdauskas L, Stefani A. Sex differences in insomnia and circadian rhythm disorders: a systematic review. *Medicina*. 2024;60(3):474. doi:10.3390/medicina60030474
2. Perger E, Silvestri R, Bonanni E, et al. Gender medicine and sleep disorders: from basic science to clinical research. *Front Neurol*. 2024;15:1392489.
3. Schwarz EI, Schiza S. Sex differences in sleep and sleep-disordered breathing. *Curr Opin Pulm Med*. 2024;30(6):593-599.
4. Haufe A, Leeners B. Sleep disturbances across a woman's lifespan: what is the role of reproductive hormones? *J Endocr Soc*. 2023;7(5):bvad036.
5. Decker AN, Fischer AR, Gunn HE. Socio-ecological context of sleep: gender differences and couples' relationships as exemplars. *Curr Psychiatry Rep*. 2022;24(12):831-840.
6. Baldi E, Meneo D, Cerolini S, Gelfo F, Baglioni C. Sleep health and psychological wellbeing in adult women: a specific focus on endometriosis—a survey study. *J Clin Med*. 2025;14(6):2103.
7. Patterson CJ. Linking stressful experiences to health disparities among sexual and gender minority individuals: the sleep deficiency pathway. *Health Psychol*. 2025;44(3):207-210.
8. Liu KA, Mager NA. Women's involvement in clinical trials: historical perspective and future implications. *Pharm Pract (Granada)*. 2016;14(1):708.
9. Auer M, Frauscher B, Hochleitner M, Högl B. Gender-specific differences in access to polysomnography and prevalence of sleep disorders. *J Womens Health (Larchmt)*. 2018;27(4):525-530.
10. Patiño MC, Bueno Florez SJ, Gallo L, et al. Gender and polysomnographic profiles findings in obstructive sleep apnea syndrome patients living in high altitude. *Nat Sci Sleep*. 2021;13:547-556.
11. Kravitz HM, Zheng H, Bromberger JT, Buysse DJ, Owens J, Hall MH. An actigraphy study of sleep and pain in midlife women: the Study of Women's Health Across the Nation Sleep Study. *Menopause*. 2015;22(7):710-718.
12. Lucena L, Andersen ML, Tufik S, Hachul H. Effects of insomnia symptoms on quality of life and mood in women: EPISONO cohort study. *J Health Psychol*. 2025;13591053251337829.
13. Bei B, Coo S, Baker FC, Trinder J. Sleep in women: a review. *Aust Psychol*. 2015;50(1);14-24.
14. Crowley SJ, Carskadon MA. Sleep and puberty: a dynamic relationship. *J Endocr Soc*. 2021;5(1):bvab167.
15. Mozafarian N, Yazdi M, Hashemipour M, Hovsepian S, Maracy MR. Association between sleep duration and early pubertal timing in children and adolescents: a

systematic review and meta-analysis. *Curr Pediatr Rev.* 2023;19(3):318-328.

16. Lawson A, Murphy KE, Sloan E, Uleryk E, Dalfen A. The relationship between sleep and postpartum mental disorders: a systematic review. *J Affect Disord.* 2015;176:65-77.
17. Khan-Afridi Z, Ruchat SM, Jones PAT, et al. Impact of sleep on postpartum health outcomes: a systematic review and meta-analysis. *Br J Sports Med.* 2025;59(8):584-593.
18. Ran-Peled D, Horwitz A, Finkelstein O, Atzaba-Poria N, Tikotzky L. A longitudinal study of postpartum maternal sleep and sensitivity: examining depressive symptoms and social support as moderators. *J Sleep Res.* 2025;e70056.
19. d'Ettorre G, Ceccarelli G, Santinelli L, et al. Post-traumatic stress symptoms in healthcare workers dealing with the COVID-19 pandemic: a systematic review. *Int J Environ Res Public Health.* 2021;18(2):601.
20. Firew T, Miranda M, Fray N, et al. Examining how gender, race/ethnicity, and clinical roles moderate the association between sleep and burnout. *J Am Coll Emerg Physicians Open.* 2025;6(1):100004.
21. Ntikoudi A, Owens DA, Spyrou A, Evangelou E, Vlachou E. The effectiveness of cognitive behavioral therapy on insomnia severity among menopausal women: a scoping review. *Life (Basel).* 2024;14(11):1405.
22. Jeon GH. Insomnia in postmenopausal women: how to approach and treat it? *J Clin Med.* 2024;13(2):428.
23. Frange C, Banzoli CV, Colombo AE, et al. Women's sleep disorders: integrative care. *Sleep Sci.* 2017;10(4):174-180.
24. McArdle N, King S, Shepherd K, et al. Study of a novel APAP algorithm for the treatment of obstructive sleep apnea in women. *Sleep.* 2015;38(11):1775-1781.
25. Libman E, Bailes S, Fichten CS, et al. CPAP treatment adherence in women with obstructive sleep apnea. *Sleep Disord.* 2017;2017:2760650.
26. Baron KG, Gunn HE, Wolfe LF, et al. Relationships and CPAP adherence among women with obstructive sleep apnea. *Sleep Sci Pract.* 2017;1:10.

SECTION II

Sleep Disorders and Disorders That Affect Sleep

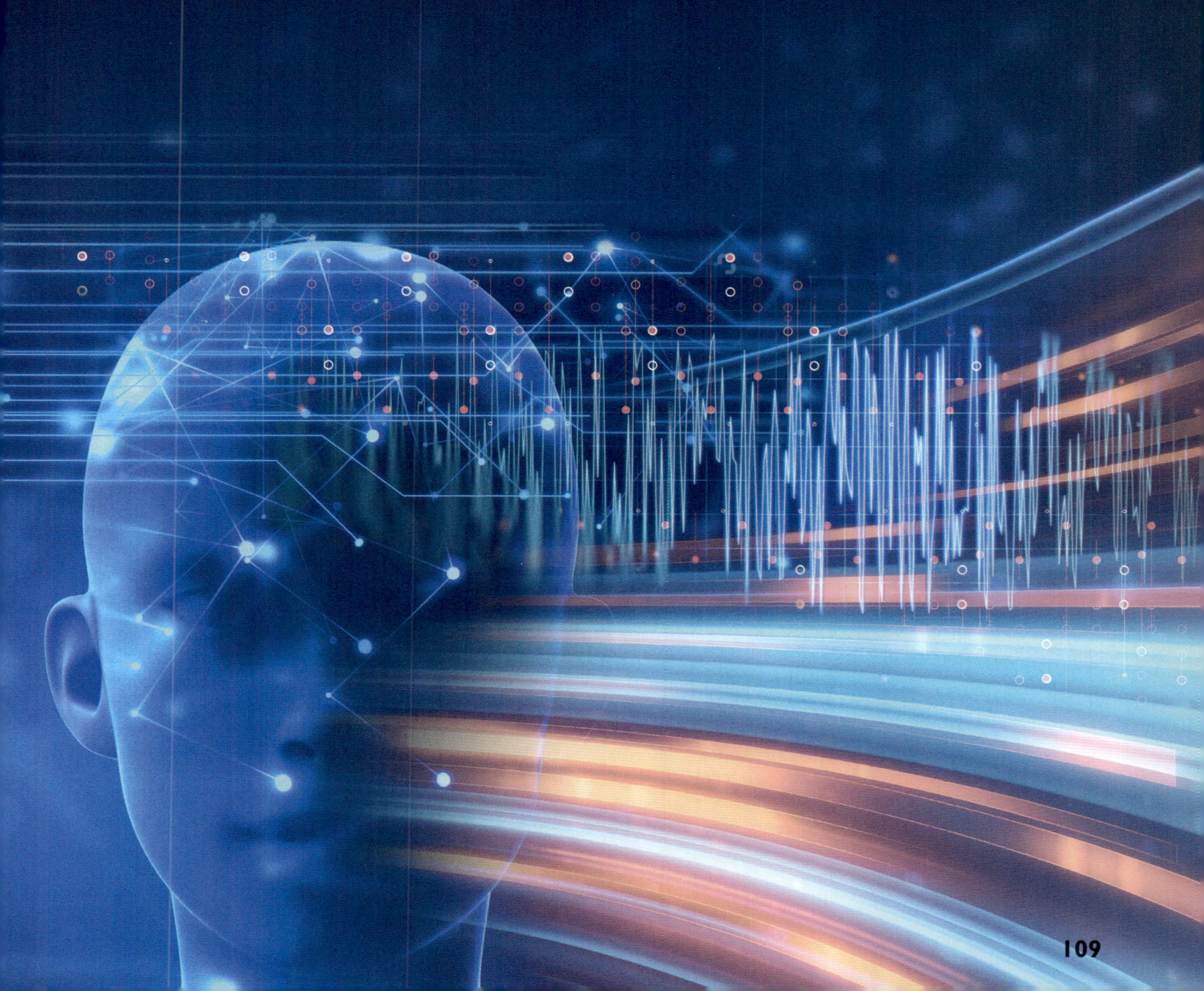

Chapter 10
Obstructive Sleep Apnea

ELISE A. MAHER

KEY CONCEPTS/LEARNING OBJECTIVES

The key concepts for this chapter include a review of the symptoms, risk factors, and associated comorbid conditions seen with obstructive sleep apnea (OSA), the polysomnographic patterns associated with sleep-disordered breathing, and the major treatments used for OSA.

KEY TERMS

Apnea
Arrhythmias
Craniofacial structure
Continuous positive airway pressure (CPAP)
Excessive daytime sleepiness (EDS)
Hypopnea
Continuous positive airway pressure (CPAP)
Obstructive sleep apnea
Pharynx
Sleep disordered breathing (SDB)
Upper airway resistance syndrome (UARS)

Obstructive sleep apnea (OSA) is a repetitive pattern of upper airway obstruction that occurs during sleep and is associated with sleep fragmentation and/or oxygen desaturation. The combination of sleep fragmentation, oxygen desaturation, and the other pathophysiologic changes causes daytime impairment, particularly excessive daytime sleepiness (EDS), and cardiovascular disease (1). There is a gradient of airway closure in OSA ranging from mild and partial obstruction to a complete and sustained blockage of the upper airway. An event with complete obstruction is called an "apnea," whereas the one with partial obstruction is called a "hypopnea." A milder respiratory disturbance called a respiratory effort–related arousal (RERA) fragments sleep with even minimal increases in upper airway resistance. The clinical syndrome has variously been called OSA syndrome, and the obstructive sleep apnea/hypopnea syndrome (OSAHS). The current terminology recommended by the *International Classification of Sleep Disorders*, 3rd edition (2), and used in this chapter, is OSA. Partial obstruction or hypopnea is frequently seen in the syndrome, and so the term OSAHS is used interchangeably with OSA.

Mild obstruction of the upper airway causes turbulent airflow that leads the tissues to vibrate and creates snoring and sometimes choking sounds. The sound levels resulting from snoring range from soft to decibel levels loud enough to be considered unsafe in the workplace (>80 dB). Obstructive events can last from 10 seconds to as long as 2 minutes, after which a brief central nervous system arousal from sleep restores the patency (opening or unblocking) of the airway. Severity is defined by the number of breathing disruptions per hour, or apnea-hypopnea index (AHI). Some authors use the term "respiratory disturbance index" (RDI) interchangeably with AHI; however, the American Academy of Sleep Medicine (AASM) *Manual for the Scoring of Sleep and Associated Events* defines RDI as the number of apneas + hypopneas + RERAs per hour of sleep. An AHI below 5 is considered normal in adults. Mild OSA is in the range of 5 to 14; moderate, 15 to 30; and severe, more than 30. The number of times that a patient's oxygen level drops below the minimum normal saturation of 88% to 90% is another indicator of severity, with greater stress on the cardiovascular system and increased risk of cardiovascular disorders related to the more frequent and larger desaturation.

SLEEP AND BREATHING

Most body systems slow down during sleep. The breathing rate slows, and tidal volume is reduced as breaths become shallower, resulting in mild hypoventilation (2-8 mm Hg increase in Pa_{CO_2}). At the same time, the heart rate slows down, and oxygenation levels dip a little below waking levels. Muscles relax and the airway narrows, leading to an increase in upper airway resistance in the pharynx (the soft tissue pathway starting from the nasal and oral airways that leads down to the larynx; Figure 10-1). The anatomic and neuromuscular systems that keep the airway open for normal breathing during wakefulness are not as active during sleep and can fail to compensate for the changes that occur in sleep.

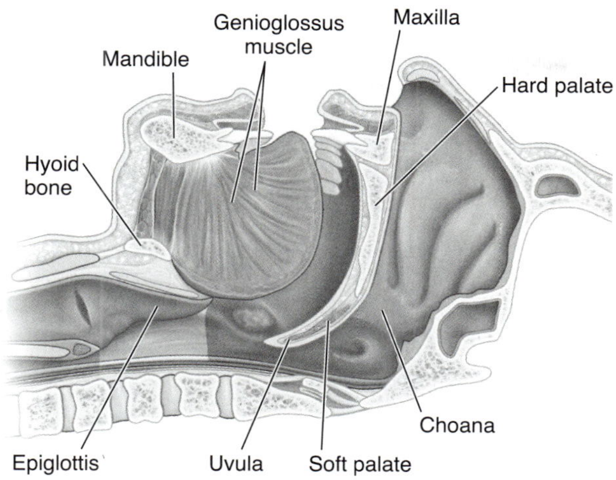

Figure 10-1 This is a sagittal section through the pharyngeal airway of a normal human. The opening to the nose is just above the **maxilla**. The other structures of the airway include the **mandible**, **hard palate**, **soft palate**, and **uvula**. The body of the tongue is the **genioglossus muscle**. Pharyngeal collapse in apneic patients occurs somewhere between the **choana** and the **epiglottis**, usually behind the uvula and the soft palate, behind the tongue, or some combination of these sites. In humans, the hyoid bone is not firmly attached to bony structures, thus increasing dependency on the upper airway muscles to keep the airway open. (Modified with permission from Moore KL, Dalley AF II, Agur AMR. *Clinically Oriented Anatomy*. 7th ed. Wolters Kluwer Health/Lippincott Williams & Wilkins; 2014. Figure 7.83.)

The human airway is anatomically at greater risk than other animals. The hyoid bone that anchors the pharyngeal muscles is not rigidly attached in humans as it is in other mammals, which allows us wide-ranging vocalizations needed for speech. However, this feature makes the upper airway more collapsible when the many muscles responsible for dilating and maintaining the airway are not fully functioning during sleep. The areas of obstruction differ considerably, depending on body position, craniofacial structure, and weight distribution. It has been shown that obese patients tend to have collapse of the velopharynx (soft palate and sidewalls of the pharynx), whereas nonobese patients with a recessed chin showed collapse in the oropharynx and velopharynx (3).

The typical reclining sleeping posture causes a gravitational effect on the soft tissue of the upper airway, promoting collapse. This positional effect is at its worst when patients are sleeping on their back (supine). Patients sometimes unknowingly self-treat their OSA by preferring to sleep propped up with extra pillows or in a recliner. In rapid eye movement (REM) sleep, the upper airway can collapse further when dilator muscle activation, reduced the greatest amount compared with waking levels, is chemically blocked.

EPIDEMIOLOGY

It is difficult to accurately determine the prevalence of OSA in the population because of the various ways that breathing obstructions in sleep are defined and measured, how individuals are screened, and how they are tested. A widely referenced study found that the occurrence of more than five obstructive events per hour during sleep is high, reported at 24% in men and 9% in women aged 30 to 60 years. The same study found the prevalence of OSA, defined as more than five obstructive events per hour *and* symptoms of sleepiness, was 2% in women and 4% in men aged 30 to 60 years (4). This seminal study was published in 1993 and likely underestimates the prevalence of OSA because of the rapid increase in obesity in the general population since that time. More recent studies suggest prevalence rates of 5% in women and 14% in men, with higher rates associated with older age and higher weight (5).

RISK FACTORS

There are multiple and often intertwined risk factors that predispose to OSA. Longitudinal studies have found that the most significant independent risk factor for OSA is being overweight (5-7). There is a 4-fold risk for OSA associated with a body mass index (BMI) increase of one standard deviation (this amount of change in BMI is approximately the difference between normal and overweight or between overweight and obese) (1). Even a 10% weight reduction can lower the AHI by an average of 26% (6). For patients with mild OSA, AHI may be objectively reduced to normal levels after significant weight loss. In a 2009 study that had patients follow a very low-calorie diet, the AHI was brought below 5 when patients lost an average of 10.6% of initial weight (8).

Gender plays a large role in the relative expression of OSA symptoms and health consequences, with males having a reported 2:1 or 3:1 prevalence over females. Hormones and fat distribution both predispose males toward a more collapsible airway. Interestingly, the ratio of males to females who present to the sleep center for testing is closer to 8:1. Males may tend to be identified more readily by primary care doctors as being candidates for OSA or may be prompted more often by female partners to seek treatment (9). The gender difference in prevalence starts to equalize post menopause.

There is a linear relationship between age and risk for OSA, which starts in middle age and plateaus at about age 65 (10). In women, there is a marked increase in OSA after menopause when the protective effects of progesterone on the respiratory system diminish (11). Although the incidence of OSA is higher in old age than in middle age, at 70% for men and 56% for women, the symptoms and risk factors are different (12). The AHI is not as strongly correlated with obesity (10), EDS, cognitive dysfunction, or hypertension (13,14) in older individuals. Snoring, one of the main complaints in middle age, subsides in old age. This could be because of hearing loss or because a central component of respiration emerges (15).

Race is a risk factor for OSA, although not as widely researched as weight, gender, age, or other factors. African Americans younger than 25 and older than 65 have an elevated risk over African American males between 25 and 65 or males of other races (16,17). Asians have similar rates of OSA as those in Western cultures. However, BMI rates are lower, and craniofacial features may be the determining factor. Chinese males, for example, have a shorter cranial base, maxilla (upper jaw), and mandible (lower jaw), causing more crowding of the airway (18).

Craniofacial features can have a large impact on the airway, particularly during sleep when muscle relaxation, body position, and gravity can compromise the airway patency of susceptible individuals. There are two types of features that impact potential upper airway obstruction: soft tissue and bone structure. Soft tissue from large turbinates, a deviated septum, occluded sinuses, polyps, a large tongue or uvula, enlarged tonsils or adenoids, or an elongated soft palate can crowd the oronasal airway and cause obstruction and reduced airflow. A large neck size (>17 inches in men and >16 inches in women) is one of the most predictive features of OSA (2). The larger the volume of tissue surrounding the airway, whether fatty or muscular, the more prone it is to partially or fully collapse.

A receding (retrognathic) or small (micrognathic) chin or narrow/high arched palate can be problematic and cause OSA in nonobese patients. Congenital conditions that impact facial bones and soft tissue of the upper airway are associated with increased risk of OSA that can be especially difficult to treat. Features of Down syndrome include a large tongue (macroglossia), small chin, narrow airway, and generalized hypotonia. In a 2009 study, 94% of Down syndrome patients were found to have at least mild OSA, and 69% were in the severe range (19). Pierre Robin, Marfan syndrome, and achondroplasia are some of the other genetic disorders that result in decreased airway size and predispose to OSA.

Familial incidence of OSA increases an individual's risk of OSA . There is a direct increase in risk of OSA for each diagnosed family member (20). This may be because of a combination of genetic and environmental factors. For instance, obesity is an independent risk factor and can be affected by familial lifestyle and dietary factors.

Smoking and sedative use (including alcohol), particularly near bedtime, are additional predisposing factors. Smoking may affect the function of upper airway tissue because of inflammation and toughening from prolonged smoke exposure. One study showed that active smokers are 3 times more likely to have OSA than nonsmokers (21). Sedatives act as muscle relaxants and also reduce reactivity in the respiratory control system. Sedatives can induce apneas and snoring in people without OSA and worsen respiratory events in symptomatic patients (22-24).

Other clinical conditions that affect airway size or airway muscle function are risk factors for OSA, including polycystic ovary syndrome, hypothyroidism, and pregnancy. Although hormones can have a protective effect on the airway in sleep, gestational weight gain and pressure on the thoracic cavity can cause or increase snoring and apneas. Apneas during pregnancy that are associated with hypoxemia can be associated with low fetal birth weight and lower Apgar scores (25).

CARDIOVASCULAR DISEASE

Cardiac disease and progression frequently coexist with OSA. Patients with OSA are at increased risk for hypertension, arrhythmias, myocardial infarction (MI), coronary artery disease, pulmonary hypertension, stroke, and sudden cardiac death. Cardiac arrhythmias are more common in patients with OSA as a result of sympathetic nervous system activation (which causes vasoconstriction and increased blood pressure), hypoxia (low oxygen levels), hypercapnia (elevated carbon dioxide levels), and increased fluctuations in intrathoracic pressure. The increase in negative intrathoracic pressure during an obstructive event negatively affects left ventricular function and decreases stroke volume and cardiac output. Many patients with OSA develop a brady-tachy heart rate pattern, in which bradycardia occurs during the apneic phase and tachycardia occurs when breathing returns (26).

Of note, the Sleep Heart Health Study (SHHS) showed that hypopneas accompanied by an oxyhemoglobin desaturation of more than or equal to 4% were associated with prevalent cardiovascular disease independently of confounding covariates (27). In contrast, no association was observed between cardiovascular disease and hypopneas associated with milder desaturation or arousals.

Hypertension

Analysis of data from more than 6,000 adults participating in the SHHS showed that those in the upper quartile of AHI (≥11.0 events per hour) had 42% greater odds of cardiovascular disease than those in the lowest quartile (AHI <1.3 events per hour) (28). Patients with hypertension have an increased incidence of OSA (30%), and

50% of patients with OSA have hypertension (29,30). Hypertension is strongly associated with OSA, even when mild (31).

The SHHS showed a linear relationship between increasing AHI and incidence of hypertension. Prevalence rates of hypertension in increasing AHI categories were 43% (<1.5 per hour), 53% (1.5-4.9 per hour), 59% (5-14.9 per hour), 62% (15-29.9 per hour), and 67% (≥30 per hour) (32). It is likely that hypertension itself increases the risks of other types of cardiac disease.

Arrhythmias

Arrhythmias are more common in patients with OSA, even in the absence of structural or electrical heart conduction problems. The higher incidence of abnormal rhythms is most likely caused by a combination of hypoxemia, the vagal response to obstructed breathing, increased sympathetic activation, acute increases in blood pressure, and rapid changes in intrathoracic pressure.

Cardiac variability is commonly seen in OSA patients with repetitive alternations between bradycardia and tachycardia in synchrony with obstructive events. Bradycardia is caused by the vagal response to apnea and is followed by an overshoot to tachycardia during the hyperpneic (recovery) phase of breathing. Decreased heart rate variability in response to repetitive apneas is a marker for subsequent development of hypertension because of excessive sympathetic activity and potential loss of vagal control (33).

Other bradycardic patterns, including second- and third-degree atrioventricular (AV) blocks and sinus pauses, are frequently seen in OSA patients. In the absence of any electrophysiologic abnormalities of the sinus or AV node, heart block was found in 10% of patients with OSA. The blocks included AV block type II (Mobitz), third-degree block, and sinus pauses and occurred more often in REM sleep and during 4% or greater oxygen desaturations (34). Sinus pauses of up to 12 seconds can be seen in REM sleep and during long apneas with desaturation.

Ventricular ectopy is also frequently seen in patients with OSA and increases in frequency along with increasing AHI. Individuals with sleep disordered breathing (SDB) had 3 times the odds of nonsustained ventricular tachycardia and almost twice the odds of complex ventricular ectopy (nonsustained ventricular tachycardia with bigeminy, trigeminy, or quadrigeminy) (35). In a study of 400 OSA patients conducted by Guilleminault et al (25), premature ventricular contractions were noted in 193 (48%) of subjects. The common arrhythmias seen in patients with OSA without known cardiac history often occur during sleep (35,36). Positive airway pressure (PAP) therapy has been shown to decrease ventricular ectopy in patients with heart failure and OSA (37).

There is a 4-fold increase in atrial fibrillation in patients with OSA (35). There is also a higher recurrence of atrial fibrillation after cardioversion in patients with untreated SDB and atrial fibrillation than in patients without a known SDB diagnosis (38).

Congestive Heart Failure

Congestive heart failure (CHF) is strongly associated with Cheyne-Stokes respiration, a type of central sleep apnea (CSA). However, many patients with CSA also have an obstructive component, and there is increased risk of heart failure with OSA as well. In a sample of 81 male patients with CHF, 40% had CSA and 11% had OSA (39). Patients with OSA were heavier, on average, than those with CSA. There is a high frequency of atrial fibrillation and ventricular arrhythmias in patients with both OSA and CHF. The SHHS reported that OSA is associated with a relative odds ratio of 2.38 for heart failure, independently of other known risk factors (28,40).

Coronary Artery Disease

There is increased risk of MI in patients with OSA, reported to be about 4 times greater than in those without OSA (41-43). Additionally, OSA patients may be at higher risk for subsequent cardiovascular events after an MI, possibly because of hypoxemia (44).

Stroke

There is a high incidence of OSA in stroke patients (45,46). In the SHHS, there was a positive relationship between the history of stroke and the AHI (28). Prospective studies have shown an increased risk of stroke in patients with OSA, with an increased hazard ratio of 2.5 in those with OSA (47).

Sudden Cardiac Death

Although sudden cardiac death tends to occur between 6 and 11 AM in the general population, there is 2.5 times the risk of sudden cardiac death between 12 and 6 AM for patients with known OSA (48). Increased nocturnal arrhythmias in patients with OSA could be a contributing factor to nocturnal sudden cardiac death (35).

ENDOCRINE DYSFUNCTION

Over the past decade, a strong relationship between diabetes mellitus, other metabolic syndromes, and OSA has been increasingly defined. Although obesity is a common comorbidity in both OSA and diabetes mellitus, OSA is independently associated with altered glucose metabolism and may predispose to the eventual development of type 2 diabetes mellitus (49). The repetitive effects of cortical arousal and hypoxia can worsen insulin sensitivity and glucose tolerance (50,51).

There is evidence of an increased risk of OSA in patients with diabetes mellitus also. One in four patients diagnosed with diabetes with autonomic neuropathy also have OSA (52,53). Neuropathy may contribute to the collapsibility of the upper airway. Given the surge in diabetes mellitus in the population, it is becoming more important to treat OSA in order to help control negative health consequences. Metabolic syndrome is a cluster of health concerns that includes obesity, hyperlipidemia (high low-density lipoprotein cholesterol), hypertension, and insulin resistance. Of these conditions, insulin resistance is considered to be the core dysfunction. Metabolic syndrome, also known as Syndrome X, has become so closely associated with OSA that the term "Syndrome Z" has been proposed for patients diagnosed with both conditions (54).

Hypothyroidism is caused by reduced production of thyroid hormone and is another endocrine system dysfunction that increases the risk of OSA. This is due mainly to associated weight gain, soft tissue (especially the tongue) and facial swelling, and myopathy.

NEUROLOGIC DYSFUNCTION

Recent studies have explored a relationship between OSA and Alzheimer disease (AD). A meta-analysis of published clinical data on the overlap of OSA and AD indicates a 5-fold increased risk of AD patients presenting with OSA when compared with cognitively nonimpaired subjects of similar age (55). A 2016 study found that 50% of patients with OSA had elevated levels of amyloid beta, a peptide that is the main component of amyloid plaques found in the brains of AD patients, and individuals who experienced more apneas throughout their normal sleep period had increased levels of amyloid beta (56). These and other studies suggest that OSA may be a risk factor for AD and the possible importance of assessing older adults for OSA.

CLINICAL SYMPTOMS

The most common symptoms that OSA patients experience are habitual snoring, pauses in breathing, gasping and choking during sleep, frequent urination, and feeling excessively sleepy during the day even after having slept adequately at night. Other nighttime symptoms include difficulty falling or staying asleep, sleep fragmentation, gastric disturbance, excessive sweating, and movement during sleep. Daytime symptoms are not as obviously associated with OSA. Patients with untreated OSA often suffer from cognitive and behavioral dysfunction and can be more depressed, forgetful, impatient, irritable and suffer from morning headaches, daytime gastric reflux, and sexual dysfunction.

The primary symptom is often EDS that interferes with work, leisure activities, and relationships. However, there is no clear relationship between the severity of OSA and subjective or objective measures of sleepiness. Many patients are unaware of the profound impact of OSA on their attentiveness and performance. There may be genetic phenotypes that make some patients more resilient against sleep disturbance. Conversely, some patients with very mild OSA can suffer from EDS and benefit from treatment. Snoring is often the reason for patients seeking treatment, and bed partners play a large role in discovering the patterns of obstructed breathing and supporting testing and treatment.

COGNITIVE AND BEHAVIORAL SYMPTOMS

There are various components of cognitive function: attention, psychomotor response, vigilance, memory, decision-making, and executive function. Deficits in cognitive function are thought to be caused by sleep fragmentation and changes in cerebral blood flow from low oxygen levels (57). Executive function and vigilance have been found to be impaired in clinic-based samples of OSA patients. In a study of newly diagnosed OSA patients, 25% showed neuropsychological dysfunction on a battery of cognitive indexes that assessed constructive ability, deductive thinking, verbal attainment, and immediate memory (58). Several studies have shown that memory is impaired in untreated OSA, but improves with PAP treatment (59,60). Sustained attention may be the function most impacted by daytime sleepiness. These decreased functions have significant consequences when OSA patients are responsible for public safety, as in commercial transportation.

There is a strong association between OSA and mood disorders, particularly depression (61-63). A 2005 study of over 4 million veterans showed that 3% had sleep apnea, and more than 21% of those with OSA also had comorbid depression (64). In a recent community-based sample of 18,900 survey respondents in Europe, 17.6% of those meeting criteria for SDB also met the criteria for major depression (65). It may be clinically important to understand how many patients with depression also have OSA. Because many patients with depression are treated pharmacologically with sedative hypnotics, there could be a worsening of nighttime breathing that could compound depressive symptoms. Both depression and OSA have the symptoms of sleepiness and fatigue in common, and it can be difficult to pull apart which is primary.

Quality of life (QOL) is a subjective self-assessment of a spectrum of factors such as standard of living, life satisfaction, health, job status, and the ability to carry out daily activities. Patients with severe OSA may be the most affected in terms of QOL (66), but even those with mild OSA report difficulties. In the SHHS, an inverse relationship between OSA severity and scores on "vitality/energy" was shown, but only when oxygen desaturation was part of the severity determination (15).

CLINICAL EVALUATION

The signs and symptoms of OSA are easily recognizable by health professionals if patients are forthcoming about them or if clinicians ask the right questions (Table 10-1). Snoring, pauses in breathing, gasping or choking, restlessness, and EDS are indicators of the need to evaluate a patient for OSA. Evaluation requires a careful review of medical history, sleep habits and problems, related daytime symptoms, and a physical examination. The physical examination includes a review of respiratory, cardiovascular, and neurologic systems, with a focus on evaluation of BMI, neck size, and the anatomy of the upper airway. Physicians use the Mallampati classification to rate the size of the airway opening at the back of the throat. Scores range from I to IV, with IV being the most occluded and ≥III having an increased risk of OSA (67).

Sleep testing should be performed when moderate to severe OSA is suggested by the presence of EDS and at least two of the following three criteria: habitual loud snoring, witnessed apnea or gasping or choking, or diagnosed hypertension. Patients with EDS who report falling asleep at the wheel or having had a motor vehicle accident should be expedited for testing and treatment. Preoperative evaluation is important for risk reduction because of increased collapsibility of the upper airway during anesthesia and sedation.

Patients with conditions that are closely associated with OSA should also be proactively screened (Table 10-2). Because obesity is one of the most predictive risk factors for OSA, anyone with a BMI of more than 35 should be evaluated, as well as patients undergoing bariatric surgery. Endocrine disorders associated with excess weight, like hypothyroidism or diabetes mellitus, will also increase the risk of OSA. Certain types of cardiovascular disease and arrhythmias are increased in patients with OSA. Likewise, patients who have had cardiovascular events like stroke or MI have a much higher risk of OSA and should be screened.

Research on the relationship of OSA and cancer is starting to suggest that patients with OSA have a higher risk of dying from cancer (68). In the Wisconsin Sleep

Table 10-1 Obstructive Sleep Apnea Symptoms That Should Be Evaluated During a Comprehensive Sleep Evaluation
Witnessed apneas
Snoring
Gasping/choking at night
Excessive sleepiness not explained by other factors
Nonrefreshing sleep
Total sleep amount
Sleep fragmentation/maintenance insomnia
Nocturia
Morning headaches
Decreased concentration
Memory loss
Decreased libido
Irritability

Used with permission of American Academy of Sleep Medicine from Epstein LJ, Kristo D, Strollo PJ Jr, et al. Clinical guideline for the evaluation, management and long-term care of obstructive sleep apnea in adults. *J Clin Sleep Med.* 2009;5(3):263-276; permission conveyed through Copyright Clearance Center, Inc.

Table 10-2 Patients at High Risk for Obstructive Sleep Apnea Who Should Be Evaluated for Symptoms
Obesity (BMI >35)
Congestive heart failure
Atrial fibrillation
Treatment refractory hypertension
Type 2 diabetes
Nocturnal dysrhythmias
Stroke
Hypertension
High-risk driving populations
Preoperative for bariatric surgery

BMI, body mass index.
Used with permission of American Academy of Sleep Medicine from Epstein LJ, Kristo D, Strollo PJ Jr, et al. Clinical guideline for the evaluation, management and long-term care of obstructive sleep apnea in adults. *J Clin Sleep Med.* 2009;5(3):263-276; permission conveyed through Copyright Clearance Center, Inc.

Cohort Study, a 4-fold increase in cancer mortality was found in OSA patients compared with matched patients without OSA (69). It may be important in the future to test for and treat OSA to prescreen for cancer and slow progression of established cancer.

DIAGNOSTIC TESTING

Testing for OSA is usually performed in a sleep center, where multiple systems (brain activity, cardiac activity, breathing, and movements) are comprehensively monitored and can be correlated in time. The channels for standard polysomnography (PSG) required by AASM standards are comprehensive enough to definitively rule OSA in or out (70). To expedite diagnosis and treatment, a split-night study is often ordered, during which the first part of the night is diagnostic for SDB and the second part introduces PAP therapy when indicated. When a PAP titration is incomplete after a split-night study, the patient can return to the lab for an all-night titration or be set up on an auto-titrating PAP device at home to determine optimal therapeutic pressure.

When there is the likelihood of OSA in the absence of a set of comorbidities (moderate to severe pulmonary disease, neuromuscular disease, CHF, history of stroke and chronic opiate medication use) or other potential sleep disorders, a limited-channel portable test can be done at home or in other settings outside the sleep center. These tests have been variously labeled "out-of-center sleep tests," portable monitoring, limited-channel tests, and home sleep tests. The AASM recommends the term "home sleep *apnea* test" (HSAT) to emphasize that home testing is indicated only in evaluating obstructed breathing (presumed to be during sleep), as sleep markers are generally not recorded. Evaluation by a sleep specialist for suitability for HSAT is required to appropriately conduct and interpret these tests. HSATs can underestimate SDB, especially when a patient primarily or exclusively has arousals rather than desaturations associated with hypopneas. In addition, total recording time is used to calculate the AHI rather than total sleep time because sleep is not measured, which can artificially reduce the AHI. These factors can cause a false-negative result in an estimated 17% of tests, and patients with a high pretest likelihood of OSA should be retested with in-lab PSG if their HSAT is negative for OSA (71). The accuracy of the diagnostic method, convenience, cost, patient preference, physical/cognitive ability for self-administration, wait time, and access issues may all be considered when choosing between home and attended sleep apnea testing. When evidence of nonobstructive SDB, such as CSA, is suggested by HSAT, full PSG should be performed.

Effectiveness of treatment for OSA on sleepiness may be evaluated by a multiple sleep latency test to determine residual sleepiness or by a maintenance of wakefulness test to determine the ability to stay awake and resume work in safety-related jobs.

POLYSOMNOGRAPHY FINDINGS

The specifications for scoring SDB are outlined in the *AASM Manual for the Scoring of Sleep and Associated Events: Rules, Terminology and Technical Specifications* (70). The breathing events that indicate OSA are apneas and hypopneas that last a minimum of 10 seconds in adults (at least two missed breaths in children). An obstructive apnea is defined by the absence of breathing in the oronasal thermal channel with continued respiratory effort throughout the event. Absence of breathing is further specified to be 90% reduced for 90% of the event's duration. The recommended hypopnea definition occurs when there is a minimum of 30% reduction in the nasal pressure transducer signal associated with a minimum of 3% oxygen desaturation and/or an associated arousal. An acceptable alternate definition requires the nasal pressure transducer signal to be reduced by at least 30% with an associated 4% or greater oxygen desaturation (70).

PSG recordings of patients with OSA reveal abnormal sleep patterns related to sleep fragmentation: decreased sleep efficiency, increased stage N1, decreased stage N3, reduced REM sleep, and increased stage changes and electroencephalogram (EEG) arousals. Oxygen desaturations and resaturations related to apneas and hypopneas may be seen, as well as elevated CO_2 levels (routinely monitored during pediatric sleep studies but infrequently in adults).

With the modified lead II configuration of electrocardiogram (ECG) electrode placement used during PSG, only certain types of arrhythmias can be accurately detected. However, heart rate and regularity can be assessed as well as irregular QRS formations. The ECG can be interpreted in correlation with sleep state and breathing patterns. A pattern of bradycardia is often seen during apneic events, followed by tachycardia at the termination of the event or the hyperpneic phase of recovery breathing. Body position and body movements are recorded and can also be correlated with sleep stage and cardiorespiratory status.

Some patients have a pattern of sustained airflow limitation that can cause mild snoring and/or arousals from sleep. Some authors have called this breathing pattern, occurring along with daytime symptoms, the "upper airway resistance syndrome" (UARS). These patients have a low AHI and often a pattern of flattening or cupping of the nasal transducer signal that does not meet criteria for hypopnea. Airflow limitation can be termed a RERA when it lasts at least 10 seconds, shows progressively increasing or maintained respiratory effort, and ends in an arousal (69). RERAs are included in the RDI calculated in some sleep centers. The PSG in patients with UARS shows an AHI below 5 per hour, but there is a dominance of RERAs, resulting in an overall RDI above 5 per hour. Sao_2 is maintained to a minimum of 92%. Chronic insomnia tends to be much more common in these patients; they report nocturnal awakenings and find it difficult to return to sleep. Parasomnias are more frequently reported in younger subjects with UARS (72,73).

TREATMENT

Behavioral Management

Patients should be educated about the causes, consequences, and treatment options for OSA. Behavioral measures can reduce risk factors and improve airway patency, including weight loss and avoidance of sedatives, alcohol, and smoking. It has been shown that alcohol near bedtime increases the duration and frequency of obstructions and significantly increases desaturations in the first hour of sleep (74). Weight loss can be curative in some cases or reduce the AHI and related symptoms. Weight loss after bariatric surgery has been shown to lower the AHI (75,76).

In theory, PAP therapy would optimally correct sleep fragmentation, endocrine dysfunction, and other processes that impact energy balance and tendencies for weight gain. However, recent research shows that on average, patients on PAP therapy show a 0.4 kg increase in weight after 3 months (77). It is possible that the small uptick in weight could be explained by a reduced energy burden after the treatment of labored breathing, resulting in fewer calories burned during sleep. More studies with better controls for PAP compliance, calorie intake, and OSA severity are warranted to further investigate the relationship between treating OSA with PAP and weight change. For some patients, treating OSA can give the energy and vitality to begin an effective weight loss program; however, counseling on weight reduction strategies should go hand in hand with PAP recommendations.

For patients with positional OSA, for whom obstruction occurs predominantly while supine, positional therapy that keeps them off their back can be a treatment option. Positional therapy is indicated only when positional apnea has been established during sleep testing. Some patients only have obstructed breathing when lying on their back. For this reason, it is essential that an effort is made to get a sample of sleep in lateral and supine positions during in-lab testing. One study showed that 55.8% of patients with OSA in a large sample had twice as many respiratory events in the supine position compared with the lateral position. These patients tended to have a lower BMI and were younger than those without a positional effect (78). There are various positioning products on the market, but any object affixed to the back (tennis balls and backpack) that makes it difficult or uncomfortable to roll onto the back can reduce obstructive events for some patients.

Positive Airway Pressure Therapy

PAP, which may be in the form of continuous PAP (CPAP), bilevel PAP (BPAP), or auto-titrating PAP (APAP), is the cornerstone of treatment. PAP is created by an air blower that generates airflow, increasing positive pressure in the airway, and keeping the airway inflated and open. CPAP was the first developed and, as the name implies, provides the same continuous pressure during both inspiration and exhalation. BPAP maintains the patency of the airway at a lower pressure during exhalation than the higher pressures that are triggered by inhalation, which can be more comfortable for some patients with OSA. APAP adjusts the pressure to the minimum needed to maintain an open airway in variable conditions (ie, different positions and sleep stages, weight changes). The airflow of the various PAP modalities is delivered through a nasal or oral-nasal interface. The pressure level is predetermined by an attended PAP or APAP titration study performed to evaluate the lowest pressure that can prevent snoring and minimize obstructive events, desaturations, and flow limitation. PAP therapy can be utilized for all categories of OSA and represents first-line therapy for mild, moderate, and severe OSA. Treatment of nasal obstruction, use of lowest required pressure levels, attention to mask-fit issues, use of heated humidification for nasal dryness and nasal discomfort, patient education, and regular follow-up play important roles in acceptance and tolerance.

Improvement is dependent on effective use of PAP. Compliance with the therapy consists of acceptance and adherence. Some patients will initially refuse to accept and use PAP therapy, and others have difficulty using PAP consistently night to night or for the duration of the sleep period. Most PAP devices have built-in compliance tracking monitors that determine nightly and average usage, leak rate, and AHI. Increasingly, compliance data is updated almost continuously to cloud-based platforms and can be accessed wirelessly by providers. Patients may use web-based portals and phone apps to track their own patterns and access more information about their therapy.

Interventions to improve PAP compliance are based on patient education and behavioral principles of positive reinforcement and empowerment. These include education about OSA and the benefits of treatment, addressing patient-perceived problems, familial and/or group support, regular compliance checks, and clinic follow-ups.

Nonadherence to nasal PAP therapy can be attributed to noise, inconvenience, partner intolerance, mask leak, skin abrasions, claustrophobia, aerophagia, epistaxis, improper fit of equipment, and incomplete resolution of symptoms. Finding an interface that is well fitting, leak free, and maximally comfortable for the patient is critical to patient acceptance of PAP. Extra time should be taken to find the correct interface because a poor fitting, uncomfortable interface can cause a patient to refuse PAP therapy. Adding heated humidification has been shown to prevent discomfort and dryness and increase compliance while using nasal CPAP (79). It is important to maximize airflow through the nasal airway by treating allergies and congestion. Nasal swelling and secretions create narrowing and resistance to nasal airflow. The AHI in patients with chronic nasal congestion can be reduced with the use of topical corticosteroids (80,81).

Effective PAP therapy reduces SDB and improves nocturnal oxygenation, sleep architecture, daytime sleepiness, neurocognitive performance, driving performance, and perceived health status (82,83). Although oxygen therapy is sometimes used in conjunction with PAP therapy to address comorbid respiratory disorders, oxygen therapy alone is not an approved treatment for OSA. Although hypoxemia caused by SDB can improve from supplemental oxygen, hypercapnia can worsen in patients with respiratory disease. Additionally, the arousal response to SDB can be impeded, thus lengthening apneas (84). Cardiovascular endpoints, such as hypertension, cardiac arrhythmia, nocturnal ischemia, left ventricular function, and mortality, may also improve with PAP therapy (83). Health care utilization is also reduced in OSA patients on PAP therapy compared with untreated patients.

Oral Appliances

Oral appliances can be used in mild-to-moderate cases of OSA, with a success rate of up to 52% (85). Dentists and orthodontists who specialize in sleep medicine assess the patient for eligibility for the appliance by evaluating jaw and dental structure. The dental appliances are made after taking an impression of the bite. The appliances are worn during sleep and work by bringing the tongue and jaw forward to increase the posterior airway space and prevent airway collapse (86,87). Adjustments are made to advance the jaw forward until the patient reports improvements in symptoms. Side effects may include jaw stiffness or significant temporomandibular joint pain. The devices require some original teeth in patients with dentures for proper fit. Elderly people who have fewer original teeth will have difficulty tolerating the appliances and may not be good candidates. Because of the variable success rate, patients should have a repeat sleep study after the final adjustment to ensure satisfactory therapeutic benefit (88).

Nasal Expiratory Resistance Devices

Nasal valves that build negative back pressure to maintain patency of the airway during expiration can be trialed on patients with mild-to-moderate OSA. These nasal expiratory resistance devices adhere to the nares and restrict expiratory airflow, increasing pressure in the airway during expiration to keep the airway open and reduce snoring. There are variable results from these devices; generally, an improvement in respiratory disturbance is seen, even without improvements in objective sleep quality. Some patients find the sensation of breathing against the nasal valves uncomfortable, but when tolerated, a lowered AHI and snoring reduction or elimination can be seen. There are no known predictors of patient types that will tolerate or respond well to the device, so trials of the device and follow-up on the efficacy of the device are indicated.

Surgical Management

Surgery can be considered when there is an anatomic obstruction that compromises the airway, when other effective treatments have failed (PAP, oral appliance), or when the patient cannot accept or tolerate other therapies. It is important that the airway be examined to determine if there are sites of possible surgical correction. The risks, potential side effects, complications, and success rates must be communicated to the patient considering surgical intervention. There are three main areas of obstruction that are amenable to surgical correction: the nose, soft tissue of the upper airway (tongue, uvula, and soft palate), and jaw.

Nasal Reconstruction

Deviated septum, nasal valve collapse, and turbinate enlargement can commonly produce resistance to airflow and are amenable to surgical correction. Radiofrequency treatment of the turbinate is a short outpatient procedure. The success rate for eliminating OSA with these procedures is low, but they can also be helpful for patients who are using PAP but have compromised nasal flow because of obstruction.

Pharyngeal Surgery

In children with sleep-related breathing, there is a high surgical success rate for adenotonsillectomy. Adults with enlarged tonsils and OSA may benefit from surgical removal, but the success rate is lower. Tonsils can be so large that they actually meet in the middle and can make

PAP therapy unviable. If tonsils are still present in adulthood, they are usually removed as part of palate surgery.

The uvulopalatopharyngoplasty (UPPP), initially introduced for the treatment of snoring, is the most common OSA surgical procedure. It may also be a component of multistep procedures, which increase surgical effectiveness. The UPPP involves removal of the uvula, tonsils, and tonsillar pillars along with the lower part of the soft palate. Success rates are variable (up to 55%). Uvulopalatal flap is a more conservative surgery, with less pain during recovery (89).

Radiofrequency ablation (RFA) to reduce the size of the soft palate can be considered for patients with mild-to-moderate OSA to reduce the AHI. The average postprocedure AHI after RFA was 14.9, consistent with residual mild OSA. RFA studies have shown improvement in EDS and, in one study, QOL (90).

Genioglossus advancement and hyoid myotomy (GAHM) is a procedure that moves the tongue forward to enlarge the hypopharyngeal space. This surgery can be performed along with palatal surgery as part of phase I surgery in a multiphase process. In a study where only the GAHM was performed, 61% of patients were deemed successfully treated. If phase II is performed (maxillomandibular advancement [MMA]), the success rate rises to 97% (91).

Palatal implants are designed to stiffen the palate and reduce snoring. Dacron rods are inserted into the soft palate to make it more rigid. This procedure can be performed under local anesthesia. There are few data on the efficacy of this procedure.

Maxillomandibular Advancement

MMA is one of the most successful surgical interventions for OSA. It involves cutting and advancing the upper and lower jaw bones, which can enlarge the posterior airway space up to 12 mm. In an analysis of nine case studies following primary MMA surgery, there was an overall reduction in AHI of 87% with a mean postoperative AHI of 7.7 (91). MMA can also be considered for patients with OSA and craniofacial developmental abnormalities resulting in a small jaw (micrognathia and retrognathia).

Tracheotomy

Tracheotomy was once a primary treatment for OSA (before the invention of CPAP). According to the *AASM Practice Parameter for the Surgical Modifications of the Upper Airway for Obstructive Sleep Apnea in Adults*, "Tracheostomy has been shown to be an effective single intervention to treat OSA. This operation should be considered only when other options do not exist, have failed, are refused, or when this operation is deemed necessary by clinical urgency" (90).

Implantable Upper Airway Stimulation

An implanted nerve stimulator targeting the hypoglossal nerve is indicated to treat moderate to severe OSA. A lead in the chest monitors respiration and triggers mild stimulation of the hypoglossal nerve when inspiration is detected. This stimulation helps maintain airway patency by activating the genioglossus muscle. Presurgical evaluation includes phenotyping for the pattern of collapse that occurs during obstructed breathing, with complete concentric collapse at the soft palate a contraindication of this type of treatment. Implanting of a hypoglossal nerve stimulator (HGNS) is considered a non–first-line OSA treatment and requires an ear, nose, throat (ENT) physician for placement and management of the device along with management by the sleep specialist. Patients must be intolerant of PAP therapy to be candidates for HGNS implantation, and it is generally recommended that ideal patients have a BMI not higher than 32 to 40. A multicenter, prospective, single-group cohort design study showed that upper airway stimulation led to significant objective and subjective improvements in OSA severity (91).

NEW AREAS OF RESEARCH

Research into OSA continues in many areas. One is understanding the impact of untreated OSA on health and well-being. Active areas of study include metabolic and neurologic consequences of SDB, impact of OSA on learning and development in children, and the role of SDB in the development of visual problems. Another area is new treatment options, including new surgeries and medications as well as refinements and improvements in current treatments such as PAP.

Another exciting area is work on utilizing personalized medicine in sleep disorders. Multiple physiologic mechanisms contribute to OSA, including airway anatomy, muscle function, and individual responses to physiologic changes such as hypoxemia or hypercapnia. By identifying the specific mechanism, called "endotyping," it will be possible to apply the precise treatment option to address that mechanism, thereby improving effectiveness and tolerance of therapy. There are four categories of physiologic endotypes of OSA dysfunction: upper airway anatomic collapsibility, ventilatory control instability (high loop gain), arousal threshold, and pharyngeal muscle responsiveness. Each endotype may indicate a different treatment approach or a combination of treatments: CPAP, oral appliance or surgery to correct anatomic compromise; oxygen therapy or acetazolamide for high loop gain; carefully prescribed hypnotic sedatives for a low arousal threshold; and HGNS or myofunctional therapy (MT) for pharyngeal muscle dysfunction.

The Food and Drug Administration (FDA) has approved tirzepatide (Zepbound), a glucagon-like peptide-1 (GLP-1) and glucose-dependent insulinotropic polypeptide (GIP) receptor agonist, for the treatment of moderate to severe OSA in adults with obesity. GLP-1 medications and other methods for medical management of weight loss will only improve OSA if excess weight contributes to the cause of OSA. An adjunct therapy like CPAP may be indicated to treat symptoms until significant weight is lost.

SUMMARY

OSA is a common disorder with a huge impact on individual health and the public health system but can be managed by sleep professionals to reduce a patient's risk of death, major cardiovascular morbidity, cerebrovascular events, and motor vehicle accidents and to reduce symptoms and improve QOL.

REFERENCES

1. American Academy of Sleep Medicine. *International Classification of Sleep Disorders: Diagnostic and Coding Manual*. 3rd ed. American Academy of Sleep Medicine; 2014.
2. Watanabe T, Isono S, Tanaka A, et al. Contribution of body habitus and craniofacial characteristics to segmental closing pressures of the passive pharynx in patients with sleep-disordered breathing. *Am J Respir Crit Care Med*. 2002;165:260-265.
3. Young T, Palta M, Dempsey J, et al. The occurrence of sleep-related breathing among middle-aged adults. *N Engl J Med*. 1993;328:1230-1235.
4. Peppard PE, Young T, Barnet JH, et al. Increased prevalence of sleep-disordered breathing in adults. *Am J Epidemiol*. 2013;177(9):1006-1014.
5. Redline S. Epidemiology of sleep-disordered breathing. *Semin Respir Crit Care Med*. 1998;19:113-122.
6. Peppard PE, Young T, Palta M, et al. Longitudinal study of moderate weight change and sleep-disordered breathing. *J Am Med Assoc*. 2000;284:3015-3021.
7. Tuomilehto HP, Seppa JM, Partinen MM, et al; Kuopio Sleep Apnea Group. Lifestyle intervention with weight reduction: first-line treatment in mild obstructive sleep apnea. *Am J Respir Crit Care Med*. 2009;179:320-327.
8. Redline S, Kump K, Tishler PV, et al. Gender differences in sleep disordered breathing in a community-based sample. *Am J Respir Crit Care Med*. 1994;149:722-726.
9. Young T, Shahar E, Nieto FJ, et al. Predictors of sleep-disordered breathing in community dwelling adults: the Sleep Heart Health Study. *Arch Intern Med*. 2002;162:893-900.
10. Bixler EO, Vgontzas AN, Lin HM, et al. Prevalence of sleep-disordered breathing in women: effects of gender. *Am J Respir Crit Care Med*. 2001;163:608-613.
11. Ancoli-Israel S, Kripke DF, Klauber MR, et al. Sleep disordered breathing in community dwelling elderly. *Sleep*. 1991;14(6):486-495.
12. Ancoli-Israel S, Coy T. Are breathing disturbances in elderly equivalent to sleep apnea syndrome? *Sleep*. 1994;17:77-83.
13. Young T. Sleep-disordered breathing in older adults: is it a condition distinct from that in middle-aged adults? *Sleep*. 1996;19:529-530.
14. Young T, Peppard P, Gottlieb D. Epidemiology of obstructive sleep apnea: a population health perspective. *Am J Respir Crit Care Med*. 2002;165:1217-1239.
15. Redline S, Tishler P, Hans M, et al. Racial differences in sleep-disordered breathing in African-Americans and Caucasians. *Am J Respir Crit Care Med*. 1997;155:186-192.
16. Ancoli-Israel S, Klauber MR, Stepnowsky C, et al. Sleep-disordered breathing in African-American elderly. *Am J Respir Crit Care Med*. 1995;152:1946-1949.
17. Lee RW, Vasudevan S, Hui DS, et al. Differences in craniofacial structures and obesity in Caucasian and Chinese patients with obstructive sleep apnea. *Sleep*. 2010;33(8):1075-1080.
18. Trois MS, Capone GT, Lutz JA, et al. Obstructive sleep apnea in adults with Down syndrome. *J Clin Sleep Med*. 2009;15:317-323.
19. Redline S, Tishler PV, Tosteson TD, et al. The familial aggregation of obstructive sleep apnea. *Am J Respir Crit Care Med*. 1995;151:682-687.
20. Wetter DW, Young TB, Bidwell TR, et al. Smoking as a risk factor for sleep-disordered breathing. *Arch Intern Med*. 1994;154:2219-2224.
21. Taasan VC, Block AJ, Boysen PG, et al. Alcohol increases sleep apnea and oxygen desaturation in asymptomatic men. *Am J Med*. 1981;71:240-245.
22. Krol RC, Knuth SL, Bartlett D Jr. Selective reduction of genioglossal muscle activity by alcohol in normal human subjects. *Am Rev Respir Dis*. 1984;129:247-250.
23. Scrima L, Broudy M, Nay KN, et al. Increased severity of obstructive sleep apnea after bedtime alcohol ingestion: diagnostic potential and proposed mechanism of action. *Sleep*. 1982;5:318-328.
24. Sahin FK, Koken G, Cosar E, et al. Obstructive sleep apnea in pregnancy and fetal outcome. *Int J Gynecol Obstet*. 2008;100(2):141-146.
25. Guilleminault C, Connoly SJ, Winkle RA. Cardiac arrhythmia and conduction disturbances during sleep in 400 patients with sleep apnea syndrome. *Am J Cardiol*. 1983;52:490-494.
26. Punjabi NM, Newman A, Young T, et al. Sleep-disordered breathing and cardiovascular disease: an outcome-based definition of hypopneas. *Am J Respir Crit Care Med*. 2008;177:1150-1155.
27. Shahar E, Whitney CW, Redline S, et al. Sleep-disordered breathing and cardiovascular disease:

cross-sectional results of the Sleep Heart Health Study. *Am J Respir Crit Care Med*. 2001;163:19-25.

28. Bassiri A, Guilleminault C. Clinical features and evaluation of obstructive sleep apnea-hypopnea syndrome. In: Kryger M, Roth T, Dement W, eds. *Principles and Practice of Sleep Medicine*. 3rd ed. W.B. Saunders Company; 2000:869-878.
29. Somers V, Fletcher E. Mechanisms of hypertension in obstructive sleep apnea. In: Pack A, ed. *Sleep Apnea Pathogenesis Diagnosis and Treatment*. Marcel Dekker; 2002:353-376.
30. Hla KM, Young TB, Bidwell T, et al. Sleep apnea and hypertension. A population based study. *Ann Intern Med*. 1994;120:382-388.
31. Nieto FJ, Young TB, Lind BK, et al. Association of sleep-disordered breathing, sleep apnea, and hypertension in a large community-based study. *J Am Med Assoc*. 2000;283:1829-1836.
32. Singh JP, Larson MG, Tsuji H, et al. Reduced heart rate variability and new-onset hypertension: insights into pathogenesis of hypertension: the Framingham Heart Study. *Hypertension*. 1998;32:293-297.
33. Koehler U, Fus E, Grimm W, et al. Heart block in patients with obstructive sleep apnoea: pathogenetic factors and effects of treatment. *Eur Respir J*. 1998; 11(2):434-439.
34. Mehra R, Benjamin EJ, Shahar E, et al. Association of nocturnal arrhythmias with sleep-disordered breathing: the Sleep Heart Health Study. *Am J Respir Crit Care Med*. 2006;173:910-916.
35. Harbison J, O'Reilly P, McNicholas WT. Cardiac rhythm disturbances in the obstructive sleep apnea syndrome: effects of nasal continuous positive airway pressure therapy. *Chest*. 2000;118:591-595.
36. Ryan CM, Usui K, Floras JS, et al. Effect of continuous positive airway pressure on ventricular ectopy in heart failure patients with obstructive sleep apnoea. *Thorax*. 2005;60:781-785.
37. Kanagala R, Murali NS, Friedman PA, et al. Obstructive sleep apnea and the recurrence of atrial fibrillation. *Circulation*. 2003;107:2589-2594.
38. Javaheri S, Parker TJ, Liming JD, et al. Sleep apnea in 81 ambulatory male patients with stable heart failure. Types and their prevalences, consequences, and presentations. *Circulation*. 1998;97:2154-2159.
39. Javaheri S. Heart failure and sleep apnea: emphasis on practical therapeutic options. *Clin Chest Med*. 2003;24(2):207-222.
40. D'Alessandro R, Magelli C, Gamberini G, et al. Snoring every night as a risk factor for myocardial infarction: a case-control study. *Br Med J*. 1990;300:1557-1558.
41. Mooe T, Rabben T, Wiklund U, et al. Sleep-disordered breathing in men with coronary artery disease. *Chest*. 1996;109:659-663.
42. Mooe T, Rabben T, Wiklund U, et al. Sleep-disordered breathing in women: occurrence and association with coronary artery disease. *Am J Med*. 1996;101:251-256.
43. Kuniyoshi FH, Singh P, Gami AS, et al. Post-myocardial infarction patients with obstructive sleep apnea exhibit impaired endothelial function. *Chest*. 2011;140(1):62-67.
44. Good DC, Henkle JQ, Gelber D, et al. Sleep-disordered breathing and poor functional after stroke. *Stroke*. 1996; 27:252-259.
45. Wessendorf TE, Dahm C, Teschler H. Prevalence and clinical importance of sleep apnea in the first night after cerebral infarction. *Neurology*. 2003;60:1053.
46. Yaggi HK, Concato J, Kernan WN, et al. Obstructive sleep apnea as a risk factor for stroke and death. *N Engl J Med*. 2005;353:2034-2041.
47. Gami AS, Howard DE, Olson EJ, et al. Day-night pattern of sudden death in obstructive sleep apnea. *N Engl J Med*. 2005;352:1206-1214.
48. Punjabi NM, Polotsky VY. Disorders of glucose metabolism in sleep apnea. *J Appl Physiol*. 2005;99:1998-2007.
49. Punjabi NM, Ahmed MM, Polotsky VY, et al. Sleep-disordered breathing, glucose intolerance, and insulin resistance. *Respir Physiol Neurobiol*. 2003;136:167-178.
50. Tasali E, Mokhlesi B, Van Cauter E. Obstructive sleep apnea and type 2 diabetes: interacting epidemics. *Chest*. 2008;133:496-506.
51. Ficker JH, Dertinger SH, Siegfried W, et al. Obstructive sleep apnoea and diabetes mellitus: the role of cardiovascular autonomic neuropathy. *Eur Respir J*. 1998;11:14-19.
52. Bottini P, Dottorini ML, Cristina CM, et al. Sleep-disordered breathing in nonobese diabetic subjects with autonomic neuropathy. *Eur Respir J*. 2003;22:654-660.
53. Wilcox I, McNamara SG, Collins FL, et al. "Syndrome Z": the interaction of sleep apnoea, vascular risk factors and heart disease. *Thorax*. 1998;53(suppl 3):S25-S28.
54. Emamian F, Khazaie H, Tahmasian M, et al. The association between obstructive sleep apnea and Alzheimer's disease: a meta-analysis perspective. *Front Aging Neurosci*. 2016;8:78.
55. Beebe DW, Gozal D. Obstructive sleep apnea and the prefrontal cortex: towards a comprehensive model linking nocturnal upper airway obstruction to daytime cognitive and behavioral deficits. *J Sleep Res*. 2002; 11:1-16.
56. Sharma RA, Varga AW, Bubu OM, et al. Obstructive sleep apnea severity affects amyloid burden in cognitively normal elderly: a longitudinal study. *Am J Respir Crit Care Med*. 2018;197:933-943.
57. Naegele B, Launois SH, Mazza S, et al. Which memory processes are affected in patients with obstructive sleep apnea? An evaluation of 3 types of memory. *Sleep*. 2006;29:533-544.
58. Zimmerman ME, Arndt JT, Stanchina M, et al. Normalization of memory performance and positive airway pressure adherence in memory-impaired patients with obstructive sleep apnea. *Chest*. 2006;130: 1772-1778.
59. Borak J, Cieslicki JK, Koziej M, et al. Effects of CPAP treatment on psychological status in patients with severe obstructive sleep apnoea. *J Sleep Res*. 1996;5:123-127.

60. Flemons WW, Tsai W. Quality of life consequences of sleep disordered breathing. *J Allergy Clin Immunol.* 1997;99:S750-S756.
61. Millman RP, Fogel BS, McNamara ME, et al. Depression as a manifestation of obstructive sleep apnea: reversal with nasal continuous positive airway pressure. *J Clin Psychiatry.* 1989;50:348-351.
62. Reynolds CF III, Kupfer DJ, McEachran AB, et al. Depressive psychopathology in male sleep apneics. *J Clin Psychiatry.* 1984;45:287-290.
63. Sharafkhaneh A, Giray N, Richardson P, et al. Association of psychiatric disorders and sleep apnea in a large cohort. *Sleep.* 2005;28(11):1405-1411.
64. Ohayon MM. The effects of breathing-related sleep disorders on mood disturbances in the general population. *J Clin Psychiatry.* 2003;64:1195-1200.
65. Finn L, Young TB, Palta M, et al. Sleep-disordered breathing and self-reported general health status in the Wisconsin Sleep Cohort Study. *Sleep.* 1998;21:701-706.
66. Mallampati S, Gugino S, Desai S, et al. A clinical sign to predict a difficult tracheal intubation: a prospective study. *Can Anesth Soc J.* 1985;32:429-434.
67. Owens RL, Gold KA, Gozal D, et al. Sleep and breathing... and cancer? *Cancer Prev Res.* 2016;9:821-827.
68. Young T, Finn L, Peppard PE, et al. Sleep disordered breathing and mortality: eighteen-year follow-up of the Wisconsin sleep cohort. *Sleep.* 2008;31:1071-1078.
69. Berry RB, Albertario CL, Harding SM, et al; for the American Academy of Sleep Medicine. *The AASM Manual for the Scoring of Sleep and Associated Events: Rules, Terminology and Technical Specifications. Version 2.5.* American Academy of Sleep Medicine; 2018.
70. Collop NA, Anderson WM, Boehlecke B, et al; Portable Monitoring Task Force of the American Academy of Sleep Medicine. Clinical guidelines for the use of unattended portable monitors in the diagnosis of obstructive sleep apnea in adult patients. *J Clin Sleep Med.* 2007;3:737-747.
71. Guilleminault C, Kirisoglu C, da Rosa AC, et al. Sleepwalking, a disorder of NREM sleep instability. *Sleep Med.* 2006;7(2):163-170.
72. Guilleminault C, Palombini L, Pelayo R, et al. Sleepwalking and night terrors in prepubertal children: what triggers them? *Pediatrics.* 2003;111:e17-e25.
73. Issa FQ, Sullivan CE. Alcohol, snoring and sleep apnoea. *J Neurol Neurosurg Psychiatry.* 1982;45:353-359.
74. Guardiano SA, Scott JA, Ware JC, et al. The long-term results of gastric bypass on indexes of sleep apnea. *Chest.* 2003;124:1615-1619.
75. Rasheid S, Banasiak M, Gallagher SF, et al. Gastric bypass is an effective treatment for obstructive sleep apnea in patients with clinically significant obesity. *Obes Surg.* 2003;13:58-61.
76. Drager LF, Brunoni AR, Jenner R, et al. Effects of CPAP on body weight in patients with obstructive sleep apnoea: a meta-analysis of randomised trials. *Thorax.* 2015;70:258-264.
77. Jokic R, Klimaszewski A, Crossley M, et al. Positional treatment vs continuous positive airway pressure in patients with positional obstructive sleep apnea syndrome. *Chest.* 1999;115:771-781.
78. Massie CA, Hart RW, Peralez K, et al. Effects of humidification on nasal symptoms and compliance in sleep apnea. *Chest.* 1999;116:403-408.
79. Kiely JL, Nolan P, McNicholas WT. Intranasal corticosteroid therapy for obstructive sleep apnoea in patients with co-existing rhinitis. *Thorax.* 2004; 59:50-55.
80. Joe S, Benson A. Nonallergic rhinitis. In: Cummings CW, ed. *Otolaryngology: Head Neck Surgery.* Mosby; 2005: 996-999.
81. Weaver T. Adherence to continuous positive airway pressure treatment and functional status in adult obstructive sleep apnea. In: Pack A, ed. *Sleep Apnea Pathogenesis Diagnosis and Treatment.* Marcel Dekker; 2002;523-554.
82. Roux F, Hilbert J. Continuous positive airway pressure: new generations. *Clin Chest Med.* 2003;24(2): 315-342.
83. Epstein LJ, Kristo D, Strollo PJ Jr, et al. Clinical guideline for the evaluation, management and long-term care of obstructive sleep apnea in adults. Adult obstructive sleep apnea task force of the American Academy of Sleep Medicine. *J Clin Sleep Med.* 2009; 5(3):263-276.
84. Ferguson KA, Cartwright R, Rogers R, et al. Oral appliances for snoring and obstructive sleep apnea: a review. *Sleep.* 2006;29(2):244-262.
85. Lowe A. Oral appliances for sleep breathing disorders. In: Kryger M, Roth T, Dement W, eds. *Principles and Practice of Sleep Medicine.* 3rd ed. W.B. Saunders Company; 2000:929-939.
86. Lowe A, Schmidt-Nowara W. Oral appliance therapy for snoring and sleep apnea. In: Pack A, ed. *Sleep Apnea Pathogenesis Diagnosis and Treatment.* Marcel Dekker; 2002:555-573.
87. Ramar K, Dort LC, Katz SG, et al. Clinical practice guideline for the treatment of obstructive sleep apnea and snoring with oral appliance therapy: an update for 2015. *J Clin Sleep Med.* 2015;11(7):773-827.
88. Malhotra A, Crowley S, Pillar G, et al. Age-related changes in pharyngeal structure and function in normal subjects [Abstract]. *Sleep.* 2000;161(2):A42.
89. Aurora RN, Casey KR, Kristo D, et al. Practice parameters for the surgical modifications of the upper airway for obstructive sleep apnea in adults. *Sleep.* 2010;33(10):1408-1413.
90. Caples SM, Rowley JA, Prinsell JR, et al. Surgical modifications of the upper airway for obstructive sleep apnea in adults: a systematic review and meta-analysis. *Sleep.* 2010;33(10):1396-1407.
91. Strollo PJ Jr, Soose RJ, Maurer JT, et al; STAR Trial Group. Upper-airway stimulation for obstructive sleep apnea. *N Engl J Med.* 2014;370(2):139-149.

Chapter 11
Central Sleep Apnea

LAURA A. LINLEY

KEY CONCEPTS/LEARNING OBJECTIVES

The key concepts for this chapter include describing the clinical presentation of central sleep apnea (CSA), defining the two different conditions contributing to CSA, explaining the respiratory drive mechanisms of sleep, reviewing physiologically normal apneic events and the presentation of Cheyne-Stokes respiration, primary CSA, and treatment-emergent CSA, outlining the patient evaluation procedure/differential diagnosis and workup, reviewing the polysomnographic findings of CSA, and citing the treatment goals and options for Central Sleep Apnea Syndrome (CSAS).

KEY TERMS

Adaptive servo-ventilation
Central sleep apnea
Central sleep apnea syndrome
Cheyne-Stokes respiration
Congestive heart failure
Hypercapnia
Hypoventilation
PAP therapy
Treatment-emergent central sleep apnea

Central sleep apnea syndrome (CSAS) is a disorder of decreased breathing rate or depth during the sleep period because of a transient reduction or withdrawal of central neural output to the respiratory muscles (the diaphragm and intercostal muscles) (1,2). There is an instability of ventilation control at sleep onset, and respiratory irregularity and abnormal breathing patterns can arise during this time. The respiratory drive centers respond differently to levels of oxygen and carbon dioxide (CO_2) during sleep and wakefulness.

The prevalence of CSA in clinical practice is less than that of obstructive apnea, constituting 5% to 10% of all sleep apnea cases (except in very premature infants, in whom it is seen commonly because of their relatively immature or underdeveloped central respiratory control centers) (1). A few short central apneas (CAs) are not uncommon, particularly following a deep breath such as with a sigh or yawn.

Obstructive sleep apnea is defined as cessation of airflow for 10 seconds or more during sleep without a cessation in effort. CSA is defined as cessation of airflow and effort channels for 10 seconds or more.

SLEEP RESPIRATORY DRIVE MECHANISMS

Sleep respiratory function is driven by the bulbar respiratory center, which reacts to metabolic, mechanic, and behavioral influences. Metabolic regulation is exerted by changes in PO_2 and PCO_2: Increased PCO_2 stimulates the bulbar center, whereas a critical reduction in PCO_2 inhibits it. Ventilation drive is also increased with decreased levels of PO_2.

Mechanical (autonomic) regulation is under the control of pulmonary vagal receptors and can, if stimulated, give rise to reflex hyperventilation. Behavioral regulation of breathing is typical during the awake state. Behavioral regulation reacts to changing patterns of breathing such as seen during talking or with exercise. Ventilation will respond to behavioral inputs only during wake, not during nonrapid eye movement (NREM) sleep. It is thought that the reason for this is that the receptors for behavior regulation are in the forebrain and are not active during NREM sleep. PCO_2 during sleep decreases temporarily to below the critical level that is necessary to keep the respiratory rhythm normal.

There are many causes for loss of central respiratory impulse during sleep. Metabolic control and neuromuscular failure may cause chronic alveolar hypoventilation syndrome that worsens during sleep when the stimulating effect of wakefulness is absent (2). CSA may also be caused by a transient instability of the respiratory drive that is otherwise undamaged: When the stimulating effect of wakefulness (neural wakefulness impulse) on respiration is lacking, then the apneic episode begins and continues until the PCO_2 critical level is reached.

Sleep affects respiration primarily at sleep onset when PCO_2 oscillates around the hypocapnic threshold (3).

Thus, CSA occurs with hypocapnia, and it ceases with arousal and hyperventilation. Subsequently recurring hypocapnia leads to a new apneic episode when sleep is resumed (4,5). Post-hyperventilation CSA is less common during rapid eye movement (REM) sleep.

RISK FACTORS

Several physiologic and pathologic factors increase the risk of CSA, including age, sex, and many medical conditions. The threshold for hypocapnic CSA is higher in males, and CSA is rare in premenopausal women. Disorders such as thyroid dysfunction, cerebrovascular disease, acromegaly, renal failure, congestive heart failure (CHF), and atrial fibrillation may increase susceptibility to the development of CSA in older patients (6).

CSA comprises 40% of apneas that develop following a cerebrovascular accident (CVA). The brainstem is the primary center for ventilation control, so any damage occurring there or to the medullary area from a CVA could impact regular respiration during sleep (7). In 1997, the American Academy of Pain Medicine (AAPM) and the American Pain Society issued a joint position statement, stating, "It is now accepted by practitioners of the specialty of pain medicine that respiratory depression induced by opioids tends to be a short-lived phenomenon, generally occurs only in the opioid-naive patient, and is antagonized by pain. Therefore, withholding the appropriate use of opioids from a patient who is experiencing pain on the basis of respiratory concerns is unwarranted" (8). Ever since this statement was made, there have been multiple studies demonstrating an association of opioids with sleep apnea. Opioid use for pain management has increased, resulting in a rise in opioid-associated morbidity and mortality. The AAPM updated its statement on the *Use of Opioids for the Treatment of Chronic Pain.* Position three of that statement indicates: "Physicians should be sensitive to and seek to minimize the risks of addiction, respiratory depression and other adverse effects, tolerance and diversion." The statement cautions titration of opioid medications in patients with underlying diagnoses such as sleep apnea (specifically CSA) or end-stage respiratory disease due to the increased risk of cardiorespiratory events. CSA occurs in 30% of patients undergoing stable methadone (opioid) maintenance treatment. The concern is that some patients present with CSA without any apparent risk factors. In these cases of "idiopathic" CSA, increased chemo responsiveness or sleep state instability could be responsible for the irregularity in breathing patterns. Occasionally, these patients may have a theretofore undiagnosed metabolic or cardiac disorder (9,10). Although CAs are commonly observed during initial polysomnography (PSG), they may be absent initially and appear during continuous positive airway pressure (CPAP) titration and present as treatment-emergent CSA. Central events that persisted with the use of CPAP or bilevel devices required more advanced therapy such as adaptive servo-ventilation (ASV) (11).

ETIOLOGY AND PATHOPHYSIOLOGY

There are two general categories of disorders that cause the central nervous system (CNS) respiratory control system to decrease output to the respiratory muscles:

1. Disorders that cause defects to the system itself (CSA with abnormal respiratory control system)
2. Disorders outside the system that cause a normal system to reduce its output (CSA with normal respiratory control system) (1)

The first condition leads to hypoventilation and CSA and is found in patients with diseases involving the brainstem, neuromuscular disorders, and central hypoventilation syndromes. These disorders involve a chemical or neural change that causes a normal control system to alternate between stimulating breathing and inhibiting breathing. Patients are not apneic while awake, because the waking neural drive stimulates breathing. With sleep, loss of the CNS drive may cause CA to occur, especially in REM sleep. These CAs tend to decrease as sleep duration progresses. When the respiratory control system is impaired by brainstem disease or an abnormal chemical drive to breathe, withdrawal of the waking stimulus results in a profound decrease in neural drive. Transient CAs may occur upon initiation of sleep, when relative waking hypocapnia triggers a central apneic event.

The pathophysiology of CSA invokes two key mechanisms (9). One is a tendency for baseline hypoventilation with hypercapnia to place breathing controllers closer to the apneic threshold during NREM sleep. The second is delayed circulation time from the lung to the chemoreceptors in the carotid artery, with destabilization and overshoot of feedback control, seen in low cardiac output states. This may be associated with a destabilization of the feedback control of breathing with delayed overshoot in the ventilatory response to stimuli. Prolonged periods of CA or hypopnea (underbreathing in response to hypocapnic hyperventilation) alternate with exaggerated periods of ventilation (overbreathing and arousals in response to apnea), perpetuating a cycle of hyperventilatory overshoot and subsequent CAs. In various studies of patients with cardiac condition and with an ejection fraction of less than 45%, the prevalence of sleep apnea in patients undergoing PSG was 40% to 68%. The majority of these patients with cardiac condition exhibited CSA with high levels of sleep disruption, repetitive oxygen desaturation episodes, and more nocturnal dysrhythmias than did patients without apnea with similar levels of left ventricular dysfunction.

Excessive daytime sleepiness, as assessed by the Epworth Sleepiness Scale (ESS) and by lower scores on multiple sleep latency testing, is a common problem for patients with repetitive CSA. Over the past decade, the diagnosis and management of obstructive sleep apnea (OSA) has received considerable attention in sleep medicine. Its impact on daytime cognitive function and cardiovascular health is increasingly recognized, and its frequency in the adult population renders it the most common pathologic diagnosis in sleep centers. Patients with cardiac condition with left ventricular dysfunction and Cheyne-Stokes respiration (CSR) with CSA are also prevalent. Mounting evidence suggests that this diagnosis may have important implications for the outcome and management of chronic CHF (12).

Periodic CSR is present in about 30% to 40% of patients with CHF, worsening their prognostic outcome. Its presence indicates a shorter survival compared with patients with CHF who do not exhibit CSR. Pulmonary congestion in a recumbent position induces reflex hyperventilation, with critical reduction of P_{CO_2} that causes apneic episodes. Cessation of breathing increases blood P_{CO_2}, stimulating bulbar centers and leads to resumption of breathing (13). The slowing of blood circulation contributes to CSR as a result of the delay in blood gas concentration information reaching the respiratory center. It is, however, unclear if CSR-CSA is simply a reflection of severely compromised cardiac function with elevated left ventricular filling pressure or if CSR-CSA itself exerts unique and independent pathologic effects on the failing myocardium. Regardless of its etiology, there is evidence that CSR-CSA may have detrimental physiologic effects on the failing heart (14).

In CSA, upper respiratory airways remain patent, and apneic episodes end with a different mechanism than the arousal seen with OSA. In fact, arousals seen with CSA generally occur together with the recovery of breathing activity. Arousal occurs with hyperventilation and gives rise to a vicious circle.

Patients with OSA convert to CSA and vice versa. Deterioration of left ventricular contractile function because of OSA may create conditions that lead to the emergence of pathophysiologic CSR. In turn, CSA makes the CHF prognosis worse, even if the mechanism of this phenomenon is still unclear (15). See Figure 11-1 for an example of Cheyne-Stokes respirations.

The diagnosis of CSR requires overnight PSG performed in a sleep center. It has been reported that mortality over a 3-year period is 56% in patients with CHF and CSAS, compared with 11% in patients without CSAS, despite comparable left ventricular function. More recently, studies in 62 patients with CHF with left ventricular dysfunction demonstrated that the apnea-hypopnea index was the most powerful independent predictor of survival (15).

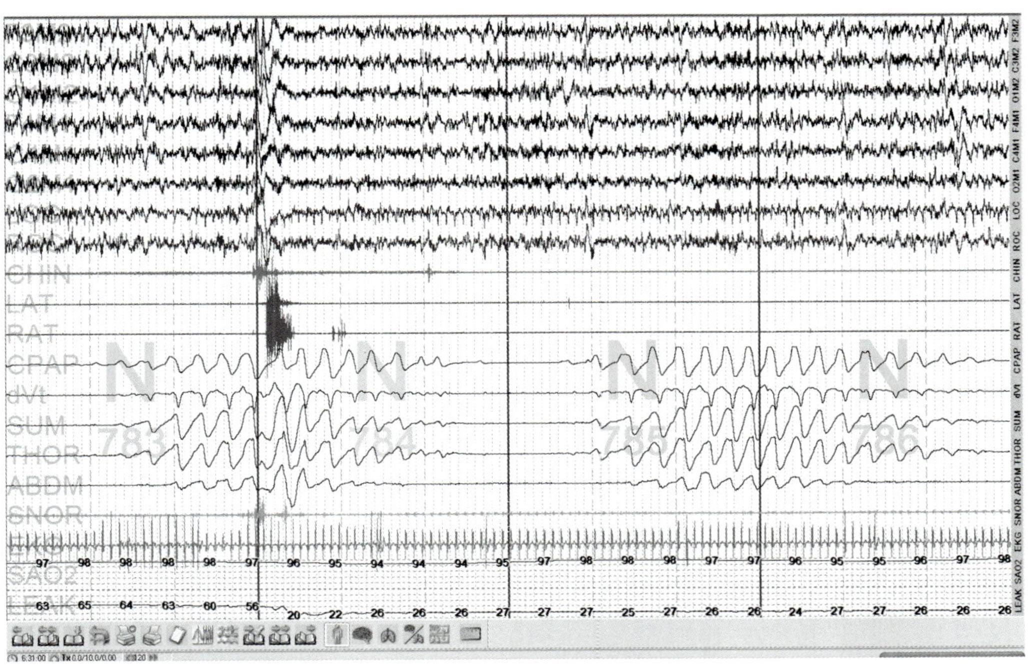

Figure 11-1 Cheyne-Stokes respirations. There is a crescendo-decrescendo breathing pattern during each breathing cycle, which drops the carbon dioxide levels below the "apnea threshold," causing central apnea.

TREATMENT-EMERGENT CENTRAL SLEEP APNEA

Treatment-Emergent Central Sleep Apnea (TECSA) is characterized by the combined phenomena of both OSA and CSA. TECSA is defined as the development of CSA in the patient with OSA during the initial CPAP titration. Patients with TECSA can have persistent sleep fragmentation and central events on CPAP treatment, predominately in N1 and N2 sleep, while breathing normalizes in N3 and REM. Note that there have been reports of treatment-emergent CSA developing with other treatment modalities for OSA, including tracheostomy, maxillomandibular advancement, and oral appliance treatment. ASV is an advanced positive pressure therapy option for normalizing central events (16).

The pathophysiology of TECSA is not clearly defined. There are multiple models to explain the cause. Some theorized mechanisms are ventilatory control instability, low arousal threshold, activation of stretch lung receptors, and prolonged circulation time. Further study is needed to verify factors that predispose a patient to developing TECSA.

CLINICAL PICTURE

The clinical features of CSAS are directly related in the cardiorespiratory and nervous systems. Figure 11-2 shows examples of CA events.

Frequent arousals cause frequent sleep disturbances. Both slow-wave sleep and REM sleep are reduced. CSA can be divided into two groups: hypercapnic CSA and nonhypercapnic CSA. Hypercapnic CSA with alveolar hypoventilation is idiopathic and is caused by diseases in the brainstem or secondary to neuromuscular

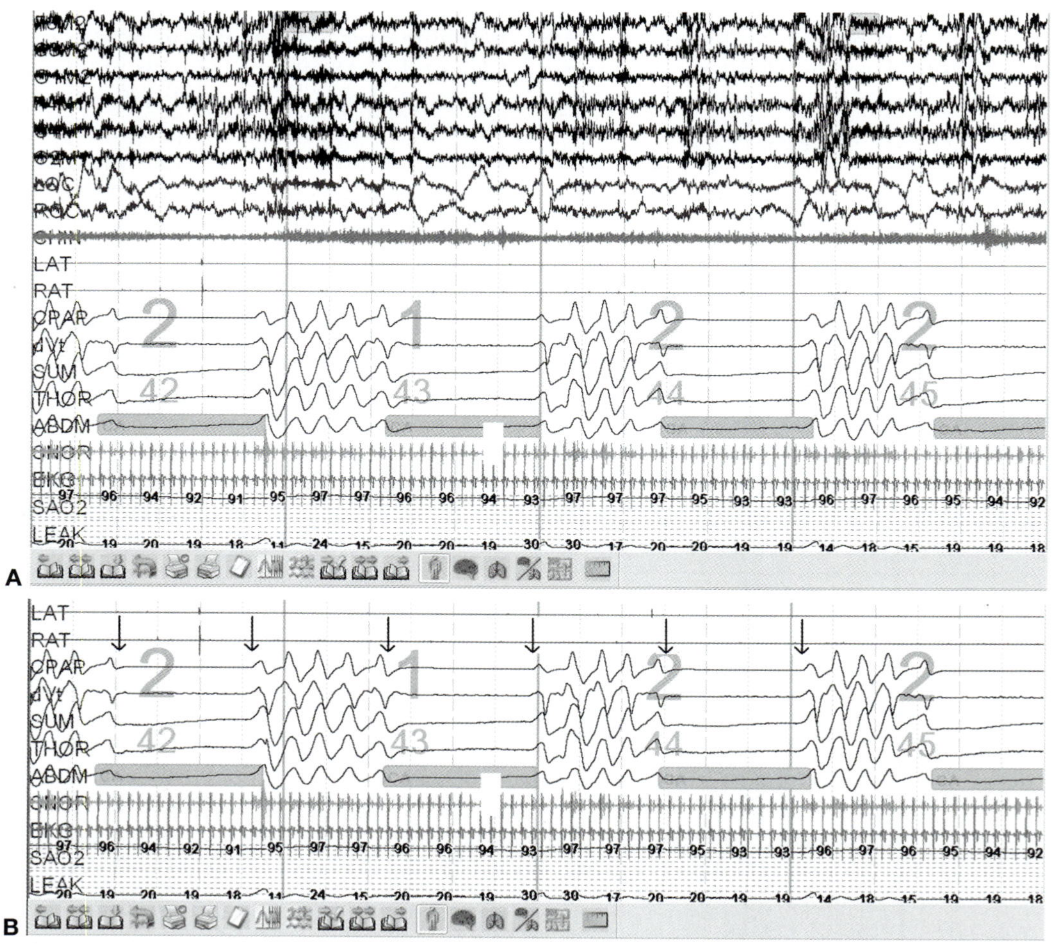

Figure 11-2 A: Central apnea. Notice the low oxygen saturation that is associated with each event. During a central apnea, there is a complete loss of diaphragmatic and intercostal activity, with resumption of activity when breathing begins. B: The arrows denote the beginning and end of the central apneic event.

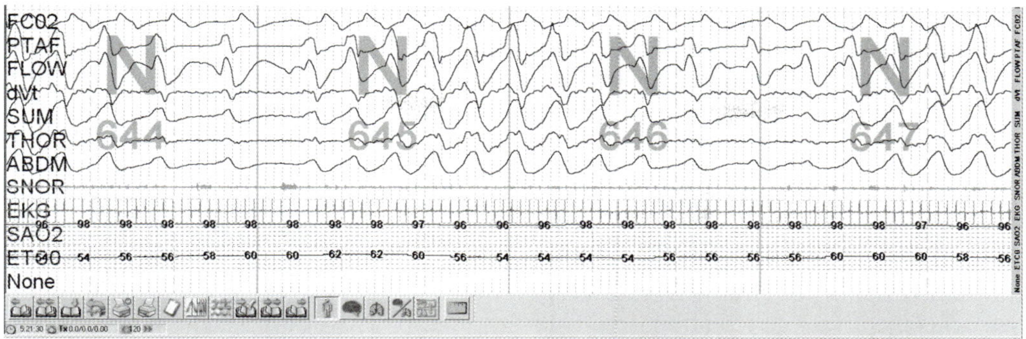

Figure 11-3 Hypoventilation verified by increasing end-tidal carbon dioxide levels.

disorders, such as myopathies, motor neuron disorders, and neuromuscular junction disorders. People with idiopathic central alveolar hypoventilation have severe daytime hypoventilation without lung disease or any known lesions in the nervous system. Chemical control of breathing is absent in these patients. People with brainstem abnormalities have no control for breathing because of disorders in the medulla, such as infarction, tumor, or hemorrhage. These may cause a true hypoventilation syndrome.

Central hypoventilation (Figure 11-3) is a disorder of decreased breathing rate or volume. This may cause daytime sleepiness and, if significant, may cause elevated blood pressure in the lungs (pulmonary hypertension) (12). There is a complete cessation of breathing during sleep with CSA. Individuals with Prader-Willi syndrome may be at increased risk for death because of a decreased neural drive for breathing.

Myopathies are neuromuscular disorders that include a large number of disorders such as muscular dystrophies and metabolic myopathies. Patients with postpolio syndrome may become symptomatic 30 to 40 years after recovering. Some apparently healthy men may develop insomnia, which can stem from a nonhypercapnic CSA.

DIAGNOSIS

CSAS diagnosis is based on technical documentation, PSG findings, and cardiorespiratory monitoring of apneic events. In this manner, it is possible to define sleep breathing characteristics and obtain indexes useful to quantify the gravity of the sleep-related clinical picture (15). These indexes, together with the underlying comorbidities, guide therapy (15).

Evaluation includes history, physical examination, and laboratory testing. Snoring, apneas, sleepiness, neurologic, cardiovascular, and renal history should be included in the patient's history. Also, symptoms of other disorders that cause sleepiness or insomnia, such as narcolepsy, periodic limb movements in sleep, insufficient sleep, and drug misuse or medication side effects, should be reviewed. During the physical examination, a general inspection of the skeletal structure of the face can be useful to observe if the upper or lower jaws are too far back (retrognathic) or too small (micrognathic). The nasal airway should also be examined for patency and for anatomic obstruction (deformity, deviation, polyps). Examination of the oral airway may give information about the size of tonsils, configuration of palate and uvula, and any other obstructing mass lesion. Cardiovascular examination can be useful to check for the presence of heart murmurs, peripheral blood hypertension, and cor pulmonale. Some tests may be needed to diagnose the medical disorders that may cause CSAS, whereas others may be needed to document the location of a CNS lesion. Apnea itself can be confirmed by a sleep study. Other tests may include imaging, chest radiographs, pulmonary function tests, and blood gases.

The American Academy of Sleep Medicine (AASM) has updated the classification of sleep disorders in the *International Classification of Sleep Disorders*, third edition (17). Within this classification, there is an expanded definition of CSA associated with other identifiable etiologies along with updated ICD-10-CM codes. These include the following:

- R06.3 Central Sleep Apnea with Cheyne–Stokes Breathing
- G47.37 Central Apnea Due to a Medical Disorder without Cheyne–Stokes Breathing
- G47.32 Central Sleep Apnea Due to a High-Altitude Periodic Breathing
- G47.39 Central Sleep Apnea Due to a Medication or Substance
- G47.31 Primary Central Sleep Apnea
- P28.3 Primary Central Sleep Apnea of Infancy
- P28.4 Primary Central Sleep Apnea of Prematurity
- G7.39 Treatment-Emergent Central Sleep Apnea

The most notable aspect of these expanded definitions is that for a diagnosis of TECSA, the presence of at least one associated sign or symptom is now required.

These symptoms include sleepiness, difficulty initiating or maintaining sleep, frequent awakenings, nonrestorative sleep, awakening short of breath, or witnessed apneas.

POLYSOMNOGRAPHY FINDINGS

CSA is characterized by a cessation or reduction of ventilatory effort and cessation of airflow during sleep and is usually associated with oxygen desaturation. Full PSG is required to properly diagnose CSAS disorders. To adequately score a CA event, there must be no recorded respiratory effort. The recommended sensor for detection of respiratory effort is esophageal manometry, dual thoracoabdominal calibrated or uncalibrated respiratory inductance plethysmography (RIP) belts, or dual thoracoabdominal polyvinylidene fluoride. If there is a complete lack of movement in the RIP channel, you can deduce that the event is central in nature (13,17). If transitional central events seem to be inhibiting sleep onset, noting this in the technical observations is important. Figure 11-4 provides an example of a sleep-onset CA.

The PSG montage should include the recording of electroencephalogram, body position, movement events, cardiac abnormalities, and respiratory events. Appropriate system calibrations, observation, and documentation by the technologist during the PSG are required. To be considered a clinical event in adults, a CA is defined as a minimum of 10 seconds of cessation of breathing effort and airflow. It is characterized by a drop in the peak breathing effort and airflow signal for more than 10 seconds, with a reduction of over 90% from the pre-event baseline, as measured by an oronasal thermal sensor during a diagnostic study or by the PAP device flow during a titration study. This event is associated with absent inspiratory effort throughout the entire period of absent airflow. Scoring central hypopneas is optional, although in patients with central syndromes, this may be important. Many Medicare local coverage determinations require reporting a central apnea-hypopnea index in order to qualify a patient for an advanced respiratory assist device such as ASV therapy. The AASM scoring manual also includes guidelines for scoring central hypopneas. According to this guideline, a central hypopnea must meet the requirements for a hypopnea: airflow decrease by 30% or more for 10 seconds associated with a 3% or 4% oxygen desaturation (rule 1.A or 1.B). To qualify as a central hypopnea, the event *cannot* have snoring, increased inspiratory flattening of the flow signal (nasal pressure or PAP), or associated thoracoabdominal paradox.

The clinical and therapeutic significance of central hypopneas is not well established in the literature. There is some increased interest in quantifying central hypopneas due to the introduction of phrenic nerve stimulator treatment for CSA. Some patients may not have clear CAs syndrome but may have central hypopneas that could theoretically benefit from phrenic nerve stimulation. The definition, quantification, and treatment of central hypopneas will continue to develop as the body of research increases.

Reporting an occurrence of Cheyne-Stokes breathing (CSB) on the PSG report is required if repetitive CAs and/or central hypopneas are present. The *AASM*

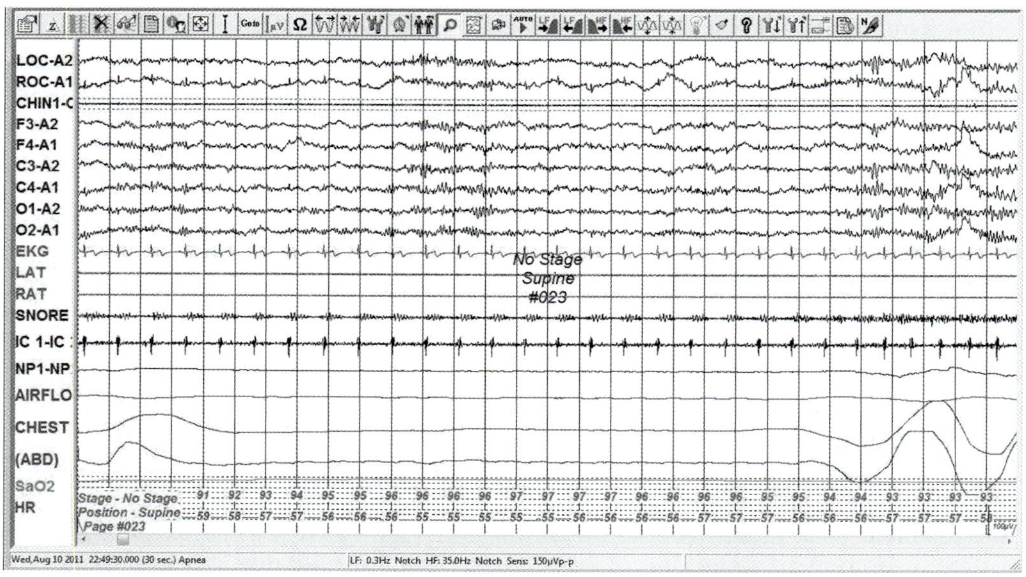

Figure 11-4 Sleep-onset central apnea. The central pauses seen in the example are related to sleep onset. The breathing pattern normalizes when the patient progresses to stage N2 sleep.

Manual for Scoring of Sleep and Associated Events (17) indicates scoring criteria for CSB (Figure 11-2). Score CSB if both of the following criteria are met:

1. Three or more consecutive CAs and/or central hypopneas separated by a crescendo and decrescendo change in breathing amplitude with a cycle length of more than 40 seconds.
2. More than or equal to five CAs and/or central hypopneas per hours of sleep associated with the crescendo/decrescendo breathing pattern recorded over more than 2 hours of monitoring (17).

TREATMENT

Treatment of CSAS can be difficult. In patients with CHF, optimize CHF treatment first. Among those with persistent CSR, various forms of CPAP have been advocated, and some patients do respond well to PAP devices. The use of CPAP has been shown to improve cardiac function and quality of life and reduce the need for organ transplantation in patients with CHF. Overall, the goal is to normalize breathing patterns, so that patients will have improved cardiac function and quality of life. Patients using PAP devices experience less fluctuation of blood gases, indicating that normalizing P_{CO_2} may normalize breathing drive. CPAP titration in these patients is usually more time-consuming, and these patients are fragile sleepers.

CSAS may respond to nasal CPAP, especially if it is combined with OSA episodes. CPAP therapy showed positive reduction of CSAS events, increasing overnight oxygen intake, lowering of norepinephrine levels, and improved cardiac ejection fraction (13). CPAP therapy corrects CSAS in some patients even if it is not accompanied by OSA. In patients with hypocapnic CSAS, CPAP may, however, increase hypocapnic status, worsening the clinical picture (18).

Some patients with hypocapnic CSAS may benefit from the use of bilevel positive airway pressure (BPAP). However, BPAP, especially when used with a high inspiratory positive airway pressure (IPAP) to expiratory positive airway pressure (EPAP) differential (delta), may exacerbate CSAS by lowering partial pressure of carbon dioxide (P_{CO_2}) levels, ultimately worsening CSA (19). An alternative to a high IPAP to EPAP differential is the use of a backup rate, which can be beneficial for patients with CSAS. BPAP has also been used in patients with CHF or Cheyne-Stokes respiration-central sleep apnea syndrome (CSR-CSAS) with variable results. Further studies are necessary to better evaluate the role of BPAP treatment in these patients.

Servo-ventilation incorporates an automatic, minute ventilation or peak flow targeted device that performs breath-to-breath analysis and adjusts pressure settings accordingly. Depending on airflow, the device will automatically adjust the amount of pressure it delivers in order to reduce hyperpneas, hypopneas, and apneas. In 2025, the AASM released an update on ASV recommending the use of ASV for patients with primary CSA, CSA due to heart failure, CSA due to medication or substance use, treatment-emergent CSA, and CSA due to a medical condition or disorder. They commented that previously research had indicated a reduced mortality in patients with a lowered ejection fraction but that the device used in the study was no longer being manufactured. There is no data available on reduced ejection fraction for any of the currently manufactured machines. The application of these recommendations is limited to the target patient populations; the ultimate judgment regarding the propriety of any specific care must be made by the clinician.

A novel approach to treating CSAS is transvenous phrenic nerve stimulation. This treatment works by stimulating the phrenic nerve to induce diaphragmatic contraction, thereby restoring normal breathing during sleep. It has been shown to improve sleep quality, oxygenation, respiratory parameters, and overall quality of life with few complications. This method may be an effective treatment for moderate to severe CSAS in adult patients, including those with heart failure (20).

However, this device is not intended for use in patients with primary OSA, and special consideration must be given to patients who require magnetic resonance imaging (MRI) (21). The patient selection pathway includes a diagnostic study for moderate to severe CSAS, documented titration studies, and a trial of CPAP and ASV treatment if appropriate. If symptoms and events persist despite CPAP and ASV treatment, phrenic nerve stimulation should be considered.

REFERENCES

1. Malhotra A, Owens RL. What is central sleep apnea? *Respir Care*. 2010;55(9):1168-1178.
2. Wellman A, Malhotra A, Fogel RB, et al. Respiratory system loop gain in normal men and women measured with proportional assist ventilation. *J Appl Physiol*. 2003;94:205-212.
3. Dunai J, Kleiman J, Trinder J. Ventilatory instability during sleep onset in individuals with high peripheral chemosensitivity. *J Appl Physiol*. 1999;87:661-672.
4. Safwan B. Central sleep apnea in patients with congestive heart failure. *Heart Fail Rev*. 2009;14:135-141.
5. Orem J, Lovering AT, Dunin-Barkowski W, et al. Tonic activity in the respiratory system in wakefulness, NREM and REM sleep. *Sleep*. 2002;25:488-496.
6. Grunstein RR, Ho KY, Berthon-Jones M, et al. Central sleep apnea is associated with increased ventilatory response to carbon dioxide and hypersecretion

of growth hormone in patients with acromegaly. *Am J Respir Crit Care Med.* 1994;150:496-502.

7. American Academy of Pain Medicine and the American Pain Society. The use of opioids for the treatment of chronic pain: a consensus statement from the American Academy of Pain Medicine and the American Pain Society. *Clin J Pain.* 1997;13(1):6-8.
8. Xie A, Wong B, Phillipson EA, et al. Interaction of hyperventilation and arousal in the pathogenesis of idiopathic central sleep apnea. *Am J Respir Crit Care Med.* 1994;150:489-495.
9. Javaheri S, Malik A, Smith J, et al. Adaptive pressure support servoventilation: a novel treatment for sleep apnea associated with use of opioids. *J Clin Sleep Med.* 2008;4:305-310.
10. Franklin KA, Sandstrom E, Johansson G, et al. Hemodynamics, cerebral circulation, and oxygen saturation in Cheyne-Stokes respiration. *J Appl Physiol.* 1997;83:1184-1191.
11. Trinder J, Merson R, Rosenberg JI, et al. Pathophysiological interactions of ventilation, arousals, and blood pressure oscillations during Cheyne-Stokes respiration in patients with heart failure. *Am J Respir Crit Care Med.* 2000;162:808-813.
12. Saunders MH. Sleep breathing disorders/central sleep apnea. In: Kryger M, Roth T, Dement W, eds. *Principles and Practice of Sleep Medicine.* 4th ed. Elsevier Saunders; 2005.
13. Farre R, Montserrat JM, Navajas D. Noninvasive monitoring of respiratory mechanics during sleep. *Eur Respir J.* 2004;24:1052-1060.
14. Yumino D, Bradley TD. Central sleep apnea and Cheyne-Stokes respiration. *Proc Am Thorac Soc.* 2008;5:226-236. doi:10.1513/pats.200708-129MG
15. Allam JS, Olson EJ, Gay PC, et al. Efficacy of adaptive servoventilation in treatment of complex and central sleep apnea syndromes. *Chest.* 2007;132:1839-1846.
16. Troester MM, Quan SF, Berry RB, et al; for the American Academy of Sleep Medicine. *The AASM Manual for the Scoring of Sleep and Associated Events: Rules, Terminology and Technical Specifications. Version 3.* American Academy of Sleep Medicine; 2023.
17. American Academy of Sleep Medicine. *International Classification of Sleep Disorders.* 3rd ed. American Academy of Sleep Medicine; 2014.
18. Lehman S, Antic NA, Thompson C, et al. Central sleep apnea: commencement of continuous positive airway pressure in patients with a diagnosis of obstructive sleep apnea–hypopnea. *J Clin Sleep Med.* 2007;3:462-466.
19. Johal A, Lenet A, Sigua NL. Blowing past the apneic threshold. *J Clin Sleep Med.* 2022;18(10):2515-2518.
20. Aurora RN, Bista SR, Casey, KR, et al. Updated adaptive servo-ventilation recommendations for the 2012 AASM guideline: "the treatment of central sleep apnea syndromes in adults: practice parameters with an evidence-base literature review and meta-analyses". *J Clin Sleep Med.* 2016;12(5):757-761. doi:10.556/jcsm.5812
21. Sagalow ES, Ananth A, Alapati R, Fares E, Fast Z. Transvenous phrenic nerve stimulation for central sleep apnea. *Am J Cardiol.* 2022;180:P155-P162.

Chapter 12
Hypoventilation Syndromes

BYRON JAMERSON

KEY CONCEPTS/LEARNING OBJECTIVES

The key concepts for this chapter include the physiology of normal ventilation and respiration, and identification of sleep-disordered breathing during sleep studies, and a review of hypoventilation and the associated pathophysiology. We will review the clinical significance of hypoventilation, how hypoventilation is identified during a sleep study, the difference between hypopneas and hypoventilation, and a review of the process for performing a diagnostic study and treatments for patients with hypoventilation.

KEY TERMS

Arterial blood gas (ABG)
Gas exchange
Minute ventilation (MV)
Noninvasive ventilation (NIV)
Pulmonary function test (PFT)
Pulmonary hypertension
Respiration
Tidal volume (V_T)
Ventilation

Hypoventilation is an impairment of the body's ability to breathe. Chronic hypoventilation may be the result of disorders that affect any part of the respiratory system. It may be caused by congenital disorders, brainstem disorders, neurologic disorders associated with signal communication from the brain through the spinal column, or neuromuscular disorders that compromise the signals in the nerves or muscles (1).

Before delving more deeply into hypoventilation, let's first discuss normal breathing and how the respiratory and circulatory systems work to deliver oxygen (O_2) to the cells of the body, and the other sleep-disordered breathing (SDB) events seen in the sleep laboratory during polysomnography (PSG).

PHYSIOLOGY OF NORMAL VENTILATION AND RESPIRATION

Ventilation or breathing is the process of moving air in and out of the lungs. Inhalation brings needed O_2 to the lungs, and exhalation removes carbon dioxide (CO_2), the waste by-product of cell metabolism.

Inhalation is initiated when the brain signals the diaphragm (the major muscle of ventilation) to contract, causing the thoracic cavity to expand. The expansion creates a pressure drop in the chest. It is this pressure gradient between the atmosphere and the chest that causes the air to pass through the nasal cavity, upper airway, bronchi, bronchioles, and ultimately to the alveoli. The alveoli are small sacks in the lungs that are surrounded by capillaries where respiration or gas exchange takes place (exchange of O_2 with CO_2).

The right side of the heart pumps blood to the lung's capillary bed, where O_2 molecules, brought to the alveoli by the inhalation process, pass through the alveolar membrane and the capillary walls into the blood. Conversely, CO_2 passes through the capillary wall and the alveolar membrane into the alveoli, where it is eliminated by exhalation. It is the concentration gradient between the gases in the alveoli and the capillaries that allows this gas exchange to take place through simple diffusion. Once the blood in the capillary bed surrounding the alveoli has less CO_2 and more O_2, the oxygenated blood is then pumped from the right side of the heart to the left side of the heart. The heart's left ventricle then pumps the oxygenated blood, through the arteries, to all the cells in the body.

The body's motivation to breathe (contract the diaphragm) is created by the amount of CO_2 in the blood. The CO_2 molecules, pumped to the brain by the heart, pass through capillaries into the spinal fluid that bathes the brain. Through a chemical process, the CO_2 molecule is turned to hydrogen ion and water. It is the hydrogen molecule that changes the spinal fluid pH, making it more acidic. This change in spinal fluid pH is detected in the hindbrain by the medulla oblongata and pons, which, in turn, signal the diaphragm to contract. CO_2 levels in the blood are the primary driver to breathe. This is the normal breathing process and how every cell in the body receives O_2 and maintains life (2).

Now let's discuss what occurs during sleep that may compromise or impair this process.

KEY TAKEAWAY: Physiology of Normal Breathing

- Normal breathing: CO_2 levels in the blood provide the primary drive to breathe. As CO_2 levels increase, the spinal fluid becomes more acidic and triggers the brain to send a signal to the diaphragm to contract and start the breathing process.
- Air is inhaled into the body when the diaphragm contracts, creating negative pressure in the lungs. This contraction creates a pressure gradient that causes air to pass through the respiratory system into the alveoli.
- Gas exchange takes place between the alveoli and the blood in the capillary beds surrounding the alveoli—CO_2 is exchanged for O_2.
- The heart pumps the blood through the arteries to the entire body exchanging the O_2 for CO_2 (a by-product of cell metabolism) to keep cells alive.
- The veins carry the CO_2 from the cells back to the right side of the heart and into the lungs to exchange the CO_2 for O_2 and start the breathing process again.

SLEEP-DISORDERED BREATHING

A polysomnogram (PSG) monitors how well a person sleeps and how well the body functions while they are asleep. A PSG records the patient's brain activity using a modified electroencephalogram (EEG), eye movement using electrooculogram (EOG), muscle tone using electromyogram (EMG), and the heart and heart rate via a modified electrocardiogram (ECG). SDB is identified by monitoring airflow, respiratory effort, oxygen saturation, and, if possible, CO_2 levels in the blood (3).

SDB disrupts the normal breathing process during sleep. This may be caused by air not getting into the lungs because of airway obstructions, the drive to breathe being affected due to the diaphragm not receiving the signal to contract or not being able to contract, or a combination of both.

Table 12-1 summarizes the categories of SDB and how they are monitored and includes short descriptions (4).

The treatment for SDB caused by airway blockage is continuous positive airway pressure (CPAP) or bilevel positive airway pressure (BPAP), applied to the airway via a mask to keep the airway open. The treatment for a patient who has a diminished drive to breathe or no drive to breathe is usually a BPAP device that includes a timed backup rate (BPAP S/T) or more sophisticated noninvasive ventilation (NIV) if needed (5).

Cheyne-Stokes Respirations (CSR) are characterized by the appearance of a crescendo-decrescendo (waxing and waning) of the breathing pattern caused by changes in the partial pressures of oxygen and carbon dioxide. CSR may be caused by cardiac failure, renal failure, narcotic poisoning, and raised intracranial pressures. CSR displays periods of increased tidal volumes and respiratory rate (blowing off CO_2) caused by increases in CO_2

Table 12-1 Description of Sleep-Disordered Breathing Categories Seen During Polysomnography

SDB Categories	Airflow	Effort	Description
Obstructive sleep apnea (OSA)/hypopnea	No airflow or reduced airflow	Effort is noted	Airway blocked, cannot get air into the lungs
Central sleep apnea (CSA)/hypopnea	No airflow or reduced airflow	No effort or reduced effort	Compromised drive to breathe
Mixed apnea	No airflow	No effort at beginning of event noted before airway opens	Starts with no drive to breathe, then airway is blocked
Cheyne-Stokes respirations (CSR)	Waxing and waning noted in the airflow channel	Waxing and waning noted in the effort channels	Drive to breathe is compromised—breathing cycles exhibit waxing and waning lasting 30 s-2 min duration
Complex sleep apnea	No airflow—central apneas appear with CPAP changes	No effort—as CPAP is increased, the obstructive apneas change to central apneas	Closure of airway is present, but the drive to breathe is compromised by the administration of CPAP, causing changes in CO_2 and decreased drive to breathe.
Hypoventilation	Airflow reduced for long periods of time—AASM rules state at least 10 min	Equal reduction in effort noted	Drive to breathe is compromised.

AASM, American Academy of Sleep Medicine; CPAP, continuous positive airway pressure; SDB, sleep-disordered breathing.

and a decrease in volume and rate, often resulting in central apnea caused by decreases in CO_2.

Treating CSR and complex sleep apnea with conventional BPAP S/T may overventilate the patient and knock out the drive to breathe even more. Servo-ventilation is the treatment of choice for these patients. By identifying the patient's peak flow or minute ventilation (MV) and applying supplemental pressure support, the patient gets only the flow that they need without overventilation (6).

KEY TAKEAWAY: Sleep-Disordered Breathing

- PSG monitors and records how well the body is working during rest and while asleep.
- SDB is identified during a PSG using airflow, effort, oximetry, and, in some cases, CO_2 monitors.
- The most common SDB identified during PSG is obstructive sleep apnea (OSA), which does not let air enter the lungs. The treatment of choice for OSA is CPAP therapy.
- Other types of SDB may be secondary to a diminished or absent drive to breathe. This can be caused by compromises in the signal to breathe: the brain not identifying the need to breathe, the signal being interrupted and not reaching the lungs, or the muscles not responding to the signal. The most common therapy is some form of BPAP or, if necessary, NIV.

HYPOVENTILATION AND ASSOCIATED PATHOPHYSIOLOGY

Hypoventilation is a state in which there is a reduced amount of air entering the alveoli that causes an increase in CO_2 levels in the blood. The primary function of the lungs is to inhale O_2 and exhale CO_2. When we discuss the needed amount of air that a person breathes, we often refer to it in terms of tidal volume (V_T) or MV. The V_T is the amount of air inhaled or exhaled during a normal breathing cycle. In a normal young adult, it is approximately 500 mL per inspiration or 7 mL/kg of ideal body mass. The MV is found by multiplying the V_T by the respiratory rate (Figure 12-1).

Some normal variables influence our V_T and therefore our MV—issues such as stress, exercise, and sympathetic nervous system activation (fight or flight). These can cause V_T and respiratory rates to increase. Conversely, when we relax by reading a book or watching TV, our V_T and respiratory rate may decrease and still be able to maintain adequate oxygenation for the body.

Another variable is the normal increase in CO_2 retention that occurs when we transition from wakefulness to sleep. There is an additional increase in CO_2 retention when we transition from nonrapid eye movement to rapid eye movement (REM) sleep. All of these are normal occurrences that elicit a decrease or increase in V_T, and all are done without conscious effort (1).

The body uses the V_T to adequately oxygenate and eliminate CO_2. In normal adults, it is not unusual for the CO_2 level to increase by 7 mm Hg from wake to sleep and to fluctuate by 10 mm Hg throughout the sleep stages. These variables should still be no higher than 50 mm Hg. This normal variability is maintained by the body taking deeper or shallower breaths as well as increasing or decreasing the respiratory rate. In addition, diminished muscle tone develops during REM sleep, which may exacerbate hypoventilation secondary to reduced respiratory effort.

Now let us discuss what happens when the body cannot maintain adequate ventilation. A very short and concise definition of hypoventilation is an increase in CO_2 and decrease in O_2. Hypoventilation is a complicated breathing pattern caused by breathing that is too shallow or too slow or that has diminished lung function.

The body/brain tries to maintain adequate ventilation in all situations. Think about when you exercise. First, you try to take deeper breaths, then you breathe faster—you do not do this consciously, the brain knows it needs to do this to keep you oxygenated. At some point, your body says enough, and you stop exercising to catch your breath. You breathe fast and deep until you reach an equilibrium and start breathing normally.

This type of breathing (fast rate, deep volume) is what happens in the body during sleep if the patient's CO_2 level increases and they try to blow off the CO_2 and get more O_2. This also occurs in patients with lung disorders that cause them to breathe with accessory muscles during the day. They increase their lung volume by raising their shoulders (to pull in more O_2) and use pursed lip breathing while exhaling, to keep oxygen in their lungs longer. When they lie down, gravity puts additional stress on their diaphragm and accessory muscles, and muscle tone is decreased. The patient's airflow and effort decrease, and their O_2 level will slowly decrease over time. During REM sleep, the patient will often have central apneas due to the lack of muscle tone—they can no longer use the accessory muscles. The patient will often have very short periods of REM (since they cannot use accessory muscles during this time–central apneas are longer) and spend most of their sleep time in nonrapid eye movement (NREM) sleep.

Remember, the brain is trying to move enough air in and out of the lungs to keep the body alive and oxygenated. These compromised breathing periods may last for a very long time. The American Academy of Sleep Medicine (AASM) states that they should be at least 10 minutes in duration for scoring purposes, but they may last much longer.

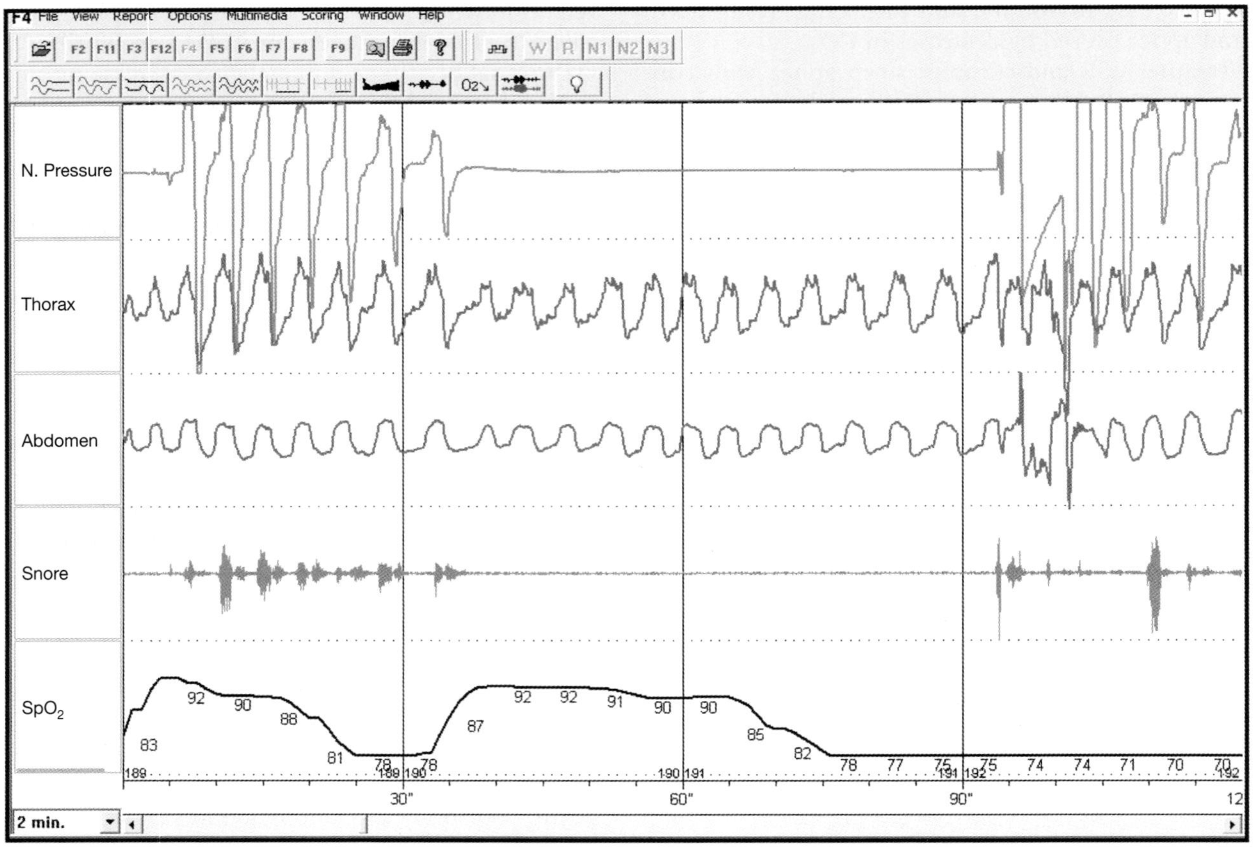

A

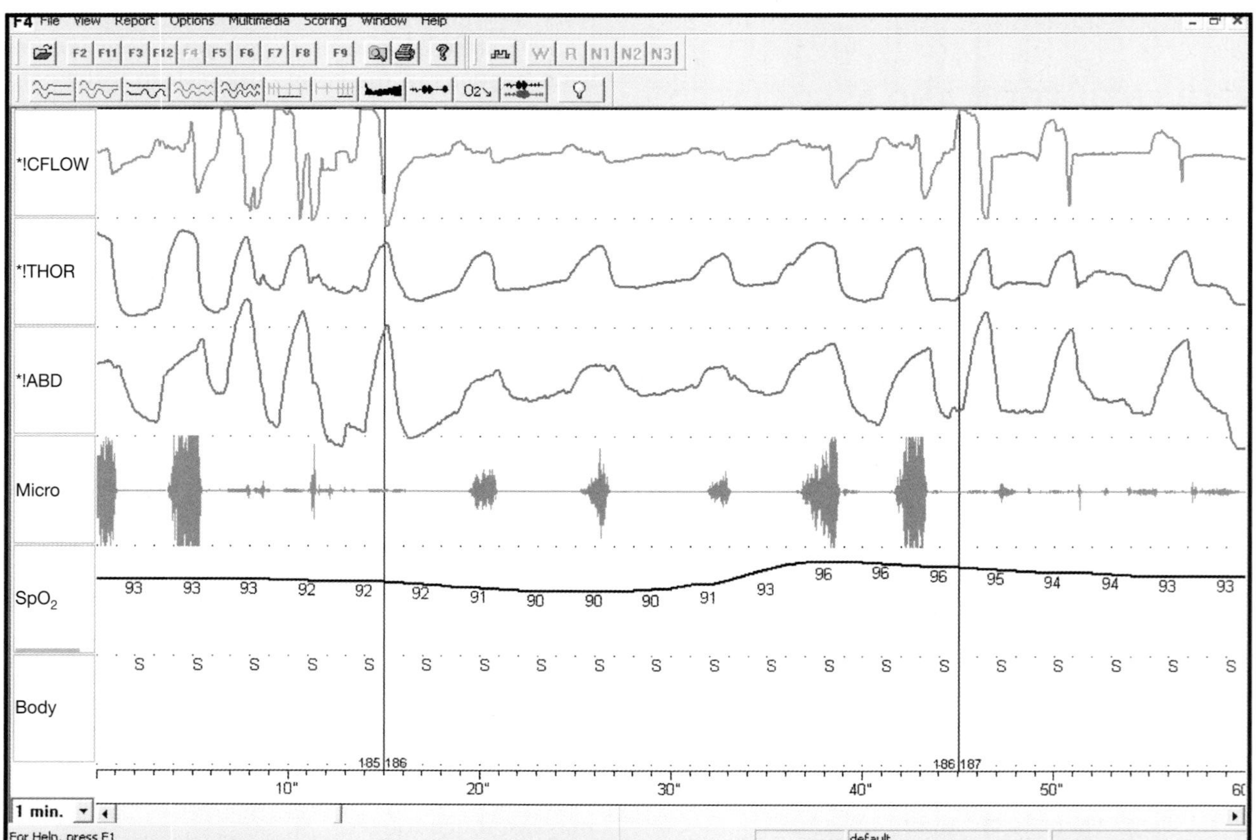

B

Figure 12-1 A: Obstructive apnea—no airflow, effort, snoring noted when airway is open, desaturations. B: Obstructive hypopnea—decreased airflow, effort, and snoring noted as well as desaturations.

CLINICAL SIGNIFICANCE OF HYPOVENTILATION

When hypoventilation occurs during sleep, the normal mechanisms to maintain adequate ventilation are unable to do their job. The lungs cannot breathe deeply enough or fast enough to maintain adequate ventilation, so the body starts to accumulate CO_2. Chronic hypoventilation during sleep may be associated with excessive daytime sleepiness, frequent awakenings resulting in poor sleep quality, enuresis, insomnia, fatigue, nightmares, morning headaches, and reduced exercise capacity. These symptoms are due to the increases in CO_2 and decreases in O_2.

What happens when there is a chronic condition that affects the lungs? The ventilatory control system attempts to compensate by increasing the drive to breathe to keep the CO_2 level in the normal range (35-45 mm Hg). It does this by increasing the respiratory rate and decreasing the V_T (decreased flow) (7).

Sleep-related hypoventilation may be an early symptom of chronic disorders.

The disorders most often associated with hypoventilation are summarized in Table 12-2.

Obesity hypoventilation syndrome (OHS) is a condition that is often seen in the sleep laboratory. OHS is defined as a combination of obesity (BMI 30 kg/m^2) and chronic hypercapnia (ie, $Pa{CO_2}$ >45 mm Hg) accompanied by SDB. These are not your typical OSA patients; their weight compresses their lungs and makes it hard to breathe, and they have extra adipose tissue in their tongue, airway, and neck. The added intra-abdominal or visceral fat makes these patients more susceptible to pulmonary hypertension, heart disease, diabetes, some cancers, and death (8).

KEY TAKEAWAY: Hypoventilation

- Hypoventilation is an impairment of the body's ability to breathe normally.
- Hypoventilation may be defined as an increase in CO_2 level and is commonly accompanied by a fall in O_2 level.
- Hypoventilation is a complicated breathing pattern caused by breathing that is too shallow or too slow or that has diminished lung function.
- Chronic hypoventilation may be the result of disorders that affect any part of the respiratory system.
- Chronic hypoventilation may be associated with excessive daytime sleepiness, poor sleep quality, enuresis, fatigue, nightmares, and morning headaches.
- OHS may present with comorbid OSA and sleep disturbances.

IDENTIFICATION OF HYPOVENTILATION DURING POLYSOMNOGRAPHY

Sleep technologists are trained to recognize all types of sleep disorders. They can identify a patient with OSA, insomnia, central sleep apnea (CSA), narcolepsy, REM behavior disorder, and all types of parasomnias.

Table 12-2 Types of Hypoventilation With Short Descriptions

Type of Disorder	Description	Diseases/Conditions
OHS	BMI >30 with weight accumulated in the thoracic region putting stress on the functionality of the lungs	OHS may also be associated with obstructive apneas and central apneas during sleep.
Congenital disorders	Genetic form of sleep apnea: Patient stops breathing when falling asleep—if undiagnosed, death may occur	Central hypoventilation syndrome, formerly known as Ondine's curse, kyphoscoliosis, or chest wall deformities
Brainstem disorders	Issue in the brainstem that controls the normal breathing process, resulting in inadequate ventilation and increased levels of CO_2	Causes of brainstem disorders include stroke, tumor, trauma, and medical conditions such as meningitis, etc.
Neurologic disorders	Disorders that affect either the signals to breathe or the signal transmission from the brain through the spinal column to the nerves in the body	Neurologic disorders include Parkinson disease, memory disorders, multiple sclerosis, and ALS.
Neuromuscular disorders	Typical features are a reduced forced vital capacity, reduced respiratory muscle strength, and, in some cases, malfunction of the neurons that control breathing.	Disorders that compromise the signals in the nerves or muscles such as myasthenia gravis, Guillain–Barré syndrome, poliomyelitis, muscular dystrophy, and Duchenne muscular dystrophy
Drug or medication induced	Caused by drugs that depress ventilatory drive or impair muscle function	Long-acting narcotics, anesthetics, sedatives, muscle relaxants, alcohol, and chronic opioid usage

ALS, amyotrophic lateral sclerosis; BMI, body mass index; OHS, obesity hypoventilation syndrome.

They can identify if a patient is having a seizure or some other medical emergency during the PSG, and they know what to do. They work all night monitoring their patients and make sure the information that is collected is complete and accurate. As Dr German Nino Murcia said, "Sleep techs are the eyes and ears of the physician."

Most of the patients who are diagnosed using PSG have OSA, and the sleep recordings verify this diagnosis. The events recorded are obstructive apneas and hypopneas with associated oxygen desaturations and electroencephalogram (EEG) arousals. These events happen all night long and are worse when the patient is in the supine sleeping position and/or in REM sleep.

Apnea events need to be at least 10 seconds in duration for scoring purposes but will often last longer. Some sleep laboratories have a general rule that if an event lasts longer than 60 to 90 seconds with associated desaturations, the patient should be awakened and started on therapy (Figure 12-1A).

According to the AASM scoring guidelines, an obstructive hypopnea is scored if there is a reduction of airflow by 30%, the reduced airflow lasts for at least 10 seconds, and there is a 3% or greater drop in oxygen saturation, or an arousal. Any of the following should also be noted (Figure 12-1B):

1. Snoring during the event
2. Flattening of the nasal pressure signal
3. Paradoxical thoracoabdominal movement

Sleep technologists may see central apneas in patients who are diagnosed with neurologic or neuromuscular disorders, severe OSA, or complex sleep apnea. These events are at least 10 seconds in duration and are associated with no airflow and no drive to breathe (flat respiratory effort signals). Central hypopneas are identified by the same criteria as obstructive hypopneas for reduction in flow and duration, but a central hypopnea must include (Figure 12-2A, B) the following:

1. No snoring
2. No inspiratory flattening of the flow signal compared with baseline
3. No associated thoracoabdominal paradoxical movement during the event

Please see the specific criteria for event scoring in the current version of the AASM Manual for Scoring of Sleep and Associated Events (9).

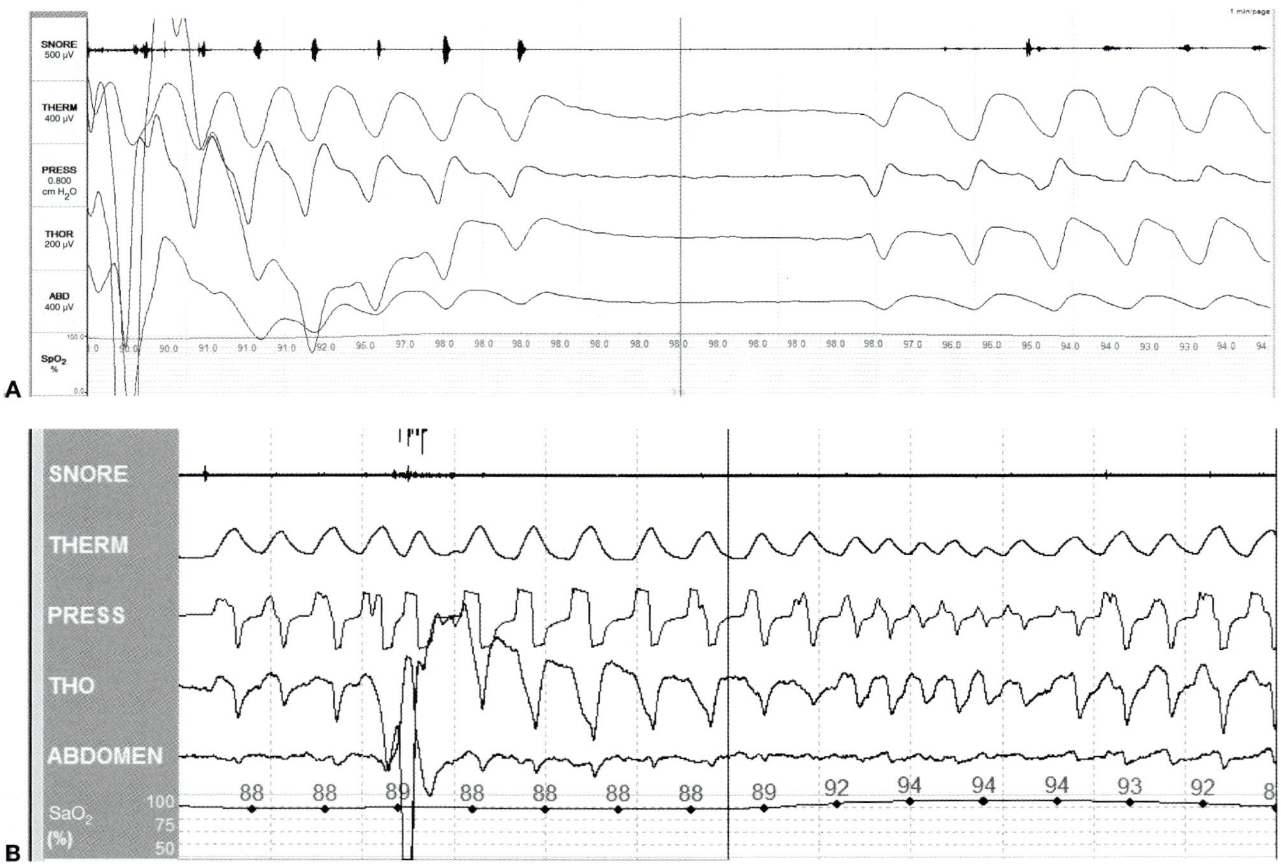

Figure 12-2 A: Central apnea 60-second epoch—no airflow, no effort. B: Central hypopnea (30-second epoch)—decreased airflow, decreased effort, no snoring, no squaring off of airflow signal, and no paradoxical movement.

In addition to sleep disorders that are diagnosed easily with a PSG, there are patients who have sleep studies because they have a condition that makes breathing during sleep difficult or impossible. These are the patients who mainly have central events and may have hypoventilation.

As previously mentioned, diseases that cause the patient to have hypoventilation and difficulty breathing when they are sleeping include central hypoventilation syndrome (Ondine curse), neurologic conditions (amyotrophic lateral sclerosis, postpolio syndrome, etc.), OHS, and narcotic abuse. Often, these patients have an exacerbation of their condition and are placed on NIV in the emergency room or intensive care unit. Once they are stable, the physician may order a PSG to verify the need for NIV and to validate the settings.

A second patient population includes those who have not been diagnosed with a disease that causes hypoventilation but who have difficulty breathing while they are sleeping. The physician may suspect that these patients have OSA or some type of CSA and study them to better understand their symptoms and identify the cause. These patients may have been diagnosed with chronic obstructive pulmonary disease or some underlying lung problem and come into the sleep laboratory to be evaluated for excessive daytime sleepiness or fatigue upon exertion. The technologist and physician may anticipate OSA or identify some type of overlap syndrome (10).

DIAGNOSTIC POLYSOMNOGRAPH FOR HYPOVENTILATION

When a patient arrives in the sleep laboratory, a review of their chart is imperative. The technologist needs to understand why the patient is having a PSG. Does the physician suspect OSA, insomnia, or some type of parasomnia, or does the patient have a condition that may cause hypoventilation? The technologist reviews the patient's comorbidities and the types of diagnostic tests the latter has had, such as arterial blood gas (ABG), stress tests, pulmonary function test (PFT), and so on.

Some of the test results that may be helpful for the sleep technologist in identifying the possibility of hypoventilation include the following:

- ABG shows the patient's Pa_{O_2} is decreased and Pa_{CO_2} is increased. If the patient's blood is compensating for the increased CO_2, high levels of bicarbonate (HCO_3) and increased pH acidity will be noted (11).
- Blood cell count shows an elevated hematocrit level (increased red blood cells)—the body does this to carry more O_2 and CO_2 to compensate for hypoventilation.
- PFT shows a measurement of maximal inspiratory and expiratory pressures, which may be useful in screening for respiratory muscle weakness and neuromuscular disorders.

For the PSG, the patient will be set up with traditional recording parameters: EEG, electrooculogram (EOG), electromyogram (EMG), electrocardiogram (ECG) airflow, abdominal and thoracic effort, oximetry, and CO_2 monitoring if available. During the daytime and while up and about, the patient that has chronic obstructive pulmonary disease (COPD) or some other breathing disorder will use accessory muscles to breathe. When they lie down, gravity plays a negative role and results in accessory muscles not being able to support adequate respirations. This causes the patient's breathing ability to deteriorate, especially if the bed is in a flat position. At home, the patient may have compensated for this deterioration in the ability to breathe by having their head of the bed elevated or by using multiple pillows to be in a sitting position. If questioned, the patient may admit that they sleep in a lounge chair with the head elevated.

A simple description of hypoventilation is inadequate ventilation leading to an increase in CO_2 and decrease in O_2. Sleep reduces MV in healthy adults, and it is much more pronounced in patients with diseases that affect lung function. Therefore, sleep-related hypoventilation may be an early manifestation of chronic hypoventilation (Figure 12-3) (1).

With sleep onset, the patient may exhibit central apneas and central hypopneas. This will last for a few minutes, and then the patient may start taking deep breaths with shorter pauses. The pauses are often too short to technically be called a central event. Eventually, when the patient goes into deeper sleep stages, the deep breathing may be replaced with shallow breaths and an increase in the respiratory rate—very consistent with hypoventilation.

It is not unusual to see hypoventilation occurring in patients who have not yet been diagnosed with some type of disorder that causes hypoventilation. The disorders are often not respiratory based but have respiratory ramifications. If CO_2 is not being monitored, a decrease in airflow and effort with slow desaturations may be noted along with increased respiratory rates.

Remember, central hypopneas show decreased airflow, decreased effort, and associated oxygen desaturations. The difference between central hypopneas and hypoventilation is the length of time before the patient takes a deep breath or begins to breathe normally. The duration of a hypopnea is at least 10 seconds but usually not more than 60 to 90 seconds. According to AASM guidelines, hypoventilation should be at least 10 minutes in duration and is often of much longer duration.

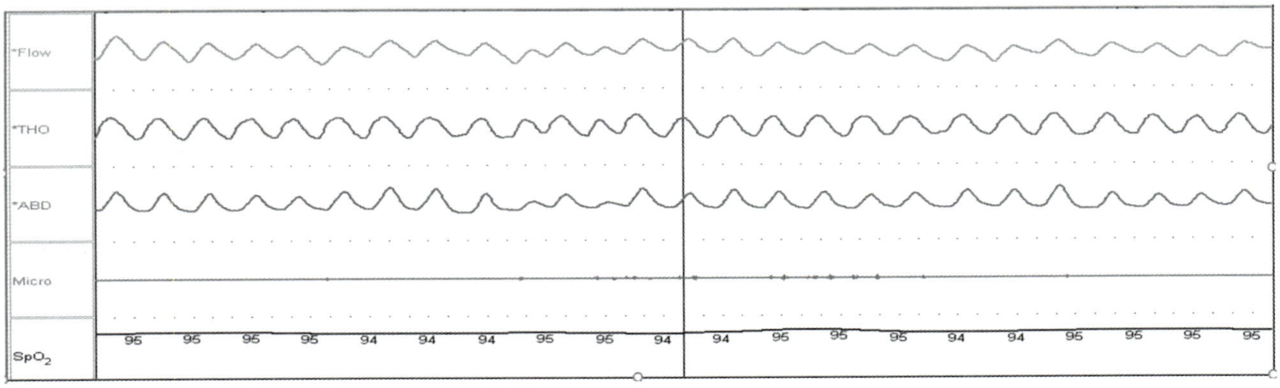

Figure 12-3 One-minute excerpt of hypoventilation showing decreased airflow, decreased effort, slight decrease in Spo_2 (as the time increases, the Spo_2 will decrease more), and increased respiratory rate 26 breaths per minute. This breathing pattern lasted for over 15 minutes, with the Spo_2 declining to 83%.

The most recent revision of the AASM scoring criteria (9) suggests scoring sleep-related hypoventilation if:

- There is an increase in the arterial Pco_2 to a value greater than 55 mm Hg for greater than or equal to 10 minutes or.
- There is an increase in arterial Pco_2 during sleep (in comparison with an awake supine value) to a value greater than 50 mm Hg for greater than or equal to 10 minutes.

Hypoventilation is usually associated with long-term oxygen desaturation, so an oxygen saturation of less than 90% for greater than 5 minutes with a nadir of less than or equal to 85% may also indicate hypercapnia and should warrant a further diagnostic workup (1).

Many of the patients who have hypoventilation syndrome may also have OSA. During the PSG, you may see obstructive apneas, central apneas, and hypoventilation. Look at the airflow and the effort. If they are both reduced and the condition lasts for 10 minutes, you are seeing hypoventilation. After the patient changes position or uses the bathroom and sleep is reinitiated, central apneas resume, changing to deep breaths with long pauses until the reduced flow and effort is displayed, indicating hypoventilation. Typically, hypoventilation-associated desaturations are very prolonged or slow, and no additional respiratory effort is apparent.

If a CO_2 monitor is not used, the patient cannot be diagnosed with hypoventilation, but a strong indication that hypoventilation is occurring can and should be made known to the physician. There needs to be a protocol available in the event that hypoventilation is suspected that indicates how and when it should be treated.

Hypoventilation puts additional stress on the body. Patients with hypoventilation are at increased risk for congestive heart failure, cor pulmonale, pulmonary hypertension, angina, etc. When possible, the cause of hypoventilation should be treated by controlling weight and decreasing the intake of opioids, etc, and ventilatory support should be administered expeditiously in the interim (8).

KEY TAKEAWAY: Polysomnography and Hypoventilation

- Hypoventilation may initially be identified or suspected during a PSG.
- At the start of the PSG, patients who have hypoventilation may have central apneas and hypopneas because of an inability to use accessory muscles effectively while lying down.
- Central hypopneas and hypoventilation have some of the same properties, but central hypopneas are usually no longer than 60 to 90 seconds, whereas hypoventilation, as defined by the AASM, must be at least 10 minutes in duration.
- Patients with OHS are unable to move enough air in and out of the lungs because of their increased girth and therefore breathe very shallow, causing decreased levels of O_2 and increased levels of CO_2.
- Hypoventilation is a complicated breathing pattern that puts the patient at risk for congestive heart failure or pulmonary hypertension.

TREATMENTS FOR HYPOVENTILATION

As stated throughout this chapter, hypoventilation is a breathing disorder that may be seen and diagnosed during a PSG. The causes vary from obesity or drug use to physiologic disorders, but the result is that the patient has difficulty breathing sufficiently while sleeping.

Treating the underlying condition by undertaking weight loss methods or weaning off opioids is the primary goal. In OHS, CPAP may be sufficient to treat the patient until sufficient weight loss is achieved. There is a subset of OHS patients for whom CPAP is unviable, and they need NIV to support their breathing during the weight loss process.

Many of the underlying conditions causing hypoventilation do not have a cure, and therefore, the symptom itself needs to be addressed. A few years ago,

Table 12-3 BPAP Titration Process for OSA and Ventilation

BPAP Setting	Titration for OSA (13)	Titration for Ventilation (14)
EPAP	Increase for apneas	Increase to open airway; airway closure may be seen at the end of a central event or may be seen by decreased or lack of flow with delivered breaths. Also used to increase oxygenation (increases the time oxygen is held in the lungs)
IPAP	Increase for hypopneas, desaturations, EEG arousals, snoring	Increase to ensure sufficient tidal volume delivered on each breath—verified by watching Sp_{O_2} and CO_2
Backup rate	Used if central events are noted on diagnostic PSG. Rate identified by the physician or should be 2-3 breaths below the patient's respiratory rate.	Backup rate set to deliver mechanical breaths during central events (the rate is usually recommended by the physician and may be around 8-10 breaths/min with the option to increase as needed to keep the oxygen and CO_2 at acceptable levels)
Volume-assured pressure support	Not used for OSA	Tidal volume delivered via pressure support so that if the patient's condition deteriorates, the set V_T is still maintained

BPAP, bilevel positive airway pressure; EEG, electroencephalogram; EPAP, expiration positive airway pressure; IPAP, inspiration positive airway pressure; OSA, obstructive sleep apnea; PSG, polysomnography; V_T, tidal volume.

the only option was a tracheostomy and volume ventilation. Since the mid-1990s, NIV with BPAP using a mask has been a very strong treatment option.

During the diagnostic PSG, the patient may present with hypoventilation, central apneas, and obstructive apneas. All these need to be considered when treating the patient. NIV is the treatment of choice for hypoventilation. This is initially delivered by using a BPAP unit with BPAP S/T or volume targeted pressure support. The settings on the device that the technologist uses during the titration support ventilation instead of only keeping the airway open (Table 12-3).

NIV has proven to improve quality of sleep, nocturnal oxygen saturation, diurnal and nocturnal Pa_{CO_2}, and quality of life in a broad spectrum of chronic hypoventilation disorders. Moreover, NIV may improve patients' survival. In addition, untreated OHS patients are more likely to require invasive ventilation and have prolonged hospital stays.

When observing central apneas, be aware of the machine-driven breaths. If an obstructive component is present during a central apnea, the machine breath cannot be delivered or is restricted, as in a hypopnea. See Figure 12-4 for examples.

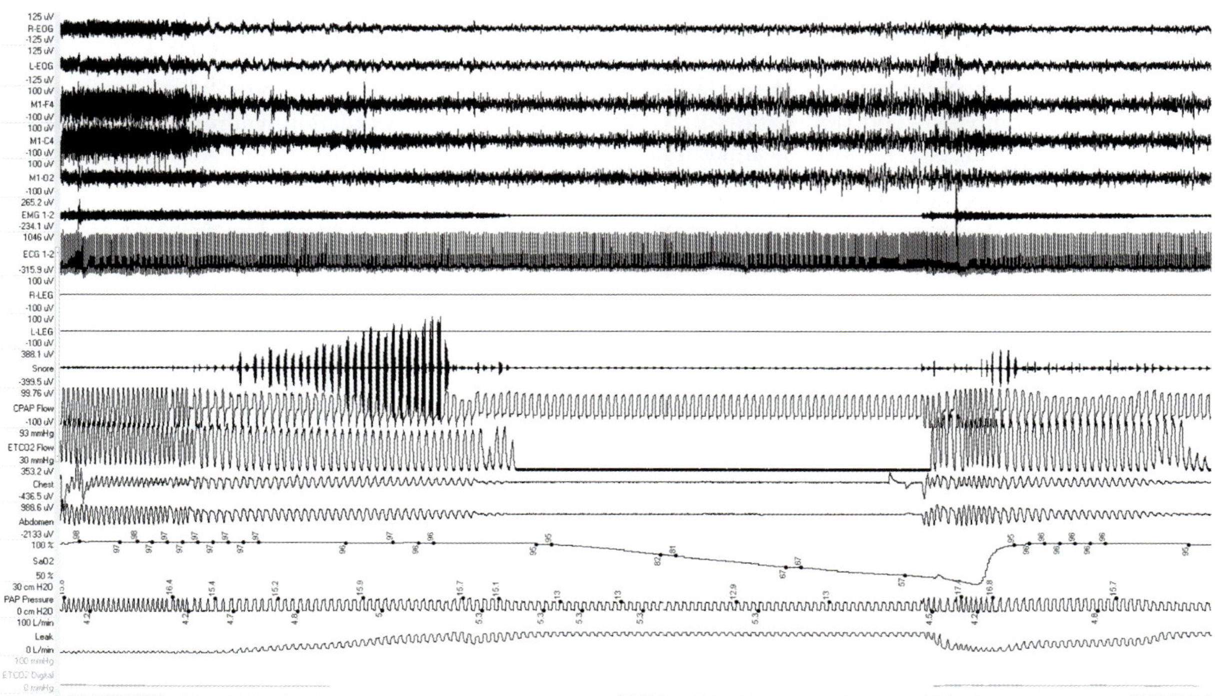

Figure 12-4 There is no effort recorded during the central events. The machine-driven breaths are indicated by the absence of flow in the end-tidal CO_2 flow channel. To correct this issue, the expiration positive airway pressure needs to be increased.

In summary, if a patient has a PSG because of excessive sleepiness or reduced functionality during the day and the study is to rule out OSA, the diagnosis of a disease process causing hypoventilation may not yet have been made. The sleep technologist may be the first to identify that the patient has hypoventilation. Everything the technologist sees needs to be well documented so that the physician can take the next step with an assurance that the information gathered is accurate.

Remember, the technologist is the eyes and the ears of the physician. This role is especially important when a patient with hypoventilation has a PSG. This may be a condition that has already been diagnosed, and the physician is gathering baseline information and verifying the therapy setting, or it may be part of a new diagnosis.

ACKNOWLEDGMENT

I wish to thank Joyce M. Black for her original contribution to this chapter. You were a friend and mentor, and you are missed in the field of Sleep Medicine.

REFERENCES

1. Böing S, Randerath WJ. Chronic hypoventilation syndromes and sleep-related hypoventilation. *J Thorac Dis*. 2015;7(8):1273-1285.
2. Egan DF. *Eagan's Fundamentals of Respiratory Care*. 5th ed. Mosby; 1990.
3. Carskadon MA, Rechtschaffen A. Monitoring and staging human sleep. In: Kryger M, Roth T, Dement W, eds. *Principles and Practice of Sleep Medicine*. 3rd ed. WB Saunders Company; 2000:1197-1214.
4. Kryger M. Monitoring respiratory and cardiac function. In: Kryger M, Roth T, Dement W, eds. *Principles and Practice of Sleep Medicine*. 3rd ed. WB Saunders Company.; 2000:1217-1229.
5. Sullivan C, Issa F, Berthon-Jones M, Eves L. Reversal of obstructive sleep apnea by continuous positive airway pressure applied through the nares. *Lancet*. 1981;1:862-865.
6. Javaheri S, Brown LK, Randerath WJ. Clinical applications of adaptive servoventilation devices part 2. *Chest*. 2014;146(3):858-868.
7. Piper AJ, Yee BJ. Hypoventilation syndromes. *Compr Physiol*. 2014;4(4):1639-1676.
8. Balachandran JS, Masa JF, Mokhlesi B. Obesity hypoventilation syndrome epidemiology and diagnosis. *Sleep Med Clin*. 2014;9(3):341-347.
9. Troester M, Quan S, Berry RB, et al; *for the American Academy of Sleep Medicine. The AASM Manual for the Scoring of Sleep and Associated Events: Rules, Terminology and Technical Specifications. Version 3.0*. American Academy of Sleep Medicine; 2023.
10. Eckert DJ, Jordan AS, Merchia P, et al. Central sleep apnea: pathophysiology and treatment. *Chest*. 2007;131(2):595-607.
11. Malley WJ. *Clinical Blood Gases*. WB Saunders Company; 1990.
12. Ozsancak A, D'Ambrosio C, Hill NS. Nocturnal noninvasive ventilation. *Chest*. 2008;133(5):1275-1286.
13. Kushida CA, Chediak A, Berry RB, et al; American Academy of Sleep Medicine Task Force. Clinical guidelines for the manual titration of positive airway pressure in patients with obstructive sleep apnea. *J Clin Sleep Med*. 2008;4(2):157-171.
14. NPPV Titration Task Force of American Academy of Sleep Medicine. Best clinical practices for the sleep center adjustment of noninvasive positive pressure ventilation (NPPV) in stable chronic alveolar hypoventilation syndromes. *J Clin Sleep Med*. 2010;6(5):491-509.

Chapter 13
Insomnia

ROBERT N. TURNER

KEY CONCEPTS/LEARNING OBJECTIVES

The key concepts for this chapter include a review of the complexity of insomnia, the prevalence, types, and potential causes of insomnia, and the sleep history and relevant self-report techniques used in the assessment of insomnia.

KEY TERMS

Depression
Hyperarousal
Pittsburgh Sleep Quality Index
Psychological testing
Sleep hygiene

Difficulties with initiating and/or maintaining sleep have been described for centuries, yet significant progress in the understanding of these problems has occurred only over the last several decades. Some cultures believed that disturbed sleep and dreams were associated with evil spirits and ghosts. Others have suggested that the gods determined poor sleep and that the severity of the condition was in proportion to one's sinful deeds. Since significant mysticism surrounded the complaint of sleep disturbances, remedies for these troubles included religious practices as well as assorted other rituals and various compounds. Disturbed sleep has long been associated with a wide variety of medical and psychological conditions. Chronic and acute pain, allergies, and various other disease processes have certainly been associated with sleep. In addition, psychiatric conditions and insomnia have long been described. An early study with groups of good and poor sleepers suggested a biologic basis for insomnia, with greater physiologic arousal, including higher electromyogram levels and a faster heart rate, among poor sleepers (1). These differences were noted both during wakefulness and during sleep.

WHAT IS INSOMNIA?

From our own lifetime experiences, most of us intuitively understand what is meant by the term "insomnia." There are criteria for diagnosis provided by the American Academy of Sleep Medicine (AASM). Short-term insomnia is considered a transient disturbance, typically lasting a few days to a few weeks, and typically not requiring treatment. Chronic insomnia persists for months or even years. The *International Classification of Sleep Disorders*, 3rd edition, text revision *[ICSD-3-TR]* (2) requires that adults and children diagnosed with insomnia report one or more of the following:

1. Difficulty initiating sleep
2. Difficulty maintaining sleep
3. Waking up earlier than desired
4. Resistance to going to bed according to an appropriate schedule
5. Difficulty sleeping without parent or caregiver intervention

In the past, subtypes of insomnia were described, but patients often failed to fit into a single category. Multiple symptoms are more common than any single symptom, with symptoms occurring simultaneously or switching from one to another over time. In addition, patients with insomnia often overestimate the time taken to fall asleep and underestimate sleep duration, indicating an altered perception of sleep (3).

Patients with insomnia vary in the amount of sleep per night. Some people feel alert, refreshed, and energized with only 6 hours of sleep, whereas other individuals feel "horrible" after such a "poor" night's sleep. In addition, some regularly require more than an hour to initiate sleep, awaken four or more times during the sleep episode, and generally sleep about 6 hours per night yet do not complain of insomnia. Others awaken early in the morning. They do not complain of poor sleep. However, some experience sleep-onset problems when requiring longer than 15 minutes to fall asleep, complain of insomnia with one or two brief awakenings during the sleep episode, and/or describe disturbed sleep if awakened earlier than usual. How do we make clinical sense of this?

First, the subjective experience of insomnia may have little to do with currently utilized objective sleep-electroencephalogram (EEG) parameters. Considerable variability obviously exists between one's perception and impression of sleep and laboratory findings (sleep latency and sleep duration). There exists a possibility that several other important measures of physiologic functioning, both during wakefulness and during sleep, which are not routinely employed in clinical evaluation settings, may more accurately reflect the subjectively experienced complaint of insomnia. As such, our current view of insomnia remains limited, and only a partial view of the entire problem is understood.

Second, people with other sleep-wake disorders may incorrectly perceive that their problem is insomnia. Consider the middle-aged, moderately overweight, "stressed-out" male who snores and awakens frequently. He may believe that his problem is insomnia, yet obstructive apnea is one of his significant problems. Another example is a 50-year-old married female with a history of recurrent depression, migraine headaches, fibromyalgia, and asthma. Upon polysomnographic evaluation, snoring with repetitive arousals and stereotypic movements of the lower extremities are observed. Diagnoses may include upper airway resistance syndrome, periodic limb movement sleep disorder, and major depressive disorder. Both patients complain of insomnia, yet objective evaluation reveals other causes, likely promoting the experience of inadequate, nonrefreshing sleep.

Third, *people may have disorders comorbid with insomnia*. In other words, the patients described previously may have obstructive apnea *and* insomnia, or, perhaps most commonly, depression *and* insomnia. In the past, primary insomnia was intended to represent discrete conditions, predicated on conditioning factors, sleep-wake processes, and other matters as well. Secondary insomnia referred to the disturbance as a symptom associated with other variables, such as personality styles, numerous illnesses and disease, and a variety of psychiatric disorders. However, the cause-and-effect relationships of these factors have been difficult to determine. The most recent version of the *ICSD* (2) uses the term "comorbid" instead of secondary, reflecting a complex interaction between insomnia and other disorders. This is evident in a variety of medical disorders, especially those associated with pain; many psychiatric disorders, especially depression; and in interactions between sleep and medications used to treat comorbid disorders.

Fourth, circadian and aging factors also require consideration. In general, variations in core body temperature are correlated with the timing and duration of sleep and alertness. Older people may exhibit a lower amplitude of temperature rhythms and may also advance the sleep-alertness phase to an earlier time than younger people. Older patients may also report more frequent awakenings during the major sleep episode and complain of sleep-maintenance insomnia, whereas younger patients may describe sleep-onset insomnia. Both circadian and aging issues require consideration of normal sleep and rhythmic processes across the lifespan.

Fifth, in order to meet *ICSD-3-TR* criteria for diagnosis (2), some degree of distress *must* be associated with the complaint. It has long been known that poor sleep can be associated with decrements in mood and performance. Consequences of poor sleep can be described in terms of interpersonal, emotional, cognitive, vocational, and/or other areas of general functioning. Resultant sleepiness during normal waking hours may or may not occur. Although these troubles can be merely annoying with short-term insomnia, data suggest the potential medical consequences of persistent difficulties initiating and/or maintaining sleep.

Sixth, chronic insomnia may be conceptualized as a disorder of hyperarousal. It is essential that one is aware of the potential 24-hour overactivation of the hypothalamic-pituitary-adrenal (HPA) axis and/or other systemic physiologic processes, because these may be primary etiologic factors. As mentioned, hyperarousal is typically present throughout the day and night (1).

To summarize, numerous factors, characteristics, and consequences are associated with insomnia. These sleep-wake disturbances require careful consideration of many potential medical/psychiatric factors in the complaint of insomnia, as well as environmental factors, primary sleep-wake pathologies, and numerous other variables.

Epidemiology

Early epidemiologic studies indicated that approximately one-third of respondents to surveys described sleep difficulties over the previous year and that at least 50% reported the experience of insomnia at some time during their lives. Severe or constant sleep troubles were reported by about 10% to 30%, and an estimated 6% meet criteria for the diagnosis of insomnia (4). The most frequent type of disturbance was sleep-maintenance insomnia, whereas sleep-onset insomnia and early-morning awakening insomnia were less common. Importantly, some individuals reported a combination of these troubles.

More recent studies have documented daytime consequences of insomnia. Patients with insomnia reported memory problems and attention/concentration impairments, as well as mood decrements and less positive experiences with interpersonal relationships. Katz and McHorney (5) found that insomnia was associated with a worsened quality of life among a variety of patients with various illnesses. Collectively, evidence indicates that insomnia is widely prevalent, associated with daytime consequences, correlated with medical and mental health conditions, and associated with a reduced quality of life.

Short-Term Insomnia

Short-term insomnia, or a brief episode of trouble falling and/or remaining asleep, affects almost everyone from time to time. Short-term insomnia is defined as a sleep problem lasting less than 3 months. During periods of stress or change (such as the loss of a loved one), individuals may exhibit time-limited difficulties with sleep. Sparingly studied through empirical methods, much remains unknown about this common problem within the general population.

According to the *ICSD-3-TR* (2), the diagnosis of short-term insomnia requires that a sleep disturbance occurs for less than 3 months and represents a clear change from the person's typical sleep-wake patterns and habits.

Numerous external factors may promote short-term insomnia. Environmental disturbances, such as light and noise, stress, problematic interpersonal circumstances, and other matters, can initiate the problem. Changing one's typical circadian sleep-wake pattern and drug initiation and/or withdrawal are also possible contributors to short-term insomnia. Other external events, internal circumstances (eg, medical problems), and short-duration pain or discomfort can also promote short-term insomnia. It is important to keep in mind that this time-limited, usually resolvable, problem can become a very significant issue in people's lives. It is well known that numerous factors can activate short-term insomnia. Personality style, genetic makeup, vulnerability to psychiatric illness, medical problems, and other issues can make the patient susceptible to persistent insomnia.

Distressing situations can impact the ability to sleep, as evidenced by sleeplessness experienced by those who lived through the COVID-19 pandemic.

Chronic Insomnia

Criteria for the diagnosis of chronic insomnia are provided in *ICSD-3-TR* (2). These problems must occur for 3 months or longer, and some degree of daytime impairment or distress is essential. The new classification system makes the diagnosis a binary decision—either yes or no. Previous insomnia subcategories may have some value in tailoring treatment plans to address primary complaints but no longer have an influence on whether or not the diagnosis is made.

A common thread in the diagnosis of chronic insomnia provided by research is the role of neuroendocrine dysregulation. Twenty-four-hour HPA axis activation has been reported among a small sample of subjects, as assessed by plasma levels of adrenocorticotropic hormone and cortisol (6). Shaver et al. (7) found elevations of morning urine cortisol levels among women with psychophysiologic insomnia. These studies suggest HPA overactivation among a proportion of patients with insomnia.

States of hyperarousal, which are often present, cause increased affective, physiologic, or cognitive activity, which can decrease the likelihood of sleep (8).

A useful model of insomnia has been provided by Spielman and colleagues, as reviewed by Espie (9). The model is often referred to as the three P model. It proposes predisposing, precipitating, and perpetuating factors as key to the development of chronic insomnia. The predisposing factors would include HPA activation and other biologic contributors to insomnia. Precipitating events typically lead to short-term insomnia, which can evolve into chronic insomnia when perpetuating factors are present. Evaluating these factors is no longer a necessary part of the diagnostic process but can be key to the choice of effective treatment options.

PREVIOUS INSOMNIA SUBCATEGORIES

In earlier editions of *ICSD*, several subcategories of insomnia were listed. The current *ICSD-3-TR* (2) has chosen to eliminate these categories because it is difficult to reliably distinguish between them, and their validity is questionable. Many of these classifications are, however, illustrative of the scope of the problem and help in framing issues with chronic insomnia. Only a brief, introductory description of selected subcategories will be presented here.

PSYCHOPHYSIOLOGIC INSOMNIA

People with psychophysiologic insomnia tend to be absorbed with their troubles initiating and/or maintaining sleep. This condition is manifested by agitation, somatized tension, and conditioning factors, which prevent sleep from occurring. Both anticipatory and performance anxiety can be significant components. Most people consciously try to fall asleep, feel frustrated and anxious, become more aroused, and subsequently experience increased trouble falling and remaining asleep. Polysomnographic studies can reveal increased wakefulness, reduced sleep efficiency, and prolonged sleep latency. This form of conditioned or learned insomnia appears to perpetuate itself.

PARADOXIC INSOMNIA

People with paradoxic insomnia are seen to sleep normally on measures observed by routine sleep-EEG measures. However, they report a reduced amount, or a complete lack, of sleep. Older terminologies referred to this condition as "pseudoinsomnia" or sleep state misperception disorder, because objective measures did not parallel the patient's subjective complaint (8). Occasionally, patients report a complete lack of sleep and will passionately debate objective, sleep-EEG data when it is presented to them. One patient described the sleep study report as a good read but a work of complete fiction. Primary psychiatric disorders, apparently, are not clearly causative.

HYPNOTIC-DEPENDENT SLEEP DISORDER

Because people can become tolerant of the effects of sedative-hypnotics, higher dosages may be required in order to achieve the same effect (a patient with insomnia may need more and more medication to fall and/or remain asleep). Following abrupt cessation of hypnotic use, severe insomnia can result. Nervousness, intense dreams or nightmares, fragmented sleep, and other physiologic symptoms (nausea and tension) can be experienced. This is sometimes called "drug-withdrawal insomnia" and is particularly common following the withdrawal of benzodiazepines with short half-lives (<4 hours).

INADEQUATE SLEEP HYGIENE

Some people engage in behavioral patterns that are inconsistent with sleeping well. Consumption of caffeine, irregular sleep-wake timing, various poor presleep habits, and numerous other factors will promote trouble falling and remaining asleep. This is seen when these variables are the most significant factors underlying the patient's insomnia.

IDIOPATHIC INSOMNIA

Idiopathic insomnia is a condition characterized by lifelong difficulties initiating and maintaining sleep. It seems to begin during infancy or early childhood and causes ongoing functional impairment or distress. Unusual sleep spindles can be seen during stage N2 sleep, and rapid eye movement (REM) sleep can contain few eye movements. Although its etiology is not completely understood, an underlying neurologic abnormality is suspected. Severity can range from mild to severe, and daytime consequences often include attention/concentration problems, irritability, depressed or anxious mood, daytime fatigue, and, perhaps, memory impairment. The course of this condition is chronic and is not better explained by another sleep, neurologic, medical, psychiatric, or substance misuse disorder (8).

CIRCADIAN RHYTHM DISORDERS AND CHRONIC INSOMNIA

Circadian rhythm disorders can initially present as insomnia. Difficulty initiating or maintaining sleep may be perceived by the patient as the primary complaint. However, patients with advanced or delayed sleep phase sleep relatively normally when time constraints are removed. Chronic insomnia may include an element of chronobiologic dysfunction (10), and patients may or may not achieve diagnostic criteria for circadian rhythm sleep disorders, as defined in *ICSD-3-TR* (2).

OTHER ASSOCIATED DISORDERS

Previously, a distinction of insomnia associated with other conditions was referred to as "secondary insomnia." The current *ICSD-3-TR* has eliminated these distinctions. It argues that even when other disorders are treated, there is often residual insomnia that must be addressed. Nevertheless, other disorders can, and do, impact insomnia and are valuable to discuss.

PSYCHIATRIC DISORDERS

Virtually any psychiatric disorder can be associated with comorbid insomnia. Most notably, generalized anxiety disorder, acute stress disorder, posttraumatic stress disorder, dysthymia, major depression, bipolar disorder, and schizoaffective disorder are all associated with sleep-alertness disorders. Abbreviated REM sleep latencies, delta sleep abnormalities (usually decreases in slow-wave sleep), increased REM densities (especially during the first third of the night), and sleep continuity disturbances can be found among patients with major depressive disorder. However, these sleep-EEG characteristics may also be found among patients with other psychiatric syndromes and personality disorders. Diagnostic and research issues with sleep and depression were discussed by Buysse (3). The interaction between insomnia and depression is complex, and the comorbidity of the two makes treatment challenging.

MEDICAL CONDITIONS

Many medical conditions or disease processes may promote secondary insomnia. Pain syndromes, asthma, chronic obstructive pulmonary disease, fibromyalgia, migraine and cluster headaches, gastroesophageal reflux disease, peptic ulcers, and scores of other medical problems can be associated with chronic disturbances of sleep initiation and/or sleep maintenance. Neurologic conditions, such as Parkinson disease and dementia, can also contribute to insomnia. Sleep research data are limited or simply not available for many medical conditions, and the impact of insomnia on patients with these problems has not been fully explored.

MEDICATIONS AND INSOMNIA

Virtually any medication can potentially promote problems falling or remaining asleep. These therapeutic agents target the treatment of medical or psychiatric conditions, but sleeplessness can be an undesirable side effect of the given compound. Stimulants and antidepressants with inhibition of serotonin uptake are known to promote insomnia in some patients. Corticosteroids, bronchodilators, and some antihypertensives can have the same effect. Insomnia can also be caused by the abrupt discontinuation of hypnotics and anxiolytics. Further details of medication are available in Chapter 56.

OTHER SLEEP DISORDERS

Other sleep-wake disorders can facilitate disturbances initiating and/or maintaining sleep. Restless legs syndrome and periodic limb movement sleep disorder, central sleep apnea, and some types of parasomnias can be associated with complaints of chronic insomnia. Even patients with narcolepsy can present with complaints of insomnia. As indicated previously, a robust kinship between any primary sleep disorder and the complaint of trouble falling and/or remaining asleep may exist.

Evaluation

Evaluation of insomnia requires the completion of several steps in order to effectively assess the problem and determine appropriate treatment strategies. Establishing a diagnosis of chronic insomnia is relatively straightforward, but because chronic difficulties initiating and maintaining sleep may be a symptom of other medical/psychiatric problems, a sleep history, a full medical history, a family history of disease, a family history of sleep disorders, and a physical examination are always indicated. Specific sleep questionnaires and sleep diaries, as well as psychological assessment measures, are also important in describing the characteristics and consequences of the patient's sleep problem(s). It is important to note that, at this writing, a standardized manner of data collection has not been clearly established, and procedures may vary from setting to setting. Some evaluation and treatment programs prefer the completion of questionnaires and other forms before the first visit, whereas others initiate the consultation first and then obtain self-report measures.

SLEEP HISTORY

The initial, crucial step in the evaluation of disturbed sleep (insomnia, sleep apnea, or any sleep-wake disorder) includes one-on-one consultation with the sleep specialist. This first appointment serves several important purposes, including information gathering and providing an environment for the description of wakefulness and/or sleep problems. Importantly, the first contact often fosters alliance with the sleep specialist, promoting a sense of security and also implying that the patient's complaint will (finally!) be taken seriously. Because the patient may or may not be aware of certain features of the disturbance, a family member or bed partner can accompany them during this visit. Sleep specialists work to build rapport, promoting a calm, trusting environment for addressing and expounding on relevant issues and complaints.

Flexibility in obtaining subjective information pertaining to the patient's sleep-wake disorder is important. Other related procedures, such as a mental status examination and general psychological evaluation interview, can be completed along with the consultation. What follows is only a general overview of some parameters assessed during the first visit. Table 13-1 describes the core elements of the sleep history.

The sleep consultation includes both open-ended questions and opportunities for straightforward, concrete "yes" or "no" responses to inquiries. Starting the interview with basic demographic information (name, date, referral source, age, birth date, and telephone number) followed by the patient's description of the reason for referral initiates the process smoothly. It is imperative that the interviewer listen carefully to the patient's perception of the problem, because *their view of the problem* will be very important to integrate later with acquired clinical information. In addition, this preliminary information can aid in establishing a reasonable treatment plan and may also provide clues to potential compliance issues.

Following the patient's open-ended response to the "Why are you here today?" inquiry, it is useful to ask about the duration of the problem as well as sleep-wake

Table 13-1 Core Elements of a Sleep History Consultation

• Ask about and define the patient's sleep-wake problem
• Determine the duration and course of the condition(s).
• Assess sleep-wake patterns, habits, and daytime sleepiness.
• Address symptoms of sleep-related breathing disorders, parasomnias, narcolepsy, and movement disorders.
• Discuss both prescription and over-the-counter drug use, as well as alcohol and other substance use.
• Address weight loss/gain, as well as cardiac, pulmonary, neurologic, psychiatric, and other system illnesses.
• Evaluate current medication schedule, current medical problems, and medical-surgical history.
• Assess other subjective characteristics of sleep-alertness disorders.
• Assess family medical and sleep disorder histories and social history.
• Review obtained information with the patient.
• Explain tentative diagnoses to the patient.
• Describe further testing and/or treatment strategies.
• Offer follow-up visit.

habits (bedtime, time in bed, perceived sleep latency, the frequency and duration of awakenings, and customary arising time). Thereafter, one may choose to ask about the tendency to arise immediately following awakenings and how they feel at that time. These data are essential in describing sleep-wake rhythms, as well as to document variations in habits and potential physiologic disturbances.

An assessment of circadian functioning is useful. Simply asking about the patient's "best time of day," if any, will allow the interviewer to ascertain whether the patient's "peak time" corresponds with established patterns and habits. An assessment of daytime sleepiness follows, determining the likelihood of sleeping while driving, at work, during social situations, at home, or during other quiet activities. An evaluation of the consequences of sleepiness is also helpful, because hypersomnia may negatively impact familial, occupational, social, and leisure functions. Additionally, problems with attention and concentration, memory functions (especially recent memory), and stability of mood are also worth exploring.

Because insomnia can be combined with a variety of sleep disorders, questions pertaining to snoring and sleep apnea are also necessary. Awakening with chest pain, brady-tachycardia episodes, and/or respiratory distress are all significant. A determination of whether apneic events have been observed by others is likewise important. An inquiry regarding sleep position preference is also helpful.

An assessment of vital signs, the physical examination, and a brief medical history may follow. The patient may report current weight and height, whether they have gained or lost weight over the past year, and whether substantial changes in weight have occurred during the previous years. Patients may be asked about hypertension, as well as a medical history that includes cardiac, pulmonary, thyroid, kidney, liver, diabetes, or other diseases. Psychiatric history and associated past treatments, including therapies for sleep disturbance, are also discussed. An evaluation of the patient's current medication schedule, as well as a history of sedative-hypnotic and other psychotropic drug use, is important. A review of current medical problems, as well as medical/surgical history, is necessary. A discussion of alcohol, caffeine, and other substance use is also indicated. Finally, a determination of when the patient last visited their doctor is critical.

An evaluation of parasomnias, movement disorders, and narcolepsy should be done. A review of the occurrence of sleepwalking, nightmares, enuresis, sleep terrors, significant somniloquy, and other potential unusual behavioral disorders of sleep is helpful. Symptoms of restless legs syndrome or periodic limb movement sleep disorder require exploration. Furthermore, addressing other potential medical conditions and sleep (gastroesophageal reflux disease, nocturnal headache, etc.) is necessary. Finally, a discussion of intentional and unintentional nap episodes, cataplexy, sleep paralysis, and both hypnagogic and hypnopompic hallucinations is important.

Toward the end of the sleep history consultation, it is beneficial for patients to describe the last time they slept well and felt alert throughout the following day. The patient's view of the severity of their problem (mild, moderate, or severe), as well as any previous treatment gains and preferences, is also important. A family medical history, addressing cardiac, neurologic, pulmonary, thyroid and other diseases, as well as diabetes and hypertension, is also necessary. The family sleep disorders history, detailing snoring, insomnia, parasomnias, and so on, is also described. When concluding the interview, the patient's relational, academic, and occupational histories round out the initial consultation.

These data provide the sleep specialist with a reasonable amount of information to assign preliminary diagnoses as well as justify the need for confirmatory testing or treatment implementation. Polysomnograms and/or multiple sleep latency tests are necessary if significant symptoms of sleep apnea, narcolepsy, or other primary sleep-wake disorders are likely on the basis of historical data. If physiologic evaluation of sleep and/

or wakefulness is not clearly indicated, an individualized sleep diary can be written with the patient. Other questionnaires and psychological evaluations can also be completed.

Before ending the consultation, it is helpful for the patient to review obtained information, discuss diagnoses, and address steps that will be taken in their evaluation and treatment. The latter is an essential part of the initial process, because this provides objective reasons for further assessment, serves to inform about procedures involved (including polysomnography and psychological testing), and establishes the groundwork for interventions. It is also important for the interviewer to respond openly and directly to patient inquiries and to do so in an appropriate fashion. Neglecting or minimizing this last portion of the initial assessment can lead to patient dissatisfaction, compliance problems, and, unfortunately, numerous other evaluation and treatment problems.

QUESTIONNAIRES/SELF-MONITORING MATERIALS ASSOCIATED WITH SLEEP AND ALERTNESS

Many questionnaires and other self-report inventories are currently available that purportedly assess the subjective aspects of disordered sleep and wakefulness. Some clinics and sleep centers may use assessment instruments that have been authored by staff members. Although these may possess some degree of validity (measure what they are intended to measure) and reliability (consistency or stability), they may not adequately describe symptoms, associated problems, or the nature and the impact of the condition on an individual's functioning. In addition, the use of inventories and/or questionnaires as a "substitute" for the more time-intensive sleep history consultation is suboptimal because interview and questionnaire procedures actually serve different, complementary purposes. At worst, many significant aspects of the ongoing sleep-wake disorder are neglected. Therefore, these self-report instruments need to be integrated with the sleep disorder consultation findings.

Two widely used assessment instruments, developed within sleep research, have been subject to psychometric evaluation. The Pittsburgh Sleep Quality Index (11), a brief clinically useful self-report inventory, evaluates subjective sleep quality and disturbance over the previous month. The Epworth Sleepiness Scale (12) measures subjective sleepiness. Reliability and validity measures have been acceptable for both. Together, these provide additional subjective information, which may support the patient's perception of the sleep-wake disturbance and provide evidence to support the diagnostic criteria. However, these instruments may not strongly correlate with objective physiologic findings and do not substitute for polysomnograms or multiple sleep latency tests in the diagnosis of other sleep disorders.

MOOD AND PERSONALITY ASSESSMENT

Although there are numerous purposes for psychological assessment, these procedures are generally concerned with utilizing various techniques and specific psychological tests in evaluating an individual's cognitive, emotional, interpersonal, and behavioral functioning, as well as providing recommendations for appropriate treatment interventions. A large number of instruments are available, focusing on several different domains of professional practice. Many self-report tests have not been used in clinical sleep medicine, but focused psychological testing can be quite valuable in clarifying areas of problematic functioning. In addition, some brief inventories or scales provide objective scores in measuring or determining the severity of depression, anxiety, anger, irritability, and other mood states or traits. Longer or more involved procedures, such as personality or neuropsychological assessment, focus on broader ranges of the person's cognitive abilities, strengths and weaknesses, emotional and adaptive functioning, interpersonal style, and behavioral tendencies. The collaborating psychologist usually determines which tests are most appropriate for use with individual patients.

As with inventories assessing sleep quality and disturbances, self-report instruments have been administered to clinical and research samples of patients. Dozens of these brief, symptom-oriented questionnaires are available, and many possess adequate validity and reliability. A few have been routinely used in sleep disorder clinics. The Beck Depression Inventory (13) is a multiple choice, 21-item device, which detects the presence of depression and accurately rates its severity. This and other scales are useful for evaluation of patients in sleep disorder clinics.

Assessment of psychopathology and personal adjustment generally requires the use of clinical interviews and structured, standardized psychological tests. This typically falls outside of the purview of the sleep center evaluation.

Polysomnography and Actigraphy

In the absence of symptoms of sleep apnea or movement disorders, the AASM recommends that "Polysomnography and daytime multiple sleep latency testing (MSLT) are not indicated in the routine evaluation of chronic insomnia, including insomnia due to psychiatric or neuropsychiatric disorders" (13). An overnight sleep study may be indicated if the patient fails treatment or if the diagnosis is uncertain. Actigraphy provides an indication of sleep timing and duration, as estimated from periods of reduced movement. "Actigraphy is indicated as a method to characterize circadian rhythm patterns or sleep disturbances in individuals with insomnia, including insomnia associated with depression" (14).

REFERENCES

1. Monroe L. Psychological and physiological differences between good and poor sleepers. *J Abnorm Psychol.* 1967;72(3):255-264.
2. American Academy of Sleep Medicine. *International Classification of Sleep Disorders*. 3rd ed, text revision. American Academy of Sleep Medicine; 2023.
3. Buysse DJ. Insomnia. *JAMA.* 2013;309:706-716.
4. Roth T. Insomnia: definition, prevalence, etiology, and consequences. *J Clin Sleep Med.* 2007;3:S7-S10.
5. Katz DA, McHorney CA. The relationship between insomnia and health-related quality of life in patients with chronic illness. *J Fam Pract.* 2002;51:229-235.
6. Vgontzas AN, Bixler EO, Lin H, et al. Chronic insomnia is associated with nyctohemeral activation of the hypothalamic-pituitary-adrenal axis: clinical implications. *J Clin Endocrinol Metab.* 2002;86(8): 3787-3794.
7. Shaver JL, Johnston SK, Lentz MJ, et al. Stress exposure, psychological distress, and physiological stress activation in midlife women with insomnia. *Psychosom Med.* 2002;64:793-802.
8. Levenson JC, Kay DB, Buysse DJ. The pathophysiology of insomnia. *Chest.* 2015;147(4):1179-1192.
9. Espie CA. Insomnia: conceptual issues in the development, persistence, and treatment of sleep disorder in adults. *Annu Rev Psychol.* 2002;53(1):215-243.
10. Khazaie H, Sharafkhaneh A, Zakiei A, Crew EC. A clinical algorithm for diagnosis and treatment of insomnia in adults: an updated review. *CNS Spectr.* 2024;29(5):463-473.
11. Buysse DJ, Reynolds CF, Monk TH, et al. The Pittsburgh Sleep Quality Index: a new instrument for psychiatric practice and research. *Psychiatry Res.* 1989;28:193-213.
12. Johns MW. A new method for measuring daytime sleepiness: the Epworth Sleepiness Scale. *Sleep.* 1997;14(6):540-545.
13. Beck AT, Ward CH, Mendelson M, et al. An inventory of measuring depression. *Arch Gen Psychiatry.* 1961;4:561-571.
14. Schutte-Rodin S, Broch L, Buysse D, et al. Clinical guideline for the evaluation and management of chronic insomnia in adults. *J Clin Sleep Med.* 2008;4(5):487-504.

Chapter 14
Central Disorders of Hypersomnolence

RUI M.DE SOUSA

KEY CONCEPTS/LEARNING OBJECTIVES

The key concepts for this chapter include a review of the types of narcolepsy, the narcoleptic tetrad, the role of hypocretin in sleep, medical disorders that may cause hypersomnia, drugs or substances that may cause hypersomnia, and psychiatric disorders that may cause hypersomnia.

KEY TERMS

Advanced sleep phase syndrome (ASPS)
Atonia
Cataplexy
Delayed sleep phase syndrome (DSPS)
Epworth Sleepiness Scale (ESS)
Hypnagogic and hypnopompic hallucinations
Hypocretin/orexin
Insufficient sleep syndrome
Kleine-Levin syndrome (KLS)
Sleep-onset REM period (SOREMP)

Hypersomnia, derived from the Greek "hyper" (over, above, too much) and the Latin *somnus* (sleep), literally refers to the condition of sleeping too much. However, in current medical terminology, both *hypersomnia* and the related word *hypersomnolence* are used more broadly to indicate long sleep duration, excessive daytime sleepiness (EDS), or both. Hypersomnolence, the state of being excessively sleepy during periods when the person should be awake and alert, is one of the most common sleep-related complaints that patients mention to their doctors.

The third iteration of the *International Classification of Sleep Disorders* (*ICSD-3*) describes eight central disorders of hypersomnolence, of which the primary complaint is overbearing daytime sleepiness not caused by disturbed nocturnal sleep or misaligned circadian rhythms. Although the *ICSD-3* does not explicitly divide these eight sleep disorders into categories, we can discern two basic groups of hypersomnias, the *primary hypersomnias* (occurring on their own, not caused by another condition) and *secondary hypersomnias* (caused by or intimately related to a different condition).

The four primary hypersomnias are those occurring independently of any other condition or effect. There are *narcolepsy type 1* and *type 2*, *idiopathic hypersomnia* (IH) and *recurrent hypersomnia*. The most salient feature is an extreme, overwhelming sleepiness during periods when the patient should be alert and awake, most often during the daytime hours. Even though the patient's nighttime sleep may seem to be of normal quality and timing, patients still feel sleepy and lethargic during the day.

A vast array of conditions can cause secondary hypersomnias. Sleep disorders like obstructive sleep apnea (OSA) or periodic limb movements (PLMS), as well as other medical conditions, disorders, and diseases as well. Drugs (whether prescribed or not) and other substances will often have side effects that cause extreme sleepiness in those who take them. Hypersomnia is often noted in psychiatric disorders. Some people will often curtail their normal nocturnal sleep on a regular basis, resulting in inappropriate daytime sleepiness.

EDS is the primary concern for many patients presenting with a sleep complaint. EDS is a significant public health problem, with prevalence in the community estimated to be as high as almost 28% (1). Yet because it is an invisible condition, there is often a stigma that often prevents the patient from seeking out help. Patients who are excessively sleepy are at greater risk for psychosocial problems, behavioral disorders, motor vehicle and workplace accidents, and obesity. Due to its insidious and pervasive nature, the clinical significance of EDS cannot be overemphasized nor its negative impact on society underestimated.

There are several objective and subjective measures at the clinician's disposal that can be used to assess and diagnose sleepiness and disorders of hypersomnolence. Polysomnography (PSG), the multiple sleep latency test (MSLT) and its variant, the maintenance of wakefulness test (MWT) are used to objectively measure sleep and propensity to sleep. Actigraphy is an adequate proxy in the absence of the PSG. Scaled questionnaires such as the Epworth Sleepiness Scale (ESS) and the Stanford Sleepiness Scale (SSS) can be used as well. Self-reported sleep diaries and detailed medical histories are also crucial tools when diagnosing or treating hypersomnia.

Some significant changes were made to the *ICSD* between the second and third editions. Specifically, the narcolepsies are no longer divided by the presence or absence of a symptom (narcolepsy with cataplexy and narcolepsy without cataplexy) but are now divided by their inferred pathogenesis (narcolepsy type 1 [no hypocretin] or narcolepsy type 2 [normal hypocretin levels]) (2). IH was streamlined, from IH with, and without, long sleep time to just simply idiopathic hypersomnia. The recurrent hypersomnias were also trimmed to just include the Kleine-Levin syndrome (KLS). The rest of this chapter will mirror the general blueprint of the hypersomnia disorders as outlined in the *ICSD-3*.

CENTRAL DISORDERS OF HYPERSOMNOLENCE: NARCOLEPSY

Introduction

Narcolepsy is a lifelong condition. It is a rare, chronic, neurologic sleep disorder with no known cure. It is characterized by EDS and a deterioration in the brain's ability to control sleep-wake cycles. There are two subtypes, *narcolepsy type-1*, with extremely low concentration of hypocretin, a neuropeptide that regulates arousal, wakefulness and appetite, and *narcolepsy type-2*, with near normal hypocretin levels. Narcolepsy is a rare disorder, its prevalence estimated to range from 40 to 160 per 100,000.

Salient Features: The Narcoleptic Tetrad

Although the severity and range of symptoms may vary, it is generally characterized by a tetrad of symptoms:

1. **Excessive Daytime Sleepiness:** EDS is the most common feature of narcolepsy and can manifest in many ways, including difficulty staying awake; irresistible microsleeps; increased napping; memory loss; cognitive problems; and struggles in work, school, or personal life. This sleepiness usually persists throughout the day regardless of the quality or quantity of sleep during the night. These naps are characteristically short but refreshing, although the normal wake state between naps will not typically last too long. The patient with this disorder will soon return to a sleepy state.
2. **Cataplexy:** Cataplexy is a medical condition in which strong emotion or laughter causes a person to suffer sudden physical collapse or an abrupt loss of voluntary muscle tone (*atonia*). It is characterized by preservation of consciousness and memory, lasting only a short duration, and a successful response to antidepressant medication. It may occur several times per day or a few times per year. Cataplexy usually develops within a few months of EDS symptoms but may develop 10 to 30 years later. Sudden positive emotional outbursts, especially laughter, is a most common instigator of cataplexy. It is believed that in cataplexy, the processes that produce paralysis during rapid eye movement (REM) sleep become inappropriately active during times of wakefulness.

   Often mild, typical examples are simple buckling of the knees, head dropping, facial muscle flickering, sagging of the jaw or weakness in the arms. Slurred speech or a complete inability to speak may also be observed. At times, it can escalate into episodes of complete muscle paralysis that can last up to several minutes. However, the patient often has sufficient warning of such "drop attacks" and can sit down or lie down in time to prevent a fall or injury. Longer episodes can sometimes evolve into sleep, often with hypnagogic hallucinations. Cataplexy has been reported to improve with age, likely after the patient has learned to better control their emotions (3). In rare cases, withdrawal from certain antidepressant or anticataplectic drugs can result in *status cataplecticus*, a state in which the patient is cataplectic for a prolonged time, often hours (3,4).

   The importance of cataplexy for the diagnosis of narcolepsy has been recognized since its first connection with narcolepsy. Historically, narcolepsy was divided into the presence or absence of cataplexy. More recently, however, this approach has been eschewed for a different model, focusing on underlying disease processes rather than witnessed symptoms. The current *International Classification of Sleep Disorders (ICSD-3)* divides narcolepsy into two distinct subgroups; *narcolepsy type 1*: those having narcolepsy with very low levels of hypocretin in the cerebrospinal fluid (CSF), often manifesting as cataplexy, and *narcolepsy type 2*: those having narcolepsy with near normal concentration of hypocretin, which does not result in cataplexy (2).
3. **Hypnagogic and Hypnopompic Hallucinations:** Hallucinations are a common characteristic of narcolepsy. They occur either as the patient is falling asleep (*hypnagogic*) or right as they are waking up (*hypnopompic*). Although the majority of hallucinations are visual, they can also be auditory or tactile (4). Like cataplexy, these hallucinations are believed to be REM phenomena (dreams) intruding into the wake state.

4. **Sleep Paralysis**: Sleep paralysis is a state in which the person is physically immobile, but fully conscious and has been reported in 20% to 50% of narcoleptics. It is experienced by patients when they are falling asleep or awakening, and it is the inability to move their limbs, lift their head, or even breathe that can often be distressing. Sleep paralysis may last up to a few minutes and is usually interrupted by noise or other stimuli (3). It is also more commonly noted with hypnagogic hallucinations. And just like cataplexy and hallucinations, sleep paralysis is likewise believed to be a particular feature of REM sleep (paralysis) manifesting in wakefulness.

   It is important to keep in mind that sleep paralysis and hypnagogic hallucinations are not specific to narcolepsy. These symptoms can occur in 15% of otherwise normal persons and can often be precipitated by sleep loss, schedule change, or alcohol consumption. These symptoms can also occur in IH. Narcoleptic hallucinations are sometimes misdiagnosed as schizophrenic ones (3,4). However, most of the narcolepsy-related hallucinations tend to be visual, while the schizophrenic ones are more likely to be auditory.

Other characteristic features of narcolepsy include objective differences in REM sleep, namely, a short latency to REM sleep and REM episodes during short naps, fragmented nocturnal sleep, automatic behavior, loss of concentration and memory, and blurry vision (5).

The presentation of this tetrad is variable in symptoms and intensity across patients and over time, and only about 10% of patients concurrently exhibit all components (6). There is no known cure for narcolepsy, and treatment is currently tailored to the individual and focused on managing symptoms with various medications and lifestyle changes.

A Brief History of Narcolepsy

Gélineau, in 1880, is recognized for giving narcolepsy its name and for recognizing the disorder as a specific clinical entity. However, he did not differentiate episodes of muscle weakness and sleep attacks triggered by emotions. The first descriptions of narcolepsy-cataplexy were reported in Germany by Westphal (1877) and Fisher (1878). Both reported irresistible sleepiness and episodes of muscle weakness triggered by excitement (7). Post World War II, at the height of psychoanalytic influence, there was a push to describe and treat narcolepsy as a psychosomatic disorder; however, work by Kleitman and Daniels refocused research to investigate a possible organic cause for narcolepsy (7). In 1960, Vogel was the first to report REM sleep at sleep onset in a narcoleptic patient, which was confirmed and expanded by Rechtschaffen and Dement a few years later. These observations led to the hypothesis that narcolepsy and REM were associated. This also led to the development of the MSLT test, discussed in more detail further on. The first narcolepsy clinic was opened in Stanford University in 1964 by Dement.

In the early 1900s, ephedrine was used until amphetamines were introduced in 1935. In 1959, Yoss and Daly used methylphenidate to treat narcolepsy, and in 1960 Akimoto, Honda, and Takahashi used imipramine (a tricyclic antidepressant) in the treatment of human cataplexy, establishing the stimulant/antidepressant model used to treat narcolepsy to this date (7). In the mid-1990s, research into the neurogenesis of narcolepsy by two separate and independent teams of researchers revealed the role of a new neuropeptide simultaneously named *hypocretin* and *orexin*. Today, both terms are used interchangeably to reference the same neuropeptide (8,9).

Prevalence of Narcolepsy

Prevalence of narcolepsy is estimated to be between 0.02% and 0.16% of the general population, with possible ethnic or genetic factors influencing the observed variance in rates. Symptoms usually appear in the midteens, but diagnosis is typically made later in life. A second, though smaller, peak is observed in the midthirties. Both genetic and environmental factors have been linked with narcolepsy. Recent mouse and human research indicates that more females may have narcolepsy than males, especially with cataplexy, although more research is needed (10).

Genetic Determinants of Narcolepsy

Although the prevalence of narcolepsy type 1 in first-degree relatives of patients with narcolepsy is only 1% to 2%, this still represents a 10 to 40 times relative risk of getting narcolepsy compared to the general population (11). Narcolepsy's strong association with the human leukocyte antigen (HLA) led the first investigators to believe that narcolepsy was an autoimmune disorder. Early genetic research into narcolepsy showed a relation with the HLA genes, more specifically, the subtypes DR2/DRB1*1501 and DQB1*06–02. Other HLA subtypes have shown a weaker association with narcolepsy. Current research focuses on the HLA DQB1*0602 allele, present in over 90% of patients with narcolepsy. However, because about 20% of the population carries this allele and only 0.05% of the population develops narcolepsy, this association is not very specific.

Although the HLA research is most well known, there are also many studies that concluded other genetic links with narcolepsy, including polymorphisms in the

T-cell-receptor-α (TCRA) locus on chromosome 14, TNFSF4 (also called OX40L), Cathepsin H (CTSH) the purinergic receptor P2RY11, the DNA methyltransferase DNMT1, and carnitine palmitoyl transferase (CPT1B) (11). Despite the genetic evidence in narcolepsy, the picture is complex and incomplete. In fact, even with monozygotic, or identical, twins, chances are that narcolepsy is *not* shared between the two.

Environmental Factors in Narcolepsy

Genetic expression is likely influenced by environmental factors, although the specific nature of these triggers are unknown. Concordance rates of 25% to 31% in monozygotic twins have been reported (12). Onset is frequently associated with nonspecific environmental factors, such as head trauma, stroke, and change in sleep-wake cycle (12). There may also be an association with streptococcal infection, HIN1 vaccination or infection, and exposure to heavy metals, insecticides, and weed killers.

Narcolepsy: A Tale of Two Types

In the past, type 1 narcolepsy was previously known as *narcolepsy with cataplexy and* type 2 narcolepsy was known as *narcolepsy without cataplexy*. This underlay the role that cataplexy has had in the history of narcolepsy and its diagnosis. However, with the discovery of the neuropeptide *hypocretin* (also known as *orexin*), and of the important role that it plays in narcolepsy, the *ICSD-3* elected to categorize narcolepsy by the absence (*type 1*) or presence (*type 2*) of hypocretin, rather than using cataplexy as a diagnostic criterion.

Diagnostic Criteria for Narcolepsy Type 1

Criteria A and B must be met (2):

A. The patient has daily periods of irrepressible need to sleep or daytime lapses into sleep occurring for greater than or equal to 3 months.
B. The presence of one or both of the following:
  - Cataplexy and a mean sleep latency of less than or equal to 8 minutes and greater than or equal to 2 sleep-onset REM periods (SOREMPs) on an MSLT performed according to standard techniques. A SOREMP (within 15 minutes of sleep onset) on the preceding nocturnal polysomnogram may replace one of the SOREMPs on the MSLT.
  - CSF hypocretin-1 concentration, measured by immunoreactivity, is either less than or equal to 110 pg/mL or less than 1/3 of mean values obtained in normal subjects with the same standardized assay.

To diagnose narcolepsy type 1, the patient must present with irresistible sleep attacks and either cataplexy and/or decreased hypocretin levels.

Narcolepsy Type 1: The Role of Hypocretin

The hypothalamic neuropeptide hypocretin (or orexin) regulates arousal, wakefulness, and appetite. Narcolepsy type 1 is caused by a lack (or significant reduction) of hypocretin in the brain due to destruction of the cells that produce it. Using immunoassay techniques, hypocretins were first discovered in 1998 (8) and their roles in sleep regulation were immediately evident. A second group of researchers simultaneously and independently found the same neuropeptides and called them orexin (9). Hypocretins are measured in the CSF, collected via a lumbar puncture, or spinal tap. When testing for narcolepsy, CSF concentration of hypocretin is either less than 110 pg/mL or less than one-third of mean values of normal subjects (2).

In the healthy population, that is, those with well-regulated sleep, hypocretins are released when awake and target neurons that promote wakefulness and suppress REM sleep. In people who have narcolepsy type 1, most (up to 95%) of the hypocretin-producing neurons die off (11). Other neurologic insults may also reduce hypocretin concentration, such as hypothalamic lesions, or vascular, inflammatory or traumatic injuries to the brain. This can affect hypocretin levels either permanently or temporarily. The consequent lack of hypocretins results in prolonged sleepiness and poor control of REM sleep. REM sleep can become so poorly regulated that the paralysis or dreaming that normally occurs only in REM sleep can intrude into wakefulness, causing cataplexy and dreamlike hallucinations. Although low levels of hypocretin can assist in diagnosing narcolepsy, one must be aware that low levels can also be observed in other neurologic disorders such as advanced Parkinson disease; Guillain-Barré syndrome and Miller Fisher syndrome; other neurologic conditions associated with lesion or dysfunction of the lateral hypothalamus.

During REM sleep, most muscles are temporarily paralyzed by processes in the lower brainstem. Cataplexy and sleep paralysis are states in which these processes become active during wakefulness. These processes are normally blocked by norepinephrine and serotonin during wakefulness. With loss of hypocretins, the levels of these two neurotransmitters may be lower, permitting paralysis to occur even during wakefulness. This observation provides the basis for treating cataplexy with antidepressants that increase brain levels of norepinephrine and serotonin.

The role of hypocretins may also explain how cataplexy may be triggered by strong emotions. The amygdala and prefrontal cortex are brain regions that regulate emotional responses. They connect with the paralysis pathways in the brainstem. Neurons in the amygdala and prefrontal cortex are active during cataplexy. Deactivating either of these regions reduces cataplexy in mice with narcolepsy (13).

Narcolepsy Type 2

Diagnostic Criteria for Narcolepsy Type 2 (2).
Criteria A—E must be met:

A. The patient has daily periods of irrepressible need to sleep or daytime lapses into sleep occurring for ≥3 months.
B. A mean sleep latency of ≤8 minutes and ≥2 SOREMPs are found on an MSLT performed according to standard techniques. A SOREMP (within 15 minutes of sleep onset) on the preceding nocturnal polysomnogram may replace one of the SOREMPs on the MSLT.
C. Cataplexy is absent.
D. Either CSF hypocretin-1 concentration has not been measured or CSF hypocretin-1 concentration measured by immunoreactivity is either >110 pg/mL or >1/3 of mean values obtained in normal subjects with the same standardized assay.
E. The hypersomnolence and/or MSLT findings are not better explained by other causes such as insufficient sleep, OSA, delayed sleep phase disorder, or the effect of medication or substances or their withdrawal.

To diagnose narcolepsy type 2, a patient must present with irresistible sleep attacks, MSLT criteria must be met, absence of cataplexy and hypocretin concentration within normal parameters, and no other explanation for the reported sleepiness.

Just as in type 1 narcolepsy, type 2 is also characterized by EDS and REM on the PSG and the MSLT. Cataplexy is always absent; however, some weakness or other unusual sensations may be reported during periods of intense emotion. Approximately 15% to 25% of all narcolepsy cases present without cataplexy. Of these, about 24% will present with abnormally low CSF hypocretin-1 levels, and almost all of these subjects will test positive for the HLA DQB1*0602 antigen (2). The procedure and interpretation of the MSLT is the same as in type 1, namely, the presence of two or more SOREMs and an average sleep-onset latency of less than 8 minutes.

Diagnosis

The first step in the diagnosis of narcolepsy is a complete and thorough sleep history from the patient and, if possible, from partners, relatives, and friends. The physical examination should be normal unless the patient is having an attack of cataplexy, in which case, muscle atonia and areflexia would be noted, lasting from a few seconds to a couple of minutes. The sleep history should reflect all or parts of the narcoleptic tetrad, most notably, EDS throughout the day, with possible episodes of sleep attacks, varying severity and frequency of cataplexy, possible hypnagogic or hypnopompic hallucinations, and probable sleep paralysis. The frequency and number of the narcoleptic tetrad symptoms vary from patient to patient, although EDS is the most persistent feature. Please note that it is no longer necessary for the patient to present with cataplexy in order to diagnose narcolepsy type 1. Even in the absence of cataplexy, low or nonexistent hypocretin levels are sufficient evidence to identify type 1 narcolepsy.

Subjective Scales of Sleepiness

The *ESS* is a self-administered questionnaire in which patients rate their likelihood of falling asleep in eight different life situations. Each situation is scored from 0 to 3, and the total score varies from 0 to 24. Epworth scores can be interpreted as follows: 0 to 5, lower normal daytime sleepiness; 6 to 10, higher normal daytime sleepiness; 11 to 12, mild EDS; 13 to 15, moderate EDS; 16 to 24, severe EDS. Deceptively simple and rudimentary, it has been validated across different clinical situations and various languages (5). Internal consistency and external validity are well established.

The *SSS* rates EDS according to the subjects' perception of their own sleepiness/alertness at a particular time. When averaged throughout the day, it was found to correlate highly with performance tasks previously tested to be sensitive to moderate amounts of sleep. The major advantages of both the Epworth and the Stanford scales are that they are rapidly taken, easily scored, and inexpensive to administer.

Objective Tools for Assessing Sleepiness

The polysomnogram (PSG). Typically, a full PSG is run overnight, recording data from the brain (electroencephalogram/EEG), eye movements (electrooculogram/EOG), muscle tone (electromyogram/EMG), heart rate (electrocardiogram/ECG), respiration, peripheral limb movements, blood oxygen and pulse using pulse oximetry, and snoring sounds. The PSG can be used to reveal other possible causes of EDS, possibly ruling out narcolepsy as a cause of the daytime sleepiness. It is also used to investigate other features of narcolepsy, such as sleep-onset REM and fragmented sleep. The PSG is most often performed the night before the MSLT. Note that the subjective scales and the objective tests do not always show a high correlation with each other and that appropriate clinical judgment and a detailed medical history must be considered as well.

The MSLT is the standard diagnostic test for narcolepsy. It is a diurnal sleep test, with designated nap times every 2 hours. Each nap can last from 20 minutes to 35 minutes, and four or five scheduled naps, 2 hours apart, are run during the day. Patients are required to stay awake between each nap opportunity and asked to try and sleep during the 20 minute nap window (14).

Various measures are recorded. Of particular interest are the length of time it takes one to fall asleep (sleep latency) and the presence of sleep-onset REM (SOREM) in each nap window. SOREMs are more common in narcolepsy than in the general population. In the MSLT, SOREM is defined as a REM period during the first 15 minutes after sleep onset. A mean sleep latency of less than or equal to 8 minutes and greater than or equal to 2 SOREMPs should be found on an MSLT. A SOREM on the preceding nocturnal PSG may replace one of the SOREMs on the MSLT. A mean sleep latency of less than 5 minutes is indicative of significant EDS and when longer than 10 minutes, is considered within normal levels of alertness. Approximately 90% of narcoleptics have a mean sleep latency of 8 minutes or less; however, SOREM still remains a more specific predictor of narcolepsy (2).

The MWT is a variant of the MSLT. Because it has been found to measure alertness rather than sleepiness, it is used predominantly in the assessment of treatment efficacy rather than the diagnosis of narcolepsy.

Genetic Testing. Although narcolepsy (HLA-DQB1 *06:02) genotyping may help rule out narcolepsy when clinical history and sleep studies are inconclusive, it is not diagnostic and should be used to help only when clinical tests and past medical history are inconclusive. Although this allele is present in a very high percentage of patients with narcolepsy, it is also present in about one in five normal individuals. This low specificity limits the diagnostic strength of this test.

Immunoassay testing of hypocretin-1 concentration in the CSF is a valid and reliable way to test for narcolepsy type 1. In short, a low concentration of hypocretin in the CSF meets diagnostic criteria for type 1 narcolepsy, even in the absence of cataplexy. Low concentration is defined as less than or equal to 110 pg/mL or less than one-third of mean values obtained in normal subjects.

Differential Diagnosis

By definition, daytime sleepiness is the common symptom underlying all hypersomnias. Although IH may share the extreme EDS that affect narcoleptics, these patients do not have cataplexy (separating them from type 1 narcolepsy). Mean sleep latency may be similar in the MSLT; however, patients with IH have fewer than the two SOREMs. Sleep efficiency tends to be higher in patients with IH, and overall sleep is better consolidated. Daytime naps also tend to be longer and less refreshing than naps of patients with narcolepsy.

Sleepiness may also be secondary to other sleep disorders, such as OSA, delayed sleep phase syndrome (DSPS), insufficient sleep syndrome, and periodic limb movement disorder (PLMD). These sleep disorders should be ruled out before a diagnosis of narcolepsy is declared. Sleepiness may also be a direct result of shift work, or the use or abuse of prescribed medications, drugs or toxins, or other substances. Other medical conditions such as chronic fatigue syndrome, multiple sclerosis, congestive heart failure, depression, and malingering should also be ruled out.

Current Treatment

There is currently no cure for narcolepsy. Treatment involves controlling and improving symptoms, especially daytime sleepiness, sleep attacks, and cataplexy. Scheduling several short (under 20 minute) naps throughout the day has been shown to reduce EDS, both subjectively and objectively, but it is not recommended as the only course of treatment. Other lifestyle strategies include maintaining a consistent sleep schedule by going to sleep and waking up at the same time every day, including weekends. Getting regular exercise and avoiding the use of tobacco, alcohol, or drugs may also help increase energy during the day. These strategies should improve sleep consolidation during the night and could lead to more daytime alertness. However, pharmacologic interventions are currently the most effective way to manage narcolepsy (Table 14-1).

The AASM recently updated the clinical practice recommendations for the pharmacologic treatment of narcolepsy. Newly approved medications have been shown to be effective in treating narcolepsy, specifically, the central nervous system (CNS) depressant *sodium oxybate (Xyrem and Xywav)*, the histamine-3 receptor antagonist (H3R) *pitolisant (Wakix)*, and dopamine-norepinephrine reuptake inhibitor (DNRI) *solriamfetol (Sunosi)*. The CNS stimulant *modafinil (Provigil)* remains a strong recommendation. Other stimulants recommended, although not as strongly, are *methylphenidate, armodafinil,* and *dextroamphetamine* (15). The AASM did not find strong evidence for the use of antidepressants in the treatment of narcolepsy. Its continued use has persisted, albeit less commonly than in the past, mostly due to a history of anecdotal evidence (11). *Mazindol (Sanorex)* is a tricyclic nonamphetamine stimulant. Although used as an appetite suppressant, recent evidence indicates an improvement in EDS and cataplexy, although it is not yet specifically recommended in the latest AASM guidelines (15,16).

Future Directions

With our deeper understanding of narcolepsy comes a renewed and exciting search for novel medications. The discovery of the role of hypocretin focuses new research on hypocretin-based therapies. Various hypocretin replacement therapies have been pursued, including *stem cell transplantation, peptide replacement* (doses of hypocretin-1), *selective hypocretin receptor-2 agonists*

Table 14-1 Current Medications for Narcolepsy

For Cataplexy, Hypnogogic Hallucinations, and Sleep Paralysis	For Excessive Daytime Sleepiness
First-line therapy	**First-line therapy**
Sodium oxybate (Xyrem)	Sodium oxybate (Xyrem)
Low sodium oxybate (Xywav)	Low sodium oxybate (Xywav)
Pitolisant (Wakix)	Modafinil (Provigil)
	Pitolisant (Wakix)
	Solriamfetol (Sunosi)
Second-line therapy	**Second-line therapy**
Dextroamphetamine (Dexedrine)	Methylphenidate (Ritalin, Concerta)
	Armodafinil (Nuvigil)
Venlafaxine (Effexor)[a]	Dextroamphetamine (Dexedrine)
Atomoxetine (Strattera)[a]	Amphetamine/dextroamphetamine (Adderall)
Fluoxetine (Prozac)[a]	
Sertraline (Zoloft)[a]	*Mazindol (Sanorex)*[a]
Protriptyline (Vivactil)[a]	
Clomipramine (Anafranil)[a]	

[a]No longer explicitly recommended on the latest AASM treatment guidelines (2025).
Maski K, Trotti LM, Kotagal S, et al. Treatment of central disorders of hypersomnolence: an American Academy of Sleep Medicine clinical practice guideline. *J Clin Sleep Med.* 2021;17(9):1881-1893.

(ORX2R), and *gene replacement therapy*. ORX2R drugs show promise. *Danavorexton* (TAK-925) is now available, and *E2086*, *TAK-861*, *TAK-925*, and *TAK 994* are all in various stages of clinical trials (7). Gene replacement therapy has shown promise, although it is still a long way off from coming to market.

Immunotherapy aims to slow down or prevent the destruction of hypocretin-producing neurons by targeting the autoimmune mechanism of narcolepsy. Trials of *immunoglobulin* (IVIG) are just beginning. *Corticosteroids* can suppress immune activity, potentially preventing further damage to hypocretin-producing neurons, and *monoclonal antibodies* may target specific pathways involved in the immune response. Although immunotherapy studies are promising, they are still in their infancy, and results are inconsistent and transient (17,18).

Research on nonhypocretin-based drugs also continues, specifically on:

1. Histamine receptor H3 antagonists/inverse agonists,
2. Monoaminergic (MAO) reuptake inhibitors that may target specific neurotransmitters,
3. Drugs developed to treat other conditions like IH or attention-deficit hyperactivity disorder (ADHD) that may target multiple reuptake sites,
4. Novel slow-wave sleep (SWS) enhancers may help consolidate disrupted night sleep,
5. Thyrotropin-releasing hormone (TRH) analogs,
6. New formulations and/or delivery systems, and
7. Adapting current medications to the pediatric population (11).

The success of pitolisant, a H3R antagonist, has started a search for other H3R antagonists for use in narcolepsy treatment, specifically *SUVN-G3031*, which is still early in clinical trials. Currently, there are at least nine H3 R antagonists in various stages of development for EDS, schizophrenia, Alzheimer ADHD, neuropathic pain, and seasonal allergies (19).

Although the selective serotonin reuptake inhibitor (SSRI) and serotonin-norepinephrine reuptake inhibitor (SNRI) antidepressant medications are no longer recommended to treat narcolepsy/hypersomnia, *solriamfetol* is a dopamine-noradrenaline reuptake inhibitor and has recently been recommended as first-line treatment for EDS in narcolepsy. Similarly, *reboxetine (AXS-12)*, a norepinephrine reuptake inhibitor (with no effect on dopamine reuptake), shows early promise in reducing cataplexy and sleep attacks (7).

CONCLUSION

Narcolepsy is a lifelong sleep disorder. It is often characterized by EDS, cataplexy, hypnagogic hallucinations, sleep paralysis, and fragmented nocturnal sleep.

Although there is no known cure, it is relatively well controlled with medication and personalized lifestyle adjustments. New research into its etiology and the novel treatments that arise may one day lead to a cure for narcolepsy.

CENTRAL DISORDERS OF HYPERSOMNOLENCE: IDIOPATHIC HYPERSOMNIA

Introduction

IH is a rare sleep disorder of unknown etiology. Evaluation of the prevalence of IH in the general population is difficult due to the limited number of patients with IH and the difficulty of making a definitive diagnosis. It has been reported to be 6× to 10× less frequent than narcolepsy (20), suggesting a prevalence in the general population between 1 in 10,000 and 1 in 50,000.

As the name suggests, IH is characterized by EDS, and the patient often wakes up with difficulty, feeling disoriented or confused, seemingly "drunk" with sleep (*sleep drunkenness*). This sleepiness is pervasive and lasts all day. The severity of sleepiness, however, may fluctuate from person to person and from day to day. Unlike narcolepsy, however, there is no evidence of cataplexy nor sleep-onset REM (SOREM) periods in the PSG and/or MSLT are rare. Compared to narcolepsy, naps in IH tend to last longer, sometimes hours, and are usually not refreshing (21). There is some recent research that suggests that type 2 narcolepsy (without cataplexy, HLA-negative) and IH may be somehow related pathophysiologically. Both are genetically similar (HLA-negative, normal, or near normal hypocretin levels), and clinical observations show an equivalent degree of severity of hypersomnia (22). Despite the similarities between narcolepsy type 2 and IH, there are still some significant features such as an absence of multiple SOREMs on the MSLT; the presence of long habitual sleep periods, long nonrefreshing naps, sleep inertia; and a high sleep efficiency on the overnight PSG (23).

Literature Review and a History of Idiopathic Hypersomnia

The term idiopathic hypersomnia was used as early as 1829 by Schindler ("die idiopathische chronische Schlafsucht") for EDS of undetermined origin. By 1928, Wilson had described several "narcolepsies" and often used the term narcolepsy to refer to any condition characterized by irresistible sleepiness. It was not until the 1976 article by Roth that IH was described in its modern definition. This work was instrumental in the definition and classification of IH in 1979 for the first International Classification of Sleep Disorders diagnostic and coding manual (*ICSD*). IH was defined as a CNS disorder that is associated with a normal or prolonged major sleep episode (nighttime sleep) and excessive sleepiness consisting of prolonged (1-2 hour) sleep episodes of NREM (daytime naps). The *ICSD* initially described two clinical forms of IH—a polysymptomatic form with nocturnal sleep and naps of abnormally long duration with sleep drunkenness on awakening and a monosymptomatic form manifested by normal nocturnal sleep times yet persistent EDS during the day. These forms were eventually described as IH with long sleep time and IH without long sleep time, respectively (24).

Today, the *ICSD-3* has since eliminated these diagnostic classifications because recent research shows there is no significant pathophysiologic or therapeutic difference between either. Comparison of patients with greater than 10 hours of sleep to those with less than 10 hours shows no differences in ESS scores, MSLT mean sleep latencies, sleep drunkenness, unrefreshing naps, hypnagogic hallucinations, or sleep paralysis. The only reported differences are that the group with long sleep is somewhat marginally younger and thinner (2). Patients with IH also tend to overestimate their total sleep time by an average of an hour. For this reason, taking a detailed medical history will be subject to these perceptual inconsistencies, making a criterion of sleep time (long vs short) almost meaningless. As research using objective measures like actigraphy becomes more commonplace, this criterion may yet be revisited. For now, however, one may continue to note sleep duration as an important clinical feature but not consider it diagnostic nor defining. Separating IH into distinct conditions must await further research and understanding of the underlying biology (2).

Salient Features

EDS is the essential feature of all hypersomnias but is especially prominent in IH. The sleepiness is pervasive, lasting throughout the day. The disorder has a significant debilitating impact on social, family, scholastic, and occupational life (21,25). Naps, when taken, are long in duration, often an hour or longer, and the patient wakes up still tired and feeling unrefreshed. Unlike narcoleptic sleep attacks, however, patients with IH can usually hold off from napping until a more convenient time. Furthermore, sleep paralysis and hypnagogic/hypnopompic hallucinations are rare (26,27).

Waking up is very difficult. The subject is overwhelmed by a sense of extreme grogginess or confusion. Known as *sleep drunkenness*, it is the clinical term for the state after awakening defined by extreme difficulty arousing, confusion, disorientation, automatic behaviors, and poor coordination. The transition from sleep to wakefulness can be long and difficult (26). Often, the subject just returns to sleep rather than waking up.

Other salient features of IH (although the same may be said for someone deeply sleep deprived) are motor hyperactivity (constantly active, talking a lot), cognitive dysfunction (memory, attention and concentration problems), hallucinations, sleep paralysis, automatic behaviors, headaches, and problems with balance (2,21).

The major sleep period (usually at night) is generally well consolidated, with low sleep fragmentation and relatively high sleep efficiency, typically above 90%. The amount of deep sleep (Stage N3) may also be elevated. This major sleep period may be very long or within normal parameters, but the overall sleep time in a 24-hour cycle is always elevated. To meet diagnostic criteria, total sleep time over the 24-hour period must be a minimum of 660 minutes (11 hours) (2).

There seems to be a small but positive family history (27). Gender ratio for IH is unknown. It is believed to be equal between males and females, although one study has reported 65% of patients were female (27). Age of onset has been reported to be in the middle to late teens and the average age of diagnosis in the low 30s (26,27). The diagnosis of IH is complicated by the fact that differentiating between excessive versus long sleep or normal versus abnormal wakefulness is often difficult, especially in the teenage population. Consequently, patients must deal with IH an average of 10 to 12 years before a diagnosis is made and effective treatment commenced.

The symptoms of IH tend to remain stable over many years, but up to 11% of patients in one study had spontaneous remission of their symptoms (26), and another more recent study showed 14% to 25% spontaneous remission. Note that narcolepsy, on the other hand, has no history of remission and is considered a lifelong disorder (25).

Diagnosis

The pathophysiology of IH is not well understood, and diagnosis requires exclusion of other more common causes of excessive sleepiness. The *ICSD-3* lists six criteria that must be met before a diagnosis of IH can be considered. First, the symptoms of excessive and irrepressible sleepiness must have persisted every day for a minimum of 3 months. Unlike narcolepsy, there is no evidence of cataplexy or of sleep-onset REM periods. In fact, when the MSLT is performed, a maximum of one SOREM can be observed. And at least one of the following must be present; a mean sleep latency on the *MSLT* of 8 minutes or less, or greater than 660 minutes of total sleep in a 24-hour period, as measured by 24-hour PSG monitoring or wrist actigraphy averaged over 7 consecutive days.

A *sleep diary* may be used to complement the actigraphy data. Although self-reported impressions of total sleep time are notoriously overestimated (by an average of about an hour per 24 hours) (27), a sleep diary may give other important information that may impact amount and quality of sleep, such as sleep hygiene. Sleep diaries can record the timing and length of naps, the episodes of sleep drunkenness, and other essential features of IH. Although not necessarily diagnostic, these are helpful in tracking indicators of IH.

The ESS can help quantify sleepiness in certain situations, and a minimum score of 10 can signify someone suffering from EDS and fighting to stay awake. Studies in IH have shown a median ESS score in the 16 to 17 range (26,27). Other well-known scales include the SSS, the Oxford sleep resistance test (OSLER), and the Pittsburgh sleep Quality index (PSQI). New scales have been developed recently that more specifically target IH symptoms, namely, the idiopathic hypersomnia severity scale (IHSS) and the hypersomnia severity index (HSI) (28).

Differential diagnosis is important in correctly diagnosing IH since IH is primarily a diagnosis of exclusion. When a patient presents with symptoms of EDS, all other known contributors to EDS must be excluded before a diagnosis of IH can be contemplated. Given the exclusionary nature of diagnosing IH, it is often overestimated because it is very difficult to always rule out all other possible contributors to daytime somnolence.

A comprehensive medical history and a battery of medical and personality tests should be performed in order to rule out insufficient sleep syndrome and other sleep, medical, or psychiatric disorders. A toxicology screen can also be ordered to rule out drug use or certain medications. A nocturnal PSG followed by an MSLT the next day will rule out narcolepsy, especially narcolepsy type 2, which closely mimics IH. OSA and PLMS must also be ruled out, as the fragmented sleep they cause will often result in EDS and fatigue. Another objective measure is the MWT. Just as the ESS, these tests are not diagnostic for IH but may help the clinician in more accurately diagnosing IH.

Treatment

Because the underlying cause of IH is unknown, the goal of treatment is symptom relief and improvement in the quality of life. When a diagnosis of IH is established, treatment is largely pharmacologic with generally good, but somewhat variable, results. The current AASM guidelines strongly recommend *modafinil*, as first-line drug therapy. Conditionally recommended drugs are *methylphenidate, clarithromycin, pitolisant,* and *sodium oxybate* (15,28). Although amphetamine-like compounds are effective in reducing the sleepiness felt during the wake period, other symptoms such as sleep inertia or sleep drunkenness persist. If amphetamine-like stimulants are prescribed, tolerance and dependence should be closely monitored as possible complications.

Self-medication is common in patients with IH due to the long time between onset of symptoms and eventual diagnosis and treatment. Case histories reveal that excessive intake of caffeine, energy drinks, and other stimulants is often used to help the subject achieve a minimum level of awareness during the day.

Behavioral therapies are typically ineffective. Nocturnal sleep is already well consolidated, and improving sleep hygiene should have very little improvement in daytime function. The daytime hypersomnolence observed in IH is independent of the length or quality of nocturnal sleep. Scheduling naps is likewise not very helpful, as patients with IH do not recover energy from napping. They wake up as tired as they were before the nap. It has been reported that some patients with IH have found cognitive behavioral therapy (CBT) to be helpful for learning coping skills (29). Patient education and sleep hygiene tailored to IH has also been helpful. Emphasis on circadian rhythms such as avoiding even minor sleep deprivation, maintaining a regular light/dark cycle and conforming to regular sleep schedules can be of benefit to many patients (28).

Although not strictly a "treatment," *support for the patient* and family through organized patient advocacy and support groups is often reported by patients to be helpful in providing information and combating the negative public perception of those who are excessively sleepy (25).

Future Directions

New medications in use with narcolepsy may prove to be useful for IH. For example, pitolisant stimulates histamine release and promotes wakefulness. It has been used with some success in patients with treatment-resistant IH (23).

Gamma-aminobutyric acid (GABA) modulators are drugs that affect the GABA receptor. Positive allosteric modulators can have sedative effects. Typical examples are benzodiazepines, barbiturates, and alcohol. Current research into negative allosteric GABA modulators shows promise. Clarithromycin, primarily known as an antibiotic, is already recommended by the AASM. Flumazenil likewise shows promise (28). Research is concentrated on testing other positive GABA allosteric modulators.

Despite current understanding that narcolepsy type 2 and IH are separate and independent sleep disorders, there are some researchers that believe narcolepsy type 2 and IH are closer in nature than what we currently understand. Symptoms of narcolepsy type 2 and IH can often overlap significantly, and there are few fundamental differences between these two disorders, prompting some to hypothesize that they are the same sleep disorder or different aspects of the same disorder. More research is needed to better understand this relationship.

CENTRAL DISORDERS OF HYPERSOMNOLENCE: RECURRENT HYPERSOMNIA

Introduction

Recurrent hypersomnias are sleep disorders that cycle between active phases and periods of remission with relatively normal sleep. During the active phase, individuals experience social, scholastic, and occupational impairments. The *ICSD-3* classifies recurrent hypersomnias under one disorder, KLS, and its subtype, menstrual-related Kleine-Levin syndrome, based on data indicating the condition is fairly homogeneous and lacking evidence for other major subcategories (2). KLS is marked by recurring severe hypersomnia along with cognitive (memory, language), psychiatric (mood, delusions, hallucinations), and behavioral (hyperphagia, hypersexuality) disturbances. These episodes are followed by remission periods with relatively normal sleep and normalized associated features. Although the cause of KLS is unknown, it usually follows a benign course, eventually leading to spontaneous remission of all symptoms with few or no lingering effects. Patients typically experience less frequent and less intense episodes toward the end of the disease and are considered cured if they do not have an episode for six or more years. Due to the typical age of onset, KLS can have long-term and unintended harmful side effects on a patient's scholastic performance throughout their life.

LITERATURE REVIEW AND A HISTORY OF KLEINE-LEVIN SYNDROME

The first account in the literature of a person with recurrent sleep episodes was reported by William Oliver in 1705. A literature review counted a total of 12 cases published between 1786 and 1924, reflecting the rarity of this sleep disorder (30). Multiple cases of recurrent hypersomnia were first collected and reported in Germany by Willi Kleine. Max Levin emphasized the association of periodic somnolence with morbid hunger in 1929 and 1936. Critchley was the first to name this Kleine-Levin syndrome, in 1942, and in 1962, he developed the fundamental features that we recognize as KLS today. He described a triad of symptoms, highlighting periodic hypersomnia, excessive and compulsive eating, and abnormal behavior. He also noted that young adolescent males are predominantly affected, that the syndrome will spontaneously disappear (30). In 1990, the diagnostic criteria for KLS were codified in the *ICSD*, where it was defined as a syndrome composed of recurring episodes of undue sleepiness lasting some days, which may or may not be associated with hyperphagia and abnormal behavior (2).

Prevalence/Etiology

The etiology of this disorder is not known or fully understood. Although many (39%) KLS patients reported no precipitating factors before their first episode, most (42%) had reported feeling sick with an infection or fever 3 to 5 days before their initial episode.

Although population-based studies reporting on KLS prevalence are not readily available, it is generally considered an exceptionally rare disorder, affecting approximately 1 in 1.0 to 1.5 million (31). By 2014, approximately 500 cases were reported worldwide in the literature (2). It usually starts in the mid-teens (median age is 15 years) and affects mostly males (2:1-3:1) (32,33). Approximately 80% of KLS cases were first observed during the second decade, and the syndrome will last on average 8 to 10 years, with only a small fraction still exhibiting symptoms after 20 years. It is very rare for an active episode to last beyond 4 weeks, and remission periods very rarely last 12 to 15 months (33). Although reported worldwide, it seems to be somewhat more frequent in Israel and in American Ashkenazi Jews (30). The preponderance of cases in this patient demographic suggests a genetic component in the disorder. It is likely that KLS is caused by the interplay of some environmental factors acting on a susceptible genetic background. Familial KLS is rarely encountered, with a low risk of occurrence in first-degree relatives (30).

Neurophysiologic Evidence

Polysomnographic (PSG) and MSLT studies were performed on 19 patients. SWS was markedly reduced during the first half of the active episode, with eventual return to normal amounts in the second half of the episode. By the last days of the episode, SWS was at near normal levels (when KLS symptoms are in remission). This improvement in SWS amount had no effect on the persistence and severity of KLS symptoms. REM sleep also changed as the days progressed during the active phase of the disorder. REM remained normal or near normal in the first half of the episode but subsequently decreased as the days progressed.

Salient Features

Hypersomnia

Hypersomnia is present in 100% of KLS cases during the active phase of the disorder. The patients have recurrent episodes of severe hypersomnia, which are often associated with compulsive overeating and hypersexuality (32). Each individual sleep period is extremely long, ranging from 12 hours to 24 hours (mean 18.62 hours) (31,33). The active phase of the disorder (periods of hypersomnia) can last for days to weeks at a time (average 10 days, range 2.5-80 days) (2) and can recur several times a year. Often, the patients remain arousable, waking up only to void and eat. Despite the prolonged sleep time, incontinence is not observed. Patients can become irritable or aggressive when they do wake up or are prevented from sleeping. Between these symptomatic periods, the disorder will enter a time of remission whereby patients will have relatively normal sleep without EDS (31). Hypersomnia itself may also change as the disorder progresses. In the early years, the hypersomnia is more intense and longer lasting, whereas in later years, it may become a "heavy fatigue" and feelings of being in a zone between awake and asleep (31) (Figure 14-1).

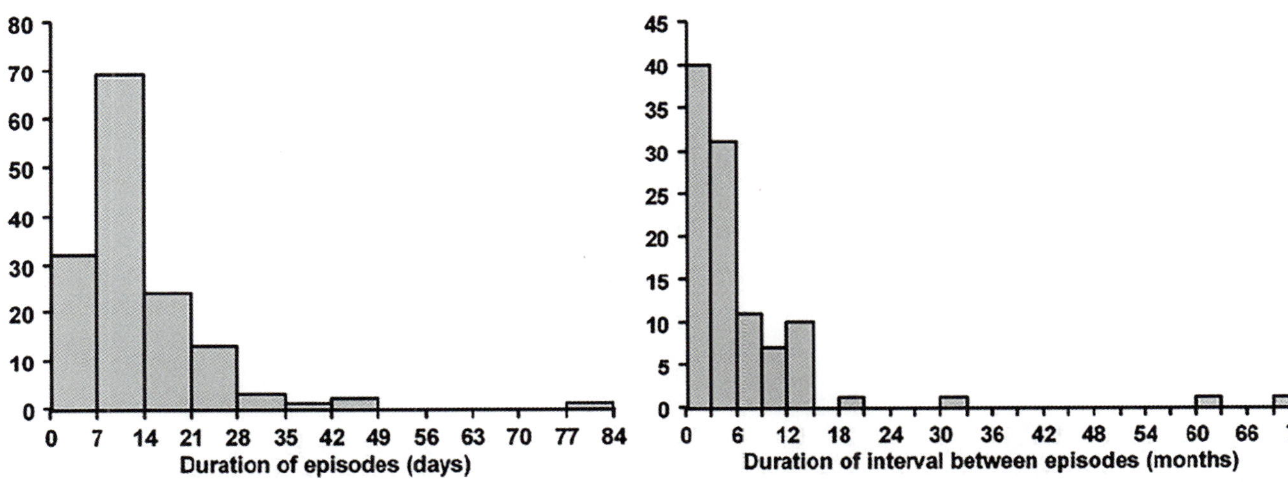

Figure 14-1 Histogram of the duration of Kleine-Levin syndrome episodes, in days (left panel), with a median of 10 days, and of the duration of the interval between episodes, in months (right panel), with a median of 3 months. (From Arnulf I, Zeitzer JM, File J, Farber N, Mignot E. Kleine-Levin syndrome: a systematic review of 186 cases in the literature. *Brain*. 2005; 128(pt 12):2763-2776. Reproduced by permission of Oxford University Press.)

Cognitive Disturbances

During an active episode, most of the patients often report feelings of confusion and difficulty with concentration, attention, and memory (31,33). Abnormal speech has also been reported in the majority of cases. Occasionally, amnesia has also been reported, with patients often not remembering events that occurred during an episode. During the remission period between active episodes, the overwhelming majority of patients reported normalized sleep and cognitive functioning. In some patients, a mild but long-lasting cognitive decline was observed, even years after the final episode (31).

Eating Disorders

The vast majority of KLS patients ate larger amounts of food than otherwise normal (megaphagia). A preference for sweets was noted in some cases. The increase in food could be mild to severe, with some patients eating up to 3 times their normal amount of food. The changes in appetite and eating were normalized after each episode.

Changes in Mood

Another common feature of KLS are the accompanying changes in mood during an episode. Depressed mood was observed in half of the patients, particularly in women. Approximately 15% of the patients reported suicidal thoughts, and two of 186 patients attempted suicide (33). A few patients report flattened affect, irritability, anxiety, and feelings of panic. Irritability and sometimes severe aggressive behavior was observed (although rare) when sleep, sexual or food drive was impeded. All mood phenomena were transient and normalized after each episode (31).

Compulsive Behaviors

Another salient feature of KLS is the presence of compulsions. They are defined as *behaviors that result* from an abnormal and uncontrollable need to perform a particular action. If the impulse is resisted, there is intense anxiety. The action is often repetitive and ritualized. The most common of these compulsions involve sexual activity. This hypersexuality is much more common in males than in females and can range from increased or overt masturbation, exposing oneself, and making unwanted and inappropriate sexual advances. Obscene language is also common, as is compulsive singing, body rocking, chewing lips, writing on walls, and even setting fires (31). Interestingly, whereas hypersexuality is more common in male patients with KLS, depressed mood is more common with female patients (2). Hypersexuality and other compulsions subside after each episode.

Perceptual Anomalies

Defined as a feeling that one's surroundings are not real, especially as a symptom of mental disturbance, derealization is a common feature in the subjective experience of patient with KLS. Almost all patients report a feeling of "unreality" or "disconnected thinking." Surroundings seem wrong somehow, distorted or unreal, as in a dream. Perception was described as strange, detached, or different. Objects were often seen to be "far away" and voices "distant bizarre, wrong or unpleasant." Some patients experienced visual or auditory hallucination (31) (Figure 14-2).

Frequency of symptoms during episodes of Kleine-Levin syndrome

Symptoms	Patients with the symptom/total	Percentage
Hypersomnia	168/168	100
Cognitive disorders	98/102	96
Abnormal speech	35/58	60
Confusion	24/47	51
Amnesia	24/50	48
Derealization	22/93	24
Hallucinations	13/93	14
Delusions	15/93	16
Eating behavior disorders	125/157	80
Megaphagia	97/125	78
Craving for sweets	15/125	12
Increased drinking	10/125	8
Binge eating	7/125	6
Decreased appetite	6/125	5
Food utilization behavior	5/125	4
Depression	41/86	48
Irritability	79/86	92
Other behavioral disorders		
Hypersexuality	67/155	43
Compulsions to sing, write, pace	17/59	29

Figure 14-2 Frequency of symptoms during episodes of Kleine-Levin syndrome.

Normality During Remission

As noted previously, KLS is characterized by recurring periods when the hypersomnia and other characteristic symptoms are present and longer periods when all symptoms are absent. During these periods of remission, the patient is essentially "back to normal," with all or most of the clinical symptoms absent.

KLS will eventually disappear spontaneously after a number of years (average range 8-12 years) for most people. Some patients may develop symptoms of irritability, impulsive behavior, hallucinations, depression, confusion, and memory problems, which may linger for years after the final episode (32).

Diagnosis

KLS is a diagnosis of exclusion, involving a thorough clinical evaluation to rule out all other possible conditions. Attention must be paid to other disorders that may closely mimic KLS. Severe depression will share periods of somnolence, overeating, and social withdrawal. The occasional brief period of hypermania (elevated energy) at the end of some episodes may mimic a manic episode of bipolar disorder. Some characteristic mood or perceptual disturbances may mimic primary psychiatric disorders. Narcolepsy, Kluver-Bucy syndrome, and temporal lobe epilepsy may also produce similar symptoms to KLS. Idiopathic recurrent stupor should also be ruled out, as well as metabolic encephalopathies (31). The use of drugs and other toxins should also be ruled out.

Although there is no single defining symptom, test, or procedure that provides a positive diagnosis, clinicians typically use the following to help with the diagnosis:

1. **Clinical Evaluation**: A comprehensive medical history and physical examination to identify characteristic symptoms and rule out other conditions
2. **Sleep Studies**: PSG and the MSLT/MWT to assess excessive sleepiness and sleep patterns
3. **Neurologic Studies**: Tests like the EEG, MRI, or CT scan to rule out structural brain abnormalities
4. **Psychiatric Evaluation**: To differentiate KLS from other psychiatric or mood disorders
5. **Questionnaires**: A questionnaire such as the **ESS or the SSS can be used** to measure daytime sleepiness

Treatment

Treatment of KLS is not standardized and is mostly pharmacologic. The goal is symptom relief and improvement in quality of life. A myriad of drugs have been used to mitigate the severity of the symptoms, from stimulants (*modafinil*) to antidepressants (*sertraline* and *lamotrigine*) and mood stabilizers (*lithium* and *valproate*), with varying degrees of efficacy. Antipsychotics, antiepileptics, antivirals, benzodiazepines, dopamine agonists, and electroconvulsive therapy have also been attempted but shown to be largely ineffective (34). At the moment, the AASM has only one recommended drug for KLS, a conditional recommendation of *lithium* (15).

Nonmedicinal approaches include *psychological support and counseling* to help patients and their families cope with the challenges of KLS and *lifestyle adjustments* such as maintaining a regular sleep schedule, identifying, and avoiding possible triggers that may induce episodes.

Special Mention

Menstrual-related hypersomnia is diagnosed when EDS occurs on a periodic basis over a few days preceding menstruation (32). This is an extremely rare disorder, with only 18 cases reported worldwide in the literature by 2014 (2). Although menstrual-related hypersomnia is currently considered a variant of KLS, a positive response to estrogen and progesterone therapy may indicate a reproductive endocrine abnormality (2).

Emerging Research

Recent research has identified potential *genetic* links, such as variations in the TRANK1 and LMOD3 genes, which may help in understanding the underlying mechanisms of KLS (35). Studies using *functional imaging* have shown abnormalities in brain activity during and between episodes, providing insights into potential therapeutic targets (35).

Studies are investigating the relationship between flu-like symptoms and onset of episodes and may shed some light on the autoimmune or inflammatory processes involved in KLS. One study found that *antibodies in the serum of patients with KLS* reacted with proteins from neural tissue, indicating a possible autoimmune response. This suggests that the immune system might mistakenly target brain proteins, contributing to the symptoms of KLS (36). Additionally, proteomic biomarker studies have identified **differentially expressed proteins** in the CSF and serum of patients with KLS, which could help in understanding the underlying mechanisms of the disorder (37).

Conclusion

KLS is a rare and little understood sleep disorder with a cyclical pattern of hypersomnia and normalized episodes. Although the clinical features are well defined and readily observed, the causes and prevalence are not well known. It is seen mostly in males, and in the second decade of life. The disorder spontaneously goes away after about 10 to 15 years in most people, with little or no lingering effects. Treatment is given for symptom relief and consists mostly of stimulants or lithium. Most other medications are deemed ineffective.

Improving social support and patient education may be an effective way to reduce the stress of KLS. Setting up contingencies during times when KLS is active and reassuring the family that this is usually a benign disorder that will eventually disappear, goes a long way toward helping patients cope with the anxiety and mystery associated with their affliction. Involvement of the school, teacher, or employer will also help mitigate long-term adverse effects. Special dispensation and a more flexible workload at school may reduce the educational burden seen when patients with KLS are still students.

CENTRAL DISORDERS OF HYPERSOMNOLENCE: HYPERSOMNIA DUE TO A MEDICAL DISORDER

Introduction

This collection of disorders identifies patients who experience hypersomnia secondary to a preexisting medical or neurologic disorder. Hypersomnia may take the form of prolonged nocturnal sleep, EDS or excessive napping. EDS may be of variable severity and may resemble that of narcolepsy (eg, refreshing naps) or IH (eg, long periods of nonrestorative sleep).

Hypersomnia and SARS CoV-2

A brief discussion regarding hypersomnia in a post–COVID-19 pandemic context. As a proposed neuroimmunologic disease, the hypersomnias may be triggered by environmental factors such as infections, viruses themselves, immune responses to vaccines, or even as a result of widespread pandemic quarantine. There is evidence of increased incidence of hypersomnia after the Spanish Flu of 1918, after administration of some H1N1 vaccines in 2010. Research is looking for any direct links between the SARS CoV-2 virus or its infection and the hypersomnias. Indirect evidence has already been found. Quarantine and home confinement itself has been implicated in immune system dysfunction likely through dysregulation of the circadian rhythm. This may lead to any of the hypersomnias. Depression or anxiety during the pandemic may have also caused or worsened existing EDS. SARS CoV-2 may result in encephalitis, which may, in turn, cause hypersomnia if the trauma affects relevant brain structures (hypothalamus, temporal lobes, hippocampus, brain stem). A COVID-19 infection may also result in exacerbating existing hypersomnias or cause a relapse of symptoms in a patient who was previously symptom free (eg, a KLS episode) (38). One study with over 500 "long-COVID" patients found eight patients who developed hypersomnias after COVID infection. Of these, four were shown to have no other comorbidities that may have caused the hypersomnia. Three patients were subsequently diagnosed with IH and one other with narcolepsy type 2 (39).

Vaccine-related incidences of hypersomnia continue to be investigated. A link between the Pandemrix H1N1 vaccine and narcolepsy has been proposed, with an adjuvant to the vaccine directly implicated. Likewise, similar research is ongoing for comparable adverse reactions to the many and varied COVID-19 vaccines used worldwide (38).

It is important to note, however, that there is currently no direct causal evidence between COVID-19 infection (nor its vaccines) and the appearance of hypersomnias. At this moment, any link is observational, theoretical, and correlational.

Narcolepsy due to a Medical Condition

This condition is diagnosed when an underlying comorbid medical disorder is the direct cause of narcolepsy. The medical condition may feature involvement of the areas of the brain responsible for REM sleep, such as the hypothalamus and pons, in hypothalamic pituitary pathology, head trauma and brain tumors, hypothalamic sarcoidosis, multiple sclerosis, and myotropic dystrophy. In addition to EDS, other features of narcolepsy may be present, such as sleep paralysis, hypnagogic hallucinations, or automatic behaviors, but if the patient also has cataplexy, or the MSLT shows two or more SOREMs, or CSF hypocretin-1 levels are low, then narcolepsy (type 1 or type 2) due to a medical condition should be diagnosed (2).

Hypersomnia Secondary to Parkinson Disease

Some patients with Parkinson disease (PD) have reported significant hypersomnolence as documented by the MSLT. The hypersomnia may be due to inadequate control of nocturnal symptoms, resulting in insufficient or poor sleep and consequent EDS. If this is the case, then the diagnosis should be an *insomnia disorder*. Although dopaminergic drugs are an effective treatment for PD, they are known to have side effects that include hypersomnolence. In this case, the diagnosis should be *hypersomnia due to a medication or substance*. Patients with PD with a disease profile consistent with narcolepsy should be diagnosed as *narcolepsy due to a medical condition*. All other cases of hypersomnia in a patient with PD should be diagnosed *hypersomnia secondary to PD* (2).

Posttraumatic Hypersomnia

Mild to moderate traumatic brain injury (TBI) often results in hypersomnia (40). The most common causes of TBI are falls, vehicle-related collisions (cars, motorcycles, bicycles, pedestrians), violence/gunshots, sports injuries, and explosive blasts/combat injuries (40). Studies have shown that sleepiness is common following

TBI, with more severe injuries often resulting in greater sleepiness. In a study of 87 patients with TBI, 11% were diagnosed with posttraumatic hypersomnia, a further 6% with narcolepsy, and 25% were found to have objectively quantified EDS as measured by an average MSLT sleep latency of less than 10 minutes (41). Although sleepiness improves in many patients, about a quarter of TBI subjects remained sleepy up to 1 year after injury.

Genetic Disorders Associated With Primary Central Nervous System Somnolence

Many genetic disorders and diseases have been associated with daytime sleepiness. Niemann-Pick type C disease and Norrie disease myotonic dystrophy, Moebius syndrome, fragile X syndrome, and Prader-Willi syndrome are known to result in EDS. Care must be taken to account for some genetic disorders that are also associated with sleep-disordered breathing, such as myotonic dystrophy and Prader-Willi syndrome. Hypersomnia due to medical disorder should only be diagnosed after adequate treatment of the sleep-disordered breathing. Smith-Magenis syndrome is a neurodevelopmental disorder characterized by a circadian reversal in melatonin secretion, where melatonin levels are high diurnally and low at night, resulting in daytime sleepiness (2).

Hypersomnia Secondary to Brain Tumors, Infections, or Other Central Nervous System Lesions

Brain tumors, infections, strokes, or neurodegenerative lesions in the brain can result in disturbances in sleep, including daytime somnolence, depending on where the assault was localized. Damage to the hypothalamus, pons, or rostral midbrain may produce daytime sleepiness. In patients with brain tumors, the sleepiness may be due to the tumor itself or the effects of treatment, in which case the diagnosis should be *hypersomnia due to a medication or substance* (2).

Hypersomnia Secondary to Endocrine Disorder

Hypothyroidism is the most recognized example of this condition (2). Case studies have shown a positive response to administration of low-dose levothyroxine in some cases of hypersomnia in subclinical or mild hypothyroidism.

Hypersomnia Secondary to Metabolic Encephalopathy

Before diagnosing a primary hypersomnia, care should be taken to eliminate toxic metabolic encephalopathies. A number of disorders caused by systemic illness such as adrenal or pancreatic insufficiency, liver disease, renal failure and heart failure, exposure to toxins, and certain inherited metabolic disorders in childhood may cause hypersomnia (2).

Residual Hypersomnia in Patients With Adequately Treated Obstructive Sleep Apnea

Some patients with sleep-disordered breathing (SDB) report persistent daytime sleepiness despite documented treatment success and adequate sleep. Before a diagnosis is made, the patient should be treated for at least 3 months and treatment success evaluated objectively by assessment of continuous positive airway pressure (CPAP) (or other PAP machine) data demonstrating optimal compliance (at least 7 hours/night). An overnight sleep study demonstrating elimination of essentially all SDB may also be warranted (2). Proposed mechanisms for continued daytime sleepiness include persistent arousals from emergent PLMS or other sleep disorders, previously undiagnosed obesity hypoventilation syndrome (OHS), or possible structural or physical damage to wake neurons (42). Hypoventilation due to OHS or other chronic obstructive lung disease will result in continued hypercapnia, which can cause EDS. Brainstem dysfunction may be the underlying cause of both lack of alertness and cardiovascular control. The possible cause of this dysfunction is unknown. However, in animal models, prolonged exposure to hypoxia-reoxygenation cycling (similar to those seen in patients with severe OSA) has been shown to irreversibly damage catecholaminergic wake neurons. Catecholamines (epinephrine/adrenaline, norepinephrine/noradrenaline, dopamine, etc.) are also involved in the arousal response, and excessive arousals over many years may cause damage to these neurons. It is likely that even after successful PAP therapy, patients may have subtle cardiac dysrhythmia and EDS due to the damage to the brainstem (42).

CENTRAL DISORDERS OF HYPERSOMNOLENCE: HYPERSOMNIA DUE TO A MEDICATION OR SUBSTANCE

Introduction

These disorders occur in patients who have hypersomnia secondary to sedating medications, alcohol, or drugs of abuse. This diagnosis also includes hypersomnolence associated with withdrawal from amphetamines and other drugs (2). A thorough medical history and a toxicology screen should be considered to implicate or eliminate the possible presence of sedating medications.

Hypersomnia due to Sedating Medications

Sedation is a common side effect of many prescription medications, including benzodiazepines, nonbenzodiazepine hypnotics, opioids, barbiturates, anticonvulsants, antipsychotics, anticholinergics, and some antidepressants and antihistamines. Sleepiness can also occur with some dopamine agonists such as pramipexole or ropinirole, and with many antiepileptic medications. Although less common, sleepiness can also occur with nonsteroidal anti-inflammatory drugs, some antibiotics, antispasmodics, antiarrhythmics, and β-blockers. Over-the-counter medications, such as valerian root and melatonin, can produce sedation (2). Natural herbs and plants can also have powerful sedating effects. These include kava kava, passionflower, poppies, hops, Jamaican dogwood, marijuana, chamomile, lavender, valerian, among others. Older patients are especially susceptible to sleepiness induced by these drugs and supplements. Some of the sedating effects of these drugs are further amplified when used in combination with other medications, complicating the managed care of patients with multiple comorbidities being treated simultaneously. Tolerance to the sedative effects can occur over time.

Hypersomnia due to Substance Abuse

Daytime sleepiness can occur with abuse of alcohol, benzodiazepines, barbiturates, gamma hydroxybutyrate (GHB), opiates, and cannabis. Similarly to sedating medications, certain substances can also cause somnolence if abused, when taken in excess or used inappropriately.

Hypersomnia due to Stimulant Withdrawal

A sudden discontinuation of stimulant use can result in an increased total sleep time, including daytime napping, and general sleepiness lasting for up to 3 weeks after withdrawal of stimulants. Despite the longer sleep time, sleep itself may be more fragmented and nonrestorative. Milder and shorter lasting sleepiness, fatigue, and inattentiveness can also occur when caffeine is withdrawn from regular coffee drinkers. It is also possible that some residual sleepiness can last for years after the discontinuation of stimulant use (2).

CENTRAL DISORDERS OF HYPERSOMNOLENCE: HYPERSOMNIA DUE TO A PSYCHIATRIC CONDITION

Introduction

Hypersomnolence can occur secondary to an underlying psychiatric disorder, such as depression, bipolar disorder, posttraumatic disorder, and panic disorder; however, the link to hypersomnia is not clear. The hypersomnolence observed is not necessarily directly caused by the psychiatric disorder. For example, a patient diagnosed with depression and hypersomnia will have both depression and hypersomnia, but whether the depression caused the hypersomnia or the hypersomnia caused the depression or whether the two are related in some other ways is neither known nor implied.

Patients may report sleeping in excess during the night, napping often or at length during the day, sleep inertia or EDS or fatigue (43). Fatigue is not usually relieved by increased sleep and may be unrelated to sleep quantity or quality. Many will also feel that sleep itself is nonrestorative, or of poor quality, often waking up just as tired as, or more tired than, before bedtime. Often, patients will have poor attendance at work or at school. They often spend days in bed several times a week. Patients may experience social withdrawal, apathy, and feelings of low energy. Women are more susceptible than men, and the typical age range is between 20 and 50 years (2).

Before a diagnosis can be made, a thorough medical history and a psychiatric consult should be considered to eliminate any possible psychiatric disorders that may have hypersomnia as a symptom. In these disorders, the diagnosis should be hypersomnia associated with mood disorder or conversion disorder.

Hypersomnia Associated With Mood Disorder

Hypersomnolence is a common feature of depression. Patients may sleep too much or have little energy during the day. Daytime function at school, work, or socially is often impaired. Similar symptoms are noted during the depressive episodes in bipolar disorder and in seasonal affective disorder (2).

Sleep complaints are very common in patients diagnosed with major depression. Depending on how it is defined, hypersomnolence will range from 5% to over 50% in patients with diagnosed major depression (2). The prevalence of insomnia alone was reported as 48%, hypersomnia alone as 14%, and co-occurrence of both as 30% (43). In fact, co-occurring insomnia and hypersomnia was associated with more severe symptoms of major depression. With major depression, hypersomnolence may persist even after the depressive episode improves, and persistent hypersomnolence is associated with increased risk of recurrent depression (2).

Bipolar disorder patients may also present with hypersomnia, noted during the depressive episodes. As opposed to symptoms of insomnia, these patients were more likely to be younger and to have shorter illness duration. Hypersomnolence also affects over 50% of patients with seasonal affective disorder (SAD), a mood disorder in which people exhibit symptoms of depression at the same time each year, most commonly in the winter (2).

Hypersomnia Associated With a Conversion Disorder or Somatic Symptom Disorder

Pseudo-hypersomnia or pseudo-narcolepsy, sometimes with pseudo-cataplexy, has been described.

Conversion disorder is a psychiatric condition in which a person has blindness, paralysis, or other nervous system (neurologic) symptoms that cannot be explained by medical evaluation. In the relevant cases, the patient will show symptoms of IH, narcolepsy, or cataplexy, without the objective support and confirmation of diagnostic testing.

Treatment

The AASM treatment guidelines for disorders of hypersomnolence do not recommend any specific pharmacologic treatment for hypersomnia associated with psychiatric disorders. Although it does recognize the use of modafinil and light therapy, it warns that the evidence is insufficient and inconclusive (15).

CENTRAL DISORDERS OF HYPERSOMNOLENCE: INSUFFICIENT SLEEP SYNDROME

Introduction

Patients with insufficient sleep syndrome (ISS) curtail their normal sleep on a regular basis by choice, causing severe sleepiness the during the day. Reasons vary but include work or school commitments, social obligations, or just personal choice. As sleep debt accumulates over many nights, daytime functioning deteriorates and extreme sleepiness is noted.

Prevalence

An estimated 2% of all sleep lab cases are diagnosed with ISS (44). Although ISS affects all ages and sexes, it seems to be more frequent in adolescence, when intrinsic sleep need is higher, yet social and scholastic pressures curtail total sleep time. Homework and studying may result in later bedtimes, and sports/extracurricular activities may require earlier wake-up times. ISS is also noted in young adults starting new jobs. Working long hours and taking on extra work may be seen as a desirable trait in the employee wanting to advance in the corporate environment. Female patients may experience additional pressures in the home even after a full day of work. Often, child-rearing and housekeeping duties (cleaning and cooking) still fall on the female patient. This usually results in later bedtimes and/or earlier wake-up times. Cultural influences may also contribute to ISS. In countries where napping, or the siesta, is commonplace, it may lead to enhanced nighttime alertness, delaying bedtime or sleep onset.

Especially salient to the sleep technologist, the shift worker may be peculiarly susceptible to ISS. Often, chores and errands are run during daytime hours, when the shift worker should be asleep. Often, there is no choice but to conform to daytime business hours, which means cutting sleep time by going to bed later than at the normal time or waking up sooner than ideal. This is especially true for long-shift workers (10-12 hours), when the demands of a 12-hour shift leave a shortened time to get all chores done and still sleep sufficient hours. These errands are often one-off occurrences and therefore not truly ISS. Sometimes, however, they are regular everyday events like taking the children to school and bringing them back,, long commute times, or going to the gym.

Salient Features

The primary symptom is daytime somnolence. The patient's ability to initiate and maintain sleep is within normal parameters. There is a noted discrepancy between the amount of sleep needed to maintain normal levels of alertness and wakefulness and the amount of sleep the patient reports getting nightly. The patient is often unaware how much their daytime sleepiness is affected by their poor sleeping choices (2). When sleep time is increased during the holidays, weekends, or vacation, daytime sleepiness is improved immediately. If sleep restriction is severe enough, the patient may experience sleep paralysis and/or hypnagogic hallucinations (2). Other features include personality changes; irritability; lack of motivation; fatigue; restlessness; and problems with memory, motor coordination, concentration, and attention. Obesity, depressed mood, increased anxiety, decline in school performance, and adolescent suicidal ideation have also been linked with ISS. Also of significance is the finding that people with severe ISS are at higher risk for getting into accidents. No other medical reason is readily apparent for the complaint of daytime sleepiness.

Diagnosis

Diagnosis is made via a detailed medical history and an elimination of other possible disorders. Actigraphy can be used in combination with sleep diaries for 2 to 3 weeks until a pattern emerges. Results would show a curtailed total time in bed, short sleep latency, short total sleep time, and high sleep efficiency. The PSG and the MSLT is not indicated in the diagnosis of ISS. After a sleep history via actigraphy and sleep diary is complete, a trial period with longer times in bed is tried. If the symptoms are alleviated, then the diagnosis of ISS is made.

Differential Diagnosis

DSPS may mimic the ISS patient who goes to bed late. Whereas patient with ISS chooses to stay up late, the patient with DSPS is just not sleepy due to their intrinsic circadian rhythm. When a patient has an endogenous *circadian* period that is much *longer* than 24 hours, they will not feel sleepy until later in the evening. Usually the wake-up time is set at a certain time (for school or for work) and is not flexible. This results in a persistent late bedtime, and an earlier than desirable wake-up time. Similarly, advanced sleep phase syndrome (ASPS) results in a constant early wake-up time. When a patient has an endogenous *circadian* period that is much *shorter* than 24 hours, they will feel sleepy earlier in the evening and wake up earlier in the morning. The patient may go to bed at a "normal" hour (which for their circadian rhythm may already be late) but then wake up too early.

ISS may also mimic the insomnias, but it is distinctly different. Patients with ISS maintain the ability to sleep normally, with sleep latency and sleep duration within normal parameters. They just choose not to. Patients with insomnia do not have a conscious choice to stay up late or curtail their sleep. Sleep initiation and/or consolidation of sleep is impaired beyond their control. Patients with ISS will sleep "normally" on vacation, holidays, or the weekend, whereas insomnia sufferers will continue to experience sleep troubles.

One must also keep in mind "long sleepers," those individuals with natural sleep requirements significantly more than the average 7 to 8 hours. In these patients, getting average amounts of sleep (eg, 7 hours/night) may not be enough. Societal pressures (work, school, family) and stigma (laziness) may prevent the patient from sleeping enough hours, and chronic sleep deprivation will incur. In this case, ISS should be diagnosed even if the patient reports an "average" full night's sleep of 7 or 8 hours.

Treatment

A therapeutic trial of a longer major sleep period can reverse the symptoms. If so, treatment would be to maintain that sleep schedule indefinitely. Sleep hygiene is also an effective tool to treat ISS. Education and adherence to proper sleep hygiene procedures will help increase total sleep time.

Conclusion

A sufficient amount of sleep is essential for optimal physical health, immune function, mental health, and cognitive function. Adults should sleep 7 to 8 or more hours per night on a regular basis for optimal sleep health. Infants, children, and teenagers require substantially more sleep than adults. However, societal, familial, entertainment, scholastic, and work-related pressures often demand more of our time than there are hours in the day. One of the first things to be sacrificed is sleep time. To deal with the epidemic of reduced sleep times, we must reemphasize the need for, and benefits of, a full night of uninterrupted sleep. The health costs of reduced sleep puts a burden not only on the patients themselves but on society as a whole.

CENTRAL DISORDERS OF HYPERSOMNOLENCE: THE LONG SLEEPER—A NORMAL VARIANT

Introduction

Long sleepers are people with natural sleep requirements significantly more than the average 7 to 8 hours, typically about 10 to 12 hours. Sleep, although long, is normal in architecture and physiology. Sleep is reportedly of a good quality, refreshing, and consistent throughout the years. It is simply much longer than what most people need (2). Long sleepers are often stigmatized as lazy or depressed. There is no definitive link between long sleepers and adverse long-term or chronic health problems (45).

Prevalence

An estimated 2% of men and 1.5% of women subjectively identify as long sleepers, reporting sleeping 10 hours per night or more. There seems to be a strong genetic heritability (44%) and a high concordance with monozygotic twins. Genome studies indicate an involvement of circadian clock and other related genes (2).

Salient Features

Long sleepers have longer than normal primary sleep periods but are not excessively sleepy in the daytime, nor are they more likely to nap. Sleep efficiency is on a par with normal sleepers; so is arousal index, total slow-wave time and REM sleep percentage. Apnea index and PLMS indexes were also comparable to average sleepers. In general, long sleepers tended to go to bed earlier and wake up later than average sleepers. Long sleepers will often function on near-average sleep times, sleeping 9 hours per night, then catch up on the weekends, sometimes sleeping 12 hours or more (2).

ISS may be common among long sleepers due to an expectation to conform to the sleep times of average adults. Although "the" average sleep may indeed be 8 hours, this would be inadequate for the long sleeper.

Diagnosis

It is critical to first rule out any of the myriad of sleep disorders that cause a patient to feel the need to sleep longer times, such as sleep apnea, any one of the hypersomnia disorders, some psychiatric disorders, physical illnesses, or drug effects.

A determination of long sleeper can be confidently made after other medical conditions have been ruled out and objective measures record at least 10 hours of sleep over a minimum of seven nights, usually by way of a sleep diary or actigraphy (2). These longer sleep times should be consistent throughout most of the individual's life and must be considered relatively high quality, with the subject waking up refreshed and not feeling sleepy during the day.

Treatment

There is no treatment as this is not, strictly speaking, a sleep disorder. However, care should be taken to ensure adequate sleep despite pressures to curtail sleep times, lest a bona fide sleep disorder develop over time.

Conclusion

Long sleepers do not differ importantly in their sleep from those reporting normal sleep times, other than the increased amount of time spent in bed and asleep. Health outcomes are normal, and no long-term adverse consequences are expected due to the longer-than-average sleep drive. Long sleepers presumably represent the high end of the normal sleep duration continuum.

REFERENCES

1. Ohayon MM, Dauvilliers Y, Reynolds CF. Operational definitions and algorithms for excessive sleepiness in the general population: implications for DSM-5 nosology. *Arch Gen Psychiatry*. 2012;69:71-79.
2. American Academy of Sleep Medicine. *International Classification of Sleep Disorders*. 3rd ed. American Academy of Sleep Medicine; 2014.
3. Nishino S. Clinical and neurobiological aspects of narcolepsy. *Sleep Med*. 2007;8(4):373-399.
4. Flygare J, Parthasarathy S. Narcolepsy: let the patient's voice awaken us! *Am J Med*. 2015;128(1):10-13.
5. Akintomide, GS, Rickards H. Narcolepsy: a review. *Neuropsychiatr Dis Treat*. 2011;7:507-518.
6. Morrish E, King MA, Smith IE, Shneerson JM. Factors associated with a delay in the diagnosis of narcolepsy. *Sleep Med*. 2004;5(1):37-41.
7. Mignot E. A hundred years of research. *Arch Ital Biol*. 2001;139(3):207-220.
8. de Lecea L, Kilduff TS, Peyron C, et al. The hypocretins: hypothalamus-specific peptides with neuroexcitatory activity. *Proc Natl Acad Sci U S A*. 1998;95:322-327.
9. Sakurai T, Amemiya A, Ishii M, et al. Orexins and orexin receptors: a family of hypothalamic neuropeptides and G protein-coupled receptors that regulate feeding behavior. *Cell*. 1998;92:573-585.
10. Slowik JM, Collen JF, Yow AG. Narcolepsy. In: *StatPearls* [Internet]. StatPearls Publishing; 2023.
11. Abad VC, Guilleminault C. New developments in the management of narcolepsy. *Nat Sci Sleep*. 2017;9:39-57.
12. Mignot E. Genetic and familial aspects of narcolepsy. *Neurology*. 1998;50(2 suppl 1):S16-S22.
13. Schwartz S, Ponz A, Poryazova R, et al. Abnormal activity in hypothalamus and amygdala during humour processing in human narcolepsy with cataplexy. *Brain*. 2008;131(pt 2):514-522.
14. Littner MR, Kushida C, Wise M, et al. Practice parameters for clinical use of the multiple sleep latency test and the maintenance of wakefulness test. *Sleep*. 2005;28:113-121.
15. Maski K, Trotti LM, Kotagal S, et al. Treatment of central disorders of hypersomnolence: an American Academy of Sleep Medicine clinical practice guideline. *J Clin Sleep Med*. 2021;17(9):1881-1893.
16. Nittur N, Konofal E, Dauvilliers Y, et al. Mazindol in narcolepsy and idiopathic and symptomatic hypersomnia refractory to stimulants: a long-term chart review. *Sleep Med*. 2013;14(1):30-36.
17. Nallu S. Narcolepsy guidelines. In: Benbadis SR, ed. *Medscape: Drugs & Diseases*. WebMD. Updated June 27, 2024. Accessed February 3, 2025. https://www.emedicine.medscape.com/article/1188433-print
18. Giannoccaro MP, Liguori R, Plazzi G, Pizza F. Reviewing the clinical implications of treating narcolepsy as an autoimmune disorder. *Nat Sci Sleep*. 2021;13:557-577. doi:10.2147/NSS.S275931
19. Harwell V, Fasinu PS. Pitolisant and other histamine-3 receptor antagonists-an update on therapeutic potentials and clinical prospects. *Medicines (Basel)*. 2020;7(9):55. doi:10.3390/medicines7090055
20. Billiard M, Dauvilliers Y. Idiopathic hypersomnia. *Sleep Med Rev*. 2001;5:351-360.
21. Billiard M, Sonka K. Idiopathic hypersomnia. *Sleep Med Rev*. 2016;29:23-33.
22. Sasai T, Inoue Y, Komada Y, et al. Comparison of clinical characteristics among narcolepsy with and without cataplexy and idiopathic hypersomnia without long sleep time, focusing on HLA-DRB1(*)1501/DQB1(*)0602 finding. *Sleep Med*. 2009;10(9):961-966.
23. Leu-Semenescu S, Nittur N, Golmard JL, Arnulf I. Effects of pitolisant, a histamine H3 inverse agonist, in drug-resistant idiopathic and symptomatic hypersomnia: a chart review. *Sleep Med*. 2014;15(6):681-687.

24. Roth T. Introduction: narcolepsy and excessive daytime sleepiness: from the bench to the bedside. *J Clin Psychiatry*. 2007;68(suppl 13):4.
25. Khan Z, Trotti LM. Central disorders of hypersomnolence: focus on the narcolepsies and idiopathic hypersomnia. *Chest*. 2015;148(1):262-273.
26. Anderson K, Phil D, Pilsworth S, et al. Idiopathic hypersomnia: a study of 77 cases. *Sleep*. 2007;30(10): 1274-1281.
27. Ali M, Auger R, Slocumb NL, Morgenthaler TI. Idiopathic hypersomnia: clinical features and response to treatment. *J Clin Sleep Med*. 2009;5(6):562-568.
28. Arnulf I, Thomas, R, Roy A, Dauvilliers Y. Update in the treatments of idiopathic hypersomnia: progress, challenges and expert opinion. *Sleep Med Rev*. 2023;69: 101766.
29. Mignot E. A practical guide to the therapy of narcolepsy and hypersomnia syndromes. *Neurotherapeutics*. 2012;9:739-752.
30. Gadoth N, Oksenberg A. Kleine-Levin syndrome; an update and mini-review. *Brain Dev*. 2017;39(8): 665-671.
31. Ramdurg S. Kleine-Levin syndrome: etiology, diagnosis, and treatment. *Ann Indian Acad Neurol*. 2010; 13(4):241-246.
32. Preda A. Primary hypersomnia. In: *eMedicine Psychiatry. Medscape*; 2009:1-22. http://www.academia.edu/550258/Primary_Hypersomnia
33. Arnulf I, Zeitzer J, Farber N, Mignot E. Kleine-Levin syndrome: a systematic review of 186 cases in the literature. *Brain*. 2005;128(12):2763-2776.
34. de Oliveira MM, Conti C, Prado GF. Pharmacological treatment for Kleine-Levin syndrome. *Cochrane Database Syst Rev*. 2016;2016(5):CD006685. doi:10.1002/14651858.CD006685.pub4
35. Qasrawi SO, BaHammam AS. An update on Kleine-Levin syndrome. *Curr Sleep Med Rep*. 2023;9:35-44. doi:10.1007/s40675-022-00246-1
36. Hamper M, Keating P, Arnulf I, Schmidt-Kastner R, Blakely R, Hartmann J. *Kleine-Levin Syndrome: Antibodies in Patient Serum and Their Reactivity with Proteins From Neural Tissue*. Department of Biological Sciences, Florida Atlantic University. Accessed January 2025. https://klsfoundation.org/what-is-kleine-levin-syndrome/kls-medical-publications/
37. Hédou J, Cederberg KL, Ambati A, et al. Proteomic biomarkers of Kleine-Levin syndrome. *Sleep*. 2022;45(9):zsac097. doi:10.1093/sleep/zsac097
38. Frange C, de Oliveira GP, Coelho FMS. COVID-19 and central nervous system hypersomnias. *Curr Sleep Med Rep*. 2022;8(3):42-49. doi:10.1007/s40675-022-00226-5
39. Morelli-Zaher C, Vremaroiu-Coman A, Coquoz N, et al. Post-COVID central hypersomnia, a treatable trait in long COVID: 4 case reports. *Front Neurol*. 2024;15: 1349486. doi:10.3389/fneur.2024.1349486
40. The Mayo Clinic. Traumatic brain injury. Published 2018. Accessed March 2, 2018. https://www.mayoclinic.org/diseases-conditions/traumatic-brain-injury/symptoms-causes/syc-20378557
41. Castriotti RJ, Wilde MC, Lai JM, Atanasov S, Masel BE, Kuna ST. Prevalence and consequences of sleep disorders in traumatic brain injury. *J Clin Sleep Med*. 2007; 3:349-356.
42. Zhu Y, Fenik P, Zhan G, et al. Selective loss of catecholaminergic wake active neurons in a murine sleep apnea model. *J Neurosci*. 2007;27:10060-10071.
43. Dauvilliers Y, Lopez R, Ohayon M, Bayard S. Hypersomnia and depressive symptoms: methodological and clinical aspects. *BMC Med*. 2013;11:78.
44. Hublin C, Kaprio J, Partinen M, Koskenvuo M. Insufficient sleep: a population-based study in adults. *Sleep*. 2001;24(4):392-400.
45. Lauderdale DS, Knutson KL, Rathouz PJ, Yan LL, Hulley SB, Liu K. Cross-sectional and longitudinal associations between objectively measured sleep duration and body mass index: the CARDIA sleep study. *Am J Epidemiol*. 2009;170:805-813.

Chapter 15
Circadian Rhythm Sleep-Wake Disorders

CHAD WHITTLEF AND KATHERINE M. SHARKEY

KEY CONCEPTS/LEARNING OBJECTIVES

The key concepts for this chapter include defining the common terms used to describe circadian physiology, describing the neurobiology of the circadian clock and the effects of light, darkness, and other factors on circadian function, identifying the clinical features of circadian rhythm sleep-wake disorders (CRSWD), circadian rhythm measurements used for clinical diagnosis of CRSWD, laboratory assessments of circadian rhythms, and the most common treatments for CRSWD, including the potential risks associated with shift work in the sleep laboratory.

KEY TERMS

Advanced sleep-wake phase disorder
Chronotherapy
Circadian rhythm sleep-wake disorders
Circadian rhythms
Delayed sleep-wake phase disorder
Dim light melatonin onset
Entrainment
Forced desynchrony
Free running
Infradian
Irregular sleep-wake rhythm
Jet lag disorder
Light therapy
Phase angle
Phase response curve
Phase shift
Shift-work disorder
Suprachiasmatic nuclei
Ultradian
Zeitgeber

FUNDAMENTALS OF CIRCADIAN RHYTHMS

Throughout history, scientists have observed that most living things have physiologic rhythms that parallel the 24-hour cycle of day and night. These are called "circadian rhythms" from the Latin "circa," meaning about, and "diem," meaning day, a term coined by Franz Halberg in 1959. Circadian rhythms are found in virtually all living things, including one-celled animals and plants. The sleep-wake cycle, rhythm of core body temperature, and hormonal rhythms that fluctuate across the 24-hour day (eg, melatonin) are examples of human circadian rhythms. Circadian rhythms are so foundational to physiology and behavior that the scientists whose work unraveled the molecular mechanisms of circadian rhythms, Jeffrey Hall, Michael Rosbash, and Michael Young, were awarded the 2017 Nobel Prize in Physiology or Medicine for their contributions to science.

In addition to circadian rhythms, there are other oscillations that are present in humans and animals. *Ultradian rhythms* are rhythms shorter than 24 hours, for instance, the rapid eye movement-nonrapid eye movement (REM-NREM) cycles that are observed in sleep. The term *infradian rhythms* refers to oscillations that are longer than 24 hours. As an example, the menstrual cycle approximates 28 days.

Typically, circadian rhythms are represented by a sine wave (Figure 15-1). Various terms are used to describe different aspects of the rhythm. The *period*, also referred to as *tau*, is the length of the rhythm. This is usually very close to 24 hours. The *amplitude* is the magnitude of the rhythm from its peak to nadir. The amplitude of different circadian rhythms is variable and can be affected by age, sex, sleep state, and so on. The *phase* refers to the circadian position at any specific instant of time. Depending on what rhythm is measured, different phase markers are used. For instance, when the circadian rhythm of core temperature is measured, the temperature minimum or maximum is commonly used as a marker of phase. When hormonal rhythms

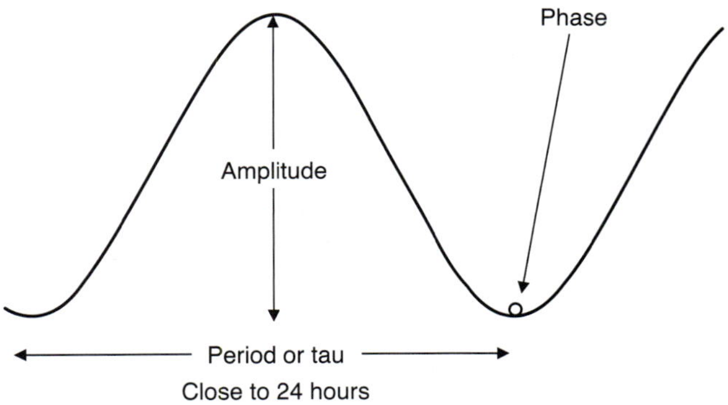

Figure 15-1 Circadian rhythms are schematically represented by a sine wave.

are measured—most commonly melatonin—the onset, offset, or peak of hormone secretion is used as a phase marker. In some cases, it is helpful to calculate a *phase angle*, which refers to the difference in timing between two cyclic rhythms. For instance, the phase angle between the time of melatonin onset and the midpoint of sleep provides information about an individual's sleep timing with respect to their internal body clock.

NEUROBIOLOGIC BASIS OF THE INTERNAL CIRCADIAN CLOCK

Circadian rhythms are endogenously driven by a master circadian clock located in the suprachiasmatic nuclei (SCN) of the anterior hypothalamus. Information about the lighting conditions of the external environment is conveyed to the SCN from the retina through the retinohypothalamic tract (Figure 15-2). The cells in the retina responsible for conveying information about light and dark are called intrinsically photosensitive retinal ganglion cells; these ganglion cells differ from the conventional ganglion cells that transmit rod and cone input to the brain for visual image formation. The SCN also receive input from the intergeniculate leaflet of the thalamus and the midbrain raphe nuclei. These two

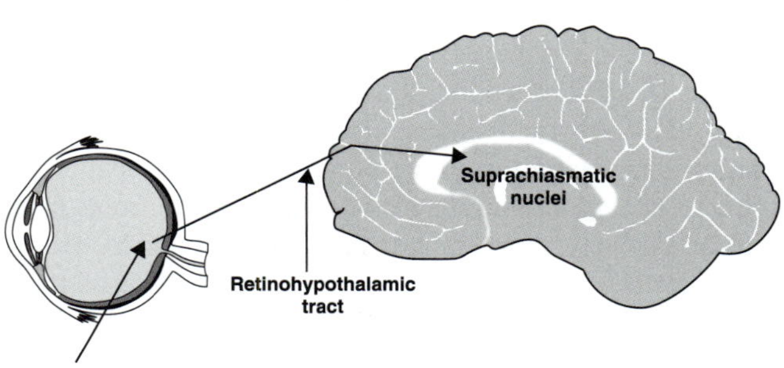

Figure 15-2 Diagram of the retinohypothalamic tract.

pathways are thought to transmit both photic (light) and nonphotic information to the circadian clock.

Most SCN projections stay within the hypothalamus, although a small fraction of SCN neurons terminate in the basal forebrain and midline thalamus. Secondary efferents from these three areas project to many brain regions, including the neocortex, hippocampus, basal ganglia, anterior pituitary, hypothalamus, reticular formation, and pineal gland. It is through this expansive network that the SCN exert control over many physiologic functions, including endocrine regulation, body temperature, the sleep-wake cycle, metabolism, autonomic regulation, psychomotor and cognitive performance, attention, memory, and emotion.

Recent progress in circadian biology has demonstrated that circadian physiology is driven by a hierarchical multioscillator system, where the SCN serves as the central circadian clock orchestrating peripheral clocks in the various organ systems throughout the body. These peripheral clocks are responsive to, and integrate, information from input outside of the SCN. For instance, circadian rhythms of liver function and metabolism are influenced by a food-entrainable oscillator located in brain regions outside the SCN.

Circadian rhythm researchers measure physiologic rhythms that are downstream outputs of the endogenous clock to infer the phase position of the circadian rhythms. The circadian rhythms of the hormone melatonin and core body temperature are common measures of circadian phase in humans.

EFFECTS OF THE LIGHT-DARK CYCLE ON CIRCADIAN RHYTHMS

As mentioned, sensory receptors in the retina provide information about the light-dark cycle to the master circadian clock in the SCN. The light-dark cycle helps the organism remain synchronized or entrained to the 24-hour day of the external environment (Figure 15-3). In the absence of a light-dark cycle and other time cues, circadian rhythms "free run" at a rate not equal to 24 hours but equal to the endogenous period length, or tau. The period (tau) is close to, but not exactly, 24 hours. Free running is observed in humans when they have no photic (light) stimuli, for instance, in people with blindness and no photoreception, or when the light-dark cycle to which they are exposed is outside of the time range of possible biologic entrainment, as occurs in orbiting astronauts who experience a "sunrise" and "sunset" every 90 minutes.

In 1979, Wever and colleagues published some of the initial experiments using bright light to entrain human circadian rhythms, confirming an important principle of human circadian rhythms: the light-dark cycle

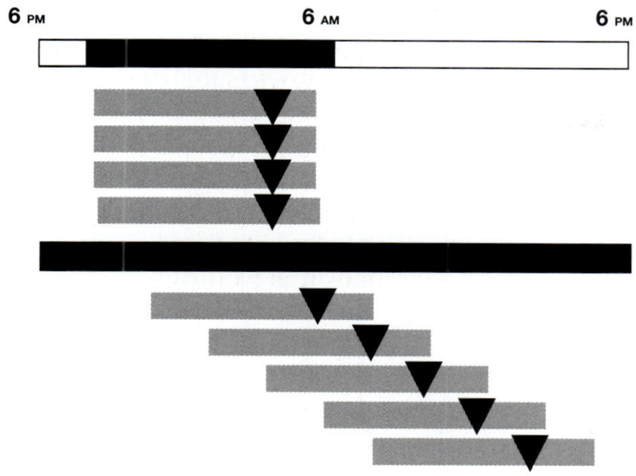

Figure 15-3 Examples of entrainment and free running. The gray bars represent time when the body temperature is low and the triangles represent the temperature minimum. The black and white bars represent the lighting conditions. The top half of the figure depicts entrainment. When a changing light-dark cycle is present, the internal circadian clock uses the photic cues to synchronize or entrain to the 24-hour light-dark cycle. The bottom half of the figure depicts free running. When there is no change in the light-dark cycle, the circadian rhythms free run at a period length (tau) determined by the endogenous circadian clock. In this case, the period length is longer than 24 hours, causing the circadian rhythms to delay (move later) because each day starts and ends at a slightly later clock time than the previous day.

is one of the most powerful synchronizers of the endogenous circadian pacemaker in humans. Studies that tested various intensities and wavelengths of light and have shown that in humans, as in animals, the brighter the light is, the stronger it is as an entraining stimulus. In addition, the circadian system is most sensitive to short-wavelength (blue-green spectrum) light.

Whether free running or entrained, circadian rhythms can be reset to a new time. This process is called "phase shifting," or "re-entrainment." Humans are frequently faced with situations in which their circadian rhythms are misaligned with the environmental light-dark cycle. This can be a result of jet lag, daylight savings time, or shift work. In these situations, circadian rhythms may (but do not always) phase shift to adapt to the new light-dark cycle. Various external stimuli, called *zeitgebers* (from the German word "time giver"), act as time cues and can affect the internal clock, causing a resetting or phase shifting of circadian rhythms. Photic information about the light-dark cycle is the strongest stimulus for resetting the biologic clock. Phase shifts differ in direction and magnitude depending on where in the circadian cycle (at what circadian phase) the zeitgeber is administered.

PHASE-SHIFTING EFFECTS OF LIGHT AND LIGHT PHASE RESPONSE CURVES

The relationships between circadian rhythms, phase shifting, and various time cues or zeitgebers are described using phase response curves (PRCs). A PRC is derived by administering a stimulus at many different circadian phases and measuring the resulting shifts in the circadian clock. The multiple phase-shift data points are then plotted to predict the magnitude and direction of a phase shift given a particular stimulus at a specific circadian phase.

A schematic PRC for light is shown in Figure 15-4. When humans are exposed to light at the end of the day and beginning of the night, circadian rhythms shift to a later time, which is called a "phase delay." In contrast,

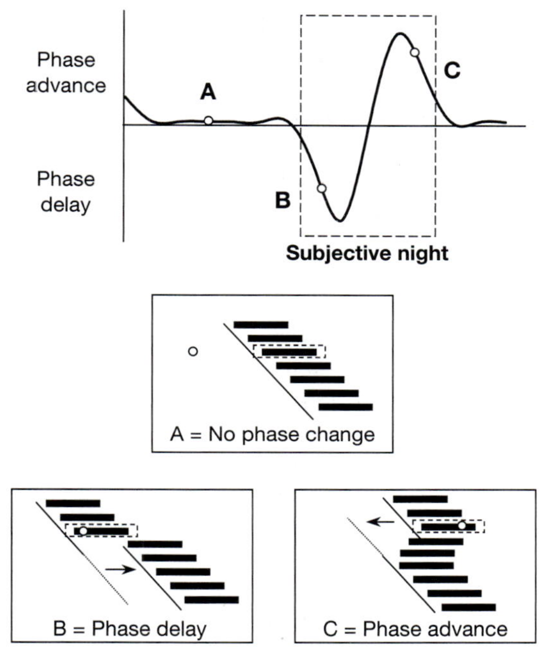

Figure 15-4 Schematic light phase response curve (PRC). The horizontal black bars in A, B, and C indicate circadian measures that occur at night, such as low core temperature or high melatonin levels. Within each inset, the effect of a single stimulus (eg, a light pulse in otherwise constant darkness) on free-running circadian measures is shown. The effects of stimuli (open circles) presented during the subjective day (A), the early part of the subjective night (B), and late in the subjective night (C) are shown. Note the very different effects that these identical stimuli have at those different phases. Those results are then plotted at the corresponding points (labeled A, B, and C) in the central diagram, which is a PRC. The boxed area represents the subjective night of the organism, and the remaining area represents subjective day. (Adapted from Czeisler CA, Richardson GS, Coleman RM, et al. Chronotherapy: resetting the circadian clocks of patients with delayed sleep phase insomnia. *Sleep*. 1981;4(1):1-21. Reproduced by permission of Oxford University Press.)

when light exposure occurs at the end of the night and early part of the day, circadian rhythms shift to an earlier time, which is called a "phase advance." Minimal phase shifting occurs when humans are exposed to light in the middle of the day. Shifts in circadian phase elicited by light are dependent not only on the timing and duration of the exposure but also on the intensity of light, which decreases as distance from the light source increases, and the wavelength of light.

PHASE-SHIFTING EFFECTS ON NONPHOTIC STIMULI

In addition to light, other nonphotic stimuli have been shown to affect circadian rhythms. For instance, exogenous administration of the hormone melatonin can lead to phase shifts in the circadian clock. Lewy and colleagues produced a PRC for melatonin that demonstrates that circadian phase delays are produced when melatonin is administered in the later hours of sleep and in the morning, and phase advances are produced when melatonin is administered in the afternoon and early evening.

Physical activity or exercise has also been shown to phase shift the human circadian clock. Phase advances in circadian rhythms occur after exercise in the evening, and phase delays are produced with exercise in the middle of the night. The magnitude of the circadian phase shifts produced with exercise appears to be related to the duration and intensity of the physical activity.

TYPES OF CIRCADIAN RHYTHM SLEEP-WAKE DISORDERS

Before describing the types of circadian rhythm sleep-wake disorders (CRSWD), it is important to note that by influencing the timing of virtually all physiologic and behavioral phenomena, circadian rhythms have an impact on health and safety that extends far beyond CRSWD. Examples of circadian variation include the timing and severity of clinical symptoms unrelated to sleep disorders and the daily pattern of critical events in the population, such as stroke, myocardial infarction, and motor vehicle accidents. In addition, the outcomes of clinical experiments, diagnostic tests, and treatments can all vary as a function of administration time. Clearly, the influence of circadian rhythms needs to be appreciated throughout the biomedical sciences.

Shift-Work Disorder

The misalignment of the sleep-wake cycle and intrinsic circadian rhythms seen in CRSWD is demonstrated in the case of shift work. Shift-work disorder (SWD) can occur when work schedules conflict with the timing and duration of an individual's habitual sleep period. Working a fixed night shift (when the circadian clock is programmed for sleep) is a primary example of such a conflict, but early morning shifts and rotating shifts can be just as difficult to tolerate because sleep timing is misaligned with respect to internal circadian rhythms.

Symptoms of SWD include reduced sleep quality and quantity as well as sleepiness during time awake. Sleep duration during the day following a night shift is typically reduced by several hours. Subjective sleep quality can be impaired, and sleep is less restorative. Impairments of sleep quality during shift work include prolonged sleep latencies, sleep maintenance difficulties, and early termination of the sleep period. Owing in part to this reduction in sleep quality and quantity, an individual typically experiences excessive sleepiness during the time of day in which they are attempting to remain awake and work. Another major factor contributing to sleepiness during a night shift is the acute reduction in alertness that usually occurs in the early morning hours. This early morning nadir of alertness is a circadian phenomenon, occurring independently of accumulated sleep loss. At the end of a night shift, sleepiness is typically high because of this reduced alerting effect in tandem with the long period of wakefulness that has elapsed since the last sleep period. This can potentially increase night shift workers' risks of accidents in the workplace and while driving home.

A number of other disturbances unrelated to sleep may be reported by shift workers. A common complaint is increased gastrointestinal disturbance. Cardiovascular disease, as well as several major risk factors for this disease—smoking, high cholesterol, hypertension, and obesity—have been found to be more prevalent among shift workers. Reproductive difficulties such as menstrual irregularities, increased time to conception, and infertility may be more prevalent in female shift workers. Night shift work has repeatedly been associated with increased risk of developing cancer and has been classified as a "probable carcinogen" by the International Agency for Research on Cancer. The psychosocial consequences of shift work can include disturbances of family and marital relationships.

Although SWD may be transient in that resuming a daytime work/nighttime sleep schedule will attenuate its symptoms, complete adaptation to late night, early morning, and rotating shifts is difficult to achieve and in most cases, does not occur. Adaptation to a nighttime work and daytime sleep schedule, however, is possible if appropriate steps are taken to reinforce a nocturnal lifestyle. This is rare among most shift workers because environmental zeitgebers, such as light, as well as social and domestic responsibilities and personal preferences, reinforce a diurnal schedule, preventing significant adaptation from occurring. In addition, maintaining a nocturnal lifestyle is not a priority for most individuals, suggesting that circadian adaptation is not only difficult but perhaps also undesirable. Figure 15-5 shows the activity of a shift worker over a several-week period, and Figure 15-6G depicts a typical phase relationship (phase angle) between the temperature minimum and the sleep period for a night shift worker.

A number of individual differences mediate tolerance to shift work. One of the most important determinants of shift-work tolerance is commitment to the work schedule. Individuals who are able and choose to alter their sleep-wake pattern by adhering to a light-dark schedule to assist in phase shifting are much more likely to adapt to shift work than those who disregard the diurnally oriented zeitgebers. Older individuals typically tolerate night shift work less well than younger individuals. Those with a short sleep requirement, as well as a relatively delayed circadian rhythm (night owls), typically tolerate night work better than those needing more sleep or who are relatively phase advanced (morning larks).

A proactive way for employers to address the increased risks associated with shift work is through the implementation of specific policies aimed at mitigating those risks. Because all sleep laboratories utilize shift work, having fatigue management policies in place should be considered a matter of professional integrity.

Jet Lag Disorder

Jet lag disorder is identified by difficulty initiating or maintaining sleep following the rapid crossing of time zones, which occurs in air travel in the east or west direction. The cause of these symptoms is a misalignment of the endogenous circadian system with the environmental time cues of the new time zone (Figure 15-6F). For example, airline flights from North America may land during the morning hours in Europe. This morning arrival time corresponds to nighttime hours in North America, and travelers are thus presented with European day at a time when their bodies are primed for night and sleep. Furthermore, when the European night arrives, travelers may have difficulty initiating sleep because the biologic clock remains entrained to North American time, where it is afternoon. Secondary to this misalignment, as well as sleep loss that comes about because of the misalignment, excessive sleepiness and decreases in alertness may ensue. Somatic complaints may also be

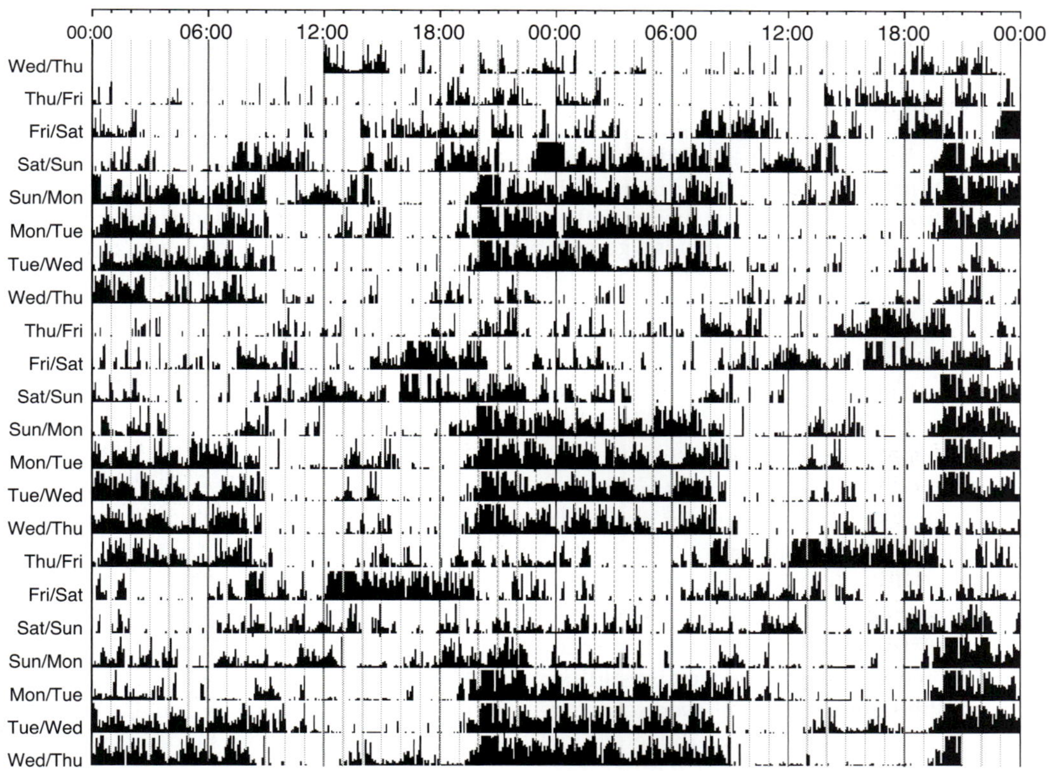

Figure 15-5 Double plot of wrist actigraphy from a middle-aged man working four consecutive night shifts. Note that when this individual is not working the night shift, he reverts to a diurnal schedule. Shift-work disorder becomes chronic because the circadian rhythms do not have enough time to fully entrain to either the weekend or the work schedule.

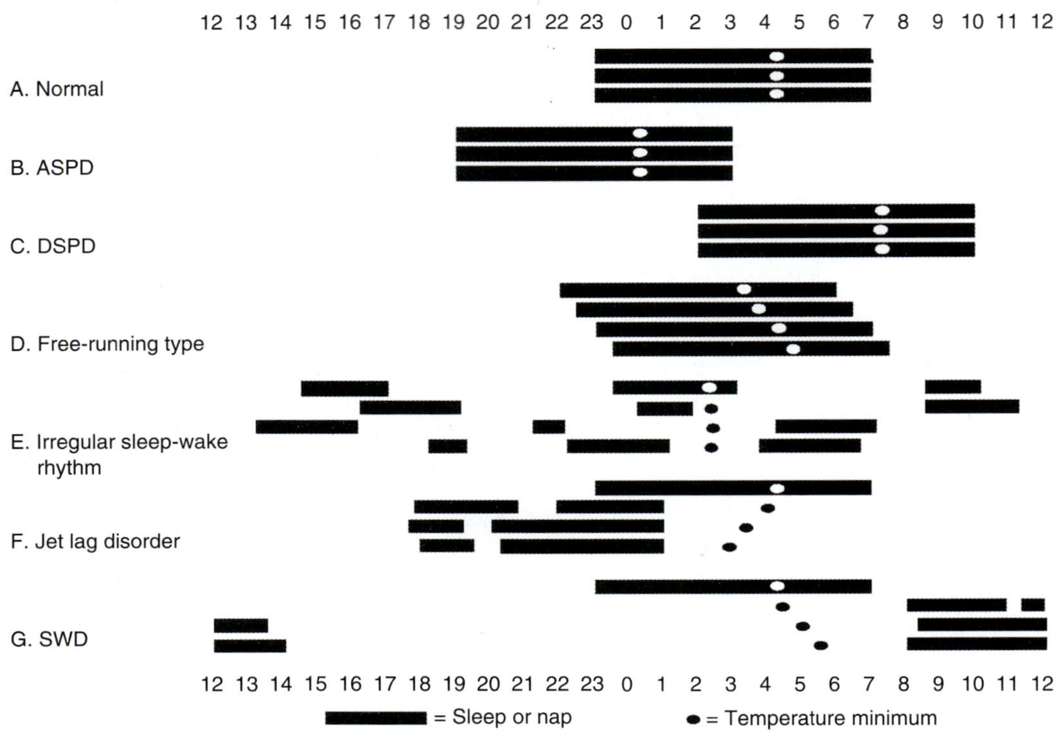

Figure 15-6 Schematic summary of the clock times of sleep periods in normal entrainment and circadian rhythm sleep-wake disorder, as well as typical phase relationships between sleep period and the temperature minimum (Tmin), which is an approximate time of peak sleep propensity. A: Normally entrained sleep. Tmin occurs 2 to 3 hours before habitual wake time. B: Advanced sleep phase disorder (ASPD). Preferred sleep onset and waking times occur at substantially earlier clock times than conventional sleep and wake times. C: Delayed sleep phase disorder (DSPD). Preferred sleep onset and wake times occur at substantially later clock times than conventional sleep and wake. D: Free-running type. Sleep and wakefulness occur at a progressively later clock time each successive day. E: Irregular sleep-wake rhythm. The normal periodicity of the sleep-wake cycle is attenuated or absent. F: Jet lag disorder. After an initial night of normal sleep, rapid transmeridian travel (as illustrated, eastward across six time zones) results in an abrupt shift of the attempted sleep period to an earlier time, and subsequent misalignment of circadian rhythms and environmental time. Tmin occurs after the scheduled wake time in the new time zone, giving rise to symptoms of sleepiness. G: Shift-work disorder (SWD). After an initial night of normal sleep, night shift workers typically attempt to work through the night during the time of peak sleep propensity, and sleep during the daytime, when increased circadian alerting can fragment and curtail sleep.

present, the most common of which is disturbance of the gastrointestinal tract. The symptoms of jet lag disorder are usually transient. Symptoms typically diminish as the endogenous circadian rhythms adapt to the local time cues of the new environment but are initially present because adaptation occurs slowly. In addition, exposure to time cues such as light at the wrong time can cause re-entrainment in the wrong direction, resulting in prolonged jet lag. Phase delays are believed to occur more rapidly than phase advances because the length of the human circadian rhythms is typically slightly more than 24 hours. This makes it easier for an individual to stay up for a period longer than 24 hours before initiating the next sleep period (delaying) than to initiate a sleep period before 24 hours have elapsed since the previous bedtime (advancing). The symptoms associated with jet lag may become chronic for individuals who frequently fly across time zones.

Several factors influence the severity of this disorder. Because of the relative ease with which individuals phase delay, traveling in the eastward direction (advancing) can produce more difficulty adjusting to the new time zone than traveling in the westward direction. The duration of symptoms is usually commensurate with the number of time zones crossed. Because entrainment to the local environment occurs at a slow pace, the larger the time difference between the home and the new environment, the longer the symptoms may be expected to persist. Although the overly simple rule of thumb is that re-entrainment occurs at a rate of approximately one time zone per day, conflicting timing of light exposure and other zeitgebers can slow this adjustment and prolong jet lag symptoms. On the other hand, strategically timed light exposure and sleep scheduling, as well as judicious use of exogenous melatonin and caffeine, can accelerate adjustment to jet lag.

Non-24-Hour Sleep-Wake Rhythm Disorder

Non-24-hour sleep-wake rhythm disorder occurs when an individual's circadian rhythms persist with a periodicity of more than 24 hours despite living in society and being exposed to the time cues that normally entrain the rhythms to the 24-hour day (Figures 15-6D and 15-7). The symptoms of this disorder result from the conflict that arises when a person with free-running rhythms attempts to adhere to a normal diurnal schedule in which sleep and wake times are relatively fixed from day to day. As the endogenous rhythms progressively shift around the clock, some nighttime sleep periods will occur when there is a normal phase relationship between the sleep period and body rhythms. On other days, attempts to initiate nighttime sleep periods at the usual environmental time will conflict with the current phase of the biologic clock. During these times of desynchronization between the circadian clock and the environment, the quality and quantity of sleep may be reduced, with accompanying increases in daytime sleepiness. In this way, free running can manifest as periodically recurring symptoms of insomnia and sleepiness.

Although the disorder has been observed in sighted individuals, most patients of non-24-hour sleep-wake rhythm disorder have some degree of blindness. This is because light is the most important environmental time cue for the entrainment of circadian rhythms in humans. Enucleated patients, totally blind patients, or patients with disrupted transmission of light information to the brain are most susceptible to free-running circadian rhythms and non-24-hour sleep-wake rhythm disorder. However, visual blindness is not necessarily associated with attenuated circadian responses because

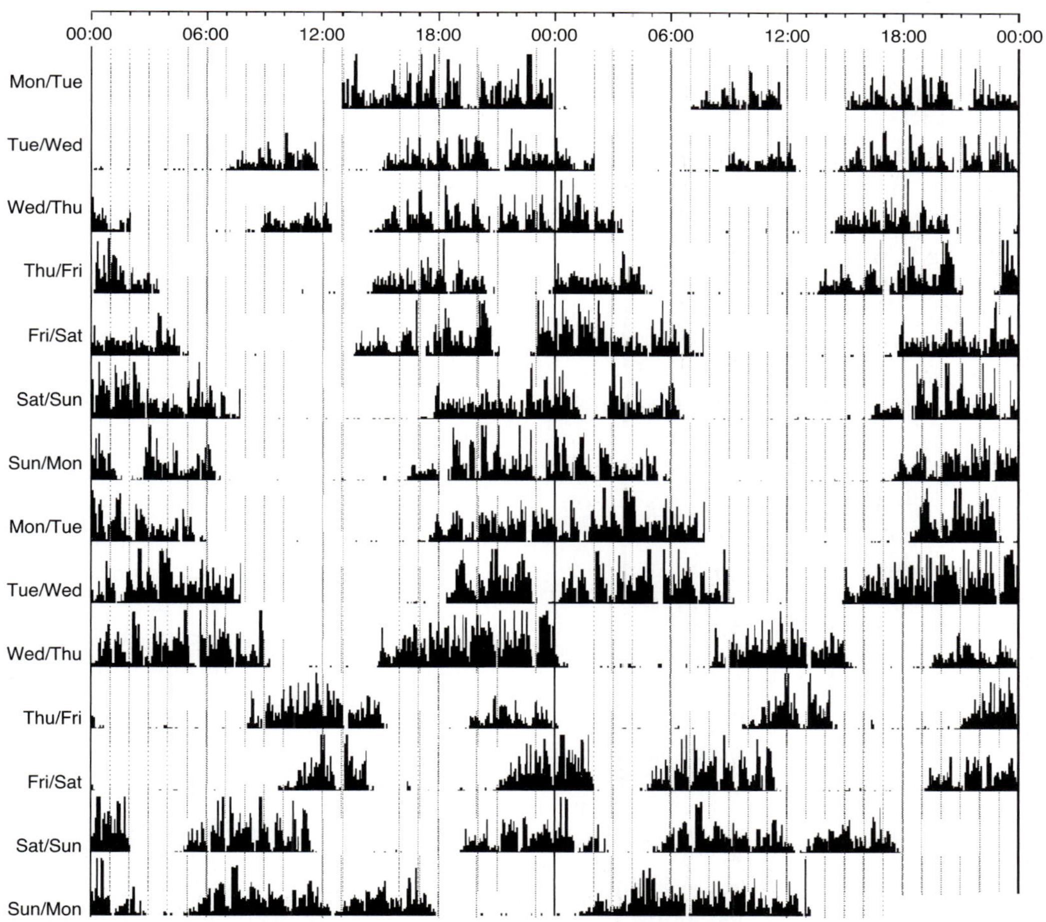

Figure 15-7 Double plot of wrist actigraphy of a patient with free-running type disorder. Note that the activity onset (the time of awakening) trends progressively later each successive day.

the photoreceptors mediating conscious vision are not necessary for the entrainment of circadian rhythms. Nonconscious ocular light perception occurring through distinct pathways may be sufficient for photic entrainment to occur.

Irregular Sleep-Wake Rhythm Disorder

Irregular sleep-wake rhythm disorder is a rare syndrome in which total sleep time within each 24-hour day may remain roughly equal to the amount that would be obtained if sleep was obtained in a single sleep period, but the sleep is distributed throughout the day and night in multiple short episodes (Figure 15-6E). This disorder is commonly observed in patients with neurologic diseases, such as children with neurodevelopmental disorders and older patients with neurodegenerative disorders such as dementia. Irregular sleep-wake patterns can also be observed in individuals not suffering from brain disease. In these rare cases, the disorder may be precipitated by a disregard for social and environmental zeitgebers. An erratic, self-perpetuating pattern of sleep and wakefulness can develop, in which nocturnal wakefulness instigates daytime naps, which then exacerbate nocturnal insomnia.

Delayed/Advanced Sleep-Wake Phase Disorders

There is variation in the times of day that any given person prefers to sleep and to be awake. Night owls feel most alert and have a relatively easy time functioning late in the day, into the evening and night, and may also experience a more difficult time awakening early in the morning. In contrast, morning larks prefer to awaken early in the morning, feel most alert early in the day, and have a relatively difficult time staying awake late at night.

Not everyone has a strong morning or evening preference. The range of preferences can be thought of as a continuum, with strong evening types on one end and strong morning types on the other. In between are degrees of each, including those who have a slight morning or evening preference or those who have no preference at all. At the extreme ends of this continuum are those patients whose morning or evening preference comes into conflict with conventional sleep-wake schedules. This conflict is the basis of both delayed sleep-wake phase disorder (DSWPD) and advanced sleep-wake phase disorders (ASWPD).

Delayed Sleep-Wake Phase Disorder

DSWPD results when a patient's biologic clock naturally begins and ends the sleep-wake period at a time of day significantly later than what is considered typical for the individual's age and social expectations. The sleep period is typically initiated between the hours of 2:00 and 6:00 AM (Figure 15-8). Sleep has normal quality and duration when the patient is allowed to maintain the late schedule preferred by the biologic clock. In DSWPD, sleep problems and the resulting difficulties occur when a person with a late sleep-wake period attempts to adhere to a conventional (earlier) sleep-wake schedule.

The symptoms of DSWPD result from the misalignment of biologically preferred and socially conventional rhythms. When attempting to initiate the sleep period at a conventional bedtime, sleep onset insomnia is prevalent. Often, sleep onset occurs at the same (late) clock time—the time at which the circadian system allows sleep to occur—regardless of the time at which a person attempts to go to sleep. Extreme difficulty awakening in the morning at a conventional time is a second prominent symptom. When awakening for work or school, individuals with DSWPD are trying to prepare for the day at a time when their circadian alerting system is at or near its minimum. For a person who copes well with a 9-AM-to-5-PM work schedule, this is akin to awakening for the day at around 3:30 or 4:00 AM, while maintaining the same bedtime.

Excessive sleepiness during the daytime occurs in DSWPD for two reasons. First, when attempting to maintain a conventional schedule, those with DSWPD will accumulate significant sleep debt from multiple nights of insufficient sleep. Second, levels of sleepiness will be high during the morning hours because the circadian system is not yet producing its alerting effects. In essence, the biologic clock of a person with DSWPD is telling the body to be asleep during the morning hours. The sleepiness caused by this type of misalignment can cause difficulty in work, school, and domestic settings. DSWPD is most common in adolescence and young adulthood.

Advanced Sleep-Wake Phase Disorder

At the other end of the morning-evening continuum are the extreme morning larks. In some cases, morning preference is so strong and conflicts with conventional sleep times to such an extent that an individual is diagnosed with ASWPD. In ASWPD, a patient has a biologic predisposition for the sleep period to occur at a time that is significantly earlier than for the typical adult. The intrinsically preferred bedtime will occur in the early evening, and a person may experience difficulty sleeping later than the very early morning hours. Consequently, the circadian alerting system often awakens a person with ASWPD between 2:00 and 4:00 AM (Figure 15-9).

As in patients with DSWPD, there appears to be nothing inherently wrong with the sleep quality or sleep architecture of an individual with ASWPD. If sleep occurs at the biologically preferable (early) time, it is usually of normal duration and quality. The conflict

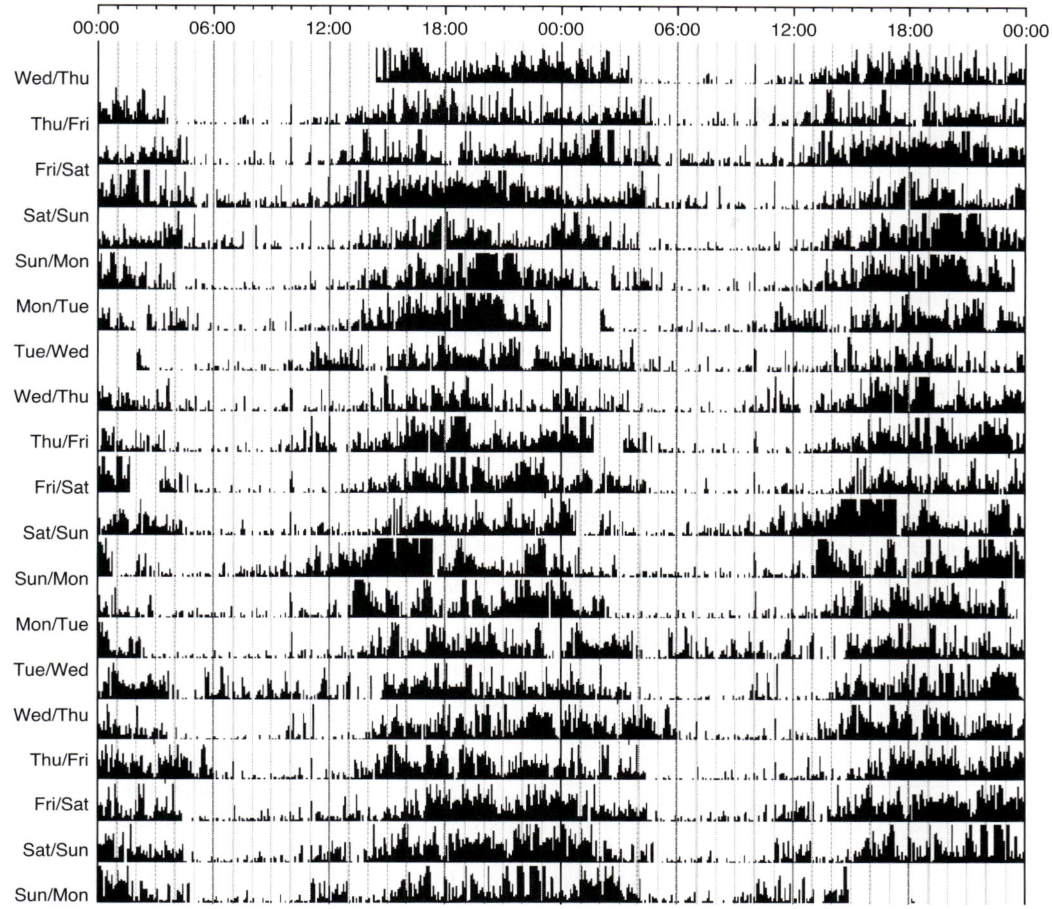

Figure 15-8 Double plot of wrist actigraphy on a patient with delayed sleep phase disorder. Note that the bedtime typically occurs from 2:00 to 4:00 AM, with wake times in the early afternoon.

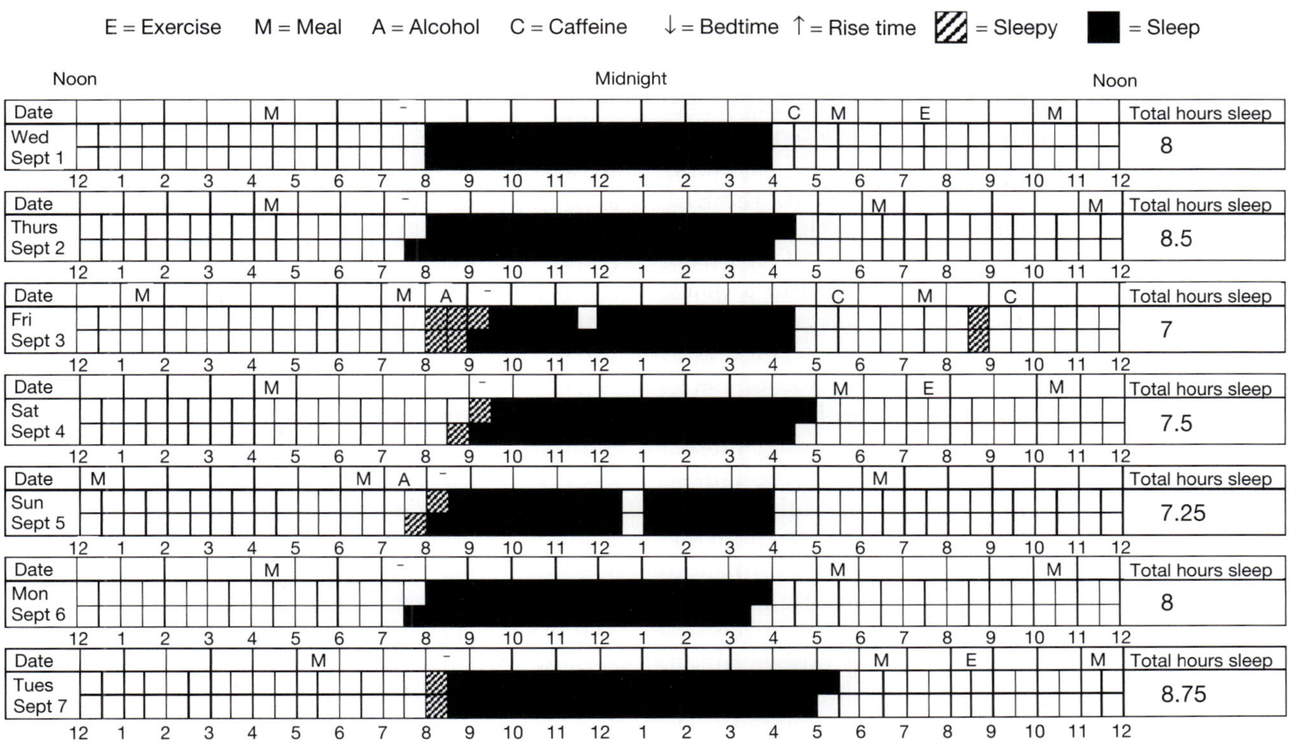

Figure 15-9 A sleep-wake diary maintained by an individual with advanced sleep phase disorder. Note that sleepiness generally ensues in the early evening hours, whereas spontaneous awakenings typically occur from 4:00 to 5:00 AM.

again arises because the early sleep period is misaligned with the socially acceptable sleep period. In the case of ASWPD, patients experience pressure to remain awake in the evening hours, often for social or domestic reasons, when the biologic clock has reduced its alerting influence, resulting in an increasing drive to sleep. In addition, early morning awakenings occur because of increased circadian alerting, resulting in wakefulness at times when most people are asleep. Therefore, patients with ASWPD can become sleep deprived and develop excessive sleepiness during their waking hours. Contrary to the occupational and academic conflicts occurring in the morning hours in DSWPD, the misalignment of circadian rhythms and social cues in ASWPD is often a source of social and family conflict, because the evening hours are typically a time one spends with family and friends. Advanced circadian rhythms are more prominent in older individuals and have also been associated with premature birth. Finally, there is evidence that human diurnal preference, including DSWPD and ASWPD, is associated with specific genetic variants.

EVALUATION OF CIRCADIAN RHYTHM SLEEP-WAKE DISORDERS

Clinical evaluation of CRSWD typically begins with a patient history by a qualified clinician. A thorough patient history includes examination of the intrinsic and extrinsic factors that may combine to precipitate the symptoms of CRSWD. Other medical or psychological problems that present with fatigue and insomnia can masquerade as CRSWD. Similar symptoms can also occur secondary to certain medical treatments or following neurologic damage and are frequently seen in other sleep disorders, such as narcolepsy, idiopathic hypersomnia, behaviorally induced insufficient sleep syndrome, and insomnia.

Evaluation of CRSWD often involves analysis of the patient's sleep-wake diary (Figure 15-9). Sleep-wake diaries provide useful and inexpensive information that, together with the patient history, can lead to a quick diagnosis. Typically, the patient maintains a sleep-wake diary for at least 2 weeks. Several parameters are documented, including the timing and duration of sleep, wakefulness, and time in bed, along with a record of medication, caffeine, alcohol, and other drug intake. Well-designed sleep-wake diaries are easy for the patient to use and provide space designated for the patient's daily comments. When a sleep-wake diary is collected from the patient, it is helpful to ascertain whether the information is representative, accurate, and understandable. Potential inaccuracies due to the patient's neglect, misunderstanding of instructions, or sleep-state misperception are the main shortcomings of the sleep-wake diary. The subjective data obtained from sleep-wake diaries can be analyzed in a manner that is similar to objective polysomnography (PSG) data. In reporting the results, ranges and averages can be utilized to summarize bedtimes, sleep latencies, total sleep times, and other relevant parameters. In addition, it is important to note the interaction of work hours and the sleep-wake schedule as well as weekend variations and other patterns that emerge. In addition to data from a sleep-wake diary, wrist actigraphy can be valuable for the diagnosis of CRSWD. Wrist actigraphy is an unobtrusive and relatively inexpensive method for collecting objective activity data, usually over the course of 2 weeks or more (Figures 15-5, 15-7, and 15-8). Daily patterns of rest and activity normally correlate with the sleep-wake cycle, providing a useful objective measure of sleep and wakefulness that can be compared with the subjective information in sleep-wake diaries. It should be recognized that wrist actigraphy may not reliably differentiate between sleep and motionless wakefulness. Thus, activity data are less reliable in the presence of insomnia or, conversely, in the presence of frequent sleep-related movements that can appear as wakefulness. Nevertheless, wrist actigraphy and sleep-wake diaries often provide ample information to detect and characterize CRSWD. Many people wear smartwatches or other personal monitoring devices that can serve as an electronic sleep diary to obtain information about sleep patterns over several days or weeks.

PSG and the multiple sleep latency test (MSLT) are of limited value in the diagnosis of CRSWD because they usually provide only a snapshot of a single sleep-wake cycle. The results of PSG in each of the different CRSWD will vary depending on the clock time and the day of PSG administration. For example, PSG performed on a patient with SWD on a day off or during a vacation may be normal, because SWD is not a problem with the patient's sleep per se but a clash between the attempted sleep schedule and the circadian clock. A daytime PSG performed after a night of shift work may show reduced total sleep time, increased wake after sleep onset, and relatively low sleep efficiency. These findings are due to the daytime alerting influence of the circadian clock, which does not change its orientation in most shift workers and disrupts and curtails daytime sleep.

PSG findings in patients with DSWPD and ASWPD reflect the altered timing of sleep in these disorders. Although PSG is not usually performed to diagnose DSWPD or ASWPD, these syndromes can coexist with other sleep disorders and may result in PSG data that require additional interpretation. If PSG is performed at conventional times, patients with DSWPD are likely to have long sleep latencies, whereas patients with ASWPD are likely to exhibit early morning awakenings because their preferred sleep and wake times are later and earlier, respectively, relative to conventional sleep and wake times. In contrast, if the start and end times of PSG are determined by the preference of patients with DSWPD and ASWPD, normal results would be expected because there is typically nothing inherently wrong with the sleep of these patients, but the conflict arises when their preferred sleep and wake times differ from conventional times.

PSG is clearly warranted when the possibility of other sleep disorders exists. When performing PSG in patients with CRSWD, it is recommended that the start time be adjusted to match the patient's routine bedtime. Likewise, MSLT schedules can be altered to begin 2 to 3 hours after the habitual rise time. This technique is particularly useful in the evaluation of CRSWD. In such cases, it may be clinically relevant to record PSG during the day and extend the MSLT schedule to cover times corresponding to both the night shift and the commute home.

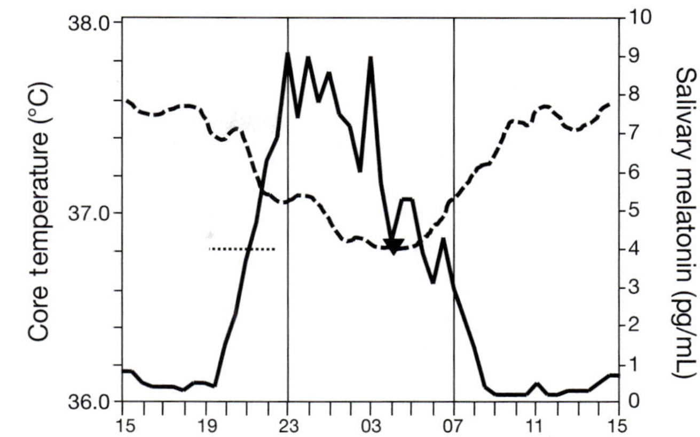

Figure 15-10 Circadian rhythms of core body temperature and salivary melatonin in a young adult male recorded in constant conditions. As shown in the solid line, temperature is high during the daytime hours and low at night. Melatonin (depicted in the dashed line) is low during the day and high at night. Two circadian phase markers are shown: the fitted temperature minimum, indicated by the black triangle, and the dim light melatonin onset (DLMO) (with DLMO threshold set at 4 pg/mL), indicated by the dotted black line.

MEASURING CIRCADIAN RHYTHMS

Circadian rhythms are measured with more precision in research situations. For instance, if a circadian phase-shift intervention is planned, the baseline circadian phase is determined in order to time the intervention correctly. Similarly, the rhythms are measured after the intervention to measure the magnitude of the shift in circadian rhythms. Rhythms are also measured when a researcher wants to demonstrate that an intervention did not affect circadian rhythms.

In humans, the master circadian clock (SCN) cannot be monitored directly; thus, marker rhythms that are controlled by this master clock are used to estimate circadian phase. Several markers are employed in studies of human circadian rhythms, including the rhythm of core body temperature, rest-activity rhythms, and hormonal rhythms (eg, melatonin, cortisol). Each of these has its advantages and disadvantages with respect to cost, invasiveness, precision, labor intensity, influences of confounding variables, and duration of monitoring.

One difficulty in measuring circadian rhythms is that rhythms can be affected by other physiologic variables and by the techniques used to measure the rhythms. This is called *masking*. For instance, as shown in Figure 15-10, human core body temperature has a robust circadian rhythm—it is high during the day, peaks in the midafternoon, and becomes lower at night, with a nadir about 2 hours before wakefulness. However, core body temperature varies because of things other than the circadian cycle. Sleep and wakefulness, activity, meals, medications, fever, and menstrual phase are a few of the factors that can alter the "true" circadian rhythm of core body temperature. These factors obscure or "mask" the endogenous temperature rhythm produced by the circadian pacemaker. There is extensive literature on mathematical and statistical techniques that can be used to "demask" data so that other physiologic variables do not interfere with measuring the "true" circadian rhythm. As with many physiologic variables, it can be difficult to measure circadian rhythms without also affecting the rhythm you are attempting to measure.

Another method for estimating circadian phase is to derive it from rhythms of hormone secretion. The onset of melatonin secretion recorded in dim light, that is, the dim light melatonin onset a.k.a., DLMO, is used frequently as a circadian phase marker (Figure 15-10), and the peak of cortisol also has been used as a measure of circadian phase. These hormonal measures, particularly DLMO, are quite reliable. Nevertheless, hormonal secretion is also subject to masking. For instance, stress can increase the amplitude of the circadian rhythm of cortisol, and light can attenuate or eliminate the circadian rhythm of melatonin. In addition, hormonal measures require assays that can be expensive and that require specialized training and equipment to perform. Hormonal measures can also be invasive depending on which body fluid (saliva, serum, or urine) is used to determine the hormone levels. Another disadvantage to measuring circadian phase using hormonal rhythms is that there is usually a time delay between data collection and determination of phase. The masking effects on circadian rhythms can be reduced by the use of constant routine (CR) protocols. The purpose of a CR is to attenuate factors that can influence the circadian rhythm(s) being measured or, when this is not possible, evenly distribute them across a circadian cycle. For example, because light exposure can mask (suppress) the circadian rhythm of melatonin, CRs typically involve dim and/or longer wavelength light, which does not appreciably influence the melatonin rhythm. Also, because body temperature decreases during sleep and increases with physical activity, CRs may incorporate constant wakefulness with recumbent posture to eliminate the masking influence of sleep and activity when the circadian temperature rhythm is being measured. In most situations, other factors such as eating and drinking cannot ethically be reduced or eliminated when dealing with human participants. CR protocols deal with this by including small identical snacks and liquid portions at regular intervals (eg, every hour) or by using intravenous feeding methods so that the possible influence of eating and drinking on the rhythms being measured is distributed evenly over the circadian cycle. CR protocols for determining circadian phase position are usually used in a research setting in which participants stay in the laboratory for a complete circadian cycle or more.

Another circadian rhythm research technique is the forced desynchrony (FD) protocol. FD protocols are utilized to separate the circadian and homeostatic components to a variable being measured. For example, sleep and alertness are influenced by both circadian and homeostatic factors, such that the homeostatic drive for sleep increases across the normal waking day and dissipates when sleep occurs at night, whereas the circadian drive for sleep is low across the normal waking day and increases when sleep occurs at night. During a normal day and night, the homeostatic and circadian contributions to sleep interact in a coordinated manner, producing consolidated wakefulness during the day and consolidated sleep at night. During an FD protocol, individuals stay in the laboratory for several circadian cycles, and the laboratory light-dark cycle is manipulated in such a way that the internal circadian clock cannot adjust (or entrain). For example, an FD protocol could involve 20-hour "days," in which a participant stays awake for 13.3 hours and then has a 6.7-hour sleep opportunity. A 20-hour "day" is outside the "range of entrainment" of the internal biologic clock, meaning that the clock cannot adjust to a schedule that is so different in cycle length from its own, and instead the internal clock will continue to drive circadian rhythms at its endogenous cycle length, which is typically about 24 hours. When this occurs, the imposed sleep-wake rhythm (20 hours) becomes dissociated (or desynchronized) from the endogenous circadian rhythms (~24 hours), and each persists with its own cycle length. As this desynchronization persists over the course of days or weeks, the time of scheduled sleep and wakefulness is eventually distributed across all circadian phases. This permits dependent variables (eg, sleepiness, performance, or mood) to be measured with respect to either factor, while controlling for the other. For example, performance on a reaction time task can be measured upon awakening from every sleep episode. Because each sleep episode ends at a different circadian phase, the circadian influence on performance can be assessed while controlling for the homeostatic drive for sleep. The homeostatic drive for sleep is thought to be held relatively constant because the sleep opportunity preceding each performance test is thought to satiate the homeostatic sleep drive. FD protocols thus provide paradigms that can separate the circadian and homeostatic modulation of behavior and physiology to examine specific research questions.

Many of these specialized circadian rhythm measurement techniques fall outside the range of most clinical sleep disorders services, but it is important to be aware of them. The correct interpretation of these data is dependent on accurate and valid sampling techniques in the setting of a strictly controlled environment, as well as an understanding of statistical techniques for analyzing circadian rhythms data. For unusual cases of CRSWD that warrant additional testing, referral to a specialized laboratory may be advisable.

TREATMENT OF CIRCADIAN RHYTHM SLEEP-WAKE DISORDERS

In most cases, the key to treating CRSWD is the correct utilization of PRCs. According to the 2015 Clinical Practice Guideline for the Treatment of Intrinsic Circadian Rhythm Sleep–Wake Disorders published by the American Academy of Sleep Medicine (AASM), administration of light therapy in accordance with the PRC is the preferred first-line treatment for ASWPD and irregular sleep-wake rhythm disorder (ISWRD) (Figure 15-4). CRSWD treatment may also involve controlled exposure to light, darkness, and other time cues. A patient might be given a "prescription" to actively seek and avoid light at appropriate times. In suitable climates and weather conditions, artificial therapeutic light sources may be unnecessary. For example, a regular walk outside in sunlight immediately upon awakening could benefit a patient with DSWPD because bright light exposure at that time would likely fall on the phase advance portion of their light PRC, resetting the circadian clock to a relatively earlier time. Conversely, bright light exposure in the evening and the first half of the night, falling on the phase delay portion of the light PRC, would exacerbate a delayed sleep schedule. Thus, actively seeking morning light and avoiding bright evening light are behavioral strategies used to treat delayed sleep phase disorder (DSPD). On the contrary, avoiding early morning light and seeking bright light in the evening can help patients with ASWPD.

Light exposure at inappropriate times can prevent phase shifts in a desired direction or even induce shifts in the opposite direction. In individuals working night shifts, wearing low-transmission, blue-wavelength blocking sunglasses during the morning commute and avoidance of light during the daytime sleep period by the installation of blackout shades for bedroom windows can promote phase delays. These practices reduce morning light exposure, which is beneficial if adaption to the night shift is desired because morning light typically falls on the phase advance portion of the light PRC and will thus hinder any phase delays that might occur when working consecutive night shifts. Jet lag sufferers can be directed to printed resources or websites that provide customized instructions for the manipulation of zeitgebers to promote entrainment to the new time zone.

PRCs for exogenous melatonin are also utilized therapeutically. For example, in patients with DSWPD, it is recommended that melatonin administration occur in the late afternoon or early evening, when it is expected to promote a phase advance. Appropriately timed melatonin administration is recommended in the AASM Clinical Practice Guidelines for the treatment of intrinsic CRSWD for DSWPD, non-24-hour sleep-wake rhythm disorder, and treatment of Irregular Sleep-Wake Rhythm Disorder (ISWPD) in children and adolescents with neurologic disorders. Because of scant evidence for benefit and possible increases in depressed mood, however, melatonin for ISWPD is not recommended in older patients with dementia. Consumption of morning melatonin produces a phase delay, but this approach is less well studied and may have limited clinical utility because melatonin may have a soporific effect in diurnal mammals such as humans. Exogenous melatonin is particularly useful in some blind or enucleated patients with free-running type disorder as a nonphotic method of achieving circadian entrainment to the 24-hour day. In the United States, melatonin is classified as a dietary supplement and available without prescription in a wide range of doses, many of which produce melatonin concentrations much higher than normal endogenous levels. There is little evidence indicating that larger doses of melatonin produce a larger phase shift. To the contrary, data from blind patients indicate that high doses of exogenous melatonin may attenuate the size of a phase shift and that a lower dose can result in a larger net phase shift of the circadian clock. The routine use of melatonin for unsound reasons should be discouraged. Long-term safety data for melatonin are sparse, and in some countries, the drug is available only by prescription.

Chronotherapy is another technique utilized for treating highly motivated patients with DSWPD. This technique utilizes the relative ease with which individuals are able to progressively delay their sleep periods by 1 or 2 hours/d. Over the course of several days, the sleep period is shifted around the clock until the desired bedtime is reached, and a rigid sleep schedule is introduced. After the desired sleep schedule has been reached, bright light upon awakening in the morning is utilized to maintain entrainment to the earlier schedule.

Several other treatments are available for CRSWD. Hypnotics and stimulants are used to treat the symptoms of CRSWD, yet these treatments do not address the cause of the disorder, which is circadian misalignment. In some cases, the best solution to CRSWD is accommodation of the patient's circadian tendencies through lifestyle adaptation.

SUMMARY

Circadian rhythms are internally generated daily cycles in physiology and behavior that are characteristic of life on Earth. In time isolation, human circadian rhythms normally persist with a period slightly more than 24 hours. Examples of circadian rhythms include such diverse phenomena as hormone secretion, body temperature, alertness, and performance. The circadian rhythms most commonly recorded in the clinical sleep laboratory are those of sleep and activity.

Typically, circadian rhythms are synchronized with the 24-hour terrestrial day by continuously adjusting in response to time cues known as zeitgebers. The process of resetting circadian time is known as entrainment. Light is the most effective zeitgeber for the entrainment of circadian rhythms in sighted humans. Other potential zeitgebers include physical activity and social cues. Administration of exogenous melatonin has also been shown to influence the timing of circadian rhythms. The change in circadian timing elicited by a zeitgeber is known as a phase shift. The magnitude and direction of a phase shift evoked by a zeitgeber varies with the time of day. This relationship is expressed in a PRC.

When circadian rhythms are disrupted, the resulting symptoms of insomnia and/or excessive daytime sleepiness may be categorized as a CRSWD. In most cases, CRSWDs arise from a combination of intrinsic and extrinsic factors. The types of CRSWDs are summarized in Figure 15-6. Clinical sleep laboratories routinely collect and analyze the data necessary for the diagnosis and treatment of CRSWDs, primarily through sleep diaries and wrist actigraphy. PSG and MSLT are used less frequently in the diagnosis of CRSWD, primarily for the detection of comorbid sleep disorders. Some specialized sleep laboratories record additional circadian parameters, such as body temperature and melatonin concentration. The most common treatments for CRSWD include carefully timed light therapy, exogenous melatonin administration, and lifestyle adaptation.

ACKNOWLEDGMENT

Special thanks to Mark R. Smith, PhD, for his contributions to earlier editions of this chapter.

SUGGESTED READINGS

Cirelli C, ed. *Fundamentals of Sleep and Circadian Science*. 3rd ed. Oxford Academic; 2025.

Burki T. Nobel prize awarded for discoveries in circadian rhythm. *Lancet*. 2017;390(10104):e25.

Hastings MH, Maywood ES, Brancaccio M. Generation of circadian rhythms in the suprachiasmatic nucleus. *Nat Rev Neurosci*. 2018;19(8):453-469. doi:10.1038/s41583-018-0026-z

Honma S. The mammalian circadian system: a hierarchical multi-oscillator structure for generating circadian rhythm. *J Physiol Sci*. 2018;68:207-219.

Lockley SW, Arendt J, Skene DJ. Visual impairment and circadian rhythm disorders. *Dialogues Clin Neurosci*. 2007;9(3):301-314. doi:10.31887/DCNS.2007.9.3/slockley

Blume C, Garbazza C, Spitschan M. Effects of light on human circadian rhythms, sleep and mood. *Somnologie*. 2019;23:147-156. doi:10.1007/s11818-019-00215-x

Skene DJ, Arendt J. Human circadian rhythms: physiological and therapeutic relevance of light and melatonin. *Ann Clin Biochem*. 2006;43(pt 5):344-353. doi:10.1258/000456306778520142

Lockley SW, Brainard GC, Czeisler CA. High sensitivity of the human circadian melatonin rhythm to resetting by short wavelength light. *J Clin Endocrinol Metab*. 2003;88:4502-4505.

Lewy AJ, Ahmed S, Jackson JML, et al. Melatonin shifts human circadian rhythms according to a phase–response curve. *Chronobiol Int*. 1992;9:380-392.

American Academy of Sleep Medicine. *International Classification of Sleep Disorders*. 3rd ed. American Academy of Sleep Medicine; 2014.

Arlinghaus A, Bohle P, Iskra-Golec I, Jansen N, Jay S, Rotenberg L. Working Time Society consensus statements: evidence-based effects of shift work and non-standard working hours on workers, family and community. *Ind Health*. 2019;57(2):184-200. doi:10.2486/indhealth.SW-4

Hulsegge G, Coenen P, Gascon GM, et al. Adapting shift work schedules for sleep quality, sleep duration, and sleepiness in shift workers. *Cochrane Database Syst Rev*. 2023;9(9):CD010639. doi:10.1002/14651858.CD010639.pub2

Morgenthaler TI, Lee-Chiong T, Alessi C, et al. Practice parameters for the clinical evaluation and treatment of circadian rhythm sleep disorders. *Sleep*. 2007;30:1445-1459.

Auger RR, Burgess HJ, Emens JS, Deriy LV, Thomas SM, Sharkey KM. Clinical practice guideline for the treatment of intrinsic circadian rhythm sleep-wake disorders: advanced sleep-wake phase disorder (ASWPD), delayed sleep-wake phase disorder (DSWPD), non-24-hour sleep-wake rhythm disorder (N24SWD), and irregular sleep-wake rhythm disorder (ISWRD). An update for 2015. *J Clin Sleep Med*. 2015;11(10):1199-1236.

Meyer N, Harvey AG, Lockley SW, Dijk DJ. Circadian rhythms and disorders of the timing of sleep. *Lancet*. 2022;400(10357):1061-1078. doi:10.1016/S0140-6736(22)00877-7

Chapter 16
Parasomnias

AMANDA MOORE

KEY CONCEPTS/LEARNING OBJECTIVES

The key concepts for this chapter include a basic understanding of nonrapid eye movement and rapid eye movement parasomnias; recognition of issues that require a technologist response; and identifying, differentiating, and documenting the clinical presentation of parasomnias that occur during the polysomnographic recording in children and adults.

KEY TERMS

Arousal disorders
Atonia
Confusional arousals
Hallucinations
REM sleep behavior disorder (RBD)
Sleep inertia
Sleep terrors
Sleep-related eating disorder (SRED)
Sleepwalking (Somnambulism)

Parasomnias are defined as undesirable physical phenomena that occur predominantly or exclusively during the sleep period (1,2). Classification by the *International Classification of Sleep Disorders*, 3rd edition (*ICSD-3*) is as follows (Figure 16-1):

1. During nonrapid eye movement (NREM) sleep
2. Associated with rapid eye movement (REM) sleep
3. During the transition from wakefulness to sleep and from sleep to wakefulness

The pathophysiology of parasomnias is variable. Researchers suggest that the simultaneous occurrence or rapid transition between the brain's states of wakefulness, NREM sleep, and REM sleep may result in the blending of elements from these states. Consequently, a combination of wakefulness and NREM sleep can lead to disorders of arousal (DOA), while the interplay between REM sleep and certain aspects of wakefulness may give rise to REM behavior disorder (RBD) (3).

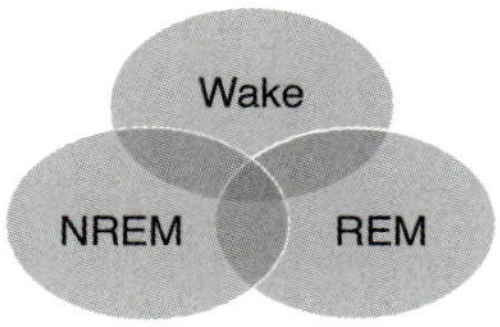

Figure 16-1 Human consciousness is traditionally categorized into three distinct states: wake, nonrapid eye movement (NREM), and rapid eye movement (REM) sleep. As humans transition from one state of consciousness into another, there exists a state that is not fully declared. This temporary and unstable period is known as the *state of dissociation* (dark intersection). Parasomnias are often a result of this period of sleep, which is a combination of one or more states of consciousness.

Parasomnias are particularly prone to occur during transition between different sleep states and may involve complex, seemingly purposeful behaviors. Upon awakening, patients often do not recall these actions, which are frequently referred to as automatisms, occurring without conscious intent or control. Individuals may suffer from multiple parasomnias. In some patients, the overlapping characteristics of nocturnal seizures may present an added difficulty in differential diagnosis (4).

DISORDERS OF AROUSAL (FROM NONRAPID EYE MOVEMENT SLEEP)

DOA occur during the transition between sleep and wakefulness. DOAs typically occur during NREM sleep, in the first third of the night and most commonly, during NREM stage 3 sleep. DOA are characterized by unusual behaviors, and typically, the patient is unresponsive to redirection. Frequently, the patient is amnestic of the event (5).

These disorders most commonly occur during childhood and often diminish with increasing age. These disorders are believed to result from abnormal arousal processes, when motor activity is restored without full consciousness and can be exacerbated by external factors such as sleep deprivation or stress. Individuals with

DOA may walk, talk, or perform activities during an event that can last from seconds to hours. DOA include confusional arousals, sleepwalking (somnambulism), or sleep terrors. A sleep study is not typically required for the diagnosis of DOA as it can be diagnosed based on the physician interview and clinical history if there is no suspicion of other sleep disorders (5). Often, there is a familial history of DOA.

Confusional Arousals

Confusional arousals (CA), also termed "sleep drunkenness," are a type of DOA that are seen more commonly during the first third of the night, when NREM stage 3 sleep is most prevalent or during the morning awakening (1). Confusional arousals are characterized by diminished vigilance, excessive sleep inertia, unclear thoughts, and slowed speech. Behaviors tend to demonstrate a lack of orientation to the environment. For minutes to hours, the person may react inappropriately, be resistive, and even be violent; attempts at redirection may cause more agitation.

Confusional arousals may be exacerbated by idiopathic hypersomnia, sleep deprivation, the use of central nervous system (CNS) depressants, neurologic disorders, or forced awakenings from deep sleep. Parasomnias such as confusional arousals are most prevalent in young children and less common in adults, with no notable gender differences observed. During an episode of confusional arousal, polysomnographic (PSG) findings may include alpha rhythm, repetitive microsleeps, and NREM stage 1 sleep (4).

Treatments may include sleep extension, scheduled awakenings, avoidance of sleep deprivation, psychotherapy, or drug therapy (eg, tricyclic antidepressants or benzodiazepines) (6). Treatment for children may not be required as the disorder may resolve with age (4).

Sleepwalking

Sleepwalking, also referred to as somnambulism, is characterized by ambulation that occurs during sleep. Somnambulism is considered a DOA and is most commonly observed in the first third of the night, when NREM stage 3 sleep is more prominent. The episode will often start with the person sitting up in bed, followed by walking or running. The sleepwalker may return to bed without waking or awaken elsewhere. Behaviors exhibited may occasionally be inappropriate, or dangerous, such as driving a car over long distances. It is characterized by highly elaborate behaviors with amnesia of the event. The sleepwalker's eyes are usually open but attempts to communicate are usually unsuccessful. Episode duration varies widely from several minutes to hours. It is most prevalent in young children and less common in adults (7,8). Familial occurrences are common (9,10).

Episodes generally follow an arousal from NREM stage 3 sleep. PSG patterns seen in adults with injurious sleepwalking and sleep terrors include (1) diffuse, rhythmic delta activity, (2) diffuse delta and theta activities, and (3) prominent alpha and beta activities. Abrupt heart rate acceleration may be noted post arousal (11,15).

Treatment may include hypnosis, scheduled awakenings, or medication (eg, tricyclic antidepressants or benzodiazepines) (6). In children, time and protection from harm may be all that is required for these events to resolve (4).

Sleep Terrors

Sleep terrors, also referred to as "night terrors or pavor nocturnus," are one of the most dramatic forms of arousal disorders. Sleep terrors are seen most often in the first third of the night, when stage N3 sleep is more prevalent. Sleep terrors occur more commonly in children, but adults can also suffer from sleep terrors throughout the night. They are characterized by crying or loud screaming and a general sense of fear. Autonomic responses, such as tachycardia, tachypnea, diaphoresis, and increased muscle tone, can be noted. Patients are inconsolable and have amnesia of the event.

PSG features include a reduction in sleep efficiency, more frequent arousals, and greater wake time after sleep onset. There is often a decrease in NREM stage N2 sleep and an increase in stage N3 sleep.

Therapy may include sleep extension, avoidance of sleep deprivation, scheduled awakenings, hypnosis, or medications (eg, benzodiazepines or L-5-hydroxytryptamine) (6). In children, treatment may not be needed because the disorder will often resolve over time (4). The physician should consider other sleep disorders, such as obstructive sleep apnea (OSA), that could be causing the night terrors. If the night terrors are secondary to another issue, the physician will identify and treat the underlying disorder first (4).

OTHER PARASOMNIAS

Sexsomnia

Sexsomnia is an NREM parasomnia in which the patient has atypical sexual manifestations during sleep, such as vocalizations, fondling, kissing, masturbation, and full sexual intercourse without recall after awakening followed by morning amnesia (1,12). Sexsomnia can occur as part of overlap syndrome combined with other parasomnias: REM behavior disorder, confusional arousals, sleepwalking, and sleep terrors may be accompanied by OSA. The differential diagnosis could include seizures or REM sleep behavior disorder (1).

PSG data will demonstrate sudden spontaneous arousals from non-REM slow-wave (N3) sleep (12).

While not a disorder of arousal, the *ICSD-3* considers sexsomnia a type of "confusional arousal." Terms used in the literature are "atypical sexual behavior during sleep," "sexsomnia," or "sleep sex." Sexsomnia is a recently reported variation of NREM arousal parasomnias (1,4). These behaviors often occur during confusional arousals and have also been reported during somnambulism (somnambulistic sexual behavior) (1). Most people reporting sexsomnia have had past episodes of sleepwalking (12). Sleepwalking does not present with sexual arousal; however, sexsomnia is associated with the engorgement of the sexual organs, lubrication, and ejaculation. Males are described as being more physical, with sexual fondling and intercourse often occurring, while females are more likely to present with masturbation and vocalization of a sexual nature (12).

Sexsomnia can be quite disturbing for all parties involved. It can make relationships and marriages difficult and strained. There is some evidence that alcohol and drug misuse may be factors in some sexsomnia cases in addition to stress and sleep deprivation. Past trauma may also be a factor. Multiple polysomnograms may need to be performed to capture these episodes.

Treatments for this parasomnia include serotonin reuptake inhibitors, benzodiazepines (eg, clonazepam), and antidepressant medications (6,12). Sleep hygiene issues should be addressed with these patients, and stress management for those with depression or anxiety is often indicated.

Sleep-Related Dissociative Disorders

Dissociative disorder can emerge throughout the sleep period (1). Nighttime episodes can consist of violent or sexualized behavior, self-mutilation, screaming, running, eating, or driving a car. There is generally amnesia for the event. Dissociative disorders can result in injuries. The disorder is more prevalent in females, and episodes may be sporadic or may slowly increase across time (4). Patients also usually present with daytime dissociative disorders, which may be associated with a history of trauma, physical abuse, or sexual abuse (4).

PSG reveals sustained EEG wakefulness during these episodes. Treatment may require psychiatric intervention because this parasomnia is often associated with past traumatic events (4).

Sleep Enuresis

Sleep enuresis (SE) is recurrent, involuntary bed-wetting occurring during sleep in a child older than 5 years. Most children achieve bladder control at night by 3 years of age. Although it can arise throughout the night, enuresis tends to occur most commonly early during sleep in the first third of the evening. There are two classifications of enuresis: primary and secondary. In primary enuresis, the child must be 5 years or older and have never been consistently dry during a sleep period and exhibit involuntary bed-wetting at least twice a week for at least 3 months. Children with primary enuresis often have a positive family history among their siblings or parents. Spontaneous cure rate in children with primary SE is estimated at 15% annually. In secondary cases, the child must be 5 years or older, exhibit recurrent involuntary bed-wetting during sleep at least twice a week for 3 months but has been consistently dry for at least 6 months. Secondary SE can occur at any age and accounts for approximately 5% to 10% of cases. SE can be seen during adolescence and in about 1% to 3% of adult patients with primary nocturnal enuresis (4).

PSG typically demonstrates normal sleep architecture. Treatment may include "bed-wetting alarms," bladder training, medications (eg, desmopressin, oxybutynin, or imipramine) (4,12). In secondary SE, the physician should diagnose and treat any underlying cause that may be present before treating the SE.

Sleep-Related Groaning (Catathrenia)

Sleep-related groaning (catathrenia) is defined as groaning during exhalation in sleep (mostly during REM sleep). The person with this disorder is often unaware of the episodes; however, the bed partner is often disturbed because of the loud vocalizations. There is no known cause of sleep-related groaning, and there is no problem related to breathing that causes the events (5). PSG may demonstrate episodes of bradypnea, and loud expiratory groaning sounds occurring in clusters that recur several times throughout the night. Sleep architecture and oxygen saturation are normal.

Exploding Head Syndrome

Exploding head syndrome is characterized by a sudden, loud imagined noise or explosion in the head occurring during the transition between wakefulness and sleep. A flash of light, myoclonic jerk, and sense of fear or concern may accompany the experience and can cause an elevated level of distress to the individual. The frequency of attacks varies significantly among individuals. Frequent attacks can give rise to complaints of insomnia.

PSG features of the disorder are sudden arousals occurring during the sleep-wake transition, with the EEG demonstrating alpha and theta activity. Treatment is not needed because the disorder is of a benign nature and because these episodes often resolve over time (4).

Sleep-Related Eating Disorder

Sleep-related eating disorder (SRED) is characterized by recurrent episodes of drinking and eating during arousals from sleep. This disorder frequently arises in individuals experiencing significant stress, those who have recently quit smoking, or individuals recovering from alcohol or substance misuse.

Affected individuals are unaware or only partly conscious of abnormal behavior. Episodes can be observed anytime during sleep, and episodes may occur many times every night. In many instances, the awakenings appear to be triggered by learned behavior and not by real hunger or thirst.

PSG may show multiple arousals, typically from NREM stage N3 sleep but occasionally from REM sleep as well. Treatment may include treating an underlying sleep disorder causing frequent arousals, for example, leg movements and OSA (4).

Sleep-Related Hallucinations

For some, hallucinations may occur during sleep-wake transitions. They can manifest either at sleep onset (hypnagogic hallucinations) or during awakening (hypnopompic hallucinations). These experiences can encompass a range of forms, including visual, auditory, or tactile phenomena. The hallucinations are often associated with sleep paralysis, and while more prevalent in individuals with narcolepsy, they can also be experienced by anyone. PSG demonstrates events occurring predominantly during sleep-onset REM periods, but these episodes can also arise during NREM sleep. Hypnagogic and hypnopompic hallucinations may be benign or tolerable for some individuals, but narcolepsy should be considered in patients presenting with these symptoms because it may be the underlying cause, and treatment of narcolepsy would be indicated (4).

Parasomnia Because of Medical Condition

This diagnosis is indicated when a parasomnia (eg, RBD) is associated with an underlying neurologic or medical condition. Sleep paralysis and sleep hallucinations may also be related to ongoing neurologic disorders.

Parasomnias Because of Medications or Substances

Association between medications or other substances and the induced parasomnia is increasingly recognized. Parasomnias may be associated with the use or withdrawal of a substance, often a medication, and the associated nonconscious behaviors can occur during NREM or REM sleep. The *ICSD-3* does not list substances that cause this specific disorder. The literature does cite cases, and this is a cursory overview of some of these cases.

Zolpidem (Ambien), zaleplon (Sonata), and eszopiclone (Lunesta) are benzodiazepine receptor agonists that react with a1-gamma-aminobutyric acid $(GABA)_A$ receptors, thought to eliminate sedative, amnesic, and motor impairment actions associated with benzodiazepines that react at other GABA receptor sites (13). Zolpidem states, on its packaging materials, that alcohol or other CNS depressants taken together may increase the risk of associated parasomnias. The behaviors or automatisms involved, such as sleep driving and sleep shopping, are parasomnias associated with DOA, RBD, or parasomnia overlap disorder (4,13). Sexsomnia, somnambulism, and sleep-eating can also be seen because of medication or substance use.

Somnambulism was reported in a case study where bupropion's use may have initiated somnambulism episodes; when the medication was discontinued, the sleepwalking was curtailed (14). The bupropion (a noradrenaline and dopamine reuptake inhibitor) was prescribed for use during smoking cessation; however, because of nicotine withdrawal, bupropion could not be assumed causal in this case (14). Another case report describes a patient prescribed bupropion for depression, who about 2 weeks later was discovered to be leaving her bed, making phone calls, and bringing back food that she hid under her pillow. Bupropion was stopped, and that night so did the parasomnia. Months later, another physician prescribed bupropion, and the parasomnia returned in about 2 weeks. Again, the parasomnia went away the first night she stopped taking the bupropion. Bupropion increases slow-wave sleep and total duration, density, and latency of REM sleep (14).

New classes of sleep medications and substances that have been around for years (eg, alcohol) can be the cause of parasomnias. The use of these substances is increasing, and more reporting has indicated a likely relationship between their use and some parasomnias.

Although we would normally expect to see a short interval between starting a new medication and seeing a reaction to it, many medications take weeks for their full effects to be established. Polypharmacy presents confounding evidence of what medication may be causing a parasomnia. The drug or drugs used to treat an original disorder may cause the problem, but it may also be an interaction between several medications that is the cause. Patients can be taking large numbers of drugs for comorbid and morbid conditions unrelated to sleep. It has been postulated that parasomnias, such as sexsomnia, may emerge because of medication initiation or withdrawal (4).

These parasomnias may be quite dangerous and yet unknown to the patient for a time before they or their physician are able to put the pieces together and identify that they have a sleep disorder. RBD, discussed later in this chapter, can be associated with the use of medications and biologic substances and is an example of a disorder that can be dangerous to the patient or others in the proximity of the patient having an episode.

Treatment of these parasomnias may consist of removal of the offending medication or substance. Changes in dosage and timing of medication may also prove beneficial.

Parasomnias Usually Associated With Rapid Eye Movement Sleep

Rapid Eye Movement Sleep Behavior Disorder

Two unique characteristics of REM sleep include increased reports of dreaming and muscle atonia. Atonia is important during REM sleep as it prevents us from acting out our dreams, but people with RBD lack atonia during REM and may therefore act out their dreams. These dangerous episodes can lead to injury to themselves or others (15), and in some cases, it may be advised that the patient with RBD sleep alone. RBD episodes are more common during the second half of the night (early morning hours), when REM sleep is more prevalent. Behaviors associated with RBD range from simple motions to highly complex actions (screaming, punching, kicking, or running). The episode typically ends with a rapid awakening and full alertness. RBD most often occurs in the sixth or seventh decade of life and is most prevalent in males. Neurologic disorders (dementia, Parkinsonism, or narcolepsy) are predisposing factors.

Between 70% to 90% of patients who suffer from RBD will develop a neurologic disorder such as Parkinson disease (PD), Lewy body dementia (LBD) or multiple system atrophy (MSA) (5). RBD is linked to PD as 50% to 60% of people with RBD also have PD (5).

PSG must be performed to establish the diagnosis of RBD. PSG can demonstrate an augmentation of electromyographic (EMG) activity and the presence of body movements during REM sleep. Mild RBD may present with nothing more than arm movement or flailing; however, more violent activities such as slapping, punching, kicking, leaping from the bed, and running have been documented during PSG. Time-synchronized video recording is essential. More than one study may be required to capture an episode. Additional EMG monitoring of the upper extremity muscles (flexor digitorum) is useful for capturing upper limb movements during REM.

The technologist must consider the safety of the patient, themselves, and others when studying these patients. The technologist should be mindful of dangers within the testing room to prevent injurious nocturnal behaviors. Furniture with sharp corners should be moved away from the bed, the headboard may need to be padded and covered, lamps or TV remotes should be removed to create a safe sleeping environment.

Common treatment includes ensuring a safe sleeping environment and treatment with melatonin or clonazepam (4,6).

Recurrent Isolated Sleep Paralysis

Sleep paralysis is a REM-related parasomnia involving paralysis of skeletal muscle either at sleep onset (hypnagogic) or upon waking from sleep (hypnopompic). During a sleep paralysis event, the patient becomes conscious while the body remains unable to move or speak due to REM sleep–related atonia. This can be quite frightening for the individual to experience. Atonia during the event affects the head, body, and limbs, but the eye and respiratory muscles remain unaffected. Paralysis can last from several seconds to a few minutes. Consciousness remains intact, and individuals may recall dream imagery. The onset typically occurs during adolescence and can affect both genders equally. Most cases are isolated, although some may occur within families or in individuals with narcolepsy (16). Factors such as lack of sleep and poor sleep hygiene can increase the likelihood of experiencing paralysis.

PSG recordings are characterized by abundant alpha electroencephalogram (EEG) activity and persistence of muscle atonia into wakefulness (17). Treatment may include REM sleep suppression with medication (eg, antidepressants) (4).

Nightmare Disorder

Nightmares are unpleasant and frightening dreams that occur during REM sleep. Episodes typically occur in the latter half of the night, when REM sleep is more prevalent. Dream content is disturbing and often relates to imminent physical danger to the patient. The patient can often describe the nature of the nightmare on waking, and there is little, if any, confusion, which differentiates nightmare disorder from night terrors. Nightmares often occur after periods of REM sleep deprivation and can be precipitated by illness, traumatic experiences, acute alcohol ingestion, and certain medications (18). Occasional nightmares occur during childhood and generally become less frequent during adulthood (19). Recurring nightmares can result in insomnia, sleep avoidance because of fear of falling asleep, excessive daytime sleepiness, and anxiety.

PSG demonstrates abrupt awakenings from REM sleep. REM sleep abnormalities, including a reduction in REM sleep latency, an increased REM density, and an increased percentage of REM sleep, may be observed. Treatment may include sleep hygiene, comfort, image rehearsal, psychotherapy, and medications for REM suppression (6).

EVALUATION OF PARASOMNIAS

Clinical evaluation of a patient presenting with a possible parasomnia involves an interview with the patient, the spouse, and other family members. A comprehensive sleep questionnaire is valuable (Figure 16-2). Neurologic and psychiatric examinations and complete psychological testing may also be indicated using psychological measurement tools such as the Minnesota Multiphasic Personality Inventory or Beck Depression Inventory.

Please answer the following questions using this scale. (Consult bed partner.)

0 = never; 1 = rarely; 2 = sometimes; 3 = often; 4 = frequently; 5 = always

0 1 2 3 4 5	I have been told that I walk in my sleep
0 1 2 3 4 5	I wet the bed as an adult
0 1 2 3 4 5	I move my arms, legs, and/or body during sleep
0 1 2 3 4 5	I have been told that I act out my dreams
0 1 2 3 4 5	I cannot tell dreams from reality
0 1 2 3 4 5	I make loud, unusual sounds during my sleep
0 1 2 3 4 5	I have been told that I talk, shout, or groan in my sleep
0 1 2 3 4 5	I have unusual behaviors during my sleep
0 1 2 3 4 5	I have vivid dream-like scenes upon falling asleep
0 1 2 3 4 5	I have experienced violent behaviors during my sleep
0 1 2 3 4 5	I hurt myself or my bed partner during my sleep
0 1 2 3 4 5	I have experienced night terrors with shouting or loud screaming
0 1 2 3 4 5	I eat or drink during my sleep
0 1 2 3 4 5	I have awakened in the morning feeling bloated, sick to my stomach and do not want to eat breakfast
0 1 2 3 4 5	I have initiated unusual or hurtful sexual behaviors during my sleep, either by myself or with my bed partner
0 1 2 3 4 5	I have had episodes of muscle paralysis while falling asleep or waking up
0 1 2 3 4 5	I have recurrent nightmares
0 1 2 3 4 5	I have now or in the past had seizures during my sleep

Figure 16-2 Parasomnia questionnaire.

A sleep study is not always required for the diagnosis of a parasomnia; however, if a patient is having a sleep study, and a parasomnia occurs, the sleep technologist should record the time and describe the event. For direct observation of the event, the technologist might need to go into the patient's room and do the following: document whether the eyes are open or closed and whether the eyes appear alert or "glassy," whether the patient appears to be asleep in a dreaming or nondreaming state or awake, and the level of consciousness during the event. The technologist should ask the patient about dream recall associated with the parasomnia event if they awakens and note the emotional state of the patient.

The sleep technologist must be prepared to intervene at once and enter the room if the patient exhibits behavior that may cause injury. Simultaneous digital video recording is required during the PSG. This makes it possible to correlate the parasomnia event with activity on the PSG tracing. PSG features of the various parasomnias are described in Table 16-1. Indications for PSG are outlined in Table 16-2.

Table 16-1 Polysomnographic Features of Parasomnias

Parasomnia	Observation
Confusional arousals	Arise while in the bed from SWS, REM with apnea, often sitting up in bed looking around confused
Sexsomnia	Arousals seen in transitions between sleep-wake or between differing sleep stages, SWS
Parasomnias due to medications or substances	Altered motor control during sleep, arousals
Sleepwalking	Persistence of sleep while leaving the bed, arousal from SWS, ambulation, normal muscle atonia in REM, amnesia for event, automatic behaviors that are inappropriate, disoriented with slow speech
Sleep terrors	Arousal from SWS, screaming, autonomic activation, RBD, and seizures need to be ruled out; adults may have overlap with other arousal disorders

Table 16-1 Polysomnographic Features of Parasomnias (*continued*)

Parasomnia	Observation
RBD	Loss of atonia in REM, excessive submental EMG activity in REM, disruptive or abnormal REM sleep behaviors ranging from mild limb movements in REM to getting out of bed and acting out dreams
Recurrent isolated sleep paralysis	REM sleep atonia continuing into wake, alpha intrusion into REM sleep, EMG shows atonia during the paralysis
Nightmare disorder	Nightmares generally in REM, little confusion, there is dream recall usually with fear or anxiety, return to sleep may be difficult, occur in the latter half of the night
Sleep-related dissociative disorders	Emerge from sustained EEG of wakefulness, self-mutilation, repeated injury of self or others
Sleep-related groaning	Groaning recorded during (predominantly) REM sleep
Exploding head syndrome	Patient perceives sudden loud noise (explosion) in their head during wake-sleep or sleep-wake transitions, absence of significant pain.
Sleep-related eating disorder	Waking concurrent EEG pattern, multiple confusional arousals with various levels of consciousness achieved
Sleep-related hallucinations	Hallucinations before sleep onset or awakening, usually visual

EEG, electroencephalogram; EMG, electromyogram; OSA, obstructive sleep apnea; PSG, polysomnography; RBD, REM behavior disorder; REM, rapid eye movement; SWS, slow-wave sleep.

Table 16-2 Indications for Polysomnography

Parasomnia Type	When Disorder Is Uncomplicated and Noninjurious	Forensic Considerations, Injury or Atypical Behavior, Age, Time, Duration, Frequency, or Motor Patterns
Confusional arousals	No	Yes
Sexsomnia	No	Yes
Confusional arousals	No	Yes
Sexsomnia	No	Yes
Parasomnia due to medications or substances	No	Yes
Sleepwalking	No	Yes
Sleep terrors	No	Yes
REM behavior disorder	Yes	Yes
Recurrent isolated sleep paralysis	No	Yes
Nightmare disorder	No	Yes
Sleep-related dissociative disorders	No	Yes
Sleep-related groaning	No	Unusual
Exploding head syndrome	No	Unusual
Sleep-related hallucinations	No	Yes
Sleep-related eating disorder	No	Unusual

REM, rapid eye movement.

SUMMARY

Parasomnias are common clinical complaints. Formal sleep evaluation, including PSG, is indicated for parasomnias that are injurious; disruptive to the bed partner or other household members; associated with daytime sleepiness; or related to medical, psychiatric, or neurologic disorders (2). The initial assessment usually starts with the patient interview and discussion of the presenting sleep complaint and a patient history. Often, more information may be obtained through further discussions with the bed partner, caregivers, or others familiar with the sleep complaints. Parasomnias must be distinguished from nocturnal seizures, both of which may manifest as unusual and inappropriate movements and behaviors. It is important for the sleep technologist to provide an environment that is safe for both the patient and technologist. Furniture, room decor and accessories as well as weapons can all pose a threat of injury.

REFERENCES

1. American Academy of Sleep Medicine. *International Classification of Sleep Disorders*. 3rd ed. American Academy of Sleep Medicine; 2014.
2. Mahowald MW. Arousal and sleep-wake transition parasomnias. In: Lee-Chiong TL, Sateia MJ, Carskadon MA, eds. *Sleep Medicine*. Elsevier; 2002:207-213.
3. Mahowald MW. Parasomnias. *Med Clin North Am*. 2004;88(3):669-678.
4. Thorpy MJ, Plazzi G. *The Parasomnias and Other Sleep-Related Movement Disorders*. Cambridge University Press; 2010.
5. American Academy of Sleep Medicine. ICSD-3 TR: Parasomnias. 2022. https://aasm.org/wp-content/uploads/2022/05/ICSD-3-TR-Parasomnias-Draft.pdf
6. Lee-Chiong T. *Somnology*. On-Demand Publishing LLC; 2010.
7. Ohayon MM, Guilleminault C, Priest RG. Night terrors, sleepwalking, and confusional arousals in the general population: their frequency and relationship to other sleep and mental disorders. *J Clin Psychiatry*. 1999;60:268-276.
8. Joncas S, Zadra A, Paquet J, et al. The value of sleep deprivation as a diagnostic tool in adult sleepwalkers. *Neurology*. 2002;58(6):936-940.
9. Kales A, Soldatos CR, Bixler EO, et al. Hereditary factors in sleepwalking and night terrors. *Br J Psychiatry*. 1980;137:111-118.
10. Abe K, Amatomi M, Oda N. Sleepwalking and recurrent sleep talking in children of childhood sleepwalkers. *Am J Psychiatry*. 1984;141:800-801.
11. Schenck CH, Pareja JA, Patterson AL, et al. Analysis of polysomnographic events surrounding 252 slow-wave sleep arousals in thirty-eight adults with injurious sleepwalking and sleep terrors. *J Clin Neurophysiol*. 1998;15(2):159-166.
12. Bejot Y, Juenet N, Garrouty R, et al. Sexsomnia: an uncommon variety of parasomnia. *Clin Neurol Neurosurg*. 2010;112(1):72-75.
13. Gibson CE, Caplan JP. Zolpidem-associated parasomnia with serious self-injury: a shot in the dark. *Psychosomatics*. 2011;52(1):88-91.
14. Oulis P, Kokras N, Papadimitriou GN, et al. Bupropion-induced sleepwalking. *J Clin Psychopharmacol*. 2010;30(1):83-84.
15. Olson EJ, Boeve BF, Silber MH. Rapid eye movement sleep behaviour disorder: demographic, clinical and laboratory findings in 93 cases. *Brain*. 2000;123(pt 2):331-339.
16. Buzzi G, Cirignotta F. Isolated sleep paralysis: a web survey. *Sleep Res Online*. 2000;3(2):61-66.
17. Takeuchi T, Miyasita A, Sasaki Y, et al. Isolated sleep paralysis elicited by sleep interruption. *Sleep*. 1992;15(3):217-225.
18. Pagel JF, Helfter P. Drug induced nightmares—an etiology based review. *Human Psychopharmacol*. 2003;18(1):59-67.
19. Germain A, Nielsen TA. Sleep patho-physiology in posttraumatic stress disorder and idiopathic nightmare sufferers. *Biol Psychiatry*. 2003;54(10):1092-1098.

Chapter 17

Restless Legs Syndrome and Periodic Limb Movement Disorder

MICHAEL FURGASON AND RICHARD JOHANNES HERSTEIN

KEY CONCEPTS/LEARNING OBJECTIVES

The key concepts for this chapter include defining the clinical syndrome of restless legs syndrome (RLS), identifying the characteristic polysomnographic features of periodic limb movement disorder (PLMD), differentiating between periodic limb movements and movements related to respiratory and other sleep-related events, and recognizing the relationship and differences between PLMD and RLS.

KEY TERMS

Accelerometry
Augmentation
Fasciculations
Impedance
Myoclonus
Periodic limb movement disorder (PLMD)
Physiologic
Restless legs syndrome (RLS)

Restless legs syndrome (RLS) and periodic limb movement disorder (PLMD), while sometimes associated with each other, it is important to note that they are two distinct clinical entities. RLS, also known as Willis-Ekbom disease, is characterized by an uncontrollable urge to move the legs, typically in response to uncomfortable sensations. PLMD, on the other hand, involves repetitive limb movements during sleep, which can disrupt sleep quality. RLS is a neurosensory motor disorder that occurs during wakefulness and may significantly impact sleep onset in the first half of the night as patients often must stretch, move, or walk to provide relief, resulting in a significant disruption to sleep quality. RLS is reported by about 10% of North American and northern European adults, with 2% to 3% having moderate-to-severe RLS (1). Periodic limb movements of sleep (PLMS) are physiologic signals that represent rhythmic movement of the lower extremity that are measured during sleep, which may or may not have clinical relevance. Periodic limb movements can also present in the upper extremities during sleep.

RLS is diagnosed through a patient interview and appropriate questionnaires. A polysomnogram (PSG) is not a requirement for diagnosis. In contrast, PLMD requires not only a patient interview confirming clinical sleep disturbances but also monitoring via a PSG of specific limb movement activity. By convention, periodic electromyographic (EMG) activity recorded from bilateral anterior tibialis muscles defines PLMS. Movements of the upper limbs may also be sampled, if clinically indicated. Other techniques such as accelerometry of the toe, foot, or leg have also been used to measure movements in sleep. PLMS can be monitored in numerous muscle groups, including extensors and flexors of the toe, foot, knee, hip, finger, hand, elbow, and shoulder. The EMG of the anterior tibialis muscle provides a robust signal, and it was chosen by earlier researchers for measurement of limb movement activity, thereby becoming the standard.

The recording technologist must recognize that movements during sleep arise from multiple factors and that the clinical relevance of a movement is based on the degree of arousal, which is usually defined by a 3-second or longer abrupt shift in electroencephalograph (EEG) frequency, although new research has additionally focused on cardiovascular measures of autonomic arousal from PLMS.

BRIEF HISTORY OF RESTLESS LEGS SYNDROME AND PERIODIC LIMB MOVEMENT DISORDER

The first known medical description of RLS and PLMD was by Sir Thomas Willis in 1672 ("...arms and legs, leapings and contractions of the tendons ensued... [making the bed into] a place of the greatest torture") (2).

In 1945, Karl-Axel Ekbom (1907-1977) provided a detailed and comprehensive report of this condition in his doctoral thesis and a subsequent publication (3).

The first published report of periodic movements in sleep was by Symonds in 1953 (4). He used the term *nocturnal myoclonus* to describe the movements, but the term is best avoided because the characteristic movement of myoclonus is different from that of PLMS. Lugaresi and colleagues (5) in Italy described the association between PLMD and RLS in 1965. Coleman (6), working at Stanford University, described the technique for recording and scoring of PLMS in 1982 that continues to be utilized (with modification) today.

Recently, significant advancements have been made in the understanding, diagnosis, and management of RLS and PLMD. For example, the pathophysiology of RLS has been increasingly linked to dysfunctions in dopaminergic pathways and iron metabolism in the central nervous system, leading to the widespread use of dopamine agonists and iron supplementation as first-line treatments. Genetic studies have identified several risk loci associated with RLS, highlighting a hereditary component, which displays an autosomal dominant inheritance pattern. PLMD, while often comorbid with RLS, is now recognized as a distinct condition, primarily diagnosed through PSG. Updated diagnostic criteria outlined by the *International Classification of Sleep Disorders*, third edition (*ICSD-3*) have refined the differentiation between these disorders. Moreover, the understanding of the impact of RLS and PLMD on cardiovascular health, behavioral health/mood disorders, and overall sleep quality has expanded, prompting more comprehensive approaches to treatment that address both neurologic and systemic health. Emerging research continues to explore novel therapeutic targets, including adenosine signaling pathways and nonpharmacologic interventions such as cognitive-behavioral therapy (CBT) and transcranial magnetic stimulation (TMS), reflecting the evolving landscape of care for these conditions.

Various investigators have shown that PLMS predominate during the first half of the night and tend to increase in frequency over each decade of life, with children under 10 years rarely having PLMS and many adults aged 60 years or above having more than 15 limb movements per hour of sleep (7). Zucconi et al. (8) at the National Institutes of Health demonstrated that PLMS arise from regulatory motor neurons in the spine.

The reader should be aware that generalized body movements and limb movements during sleep can have multiple causes, including sleep-disordered breathing. In particular, limb movements presenting 0.5 seconds before or after increased upper airway resistance, and subsequent respiratory effort–related arousals may be misinterpreted as PLMS. Conversely, PLMS, or other sleep-related movements, may cause changes in breathing patterns or create artifacts in the respiratory channels that can resemble sleep-disordered breathing. A careful examination of all relevant PSG data is essential for differentiating PLMS from other sleep-related events. Current consensus identifies PLMS as a relatively infrequent cause of insomnia or hypersomnia, the clinical symptoms that are required to arrive at a diagnosis of PLMD.

OVERVIEW OF MOVEMENTS IN SLEEP

Motor activity in sleep is common, as any arousing event may cause movement. Movement represents the primary reason for abrupt changes in any PSG signal. Isolated movements of the arms and legs typically occur 50 to 100 times during 7 to 8 hours of sleep. Axial changes of body position occur 5 to 7 times during an average night and will often cluster in the 10 minutes before or after rapid eye movement (REM) sleep. During REM sleep, muscle twitching is common and may be recorded as brief fasciculations in the limb EMG channels.

Generalized movements in sleep may be exacerbated by a wide variety of sleep-related disorders, such as physical pain or discomfort, psychological disturbances, and environmental factors. In contrast to these, PLMS exhibit a stereotypical pattern of independent limb movements that meet specific criteria as described in the Movement Rules section of the *AASM (American Academy of Sleep Medicine) Manual for the Scoring of Sleep and Associated Events: Rules, Terminology and Technical Specifications,* version 3.0 (9).

RLS often causes patients to shift and move as they attempt to relax into sleep. This restlessness can be particularly problematic in the confined environment of the recording room, where the sensation of restlessness and the urge to move the legs may be heightened.

Normally, patients will be able to report to the technologist that their legs are making it "difficult to settle." Some patients show heightened anxiety as RLS symptoms increase.

It occasionally proves to be a challenge for the technologist to decide whether anxiety is the principal reason for difficulty with sleep onset or whether the restriction of movement in the patient with RLS is worsening their anxiety. It is common to observe periodic limb movements of wakefulness (PLMW) appearing in a regular manner in the anterior tibialis recording as the patient with RLS falls asleep.

In some sleep centers, an average of five or more independent periodic leg movements per hour of sleep can be seen in 25% to 40% of adult patients undergoing clinical PSG. Only one-tenth to one-fifth of these PLMS lead to EEG-defined arousals of 3 seconds or more. Frequently, limb movements with arousals are secondary to the termination of breathing-related events.

DEFINITION OF RESTLESS LEGS SYNDROME AND PERIODIC LIMB MOVEMENT DISORDER

The *ICD-3* lists three clinical criteria for the diagnosis of RLS (11). Testing to establish the diagnosis is not required, and all three criteria must be met.

A. The patient must provide a history of an urge to move the legs that may or may not include an abnormal sensation in the affected limb(s).
   1. Begins or worsens at rest or inactivity.
   2. Is partially or completely relieved by movement, like walking or stretching.
   3. Occurs predominantly or exclusively in the evening or night.
B. The symptoms are not related to another medical or behavioral condition.
C. These symptoms must cause distress, sleep disruption, or functional impairment.

To assist in the recall of the primary criteria for the diagnosis of RLS, the acronym URGE is suggested:

U—urge to move
R—rest worsens the urge
G—gyration (movement) relieves the urge
E—evening or night worsening of the urge

PLMS are defined as a burst of EMG activity in the anterior tibialis muscle with a duration of at least 0.5 seconds, but not longer than 10 seconds. Quantitatively, the burst should be 8 μV greater than the resting baseline EMG amplitude. Periodicity is defined when there are four or more consecutive movements that occur with intermovement intervals of between 5 and 90 seconds. The movement onset is defined as the starting point of the movement that produces an 8 μV increase above resting EMG, and the movement offset is defined as the decline of EMG to less than 2 μV of resting EMG. Leg movements occurring in both legs that are separated by less than 5 seconds between movement onsets are counted as a single-leg movement (10).

Traditionally, a mean total of five or more PLMS per hour of sleep has been considered abnormal, especially if the movements are accompanied by an EEG arousal. The World Association of Sleep Medicine and the International Restless Legs Syndrome Study Group reviewed the methodology and clinical relevance of PLMS, proposing that the normal number of PLMS may be as high as 15/h in the older patients (7).

To score an EEG arousal associated with a limb movement, the movement must be accompanied by an abrupt shift in EEG frequency of at least 3 seconds duration, occurring within the 2 seconds before or after the limb movement.

METHODOLOGY AND RECORDING TECHNIQUES

PLMS are monitored during clinical PSG. Proper skin preparation of the recording site over the body of the anterior tibialis muscle is essential for a quality recording. Preparation is similar to that for an EEG recording. The prepped area for each electrode should be no larger than the size of the electrode used to monitor for PLMS. To ensure quality signals, excess hair may need to be shaved over the monitoring site to prevent electrode slippage throughout a full night of monitoring. A standard EEG electrode should be used and taped over the body of the muscle to be monitored, with a strain relief loop.

To define the body of the muscle, instruct the patient to flex the foot and then place the electrodes over the middle of the anterior tibialis muscle 2 to 3 cm apart or 1/3 the length of the muscle, whichever is shorter. Impedance below 5,000 Ω is ideal, but impedance of less than 10,000 Ω will generally allow for an adequate signal. The EMG channel should be filtered according to the standard EMG configurations, typically with a low-frequency filter setting of 10 Hz and a high-frequency filter setting of 100 Hz. Of equal importance is to complete biocalibrations by asking the patient to flex each foot/raise the toes on each foot separately, 5 times, to confirm adequate signal before lights off (Figure 17-1).

Recording of PLMS can be done in two ways:

1. Two electrodes on each leg that are referenced to each other by placing them longitudinally and symmetrically across each anterior tibialis muscle; this allows for two separate leg channels and is the preferred recording method.
2. Two electrodes on each leg muscle with the signals "tied" to one channel. The "tied" method can be used to conserve channels; however, this may result in a change in the number of limb movements that are detected.
3. Movements of the upper limbs may be sampled, if clinically indicated. The recommended upper limb muscles include the flexor digitorum superficialis and the extensor digitorum communis.

EXAMPLES OF INDEPENDENT AND SECONDARY PERIODIC LIMB MOVEMENT DISORDER

- Proper biocalibration signals for left and right limb movements (Figure 17-2)
- Periodic limb movements without arousal (Figure 17-2A, B)
- Periodic limb movements with arousal (Figures 17-3 and 17-4)

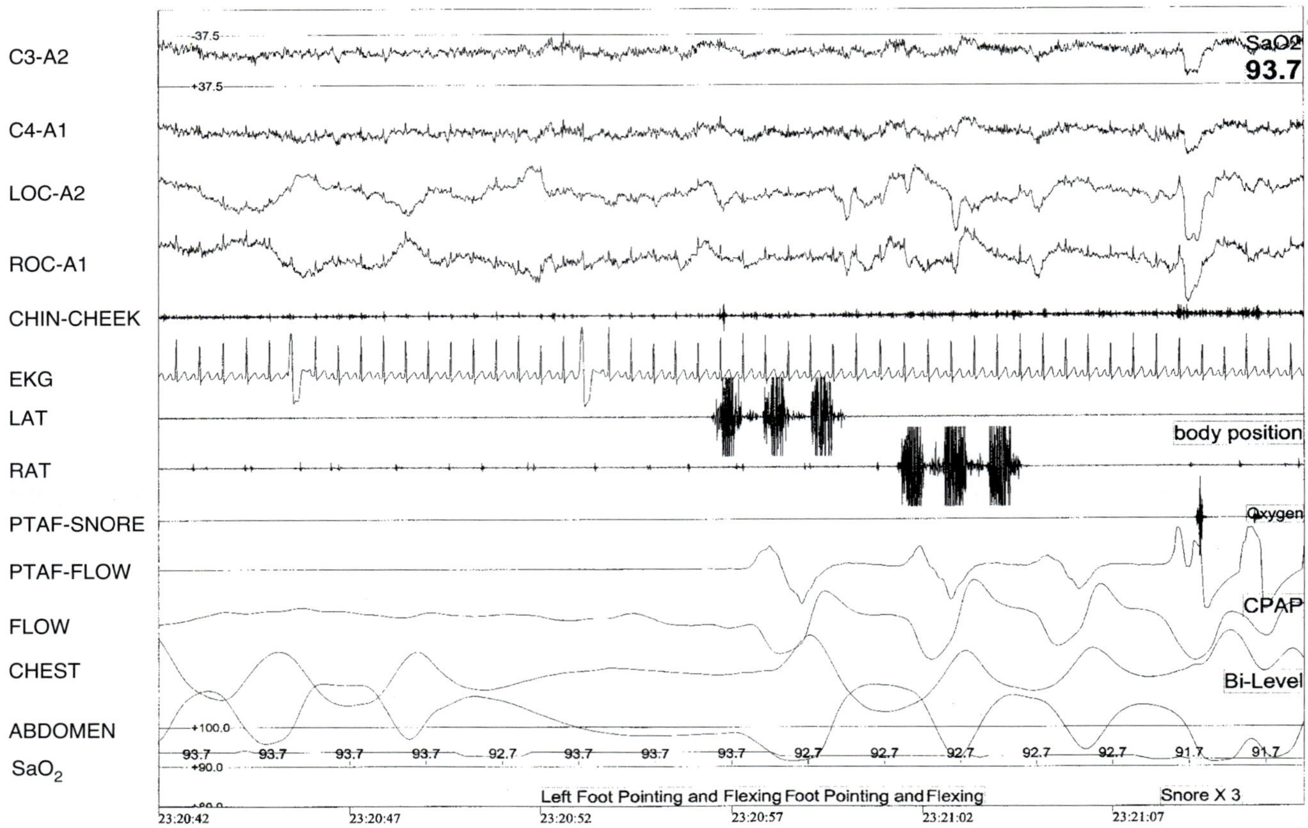

Figure 17-1 A 30-second recording. Correct biocalibration signals are used as a benchmark measure for proper scoring of periodic limb movements of sleep. The patient's electroencephalograph shows wakefulness, as he follows the technologist's instruction to flex the left foot 3 times, then the right foot 3 times.

- Muscle fasciculations and other movements that do not meet criteria for PLMS (Figures 17-5 to 17-7)
- Leg movements secondary to obstructive apneas or hypopneas (Figure 17-8A, B)
- Other movements (Figures 17-9 to 17-12)

RELATIONSHIP BETWEEN PERIODIC LIMB MOVEMENT DISORDER AND RESTLESS LEGS SYNDROME

RLS and PLMD are independent medical disorders, although RLS has a strong association with PLMS. PLMS do not establish the diagnosis of RLS, although they can support the clinical diagnosis.

In contrast, 80% or more of patients with RLS will have five or more PLMS per hour of sleep on a single night of testing (10), and most of the limb movements will be seen in the first half of the night. Although an EEG arousal, as defined by the AASM arousal rule, results in limited sleep disturbances from PLMS, the majority of PLMS in patients with RLS are arousing when other definitions of arousal are used, such as delta EEG spectrum enhancement and heart rate or other cardiovascular variables. RLS can be diagnosed only by patient interview (11).

Most cases of RLS are primary, with the exact cause still not completely understood. Secondary RLS develops as a result of other conditions, such as pregnancy, renal failure, and iron deficiency. Given that iron deficiency can contribute to RLS, measurement of serum ferritin level and iron studies are recommended (11). Also of note is that certain medications, such as antinausea medications and antidepressants, may contribute to RLS. It is also important to consider renal disease, myelopathy, and pregnancy as a cause to avoid misdiagnosis.

Although the exact cause of primary RLS remains unclear, research indicates a strong genetic component, with the condition frequently running in families, particularly when symptom onset begins before the age of 40. RLS is believed to follow an autosomal dominant inheritance pattern in many familial cases, with only one copy of the altered gene from either parent needed to cause the condition. Genome-wide association studies (GWASs) have identified several genetic variants linked to RLS, including *MEIS1*, *BTBD9*, *MAP2K5/LBXCOR1*, and *PTPRD*.

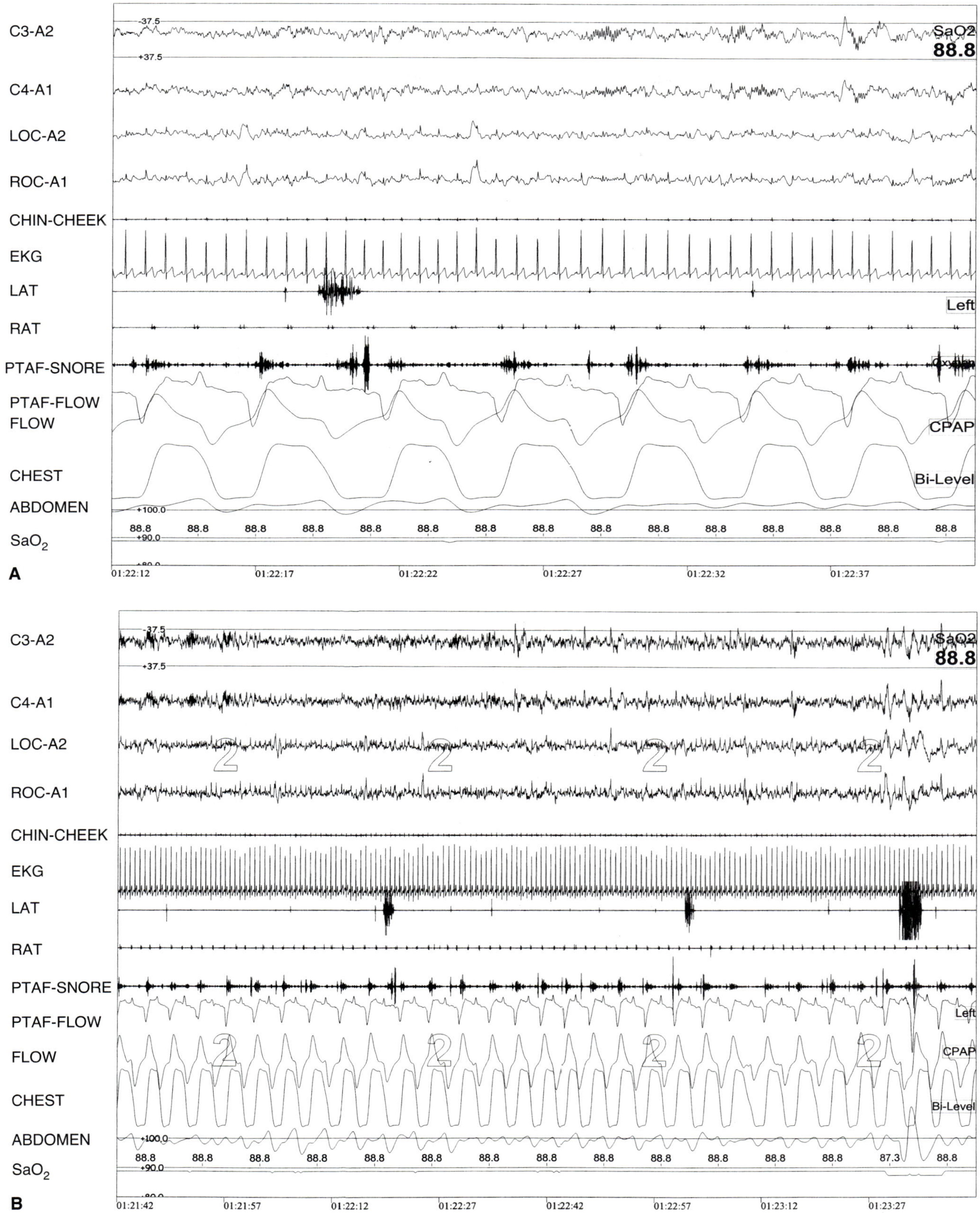

Figure 17-2 Sequence of periodic limb movements recorded in the left anterior tibialis (LAT) channel without evidence of cortical arousal in the electroencephalograph. A: 30 seconds. B: 120 seconds.

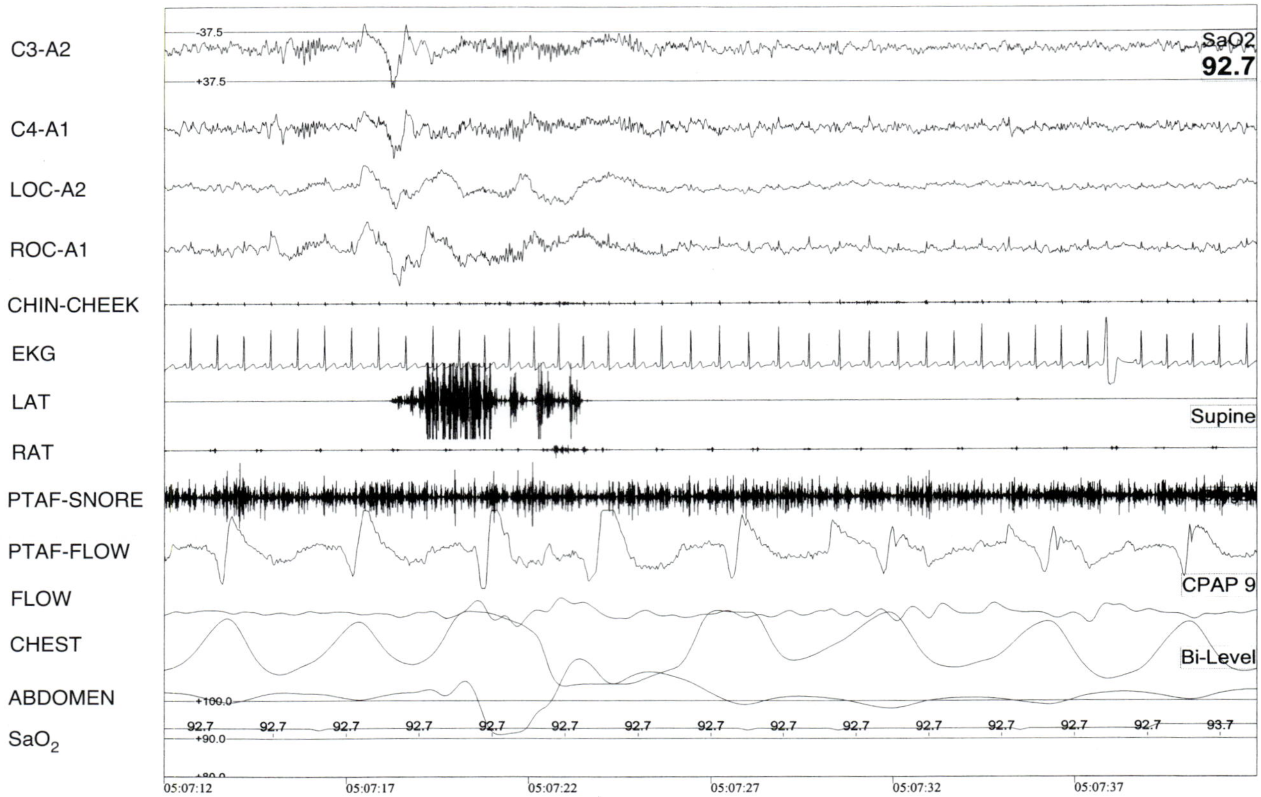

Figure 17-3 A 30-second recording. Movement in the left anterior tibialis (LAT) electromyographic channel, followed by at least 3-second arousal, demonstrated by increased alpha activity in the electroencephalograph following an initial K complex (a "K-arousal").

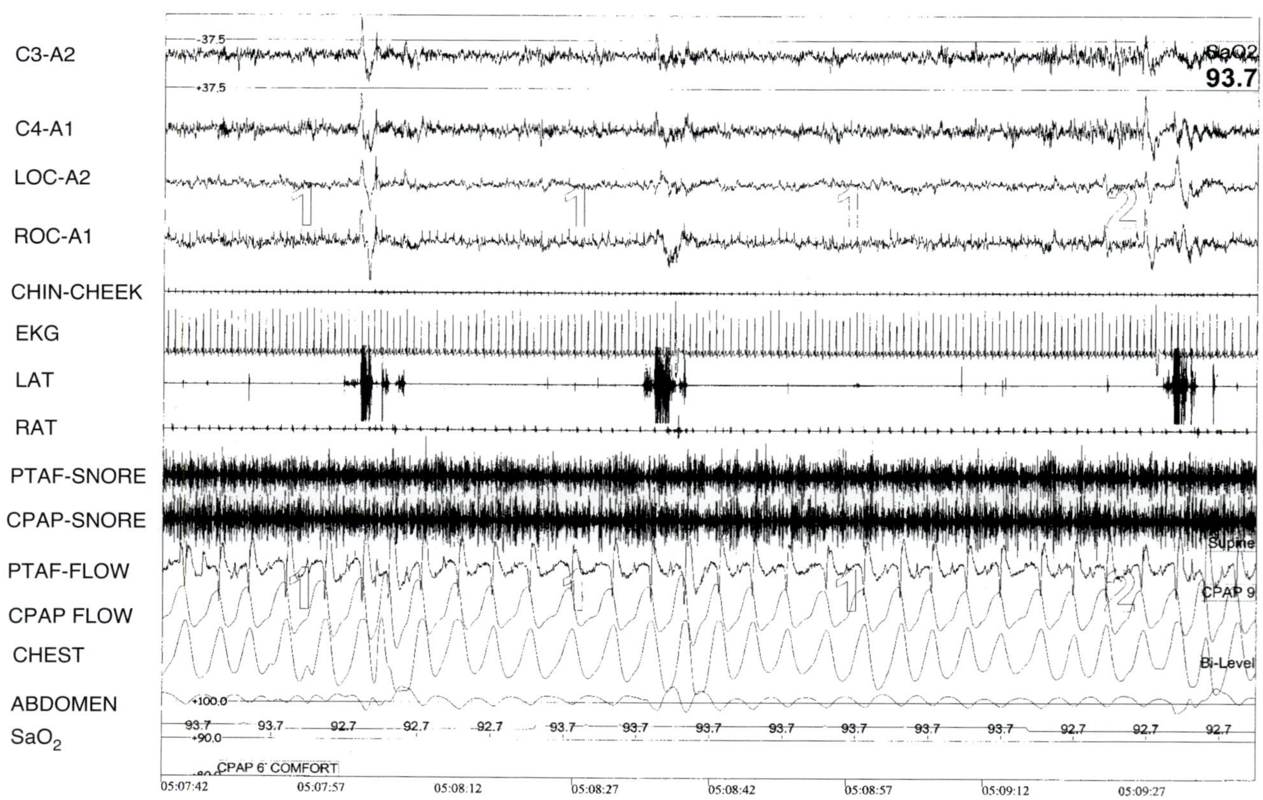

Figure 17-4 A 90-second recording. Periodic limb movements occurring at 40- to 60-second intervals with arousal.

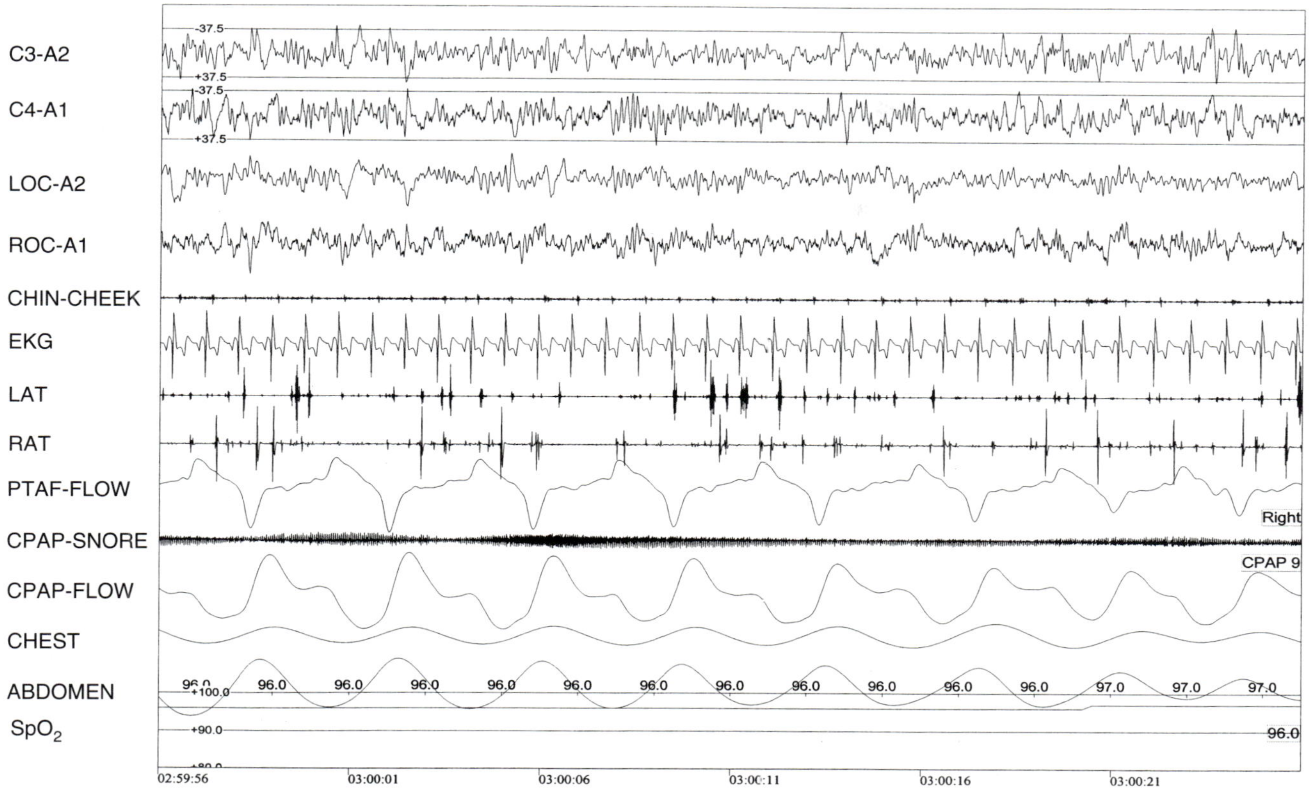

Figure 17-5 A 30-second recording. Muscle twitching activity is present in both leg channels, but these do not meet the requirements for scoring periodic limb movements of sleep.

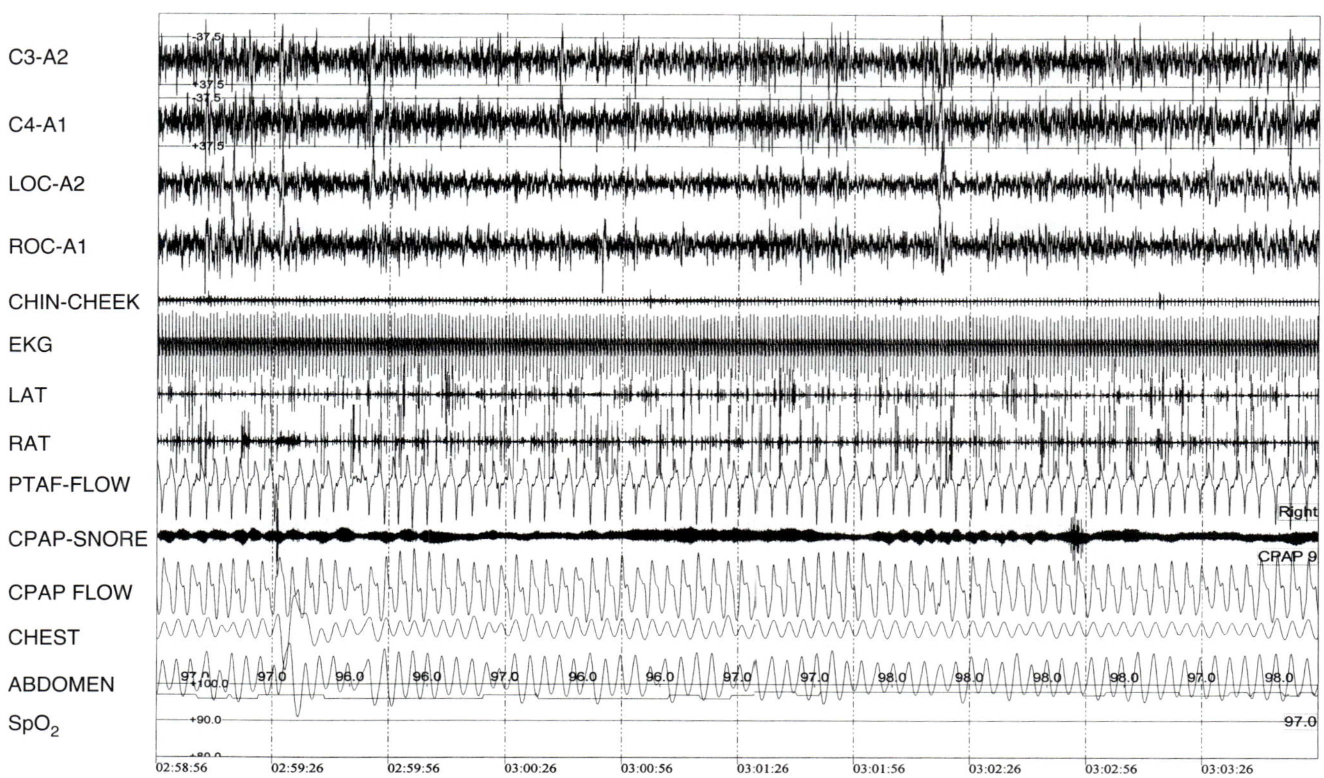

Figure 17-6 A 300-second recording. Muscle twitching recorded throughout the printout. The patient had insulin-dependent diabetes and a history of peripheral neuropathy.

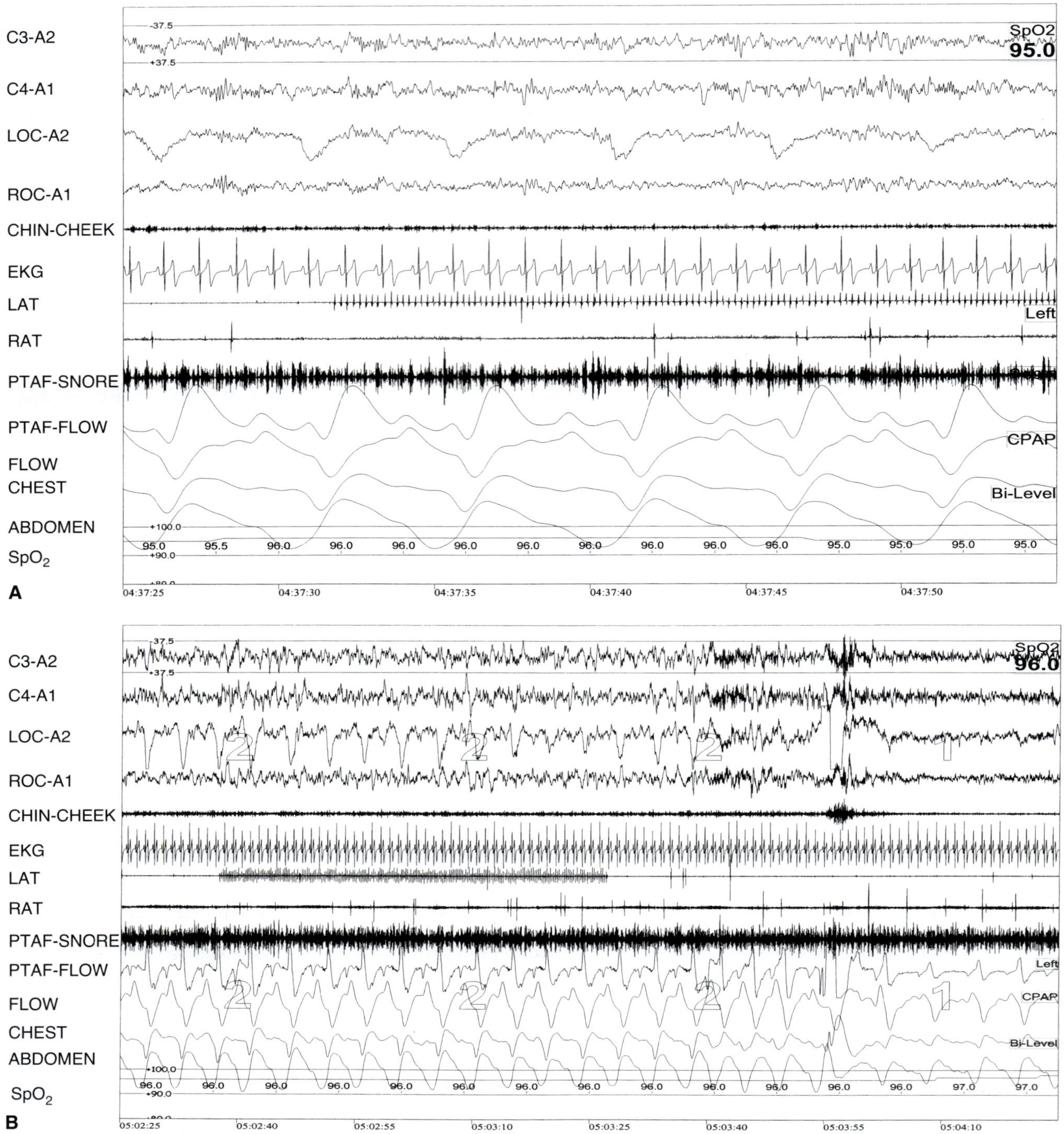

Figure 17-7 Different time intervals (A: 30 seconds; B: 120 seconds; C: 300 seconds), recorded from the same patient of sustained motor bursts that last over 30 seconds and then repeat. Although these appear periodic, the electromyographic activity continues far too long to meet standard criteria for periodic limb movements of sleep. This activity represents fragmentary myoclonus.

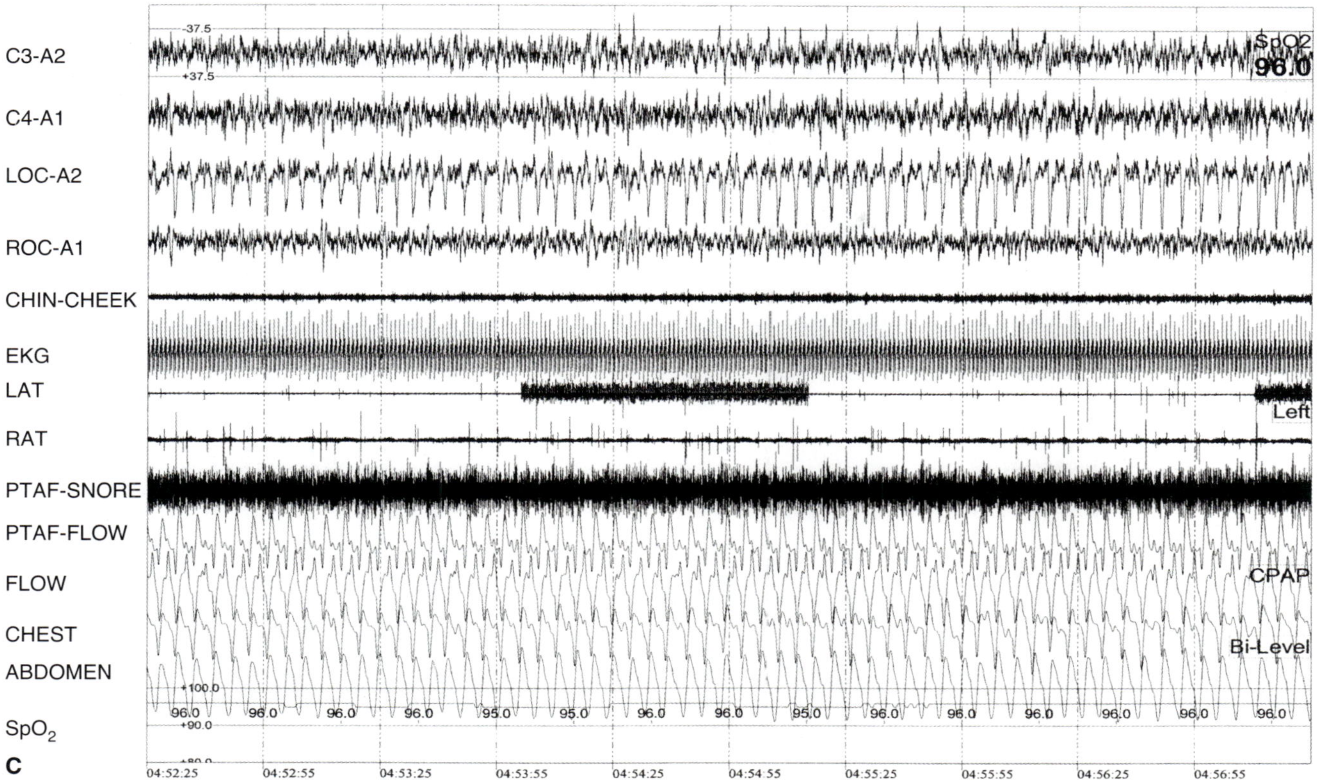

Figure 17-7 (*continued*)

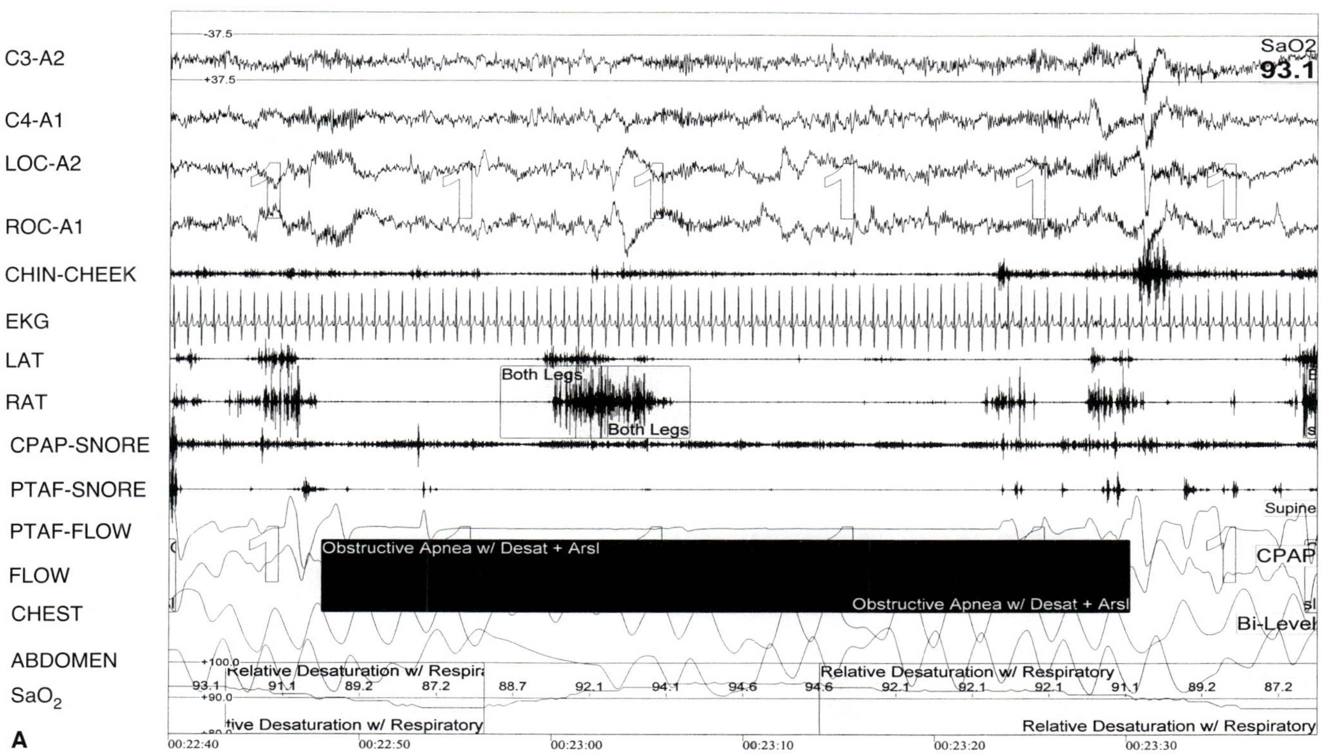

Figure 17-8 A: A 30-second recording. An independent leg movement as well as a movement occurring after an apnea/hypopnea event. It is important to avoid scoring leg movements that occur at the end of respiratory events as periodic limb movements of sleep. B: A 300-second recording from the same patient shows the respiratory events causing leg movements at the termination of the apnea or hypopnea events. In the middle of the obstructive respiratory events, note the presentation of independent limb movements, only a few of which are associated with arousal.

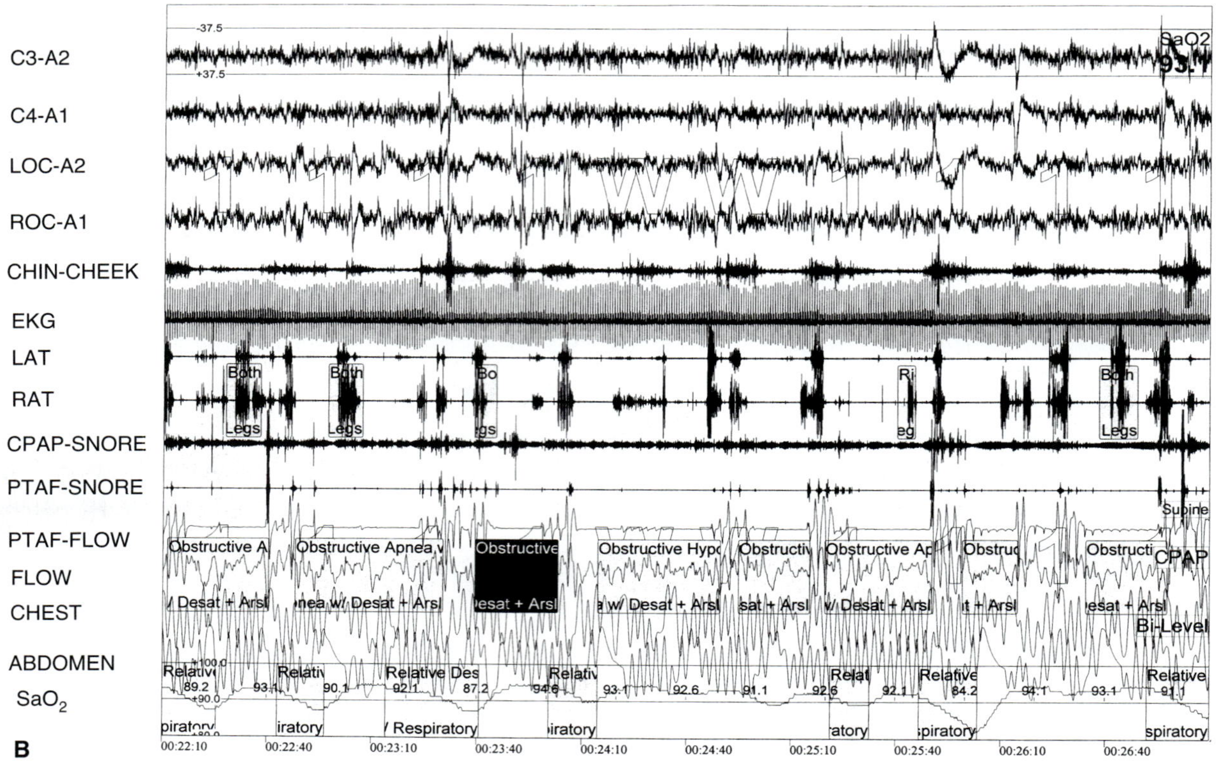

Figure 17-8 *(continued)*

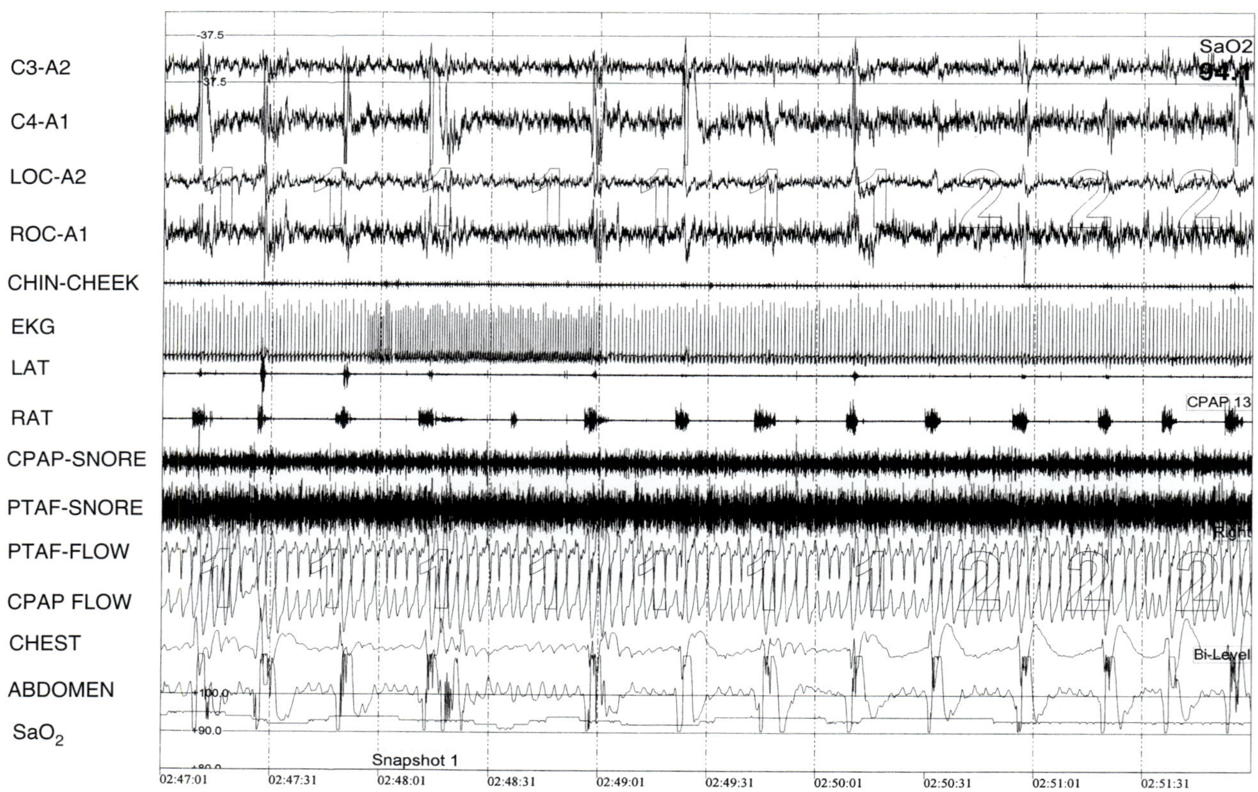

Figure 17-9 A 300-second recording. Patient on CPAP at 13 cm H_2O. Periodic limb movements of sleep (PLMS) are seen in the right anterior tibialis (RAT) channel, but there are also minor changes in the respiratory belt and airflow channels, with mild O_2 desaturations. The limb movements were scored as PLMS, along with intermittent respiratory events. The limb movements did not appear to be related to the respiratory events because increased continuous positive airway pressure (CPAP) levels, as high as 10 cm H_2O, did not change the limb movements.

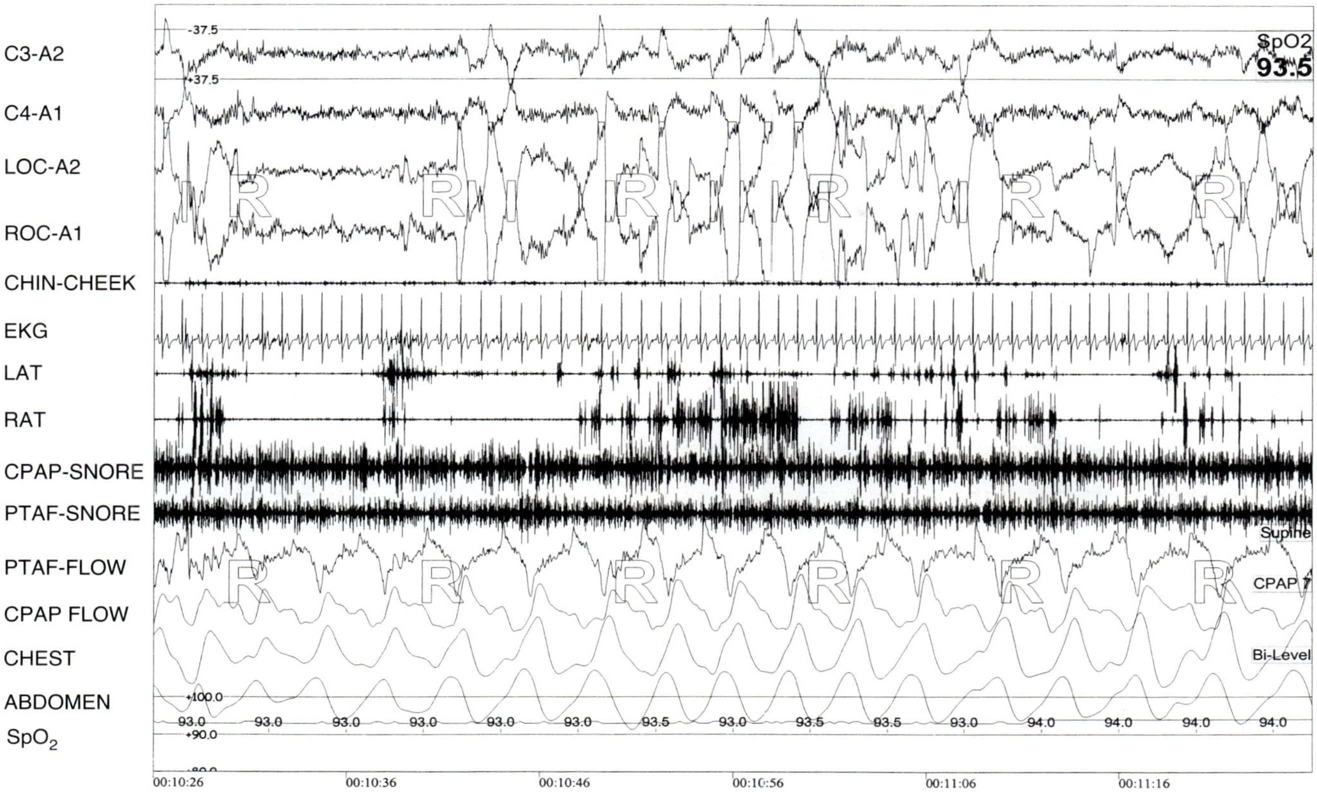

Figure 17-10 A 60-second recording. Patient effectively treated with continuous positive airway pressure (CPAP) at 7 cm H_2O who had rapid eye movement (REM) sleep rebound. Increased motor activity is seen during REM sleep, but the movements do not appear to be stereotypical periodic limb movements of sleep.

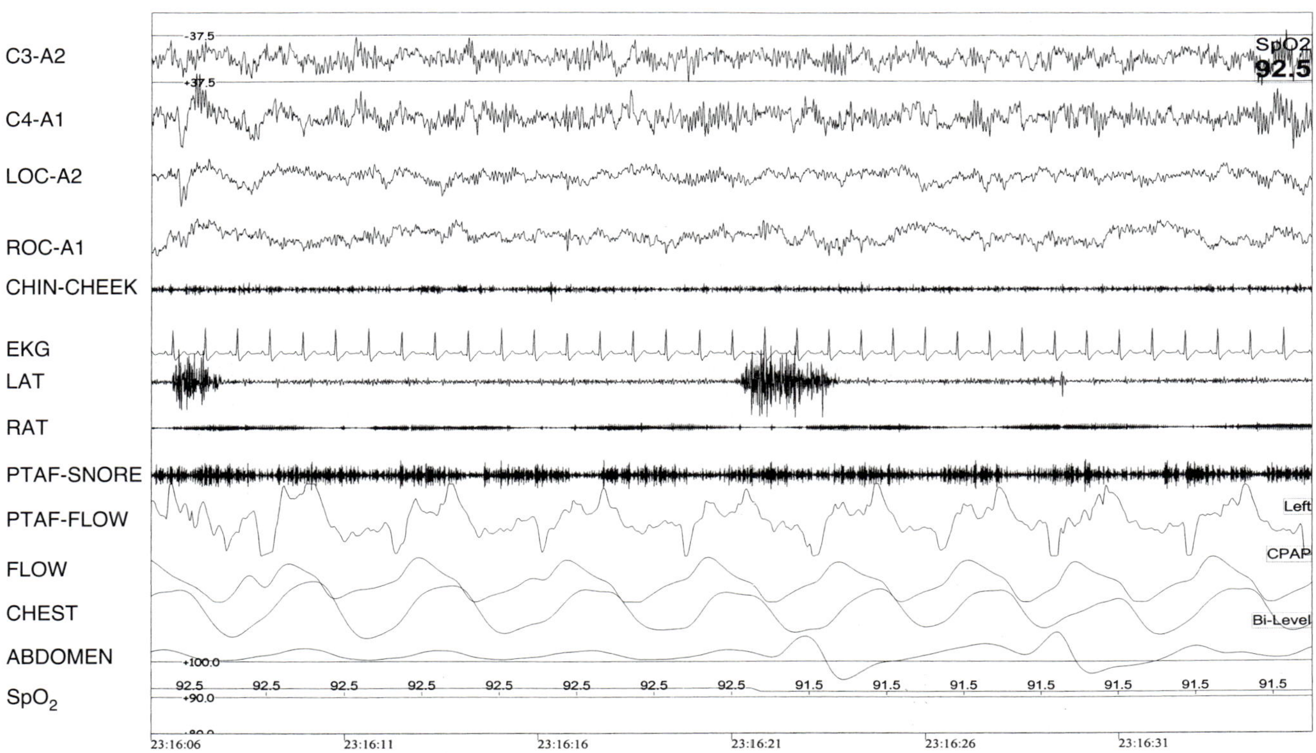

Figure 17-11 A 30-second recording. Periodic limb movements of sleep with mild to moderate alpha intrusion with sleep recorded in the electroencephalograph. The movements were classified as nonarousing events, even with the occurrence of alpha activity because the alpha activity did not change in frequency or amplitude with the anterior tibialis movements.

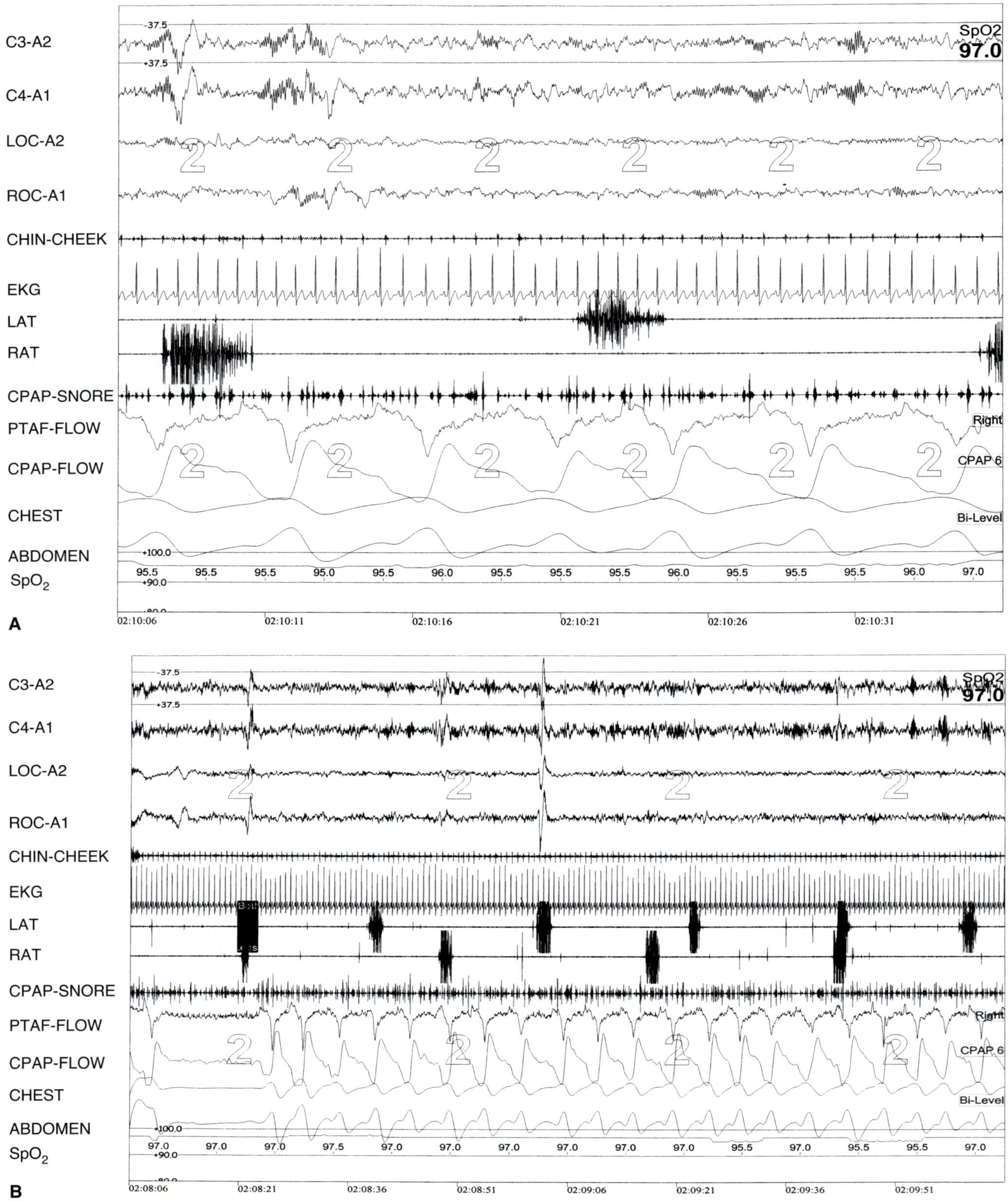

Figure 17-12 A: 30 seconds. B: 120 seconds. Limb movements alternating between the left anterior tibialis (LAT) and the right anterior tibialis (RAT), with some causing arousals and others not. All the movements meet criteria for periodic limb movements of sleep and should be scored accordingly. In B, note the difference in intermovement intervals of the movements seen on the LAT (15 seconds) and the RAT (25 seconds).

The *MEIS1* gene is considered one of the most significant genetic factors associated with RLS and plays a crucial role in the development of neurons and the regulation of genes essential for nervous system function. MEIS1 influences the formation of circuits in the central nervous system that may affect dopaminergic pathways, which are critical in the pathophysiology of RLS. Disruptions in dopamine signaling are believed to lead to the abnormal sensations and the urge to move the legs that characterize RLS.

In addition to its role in dopamine regulation, MEIS1 has been linked to genes that regulate iron homeostasis. Variations in MEIS1 may impair iron transport or utilization in the brain, subsequently affecting dopamine synthesis, as iron is a necessary cofactor for dopamine production. Furthermore, gene expression studies have demonstrated that individuals with RLS exhibit altered expression of MEIS1 in certain brain regions, particularly the substantia nigra. Reduced expression of MEIS1 in this region may disrupt normal neuronal function, resulting in the sensory and motor symptoms observed in RLS.

Understanding the role of MEIS1 in RLS opens new possibilities for genetically targeted treatments that could address the underlying molecular mechanisms rather than merely managing symptoms.

An electrophysiologic monitoring technique, termed the *suggested immobilization test*, can be used to measure PLMW in the 1 hour prior to beginning a PSG (12). The patient sits up in bed with legs outstretched and is instructed to remain still during the recording ("Do not move during the test."). EMG is recorded over the bilateral anterior tibialis muscles. Every 5 minutes during the 1-hour test, the patient is asked to document the severity of any urge to move their legs.

Most patients with RLS discover that the urge to move increases in the last 30 minutes of the test. Occasionally, the most severe patients will terminate the study before 60 minutes of recording have been completed. PLMW are periodic in presentation, but the motor activity recorded by the EMG may last for up to 10 seconds. Patients will often report that the "jerking" is involuntary. Control subjects without RLS have fewer than five PLMW per hour, whereas patients with RLS with moderate or severe disease show 10 or more PLMW per hour. A higher PLMW rate is seen in more severe cases of RLS.

TREATMENT OF RESTLESS LEGS SYNDROME AND PERIODIC LIMB MOVEMENT DISORDER

Treatment options for RLS and PLMD are similar (12). Published guidelines from the AASM (13) and the Medical Advisory Board of the RLS Foundation (13) support the use of dopaminergic agents as first-line treatment in most patients. The approved agents considered "standard of care" for the treatment of RLS include ropinirole (Requip), rotigotine (Neupro), and pramipexole (Mirapex). Other treatment options considered within the "guidelines" of the AASM practice parameters include gabapentin enacarbil (Horizant) and levodopa. Although clonazepam (Klonopin), opioids, and clonidine have been used for many years, it is recommended that these potentially addictive agents be closely monitored and used only after first-line therapy with U.S. Food and Drug Administration–approved medications has failed.

Dopaminergic therapy infrequently causes side effects such as nausea or vomiting, excessive sleepiness, muscle or joint achiness, headaches, lightheadedness, edema, or impulsive behaviors (ie, gambling), thereby limiting their continued usage. One of the long-term risks of dopaminergic therapy is the development of augmentation, a worsening of RLS symptoms. After some months of therapy, patients who develop augmentation report that they need increasing amounts of the dopaminergic medication because of increased RLS symptoms that present earlier in the day, sometimes including a spread of symptoms into the arms or other body parts. There is no specific recommendation for pharmacotherapy for PLMD alone (14).

The discovery of the *MEIS1* gene involvement in RLS has opened new possibilities for targeted treatments that go beyond simply symptom management. One promising area is personalized medicine, where treatments are tailored based on an individual's genetic profile. Since MEIS1 influences both dopamine regulation and iron metabolism, understanding a patient's genetic makeup can guide more effective interventions. Early intervention strategies could also benefit individuals with high-risk MEIS1 variants, especially those with a family history of early-onset RLS, potentially preventing the progression of symptoms.

Another avenue of exploration involves targeting iron deficiency in the brain. As MEIS1 plays a role in iron homeostasis, researchers are investigating innovative ways to deliver iron directly to the brain, bypassing the blood-brain barrier. Emerging therapies include intravenous iron treatments, such as ferric carboxymaltose injections (Injectafer), which have shown promise in addressing low brain iron levels. In addition, novel compounds designed to enhance MEIS1-regulated iron uptake in the brain are currently under investigation.

Beyond traditional dopamine agonists like pramipexole and ropinirole, research is uncovering novel drug approaches with defined targets and fewer negative side effects. One such approach includes the exploration of drugs targeting dysfunction in adenosine pathways, which has been linked to RLS. Glutamate inhibitor, targeting the elevated glutamate levels in patients with RLS, is another approach that is currently being studied.

The role of MEIS1 in neural circuits has also spurred interest in neuromodulation therapies. TMS, a noninvasive brain stimulation technique, may help normalize brain activity related to RLS. In addition, spinal cord stimulation (SCS) is being investigated for its potential to manage severe cases by altering abnormal sensory signals, especially given the spinal involvement in PLMS.

Nonpharmacologic approaches are also gaining attention, particularly those influenced by genetics. For example, CBT tailored for RLS-related insomnia may benefit patients whose MEIS1-related genetic factors predispose them to disrupted sleep. Physical therapy interventions, such as leg exercises, have been shown to alleviate symptoms, with future approaches potentially customizing exercise programs based on individual genetic profiles. Although still in the early stages, gene-editing technologies like CRISPR hold the potential to correct dysfunctional *MEIS1* gene variants, offering the possibility of a cure rather than merely managing symptoms (15).

SUMMARY

RLS and PLMS are common, affecting up to 10% of adults. Although they are two separate disorders, patients with RLS usually have PLMS, but an individual with PLMS on a PSG probably does not have RLS. Because a PSG is commonly recorded in older individuals, PLMS may occur in 25% or more of those undergoing PSG. To determine whether PLMS are significant, an EEG must be simultaneously recorded to identify movements that result in significant EEG disturbances.

Ongoing research is underway that may determine whether PLMS have cardiovascular consequences, including higher rates of hypertension. The clinical relevance of PLMS continues to be studied, although current opinion suggests that symptoms of insomnia or hypersomnia do not frequently become clinically significant when other sleep disorders such as apneas are excluded. Dopamine agonists are considered to be the first-line treatment for RLS and will also reduce PLMS. Looking ahead, the link between MEIS1 and RLS is driving a shift from one-size-fits-all treatments to personalized, precision medicine that addresses the underlying causes of the disorder. This evolution in care promises fewer side effects, better long-term outcomes, a reduced risk of augmentation, and, ultimately, an improved quality of sleep and life for patients.

REFERENCES

1. Allen RP, Picchietti D, Hening WA, et al. Restless legs syndrome: diagnostic criteria, special considerations, and epidemiology: a report from the restless legs syndrome diagnosis and epidemiology workshop at the National Institutes of Health. *Sleep Med.* 2003;4(2):101-119.
2. Coccagna G, Vetrugno R, Lombardi C, et al. Restless legs syndrome: an historical note. *Sleep Med.* 2004;5(3):279-283.
3. Ekbom KA. Restless legs syndrome. *Acta Med Scand.* 1945;158(suppl):122.
4. Symonds CP. Nocturnal myoclonus. *J Neurol Neurosurg Psychiatry.* 1953;16(3):166-171.
5. Ambrosetto C, Lugaresi E, Coccagna G, et al. Clinical and polygraphic remarks in the syndrome of restless legs. *Riv Patol Nerv Ment.* 1965;86(2):244-252.
6. Coleman RM, Bliwise DL, Sajben N, et al. Daytime sleepiness in patients with periodic movements in sleep. *Sleep.* 1982;5(suppl 2):S191-S202.
7. Bara-Jimenez W, Aksu M, Graham B, et al. Periodic limb movements in sleep: state-dependent excitability of the spinal flexor reflex. *Neurology.* 2000;54(8):1609-1616.
8. Zucconi M, Ferri R, Allen R, et al. The official World Association of Sleep Medicine (WASM) standards for recording and scoring periodic leg movements in sleep (PLMS) and wakefulness (PLMW) developed in collaboration with a task force from the International Restless Legs Syndrome Study Group (IRLSSG). *Sleep Med.* 2006;7(2):175-183.
9. Troester MM, Quan SF, Berry RB, et al; for the American Academy of Sleep Medicine. *The AASM Manual for the Scoring of Sleep and Associated Events: Rules, Terminology and Technical Specifications: Version 3.* American Academy of Sleep Medicine; 2023.
10. Michaud M, Paquet J, Lavigne G, et al. Sleep laboratory diagnosis of restless legs syndrome. *Eur Neurol.* 2002;48(2):108-113.
11. American Academy of Sleep Medicine. *International Classification of Sleep Disorders.* 3rd ed. American Academy of Sleep Medicine; 2014.
12. Montplaisir J, Boucher S, Nicolas A, et al. Immobilization tests and periodic leg movements in sleep for the diagnosis of restless leg syndrome. *Mov Disord.* 1998;13(2):324-329.
13. Littner MR, Kushida C, Anderson WM, et al. Practice parameters for the dopaminergic treatment of restless legs syndrome and periodic limb movement disorder. *Sleep.* 2004;27(3):557-559.
14. Vignatelli L, Billiard M, Clarenbach P, et al. EFNS Task Force: EFNS guidelines on management of restless legs syndrome and periodic limb movement disorder in sleep. *Eur J Neurol.* 2006;13(10):1049-1065.
15. Aurora RN, Kristo DA, Bista SR, et al. The treatment of restless legs syndrome and periodic limb movement disorder in adults—an update for 2012: practice parameters with an evidence-based systematic review and meta-analysis. *Sleep.* 2012;35(8):1039-1062.

Chapter 18
Movement Disorders

MATTHEW UHLES

KEY CONCEPTS/LEARNING OBJECTIVES

The key concepts for this chapter include an understanding and classification of different motor events, behaviors, or phenomena that may occur in sleep, polysomnographic findings of these conditions and their utility in diagnosis and differential diagnosis, and the importance of video-polysomnography and other laboratory tests.

KEY TERMS

Motor events
Polysomnography (PSG)
Video-polysomnography (vPSG)

In recent years, it has been increasingly recognized that several different kinds of movements, behaviors, or phenomena may occur in sleep. These can range from various physiologic to pathologic conditions with various manifestations. Some behaviors or movements are more likely to be associated with a specific state or stage of sleep. This chapter includes a fundamental approach to a patient who presents with abnormal events or behaviors in sleep. It focuses predominantly on the roles of polysomnography (PSG) or video-polysomnography (vPSG) and that of the technologist in the differential diagnostic process of "motor events in sleep."

APPROACH TO A PATIENT WITH MOVEMENT DISORDER IN SLEEP

Because many of the disorders associated with motor movements during sleep are sporadic, accurate identification and diagnosis can be clinically challenging. As a result, a detailed sleep and medical history, including general medical, neurologic, psychiatric, social, and family history, all form the foundation for assessing patients with complaints of movement disorders during sleep. Particular attention should be given to the age of onset, time of night, pattern, duration, and frequency of the abnormal motor movement or behavior (1). In most cases, the patient is asleep and unaware during and after the motor event. Therefore, it is often beneficial to include the patient's bed partner or parent (in the case of a child) at the time of the clinical interview. Usually, the observer can provide more detailed observations regarding the motor event and the patient's state of mind immediately following the event.

With the wide availability of personal video recorders capable of low-light recording, home recording may provide the clinician with a detailed illustration of the motor event within the patient's home. Beyond the cost savings and convenience, home recordings offer many advantages over vPSG, including capturing multiple episodes over a longer period of time (2). Numerous studies have reported that trained observers can correctly distinguish between parasomnias or seizure events associated with major body movements using video recording alone. Although most patients/caregivers can produce decent quality videos, the utility is increased when patients or caregivers are instructed on how to best obtain the videos. Instructing them on proper illumination and visibility, as well as recording patient responses after the events, is shown to not only improve the accuracy of diagnosis but also lower family stress levels (2-4). Incorporating motion-activated home security infrared cameras to capture the events also aided in capturing the initiation of the nocturnal events, which are often missed with the use of smartphone video alone (5).

The *International Classification of Sleep Disorders*, third edition Text Revision (*ICSD-3-TR*) lists 10 core categories of parasomnias; however, only one, rapid eye movement (REM) behavior disorder (RBD), requires vPSG as an essential diagnostic requirement (5). Even so, vPSG is useful in distinguishing parasomnias such as sleepwalking or RBD from other disorders such as sleep-related hypermotor epilepsy (SHE) or potentially injurious or atypical behaviors (ie, unusual age of onset, duration, frequency, or occurrence) (1). vPSG should be considered for patients with unusual nocturnal events that are potentially harmful or suggestive of another underlying disorder. Since benzodiazepines or antidepressants may inhibit clinical manifestations, consider weaning patients from these medications before vPSG.

The correlation of an event with the time of the night and the correct sleep stage is essential for the accurate diagnosis of motor events. For example, arousal disorders typically occur in the first third of the night during stage N3 slow-wave sleep (SWS); RBD occurs during REM sleep, usually in the last half to third of the night; epileptic seizures are more common during nonrapid eye movement (NREM) sleep; and rhythmic movement disorder (RMD) usually occurs during sleep-wake transitions.

Today, most commercially available PSG systems provide digital video recordings synchronized with the PSG signals, which helps time-lock motor events to the PSG signals. It also allows for a segment of PSG to be reviewed at varying paper speeds (window durations), filters, sensitivities, and montages, which help detect abnormalities and differentiation from artifacts. The infrared camera is useful for recording nighttime events. Double cameras may be used to capture the face and body simultaneously. The camera should be mounted on the wall or ceiling across from the head end of the bed. An intercom with a microphone near the patient must be available for audio recordings. The monitoring station should have a remote control to zoom or tilt the camera for adequate viewing. Video recordings can be played back in real time or at a slower speed to better visualize and analyze the section of interest. Digital video recordings are the preferred method for synchronized PSG and video data storage for later recall and review. Although the minimum required by the American Academy of Sleep Medicine (AASM) is one frame per second, the digital video should be recorded with sufficient resolution and increased frame rate to allow for adequate visualization during review to differentiate subtle movements and establish proper temporal relationship (6). The standard indications for PSG are outlined in the published guidelines by the AASM. Table 18-1 lists the indications for vPSG (7).

In routine PSG recordings, most laboratories utilize six electroencephalography (EEG) channels (F3-M2, F4-M1, C3-M2, C4-M1, O1-M2, and O2-M1), with electrodes placed in these locations according to the International 10-20 System of Electrode Placement (6). Although the EEG electrodes routinely used in PSG are typically insufficient to accurately identify and localize abnormal EEG activity, abnormal motor activity is often observed in cases where the patient's clinical history does not indicate the possibility of this activity. In these cases, it may be helpful to re-reference from the standard contralateral derivation (F3 referenced to M2) to ipsilateral deviations (F3-M1). This allows for better verification and possible localization of the epileptiform activity. Extending the scalp leads to include the full 10-20 EEG, which is typically required to better identify patients whose motor movements are due to epileptiform activity.

vPSG combines video recording with an extended EEG montage, PSG monitoring, and, at times, additional electromyographic (EMG) electrodes. It is superior to conventional PSG for evaluating parasomnias, nocturnal seizures, and other motor events in sleep because of the increased capability to correlate the observed motor behavior with EEG and PSG variables. The specific montage used varies depending on the indication for the study, the number of channels available for EEG, and the need to record additional PSG parameters. Table 18-2 lists a few sample recording montages that can be further customized as required (8). A study exploring the accuracy of adding T3 and T4 electrodes to the existing six EEG electrodes routinely recorded in standard PSG showed the abbreviated eight-channel montage was only slightly inferior to the 18-channel montage regarding interpreter agreement distinguishing seizure activity from

Table 18-1 Indications for Video-Polysomnography

• Unusual and complex arousal disorders
• Complex behaviors suspicious of RBD but not absolutely certain based on the history
• Behavior and motor events at night suggesting possible nocturnal seizure disorder
• Excessive daytime sleepiness in patients with epilepsy to determine if excessive sleepiness is due to repeated nocturnal seizures, an undesirable side effect of antiepileptic medications, or an associated sleep disorder (eg, sleep apnea)
• Suspected psychogenic dissociative disorder
• Other motor parasomnias, which may be mistaken for nocturnal seizures, for example, rhythmic movement disorder, bruxism
• Involuntary diurnal movement disorder persisting during sleep
• Coexisting second sleep disorder, for example, narcolepsy, RBD, obstructive sleep apnea, or sleepwalking
• For medicolegal purposes, when the patient presents with violent behavior during sleep, video-polysomnography studies are mandatory to evaluate such patients for making a correct diagnosis of parasomnias or seizure disorders.

RBD, REM behavior disorder.
Reprinted from Chokroverty S. Polysomnography and related procedures. In: Hallett M, ed. *Handbook of Clinical Neurophysiology: Movement Disorders*. Vol 1. Elsevier; 2003:145.

Table 18-2 Sample Electroencephalographic-Polysomnographic Montages

Indication	Montage
Arousal disorder, possible nocturnal seizures (36 channels)	F3-M2, F4-M1, C3-M2, C4-M1, O1-M2, O2-M1, Fp1-F7, F7-T3, T3-T5, T5-O1, Fp1-F3, F3-C3, C3-P3, P3-O1, Fp2-Fp8, F8-T4, T4-T6, T6-O2, Fp2-F4, F4-C4, C4-P4, P4-O2, Fz-Cz, Cz-Pz, LEOG-M2, REOG-M1, Chin EMG, LAT EMG, RAT EMG, snoring, PTAF, thermistor, thoracic effort, abdominal effort, ECG, Sao_2
RBD, possible nocturnal seizures (28 channels)	F3-M2, F4-M1, C3-M2, C4-M1, O1-M2, O2-M1, Fp1-F7, F7-T3, T3-T5, T5-O1, Fp2-Fp8, F8-T4, T4-T6, T6-O2, LEOG-M2, REOG-M1, Chin EMG, LAT EMG, RAT EMG, LED EMG, RED EMG, snoring, PTAF, thermistor, thoracic effort, abdominal effort, ECG, Sao_2
RBD, possible nocturnal seizures (38 channels)	F3-M2, F4-M1, C3-M2, C4-AM1, O1-M2, O2-M1, Fp1-F7, F7-T3, T3-T5, T5-O1, Fp1-F3, F3-C3, C3-P3, P3-O1, Fp2-Fp8, F8-T4, T4-T6, T6-O2, Fp2-F4, F4-C4, C4-P4, P4-O2, Fz-Cz, Cz-Pz, LEOG-M2, REOG-M1, Chin EMG, LAT EMG, RAT EMG, LFD EMG, RFD EMG, snoring, PTAF, thermistor, thoracic effort, abdominal effort, ECG, Sao_2
PLMS, extended limb coverage (24 channels)	F3-M2, F4-M1, C3-M2, C4-M1, O1-M2, O2-M1, LEOG-M2, REOG-M1, Chin EMG, LAT EMG, RAT EMG, LPT EMG, RPT EMG, LED EMG, RED EMG, LFD EMG, RFD EMG, snoring, PTAF, thermistor, thoracic effort, abdominal effort, ECG, Sao_2

ECG, electrocardiogram; EMG, electromyogram; EOG, electrooculogram; L, left; LAT, left anterior tibialis; LED, left extensor digitorum; LFD, left flexor digitorum; LPT, left posterior tibialis; PTAF, pressure transducer airflow; R, right; RAT, right anterior tibialis; RED, right extensor digitorum; RFD, right flexor digitorum; RPT, right posterior tibialis.

Modified with permission of Elsevier Science & Technology Journals from Malow BA, Aldrich MS. Polysomnography. In: Chokroverty S, Hening WA, Walters AS, eds. *Sleep and Movement Disorders*. Butterworth-Heinemann; 2003:128; permission conveyed through Copyright Clearance Center, Inc.

nonepileptic activity (78% agreement for eight-channel montage and 84% agreement for 18-channel montage). The eight-channel montage, however, was not as effective in localizing the seizure activity as the 18-channel montage (27% and 49%, respectively), especially in the temporal and parieto-occipital regions (9).

Adjunct EMG channels to record from additional muscles are recommended in some cases. In patients with a preliminary diagnosis of RBD, adding electrodes over the forearm flexor and extensor muscles aids in detecting upper extremity movements. These electrodes are placed 2 to 3 cm apart in line with the lateral edge of the belly of the forearm flexor digitorum superficialis (outside the underside of the forearm) and belly of the forearm extensor digitorum communis (center of the topside of the forearm) (Figures 18-1 and 18-2).

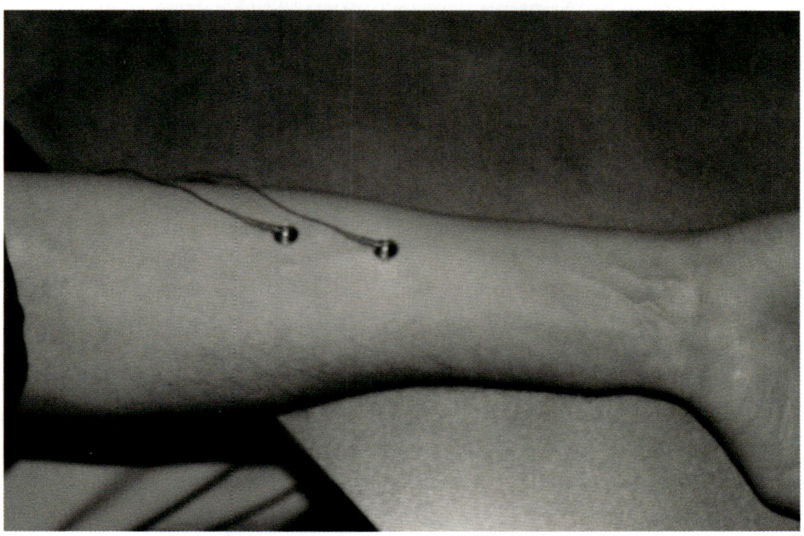

Figure 18-1 Proper placement of electrodes on the forearm flexors, 2 to 4 cm apart in line to the lateral edge of the belly of the forearm flexor (outside the underside of the forearm).

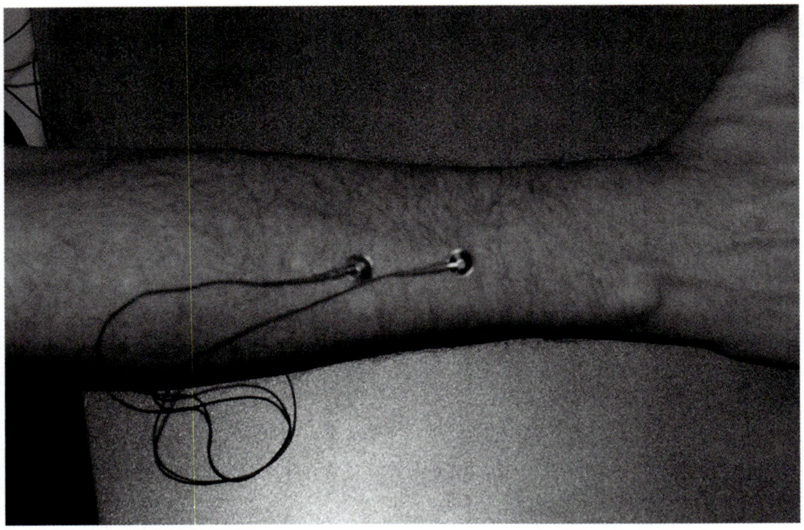

Figure 18-2 Proper placement of electrodes on the forearm extensors for evaluation of parasomnia during a sleep study.

Proper placement can be verified by asking the patient to bend their hand only at the base of the fingers, avoiding bending at the distal joints, toward the palm, and extending the fingers backward without moving the wrists to identify the flexor and extensor muscles, respectively.

Although bruxism can be accurately identified with standard mentalis and submentalis muscles EMG recording, the addition of at least one masseter electrode aids in accurately identifying sleep bruxism (SB). The masseter muscle is best located by palpating the belly of the muscle several centimeters in front of the ear while the patient clenches their teeth. The recording pair can be either a single electrode placed over the center of the belly of the masseter referenced to one of the standard chin EMG leads or two masseter electrodes placed 2 to 3 cm apart in line with the direction of the muscle fibers referenced to one another.

In cases of propriospinal myoclonus (PSM), placing a pair of electrodes along the back of the neck over the paraspinal muscles may be helpful when a RMD is suspected (6). Finally, additional EMG electrodes (sternocleidomastoid, intercostal, deltoid, orbicularis oculi, and rectus abdominis) to record the progression of muscle activation can be helpful in differentiating between organic and psychogenic etiologies.

vPSG may help define and classify abnormal nocturnal motor events and behaviors into different diagnostic entities, as listed in Table 18-3. Frequently, many nocturnal motor events may be mistaken for seizures based on history alone, for example, confusional arousals, sleep terrors, bruxism, RMD, or RBD. These conditions can be diagnosed and differentiated from one another through characteristic clinical features combined with vPSG. Major disadvantages of vPSG are the cost and availability of the study.

INDICATIONS FOR VIDEO-POLYSOMNOGRAPHY

Observation of the EEG and EMG patterns preceding, during, and following the events is important to enhance accurate diagnosis. Unfortunately, because of their sporadic and unpredictable occurrence, nocturnal motor spells are difficult to capture within the controlled environment of the sleep center. The chance of capturing a motor event increases with the increasing frequency of home occurrence of the abnormal motor event. For these reasons, as well as the alterations in naturally occurring sleep patterns of "first night effect," it has been suggested that one night in the sleep center is insufficient for diagnostic purposes for suspected nocturnal motor events. It was reported that a minimum of three nights recorded at home was required to capture at least one nocturnal event (10). Therefore, some sleep centers schedule patients for two consecutive nights to maximize the yield of recording an event when performing home monitoring.

Several studies have reported increasing the likelihood of capturing a nocturnal motor spell during vPSG by priming the patient using a variety of means, including sleep deprivation, medication, alcohol, noise, and baiting (11). Sleep deprivation has long been a standard tool in increasing the yield of documenting abnormal EEG activity in patients with seizure. Due to SWS and REM rebound observed on nights following sleep deprivation, it is suggested that intentional sleep deprivation may increase the likelihood of capturing parasomnias like sleepwalking, talking, or RBD in the sleep center. Blanchette-Carriere et al. demonstrated that sleep deprivation significantly increased the number of sleepwalking episodes captured in the sleep center during recovery sleep. It appears that the younger the age and the more

Table 18-3 Movement Disorders Stage and Characteristics

Disorder	Stage of Sleep	Other Characteristics
Confusional arousals	Predominantly N3, but any NREM	↑ Arousal out of N3/N1 theta/poorly reactive alpha
Sleep terrors	Predominantly N3, but any NREM	↑ Arousal out of N3/often associated with ≠ heart and respiratory rate. Limited recall
Sleepwalking	Predominantly N3, but any NREM	↑ Arousal out of N3/N1 theta/poorly reactive alpha. Limited recall
Nightmare	REM sleep	↑ REMs and mild ≠ heart and respiratory rate. Often associated dream recall
REM behavior disorder	REM sleep	↑ Tonic or phasic activity during REM. Often associated with dream recall
Dissociative disorder	Wakefulness	Wakefulness before, during, and after event
Sleep-related eating disorder	Predominantly N3, also NREM/REM	↑ Arousal out of N3
Bruxism	All stages	Typical electromyographic artifact/audible tooth grinding
Rhythmic movement disorder	Typically transitional sleep, but any stage	Repetitive/stereotyped rhythmic movement
Epileptic seizures	NREM > REM	Sharps, spikes, or slow waves on EEG
Pseudoseizures	Wakefulness	No epileptiform activity noted
Propriospinal myoclonus	Sleep onset	Muscular jerks during transition from wakefulness to sleep
Excessive fragmentary myoclonus	All stages	Brief myoclonic potentials lasting >10 min
Sleep starts	Sleep onset	Sudden, brief, simultaneous contractions
Hypnagogic foot tremor	Sleep onset, N1, and N2	Rhythmic movement of feet and toes
Alternating leg muscle activation	All stages	Brief alternating leg movements
Myoclonus of infancy	All stages	Bilateral large myoclonic jerks in infants

↑=increase in designated measurement or observation; ↓=decrease in designated measurement or observation.
EEG, electroencephalography; NREM, nonrapid eye movement; REM, rapid eye movement.

frequent the occurrence of episodes at home were positively associated with sleep deprivation triggering an episode in the sleep center. Interestingly, they also reported that those who slept walked had greater SWS fragmentation during their recovery sleep (12).

Although there are no controlled studies to date using medications or alcohol to elicit motor events, there are many published as well as anecdotal reports of medications and/or alcohol use associated with sleep-related movement disorders. Presentation of a loud sound during stage N3 sleep for NREM motor events and during REM for REM-related motor events has been reported to trigger motor events (13). Albeit a small sample, the combination of a loud stimulus with sleep deprivation elicited sleepwalking spells in all 10 of the patients in which this technique was attempted (14). In the case of sleep-related eating disorder (SRED), placing a table with the patient's preferred food and drink beside the bedside was demonstrated to evoke episodes of documented sleep eating in 26 out of 35 patients (15).

TECHNICAL CONSIDERATIONS

Patient Safety

The increased risk of injury in patients with unexplained nocturnal motor activity requires that appropriate precautions be incorporated to ensure the patient's safety during a PSG. The most significant risk of patient injury is a sudden motor movement with the patient leaping or falling out of bed. Therefore, the monitoring technologist should remain alert and attentive throughout the recording, remaining vigilant to intervene immediately if they perceive a potential risk to the patient. To reduce response time, locating the patient in the room closest to the technologist monitoring area is recommended. Unfortunately, it is not always feasible for the technologist to react in time to prevent an injury to the patient. Therefore, universal seizure precautions are recommended. These precautions include keeping the bed as low to the floor as possible, removing unnecessary equipment from the room, and maintaining constant observation. Some sleep centers recommend using bed rails or pillows to restrict the patient's mobility during a nocturnal spell. Although these measures can impede the patient from leaving the bed, they can also trip the patient or (in the case of bed rails) even increase the height from which the patient jumps out of bed. Thus, in some instances, these safety precautions may actually increase the likelihood of a patient injury (16). Individual sleep centers must develop their own policy regarding using rails or pillows. Patient injuries from striking sharp furniture corners can be minimized by padding them with foam corners commercially available for nurseries. Any breakable item in the room (lamps, vases, etc.) that may injure the patient should be removed. In extreme cases, such as a history of the patient diving out of bed, padding or a second mattress placed on the floor next to the patient's bed may further reduce the risk of injury.

Technologist Interactions

It is imperative for the technologist to provide detailed notes regarding their direct observation of the motor event. The observation notes should document the stage of sleep in which the event occurred and whether it was elicited or preceded by an arousal or any other stimulus. The technologist should refrain from drawing any conclusions in the notes but should objectively describe the observed behavior. It is helpful to describe the onset, progression, and duration of the event. Describing if the movement was repetitive, stereotypical, or unique is also helpful. If time allows, adjusting the camera to further isolate and highlight the motor event can facilitate classification. Because motor movement cases are sometimes associated with injuries to others, these cases sometimes result in medical-legal issues. Often, the sleep evaluation may precede the injury by months or even years. Therefore, the technologist should approach documentation in these cases with the same detail and rigor as if every case is a forensic one.

Often, the technologist's assessment and documentation of the patient's conscious state after the motor event is the key diagnostic component in accurately differentiating one motor event from another. Immediately following a motor event, the technologist should assess and document the patient's mental status and awareness without posing leading questions that may alter the patient's self-report. For example, following a motor event, the technologist should not ask, "What were you dreaming about?" Instead, the technologist could ask the more open-ended question, "What thoughts or images were you just thinking before I entered the room?"

CHARACTERISTIC POLYSOMNOGRAPHY FINDINGS IN "MOTOR EVENTS IN SLEEP"

Disorders of Arousal (From Nonrapid Eye Movement Sleep)

Disorders of arousal (DoAs), confusional arousals, sleepwalking, sleep terrors, and SRED typically occur during stage N3 sleep. Thus, they are most common in the first third of nocturnal sleep and are more common in children, although they persist into adulthood in approximately 7% of individuals (4). Diagnosis of a DoA is typically based primarily on clinical patient interviews. Patients suffering from DoA generally do not recollect their motor activity and do not usually report dream content correlating with their motor activity during sleep. Due to the potential of amnesia obscuring the patient's recall of the event, interviewing the bed partner or parents is typically helpful. Adults tend to have better recall after an episode than children. In recent years, several questionnaires to support the screening and identification of DoA have been developed and validated.

vPSG is often indicated if the patient has a history of nocturnal injury or to differentiate them from RBD or nocturnal seizures, or if the patient has suspicion of other sleep disorders. Complex motor activity, such as talking, eating, driving, and sexual activity, has been shown to occur during NREM sleep parasomnias. Eyes are usually open during the event, although the patient may appear clumsy and confused (5).

Often, during a DoA, the EEG will be difficult to interpret secondary to artifact from movement, although the event in question should be preceded by NREM sleep. If the EEG is readable, it can continue to show a slow-wave pattern (delta waves) (Figure 18-3). The EEG may also show NREM stage N1 theta patterns, repeated microarousals, or diffuse, slow, poorly reactive alpha rhythm, all indicating incomplete awakening (Figure 18-4).

Confusional arousals are episodes of mental or behavioral disorientation while the individual remains in bed. These episodes typically last less than 5 minutes but can occasionally be more prolonged. If the individual gets out of bed, the episode becomes sleepwalking and often consists of inappropriate behaviors, such as placing their cell phone in the fridge. This may even lead to some dangerous behaviors like walking out into the street into traffic, operating hazardous equipment, or even harming themselves or others. Attempting to awaken the sleepwalker is difficult and may lead to increased disorientation. Sleep terrors are sudden episodes of terror occurring out of NREM sleep initiated by a cry or loud scream and accompanied by fear, confusion, and autonomic symptoms (rapid heart rate, rapid

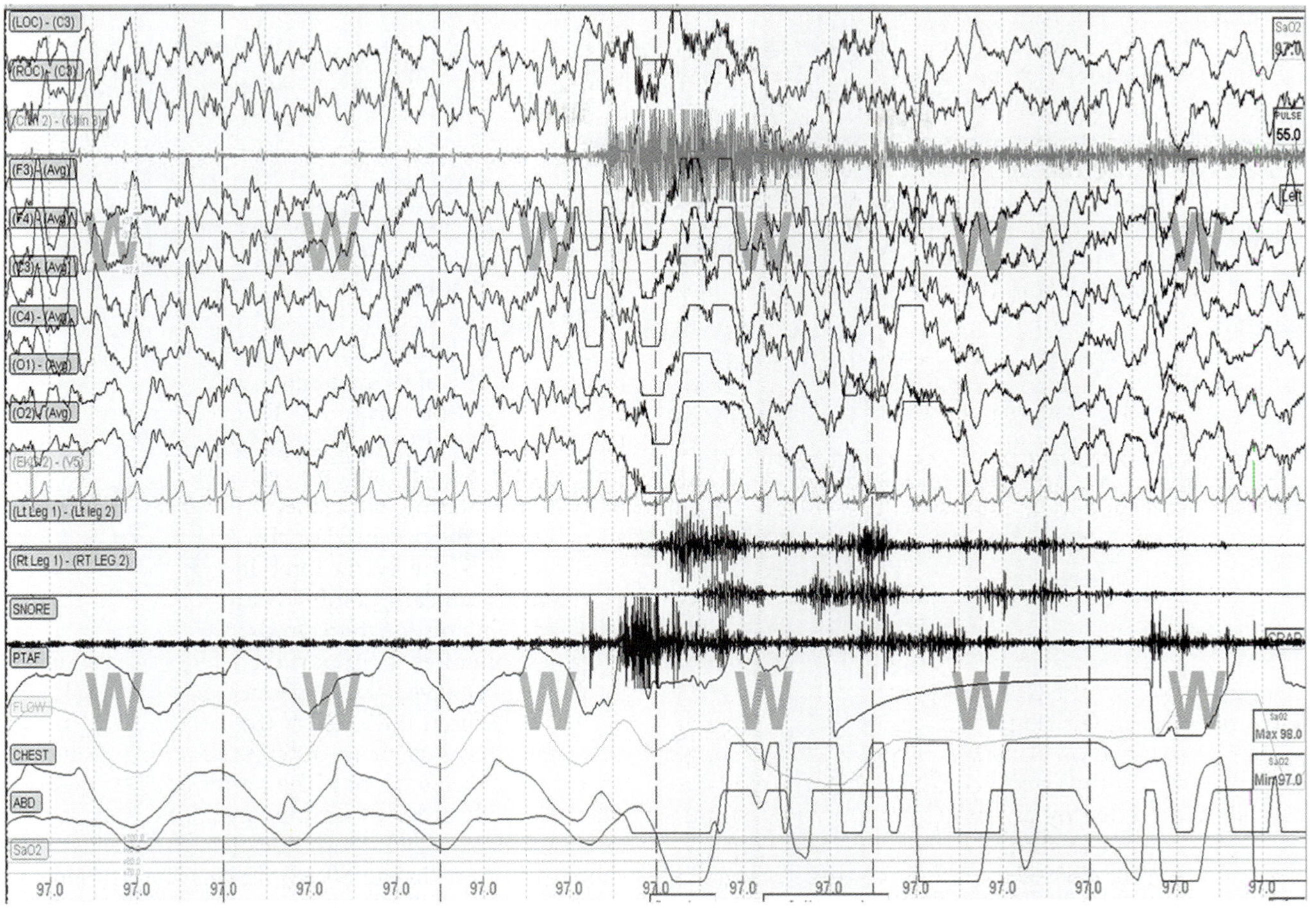

Figure 18-3 A 26-year-old female with a chief complaint of an increase in episodes of sleepwalking, later found to be related to exacerbating factors of stress, sleep deprivation, and drug use. During overnight polysomnography (PSG), an event is captured where she awakens from stage N3 sleep and sits up in bed before later trying to get out of bed to walk. This 30-second PSG fragment is an example of electroencephalogram (EEG) findings that can be seen during a sleepwalking episode. Delta slowing on EEG is seen before the event and persists even as the patient is sitting up in bed and getting ready to sleepwalk.

respiratory rate, and sweating). On PSG, sleep terror, in particular, is associated with tachycardia and increased respiratory rate in addition to the abovementioned EEG findings, which can also be found in other arousal disorders. In contrast to the other DoAs, STs are potentially caused by a dysfunction of the transition between SWS and REM sleep (17).

As one individual may have a history of several different types of DoAs, viewing them on a continuum is suggested. In an attempt to better classify the motor movements associated with DoA, the following classification system has been proposed, looking at simple arousal movements (SAMs), rising arousal movements (RAMs), and complex arousal movements (CAMs). SAMs involve a basic arousal where the patient remains in bed and are further subdivided into (A) head flexion/extension, (B) head flexion/extension and limb movements, and (C) head flexion/extension and partial trunk flexion/extension. The primary feature of RAMs is the patient sitting up with feet in or out of bed. CAMs are characterized by the patient getting up out of bed and walking (19).

Even if the typical episode of motor activity does not occur during the attended sleep study, a PSG is still helpful for identifying arousal disorders by displaying NREM sleep instability or long blocks of stage N3 sleep ending in spontaneous arousals. The association of excessive SWS fragmentation and the abnormal persistence of SWS despite arousals with DoA episodes has led to attempts to quantify SWS patterns predictive of DoAs. Slow Wave Sleep Fragmentation Index (SWSFI) is a proposed index that quantifies the number of AASM arousals that occur per hour of SWS (4). It is proposed that 6.8 or more SWS interruptions per hour for adults and 4.1 per hour for children correlate with a DoA diagnosis. More research is required to confirm

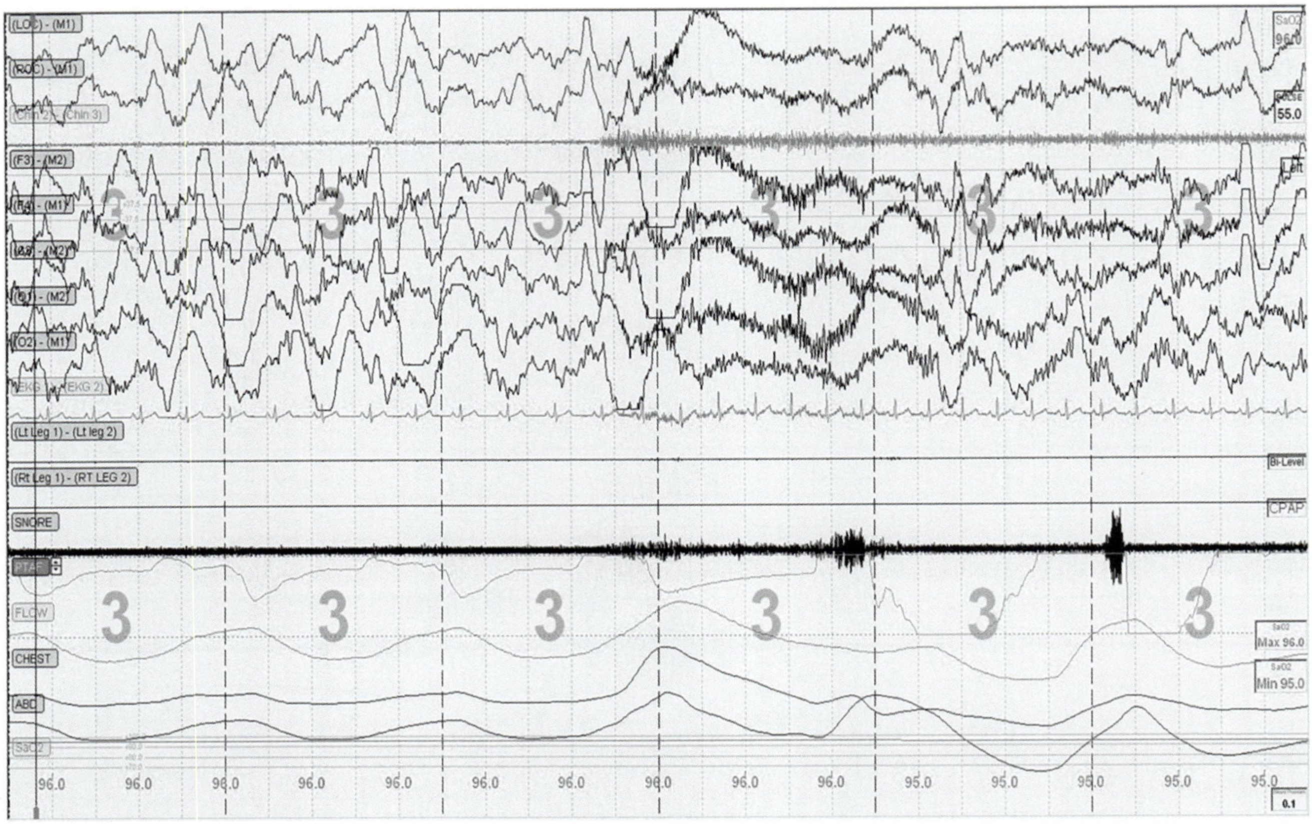

Figure 18-4 A 30-second video-polysomnography fragment is taken from a 30-year-old with a history of confusional arousals. Electroencephalogram during this episode of confusional arousal shows a change from preceding delta slowing to a mixed theta and alpha rhythm during the event, which can also be seen in arousal disorders.

the predictive properties of SWSFI, as other research has failed to show the same connection between arousals from SWS and DoAs. Furthermore, some studies have reported obstructive sleep apnea (OSA) may also be associated with a high SWSFI, but no DoAs (18). The PSG is also helpful in evaluating possible underlying sleep disorders (OSA and periodic limb movement disorder [PLMD]) that could be fragmenting sleep and precipitating the arousal disorder (Figure 18-5).

Sleep-Related Eating Disorder

SRED consists of recurrent episodes of involuntary eating and drinking during arousals from sleep with problematic consequences. Stress, medical disorders, or drug use or withdrawal can trigger episodes. Common characteristics include eating high-calorie foods, binge eating, and sloppy preparation. It can also include eating peculiar combinations of food or even toxic or inedible substances. The most common PSG findings are multiple confusional arousals, with or without eating, arising predominantly from stage N3 sleep but also from all NREM sleep stages and rarely from REM sleep. Sleep architecture is generally preserved, although reduced sleep efficiency has been reported (5). PSG evaluations have been diagnostic of a primary sleep disorder in 80% of SRED cases. The sleep disorder most commonly associated with SRED is restless legs syndrome (RLS). RLS was reported in as high as 77% of patients with SRED, and one study in patients with RLS reported that 33% had SRED. NREM sleep parasomnias (sleepwalking, sleep terrors, confusional arousals), obstructive sleep apnea syndrome (OSAS), and PLMD are other sleep disorders often observed with SRED (17). Another possible trigger is the use of hypnotics, such as zolpidem. Primary SRED is associated with younger patients, with a higher trend toward total amnesia of the episode as opposed to medication-induced episodes. SRED needs to be distinguished from night eating syndrome (NES), which occurs out of wakefulness, with full recollection of the events by the patient. However, a patient may have both SRED and NES (5).

Parasomnias Usually Associated With Rapid Eye Movement Sleep

RBD is characterized by abnormal motor behaviors during REM sleep that lead to sleep disruption or even injury to the patient or bed partner. RBD typically occurs during the second half of nocturnal sleep when REM

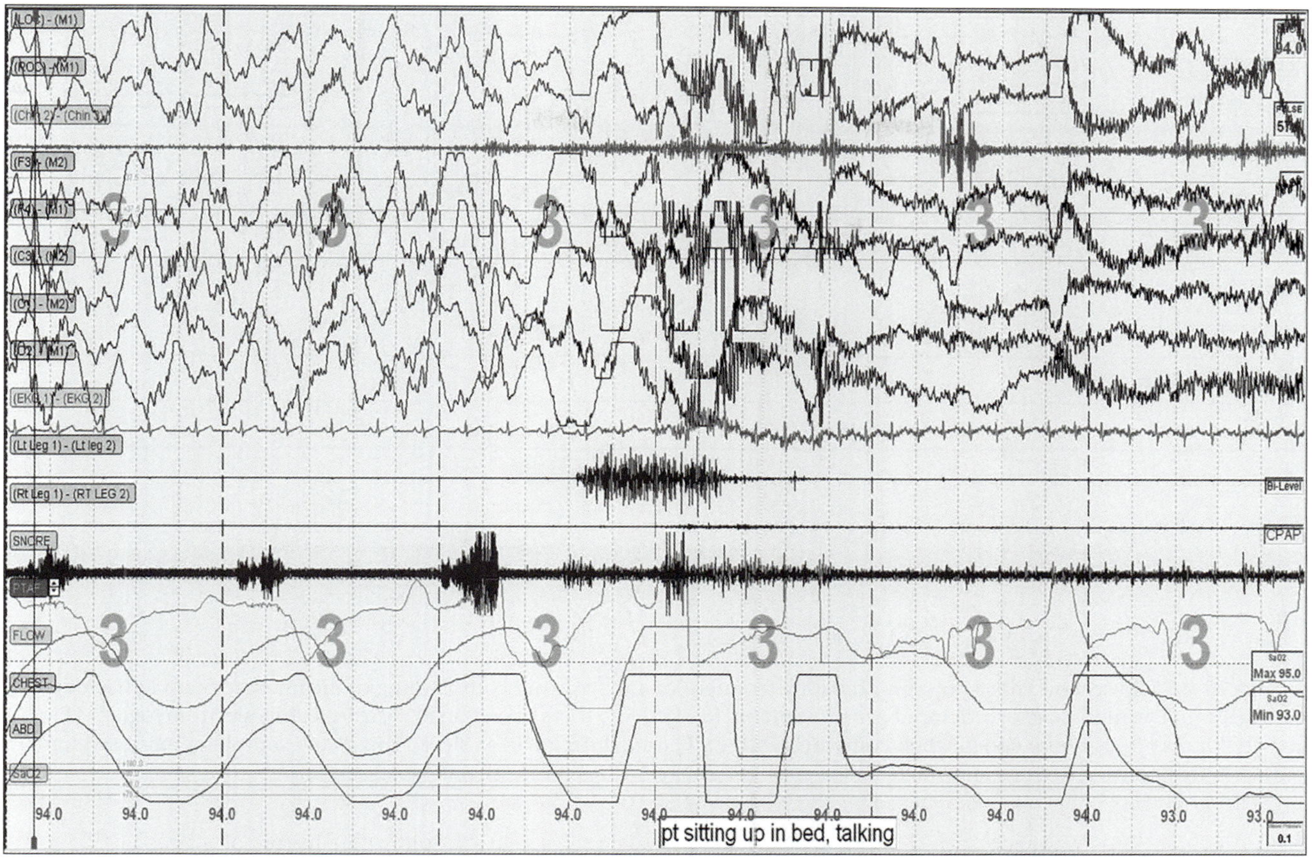

Figure 18-5 A 30-second video-polysomnography fragment of a 24-year-old patient with a history of sleepwalking and snoring. It displays an obstructive respiratory event (respiratory effort–related arousal) leading to arousal from stage N3 sleep and subsequent sleep talking and motor activity. Once the obstructive sleep apnea was treated with continuous positive airway pressure (CPAP), sleepwalking events disappeared in this patient.

sleep is more prevalent. In contrast to DoAs, the patient will often remember dream content related to the motor activity displayed. The episodes are typically brief with rapid return to alertness or sleep. The characteristic abnormal behavior emerges from REM sleep, and the video may capture excessive limb movements, which may be rhythmic or arrhythmic. Common RBD actions during sleep include laughing, yelling, swearing, grabbing, punching, kicking, jumping, or running during sleep. The eyes are usually closed during the event, and the patient rarely leaves the bedroom during an event. Episodes can vary in frequency from once every several months to as many as several times during the night (5).

A PSG may document an excessive amount of sustained EMG activity (tonic activity) in the chin or limbs when there is an epoch of REM sleep with at least 50% chin EMG amplitude greater than the minimum amplitude seen in NREM sleep (Figure 18-6). Other times, tonic activity is normal, but excessive transient muscle activity (phasic activity) in REM sleep is abnormally high (Figure 18-7). This is defined when at least 50% of "mini-epochs" (3 seconds in duration) contain bursts of muscle activity lasting 0.1 to 5 seconds in duration, with EMG being at least 4 times higher than background EMG activity (6). Some patients almost exclusively have arm and hand movements during REM sleep, indicating the need for both upper extremity and lower extremity EMG monitoring for complete evaluation of RBD. The anterior tibialis, extensor digitorum, and forearm flexor muscles are typically used when measuring EMG from four limbs.

To meet the criteria for RBD, the abovementioned PSG findings must be in addition to either a clinical history of dream enactment behavior or complex motor behaviors noted during an overnight attended sleep study. When suspicious PSG findings without the aforementioned clinical history or complex behaviors are pointed out during the recording, it is consistent with REM sleep without atonia, also referred to as "subclinical" or "prodromal" RBD. Many of these patients (at least 25%) will eventually develop RBD (5). The use of antidepressants such as serotonin reuptake inhibitors and tricyclic antidepressants can cause PSG findings of REM sleep without atonia. REM sleep percentage and latency

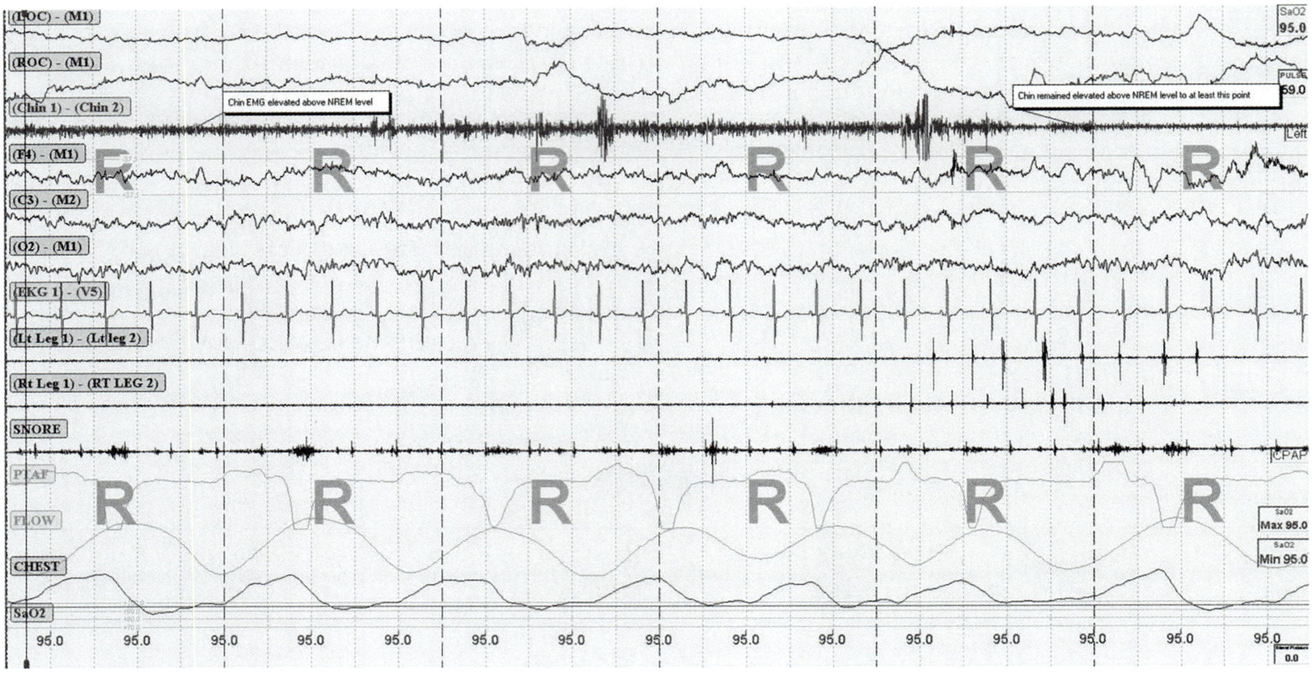

Figure 18-6 A 30-second video-polysomnography fragment of a 62-year-old complaining of dream enactment behavior during sleep. During this epoch of rapid eye movement (REM) sleep, there is sustained increased chin electromyogram (EMG) activity for over 50% of the epoch when compared with EMG tone during NREM sleep. This is an example of increased tonic muscle activity during REM sleep, which can be seen in patients with REM sleep behavior disorder.

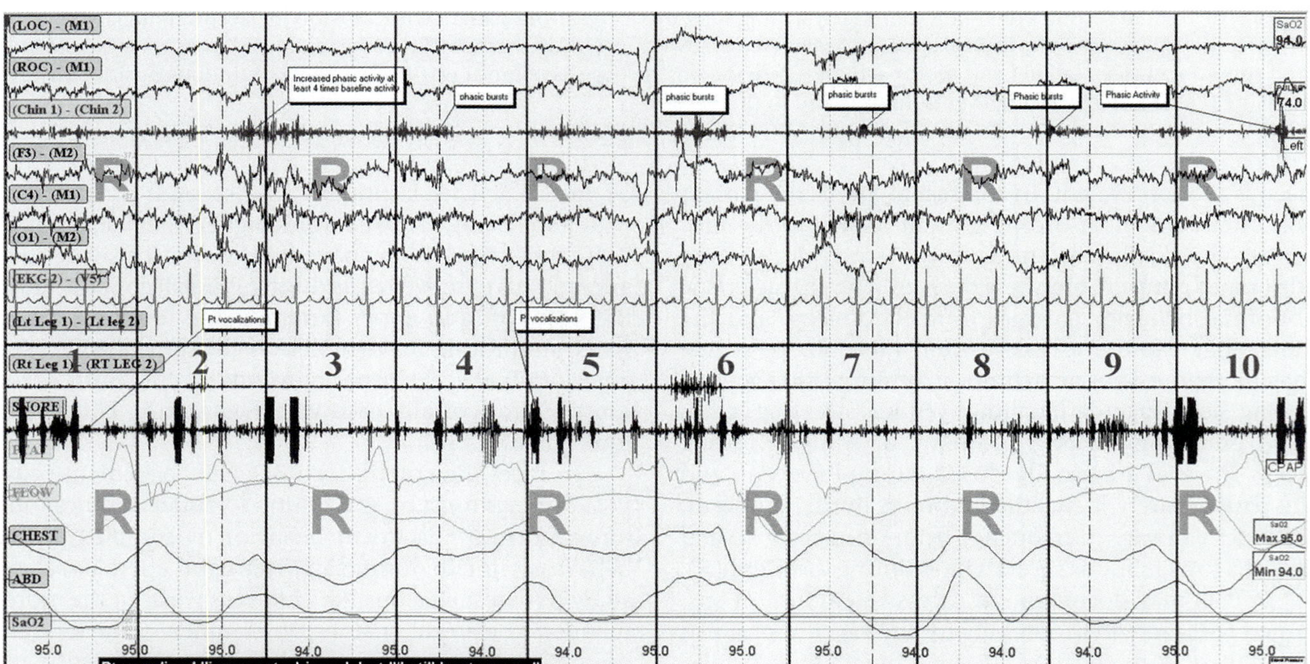

Figure 18-7 A 30-second video-polysomnography fragment from a 58-year-old with dream enactment behavior and vocalizations during sleep. There is an increase in excessive transient muscle activity during rapid eye movement (REM) sleep noted in this epoch, consistent with increased phasic muscle activity during REM sleep, which can be seen in patients with REM sleep behavior disorder. Electromyogram (EMG) tone was greater than 4 times the background EMG tone accompanied by vocalizations from the patient. The epoch has been segmented into 10 (3 seconds) fragments for better visualization of the scoring rules.

are usually preserved, although many patients with RBD have a higher percentage of stage N3 sleep. Autonomic nervous system activation is uncommon during REM sleep in RBD. Approximately 75% of patients with RBD have periodic limb movements in sleep (PLMS) during NREM sleep (5).

Polysomnography Findings in Sleep-Related Movement Disorder

Sleep Bruxism

Sleep bruxism (SB) is defined in the *ICSD-3-TR* as the presence of regular or frequent tooth-grinding sounds occurring during sleep with the presence of either abnormal tooth wear consistent with teeth grinding or transient morning jaw muscle pain or fatigue, headache, or jaw locking upon awakening. It can also cause sleep disturbance for the patient and the bed partner, as the tooth-grinding sounds can be loud. There is high individual variability in the intensity and length of bruxism during sleep. However, the intensity and frequency do not correlate with clinical signs and symptoms, such as headaches or jaw pain. There is evidence suggesting a correlation between bruxism and stress and anxiety in both adults and children. Caffeine or cigarette use in the hours before sleep also increases the chance of bruxism. Bruxism is more common in childhood (14%-17%) and decreases in prevalence over the lifespan. SB does tend to run in families, with 20% to 50% of affected individuals having at least one direct family member affected (5).

The diagnosis of SB is based on history and an orofacial examination. Still, a PSG may be indicated to demonstrate the disorder or exclude associated respiratory disturbance, RBD, night terrors, faciomandibular myoclonus, or epilepsy. In routine PSG recordings, bruxism is suggested by a typical EMG artifact recorded on EEG derivations, especially those referred to ear or mastoid electrodes. In addition to the routine chin EMG leads placed, masseter EMG electrodes may be added to identify bruxism better.

Traditionally, in routine PSG recordings, bruxism episodes have not been quantified but instead were reported by the technologist's comments and description. Current criteria define bruxism events as either phasic (brief) or tonic (sustained) increases in the chin EMG activity, which is at least double the existing background activity of the chin EMG channel. If the events are phasic, at least three bursts of increased activity, each 0.25 to 2 seconds in duration. These phasic events are also called "rhythmic masticatory muscle activity" (Figure 18-8). For tonic bruxism episodes, the chin EMG activity must be maintained for at least 2 seconds in duration (6). Care should be given to distinguish sustained increases in chin EMG because of bruxism events as opposed to sustained chin EMG activity due to arousals. The technologist can further clarify by documenting

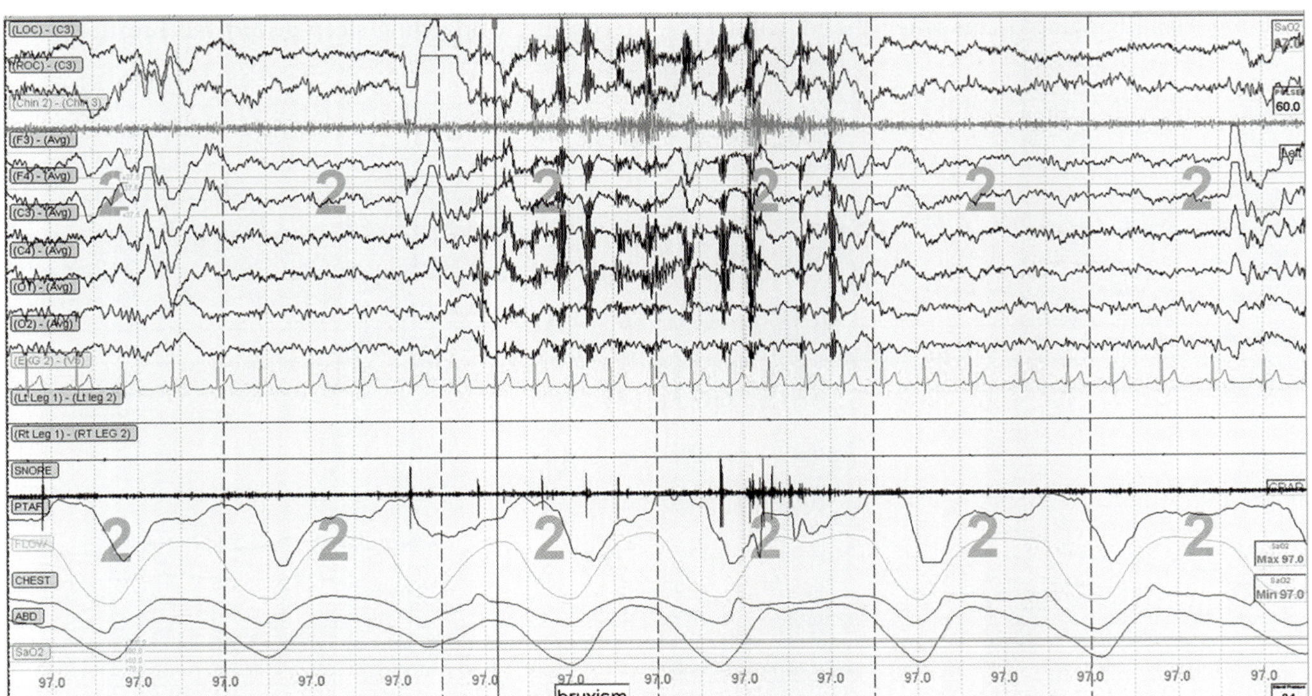

Figure 18-8 A 30-second video-polysomnography fragment showing rhythmic masticatory muscle activity of bruxism. There are several bursts of increased chin electromyogram activity, each lasting 0.25 to 2 seconds in duration. Audible teeth grinding was noted by the technician.

audio or video verification of teeth grinding. Whether they are phasic or tonic bruxism events, the criteria require at least 3 seconds of stable reduced EMG activity before scoring another episode of bruxism. Bruxism can be scored reliably by audio in combination with a PSG by at least two audible tooth-grinding episodes per night in the absence of epilepsy. SB can occur during all sleep stages but is most common in stages N1 and N2 sleep (6). There is sometimes an increase in respiratory amplitude preceding the bruxism. Monitoring SB with ambulatory recordings has also been described (19).

Sleep-Related Rhythmic Movement Disorder

This disorder consists of repetitive, stereotyped, and rhythmic motor behaviors (not tremors) that involve large muscle groups and occur predominantly during drowsiness or sleep (5). In susceptible individuals, they may also occur during quiet relaxation. It is typically seen in infants and children and usually resolves by 10 years of age. It can persist in older individuals, especially those with developmental disabilities or other neurologic disorders, and has been associated with attention deficit disorder. There is a male predominance and a childhood prevalence of 5% to 15%. It comprises several subtypes, for example, body rocking, head banging, or head rolling. Leg-banging and leg-rolling types and combinations of the subtypes mentioned earlier are also described. Body rocking consists of whole-body or torso rocking when the individual is on their hands and knees or sitting. Head banging occurs when the individual is prone to repeatedly lifting the head and often banging the head on a pillow, mattress, or headboard. These may rarely result in severe injuries, including fractures, subdural effusions, and eye injuries. Head rolling usually occurs while the patient is supine with side-to-side head movements. The behaviors are usually more disruptive to family members or bed partners because of the noise and disruption to their sleep. The movements typically occur near sleep onset, although they may occur at other times of quiet wakefulness during the day (5).

The movements occur in clusters, with rhythmic movements repeating at a frequency of 0.5 to 2.0 per second with a minimum amplitude of 2 times the background EMG activity. There must be a minimum of four individual movements to make a cluster. A cluster usually lasts less than 15 minutes (Figure 18-9). If head banging is suspected, surface EMG electrodes can be placed on the paraspinal muscles on the back of the neck. Subjects are usually unresponsive during the episodes and amnestic of their occurrence on awakening. In infants and very young children, it may need to be differentiated from bruxism or thumb sucking. Rarely, PLMD produces similar features. Sleep-related RMD needs to be differentiated from seizures, which can be difficult by history alone. PSG recording shows the presence of rhythmic movement artifact primarily in the immediate presleep period and during light NREM sleep stages, particularly in association with stage N2 sleep. The activity has rarely been recorded in stage N3 sleep or REM sleep (5). The diagnoses can be confirmed by vPSG recording. Underlying sleep-disordered breathing may

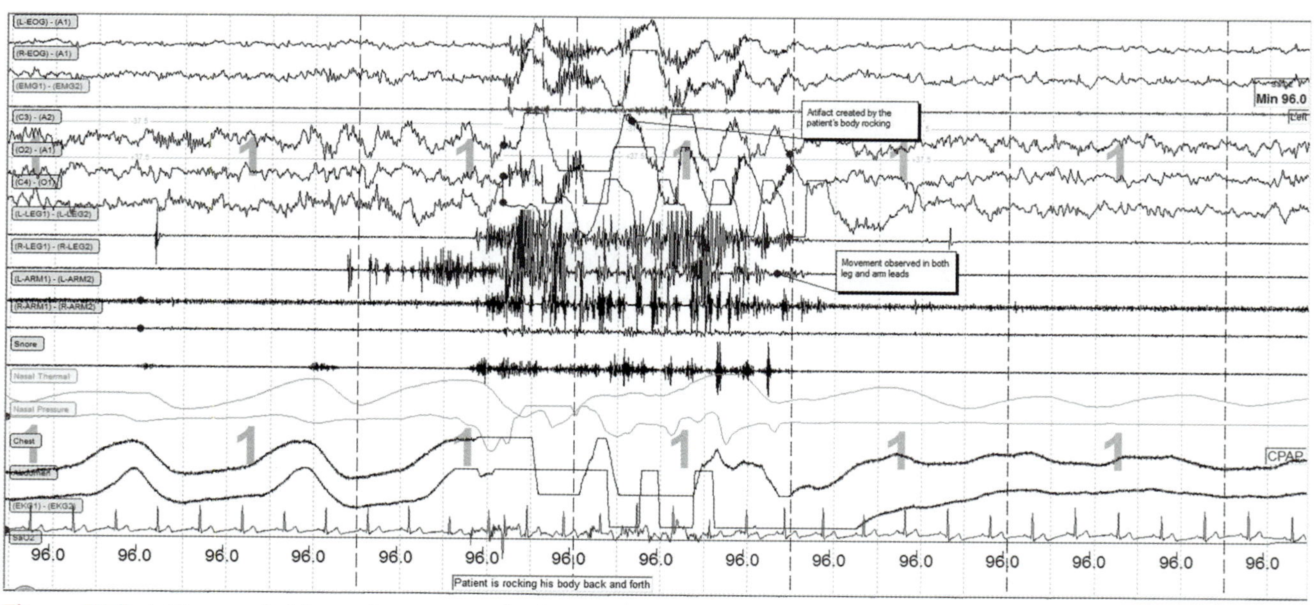

Figure 18-9 A 30-second video-polysomnography fragment in a 45-year-old male patient with a history of snoring and daytime sleepiness. The tracing displays one of many episodes of the patient rocking back and forth during brief arousals from sleep. These episodes were noted to occur out of stage N1, N2, and even rapid eye movement sleep. Episodes typically lasted from 3 to 15 seconds, although there were longer periods of rocking associated with prolonged wake periods.

also contribute to RMD, and continuous positive airway pressure treatment may reduce the motor activity. RMD can also be seen in patients with RLS as a means to help relieve leg discomfort or in patients who are narcoleptic who are trying to end episodes of sleep paralysis.

Polysomnography Findings in Epileptic and Nonepileptic Seizures

Epileptic Seizures

The close relationship between sleep and epilepsy has long been realized, and seizures were even classified according to the time of the occurrence into diurnal, nocturnal, and diffuse types. Several mechanisms have been proposed to explain this relationship, including the widespread neuronal synchronization in NREM sleep, which is conducive to the generation and propagation of discharges, the arousal mechanisms that may facilitate seizures by exacerbation of cortical hyperexcitability (as seen in juvenile myoclonic epilepsy and generalized tonic-clonic seizures on awakening, where seizures occur shortly after awakening), and, finally, the role of the anatomic substrate (eg, in patients with frontal lobe epilepsy, most seizures occur in sleep, whereas in patients with temporal lobe epilepsy, most seizures occur in wakefulness). A seizure that occurs primarily or exclusively during sleep is called sleep-related epilepsy (SRE). SRE can be subdivided into sleep-associated epilepsies (those that occur exclusively or almost exclusively during sleep), sleep-accentuated epilepsies (those that consistently show increased epileptiform activity during sleep), and awakening epilepsies (those that occur during the period immediately after an awakening). Interestingly, REM sleep appears to have a protective mechanism for epilepsy, as it is extremely rare to observe epileptiform activity during REM sleep.

The diagnostic pathway to differentiate suspected nocturnal motor behavior of epilepsy origin begins with a thorough clinical history, followed by questionnaires and the patient or caregiver maintaining a diary documenting bedtimes, time of events and descriptions, any observed potential triggers, recall after the event, and wake-up times. Home video monitoring can be exceptionally useful and ultimately a night in the sleep center with a montage that includes additional scalp leads and arm leads (3).

Description of Different Types of Seizures

Sleep-Associated Epilepsies

Sleep-Related Hypermotor Epilepsy

SHE, formerly known as nocturnal frontal lobe epilepsy (NFLE), was renamed since not all SHE episodes originate from the frontal lobe. SHE may present as brief stereotypical movements predominantly during sleep or after an arousal. It predominates in males, and seizures are typically observed between 10 and 16 years of age (20). Seizures occur mainly during stages N1 and N2 sleep, typically lasting 1 to 2 minutes. Sleep EEG only detects ictal and interictal epileptiform discharges in approximately 50% of patients (3). Marked autonomic activation is a common finding during seizures. The motor movements range from resembling simple arousal to more involved movements like sudden arousal from sleep with eye-opening, head raising, sitting up in bed with a frightened expression, and even the utterance of a scream. As such, they are frequently misdiagnosed as parasomnias (confusional arousals, sleepwalking, and sleep terrors), particularly in children. DoA episodes typically occur in the first third of the night when SWS is greatest. In contrast, SHE episodes occur more evenly distributed throughout the night, and the motor movements are more highly stereotyped (21). The other differential diagnostic considerations include panic attacks and RBD. vPSG is mandatory to confirm the diagnosis (Figure 18-10).

Self-Limited Epilepsies

Self-limiting epilepsies are referred to as self-limiting because almost all seizures will cease within 1 to 2 years of onset.

Self-limited epilepsy with centrotemporal spikes (SeLECTs), formerly known as benign epilepsy of childhood with centrotemporal spikes or benign Rolandic epilepsy, is the most common partial epilepsy in children. Seizures begin between 4 and 10 years of age, are seen predominantly in drowsiness and NREM sleep, are characterized by focal clonic twitching, and are often preceded by tingling, burning, or numb sensation around the mouth area. Consciousness is usually preserved. EEG reveals characteristic centrotemporal spike and wave discharges. The spike activity is enhanced by sleep, and approximately 30% may be present only in sleep. The prognosis is excellent, and seizures generally stop by 15 to 20 years of age without neurologic sequelae.

Self-limited epilepsy with autonomic seizures (SeLEAS), formerly known as Panayiotopoulos syndrome (PS) or early-onset benign occipital epilepsy, is the second most common partial epilepsy in children. In all, 70% of these seizures occur during sleep. Onset is usually around 3 to 8 years of age. Seizures are predominantly characterized by prominent autonomic symptoms such as sweating, vomiting, diarrhea, tachycardia, and hypotension. Eye-opening or generalized tonic-clonic movements may also accompany seizures.

Sleep-Accentuated Epilepsies

Electrical Status Epilepticus of Sleep

Electrical status epilepticus of sleep (ESES), also known as continuous spikes and waves during slow-wave sleep (CSWS), is characterized by generalized spike-wave complexes at 2 to 2.5 Hz present for 85% to 90% of

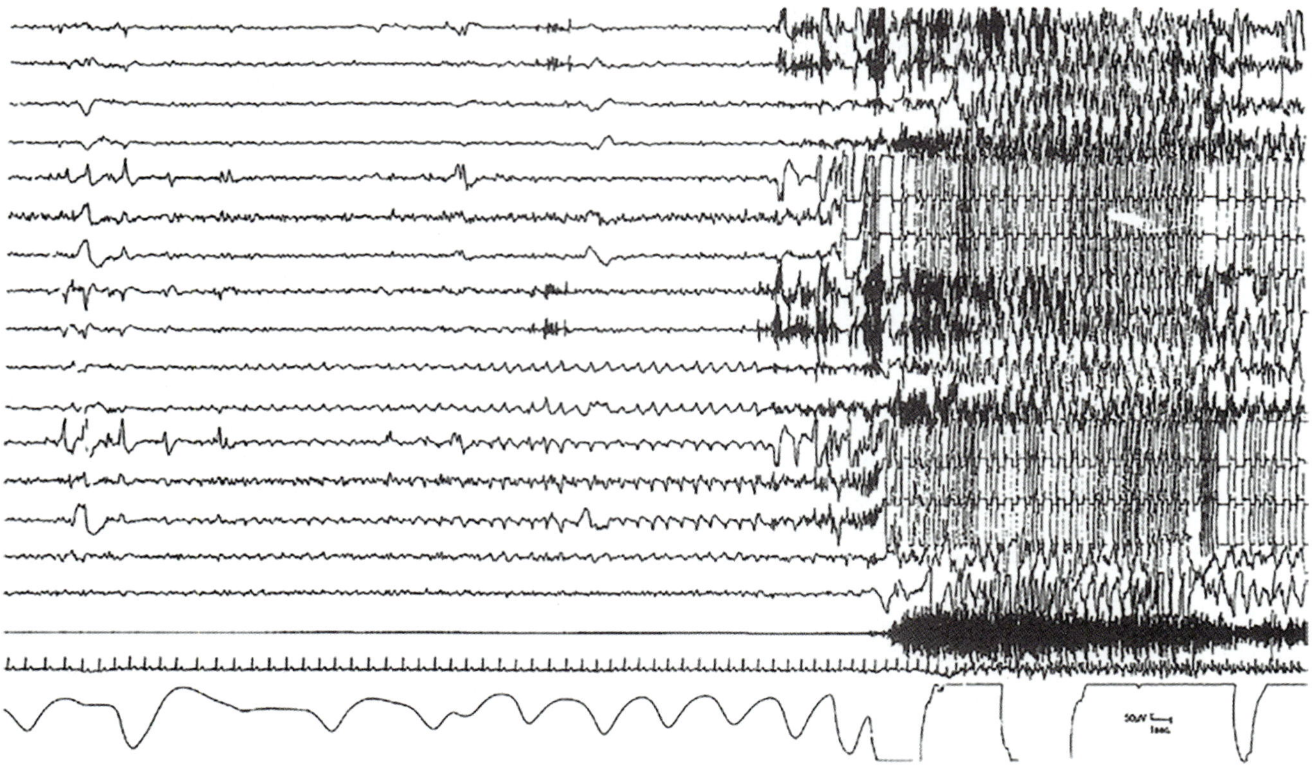

Figure 18-10 Nocturnal paroxysmal dystonia in nocturnal frontal lobe epilepsy. A 14-year-old girl presented with nocturnal episodes since age 12, characterized by head rising and complex motor automatism involving legs, arms, and trunk with dystonic postures. Seizures recurred several times a night, 2 to 3 times per month. Video-polysomnography recordings showed that at the beginning of the seizure, the patient opens her eyes, presents a deep inspiration while raising her head, then abducts her hyperextended upper limbs and presents rhythmic movements of limbs and trunk with back arching. The polysomnographic tracing shows this seizure arising from stage N2 sleep. The motor manifestation is preceded for 10 to 15 seconds by repetitive sharp waves on left anterior electroencephalogram (EEG) channels; then paroxysmal EEG activity is almost completely masked by muscle artifacts. During the seizure, tachycardia and modification of respiration occur. R. + L. Tib. Ant., right and left tibialis anterior; SO, supraorbital electrode; Sph, sphenoidal electrode; Thor. Resp, thoracic respiration. (Reprinted from Zucconi M, Montagna P, Chokroverty S. Sleep and epilepsy. In: Chokroverty S, Thomas RJ, Bhatt M, eds. *Atlas of Sleep Medicine*. Butterworth-Heinemann; 2005:213. Copyright © 2005 Elsevier. With permission.)

SWS and relatively suppressed during REM sleep and wakefulness. Seizures may have a variable presentation, manifesting as nocturnal focal motor, generalized tonic-clonic, atypical absence, or myoclonic seizures. The emergence of CSWS is associated with neuropsychological regression, and the disappearance of CSWS is associated with an improvement in neuropsychological function. The disorder may be of uncertain origin or result from various central nervous system lesions. These seizures are usually responsive to antiepileptic drugs and remit by the middle teenage years.

Lennox-Gastaut Syndrome

Lennox-Gastaut syndrome (LGS) is a severe form of epilepsy characterized by tonic seizures, predominantly during SWS. Motor presentation during the seizure may be as subtle as eyes opening or rolling, but there may also be vocalization or limb movements. In addition to the tonic seizures, they also must have at least one of the following additional types of seizures: atonic, myoclonic, atypical absence, and even generalized seizures. It typically develops between 2 and 8 years of age and continues throughout their lives. Developmental disabilities often accompany it.

Awakening Epilepsies

Juvenile Myoclonic Epilepsy

The typical presentation consists of generalized tonic-clonic seizures, which often occur in the first 1 or 2 hours after awakening and are rare at other times of the day. Bilaterally synchronous myoclonic jerks occur frequently, particularly on awakening, although patients may not easily notice them. The age of onset is usually between 8 and 9 years or between 25 and 40 years. The characteristic EEG abnormality consists of generalized 3- to 5.5-Hz spike-wave and polyspike-wave complexes that occur increasingly at sleep onset and following awakening but are virtually nonexistent during the rest of the sleep cycle (5).

Psychogenic Nonepileptic Seizures

Psychogenic nonepileptic seizures (PNES), also known as pseudoseizures, occur most commonly in young adults and are 3 times more common in women than in men. Uncoordinated nonsynchronous bizarre motor movements, for example, pelvic thrusting, side-to-side head movements, and backward arching of the body, typically characterize the episodes. Screaming or talking during episodes may also occur. The spells are commonly emotionally triggered with a gradual onset and termination. They may last for several minutes or even hours and may lack the postictal confusion seen in epileptic seizures. Nonepileptic seizures are not common during sleep but may rarely occur on awakening from sleep at night. It is essential to realize that certain features suggestive of autonomic activation and generally associated with epileptic seizures may also accompany nonepileptic seizures, for example, pupillary dilatation, Babinski responses, autonomic cardiorespiratory changes, injury, and urinary and fecal incontinence (22).

Interictal EEG recordings have limited utility in the diagnosis or exclusion of nonepileptic seizures. EEG recording during a spell is useful in documenting the absence of epileptiform discharges associated with the movements and the absence of postictal slowing. However, the EEG may frequently be obscured because of muscle and movement artifacts. Long-term video-EEG recording is usually necessary to properly evaluate nonepileptic spells. Frequently, epileptic and nonepileptic seizures may coexist in the same person, and definite diagnosis requires video-EEG of all seizure types experienced by the patient. Furthermore, malingering and factitious seizures may present similarly and need to be differentiated with the help of history.

Polysomnography Findings in Other Sleep-Related Issues

Propriospinal Myoclonus at Sleep Onset

PSM at sleep onset consists of sudden muscular jerks occurring in the relaxation period during the transition from wakefulness to sleep, mainly involving the abdomen, neck, and trunk. Owing to their association with sleep onset, these movements can result in insomnia or be associated with RLS. PSG demonstrates brief myoclonic EMG bursts recurring nonperiodically, mainly with alpha activity present on the EEG. The jerks disappear with the onset of stage N2 sleep or with mental activation. PSG has demonstrated that the jerks arise first in the spinal-innervated muscles (usually thoracic or cervical spinal segments) and then spread to more rostral and caudal muscles according to a propriospinal propagation pattern. Recording bilateral muscle groups will help demonstrate the lateral synchronization of the muscle movements. Magnetic resonance imaging (MRI) of the spine in these patients can be abnormal in up to 20% of patients with focal abnormalities (5).

Excessive Fragmentary Myoclonus

Excessive fragmentary myoclonus (EFM) is characterized by small movements of the fingers, toes, or corners of the mouth or small muscle twitches resembling fasciculations. These movements are typically too small to be visible. Episodes of these myoclonic potentials typically last from 10 minutes to several hours. They often appear at sleep onset, continue through the NREM stages, and persist during REM sleep. On PSG, the motor activity consists of recurrent, brief (75-150 ms) EMG potentials in various muscles of the face, trunk, arms, and legs, occurring asynchronously and asymmetrically on the two sides in a sustained manner. Electromyographically, they resemble physiologic phasic REM twitches but occur irregularly and not in clusters. More than five potentials per minute must be sustained for at least 20 minutes of NREM sleep. The clinical significance of EFM remains uncertain as there are no consistently reported clinical consequences, and it can be seen in patients with a variety of sleep disorders as well as in normal individuals (5). Recent data suggest that it may be a sign of peripheral nerve pathology, requiring patients to undergo neurophysiologic evaluation (nerve conduction studies/EMG) (23). It may occur in isolation or may be associated with other sleep disorders. EFM is typically differentiated from PLMS because of its significantly shorter duration and lack of stereotypical periodicity, which defines PLMS. REM-related phasic twitches are confined to REM sleep, whereas EFM is observed during a minimum of 20 minutes of NREM sleep. Scoring and documentation of EFM are considered optional by AASM standards (6).

Sleep Starts (Hypnic Jerks)

Sleep starts are sudden, brief, simultaneous contractions of the body or one or more body segments occurring at sleep onset. They are common occurrences in the normal population, reported in as high as 70% of the general population, and considered normal physiologic events. They may be accompanied by sensory feelings of falling into a void, a flash of light, unexplained fear, an electric shock–like sensation, or a dream. Purely sensory sleep starts in the absence of a body jerk, as has been described. Sleep starts may become more frequent with stimulant use, sleep deprivation, or emotional or physical stress. Occasionally, these are intensified in frequency or magnitude sufficiently to impair sleep onset or maintenance, which is considered pathologic and termed "intensified hypnic jerks." EMG recordings of the involved muscles show brief, myoclonic (generally 75-250 ms), high-amplitude potentials, either singly or in succession. The EEG typically shows stage N1 sleep, sometimes accompanied by a vertex sharp wave. Sleep starts may be mistaken for epileptic myoclonus, EFM, PSM, startle disease, or PLMS. Hypnic jerks can be differentiated from EFM in that EFM consists of repetitive brief jerks that occur not only at sleep onset but also throughout other sleep stages. The motor movements associated with PLMS are typically longer in duration and occur with the periodicity associated with PLMS observed during sleep. Purely sensory hypnic jerks may lead to an erroneous diagnosis of epileptic seizures or a psychiatric disorder. The history of occurrence, limited to sleep onset and PSG evaluation, is helpful in differentiation (5).

Hypnagogic Foot Tremor and Alternating Leg Muscle Activation

Hypnagogic foot tremor (HFT) is a rhythmic movement of feet or toes (similar to nervous jiggling of the foot with legs crossed) that occurs at the transition between wake and sleep or during light NREM sleep (stages N1 and N2). In HFT, the leg movements cannot be better explained by any other sleep disorder (5).

Alternating leg muscle activation (ALMA) is a PSG pattern with unknown clinical significance. ALMA consists of brief activation of the tibialis anterior muscle in one leg in alternation with similar activation in the other leg during sleep or arousals from sleep. The pattern in ALMA is as if the patient was marching left, right, left, right, and so on. Owing to the alternating pattern in ALMA, recording left and right leg EMG independently is mandatory. As shown in Figure 18-11, ALMA is usually associated with arousals, occurring either immediately before or after the arousal (6). ALMA, however, may occur during any stage of sleep, independent of arousals, and is seen more often in patients taking antidepressants (5). HFT and ALMA are considered together because of the similarities in their features. Scoring for both HFT and ALMA is considered optional by AASM standards (6).

In HFT, PSG demonstrates trains of recurrent 0.3- to 4-Hz EMG potentials or movements in one or both feet. In ALMA, PSG demonstrates a pattern of brief, repeated activation of the anterior tibialis in one leg alternating with similar activation in the other leg, occurring at a frequency of 0.5 to 3 Hz (usually 1-2 Hz). Like PLMS, HFT and ALMA have a minimum series of at least four muscle bursts. In contrast with PLMS, both HFT and ALMA have a much shorter interval between individual movements. Their maximum intervals of

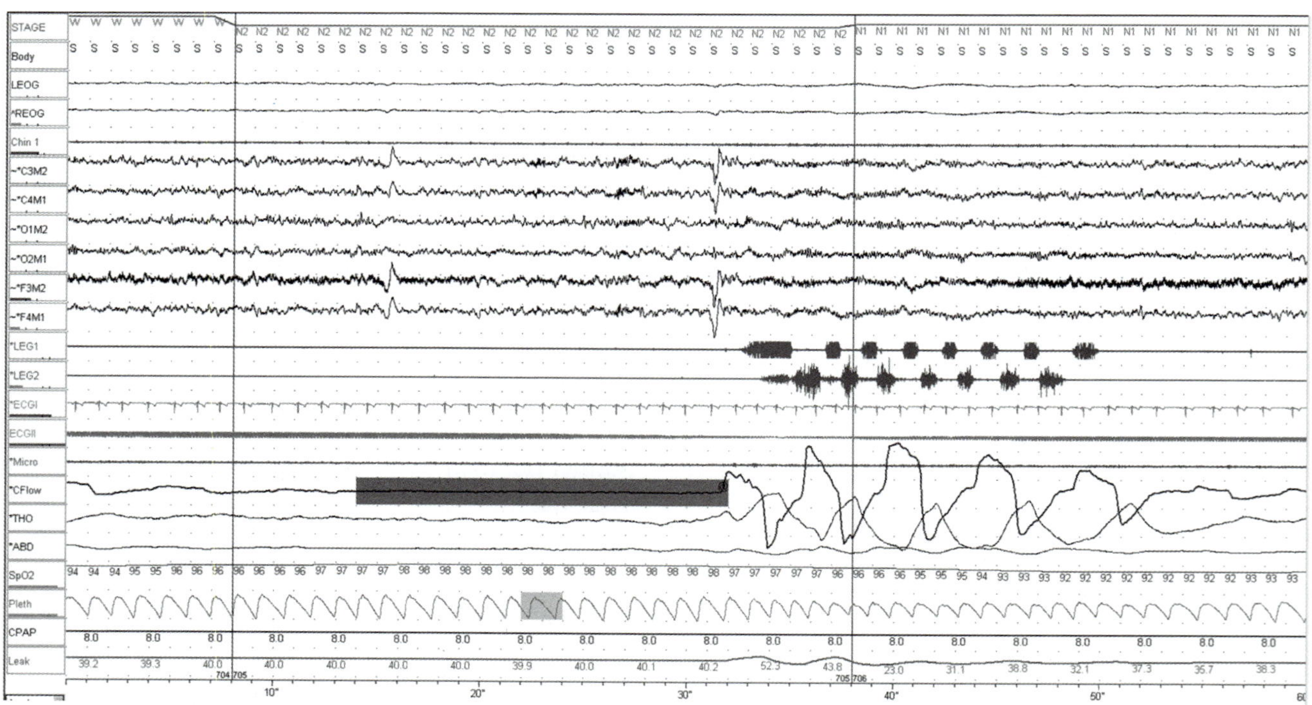

Figure 18-11 A 60-second video-polysomnography fragment showing a period of alternating leg muscle activation with electromyographic activity alternating between the left and right legs during arousal as a result of an apnea. The leg movements cease once the patient returns to sleep.

Table 18-4 Summary of Polysomnography Findings in Movement Disorders

Motor Event	Minimum No. in Series	Interval Between Movements (seconds)	Duration of Movement (seconds)	Scoring
PLMS	4	5-90 (0.01-0.2-Hz)	0.5-10	Recommended
RBD	50%	3	0.1-5	Recommended
HFT	4	0.2-1	0.25-3	Optional
Bruxism	3	3	0.5-2	Recommended
RMD	4	2	0.5-2	Recommended
HFT	4	0.25-3.3 (0.3-4 Hz)	0.25-1	Optional
ALMA	4	0.3-2 (0.5-3 Hz)	0.1-0.5	Optional

ALMA, alternating leg muscle activation; HFT, hypnagogic foot tremor; PLMS, periodic limb movements in sleep; RBD, rapid eye movement behavior disorder (RBD); RMD, rhythmic movement disorder.

3.3 and 2 seconds, respectively, are shorter than the minimum 5-second interval associated with PLMS. Their minimum intervals are almost equal at 0.25 seconds for HFT and 0.3 seconds for ALMA (Table 18-4) (6).

Benign Sleep Myoclonus of Infancy

Benign sleep myoclonus of infancy is characterized by repetitive myoclonic jerks that occur during infant sleep. The jerks are often bilateral and massive, typically involving large muscle groups, appearing exclusively in sleep. Onset is usually between birth and 1 month of age and resolves in the vast majority by 1 year of age. It is twice as likely in males versus females. vPSG has shown paroxysmal muscle activity without ictal or interictal EEG abnormalities. It occurs predominantly during NREM sleep but may also be present during REM sleep. The jerks are usually seen in clusters of four or five jerks per second, each jerk lasting 40 to 300 ms. Awakening the infant leads to prompt, abrupt, and consistent cessation of the movements (5). Benign sleep myoclonus of infancy must be distinguished from myoclonic seizures, as misdiagnosis can lead to unnecessary treatment.

OTHER DIAGNOSTIC TESTS

Ambulatory Polysomnography

In the laboratory attended, vPSG is the accepted and gold standard test for the evaluation of patients with motor events in sleep. The utility of ambulatory PSG is also under consideration, given the lower cost. Ambulatory PSG systems are available today that can record extended EEG-PSG with synchronized video recordings. The major disadvantage of ambulatory vPSG is the absence of a technologist. The technologist cannot make the necessary technical adjustments as may be required during the study for complete and meaningful data acquisition. In addition, the technologist cannot document the clinical aspects of the motor event or behavior and assess the patient's status after the event, which, as previously discussed, can significantly aid in the diagnostic process.

Actigraphy

Actigraphy is a technique of motion detection used to record activity during sleep and waking. It is very useful in diagnosing circadian rhythm sleep disorders, insomnias, and, sometimes, PLMS. Actigraphy allows the continuous recording of rest/activity for extended periods. The limitations of actigraphy are the relative inability to differentiate between resting wakefulness and sleep periods and the failure to discriminate and differentiate between the origins of various motor movements in sleep, for example, those resulting from PLMS, seizures, or dyskinesias. Current AASM Clinical Practice Guidelines do not recommend the use of actigraphy for the evaluation of sleep-related movement disorders or parasomnias (24).

24-Hour Ambulatory Electroencephalography Recording

Ambulatory EEG recordings allow 24 hours of continuous EEG recording during a subject's routine activities. Recordings can be extended to 48 or 72 hours as necessary. Extended recording increases the possibility of capturing abnormal epileptiform activity. The major disadvantage is the absence of video documentation and clinical description in the event of a seizure.

Neuroimaging

A neuroimaging study, in particular, an MRI of the brain, is indicated when a neurologic illness or structural lesion is suspected as the underlying cause of abnormal motor events in sleep. All adults with new-onset seizures and children without characteristic epilepsy syndromes typically require a brain MRI to exclude the possibility of structural brain disorders. If someone presents with an abrupt-onset motor activity or has other concerning symptoms or signs on examination suggestive of a central nervous system lesion (headaches, focal weakness, or sensory findings), imaging is indicated.

CONCLUSION

Abnormal movements, behaviors, or events in sleep pose a challenge to clinicians because of a frequent lack of adequate information from patients who may be unaware or amnestic of the events. This is further compounded when there is a lack of testimonial information from a bed partner or eyewitness. Such events, therefore, frequently remain misdiagnosed or undiagnosed and untreated or incorrectly treated for a long time. The use of digital vPSG has revolutionized the field and has brought new light to the subject. vPSG provides an opportunity to obtain an audio video recording of the event in addition to simultaneous and synchronous measurement of other PSG features, such as extended EEG, EMG, and cardiorespiratory parameters.

This chapter has outlined an approach for a patient with abnormal movements and behaviors in sleep, provided a practical classification for motor events in sleep, and discussed the utility of vPSG and related tests in the diagnosis and differential diagnosis of these conditions.

REFERENCES

1. Kushida CA, Littner MR, Morgenthaler T, et al. Practice parameters for the indications for polysomnography and related procedures: an update for 2005. *Sleep*. 2005;28(4):499-521.
2. Mainieri G, Loddo G, Provini F, Nobili L, Manconi M, Castelnovo A. Diagnosis and management of NREM sleep parasomnias in children and adults. *Diagnostics (Basel)*. 2023;13:1-24.
3. Ricci L, Boscarino M, Assenza G, et al. Clinical utility of home videos for diagnosing epileptic seizures: a systematic review and practical recommendations for optimal and safe recording. *Neruol Sci*. 2021;42:1301-1309.
4. Nobili L, DeWeerd A, Rubboli G, et al. Standard procedures for the diagnostic pathway of sleep-related epilepsies and comorbid sleep disorders: a European Academy of Neurology, European Sleep Research Society and International League against Epilepsy-Europe consensus review. *J Sleep Res*. 2020;29(6):1-18.
5. Amin U, Primiani C, MacIver S, Rivera-Cruz A, Frontera A, Benbadis S. Value of smartphone videos for diagnosis of seizures: everyone owns half an epilepsy monitoring unit. *Epilepsia*. 2021;62:135-139.
6. American Academy of Sleep Medicine. *International Classification of Sleep Disorders*. 3rd ed, Text Revision. American Academy of Sleep Medicine; 2023.
7. Troester MM, Quan SF, Berry RB, et al. *The AASM Manual for the Scoring of Sleep and Associated Events: Rules, Terminology and Technical Specifications: Version 3*. American Academy of Sleep Medicine; 2023.
8. Chokroverty S. Polysomnography and related procedures. Hallett M, ed. *Handbook of Clinical Neurophysiology: Movement Disorders: Volume 1*. Elsevier; 2000:145.
9. Malow BA, Aldrich MS. Polysomnography. In: Chokroverty S, Hening W, Walters A, eds. *Sleep and Movement Disorders*. Butterworth-Heinemann; 2003:128.
10. Foldvary-Schaefer N, De Ocampo J, Mascha E, Burgess R, Dinner D, Morris H. Accuracy of seizure detection using abbreviated EEG during polysomnography. *J Clin Neurophysiol*. 2006;23(1):68-71.
11. Lopez R, Barateau L, Chenini S, Rassu A, Dauvilliers Y. Home nocturnal infrared video to record non-rapid eye movement sleep parasomnias. *J Sleep Res*. 2022; 32(2): e13732. doi:10.1111/jsr.13732
12. Pressman M. Factors that predispose, prime and precipitate NREM parasomnias in adults: clinical and forensic implications. *Sleep Med Rev*. 2007;11:5-30.
13. Blanchette-Carriere C, Montplaisir J, Boucetta S, Desautels A, Zadra A. Differential effects of sleep deprivation on sleepwalking: role of demographic and clinical profiles. *Sleep Med*. 2024;121:144-150.
14. Dumont S, Bloch V, Lill-Lelouet A, Le Beller C, Geoffroy PA, Veyrier M. Parasomnias and sleep-related movement disorders induced by drugs in the adult population: a review about iatrogenic medication effects. *J Sleep Res*. 2024;34(2):1-15.
15. Pilon M, Montplaisir J, Zadra A. Precipitating factors of somnabulism: impact of sleep deprivation and forced arousals. *Neurology*. 2008;70:2284-2290.
16. Vertugno R, Manconi M, Ferini-Strambi L, Provini F, Plazzi G, Montagna P. Nocturnal eating: sleep-related eating disorder or night eating syndrome? A videopolysomnographic study. *Sleep*. 2006;29(7): 949-954.
17. Capezuti E, Maislin G, Strumpf N, Evans LK. Side rail use and bed-related fall outcomes among nursing home residents. *J Am Geriatr Soc*. 2002;50(1):90-96.
18. Irfan M, Schenck CH, Howell MJ. NonREM disorders of arousal and related parasomnias: an updated review. *Neurotherapeutics*. 2021;18:124-139.
19. Loddo G, Sessagesimi E, Mignani F, et al. Specific motor patterns of arousal disorders in adults: a video-polysomnographic analysis of 184 episodes. *Sleep Med*. 2018;41:102-109.
20. Hrozanova M, Morrison I, Riha R. Adult NREM parasomnias: an update. *Clocks Sleep*. 2018;1(1):87-104.
21. Sakuma T, Yamaguchi T, Maeda M, et al. Comparison of the occurrence of sleep bruxism under accustomed conditions at home and under polysomnography

conditions in a sleep laboratory. *J Prosthodont Res*. 2022;66(4):630-638.

22. Lam N, Verravigrom M. Sleep-related rhythmic movement disorder in children: a mini-review. *Front Neurol*. 2023;14:1-5.
23. Mutti C, Bernabe G, Barozzi N, et al. Commonalities and differences in NREM parasomnias and sleep-related epilepsy: is there a continuum between the two conditions? *Front Neurol*. 2020;11:1-14.
24. International League Against Epilepsy. Epilepsy Diagnosis.org. 2025. https://www.epilepsydiagnosis.org

Chapter 19
Sleep and Respiratory Disorders

ALESHIA L. DORST

KEY CONCEPTS/LEARNING OBJECTIVES

The key concepts for this chapter include describing restrictive and obstructive respiratory disorders, the changes in respiratory function during sleep, and the prevalence, etiology, pathophysiology, diagnosis, treatment, and prognosis of patients with chronic obstructive pulmonary disease (COPD) in relation to sleep, and describing overlap syndrome (OVS), defining and describing asthma, interstitial lung disease (ILD), and neuromuscular disease (NMD) in relation to sleep.

KEY TERMS

Chronic obstructive pulmonary disease (COPD)
Continuous positive airway pressure (CPAP)
Hyperventilation
Hypoventilation
Interstitial Lung disease (ILD)
Neuromuscular disease (NMD)
Noninvasive ventilation (NIV)
Obesity hypoventilation syndrome (OHS)
Overlap syndrome (OVS)
Pulmonary function test (PFT)

TYPE OF RESPIRATORY DISORDERS

Restrictive Versus Obstructive Classifications

There are several different types of respiratory disorders that can primarily be described as either restrictive or obstructive: a restrictive disorder, such as interstitial lung disease (ILD) and obesity hypoventilation syndrome (OHS); an individual has an inability to expand the lungs to the needed volume to properly ventilate (1,2). Restrictive disorders can also be a consequence of pulmonary scarring because of diseases such as idiopathic pulmonary fibrosis, which will result in failure of lung expansion. Diseases that would be considered obstructive include chronic obstructive pulmonary disease (COPD), asthma, and bronchiectasis. Obstructive disorders are more common than restrictive and share the characteristics of blocked airways. Some similarities are noted with obstructive and restrictive disorders, such as symptoms, signs, diagnosis, and treatment methods (1), and there are a wide variety of respiratory disorders that range in severity and have fluctuating treatments.

Respiratory Disorders and Sleep

Given the prevalence of sleep-disordered breathing (SDB) as well as respiratory disorders, it is not uncommon to see them in association with each other. The unfortunate consequences of both diagnoses increase the severity of these diseases and, in turn, could lead to higher morbidity, exacerbation frequency, and mortality rates (3).

People with respiratory disorders such as COPD and ILD often report increased sleep complications, including difficulty initiating and/or maintaining sleep (insomnia), as well as limited sleep and daytime fatigue; this symptom overlap can result in underdiagnosed obstructive sleep apnea (OSA) in these populations (3).

When the body makes the shift from wake to light sleep—nonrapid eye movement (NREM)—a reduction in ventilatory drive occurs, due to disruptions in the respiratory control, respiratory muscle function, and lung mechanics. A change in ventilatory response follows, due to a reduction in chemoreceptor sensitivity, which is vital to breathing stability since it is sensitive to blood level oxygen and carbon dioxide (3). Other physiologic respiratory adaptations that occur include diminished respiratory drive and reduced skeletal muscle activity that is particularly relevant to accessory muscle contraction; further changes to lung mechanics, such as reduced functional residual capacity or a reduced amount of air in the lungs after exhalation, adversely affect ventilation-perfusion relationship, impacting oxygen and blood circulation. These adaptations would not normally result in significant changes to gas exchange in a healthy individual but have been shown to result in major oxygen desaturations in an individual with a respiratory disorder such as COPD (4). When transitioning from NREM to rapid eye movement sleep (REM), atonia occurs; this loss of muscle tone will result in the diaphragm being the main muscle contributing to breathing, resulting in a decrease in tidal volume and respiratory rate. Respiratory disturbances during REM are strongly associated with negative health outcomes such as atrial fibrillation (5). Due to these changes that occur during NREM and REM, it is obvious to see why a person with a restrictive or obstructive lung disease would be more susceptible to airflow obstructions during sleep (3).

OSA is the most prevalent sleep disorder and has been shown to have negative consequences for a person's health, because it affects their ability to properly perform gas exchange—carbon dioxide (CO_2) and oxygen—while asleep. OSA can be a result of anatomic and physiologic factors that contribute to airway collapse. Nearly every organ system is at risk of dysfunction from the continued impact of untreated OSA, with an obvious emphasis on organs in the thoracic cavity, as they are especially vulnerable, due to the consequences of large fluctuations in pressure in the chest cavity called wide intrathoracic pressure swings (6). Sleep apnea is defined by a person's apnea-hypopnea index (AHI), which correlates with how frequently an apnea or hypopnea is noted during sleep. During an apneic event, there is a reduction in the airway when the pharynx collapses, resulting in reduced airflow or hypopnea event, while a completely obstructed airway refers to an apnea event. Specifically, the American Academy of Sleep Medicine defines an apnea as a 90% reduction in airflow for 10 seconds, while a hypopnea would be a 30% reduction in airflow, with an associated 3% to 4% oxygen desaturation. Mild sleep apnea requires an AHI of 5 or more, while moderate sleep apnea shows an AHI of 15 or more, and, finally, severe sleep apnea is diagnosed when 30 or more events are noted per hour (7). The frequency and the severity of these events typically depend on anatomic and neural factors. AHI does not, however, reflect the hypoxic burden, or other factors such as length of events, that can increase negative outcomes. When there is a reduction or cessation of airflow, the oxygen provided to the body is reduced, and body's neurochemical receptors are notified that the body has gone into a hypoxic state, which can lead to hypercapnia because of inefficient exchange of gases. The negative effects of sleep apnea underscore the importance of diagnosis and treatment. Individuals with sleep apnea are more likely to have comorbidities, including obesity, gastroesophageal reflux disease (GERD), heart failure, or high blood pressure (6).

DIAGNOSING RESPIRATORY DISORDERS WITH PULMONARY FUNCTION TESTING

Diagnosis of lung disorders is similar in restrictive and obstructive disorders. A person presenting with symptoms of cough, wheezing, and shortness of breath would have spirometry testing. Spirometry is relatively quick and inexpensive. Spirometers measure how much air an individual can breathe out and how quickly. How well the lungs deliver oxygen to the blood can also be measured by simply breathing into a spirometer. Other means of diagnosing and marking the severity of lung disorders are by checking arterial blood gases, a 6-minute walk test, or by performing a chest x-ray or computed tomography (CT) of the chest to evaluate signs of damage and determine their origin (5,8,9).

SLEEP-RELATED HYPOXEMIA

Sleep-related hypoxemia is classified as sustained periods of low oxygen during sleep. Typically, during sleep, the parasympathetic nervous system controls breathing, resulting in deep breaths; this ensures adequate tidal volume and gas exchange. The physiologic respiratory shift that occurs from wake to NREM is intensified by respiratory disorders that impact the lungs' ability to reach the needed tidal volume to allow the needed amount of oxygen to distribute through the body, which is further complicated in REM due to the reduced ability of the diaphragm to contract (3). Low oxygen levels can be a result of hypoventilation, reduced functional residual capacity, and elevation. These symptoms can be increased by alcohol, depressants, and sedatives, as we see in other respiratory disorders. Patients with severe respiratory diseases (COPD, obesity hypoventilation disorder) are at a higher risk of developing sleep-related hypoxia (4).

SLEEP-RELATED HYPOVENTILATION

Sleep-related hypoventilation is described as insufficient gas exchange that results in hypercapnia or increased partial pressure of carbon dioxide (Pa_{CO_2}). This is the result of slow and shallow breaths, which are inadequate in inhaling sufficient oxygen and exhaling the needed amount of CO_2. Sleep-related hypoventilation is not always in association with other lung or airway diseases and does not require associated disorders for diagnosis. Sleep-related hypoventilation is diagnosed by monitoring Pa_{CO_2} during a polysomnography, using transcutaneous or end-tidal CO_2 monitoring. Daytime

CO_2 values measured by arterial blood gas testing can be a predictor for hypoventilation (5,6). The development of OSA is often present in these situations due to ventilatory control instability, or elevated loop gain; indicating the instability of the respiratory system results in amplified disturbances to breathing, which increases chemoreceptors sensitivity to hypercapnia and hypoxia (2). Another form of sleep apnea, called central sleep apnea (CSA), can occasionally result from increased chemoreceptor sensitivity. During heightened chemoreceptor sensitivity, the body will respond to hypercapnia by hyperventilating, bringing the level of CO_2 too far down, resulting in a pause in breathing when the body tries to compensate and hold in CO_2. This often results in a cyclic pattern of poor overcompensation, followed by undercompensation.

SLEEP PROBLEMS IN OVERLAP SYNDROME—OBSTRUCTIVE SLEEP APNEA + CHRONIC OBSTRUCTIVE PULMONARY DISEASE

Chronic obstructive pulmonary disease (COPD) and OSA are two of the most common prevalent chronic respiratory disorders and have been termed "overlap syndrome" (OVS), a term that was first introduced by D.C. Flenly in 1985. (10) OVS was originally used to describe the combination of any respiratory disease with sleep apnea but is now an exclusive term referring to the relationship between COPD and OSA due to its high prevalence (6). Currently, millions of individuals across the world have been diagnosed with OVS; there is still an underestimation of the prevalence of OVS due to the limitations in diagnosing patients with COPD and OSA. The relationship between OSA and COPD has been proven to impact epidemiology, comorbidities, and survival due to local and systemic inflammation (3). In a study designed to test different treatments on patients with COPD and OSA, it was found that those who shared the two diagnoses presented with a higher AHI and a higher oxygen desaturation index. Patients with COPD alone still showed longer periods of low saturations classified as below 90% and 80%, showing the correlation between increased nocturnal hypoxemia and COPD (7).

Factors of Chronic Obstructive Pulmonary Disease That Predispose to Obstructive Sleep Apnea

Due to COPD having a spectrum of phenotypes, there are a combination of positive and negative impacts on OSA. Emphysema, for instance, is diagnosed when the walls between alveoli are damaged, while bronchitis diagnosis involves the walls of the airways being constantly irritated and inflamed, typically resulting in thick mucus in the airways. In COPD individuals with emphysema, average presentation is low BMI and showing relatively well-preserved gas exchange, with a primary symptom of dyspnea, although an individual with bronchitis will be associated with higher BMI and cor pulmonale while having a primary symptom of productive cough. Patients diagnosed with bronchitis are noted to have lower respiratory drive leading to hypoxemia and hypercapnia (10). Additional COPD factors that can predispose to OSA include tobacco smoke causing upper airway inflammation and medications like inhaled corticosteroids due to their tendency to cause weight gain or fat redistribution to the neck area (11). Some COPD factors can protect against OSA. These include lung hyperinflation, advanced age, reduced REM sleep, and medications such as theophylline (3).

The relationship between COPD and OSA has been described as complex and bidirectional, in that the worsening of one disease process leads to the deterioration of the other. The oxidative stress imposed by OSA on the airways can be compounded by inflammation such as allergic inflammation from tobacco airway damage, environmental pollution, dust, chemicals, and bad air quality (6).

Undiagnosed OVS patients have been found to show a higher 30-day readmission rate and also increased severity of hypoxemia, leading to a higher risk of pulmonary hypertension and cor pulmonale (6). Additionally, research on individuals with OVS indicated a greater carotid artery stiffness (CCA), with higher depression scores and lower executive function-processing speed than individuals with either disorder alone. Elevated CCA stiffness results in increased pulsatile pressure and flows into the cerebral microcirculation, which is associated with the development of ischemic damage in the brain, likely contributing to the development of cognitive impairment. This demonstrates the fact that OVS has detrimental effects on organs outside of the respiratory system as well and leads to elevated cardiovascular disease risk (5).

Treating Chronic Obstructive Pulmonary Disease and Overlap Syndrome

In all cases of respiratory disorders and diseases, the first suggestion to reduce symptoms is to quit smoking and reduce smoke exposure along with exposure to other irritants. The treatment goals for COPD are to manage COPD and reduce admissions due to exacerbations. Treatment involves reducing hypoxemia and hypercapnia. Continuous positive airway pressure (CPAP) is the gold standard in treating OSA and SDB; it has also been shown to improve COPD exacerbation, ER visits, and hospitalizations. CPAP has been shown to reduce the work of breathing, although biLevel PAP therapy might be a more appropriate form of treatment since it is a form of noninvasive ventilation (NIV), which promotes proper gas exchange. This, in turn, is proven to reduce hypoxemia and hyperventilation. Oxygen treatment is a first-step treatment in patients with COPD and is commonly used in OVS, although it can have a negative impact on OSA since it may result in longer durations of obstructive events when the oxygen does not drop enough to trigger a breath; furthermore, this can result in worsening hypercapnia. Alternatively, high-flow long-term oxygen therapy (LTOT) has shown positive impacts on gas exchange and reduction of obstructive events (3). The diagnosis and treatment of OVS can lead to improved spirometry, pulmonary artery pressure, and sleep architecture (6). No matter the type of treatment prescribed, it is clear that the early detection and long-term adherence to therapy are key in reducing disease progression and subsequent mortality (8).

ASTHMA AND OBSTRUCTIVE SLEEP APNEA

Asthma is defined as a chronic inflammatory disorder of the airways. Asthma presents in various forms, including intermittent, persistent, exercise-associated, aspirin-sensitive, or severe. Although there are various forms of asthma, the disease is typically categorized as acute or chronic. Patients with asthma present with symptoms such as wheezing, breathlessness, chest tightness, dyspnea, and coughing. Asthma has been described as an allergic response, although nonallergic asthma is prevalent. The airway can be irritated by several outside factors: air pollution, postnasal drip, gastroesophageal reflux disease, smoke, dandruff or pet dander, and many others.

An "asthma attack" is, in fact, a series of complex interactions between inflammatory cells and mediators in reaction to the irritants previously noted. More specifically, when an irritant is introduced into the body, the body starts an immune response by producing antibodies called "immunoglobulin E" (IgE) (12). The IgE will seek out the mast cell to release histamine; the histamine responds strongly and results in swelling of the airway and glands overproducing mucus.

Patients with asthma often experience airway constriction because of bronchoconstriction in response to exposure to stimuli. Airway edema can result from long-term inflammation to the airway and progression of asthma. A patient with asthma has an airway with thickened muscle walls as well as a swollen mucus layer and increased mucus production, which results in a smaller lumen, reducing airflow. All of these symptoms can make life with asthma painful.

OSA and asthma are closely related, and due to the increased co-occurrence, the symptoms of each can be difficult to control (6). OSA and asthma have shared risk factors such as GERD, rhinitis, and obesity (11). A bidirectional relationship is seen since asthma increases the risk of OSA likely due to inflammation and OSA has been linked to poor asthma outcomes since obstructive apneas increase cholinergic tone, activating muscarinic receptors in the airways leading to bronchoconstriction (6,11). Recent analysis has shown a 2 to 3 times higher prevalence of OSA in individuals with asthma, leading to higher frequency of annual emergency room visits and use of inhaled corticosteroids (11). Asthma symptoms worsen at night, leading to frequent arousals and poor sleep quality. This may be because cortisol levels are lowest during the early morning hours and can result in increased airway inflammation and hyperresponsiveness. These factors in combination with OSA increase ventilatory instability. In a recent experiment CPAP therapy was shown to improve daytime and nighttime symptoms of asthma, reduce bronchodilator use, reduce exacerbations, and improve quality of life (11).

The treatment for asthma can depend on the status of acute versus chronic as well as the patient's lifestyle. The most common treatments are bronchodilators to reduce bronchoconstriction and avoid irritants. Asthma is very prevalent in society and managed through medications as well as lifestyle changes. In the long term, asthma can cause airway remodeling or permanent structural changes such as thickening of the sub-basement membrane and airway smooth muscle hypertrophy and hyperplasia (12).

INTERSTITIAL LUNG DISEASE AND OBSTRUCTIVE SLEEP APNEA

ILD is a lung disorder that causes inflammation and scarring to the tissues around the air sacs in the lungs, leading to difficulty breathing and distributing oxygen to the bloodstream. Individuals with ILD show reduced muscle mass, lung volumes, and gas exchange, leading to increased work of breathing. Other factors contributing to the diagnosis of OSA in patients with ILD are corticosteroids being a common form of treatment, which was previously noted to increase fat distribution to the neck area. All these factors contribute to OSA being one of the most common comorbidities in individuals with ILD (2). Similarly to other respiratory disorders, ILD has a bidirectional relationship with OSA, since OSA shows a progression in lung injury due to repetitive micro aspirations from GERD and oxidative stress, due to intermittent hypoxia. Unlike other respiratory disorders associated with OSA, CPAP does not appear to be the most effective treatment in patients with ILD and OSA, because due to the progression of the disease, there is a need to continually change pressure settings and even modes of PAP therapy, making it difficult for an individual to be compliant with long-term treatment (6). Alternatively, individuals with ILD are recommended to undergo pulmonary rehabilitation as a form of therapy, which has shown improvement in dyspnea, functional exercise capacity, quality of life, and a reduction in AHI (2). Although the prevalence of this association between ILD and OSA seems to be rising, there is still much needed research to be done on the impacts on progression and optimal treatment options.

NEUROMUSCULAR DISEASE AND SLEEP

NMD is a progressive disorder in which the patient will present with symptoms of muscle weakness in addition to stiffness and cramping in the extremities and demonstrate problems with speech, swallowing, and, occasionally, breathing. According to the National Institute for Health and Care Excellence, shortness of breath being present at diagnosis will shorten life expectancy. These symptoms are commonly noticed initially as unexplained instances of falls or tripping, when the patient is truly suffering from increased muscle weakness. NMD is associated with a high mortality rate. The most common form of this disease is amyotrophic lateral sclerosis (ALS). The cause of NMD is unknown, although a correlation in family history has been recognized (13).

Diagnosis of an NMD needs to come from a neurologist, with common routes of assessing NMD involving oximetry testing, forced vital capacity, and sniff nasal inspiratory pressure, to obtain a respiratory baseline for the patient. Once a patient is diagnosed with NMD, several levels of care are initiated. Medications can be given to alleviate muscle cramps and pain, although not only will patients need help with the physical effects of the diagnosis, but the emotional effects of the diagnosis will also require additional support (13).

NMD often results in upper airway dysfunction and central respiratory control abnormalities, potentially leading to obstructive apneas during sleep; this increases the risk of hypercapnic respiratory failure (6).

Similarly to OVS, NIV can also be offered as a treatment for patients showing increased breathing difficulty due to NMD. Although NIV treatment can improve symptoms of respiratory distress and decrease mortality rate in patients with NMD, there is, unfortunately, no cure at this time. The main goal of treatment of NMD is to increase quality of life and maintain functional ability (13).

REFERENCES

1. Martinez-Pitre PJ, Sabbula BR, Cascella M. Restrictive lung disease. In: *StatPearls* [Internet]. StatPearls Publishing; 2025. Retrieved April 18, 2025. https://www.ncbi.nlm.nih.gov/books/NBK560880/
2. Khor YH, Ryerson CJ, Landry SA, et al. Interstitial lung disease and obstructive sleep apnea. *Sleep Med Rev*. 2021;58:101442. doi:10.1016/j.smrv.2021.101442 PMID: 33561604.
3. van Zeller M, McNicholas WT. Sleep disordered breathing: OSA-COPD overlap. *Expert Rev Respir Med*. 2024;18(6):369-379. doi:10.1080/17476348.2024.2373790 PMID: 38932721.
4. Du W, Liu J, Zhou J, et al. Obstructive sleep apnea, COPD, the overlap syndrome, and mortality: results from the 2005–2008 National Health and Nutrition Examination Survey. *Int J Chron Obstruct Pulmon Dis*. 2018;13:665-674. doi:10.2147/COPD.S148735
5. Luehrs RE, Moreau KL, Pierce GL, et al. Cognitive performance is lower among individuals with overlap syndrome than in individuals with COPD or obstructive sleep apnea alone: association with carotid artery stiffness. *J Appl Physiol (1985)*. 2021;131(1):131-141. doi:10.1152/japplphysiol.00477.2020 PMID: 33982592; PMCID: PMC8325616.
6. Locke BW, Lee JJ, Sundar KM. OSA and chronic respiratory disease: mechanisms and epidemiology. *Int J Environ Res Public Health*. 2022;19(9):5473. doi:10.3390/ijerph19095473 PMID: 35564882; PMCID: PMC9105014.
7. Economou NT, Ilias I, Velentza L, et al. Sleepiness, fatigue, anxiety and depression in chronic obstructive pulmonary disease and obstructive sleep apnea-overlap-syndrome, before and after continuous positive airways pressure therapy. *PLOS One*. 2018;13(6):e0197342. doi:10.1371/journal.pone.0197342
8. Hansson D, Andersson A, Vanfleteren LEGW, et al. Clinical impact of routine sleep assessment by peripheral arterial tonometry in patients with COPD. *ERJ Open Res*. 2023;9(2):00458-2022. doi:10.1183/23120541.00458-2022 PMID: 37101736; PMCID: PMC10123515.
9. Sanchez-Azofra A, Gu W, Masso-Silva JA, et al. Inflammation biomarkers in OSA, chronic obstructive pulmonary disease, and chronic obstructive pulmonary disease/OSA overlap syndrome. *J Clin Sleep Med*. 2023;19(8):1447-1456. doi:10.5664/jcsm.10600 PMID: 37082823; PMCID: PMC10394367.

10. McNicholas WT. COPD-OSA overlap syndrome: evolving evidence regarding epidemiology, clinical consequences, and management. *Chest*. 2017; 152(6):1318-1326. doi:10.1016/j.chest.2017.04.160 PMID: 28442310.
11. Prasad B, Nyenhuis SM, Imayama I, Siddiqi A, Teodorescu M. Asthma and obstructive sleep apnea overlap: what has the evidence taught us? *Am J Respir Crit Care Med*. 2020;201(11):1345-1357. doi:10.1164/rccm.201810-1838TR PMID: 31841642; PMCID: PMC7258643.
12. Sundborn F, Janson C, Malinovschi A, et al. Effects of coexisting asthma and obstructive sleep apnea on sleep architecture, oxygen saturation, and systemic inflammation in women. *J Clin Sleep Med*. 2018;14(2):253-259.
13. Dawoud D; Guideline Development Group. NICE motor neuron disease: assessment and management. NICE guideline [NG42]. 2019. Retrieved April 18, 2025. https://www.nice.org.uk/guidance/ng42

Chapter 20 Impact of Vascular Disorders on Sleep

JENNIFER PARR-CHRISTMAS, MONICA M. HENDERSON, JAMES D. GEYER, AND PAUL R. CARNEY

KEY CONCEPTS/LEARNING OBJECTIVES

The key concepts in this chapter include the autonomic physiology of sleep, the relationship between sleep and hypertension, the relationship between sleep and stroke, the relationship between sleep and heart failure, and the effect of treatment with positive airway pressure on vascular disease.

KEY TERMS

Arrhythmia
Catecholamines
continuous positive airway pressure (CPAP)
Heart failure
Hypertension
Metabolic syndrome
Myocardial infarction
Parasympathetic
Sympathetic

VASCULAR DISORDERS AND SLEEP

Vascular diseases, including myocardial infarction, stroke, cerebrovascular disease, heart failure, and cardiac arrhythmias, are the most common causes of morbidity and mortality in industrialized countries. Sleep-related breathing disorders are also widespread and increasing in prevalence because of the obesity epidemic, with approximately 1 billion people worldwide (1) suffering from obstructive sleep apnea. Given the frequency of the two diseases, sleep disorders and vascular disorders, it is not surprising that they often coexist. The interactions between the obstructive sleep apnea/hypopnea syndrome and vascular diseases are much more complex than originally thought, and their comorbidity is more than mere coexistence. Sleep-related breathing disorders, insomnia, and even normal autonomic changes associated with rapid eye movement (REM) sleep can adversely affect vascular diseases. This chapter will review the normal autonomic processes that are seen in sleep and discuss the role that sleep disorders may play in heart disease, hypertension, and stroke.

NORMAL AUTONOMIC PHYSIOLOGY OF SLEEP

The autonomic nervous system regulates the involuntary, automatic functions of the visceral organs. It is comprised of the parasympathetic and sympathetic divisions, two opposing systems, the balance of which determine autonomic function. The sympathetic system has a stimulant effect and is responsible for the "fight or flight" response. Its primary neurochemical mediator is noradrenaline, an adrenaline-like substance that produces an increased heart rate; increased respiratory rate; vasoconstriction of blood vessels in visceral organs with vasodilatation of blood vessels in skeletal muscles; increased blood pressure; pupillary dilation; plus inhibition of digestion, urination, and defecation. In contrast, the parasympathetic system counterbalances these effects. Its primary neurotransmitter is acetylcholine, and its effects include slowing of the heart rate and respiration, vasodilatation of visceral organs with decreased blood pressure, pupillary constriction, increased peristalsis, plus emptying of the bladder and the rectum. Since vasoconstriction and hypertension are major contributors to myocardial infarction and stroke, it is useful to examine the body's normal sympathetic and parasympathetic responses during sleep.

In general, at sleep onset, there is a decrease in sympathetic tone and a concomitant increase in parasympathetic tone, which causes a lowering of the heart rate, blood pressure, respiration rate, and tidal volume, which continues during non-REM (NREM) sleep (2). With the transition to tonic REM sleep, the parasympathetic activity continues to increase, and the sympathetic activity is further suppressed. During phasic REM sleep, there are bursts of sympathetic activity (2). Heart rate variation during NREM sleep follows a sinusoidal pattern (2).

A normal respiratory sinus arrhythmia is produced by the normal respiratory activity coupled with cardiorespiratory center activity. During normal inspiration, the heart rate briefly accelerates to accommodate venous return and increased cardiac output (2). During expiration, there is a progressive decrease in heart rate. This normal cardiac rhythm variability is a marker for cardiac health, and its absence is associated with increasing age and possible cardiac disease. During REM sleep, it is normal for the heart rate to become increasingly variable, with episodes of moderate tachycardia and bradycardia. Respiratory patterns are also irregular and may result in mild oxygen desaturations. The neurons controlling the principal diaphragmatic respiratory muscles are typically not inhibited during REM sleep, but accessory muscles in the ribcage (the intercostal muscles) and neck may have partial muscle atonia. This causes the diaphragm to bear most of the load of respiration, which leads to partial diaphragmatic fatigue, hypoventilation, and decreased oxygenation over a period of several minutes. These episodes are referred to as REM sleep hypoventilation episodes and should be scored as hypopneas if they produce an oxygen desaturation of four points or greater over a period of 10 seconds or more (2).

There may be a transient 35% increase (3) in the baseline heart rate, especially during phasic REM sleep, due to a burst of sympathetic activation. β-blockers such as atenolol tend to reduce this phenomenon. Increased parasympathetic activity during NREM sleep contributes to cardiac electrical stability and helps decrease cardiac metabolic activity, decreasing the risk of cardiac arrhythmia. The decreased blood pressure produced by the parasympathetic system during NREM sleep, however, can contribute to decreased blood flow to the coronary arteries and result in myocardial hypoperfusion, increasing the risk of infarction in patients with significant coronary atherosclerosis (2). The surges in autonomic activity and increased heart rate during REM sleep increase the risk for ventricular arrhythmias. Sympathetic activity results in increased oxygen consumption by the cardiac muscle but also produces coronary vasoconstriction, decreasing the blood flow to the heart, thus increasing the risk of cardiac ischemia. It has been documented that a significant number of myocardial infarctions occur in the early morning hours, on awakening, or shortly after awakening; however, the relationship among sleep state, cardiac ischemia, and myocardial infarction is incompletely understood at this time.

Cerebral blood flow is, of course, closely linked to cardiac output, and the factors described previously also impact blood flow to the brain. In addition, during REM sleep, there is an increase in blood flow to the limbic system and the brainstem, with circulation to these structures decreasing during NREM sleep. As brain activity increases during REM sleep, the cerebral requirements for glucose and oxygen both increase, and a compensatory increase occurs in oxygenated hemoglobin delivery accompanying the transition from NREM sleep to REM sleep. Mild hypercapnea develops during NREM sleep and appears to counteract the circulatory effect of the decreased cerebral metabolic rate during NREM sleep. $Paco_2$ is an important determinant of respiration and hence cerebral blood flow during sleep in obstructive sleep apnea and other related disorders (2).

VASCULAR PATHOLOGY AND SLEEP

Hypertension

The Sleep Heart Health Study was designed as a prospective cohort study to investigate obstructive sleep apnea and other sleep-disordered breathing as a risk factor for the development of hypertension and cardiovascular disease (4). The results of the study suggest that the elevated sympathetic activity associated with sleep-related breathing disorders likely represents the primary mechanism in the pathogenesis of developing subsequent hypertension. This would typically begin as a loss of nocturnal dipping, the normal drop in blood pressure that occurs during sleep (5). Following the loss of nocturnal dipping, some patients develop elevated nocturnal arterial blood pressure, which can then progress to an elevated daytime blood pressure. Obstructive sleep apnea is an independent risk factor for the development of both nocturnal and daytime arterial hypertension (6). There appears to be a linear association between the severity of obstructive sleep apnea and the likelihood of developing subsequent hypertension. According to the Wisconsin Sleep Cohort Study, a patient with an apnea-hypopnea index greater than 15 events per hour has a 2.9-fold relative risk of developing hypertension compared to the normal patient population. This implies that many patients thought to have essential hypertension actually have hypertension secondary, at least in part, to obstructive sleep apnea.

The Joint National Committee on Prevention, Detection, Evaluation and Treatment of High Blood Pressure has recommended that obstructive sleep apnea be excluded as a contributing cause of medically refractory hypertension. With the new tighter controls recommended for hypertension, screening for these contributing causes becomes increasingly important, especially in patients who have already had a heart attack or stroke.

Nasal continuous positive airway pressure (CPAP) in patients with hypertension and moderate to severe obstructive sleep apnea leads to a significant reduction in arterial blood pressure (7,8). The effect of CPAP on hypertension is more pronounced in patients with severe obstructive sleep apnea. Patients with only a 50% reduction in apnea on the apnea-hypopnea index did not have a significant reduction in blood pressure. This underscores the importance of good control of apnea and hypopnea, followed by excellent patient compliance with CPAP.

Heart Failure

Heart failure (HF) occurs when cardiac dysfunction requires the body to make compensatory changes to maintain adequate cardiac output. The failure of the heart to pump effectively results in venous congestion, which produces many of the symptoms of HF. The clinical features include dyspnea on exertion, orthopnea (dyspnea when lying down), and paroxysmal nocturnal dyspnea (sudden episodes of shortness of breath during sleep). Patients with HF have a significantly increased risk of sleep-disordered breathing, with obstructive sleep apnea occurring in 11% to 37% of patients, and patients with obstructive sleep apnea often have coexisting central sleep apnea (9,10). Central apnea, periodic breathing, and Cheyne-Stokes breathing are also frequently associated with HF. The Sleep Heart Health Study identified a 2.38-fold increased relative risk for the development of HF in patients with obstructive sleep apnea that was independent of all other recognized risk factors for HF. Symptoms classically associated with HF such as paroxysmal nocturnal dyspnea may, in fact, be related, in part, to obstructive sleep apnea.

Central sleep apnea occurs more frequently in patients with severe HF and may in some cases contribute to the progression of the HF. Patients with HF and central sleep apnea have higher levels of catecholamines such as adrenaline than do patients with HF without central sleep apnea. This catecholamine effect would have further negative effects on cardiac function.

In patients with HF, aggressive treatment of concomitant obstructive sleep apnea results in both a reduction in systolic blood pressure and an improvement in left ventricular function. Treatment of obstructive sleep apnea with CPAP in patients with HF can improve the left ventricular ejection fraction and left ventricular end systolic diameter and augment the heart's stroke volume (11). Furthermore, the risk of ventricular tachycardia decreases, as does the frequency of premature ventricular contractions (PVCs).

Cardiac Arrhythmias

Tachyarrhythmias commonly occur with obstructive sleep apnea, usually occurring at the end of an apnea or hypopnea episode during the period of hyperpneic breathing and often in association with an EEG arousal. Several studies have indicated that the frequency of atrial fibrillation is increased in patients with obstructive sleep apnea and other sleep-related breathing disorders (12). Ventricular tachycardia becomes more likely as oxygen saturation falls below 60% (2).

Bradyarrhythmias are also frequently associated with obstructive sleep apnea. Sinus bradycardia, which can be severe, is common during apnea or hypopnea. Rarely, patients may develop sinus arrest or atrioventricular block. Patients with nocturnal bradycardia should be screened for obstructive sleep apnea.

COAGULATION AND PLATELET ACTIVITY

Thrombus formation is the most common clinical event that leads to myocardial infarction. It also plays a significant role in stroke. The process of clot formation is a complex one that involves the interaction of platelets, circulating coagulation factors, and the surface of endothelial cells that line blood vessels. When a blood vessel is injured, circulating platelets adhere to the wall, forming a loose aggregate that occludes the lumen of the vessel. The platelet aggregate then activates the coagulation cascade, resulting in the production of fibrin, a molecular "glue" that strengthens the loose aggregate, thereby forming a thrombus (blood vessel blockage). The tendency for platelets to aggregate increases with obstructive sleep apnea, mediated, at least in part, by the increased levels of catecholamines in these patients (13,14). Furthermore, these patients may also have abnormally increased daytime levels of fibrinogen, the precursor to fibrin.

Hematocrit is defined as the volume percent of erythrocytes, or red blood cells, in whole blood. The higher a patient's hematocrit, the more red cells there are in circulation. While plasma, or the liquid component of blood, can flow freely, the cellular components of blood produce increased blood viscosity with a decreased rate of flow, especially in small blood vessels and in arteries narrowed by atherosclerotic plaque. As the rate of flow decreases, the tendency to form circulating platelet aggregates increases, increasing the risk of thrombosis. When patients with moderate to severe obstructive sleep apnea experience chronic nocturnal hypoxia, the body tries to compensate by producing more erythrocytes and increasing the oxygen-carrying capacity of the blood. This produces a state of hyperviscosity, which, when coupled with the increased tendency to produce platelet aggregates, places these patients at greatly increased risk for heart attack and stroke.

There is evidence that treatment of obstructive sleep apnea with CPAP can improve the nocturnal hypoxemia and therefore help decrease hematocrit and blood viscosity. Furthermore, lessening the episodes of catecholamine release would reduce the relative increase in platelet aggregation. CPAP may also reduce the activity of some circulating clotting factors.

METABOLIC SYNDROME X

Metabolic syndrome X is a recently recognized constellation of metabolic abnormalities that are associated with an increased risk of vascular diseases. The symptoms include central obesity with fat deposits centered around the abdomen, glucose intolerance/insulin resistance, hypertension, hypercholesterolemia, and abnormalities in clotting of blood. Although syndrome X is not a vascular disease, it greatly increases a patient's risk of heart attack and stroke and is included for discussion in this chapter. We have previously discussed the possible role sleep-related breathing disorders may have on hypertension with an increased tendency to form blood clots. We will now examine the possible role of sleep disorders and two of the other components of the syndrome: glucose intolerance and obesity.

Obstructive sleep apnea has been shown to produce glucose intolerance, with the severity of the apnea correlating with the degree of insulin resistance (15). Obstructive sleep apnea is associated with higher blood glucose, higher insulin levels, and higher glycosylated hemoglobin levels, a laboratory finding seen in poorly controlled diabetes. Unfortunately, treatment of obstructive sleep apnea with CPAP has not resulted in consistent improvement of glucose tolerance. Further study of the exact metabolic effects of CPAP is needed.

There may also be an association between obstructive sleep apnea and obesity. Leptin is a hormone produced by fat cells that is seen in increased levels in patients with higher weight. Males with obstructive sleep apnea have relatively higher levels of leptin than do males without obstructive sleep apnea. This may be secondary to leptin resistance. Leptin may increase the production of platelet aggregation and may serve as an independent marker for the risk of vascular disease. Studies have shown that leptin levels fall following treatment with CPAP, and therapy for obstructive sleep apnea may not only improve the patient's difficulty with weight gain but may also decrease the risk of heart attack and stroke by decreasing the tendency of platelet aggregation (16).

ISCHEMIC HEART DISEASE

Obstructive sleep apnea and coronary artery disease frequently coexist, with at least 50% of patients with heart disease having significant obstructive sleep apnea. Obstructive sleep apnea is an independent risk factor for myocardial infarction similarly to hypertension and smoking. The sympathetic activity of the autonomic nervous system during normal REM sleep increases blood pressure and heart rate with a concomitant increase in cardiac oxygen consumption (12). Significant oxygen desaturations in a patient with obstructive sleep apnea further contribute to nocturnal angina and nocturnal ischemic changes in the electrocardiogram (ECG).

Treatment of obstructive sleep apnea with CPAP has been shown to improve ECG changes. There is also evidence of fewer incidences or a lower degree of nocturnal angina, but large clinical trials are lacking. Outcome following myocardial infarction is worse in patients with obstructive sleep apnea, with a higher mortality in patients with untreated obstructive sleep apnea and coronary artery disease (38%) than in patients with cardiac disease but without obstructive sleep apnea (9%).

CEREBROVASCULAR DISEASE

Annually, more than 750,000 strokes occur in the United States, with approximately 150,000 fatalities. Tremendous resources are required to care for the over 3 million stroke survivors in the United States alone. Numerous studies have demonstrated that 31% to 54% of strokes occur during sleep, and the most common time of onset during wakefulness is in the first several hours following awakening. The Sleep Heart Health Study identified an increase in the prevalence of strokes in patients with concomitant obstructive sleep apnea, and other studies have shown the frequency of coexisting sleep apnea and stroke in 62.5% to 80% of stroke patients (17,18).

Cerebral autoregulation is the process by which the brain attempts to control intracranial blood pressure to maintain adequate blood flow. Obstructive sleep apnea interferes with this process. While the change has not been shown to cause stroke, the inability of the brain to change pressures to ensure adequate circulation may produce decreased cerebral perfusion and result in enlargement of an acute stroke that originated from other causes. Treatment of obstructive sleep apnea with CPAP results in improvement of the cerebral autoregulation and overall cerebral blood flow measured by transcranial Doppler ultrasound.

The sleepiness and snoring associated with obstructive sleep apnea are frequently the presenting symptoms and those with which the patients are most concerned. Sleep apnea has a major impact on a variety of vascular disorders. Identification and aggressive treatment of sleep-related breathing disorders not only decreases vascular risk but also improves functional status. This medical information can also be used to encourage the patient toward better CPAP compliance. Given the importance of effective treatment, patient compliance with CPAP therapy should be monitored closely.

REFERENCES

1. Lyons MM, Bhatt NY, Pack AI, Magalang UJ. Global burden of sleep-disordered breathing and its implications. *Respirology*. 2020;25(7):690-702. doi:10.1111/resp.13838 PMID: 32436658.
2. Carney P, Berry R, Geyer J, eds. *Clinical Sleep Disorders*. Lippincott, Williams & Wilkins; 2005.
3. Fultz NE, Bonmassar G, Setsompop K, et al. Coupled electrophysiological, hemodynamic, and cerebrospinal fluid oscillations in human sleep. *Science*. 2019;366(6465):628-631. doi:10.1126/science.aax5440 PMID: 31672896; PMCID: PMC7309589.
4. Punjabi NM, Shahar E, Redline S, Gottlieb DJ, Givelber R, Resnick HE. Sleep disordered breathing, glucose intolerance, and insulin resistance: the Sleep Heart Health Study. *Am J Epidemiol*. 2004;160(6):521-530.
5. Johnson DA, Thomas SJ, Abdalla M, et al. Association between sleep apnea and blood pressure control among blacks. *Circulation*. 2019;139(10):1275-1284. doi:10.1161/CIRCULATIONAHA.118.036675 PMID: 30586763; PMCID: PMC6428682.
6. Crinion SJ, Kleinerova J, Kent B, et al. Non-dipping nocturnal blood pressure correlates with obstructive sleep apnoea severity in normotensive subjects and may reverse with therapy. *ERJ Open Res*. 2021;7(3):00338-2021. doi:10.1183/23120541.00338-2021 PMID: 34409095; PMCID: PMC8365144.
7. Salman LA, Shulman R, Cohen JB. Obstructive sleep apnea, hypertension, and cardiovascular risk: epidemiology, pathophysiology, and management. *Curr Cardiol Rep*. 2020;22(2):6. doi:10.1007/s11886-020-1257-y PMID: 31955254.
8. Sánchez-de-la-Torre M, Gracia-Lavedan E, Benitez ID, et al. Adherence to CPAP treatment and the risk of recurrent cardiovascular events: a meta-analysis. *JAMA*. 2023;330(13):1255-1265. doi:10.1001/jama.2023.17465 PMID: 37787793; PMCID: PMC10548300.
9. Yeghiazarians Y, Jneid H, Tietjens JR, et al. Obstructive sleep apnea and cardiovascular disease: a scientific statement from the American Heart Association. *Circulation*. 2021;144(3):e56-e67. doi:10.1161/CIR.0000000000000988 Erratum in: *Circulation*. 2022;145(12):e775. doi:http://doi.org/10.1161/CIR.0000000000001043 PMID: 34148375.
10. Mehra R. Sleep apnea and the heart. *Cleve Clin J Med*. 2019;86(9 suppl 1):10-18. doi:10.3949/ccjm.86.s1.03 PMID: 31509499.
11. Masip J, Peacock WF, Price S, et al; Acute Heart Failure Study Group of the Acute Cardiovascular Care Association and the Committee on Acute Heart Failure of the Heart Failure Association of the European Society of Cardiology. Indications and practical approach to non-invasive ventilation in acute heart failure. *Eur Heart J*. 2018;39(1):17-25. doi:10.1093/eurheartj/ehx580 PMID: 29186485; PMCID: PMC6251669.
12. Linz D, McEvoy RD, Cowie MR, et al. Associations of obstructive sleep apnea with atrial fibrillation and continuous positive airway pressure treatment: a review. *JAMA Cardiol*. 2018;3(6):532-540. doi:10.1001/jamacardio.2018.0095 PMID: 29541763.
13. Guardiola JJ, Matheson PJ, Clavijo LC, Wilson MA, Fletcher EC. Hypercoagulability in patients with obstructive sleep apnea. *Sleep Med*. 2001;2(6):517-523.
14. Kovbasyuk Z, Ramos-Cejudo J, Parekh A, et al. Obstructive sleep apnea, platelet aggregation, and cardiovascular risk. *J Am Heart Assoc*. 2024;13(15):e034079. doi:10.1161/JAHA.123.034079 PMID: 39056328.
15. Giampá SQC, Lorenzi-Filho G, Drager LF. Obstructive sleep apnea and metabolic syndrome. *Obesity (Silver Spring)*. 2023;31(4):900-911. doi:10.1002/oby.23679 PMID: 36863747.
16. Lee JH, Cho J. Sleep and obesity. *Sleep Med Clin*. 2022;17(1):111-116. doi:10.1016/j.jsmc.2021.10.009 PMID: 35216758.
17. Sun B, Ma Q, Shen J, Meng Z, Xu J. Up-to-date advance in the relationship between OSA and stroke: a narrative review. *Sleep Breath*. 2024;28(1):53-60. doi:10.1007/s11325-023-02904-2 PMID: 37632670.
18. Bassetti C, Aldrich MS. Sleep apnea in acute cerebrovascular diseases: final report on 128 patients. *Sleep*. 1999;22(2):217-223. doi:10.1093/sleep/22.2.217 PMID: 10201066.

Chapter 21
Sleep and Other Medical Disorders

IAIN DUNCAN

KEY CONCEPTS/LEARNING OBJECTIVES

The key concepts for this chapter include the bidirectional influences of various respiratory, neurologic, gastrointestinal, endocrine, rheumatologic, renal, and infectious diseases on sleep and sleep disorders.

KEY TERMS

Asthma
Chronic obstructive pulmonary disease
Cystic fibrosis
Endocrine disorders
Fibromyalgia
Gastrointestinal disorders
Infectious diseases
Neuromuscular disorders
Renal disease
Rheumatologic disorders

RESPIRATORY DISORDERS

Asthma

Asthma is an inflammatory disease of the airways that occurs in about 5% of the population. It is characterized by episodic dyspnea and wheezing, reversible episodes of bronchoconstriction, and airway hyperreactivity to a variety of specific and nonspecific stimuli.

In a survey of patients with asthma, 74% of subjects reported nocturnal awakenings at least once a week, and 64% experienced nocturnal awakenings 3 times per week. In another, general population sample of patients with asthma, nocturnal symptoms occurred less than once a week in 16% to 23% and at least once a week in 5% to 15% of subjects (1).

Patients with nocturnal asthma experience poor sleep quality with frequent arousals, and report sleep deprivation, irritability, and fatigue. Worsening of asthma at night or in the early morning occurs in over two-thirds of patients with asthma, indicating nighttime bronchoconstriction. Besides normal sleep-related decreases in functional residual capacity (FRC), minute ventilation, and tidal volume, patients with asthma have further abnormal reductions in these parameters during sleep that are attributed to increased airway responsiveness; increased airway secretions; and circadian changes in vagal tone, body temperature, cortisol, epinephrine, and inflammatory mediators (2). Bronchoalveolar lavage fluid in patients with nocturnal asthma may show an increase in total leukocyte count, neutrophils, and eosinophils.

Polysomnographic (PSG) features of subjects with asthma demonstrate increased wake time, less total sleep time, reduced sleep efficiency, increased number of awakenings, and greater wake time after sleep onset compared with normal subjects. People with nocturnal asthma who snore or have obstructive sleep apnea (OSA) show increased frequency of nocturnal asthma attacks. Although they are two distinct disease processes, nocturnal asthma and OSA often share overlapping symptoms of choking, coughing, and dyspnea. Continuous positive airway pressure (CPAP) therapy has been shown to improve asthma control and increase peak expiratory flow rate in this group of patients (3).

Chronic Obstructive Pulmonary Disease

Chronic obstructive pulmonary disease (COPD) (also called "chronic obstructive lung disease") is a disease state characterized by airflow limitation that is relatively irreversible. The airflow limitation is usually associated with an abnormal inflammatory response of the lungs to noxious particles or gases and is progressive in nature (4). The inflammatory response of the lungs results in pathologic changes in the small airways and alveoli. Emphysema results when there is a predominance of alveolar destruction, whereas chronic bronchitis is the result of progressive airway narrowing because of excessive secretions blocking the lumen of the airways. Dyspnea and chronic cough are the chief complaints with which patients with COPD usually present. Respiratory failure can complicate advanced cases, with hypoxemia and hypercapnia occurring during both wakefulness and sleep. The World Health Organization states in November 2024 that chronic obstructive pulmonary disease (COPD) is the fourth leading cause of death worldwide, causing 3.5 million deaths in 2021, approximately 5% of all global deaths.

Clinicians distinguish between two subtypes of patients with COPD: blue bloaters and pink puffers. Blue bloaters have lower baseline arterial oxygen saturation ($Sa{O_2}$), and, hence, their blood will be bluer, and they will experience larger falls in $Sa{O_2}$ (especially during rapid eye movement [REM] sleep), more episodes of oxygen desaturation, and longer durations of oxygen desaturation while asleep than will pink puffers.

Patients with COPD sleep poorly compared with healthy subjects (5). The incidence of sleep complaints is related to the rates of respiratory symptoms in patients with COPD. In the Tucson Epidemiologic Study of Chronic Lung Diseases, 28% of subjects with asymptomatic COPD reported insomnia and 9% daytime sleepiness. Among subjects with one respiratory symptom, either cough or wheezing, 39% reported insomnia and 12% daytime sleepiness. When both cough and wheezing were present as respiratory symptoms, sleep complaints increased in patients, with 52% of them reporting insomnia and 22% daytime sleepiness (6).

PSG features show reduced total sleep time, increased sleep stage changes, and increased arousal frequency. Arousals may or may not be related to hypoxemia. Plywaczewski et al. showed that reversal of hypoxemia with supplemental oxygen did not diminish arousal frequency. Oxygen therapy may or may not affect sleep quality (6).

During sleep, patients with COPD may develop significant oxygen desaturation, with the most severe desaturations occurring during REM sleep (5). Sleep-related hypoxemic episodes are more common among blue bloaters than among pink puffers and occur during periods of hypoventilation, typically during REM sleep, because of the relative atonia of the intercostal muscles that occurs during REM sleep. Ventilatory abnormalities associated with decreased lung volumes (because of, for instance, obesity) also contribute to hypoxemia during sleep (4).

Overlap syndrome, also referred to as OLDOSA (obstructive lung disease and obstructive sleep apnea), is a term used for patients with coexisting COPD and/or asthma and OSA. A more severe course of sleep-disordered breathing is noted in subjects with coexisting COPD (7). Sleep studies are usually indicated in COPD when there is a possibility of sleep apnea or obesity-hypoventilation syndrome (8,9). A triad of respiratory alterations contributes to the physiologic derangements seen in overlap syndrome:

1. Increase in upper airway resistance: in addition to the excessive soft tissue and oropharyngeal anomalies seen in OSA, upper airway luminal narrowing may be further compromised by COPD processes such as mucosal inflammation, chronic rhinitis and bronchitis, and reduced cough reflex.
2. Sleep alterations in lung volumes: REM skeletal muscle atonia, thoracic restrictions related to body position, and consequent tidal volume reduction result in FRC reduction, even in normal subjects. In patients with COPD, functional lung volumes are further compromised by alveolar air trapping or hyperinflation.
3. Changes in central mediators of respiratory effort: during wakefulness, chemoreceptor responses to hypoxemia and hypercapnia regulate respiratory rate and depth. These chemoreceptor responses are blunted during sleep, impacting both ventilatory and arousal responses.

Several studies have shown that patients with COPD and OSA have more profound nocturnal oxygen desaturations and sleep disturbances compared with either disease alone. Additionally, reports from observational studies suggest increased mortality in overlap syndrome compared with COPD and OSA alone (Table 21-1) (10).

Although supplemental oxygen is the mainstay for COPD and sleep-associated desaturation alone, positive airway pressure, either CPAP or bilevel positive airway pressure (BPAP), combined with supplemental oxygen, is required for the overlap syndrome (11,12). Some patients may respond better to BPAP than to CPAP.

Table 21-1 The Cardinal Symptoms of Chronic Obstructive Pulmonary Disease and Obstructive Sleep Apnea With Potential Overlapping Symptoms Highlighted in the Center

OSA Symptoms	COPD Symptoms
Snoring	Wheezing
Respiratory pauses	Sputum production
Daytime sleepiness	Dyspnea
Overlapping Symptoms Poor sleep quality Insomnia Nocturnal cough/gasp Persistent fatigue Mood changes	

COPD, chronic obstructive pulmonary disease; OSA, obstructive sleep apnea.
Adapted from Mieczkowski B, Ezzie ME. Update on obstructive sleep apnea and its relation to COPD. *Int J Chron Obstruct Pulmon Dis.* 2014;9:349-362. Reprinted by permission of Informa UK Limited, trading as Taylor & Francis Group, www.tandfonline.com. © 2014 Mieczkowski and Ezzie.

Cystic Fibrosis

Cystic fibrosis (CF) is a multisystem genetic disorder that affects, primarily, Caucasian infants, children, and young adults. It is characterized by abnormal transport of sodium and chloride across the epithelium in all exocrine tissues, leading to an increase in sweat sodium and chloride concentration. This inability to move salt and chloride in and out of cells results in thick viscous secretions in the lungs, pancreas, intestine, liver, and reproductive tract. Consequently, patients with CF develop bronchiectasis and progressive lung disease, exocrine pancreatic insufficiency, intestinal dysfunction, abnormal sweat gland function, and urogenital dysfunction (13,14).

Patients with CF have poor sleep quality (15). Nonetheless, sleep latency and sleep efficiency are often normal in patients with CF despite poor sleep quality (15). Exacerbations of lung disease in adults with CF adversely affect sleep and neurobehavioral performance regardless of underlying disease severity. A study of 40 children with CF in stable condition showed an early occurrence of OSA associated with a mild level of sleep disruption. Early routine nocturnal respiratory monitoring is advised in children with CF (16).

Cough, sleep fragmentation, medication side effects such as β-agonists, increased work of breathing, and hypoxemia have all been documented during sleep in patients with CF. Episodic nocturnal hypoxia may lead to the development of pulmonary hypertension and cor pulmonale. Poor daytime function and quality of life have also been reported (17). Noninvasive ventilation has been proposed as a means to temporarily reverse or slow the progression of worsening respiratory failure in CF (18).

Restrictive Lung Diseases

Restrictive lung diseases are characterized by reduced lung volumes, either because of an alteration in the lung parenchyma or because of diseases of the chest wall, pleura, or neuromuscular apparatus. In the early stages, the patient may be totally asymptomatic, but with disease progression, exertional dyspnea, followed by dyspnea at rest, is commonly encountered. Restrictive lung diseases commonly associated with sleep-disordered breathing are obesity, kyphoscoliosis, interstitial lung disease, and pregnancy.

Patients with restrictive lung disease exhibit a wide range of respiratory and oxygenation abnormalities during sleep. The combination of restrictive severity (intrapulmonary as well as extrapulmonary) and confounding factors, such as obesity, age, and gender, determines the degree of disturbed nocturnal physiology (19). These patients often complain of disrupted sleep and excessive daytime sleepiness, often even before waking respiratory symptoms become discernible. Other sleep-related symptoms include apneas, awakenings, choking, unrefreshing sleep, and morning headaches (20).

PSG suggests that OSA is present in more than 50% of patients with restrictive lung diseases and nocturnal hypoventilation in more than 29% of individuals with severe obesity (21,22). REM sleep percentage and sleep efficiency are decreased in patients with obesity, but sleep-onset latency and REM latency can remain normal (21).

In patients with kyphoscoliosis, a spectrum of breathing abnormalities can be found, ranging from no abnormalities to obstructive apneas/hypopneas and central apneas (23). Patients with interstitial lung disease often demonstrate transient or sustained nocturnal desaturation during REM sleep, disturbances in sleep quality, increase in stage N1 sleep, reduction in REM sleep, and an increase in the number of arousals (24,25). During pregnancy, sleep quality is poor, with reduced sleep efficiency, increased nocturnal awakenings, increased stage N1 sleep, reduced REM sleep, increased daytime fatigue, and louder or more frequent snoring (26-28).

NEUROMUSCULAR DISORDERS

The neuromuscular disorders most commonly associated with sleep-disordered breathing are muscular dystrophy (MD), myotonic dystrophy (DM), amyotrophic lateral sclerosis (ALS), poliomyelitis, and myasthenia gravis. Neuromuscular disorders may be caused by defects in the neurons or the muscle itself. Motor neurons extend from the brain to the spinal cord (upper motor neurons), from where they reach muscle fibers throughout the body (lower motor neurons). In neuromuscular disorders, the neurons are damaged and are unable to relay neural information or innervate muscle activity. The damage may occur in the brain, along the axon, or at the axon terminals (neuromuscular junctions). The principal consequence of a neuromuscular dysfunction in a sleeping individual is compromise of the ventilatory mechanism (ie, lower motor neuron, neuromuscular junction, or muscle) (29). Nocturnal breathing abnormalities or sleep-related breathing disorders frequently precede respiratory failure during wakefulness by months or even years (30).

Subjective sleep complaints include air hunger, intermittent snoring, orthopnea (difficulty breathing except when in an upright position), cyanosis (a bluish or purplish discoloration of the skin due to deficient oxygenation of the blood), restlessness, and insomnia. Daytime symptoms such as morning drowsiness, frequent morning headaches, and excessive daytime sleepiness have been described in patients with neuromuscular diseases.

MD is a group of genetic diseases characterized by progressive weakness and degeneration of skeletal muscles. Age of onset, extent and distribution of weakness, and rate of progression vary by MD type. Duchenne MD (DMD) is the most common form of MD and is seen primarily in boys. It is caused by the absence of the protein dystrophin. Dystrophin is found in muscle cell membranes and facilitates muscle cell self-repair. Muscle degeneration leads to loss of ambulation in adolescence and progresses to respiratory impairment, eventually requiring ventilatory support. The PSG of patients with DMD may reveal an increased number of arousals during the night, reduced REM sleep, and both central and obstructive apneas (31-33). Nocturnal noninvasive ventilation may improve daytime respiratory muscle function.

Patients with DM have disrupted sleep, apneic as well as hypopneic events, and hypoventilatory oxygen desaturation during REM sleep (34,35). Central nervous system (CNS) lesions may contribute to the hypersomnia without an accompanying sleep-disordered breathing or decrease in central respiratory drive (36).

ALS is a progressive and ultimately fatal neurodegenerative disorder, which affects neurons in the brain and spinal cord, eventually causing neural cell death. Loss of muscle-activating impulses and consequent muscle function leads to muscle weakness and eventual muscle atrophy. The diaphragm and chest wall muscles are not spared, and when they fail to function adequately, mechanical ventilatory support is required. Patients with ALS may have obstructive apneic and hypopneic events, with the majority of respiratory events occurring during REM sleep (37,38). Patients with ALS and diaphragmatic dysfunction have significant nocturnal desaturation secondary to hypoventilation as well as reduced REM sleep compared with those patients with preserved diaphragmatic function. Disruption of sleep is also attributable to physical symptoms such as muscle cramps, pain, reduced mobility, spasticity, mucus retention, and restless legs syndrome (RLS). Depression and anxiety may contribute to insomnia, and in a small subset of patients, REM sleep behavior disorder may be present (39).

Poliomyelitis is an infectious viral disease affecting mainly young children. It is preventable through vaccination but not curable. The manifestations may be subclinical, nonparalytic, or paralytic. The enterovirus enters the body through the fecal-oral route, begins an alimentary phase, enters the bloodstream, and may eventually cross the blood-brain barrier, invading the nervous system. Polio is a lower motor neuron disease, which can involve the motor nuclei of the brainstem and respiratory motor nuclei, resulting in respiratory muscle dysfunction and/or paralysis, including that of the diaphragm. These patients may develop sleep-disordered breathing, including obstructive apneic and hypopneic events, nocturnal hypoventilation, reduced sleep efficiency, increased arousals, increased stage N1 sleep, and reduced REM sleep (40,41).

Decades after surviving paralytic poliomyelitis, survivors may develop symptoms of postpolio syndrome (PPS): fatigue, heat or cold intolerance, slowly progressive muscle weakness/atrophy, fasciculations, and muscle and joint pain. Although the cause of PPS is unknown, it is believed that excessive metabolic stress on those muscles initially damaged results in the loss of nerve terminals and, eventually, of motor neurons themselves (42). The stressors include illness, weight gain, and the aging process. Patients with PPS may suffer from weakness of the diaphragm and respiratory muscles sufficient to cause resting and/or exertional dyspnea and hypercapnia. PSG should be used to rule out obstructive, central, and mixed apneas as well as nocturnal hypoxemia and hypercapnia. Nocturnal noninvasive ventilation may improve sleep quality, symptoms of daytime fatigue, and daytime respiratory muscle function.

Myasthenia gravis is a chronic autoimmune disease characterized by varying degrees of skeletal muscle weakness. It is caused by a defect in the transmission of nerve impulses across the neuromuscular junction to the target muscles. The neurotransmitter acetylcholine is blocked from binding to the muscle by the body's own antibodies. Patients with myasthenia gravis have a higher incidence of both central and obstructive apneas and hypopneas that are associated with significant oxygen desaturation and that occur predominantly during REM sleep (43,44).

DM is a genetic multisystemic disease characterized by progressive muscular weakness, myotonia, and involvement of the CNS, eyes, heart, respiratory function, and endocrine systems (45). There are two major forms: DM1, also known as Steinert disease, which may have congenital, juvenile, or adult onset, and DM2, which presents in adulthood and is often less severe. DM1 is more prevalent.

The manifestations of DM1 include neuromuscular, behavioral, emotional, and cognitive disturbances. The daily activities and social roles of this population are compromised, and life expectancy is shortened. Respiratory failure results from respiratory muscle weakness and myotonia, culminating in alveolar hypoventilation and chronic hypercapnia and hypoxemia.

Diaphragm Paralysis

The diaphragm is the primary muscle of ventilation. When contracted, the diaphragm descends, increasing thoracic volume while decreasing intrapleural pressure. The change in intrapleural pressure creates a pressure gradient and allows air to flow into the lungs. A single anatomic structure, the diaphragm has two halves individually innervated by branches of the phrenic nerve. The individual nerve supply allows each half to function independently of the other, although in normal diaphragmatic function, both halves move synchronously.

The most common causes of bilateral diaphragmatic paralysis are high spinal cord injury, thoracic trauma, multiple sclerosis, anterior horn disease, and MD. Unilateral paralysis of the diaphragm is much more common than is bilateral paralysis and may be caused by phrenic nerve damage because of trauma, surgery, radiation, tumor, or neuropathy. Unilateral diaphragmatic paralysis is associated with nocturnal hypoxemia, but, in the absence of systemic lung disease, it does not generally lead to chronic respiratory failure or cor pulmonale.

During REM sleep in normal persons, ventilation depends primarily on diaphragm function. In patients with diaphragm dysfunction, during both REM sleep and wakefulness, electromyographic activity of the extradiaphragmatic respiratory muscles is higher than normal as a compensation for diaphragm weakness (46). Patients with diaphragmatic paralysis have reduced REM and stage N3 sleep. Patients with unilateral diaphragm dysfunction are at risk of developing sleep-disordered breathing during REM sleep (46). Bilateral diaphragmatic paralysis can be associated with sleep apnea. Watanabe et al. reported a case of central sleep apnea (CSA) accompanied by bilateral paralysis of the diaphragm after pediatric cardiac surgery. Hoffstein and Taylor described a rapid development of OSA following hemidiaphragmatic and unilateral vocal cord paralysis as a complication of mediastinal surgery.

It had been hypothesized that patients with bilateral diaphragmatic paralysis might not be able to sustain REM sleep. However, Bennett et al. observed that patients with bilateral diaphragmatic paralysis had a normal quantity of REM sleep achieved by inspiratory recruitment of extradiaphragmatic muscles in both tonic and phasic REM, suggesting brainstem reorganization (47).

GASTROINTESTINAL DISORDERS

Gastroesophageal Reflux

Gastroesophageal reflux (GER) is caused by a backflow of gastric acid and other gastric contents into the esophagus because of incompetent barriers at the gastroesophageal junction. The pathogenesis of GER is multifactorial, involving transient lower esophageal sphincter (LES) relaxation as well as other LES pressure abnormalities. Other factors contributing to the pathophysiology of GER include the presence of a hiatal hernia, poor esophageal clearance, delayed gastric emptying, and impaired mucosal defensive factors.

Regurgitation of gastric contents into the mouth and heartburn are the characteristic symptoms of GER. Reflux of acidic stomach contents into the pharynx, larynx, and tracheobronchial tree can cause chronic cough, bronchoconstriction, pharyngitis, laryngitis, bronchitis, or pneumonia. Morning hoarseness may be noted. Recurrent pulmonary aspiration can cause aspiration pneumonia, pulmonary fibrosis, or chronic asthma. Reflux in the sleeping horizontal person is exacerbated by delayed acid clearance secondary to decreased esophageal motility and reduced salivation and swallowing.

Several studies have reported an association between OSA and gastroesophageal reflux disease (GERD). On the one hand, GERD may play a role in the development of OSA by causing upper airway inflammation and obstruction. Acid suppression with proton pump inhibitors resulted in improvement of the apnea index in patients with OSA in a small nonrandomized study. On the other hand, OSA may lead to GERD because of increased intrathoracic pressure, and treatment with CPAP has been shown to improve nocturnal heartburn and regurgitation, as well as distal esophageal acid exposure and frequency of acid reflux episodes (48).

The negative impact on quality of life may be greater in nocturnal GER than in daytime GER. In a large nationwide telephone survey in the United States, having heartburn symptoms at night was reported by 79% of respondents, of whom 75% stated that their sleep was affected by heartburn and 63% noted that heartburn had an impact on their ability to sleep well (49). Farup et al found a prevalence of 10% for nocturnal GER, with 74% of respondents who reported frequent GER symptoms having nocturnal GER.

GER is estimated to be present in 50% to 60% of children with asthma and 60% to 80% of adults with asthma (50). A study conducted by Wasilewska and colleagues reported a possible association between nocturnal GER and sleep-related breathing disorders in children. Higher numbers of apneas and hypopneas during REM sleep were found in children with nocturnal GER. Demeter et al (51) noted that in patients with severe OSA, erosive reflux disease is more frequent, and a positive correlation between severity of reflux disease and sleep apnea has been reported by some, but not all, investigators (52).

PSG findings in patients with GERD include an increased arousal index and decreased duration spent in the deeper stages of sleep.

Functional Bowel Disorders

Functional bowel disorders are characterized by chronic gastrointestinal tract symptoms without significant anatomic, metabolic, or infectious abnormalities. They can affect the entire digestive tract. These disorders include functional dyspepsia (FD), diarrhea, constipation, abdominal bloating, abdominal pain syndrome, and irritable bowel syndrome (IBS).

Patients with functional bowel disorders have a high incidence of sleep complaints as well as abnormalities of autonomic functioning. The measurement of autonomic functioning during sleep can differentiate the patients with functional bowel disorders from normal controls (53). Patients reported significantly more dissatisfaction with their sleep quality and increased daytime fatigue as a result of both insomnia-type symptomatology and nonrestful sleep (54).

A significant proportion of patients, particularly those with IBS and dyspepsia, reported nighttime gastrointestinal symptoms (54). In a study on patients with functional bowel disorders by Vege et al, sleep disturbances were reported by 68% of those with FD, 50.2% with IBS, 71% with IBS and FD, and 55% of normal subjects. Vege et al, reported that in patients who suffered from sleep disorders, there was a prevalence of 33.3% for IBS and 21.3% for FD (55). Although both IBS and FD are prevalent in those with self-reported sleep disturbance, the presence of objective sleep abnormalities may be more difficult to detect. Elsenbruch et al (54), observed no significant differences in PSG parameters, such as sleep efficiency, sleep latency, number of arousals, and percentage of N3 sleep in patients with IBS compared with controls. In another study, women with IBS and significant depressive symptoms had increased sleep latency.

ENDOCRINE DISORDERS

Sleep Deprivation and Hormonal Alterations

Sleep deprivation has been linked to a wide variety of hormonal and metabolic alterations. The onset and severity of diabetes, hypertension, and obesity may be impacted by chronic sleep loss (56). Hormonal release by the pituitary is profoundly affected by sleep and may be either activated or inhibited through two pathways: the hypothalamic-pituitary axes and the autonomic nervous system. Modulation of hypothalamic releasing or inhibiting factors controls pituitary function, affecting growth hormone (GH) and corticotropin. The autonomic pathway impacts the hormonal control of carbohydrate metabolism. With chronic partial sleep loss, the body's ability to secrete and respond to insulin is reduced, causing alterations in glucose metabolism, and is a characteristic early marker of diabetes. Sleep loss alters the ability of leptin, a satiety hormone, and ghrelin, an appetite-stimulating hormone, to accurately signal caloric need and appetite control (57). Poor appetite control, altered glucose metabolism, and insulin resistance are predisposing factors for obesity and diabetes. In a study of 11 healthy young men over 16 consecutive nights, sleep deprivation was found to dampen the secretion of thyroid-stimulating hormone and increase blood levels of cortisol, especially during the afternoon and evening.

Hypothyroidism and Hyperthyroidism

The two main hormones produced by the thyroid, T3 (triiodothyronine) and T4 (thyroxine), are metabolism-regulating hormones essential for growth and development and maturation of the body's nervous system. Hypothyroidism refers to an underactive thyroid that produces insufficient levels of thyroid hormone. The effect is metabolic lowering, which leads to symptoms of weight gain and fatigue. Marked reduction in slow-wave sleep (SWS) has been seen in patients, which is reversible with treatment (58). OSA has been reported to occur frequently in patients with untreated hypothyroidism, especially when myxedema (dry skin and hair, loss of mental and physical vigor) is present. Pathogenesis appears to involve both myopathy and upper airway edema. Unfortunately, indices of sleep apnea severity do not diminish significantly in all patients following attainment of a euthyroid state (normal thyroid hormone levels). In addition, therapy of hypothyroidism with thyroxine in this patient group may be complicated by the development of nocturnal angina and ventricular arrhythmias.

In contrast, thyroid overactivity results in excessive thyroid hormone production. Symptoms of hyperthyroidism include fatigue but difficulty sleeping, mood impairment, difficulty concentrating, muscle weakness, tachycardia, and heat intolerance.

Acromegaly

Acromegaly is a chronic metabolic disorder in which there is excessive GH production after the skeleton and other organs have finished growing. The abnormal GH release is caused by pituitary gland dysfunction, usually a pituitary adenoma. Symptoms include enlarged facial bones, feet, hands, sebaceous glands, tongue (macroglossia), and jaw (prognathism). Somnolence and sleep apnea are part of the clinical spectrum in patients with acromegaly.

OSA is common in acromegaly, with prevalence rates ranging from 13.2% to 75% in this population (59,60). Sleep apnea is more likely to occur with greater severity of acromegaly, older age, greater neck circumference, greater initial tongue volume, alterations in craniofacial dimensions (predominantly of the mandible), and upper airway narrowing because of changes in pharyngeal soft tissues (60). Other factors that could contribute to the development of OSA are facial bone deformity, mucosal edema, hypertrophy of the pharyngeal and laryngeal cartilages, and the presence of nasal polyps (61).

There appears to be no correlation between OSA and biochemical parameters of disease activity such as GH and insulin-like growth factor 1 (IGF-1) levels (62). Improvements in the indices of OSA severity have been reported following therapy of acromegaly with bromocriptine, octreotide (a long-acting somatostatin analog), and pituitary surgery (adenomectomy or hypophysectomy). Nonetheless, OSA may still persist despite normalization of GH levels during therapy (63,64). In one report, the frequency of sleep apnea in patients with treated acromegaly was estimated to still be at least 21%.

CSA is also common and is associated with higher random GH and IGF-1 levels than in OSA. Possible mechanisms for the development of CSA in patients with acromegaly include central respiratory control dysfunction, reflex inhibition of the respiratory center as a result of upper airway narrowing, or an increase in the ventilatory carbon dioxide response of the respiratory center (61).

PSG features of acromegaly include a reduction in REM sleep and delta sleep, both of which can increase following normalization of GH levels.

Cushing Syndrome

Patients with Cushing syndrome (CS) have an excess of adrenocorticosteroid hormones, usually the hormone cortisol. Cortisol is normally released in response to stress and controls metabolism of carbohydrates, fats, and proteins. The most common cause is long-term use of exogenous corticosteroid medication, often prescribed for its anti-inflammatory effects in rheumatoid arthritis, transplant organ rejection, lupus, and asthma. Endogenous cortisol excess may be due to the overproduction of cortisol by the adrenal gland or the overproduction of the cortisol-regulating adrenocorticotropic hormone. These dysregulations are often caused by tumors of the adrenal or pituitary glands, respectively.

Symptoms include progressive obesity with hallmark fatty depositions between the shoulders (buffalo hump), on the face (moon face), midsection, and upper back. Skin changes often seen are acne, skin thinning with easy bruising, and dark purple-red striae on the abdomen, thighs, and breasts.

Sleep complaints are common and include an increased incidence of sleep apnea of approximately 32% in patients with CS and Cushing disease (CD). Parapharyngeal fat deposition may be contributory to the pathogenesis of OSA. In addition, patients without sleep apnea may present with snoring or may have changes in sleep architecture, including more fragmented sleep, poorer sleep continuity, shortened REM latency, and an increased REM density (65).

Addison disease is a rare, chronic disorder caused by adrenal gland failure, resulting in insufficient production of adrenal hormones, including cortisol, aldosterone, androgens (male), and estrogen (female). Patients with primary adrenal insufficiency or Addison disease may present with complaints of weakness, fatigue, anorexia, gastrointestinal symptoms, weight loss, hyperpigmentation, and hypotension. Owing to the nonspecific and slowly progressive nature of the symptoms, the disease is usually not apparent until the adrenal cortex is severely damaged. Hormone replacement therapy is the treatment for Addison disease.

In one study, weekly sleep disturbances were reported in 34% of patients with Addison disease, including difficulties falling asleep (13%), repeated awakenings (14%), and early morning awakenings (20%) (66). Bedtime administration of hydrocortisone in patients with Addison disease can lead to a significant reduction in REM latency, an increase in REM sleep time, and greater wake time after sleep onset (67).

RHEUMATOLOGIC DISORDERS

Acute and Chronic Pain Syndromes

Rheumatologic disorders are chronic debilitating diseases of the muscles, tendons, connective tissue, bones, and joints causing stiffness, pain, and limited mobility. There is a multitude of such disorders, the most common being gout, juvenile arthritis, fibromyalgia (FM), osteoarthritis, and rheumatoid arthritis.

Acute and chronic pain can disrupt sleep, and poor sleep can magnify perceived pain intensity, leading to a vicious cycle of increasing pain and increasing sleep disturbances. Pain can give rise to insomnia, including sleep-onset insomnia, multiple awakenings (sleep fragmentation), and early morning awakenings (waking up too early and not being able to go back to sleep) (68). PSG studies of patients with acute pain may reveal shortened and fragmented sleep, reduced SWS, and reduced REM sleep. In one study, depressive symptoms were predictive of the severity of sleep disturbances in patients with chronic pain (69).

Fibromyalgia

FM has been defined by the American College of Rheumatology as the presence of widespread pain in combination with tenderness at 11 or more of 18 specific tender point sites (70). There may be complaints of tension headaches, fatigue, sleep, memory, and mood issues. Unlike other rheumatologic disorders in which pain is caused by tissue inflammation, the painful tissues in FM are not inflamed. As a result, FM does not cause tissue/organ damage or joint deformity. It is more prevalent among women than men. Symptoms may be precipitated by a single triggering event such as infection, psychological stress, or physical trauma, or they may gradually accumulate over time.

Sleep complaints, including insomnia, early morning awakenings, less satisfying sleep, and nonrestorative sleep, have been reported. A relationship between poor sleep quality, pain intensity, and perception of pain may exist in patients with FM; among patients with FM, poorer sleepers tend to report significantly more pain, and more daytime pain leads to poorer nighttime sleep.

PSG features of FM include an increased number of electroencephalogram (EEG) arousals, increased stage N1 sleep, fewer sleep spindles in stage N2 sleep, reduced SWS, and reduced REM sleep (71,72).

An alpha frequency rhythm, referred to as an alpha-delta sleep anomaly, has been described. Alpha activity (8-13 Hz), which is typically present only during relaxed wakefulness and brief arousals, is superimposed onto the delta waves of nonrapid eye movement (NREM) sleep. There are three patterns of alpha EEG sleep in patients with FM: phasic alpha (simultaneous with delta activity), tonic alpha (continuous throughout the low voltage, mixed EEG patterns of NREM sleep), and low alpha activity. A phasic alpha sleep activity has been correlated with poor sleep, less total sleep time, lower sleep efficiency, less SWS, worsening of pain after sleep, a postsleep increase in the number of tender points, and a longer duration of FM pain compared with the other patterns of alpha intrusion. The alpha-NREM sleep anomaly has also been observed in other patient groups, including those with chronic pain syndromes and depression. Furthermore, the alpha-NREM sleep anomaly is not only nonspecific for FM, but also not universally present in all patients with FM. Some investigators doubt that the alpha-NREM sleep anomaly is abnormal. Mahowald et al, suggest that the alpha-delta NREM sleep EEG pattern is nonspecific and might actually represent a "sleep maintaining process," although others believe it to be a sign of poor quality, nonrestorative sleep (73).

RENAL DISEASE

Chronic Renal Failure (End-Stage Renal Disease)

The kidneys' functions are to regulate blood composition by removing toxic waste such as urea, ammonia, and drugs from the blood; preserve blood pressure by regulating water volume; and maintain the body's acid/base levels.

During metabolism, far more acids are produced than bases. Acids break down into hydrogen ions, are filtered through the kidneys, and are excreted. The concentration of hydrogen ions (pH) in the blood is a balance of hydrogen ions, H^+, and sodium bicarbonate, HCO_3. Carbon dioxide (CO_2), a by-product of cellular respiration, combines with water to form carbonic acid, H_2CO_3, which separates into $H^+ + HCO_3$:

$$CO_2 + H_2O \Leftrightarrow H_2CO_3 \Leftrightarrow H^+ + HCO_3$$

The equation is bidirectionally driven on the basis of an excess of CO_2 or HCO_3. The renal response to excess CO_2 as seen in hypoventilation (respiratory acidosis) is to increase blood plasma levels of HCO_3. Conversely, an excess of HCO_3 (metabolic alkalosis) results in CO_2 retention in order to maintain a neutral pH level of 7.4. The respiratory response to metabolic alkalosis is hypoventilation, whereas metabolic acidosis is compensated through hyperventilation.

As renal failure progresses, the kidneys lose their ability to effectively maintain a normal blood pH and filter metabolic wastes, causing toxic accumulation in the blood. Chronic renal failure occurs with the gradual and usually permanent loss of kidney function over time. This failure may be caused by primary diseases of the kidneys, but the major causes are diabetes and hypertension. Chronic renal failure is incurable and will progress until dialysis or kidney transplantation is needed. Proper dietary management may help slow the progression and reduce complications.

Sleep disturbances are reported by up to 80% of patients on dialysis for end-stage renal disease (ESRD), with sleep apnea, RLS, and periodic limb movement disorder (PLMD) being more prevalent than in the general population. PSG features include reduced total sleep times and sleep efficiency (74).

In one study, 63% of patients on maintenance hemodialysis (HD) for ESRD reported sleep disturbances, including diminished sleep efficiency and more fragmented sleep. In another report, 83.3% of patients on chronic HD had sleep-wake complaints, with 51% reporting disturbed sleep, 46% having delayed sleep onset, and 35% describing frequent awakenings. There appear to be no differences in the characteristics of sleep problems between HD and continuous peritoneal dialysis.

Excessive daytime sleepiness is an important problem. In patients with ESRD, it can be caused by sleep apnea, PLMD, metabolic disturbances, including uremia, dialysis treatments (with accompanying changes in serum electrolytes, osmolarity, and acid-base balance), and the production of somnogenic substances, such as interleukin-1 and tumor necrosis factor alpha during dialysis (75).

Sleep apnea is estimated to be 10 times more prevalent in patients with ESRD than in the general population and is improved by HD (75). There is also a higher prevalence of RLS and PLMD in this patient population. In a study by Winkelman et al, 23% of patients with ESRD reported moderate-to-severe RLS symptomatology. Symptoms of RLS were associated with premature discontinuation of dialysis (76). Improvements in sleep quality have been reported in patients with ESRD, RLS, and anemia treated with recombinant human erythropoietin (a hormone-like substance that stimulates the formation of red blood cells). Correction of anemia was associated with reductions in the number of arousing periodic limb movements and sleep fragmentation.

INFECTIOUS DISEASES

Human Immunodeficiency Virus Infection

Sleep disturbances, including complaints of insomnia, recurrent nighttime arousals, and excessive daytime sleepiness, are among the most commonly reported sleep-related symptoms in human immunodeficiency virus (HIV)–seropositive patients (77-81). An estimated 35% of HIV-infected subjects have alterations in their sleep-wake patterns.

Sleep quality was related to a number of variables, including duration of HIV disease and HIV-related symptoms, depression, state anxiety, daytime sleepiness, fatigue, pain, functional status, and environmental factors. The prevalence of insomnia is higher in those with cognitive impairment, an acquired immunodeficiency syndrome–defining illness, drug use, or depression. Psychological morbidity is a major determinant of insomnia in HIV infection (79). Impaired functional status and longer duration of living with HIV disease were associated with worse sleep quality (82). Immune status among HIV-seropositive patients may influence sleep quality, because lower T-cytotoxic/suppressor ($CD3^+/CD8^+$) cell counts are associated with greater sleep disturbances.

Sleep fragmentation is commonly seen in advanced HIV disease. There is an increase in the total percentage of SWS, SWS in the later sleep cycles, stage N1 shifts, REM periods and arousals, and a reduction in sleep latency and total percentage of stage N2 sleep.

Antiviral therapy used for HIV infection can also give rise to sleep disruption. Efavirenz therapy produces a number of neuropsychiatric adverse reactions, such as abnormal dreams, nocturnal awakenings, and insomnia. Patients receiving efavirenz have been reported to have longer sleep latencies and shorter durations of deep sleep (81). Antiretroviral regimens may cause lipodystrophy, leading to fat deposition in the neck that impinges on the airway as well as fat deposition in the thorax and abdomen, increasing respiratory effort. Evidence has also demonstrated higher rates of sleep apnea with the use of opioid medications; many of these patients may be on opioids for chronic pain or for the treatment of opioid dependence (ie, methadone maintenance therapy) (83).

Lyme Disease

Lyme disease is a tick-borne spirochetal illness with clinical symptoms of fatigue, headache, chills, torticollis, nausea, and vomiting (84). Left untreated, Lyme disease can cause chronic joint inflammation, neurologic symptoms of facial palsy and neuropathy, impaired memory and other cognitive defects, and cardiac arrhythmias. Patients with Lyme disease typically report sleep disturbances. Sleep-related complaints include sleep-onset insomnia, frequent awakenings, excessive daytime sleepiness, and restless legs/nocturnal leg jerking. PSG may demonstrate increased sleep latency, reduced sleep efficiency, increased arousals, and greater sleep fragmentation. Alpha wave intrusion into NREM sleep may be observed in some patients. Mean sleep-onset latency during multiple sleep latency tests is typically normal (85). Sleep difficulty may persist for several years in patients with previous Lyme disease, particularly those with facial palsy who did not receive antibiotics for acute neuroborreliosis.

Sleeping Sickness

Sleeping sickness, or human African trypanosomiasis, is a parasitic disease caused by trypanosomes and is endemic in intertropical Africa. Following the bite of a tsetse fly, human disease evolves through two stages. Diverse clinical features such as fever, cervical adenopathy, skin lesions, facial edema, and cardiac symptoms with arrhythmia characterize the first hemolymphatic stage. This is followed by increasing neurologic symptoms in the meningoencephalitic stage with excessive daytime sleepiness, headaches, sensory deficits, and abnormal reflexes and movements. If left untreated, the infection culminates in altered consciousness, cachexia, and death.

Insomnia is not uncommon. Nocturnal PSG recordings have demonstrated reduced REM sleep latency with sleep-onset REM periods. The scarcity of vertex sharp waves, sleep spindles, and K-complexes may give rise to difficulties in scoring sleep stages. Sleep disturbances can be reversed by successful antiparasitic therapy (86,87).

SLEEP IN THE INTENSIVE CARE UNIT

Sleep is characterized by a variety of physiologic, behavioral, and EEG changes and is necessary for the restoration of cognitive, mood, and physiologic functions (88). Physiologic changes that occur during sleep play an important role in homeostasis, growth, and cellular repair. Sleep disruption in the critically ill patient may negatively impact the treatment and recovery outcomes of the underlying illness or injury. Sleep deprivation, sleep-disordered breathing, and circadian misalignment are believed to have endocrine, metabolic, and cardiovascular implications (56). Sleep deprivation may also be a risk factor for delirium in critically ill patients, linking it to higher morbidity, mortality, and length of intensive care unit (ICU) stay (89).

Normal sleep architecture is divided into two distinct states: NREM sleep and REM sleep. NREM is composed of three distinct stages on the basis of EEG criteria. Stages N1 and N2 are considered to reflect light sleep followed by stage N3 deep SWS. SWS is an anabolic state and is considered the most restorative stage of sleep for physiologic repair. REM sleep is thought to be necessary for memory consolidation (88).

In adults, approximately 50% of ICU sleep occurs during the daytime hours, with a marked shift toward light stages of sleep (89). Compared with healthy adults, studies characterizing sleep disturbances in ICU patients using PSG have demonstrated prolonged sleep latency, sleep fragmentation, reduced sleep efficiency, numerous arousals, a preponderance of stage N2 sleep, reduced or absent stage N3 ("deep") sleep, and reduced or absent REM sleep (90).

The circadian rhythm or "internal biologic clock" controls the timing and duration of daily sleep-wake cycles and influences important body functions such as hormone release, body temperature, and digestion. Exposure to light has a controlling influence on circadian regulation, synchronizing sleep-wake cycles with daily external solar light and dark cycles. Alterations in circadian rhythmicity may impair recovery by disrupting the coordinated activity of normal physiologic processes. Most immunologic functions, from leukocyte numbers, activity, and cytokine secretion, undergo circadian variations, which might affect susceptibility to infections.

Normal physiologic alterations that occur during sleep are particularly significant in patients with unstable hemodynamics, impaired defense mechanisms, and limited physiologic reserve. Body temperature and thermoregulation are regulated, in part, by sleep and circadian rhythms. During sleep, voluntary control of respiration is lost, and hypoxic and hypercapnic ventilatory drives are reduced. Responsiveness to low oxygen and high carbon dioxide levels is lowest during REM compared with NREM sleep. Dynamic cardiovascular fluctuations in blood flow and electrical activity occur and have been associated with life-threatening arrhythmias and ischemic events in patients with underlying heart disease. GH and prolactin, anabolic hormones necessary for cell differentiation and proliferation, follow the sleep-wake cycle and are suppressed during sleep restriction. Sleep deprivation alters neuroendocrine control systems and has been shown to cause increases in thyroid hormone, norepinephrine, and cortisol levels with decreases in GH levels and insulin resistance (90).

Delirium is an acute state of confusion that has been shown to occur in up to 80% of critically ill patients and to be an independent predictor of adverse ICU outcomes, including increased risk of death, longer hospital stay, and higher costs (89). In healthy volunteers, sleep deprivation has been shown to impair memory, attention, response time, and other aspects of neurologic function (90).

Numerous studies have confirmed that the development of delirium during a hospital course is associated with worse physical and cognitive status on discharge and for at least 12 months thereafter, and a higher mortality (89). Sleep disturbance and delirium in the ICU are frequently related, in part, to the shared etiology of sleep loss because of interruptions and sedatives. An imbalance in neurotransmitters and an alteration in melatonin production may contribute to the pathogenesis of both delirium and sleep disturbances. The relationship between sleep deprivation and delirium in the ICU is currently unproven. However, because sleep deprivation affects cognitive function, a connection between delirium and sleep deprivation in critically ill patients may exist (90).

In addition to the effect of preexisting sleep disorders and chronic medical disorders, patients admitted to the ICU are exposed to additional risk factors for sleep disruption such as environmental stimuli (light and noise), medications that affect sleep quality and architecture, patient-care activities (lab draws, imaging, vital signs), pain, and mechanical ventilation.

The Environmental Protection Agency recommends maximum hospital noise levels of 45 dB during the day and 35 dB at night. In the ICU setting, peak daytime and nighttime noise levels routinely exceed 80 dB, the threshold associated with sleep disruption in critically ill patients (88). Noise, particularly staff talking and patient-care activities, are clearly contributing factors and represent 40% of the source of sleep disruption (88).

Approximately 60% of patients complain of disturbed sleep related to being on a ventilator; 30% stated they felt panic and anxiety, which directly inhibited their ability to rest and sleep (88). Improper ventilator settings, mode of ventilation, and patient-ventilator dyssynchrony are factors that may contribute to sleep disruption (88). Noxious factors associated with mechanical ventilation, such as endotracheal tube discomfort, ventilator alarms, suctioning, positioning, and frequent assessments, likely contribute to sleep disruption as well, but these have not been studied.

Sedation is often used in ICU patients, to increase patient comfort, reduce anxiety and agitation, and promote amnesia and sleep, particularly in those requiring mechanical ventilation (90). Any agent that acts on or through sleep regulatory neurotransmitters, modulators, or their receptors can impact sleep architecture (88). Despite their sedative, anxiolytic, and analgesic properties, benzodiazepines and opiates are potentially disruptive to sleep. Benzodiazepines provide sedation through gamma-aminobutyric acid-ergic pathways but increase stage N2 and reduce stage N3 sleep at low doses in healthy participants. Opiates such as fentanyl and morphine promote sleep onset in healthy adults but inhibit REM, profoundly suppress stage N3 sleep, provoke nocturnal awakenings, and can precipitate central apneas. Both benzodiazepines and opiates are associated with delirium in critically ill patients, even at low doses. In critically ill patients, propofol has been shown to suppress REM sleep and to worsen sleep quality. Inotropic medications can affect sleep through their effects on adrenergic receptors. β-blockers, which are a frequently used medication in the ICU, can negatively affect sleep and may cause insomnia and nightmares because of suppressed REM sleep (90).

The use of PSG in the ICU setting is met with numerous challenges. This expensive, labor-intensive test requires skilled personnel to apply equipment and interpret the dispersion of sleep in critically ill patients throughout the day and the night to study sleep in the ICU (90).

Traditional scoring rules are difficult to apply in ICU patients (90). Renal failure, hepatic dysfunction, and sedative and analgesic use, each common among ICU patients, can be associated with significant EEG changes that make PSG interpretation problematic. Sedative-induced beta EEG activity, for example, may lead to an overestimation of wake or stage N1 sleep.

Alternatively, actigraphy is a device worn on the wrist or ankle and is a valid tool to measure rest-wake patterns and total rest time (90). Actigraphy measures a patient's movement to study sleep and has been successfully used in ICU patients to show loss of circadian rhythm and sleep disruption. Actigraphy cannot, however, be considered an accurate tool to measure sleep time in ICU patients whose movement may be restricted by neuromuscular weakness, sedatives, or restraints.

Patient and nurse assessments of sleep using questionnaires can be unreliable. The accuracy of patient self-reporting may be impacted by sedation and/or delirium. Nurse-derived assessments of sleep overestimate total sleep time and sleep efficiency and underestimate the number of awakenings compared with PSG(90). There are a number of strategies to improve sleep for patients in the ICU (Table 21-2).

Table 21-2 Strategies to Improve Sleep in Intensive Care Unit Patients

Barriers to Sleep in the ICU	Strategies to Optimize Sleep in the ICU
Noise	Limit unnecessary noise, phones, and television. If possible, liberalize alarm system and add central alarm personnel. Keep patients' door closed, when possible. Post signs regarding minimizing conversations at or near the bedside. Enforce visiting hours. At night, encourage staff to switch beepers/electronic devices to vibrate. Limit the number of visitors at once, and/or consider ear plugs. Add background, low-level, white noise. Consider monitoring decibel levels, particularly at night.
Patient-care activities	At night, minimize bathing, dressing, room changes, and other wakeful activities. Regularly review nighttime orders regarding monitoring (vital checks, blood draws, fingersticks, etc).
Circadian rhythm	Encourage daytime brighter light exposure (lights on, open curtains). Turn off lights by 10 PM.
Medications/substances	Minimize the use of benzodiazepines for sleep; consider melatonin. Consider short-acting intravenous agents, such as propofol. Avoid starting multiple medications at 1 time; minimize the use of sleep-disrupting medications.
Discomfort	Maximize pain management, particularly with procedures. Evaluate the patient for anxiety as a source of sleep disruption and treat accordingly with reorientation to the environment; nightmares, dyssynchrony with ventilator, medication effects, etc.
Ventilator	Adjust settings and the mode of ventilator to maximize patient-ventilator synchrony; avoid hyperventilation. Provide nocturnal O_2, NIPPV as appropriate; if the patient is receiving NIPPV, assess the mask fit and comfort, and maximize synchrony with the ventilator.

ICU, intensive care unit; NIPPV, noninvasive positive pressure ventilation.
Adapted from Hardin KA. Sleep in the ICU: Potential mechanisms and clinical implications. *Chest*. 2009;136(1):284-294.

MISCELLANEOUS

Fatal Familial Insomnia

Fatal familial insomnia is a rare, hereditary prion-protein disease characterized by progressive sleep disturbances, including refractory insomnia, autonomic dysregulation, and neurologic abnormalities. Caused by a genetic mutation affecting intracellular protein structure, it is similar in nature to other human prion diseases such as Creutzfeldt-Jakob. Clinical features include disrupted sleep, vivid dreaming, and increasingly frequent lapses into a dreamlike (oneiric) state with motor activity as the disease progresses.

PSG features vary depending on the stage of the disease. EEG may be normal in early stages, changing to a pattern of monomorphic flat activity with occasional 1 to 2 Hz sharp waves; absent sleep spindles, K-complexes, and delta activity; and reduced and fragmented REM sleep. REM sleep may occur without muscle atonia reminiscent of REM behavior disorder. There is no known specific treatment. The condition is rapidly progressive and is uniformly fatal (91).

REFERENCES

1. Bellia V, Pistelli R, Filippazzo G, et al. Prevalence of nocturnal asthma in a general population sample: determinants and effect of aging. *J Asthma*. 2000;37(7):595-602. doi:10.3109/02770900009090815
2. Martin RJ. Nocturnal asthma: circadian rhythms and therapeutic interventions. *Am Rev Respir Dis*. 1993;147(6 pt 2):S25-S28. doi:10.1164/ajrccm/147.6_pt_2.s25
3. Ciftci TU, Ciftci B, Firat Guven S, Kokturk O, Turktas H. Effect of nasal continuous positive airway pressure in uncontrolled nocturnal asthmatic patients with obstructive sleep apnea syndrome. *Respir Med*. 2005;99(5):529-534. doi:10.1016/j.rmed.2004.10.011
4. Vogelmeier CF, Román-Rodríguez M, Singh D, Han MLK, Rodríguez-Roisin R, Ferguson GT. Goals of COPD treatment: focus on symptoms and exacerbations. *Respir Med*. 2020;166:105938. doi:10.1016/j.rmed.2020.105938
5. Fleetham J, West P, Mezon B, Conway W, Roth T, Kryger M. Sleep, arousals, and oxygen desaturation in chronic obstructive pulmonary disease: the effect of oxygen therapy. *Am Rev Respir Dis*. 1982;126(3):429-433. doi:10.1164/arrd.1982.126.3.429
6. Plywaczewski R, Sliwinski P, Nowinski A, Kaminski D, Zieliński J. Incidence of nocturnal desaturation while breathing oxygen in COPD patients undergoing long-term oxygen therapy. *Chest*. 2000;117(3):679-683. doi:10.1378/chest.117.3.679
7. Bednarek M, Plywaczewski R, Jonczak L, Zielinski J. There is no relationship between chronic obstructive pulmonary disease and obstructive sleep apnea syndrome: a population study. *Respiration*. 2005;72(2):142-149. doi:10.1159/000084044
8. Aoki T, Akinori E, Yogo Y, Sakamaki F, Suzuki Y, Suemasu K. Sleep disordered breathing in patients with chronic obstructive pulmonary disease. *COPD J Chronic Obstr Pulm Dis*. 2005;2(2):243-252. doi:10.1081/COPD-57606
9. Mieczkowski B, Ezzie ME. Update on obstructive sleep apnea and its relation to COPD. *Int J Chron Obstruct Pulmon Dis*. 2014;9:349-362. doi:10.2147/COPD.S42394
10. Owens RL, Macrea MM, Teodorescu M. The overlaps of asthma or COPD with OSA: a focused review. *Respirology*. 2017;22(6):1073-1083. doi:10.1111/resp.13107
11. Crinion SJ, McNicholas WT. Sleep-related disorders in chronic obstructive pulmonary disease. *Expert Rev Respir Med*. 2014;8(1):79-88. doi:10.1586/17476348.2014.860357
12. De Miguel J, Cabello J, Sánchez-Alarcos JMF, Álvarez-Sala R, Espinós D, Álvarez-Sala JL. Long-term effects of treatment with nasal continuous positive airway pressure on lung function in patients with overlap syndrome. *Sleep Breath*. 2002;6(1):3-10. doi:10.1007/s11325-002-0003-6
13. Rosenstein BJ. What is a cystic fibrosis diagnosis? *Clin Chest Med*. 1998;19(3):423-441. doi:10.1016/S0272-5231(05)70091-5
14. Parisi GF, Di Dio G, Franzonello C, et al. Liver disease in cystic fibrosis: an update. *Hepat Mon*. 2013;13(8):e11215. doi:10.5812/hepatmon.11215
15. Jankelowitz L, Reid KJ, Wolfe L, Cullina J, Zee PC, Jain M. Cystic fibrosis patients have poor sleep quality despite normal sleep latency and efficiency. *Chest*. 2005;127(5):1593-1599. doi:10.1378/chest.127.5.1593
16. Spicuzza L, Sciuto C, Leonardi S, La Rosa M. Early occurrence of obstructive sleep apnea in infants and children with cystic fibrosis. *Arch Pediatr Adolesc Med*. 2012;166(12):1165-1169. doi:10.1001/archpediatrics.2012.1177
17. Shakkottai A, Nasr SZ, Hassan F, Irani S, O'Brien LM, Chervin RD. Sleep-disordered breathing in cystic fibrosis. *Sleep Med*. 2020;74:57-65. doi:10.1016/j.sleep.2020.05.031
18. Moran F, Bradley JM, Piper AJ. Non-invasive ventilation for cystic fibrosis. *Cochrane Database Syst Rev*. 2017;2(2):CD002769. doi:10.1002/14651858.CD002769.pub5
19. Won CHJ, Kryger M. Sleep in patients with restrictive lung disease. *Clin Chest Med*. 2014;35(3):505-512. doi:10.1016/j.ccm.2014.06.006

20. Resta O, Foschino Barbaro MP, Bonfitto P, et al. Low sleep quality and daytime sleepiness in obese patients without obstructive sleep apnoea syndrome. *J Intern Med*. 2003;253(5):536-543. doi:10.1046/j.1365-2796.2003.01133.x
21. Resta O, Foschino-Barbaro MP, Legari G, et al. Sleep-related breathing disorders, loud snoring and excessive daytime sleepiness in obese subjects. *Int J Obes*. 2001;25(5):669-675. doi:10.1038/sj.ijo.0801603
22. Weitzenblum E, Kessler R, Chaouat A. [Alveolar hypoventilation in the obese: the obesity-hypoventilation syndrome]. *Rev Pneumol Clin*. 2002;58(2):83-90.
23. Guilleminault C, Kurland G, Winkle R, Miles LE. Severe kyphoscoliosis, breathing, and sleep: the "Quasimodo" syndrome during sleep. *Chest*. 1981;79(6):626-630. doi:10.1378/chest.79.6.626
24. Shea SA, Winning AJ, McKenzie E, Guz A. Does the abnormal pattern of breathing in patients with interstitial lung disease persist in deep, non-rapid eye movement sleep. *Am Rev Respir Dis*. 1989;139(3): 653-658. doi:10.1164/ajrccm/139.3.653
25. Hira HS, Sharma RK. Study of oxygen saturation, breathing pattern and arrhythmias in patients of interstitial lung disease during sleep. *Indian J Chest Dis Allied Sci*. 1997;39(3):157-162.
26. Prodromakis E, Trakada G, Tsapanos V, Spiropoulos K. Arterial oxygen tension during sleep in the third trimester of pregnancy. *Acta Obstet Gynecol Scand*. 2004;83(2):159-164. doi:10.1111/j.0001-6349.2004.00289.x
27. Bourjeily G, Ankner G, Mohsenin V. Sleep-disordered breathing in pregnancy. *Clin Chest Med*. 2011;32(1):175-189. doi:10.1016/j.ccm.2010.11.003
28. Orabona R, Corda L, Giordani J, et al. Sleep-disordered breathing and pregnancy outcomes: the impact of maternal oxygen saturation. *Int J Gynaecol Obstet*. 2024;164(1):140-147. doi:10.1002/ijgo.14967
29. Bhat S, Gupta D, Chokroverty S. Sleep disorders in neuromuscular diseases. *Neurol Clin*. 2012;30(4):1359-1387. doi:10.1016/j.ncl.2012.08.010
30. Piper A. Sleep abnormalities associated with neuromuscular disease: pathophysiology and evaluation. *Semin Respir Crit Care Med*. 2002;23(3):211-219. doi:10.1055/s-2002-33029
31. Barbe F, Quera-Salva MA, McCann C, et al. Sleep-related respiratory disturbances in patients with Duchenne muscular dystrophy. *Eur Respir J*. 1994;7(8):1403-1408. doi:10.1183/09031936.94.07081403
32. Khan Y, Heckmatt JZ. Obstructive apnoeas in Duchenne muscular dystrophy. *Thorax*. 1994;49(2):157-161. doi:10.1136/thx.49.2.157
33. Hukins CA, Hillman DR. Daytime predictors of sleep hypoventilation in Duchenne muscular dystrophy. *Am J Respir Crit Care Med*. 2000;161(1):166-170. doi:10.1164/ajrccm.161.1.9901057
34. Guilleminault C, Cummiskey J, Motta J, Lynne-Davies P. Respiratory and hemodynamic study during wakefulness and sleep in myotonic dystrophy. *Sleep*. 1978;1(1):19-31. doi:10.1093/sleep/1.1.19
35. Ververs CCM, Van der Meché FGA, Verbraak AFM, Van der Sluys HCM, Bogaard JM. Breathing pattern awake and asleep in myotonic dystrophy. *Respiration*. 1996;63(1):1-7. doi:10.1159/000196508
36. Laberge L, Gagnon C, Dauvilliers Y. Daytime sleepiness and myotonic dystrophy. *Curr Neurol Neurosci Rep*. 2013;13(4):340. doi:10.1007/s11910-013-0340-9
37. Gay PC, Westbrook PR, Daube JR, Litchy WJ, Windebank AJ, Iverson R. Effects of alterations in pulmonary function and sleep variables on survival in patients with amyotrophic lateral sclerosis. *Mayo Clin Proc*. 1991;66(7):686-694. doi:10.1016/S0025-6196(12)62080-1
38. Santos C, Braghiroli A, Mazzini L, Pratesi R, Franco Oliveira LV, Mora G. Sleep-related breathing disorders in amyotrophic lateral sclerosis. *Monaldi Arch Chest Dis*. 2003;59(2):160-165.
39. Boentert M. Sleep disturbances in patients with amyotrophic lateral sclerosis: current perspectives. *Nat Sci Sleep*. 2019;11:97-111. doi:10.2147/NSS.S183504
40. Steljes DG, Kryger MH, Kirk BW, Millar TW. Sleep in postpolio syndrome. *Chest*. 1990;98(1):133-140. doi:10.1378/chest.98.1.133
41. Hsu AA, Staats BA. "Postpolio" sequelae and sleep-related disordered breathing. *Mayo Clin Proc*. 1998;73(3):216-224. doi:10.4065/73.3.216
42. Bridgens R, Sturman S, Davidson C. Post-polio syndrome—polio's legacy. *Clin Med (Lond)*. 2010;10(3): 213-214. doi:10.7861/clinmedicine.10-3-213
43. Stepansky R, Weber G, Zeitlhofer J. Sleep apnea and cognitive dysfunction in myasthenia gravis. *Acta Med Austriaca*. 1997;24(3):128-131.
44. Romanova TV. Sleep disorders in patients with myastenia gravis. *Zhurnal Nevrol Psikhiatr Im S Korsakova*. 2021;121(4 vyp 2):92-97. doi:10.17116/jnevro202112104292
45. Kaminsky P, Poussel M, Pruna L, Deibener J, Chenuel B, Brembilla-Perrot B. Organ dysfunction and muscular disability in myotonic dystrophy type 1. *Medicine (Baltimore)*. 2011;90(4):262-268. doi:10.1097/MD.0b013e318226046b
46. Steier J, Jolley CJ, Seymour J, et al. Sleep-disordered breathing in unilateral diaphragm paralysis or severe weakness. *Eur Respir J*. 2008;32(6):1479-1487. doi:10.1183/09031936.00018808
47. Bennett JR, Dunroy HMA, Corfield DR, et al. Respiratory muscle activity during REM sleep in patients with diaphragm paralysis. *Neurology*. 2004;62(1): 134-137. doi:10.1212/01.WNL.0000101719.84675.E0

48. Vela MF, Kramer JR, Richardson PA, Dodge R, El-Serag HB. Poor sleep quality and obstructive sleep apnea in patients with GERD and Barrett's esophagus. *Neurogastroenterol Motil*. 2014;26(3):346-352. doi:10.1111/nmo.12265
49. Shaker R. Nighttime heartburn is an under-appreciated clinical problem that impacts sleep and daytime function: the results of a Gallup survey conducted on behalf of the American Gastroenterological Association. *Am J Gastroenterol*. 2003;98(7): 1487-1493. doi:10.1016/s0002-9270(03)00360-5
50. Parsons JP, Mastronarde JG. Gastroesophageal reflux disease and asthma. *Curr Opin Pulm Med*. 2010;16(1): 60-63. doi:10.1097/MCP.0b013e328332ca2f
51. Demeter P, Várdi VK, Magyar P. Correlations between gastroesophageal reflux disease and obstructive sleep apnea. *Orv Hetil*. 2004;145(37):1897-1901.
52. Kim HN, Vorona RD, Winn MP, Doviak M, Johnson DA, Ware JC. Symptoms of gastro-oesophageal reflux disease and the severity of obstructive sleep apnoea syndrome are not related in sleep disorders center patients. *Aliment Pharmacol Ther*. 2005;21(9):1127-1133. doi:10.1111/j.1365-2036.2005.02447.x
53. Orr WC. Gastrointestinal functioning during sleep: a new horizon in sleep medicine. *Sleep Med Rev*. 2001;5(2):91-101. doi:10.1053/smrv.2000.0149
54. Elsenbruch S, Thompson JJ, Harnish MJ, Exton MS, Orr WC. Behavioral and physiological sleep characteristics in women with irritable bowel syndrome. *Am J Gastroenterol*. 2002;97(9):2306-2314. doi:10.1111/j.1572-0241.2002.05984.x
55. Vege SS, Locke GR, Weaver AL, Farmer SA, Melton LJ, Talley NJ. Functional gastrointestinal disorders among people with sleep disturbances: a population-based study. *Mayo Clin Proc*. 2004;79(12):1501-1506. doi:10.4065/79.12.1501
56. Sharma S, Kavuru M. Sleep and metabolism: an overview. *Int J Endocrinol*. 2010;2010:270832. doi:10.1155/2010/270832
57. Morselli L, Leproult R, Balbo M, Spiegel K. Role of sleep duration in the regulation of glucose metabolism and appetite. *Best Pract Res Clin Endocrinol Metab*. 2010;24(5):687-702. doi:10.1016/j.beem.2010.07.005
58. Shekhar S, Hall JE, Klubo-Gwiezdzinska J. The hypothalamic–pituitary–thyroid axis and sleep. *Curr Opin Endocr Metab Res*. 2021;17:8-14. doi:10.1016/j.coemr.2020.10.002
59. Mestrón A, Webb SM, Astorga R, et al. Epidemiology, clinical characteristics, outcome, morbidity and mortality in acromegaly based on the Spanish Acromegaly Registry (Registro Español de Acromegalia, REA). *Eur J Endocrinol*. 2004;151(4):439-446. doi:10.1530/eje.0.1510439
60. Weiss V, Šonka K, Pretl M, et al. Prevalence of the sleep apnea syndrome in acromegaly population. *J Endocrinol Invest*. 2000;23(8):515-519. doi:10.1007/BF03343767
61. Fatti LM, Scacchi M, Pincelli AI, Lavezzi E, Cavagnini F. Prevalence and pathogenesis of sleep apnea and lung disease in acromegaly. *Pituitary*. 2001;4(4): 259-262. doi:10.1023/A:1020702631793
62. Blanco Pérez JJ, Blanco-Ramos MA, Zamarrón Sanz C, Souto Fernández A, Mato A, Lamela López J. Acromegaly and sleep apnea. *Arch Bronconeumol*. 2004;40(8):355-359. doi:10.1016/s1579-2129(06)60320-0
63. Buyse B, Michiels E, Bouillon R, Bobbaers H, Demedts M. Relief of sleep apnoea after treatment of acromegaly: report of three cases and review of the literature. *Eur Respir J*. 1997;10(6):1401-1404. doi:10.1183/09031936.97.10061401
64. Mickelson SA, Senior BA, Rosenthal LD, Rock JP, Friduss ME. Obstructive sleep apnea syndrome and acromegaly. *Otolaryngol Head Neck Surg*. 1994;111(1):25-30. doi:10.1177/019459989411100107
65. Shipley JE, Schteingart DE, Tandon R, Starkman MN. Sleep architecture and sleep apnea in patients with Cushing's disease. *Sleep*. 1992;15(6):514-518. doi:10.1093/sleep/15.6.514
66. Løvås K, Husebye ES, Holsten F, Bjorvatn B. Sleep disturbances in patients with Addison's disease. *Eur J Endocrinol*. 2003;148(4):449-456. doi:10.1530/eje.0.1480449
67. García-Borreguero D, Wehr TA, Larrosa O, et al. Glucocorticoid replacement is permissive for rapid eye movement sleep and sleep consolidation in patients with adrenal insufficiency. *J Clin Endocrinol Metab*. 2000;85(11):4201-4206 doi:10.1210/jc.85.11.4201
68. Roehrs T, Roth T. Sleep and pain: interaction of two vital functions. *Semin Neurol*. 2005;25(1):106-116. doi:10.1055/s-2005-867079
69. Palermo TM, Kiska R. Subjective sleep disturbances in adolescents with chronic pain: relationship to daily functioning and quality of life. *J Pain*. 2005;6(3): 201-207. doi:10.1016/j.jpain.2004.12.005
70. Wolfe F, Smythe HA, Yunus MB, et al. The American College of Rheumatology 1990 criteria for the classification of fibromyalgia. *Arthritis Rheum*. 1990;33(2):160-172. doi:10.1002/art.1780330203
71. Çetin B, Sünbül EA, Toktaş H, Karaca M, Ulutaç Ö, Güleç H. Comparison of sleep structure in patients with fibromyalgia and healthy controls. *Sleep Breath*. 2020;24(4):1591-1598. doi:10.1007/s11325-020-02036-x
72. Dauvilliers Y, Touchon J. Sleep in fibromyalgia patients: clinical and polysomnography pattern. *Neurophysiol Clin*. 2001;31(1):18-33. doi:10.1016/S0987-7053(00)00240-9
73. Mahowald ML, Mahowald MW. Nighttime sleep and daytime functioning (sleepiness and fatigue) in

less well-defined chronic rheumatic diseases with particular reference to the 'alpha-delta NREM sleep anomaly.' *Sleep Med*. 2000;1(3):195-207. doi:10.1016/S1389-9457(00)00028-9
74. Parker KP. Sleep disturbances in dialysis patients. *Sleep Med Rev*. 2003;7(2):131-143. doi:10.1053/smrv.2001.0240
75. Hanly P. Sleep apnea and daytime sleepiness in end-stage renal disease. *Semin Dial*. 2004;17(2):109-114. doi:10.1111/j.0894-0959.2004.17206.x
76. Lin XW, Zhang JF, Qiu MY, et al. Restless legs syndrome in end stage renal disease patients undergoing hemodialysis. *BMC Neurol*. 2019;19(1):47. doi:10.1186/s12883-019-1265-y
77. Davis S. Clinical sequelae affecting quality of life in the HIV-infected patient. *J Assoc Nurses AIDS Care*. 2004;15(5 suppl):28S-33S. doi:10.1177/1055329004269478
78. Allavena C, Guimard T, Billaud E, et al. Prevalence and risk factors of sleep disturbance in a large HIV-infected adult population. *AIDS Behav*. 2016;20(2):339-344. doi:10.1007/s10461-015-1160-5
79. Reid S, Dwyer J. Insomnia in HIV infection: a systematic review of prevalence, correlates, and management. *Psychosom Med*. 2005;67(2):260-269. doi:10.1097/01.psy.0000151771.46127.df
80. Franck LS, Johnson LM, Lee K, et al. Sleep disturbances in children with human immunodeficiency virus infection. *Pediatrics*. 1999;104(5):e62. doi:10.1542/peds.104.5.e62
81. Gallego L, Barreiro P, Del Río R, et al. Analyzing sleep abnormalities in HIV-infected patients treated with efavirenz. *Clin Infect Dis*. 2004;38(3):430-432. doi:10.1086/380791
82. Robbins JL, Phillips KD, Dudgeon WD, Hand GA. Physiological and psychological correlates of sleep in HIV infection. *Clin Nurs Res*. 2004;13(1):33-52. doi:10.1177/1054773803259655
83. Taibi DM. Sleep disturbances in persons living with HIV. *J Assoc Nurses AIDS Care*. 2013;24(1 suppl):S72-S85. doi:10.1016/j.jana.2012.10.006
84. Mac S, Bahia S, Simbulan F, et al. Long-term sequelae and health-related quality of life associated with Lyme disease: a systematic review. *Clin Infect Dis*. 2020;71(2):440-452. doi:10.1093/cid/ciz1158
85. Weinstein ER, Rebman AW, Aucott JN, Johnson-Greene D, Bechtold KT. Sleep quality in well-defined Lyme disease: a clinical cohort study in Maryland. *Sleep*. 2018;41(5):zsy035. doi:10.1093/sleep/zsy035
86. Buguet A, Gati R, Sèvre JP, Develoux M, Bogui P, Lonsdorfer J. 24 hour polysomnographic evaluation in a patient with sleeping sickness. *Electroencephalogr Clin Neurophysiol*. 1989;72(6):471-478. doi:10.1016/0013-4694(89)90223-X
87. Sanner BM, Büchner N, Kotterba S, Zidek W. Polysomnography in acute African trypanosomiasis. *J Neurol*. 2000;247(11):878-879. doi:10.1007/s004150070077
88. Hardin KA. Sleep in the ICU potential mechanisms and clinical implications. *Chest*. 2009;136(1):284-294. doi:10.1378/chest.08-1546
89. Weinhouse GL, Schwab RJ, Watson PL, et al. Bench-to-bedside review: delirium in ICU patients—importance of sleep deprivation. *Crit Care*. 2009;13(6):234. doi:10.1186/cc8131
90. Pisani MA, Friese RS, Gehlbach BK, Schwab RJ, Weinhouse GL, Jones SF. Sleep in the intensive care unit. *Am J Respir Crit Care Med*. 2015;191(7):731-738. doi:10.1164/rccm.201411-2099CI
91. Baldelli L, Calandra-Buonaura G, Provini F, Cortelli P. Fatal familial insomnia. In: *Autonomic Nervous System and Sleep: Order and Disorder*. Sudhansu C, Pietro C, eds. Springer International Publishing; 2021:199-212. doi:10.1007/978-3-030-62263-3_18

Chapter 22
Seizures and Sleep

AMY KORN-REAVIS

KEY CONCEPTS/LEARNING OBJECTIVES

The key concepts for this chapter include the causes and classifications of seizures, clinical seizure activity, treatment options available for people who have seizures, how sleep relates to the identification and control of seizures, the appearance of seizure activity on the electroencephalogram, the appropriate response to a seizure, and when to activate Emergency Medical Services.

KEY TERMS

Epileptiform discharges
Patient safety
Seizure
Sleep

A seizure is a sudden abnormal discharge of electrical activity in the brain, usually affecting how a person acts or feels for a short time. These involuntary actions or sensations can range from a brief muscle twitch to a distorted vision to a staring spell to complete loss of consciousness with tonic-clonic activity (Table 22-1). One in 10 Americans will have a seizure at some point in their lifetime, with 3% of those developing epilepsy, or seizure disorder, by the age of 80 (1). Epilepsy is defined as two or more unprovoked seizures (2) and is the third most common brain disorder, after Alzheimer disease and stroke (3). Epilepsy affects 50 million people worldwide (3). The chances of having a seizure are greatest during early childhood or after the age of 65 and men are slightly more at risk than women.

The known causes of seizures include birth trauma, brain injury, brain tumor, cerebral hemorrhage, anoxic event, brain infection (meningitis or encephalitis), stroke, cerebral palsy, mental handicap, high fever, toxins (lead), and illegal drug use (cocaine). When no underlying cause is found for the seizure, which happens in 7 out of 10 people (3), it is referred to as idiopathic.

"EEGs are known to capture approximately 50% of people with seizures however with repeat recording and recordings that include sleep the capture rate increases to 80% to 90% range." It therefore becomes important to record patients during sleep. Many of the symptoms that are indications for a sleep study, such as sleep paralysis, memory loss, confusional arousals, and fatigue, are also symptoms of seizures. This can bring to the sleep laboratory patients who may not be aware they are having seizures. Therefore, it is essential for the technologist to be familiar with seizure activity and how to identify it on EEG and with video recording (4,5).

CLINICAL OBSERVATIONS

Clinical observations during a seizure will vary depending on the location and size of the seizure focus (area of the brain where the seizure originates) and how the seizure is classified (Table 22-2) (6,7).

Table 22-1 Terminology

Aura	A sensation experienced by some people with epilepsy before a seizure. Commonly described auras include copper taste, distorted vision, burning sensation, dizziness, headache, déjà vu, and jamais vu.
Déjà vu	A feeling that you have experienced something before
Jamais vu	The familiar seems unfamiliar
Ictal	During the time a seizure is occurring
Interictal	The time between seizures
Preictal	The time before a seizure occurs
Postictal	The time after a seizure occurs
Spike	Transient electroencephalography wave with pointed peak and duration of 20-70 ms
Polyspikes	Multiple spike complexes
Sharp wave	Same morphology as a spike but with duration of >70 and <200 ms
Spike and slow wave	Spike followed by a high-amplitude slow wave

Table 22-2 Seizure Classifications

Generalized seizures	Event begins as widespread epileptiform activity over both hemispheres of the brain associated with sudden movement or loss of consciousness.
• Tonic-clonic	Occurs without warning with loss of consciousness, can be associated with injury (tongue biting or from initial fall), usually lasts up to 2-3 min, consciousness returns slowly, respirations may be absent during the tonic phase and may be labored during the clonic phase. Confusion, sleepiness, agitation, headache, and nausea all can be present postictally.
• Absence	Most commonly seen in children aged 4-14, has a duration of 5-15 s, begins and ends abruptly, described as a blank stare, appears to be daydreaming, and can be associated with rapid eye blinking.
• Myoclonic	Abnormal brief jerk-like movements involving both sides of the body lasting a second or two
• Atonic (drop attack)	Complete loss of muscle tone, including falling to the ground, usually associated with injury and often noticed by head drop
Partial seizures	Event begins as an electrical discharge over a localized area of the brain (one hemisphere). Note: Partial seizures can evolve, spreading to involve both hemispheres.
• Simple partial	Consciousness is not impaired, memory remains intact, awareness is preserved, may exhibit face twitching, eye blinking, odd smiling, or unexplained emotions.
• Complex partial	At least one of the following is present: impaired consciousness, memory, or awareness. Presents with trance-like appearance, may appear afraid and exhibit random undirected movements like walking, lip smacking, or picking at clothing
Psychogenic nonepileptic seizures	These events are defined as clinical events that appear to be an epileptic seizure without correlating electroencephalogram changes. Other terminology used in the past for this type of activity has been pseudoseizure, psychological, or psychosomatic. It is important to recognize that many precipitating factors can lead to this diagnosis, including past or present abuse, depression, and mental disorders (6).

Location

Functions of the *frontal lobe* include speech and language skills, reasoning, and problem-solving. Seizure activity in this area may present with difficulty speaking, hollering profanities, or laughing inappropriately. *Parietal lobe* functions are perception of stimuli (touch, pressure, and taste), recognition, orientation, and motor control. Presentation may include face or upper extremity numbness or twitching. Visual processing is the primary function of the *occipital lobe* of the brain. Clinical presentations may include distorted vision or visual hallucinations. Functions of the *temporal lobe* include recognition of auditory stimuli, memory, language skills, and emotional responses. Impairments during a seizure may include not being able to respond to auditory stimuli, impaired memory, or fear. The functions of each lobe of the brain are specific, and the clinical observations indicated are simplistic and may represent other medical conditions.

Standard Nomenclature for the Description of Electroencephalogram Discharges

The American Clinical Neurophysiology Society provides specific nomenclature for documentation of discharges seen in the EEG. They are defined by the area that is affected: generalized, lateralized, bilateral independent, and multifocal. When describing discharges, document which lobes are predominant and whether the discharges are symmetric or asymmetric. During sleep study, this may be limited due to the modified Ten Twenty montage used. If there is suspected seizure activity, a full Ten Twenty setup and montage can be used.

In addition, describe the frequency and pattern of the discharge, such as rhythmic discharges, periodic discharges, or spike-and-wave discharges. The morphology and the shape of the discharge should also be described. Discharges can consist of sharp waves 70 to 200 ms, spikes 20 to 70 ms, sharp- and slow-wave complexes, and multiple spike- and slow-wave complexes that are similar to spike and slow wave but include multiple spikes associated with one or more slow waves (4), and paroxysmal slow-wave discharges. In addition to morphology, we should describe the frequency of the discharges and whether they are of sudden or gradual onset.

It can be difficult to identify these discharges using a 30-second epoch; utilize a 10-second page to assist with identification. It can also be difficult to identify interictal epileptiform discharges (IEDs). Some normal variants can be mistaken for IEDs. An example is Mu rhythm, which is a rhythmic discharge of 8 to 11 Hz that has a sharp and comb-like shape. Mu rhythm can be suppressed with movement of the contralateral limb. Positive sharp transients of sleep are 4 to 6 Hz discharges seen in the occipital region. These can be confusing with IEDs. However, most IEDs are of negative polarity. Electrocardiogram (ECG) artifact can also be mistaken for spikes. If a technologist is suspicious that a wave looks like a spike, one of the first steps would be to rule out artifacts.

There are several modifiers that also need to be added to the identification. Technologists should also be aware of interictal changes that can be seen in the EEG such as voltage attenuation or augmentation, burst-suppression activity, or electrocerebral inactivity. These patterns can occur as well and should be documented.

EEG and patient activity (video) must be recorded. IEDs can be either electroclinical in nature or purely electrographic; therefore, the behavior of the patient and what occurred pre- and postevent must be clearly documented.

SLEEP AND EPILEPSY OVERVIEW

The sleep-wake cycle significantly affects the frequency of interictal epileptiform activity (IEA) as well as epileptic seizures. The two neurophysiologic states that characterize sleep (nonrapid eye movement [NREM] and rapid eye movement [REM]) have opposite consequences on both. According to most studies, generalized discharges and clinical seizures occur mostly in NREM sleep, which may be considered a natural "convulsive agent," when brain activity is relatively more synchronous. The majority of EEG discharges are seen in stage N2, whereas REM sleep, with its asynchronous cell discharge patterns and atonia, is resistant to epileptic EEG potentials (3). NREM sleep activates IEDs in both partial and generalized syndromes.

For a patient with epilepsy presenting with excessive daytime sleepiness (EDS), several possible causes need to be considered. These include, but are not limited to, nocturnal seizure activity, side effects from medications used for seizure control, an underlying sleep disorder fragmenting sleep, or poor sleep hygiene. If multiple causes are present, one can feed the other, and the patient can be caught in a vicious cycle. For example, untreated obstructive sleep apnea is associated with increased arousals, increased NREM sleep, and decreased REM sleep. All of these lower the threshold for the appearance of seizure discharges and seizures during sleep. The disruption in sleep quality leads to daytime symptoms, which can include sleepiness, increased frequency of seizures, and memory impairment.

EPILEPTIFORM DISCHARGES DURING SLEEP IN GENERALIZED EPILEPSY

Primary Generalized Tonic-Clonic Seizures

Sleep has a well-documented influence on this class of seizure that tends to occur during NREM sleep. Generalized IEA increases in NREM (8) and is most prominent at sleep onset and during the first part of the night. Interestingly, the morphology of IEA changes during sleep. In NREM sleep, generalized bursts of spike-wave complexes may become fragmented, polyspikes may appear, and the discharges may occur in a focal distribution (usually, in a frontocentral region; Figure 22-1).

One of the concerns with generalized tonic-clonic seizures (GTCS) is the suppression that occurs postictally. This suppression of brain waves can also lead to suppression of respirations and, finally, asystole. This occurs more frequently in nocturnal GTCS and can lead to sudden death (9).

Primary Generalized Myoclonus

Primary generalized myoclonic seizures are the typical awakening seizures that occur shortly after awakening in 88% to 96% of patients. Myoclonus occurs during both spontaneous and provoked arousals. IEA is characterized by generalized polyspike and polyspike-wave discharges, more commonly at the onset of sleep and during nocturnal arousals than during awakenings. Induced arousals from NREM sleep and spontaneous morning awakening activate epileptiform abnormalities. IEA decreases markedly during REM sleep.

Juvenile Myoclonic Epilepsy

These seizures are myoclonic or generalized tonic-clonic, with an onset in adolescence or in early childhood and are idiopathic in nature. They usually occur in the morning during the first 1 to 2 hours after awakening. Some may occur on awakening from a nap but rarely at other times during the day. The EEG will show spike-and-wave complexes, typically, polyspike and wave complexes. The epileptiform discharges in juvenile myoclonic epilepsy (JME) increase markedly at sleep onset and on awakening but are virtually absent in NREM and REM sleep and during the waking state. A high proportion of patients with JME (30%-42%) demonstrate photosensitivity, which is an increase in IEA with photic stimulation (rhythmic flashing of a strobe light).

Absence Epilepsy

Absence seizures usually develop in the first decade of life and are characterized by the abrupt onset of

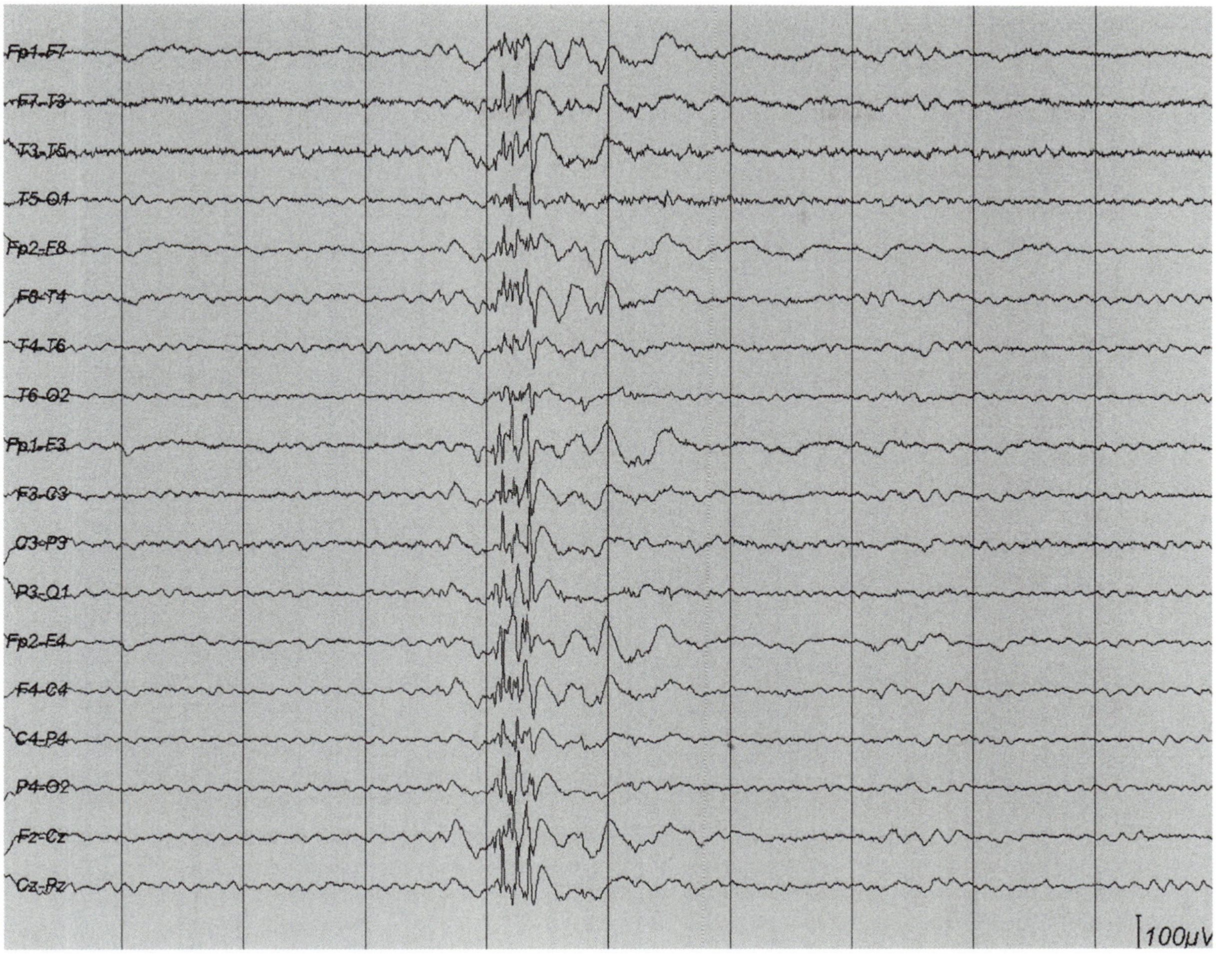

Figure 22-1 Polyspike. This is a typical generalized polyspike in a patient with an idiopathic (primary) generalized epilepsy. Note that the discharge is followed by about 2 seconds of delta activity. This aftergoing slow activity indicates substantial disruption of the background and is a significant argument to consider this discharge pathologic and not a normal variant. (Used with permission of John Wiley & Sons—Books from Benbadis SR. Introduction to sleep electroencephalography. In: Lee-Chiong TL, ed. *Sleep: A Comprehensive Handbook*. John Wiley and Sons; 2006: 1013; permission conveyed through Copyright Clearance Center, Inc.)

unresponsiveness and behavioral arrest, usually lasting 5 to 15 seconds, followed by an abrupt return to consciousness. These seizures may occur multiple times per day and may be activated by arousals from drowsiness or sleep. Clinical absence seizures are detectable only in the waking state and are usually precipitated by photic stimulation or hyperventilation. The activation of IEA is most marked in the first sleep cycle during NREM sleep. The typical EEG abnormality consists of 3-Hz spike-wave complexes in a generalized distribution (Figure 22-2). Absence-appearing seizures can also be simple partial seizures.

West Syndrome

This syndrome, with a peak age of onset at 3 to 6 months, is characterized by the triad of infantile spasms, psychomotor retardation, and EEG hypsarrhythmia, which is a typical EEG pattern consisting of multifocal and at times generalized high-voltage spikes superimposed on a disorganized and chaotic background. The infantile spasms occur infrequently during sleep (<5% of the cases). The hypsarrhythmic pattern shows a striking variation during sleep. The EEG abnormalities tend to increase in NREM sleep, and the spike–slow-wave discharges tend to become grouped, at times having a periodic appearance. During REM sleep, there is a marked attenuation or disappearance of the hypsarrhythmia pattern. In some cases, the hypsarrhythmia is observed only during sleep.

Lennox-Gastaut Syndrome

This syndrome is characterized by intractable seizures (generalized tonic-clonic, tonic, atonic, myoclonic, and atypical absence seizures), mental retardation,

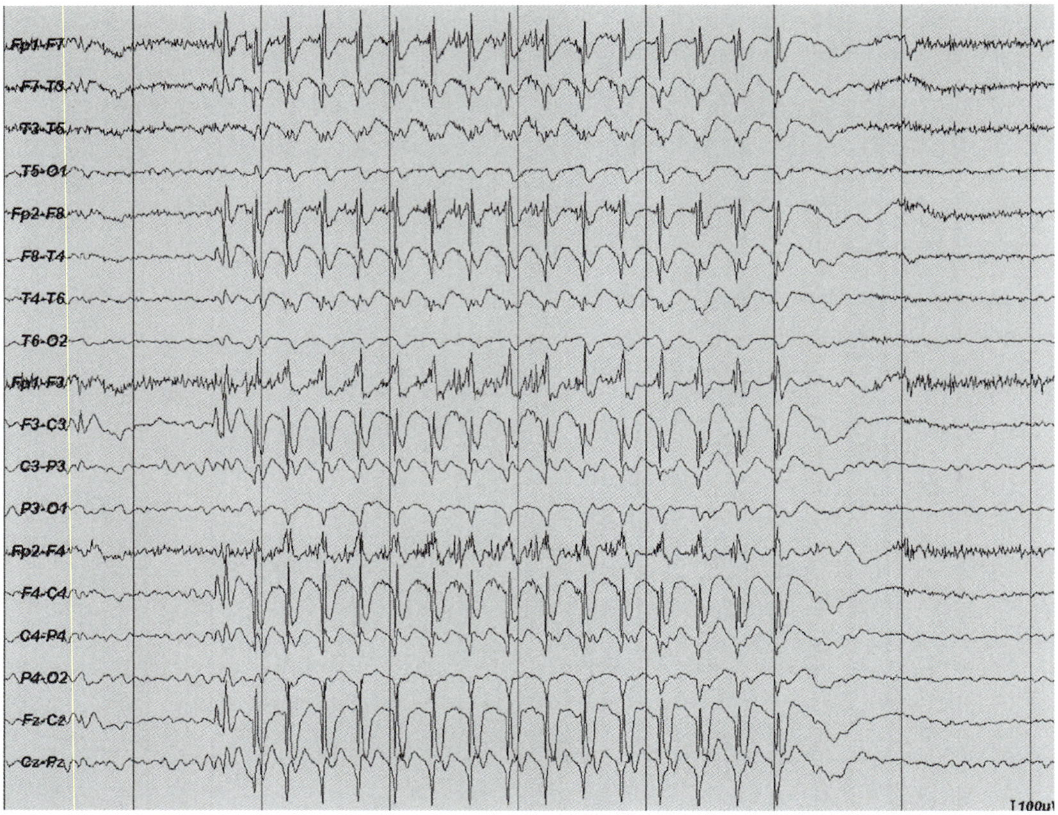

Figure 22-2 3-Hz spike-wave complexes. This shows typical 3-Hz spike-wave complexes in a patient with an idiopathic (primary) generalized epilepsy. This patient likely has absence seizures. If tested with a clicker, a discharge of this duration (about 4.5 seconds) is likely associated with a brief impairment of awareness. (Used with permission of John Wiley & Sons—Books from Benbadis SR. Introduction to sleep electroencephalography. In: Lee-Chiong TL, ed. *Sleep: A comprehensive Handbook*. John Wiley and Sons; 2006:1014; permission conveyed through Copyright Clearance Center, Inc.)

and the presence of generalized slow spike-wave complexes at a frequency of 2.5 Hz or less (Figure 22-3). An increased quantity of bursts of slow spike-wave complexes is observed in NREM sleep. The morphology of EEG discharges may change, with polyspikes becoming more prominent; also, runs of polyspikes and rhythmic bursts of rapid activity (10-20 Hz) may be observed. There may also be a burst-suppression–like pattern (high-amplitude discharges separated by very low voltage activity).

EPILEPTIFORM DISCHARGES DURING SLEEP IN FOCAL SEIZURES

Temporal Lobe Epilepsy

Studies have shown that nocturnal seizures in patients with temporal lobe epilepsy (TLE) are infrequent and usually do not cluster. Most studies of TLE have observed an increase in epileptiform discharges in NREM sleep with a decrease in REM sleep. The spike frequency is generally highest in the deep NREM sleep (N3). Morphology and distribution of IEA are often affected by sleep. Contralateral focal discharges that facilitate the secondary generalization of focal discharges may appear during NREM sleep. Secondary generalization occurs when a focal epileptiform discharge spreads broadly to both hemispheres. Isolated spikes seen during wakefulness in patients with neocortical foci may be replaced by high-frequency bursts of spikes during NREM sleep. Sleep has different effects on temporal and frontal lobe seizures (Figure 22-4).

Frontal Lobe Epilepsy

It is well known that seizures originating from the frontal lobe show a tendency to occur preferentially during sleep. They tend to have prominent motor manifestations and are likely to be recognized by the parents or bed partners. Three major clinical forms of epilepsy may be distinguished: benign focal epilepsy of childhood, supplementary sensorimotor epilepsy, and nocturnal frontal lobe epilepsy (NFLE).

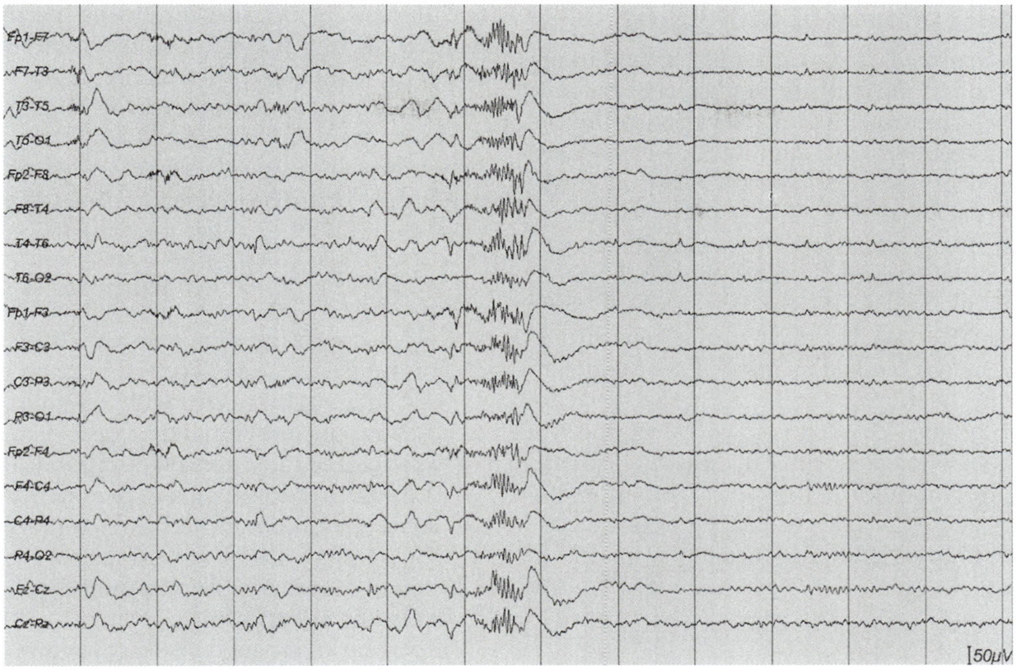

Figure 22-3 Generalized paroxysmal fast activity, followed by attenuation (electrodecrement) in a patient with a symptomatic generalized epilepsy of the Lennox-Gastaut type. This could be an interictal (asymptomatic) discharge but could also be an ictal pattern associated with a tonic-atonic seizure. (Used with permission of John Wiley & Sons—Books from Benbadis SR. Introduction to sleep electroencephalography. In: Lee-Chiong TL, ed. *Sleep: A Comprehensive Handbook.* John Wiley and Sons; 2006:1015; permission conveyed through Copyright Clearance Center, Inc.)

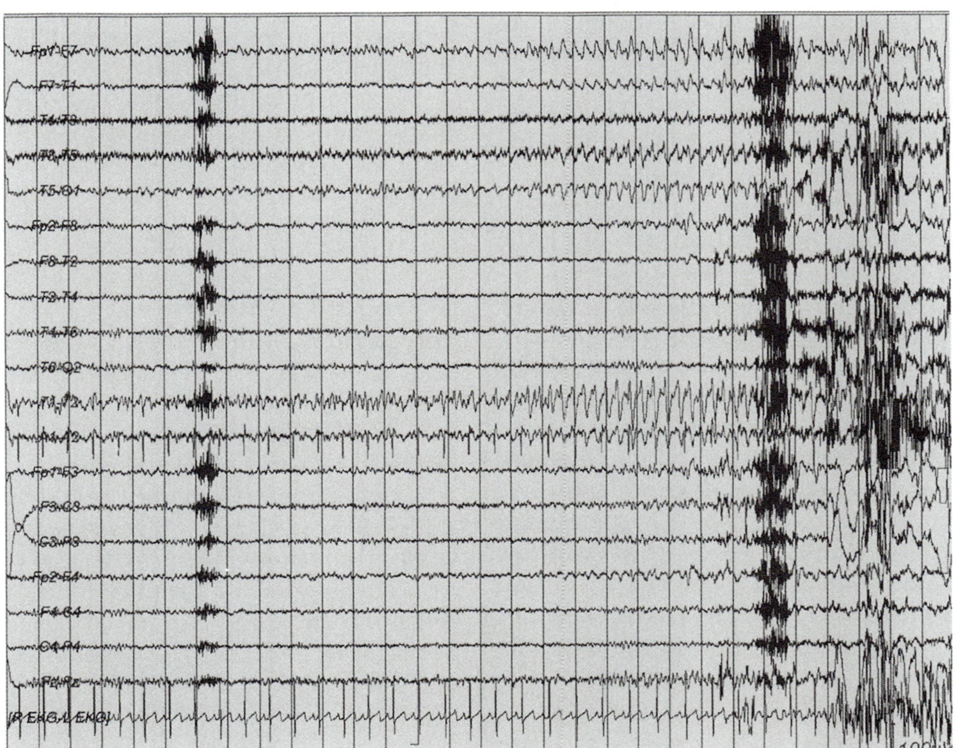

Figure 22-4 Focal seizure. Left temporal seizure (singular), showing the typical rhythmic activity that evolves (buildup). (Used with permission of John Wiley & Sons—Books from Benbadis SR. Introduction to sleep electroencephalography. In: Lee-Chiong TL, ed. *Sleep: A Comprehensive Handbook.* John Wiley and Sons; 2006:1015; permission conveyed through Copyright Clearance Center, Inc.)

Benign Focal Epilepsy of Childhood

This syndrome is also referred to as benign rolandic epilepsy or benign childhood epilepsy. Benign focal epilepsy of childhood with centrotemporal spikes is a common form of childhood epilepsy, accounting for 15% to 25% of childhood epilepsy. Approximately 75% of these seizures occur during sleep. The EEG is characterized by slow spikes or sharp waves recorded simultaneously over frontal, central, and midtemporal areas. These often appear in small clusters and may be seen in children without epilepsy. The IEA is activated by sleep; during NREM sleep, there is a marked increase in the frequency and amplitude of the interictal spike discharges, with no change in morphology. The IEA is maximal during N3 sleep. REM sleep is associated with a decrease in both the frequency and the amplitude of the spikes. Despite an increased frequency of both seizures and IEA during sleep, the sleep profile of these children is usually normal.

Supplementary Sensorimotor Area Epilepsy

This form refers to epilepsy originating from the supplemental sensorimotor area. The typical seizures are characterized by abrupt tonic posturing of the extremities. The upper extremities are usually asymmetrically involved with the abduction at the shoulders, flexion of the elbow on one side, and extension in the other extremity. The head is turned to one side, as though looking toward the flexed arm (fencing posture). The lower extremities are involved in the tonic posture, with abduction at the hips and flexion or extension at the knees. There may be associated vocalization and kicking with preserved responsiveness. Somatosensory (lateralized or diffuse) symptoms may precede the tonic contraction and consist of a feeling of pulling or heaviness or a limb sensation of moving.

The seizures tend to occur predominantly during sleep. Interictal sharp waves are usually found at the midline, maximum at the vertex, or just adjacent to the midline in the frontocentral region. It is fundamentally important to distinguish epileptiform discharges from vertex sharp transients of sleep. The appearance of sharp waves during the waking state aids discrimination between them. The ictal EEG pattern is characterized by a high-amplitude slow transient or sharp wave at the vertex, followed by low-amplitude fast activity, or an electrodecremental pattern (Figure 22-5). Following this pattern, there is a high amplitude slowing in the frontocentral regions distributed bilaterally.

Nocturnal Frontal Lobe Epilepsy

A distinct form of clear-cut attacks originating from epileptic foci located in the frontal lobe (in particular, in the mesial and orbital cortex) and emerging almost exclusively from sleep has been described (10,11). Seizures are characterized by a wide spectrum of clinical features: assumption of postures; rhythmic and repetitive movements of arms and legs; rapid uncoordinated movements, with dystonic or dyskinetic components; complex motor activities (ambulation, wandering, and pelvic thrusting); and sudden elevation of the trunk and head associated with expression of fear and vocalization. There are three subgroups of NFLE:

1. Paroxysmal arousals: characterized by a brief (<20 seconds) abrupt arousal from sleep with vocalization and motor activity consisting of head movements, sudden eye opening, head raising, or sitting up in bed, often with a frightened expression
2. Nocturnal paroxysmal dystonia: characterized by episodes of intermediate duration (20 seconds to 2 minutes) beginning as a paroxysmal arousal but subsequently associated with complex movements, including rhythmic movements of the trunk and pelvis, dystonic posturing, and vocalization
3. Episodic nocturnal wandering: characterized by episodes of longer duration (1-3 minutes) with stereotyped, paroxysmal ambulation, accompanied by screaming and bizarre, dystonic movements

Surface EEG during the attacks and interictally is often normal, uninformative, or not interpretable because of the presence of muscle artifacts (12). Deep (intracranial, sphenoidal) electrode recordings can identify ictal and/or interictal discharges (10). Various ictal EEG patterns may be observed: background flattening, rhythmic theta/delta activity, or sharp wave on the frontal regions.

Treatment for these types of seizures only results in a partial reduction of seizure activity, with events occurring most commonly during NREM sleep. This causes subsequent sleep disturbance due to the recurrence of both major seizures and more subtle arousal activities (13).

Electrical Status Epilepticus of Sleep

This syndrome is also known as epilepsy with continuous spike waves during stage N3 sleep and refers to the occurrence of continuous epileptiform activity for at least 85% of slow-wave sleep (14). The EEG is characterized by generalized spike-wave complexes at 2 to 2.5 Hz, and there is a marked attenuation of the pattern during REM sleep and in the wake state. With the onset of electrical status epilepticus of sleep (ESES), there is an associated decline in cognitive function, with improvement once the ESES has resolved. Seizures may manifest as nocturnal focal motor or generalized tonic-clonic seizures or as atypical absence or myoclonic seizures.

Landau-Kleffner Syndrome

This syndrome is a childhood disorder occurring in previously normal children, characterized by the association of loss of language skills with acquired verbal auditory agnosia and multifocal spikes and spike-and-wave

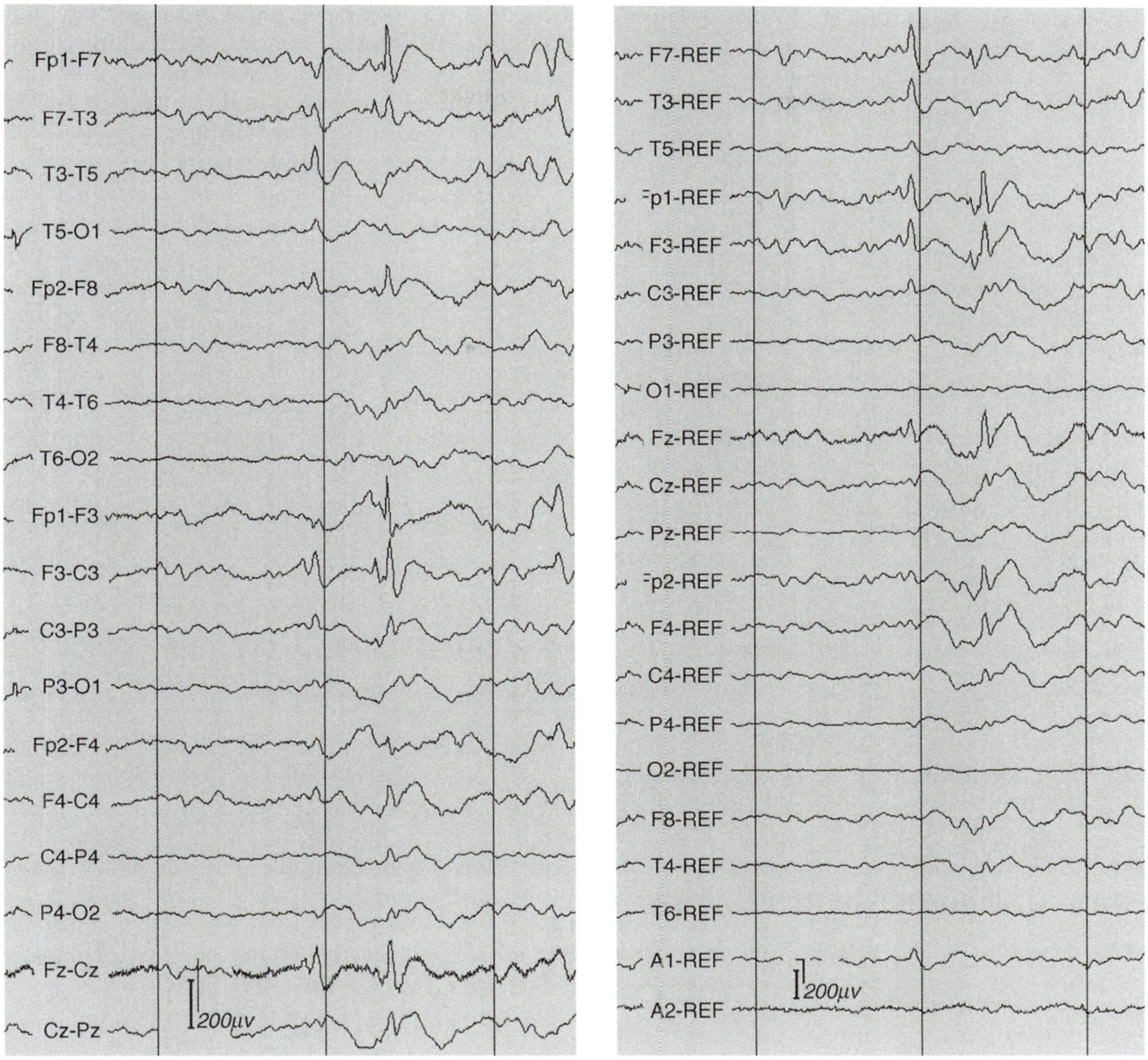

Figure 22-5 Left frontal spike in a patient with left frontal lobe epilepsy. A: Double banana. B: Referential montage showing the same sample. There are two different spikes: the first is maximum at F7 and the second at Fp1. (Used with permission of John Wiley & Sons—Books from Benbadis SR. Introduction to sleep electroencephalography. In: Lee-Chiong TL, ed. *Sleep: A Comprehensive Handbook*. John Wiley and Sons; 2006:1012; permission conveyed through Copyright Clearance Center, Inc.)

discharges localized mainly over the centrotemporal regions. There is dramatic activation of the epileptic discharges during sleep, with discharges occurring for more than 85% of slow-wave sleep, similarly to ESES. However, the occurrence of seizures is relatively rare. There is usually remission of seizures and epileptiform EEG discharges by the age of 15 years.

TREATMENT OPTIONS

Antiepileptic drugs (AEDs) are the most used treatment for seizure control (7). As with any medication, there is a risk of both side effects and adverse reactions. Side effects include, but are not limited to, nausea, vomiting, weight gain, weight loss, headaches, clumsiness, and vision change. AEDs also have an effect on sleep. For the most part, older AEDs decrease sleep latency, decrease REM sleep, and increase daytime drowsiness (15).

Newer AEDs appear to have less effect on sleep, and some increase REM sleep. Insomnia has been associated with lamotrigine, zonisamide, ethosuximide, and felbamate. Their effect on daytime sleepiness is still not well known. Keeping in mind that multiple medications are sometimes necessary for seizure control, the effects on sleep architecture from a combination of AEDs could not be found.

Commonly used medications to control seizures include carbamazepine (Carbatrol/Tegretol), valproate/valproic acid (Depakote/Depakene), phenytoin (Dilantin), felbamate (Felbatol), tiagabine (Gabitril), levetiracetam (Keppra), clonazepam (Klonopin), lamotrigine (Lamictal), pregabalin (Lyrica), primidone (Mysoline), gabapentin (Neurontin), topiramate (Topamax), oxcarbazepine (Trileptal), ethosuximide (Zarontin), and zonisamide (Zonegran).

Cannabinoids, including selective cannabinoid receptor 1 antagonists, appear to prevent seizures and are currently being researched for treatment of seizures (16). Much of this research came from the effects of cannabis on seizures and generalized convulsions.

A *vagal nerve stimulator* is also a treatment option. This is an implantable stimulator that is usually recommended when seizures cannot be adequately controlled with AEDs or the side effects cannot be tolerated. Using the pathway of the vagus nerve, the device (which is surgically implanted on the left side of the neck) delivers mild electrical pulses to the brain (7). Keep in mind that this implant will create artifact when performing a sleep study.

Surgical intervention with removal of a small specific area of the brain where the seizure activity originates is an option for some patients where other forms of treatment have not been successful.

Independently of which treatment path is being followed, maintaining regular sleep cycles, avoiding stress, and regular follow-up with physicians are important too.

GENERAL GUIDELINES FOR SEIZURE MONTAGES

Current polysomnographic (PSG) standards, in regard to assisting in the diagnosis of sleep-related seizure activity, do not mandate the use of a specific recording montage. The minimum channels required include sleep scoring channels (EEG, electrooculogram [EOG], and chin electromyogram [EMG]), EEG using an expanded bilateral montage, and EMG for body movements (anterior tibialis or extensor digitorium) (17). Audiovisual recording and documented technologist observations during the period of study are also essential (17).

The purpose of monitoring additional EEG channels is to not only identify IEA but also to be able to define the seizure focus if possible. With standard PSG monitoring, a referential montage is recorded. Incorporating a full EEG longitudinal bipolar montage can be useful in localizing seizure activity. This would require adding 12 electrodes and recording 16 channels, which is not always feasible. An abbreviated longitudinal bipolar montage is an option. Additional electrodes commonly utilized to record an abbreviated longitudinal bipolar montage include Fp1, Fp2, T3, and T4. Four additional EEG channels could be recorded: Fp1-T3, T3-O1, Fp2-T4, and T4-O2.

EMG should be recorded from all four limbs and should be performed for clinical correlation of tonic-clonic activity. If possible, each limb should be monitored independently. An alternative would be to place one electrode on each extremity and record EMG channels using left arm to right arm and left leg to right leg.

Reviewing the patient's history and considering any information the patient may share with the technologist may be prudent, as would acquiring additional EEG data using a seizure montage. Circumstances in which the technologist should consider using an expanded EEG montage include a diagnosis of epilepsy, any known cause of seizures with ongoing symptoms, witnessed rhythmic movements during sleep with nocturnal incontinence, and injury (tongue biting). As always, protocols specific to each sleep center must be followed. Be proactive for the patient, even if it means taking the time to seek approval to do additional monitoring.

VISUAL DIFFERENCES OF EPILEPTIFORM ACTIVITY ON 10- AND 30-SECOND EPOCHS

Morphology of epileptiform activity on a 10-second epoch has been documented in all previous figures. During a PSG when viewing IEA on a 30-second epoch, an abnormal burst of electrical activity is apparent, although not clearly defined until viewed on a 10-second epoch (Figures 22-6 to 22-9).

GENERAL GUIDELINES FOR RESPONDING TO INTERICTAL EPILEPTIFORM ACTIVITY

The patient's safety is always top priority when seizure activity is recognized by the technologist. If the epileptiform discharges are prolonged or frequent, it is certainly appropriate for the technologist to assess the patient and determine whether any further intervention may be required. Keeping in mind that there is a balance, that data needs to be recorded to confirm a diagnosis, and therefore, knowing when to enter the room to assess the patient is a judgment call. A review of the patient's history will aid in making these decisions, and protocols specific to each sleep center must be followed as well.

GENERAL GUIDELINES FOR RESPONDING TO A CLINICAL SEIZURE

- *Remain calm and continue recording.*
- *Protect the patient from harm*—ensure the patient does not fall out of bed, shield from hard or sharp

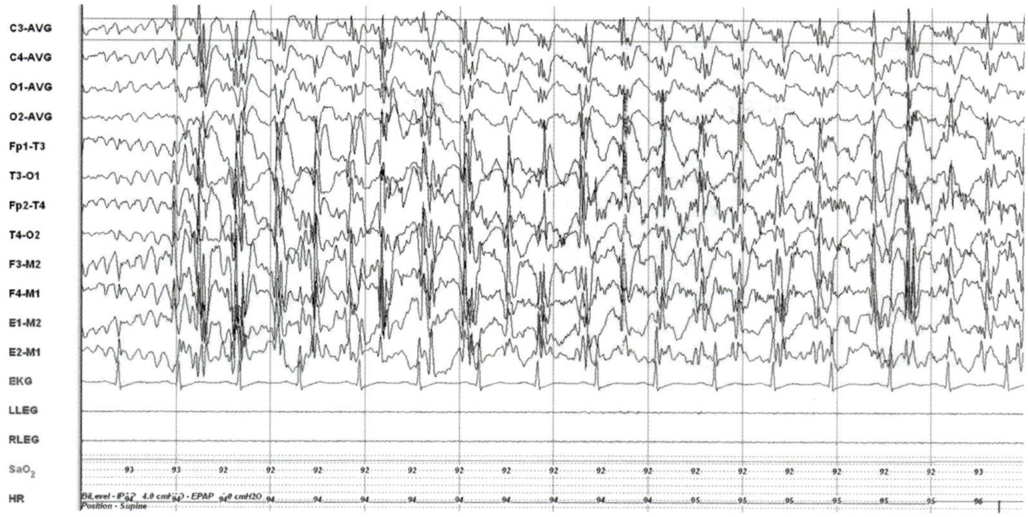

Figure 22-6 Generalized interictal epileptiform activity on a 10-second epoch.

objects, loosen anything that could become tight around the neck (clothing or electrodes), and maintain the airway, either positioning the patient laterally or turning the head to one side.

- *Time* how long the seizure lasts.
- *Do not* attempt to stop any clonic movements.
- *Do not* place objects in the patient's mouth.
- *Stay with the patient.* With the return of consciousness, the patient will need to be reassured and reoriented. During the postictal period, reorientation may need to be repeated as necessary.
- *Document* the event, including the date, time, and duration of the occurrence; a description of the event; and the actions taken by the technologist. Include a list of notifications made, the patient's vital signs following the event, and the time it took for "baseline level of consciousness" to return. All specific sleep center protocols need to be followed as well.

WHEN TO ACTIVATE EMERGENCY MEDICAL SERVICES

The following situations are medical emergencies: seizures lasting longer than 5 minutes; a second seizure starting soon after the first one has ended; consciousness not returning after clonic movements have subsided; or signs of physical distress, injury, or pregnancy. A seizure during pregnancy can be a symptom of eclampsia, and immediate evaluation is indicated.

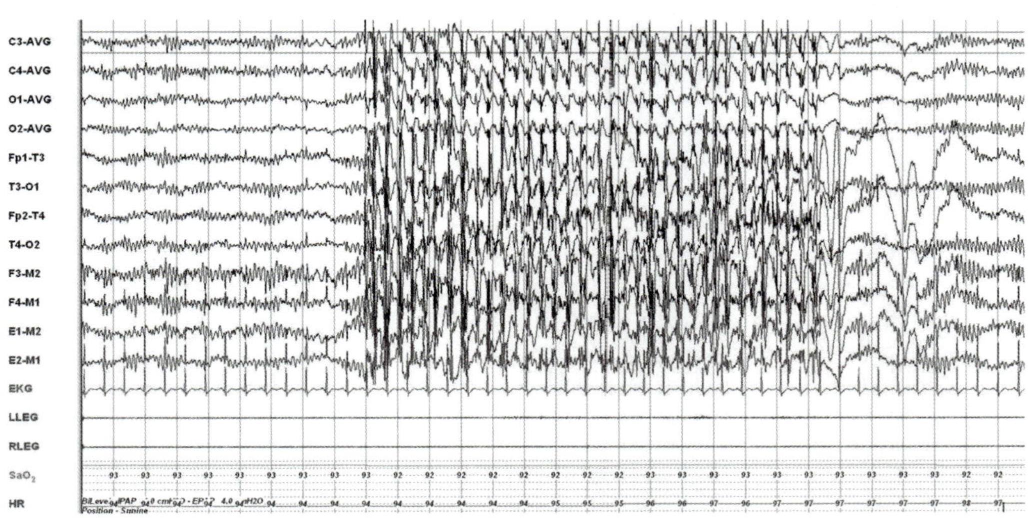

Figure 22-7 Generalized interictal epileptiform activity depicted in Figure 22-6 but on a 30-second epoch.

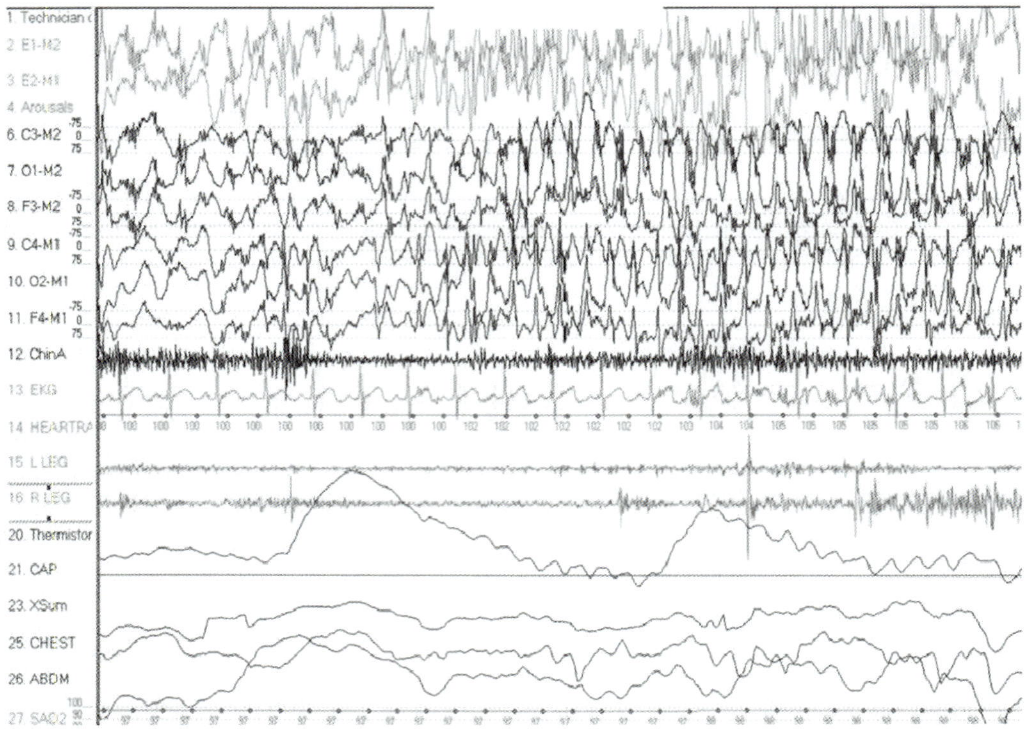

Figure 22-8 Generalized interictal epileptiform activity on a 10-second epoch.

LIVING WITH EPILEPSY

The ability to understand the impact epilepsy has on a person's life is a vital part of being able to care for the person when seizures occur. Seizures are frightening and unknown to many, and sadly, even in today's society, a stigma still surrounds epilepsy.

Sometimes, it can be a lengthy process from the initial seizure to the diagnosis and eventual management and treatment of seizures. Although AEDs are effective

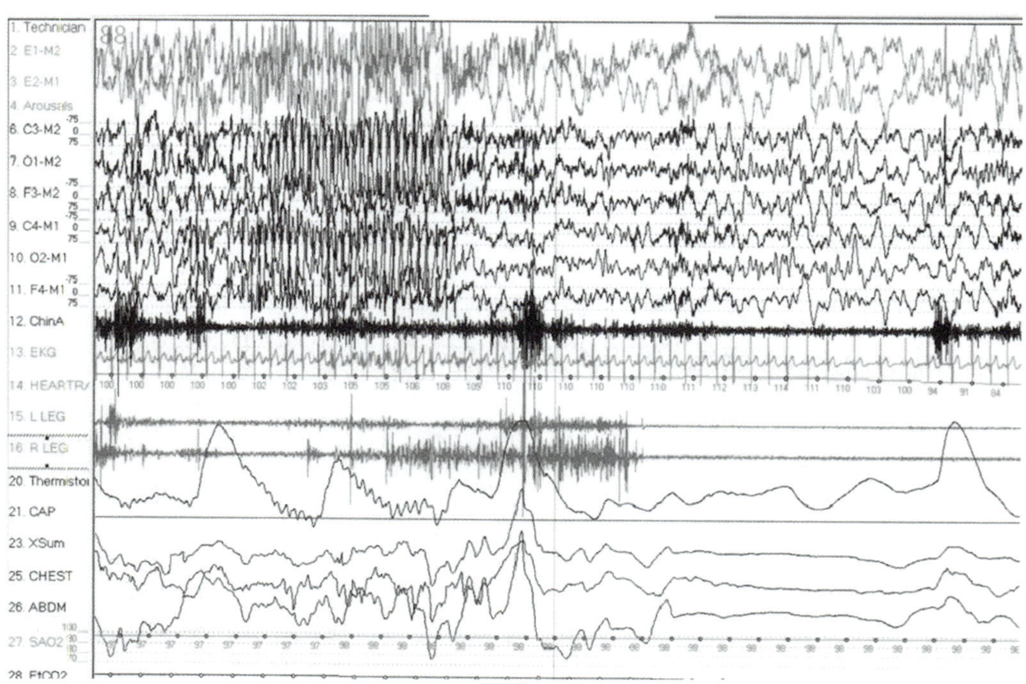

Figure 22-9 Generalized interictal epileptiform activity depicted in Figure 22-8 but on a 30-second epoch.

in a majority of cases, finding the correct medication(s) and dosage may take time. Meanwhile, employment issues, isolation, medication side effects, the possibility of invasive procedures, and loss of independence will be but a few of the hurdles these patients face. For instance, in some states, driving privileges are restricted until a person is "seizure free" for 6 months. Technologists should be aware that each patient presenting to the sleep center may be dealing with any or all of the aforementioned processes and adjust the care offered to patients experiencing seizure accordingly.

CONCLUSION

The role of the sleep technologist encompasses more than placing electrodes on a patient and recording data. Depending on patient population, nocturnal seizure activity may rarely be seen at some sleep facilities. Despite this, all sleep professionals need to understand the relationship between sleep and sleep disorders with seizure control. Reviewing the patient history may lead a technologist to question if recording additional EEG channels is warranted. Familiarity with commonly used AEDs, recognition of epileptiform activity on the EEG, and knowing how to keep a patient safe in the event of a seizure while in the sleep center are all necessary skills. All patients deserve a well-trained technologist treating them with respect and compassion. Patients put at ease by a knowledgeable technologist and a comfortable sleeping environment are quite possibly more apt to share information, likely aiding the physician in rendering a diagnosis and offering an improved individualized treatment plan.

REFERENCES

1. Centers for Disease Control and Prevention. Epilepsy facts and Stats. 2024. Accessed November 8, 2025. https://www.cdc.gov/epilepsy/data-research/facts-stats/index.html
2. National Institute of Neurological Disorders and Stroke. Epilepsy and Seizures. 2025. Accessed November 8, 2025. https://www.ninds.nih.gov/health-information/disorders/epilepsy-and-seizures
3. Lesser RP. Treatment and outcome of psychogenic nonepileptic seizures. *Epilepsy Curr*. 2003;3(6):198-200.
4. Tatum WO, Olga S, Ochoa JG, et al. American Clinical Neurophysiology Society Guideline 7: guidelines for EEG reporting. *J Clin Neurophysiol*. 2016;33(4):328-332.
5. Subbarao BS, Silverman A, Eapen BC. Seizure medications. In: *StatPearls* [Internet]. StatPearls Publishing; 2025. https://www.ncbi.nlm.nih.gov/books/NBK482269/
6. Hirsch LJ, Fong MWK, Leitinger M, et al. American Clinical Neurophysiology Society's standardized critical care EEG terminology: 2021 version. *J Clin Neurophysiol*. 2021;38(1):1-29. doi:10.1097/WNP.0000000000000806
7. National Library of Medicine–National Institutes of Health. Epilepsy. MedlinePlus. 2025. Accessed November 8, 2025. http://www.nlm.nih.gov/medlineplus/epilepsy.html#cat3
8. Montplaisir J, Laverdiere M, Saint-Hiliare JM. Sleep and epilepsy. In Gotman J, Ives JR, Gloor P, eds. *Long Term Monitoring in Epilepsy*. Elsevier; 1985:215-239.
9. Peng W, Danison JL, Seyal M. Postictal generalized EEG suppression and respiratory dysfunction following generalized tonic-clonic seizures in sleep and wakefulness. *Epilepsia*. 2017;58(8):1409-1414. doi:10.1111/epi.13805
10. Tinuper P, Cerullo A, Cirignotta F. Nocturnal paroxysmal dystonia with short-lasting attacks: three cases with evidence for an epileptic frontal lobe origin of seizures. *Epilepsia*. 1990;31:549-556.
11. Plazzi G, Tinuper P, Montagna P, et al. Epileptic nocturnal wanderings. *Sleep*. 1985;18:749-756.
12. Zucconi M, Ferini-Strambi L. NREM parasomnias: arousal disorders and differentiation from nocturnal frontal lobe epilepsy. *Clin Neurophysiol*. 2000;111(suppl 2):129-135.
13. De Paolis F, Colizzi E, Milioli G, et al. Effects of antiepileptic treatment on sleep and seizures in nocturnal frontal lobe epilepsy. *Sleep Med*. 2013;14(7):597-604. doi:10.1016/j.sleep.2013.02.014
14. Tassinari CA, Rubboli G, Volpi L, et al. Encephalopathy with electrical status epilepticus during slow sleep or ESES syndrome including the acquired aphasia. *Clin Neurophysiol*. 2000;111(suppl 2):S94-S102.
15. Epilepsy.com. Antiepileptic drugs and sleep? Epilepsy and seizure information for patients and health professionals. 2025. Accessed November 8, 2025. https://www.epilepsy.com/complications-risks/sleep/asms
16. Malyshevskaya O, Aritake K, Kaushik MK, et al. The relationship between sleep, cannabinoids and seizures. *Sleep Med*. 2017;40(suppl 1):e207-e208. doi:10.1016/j.sleep.2017.11.607
17. American Academy of Sleep Medicine. Practice parameters for the indications for polysomnography and related procedures. *Sleep*. 2005;28(4):512.

Chapter 23
Impact of Degenerative Disorders on Sleep

MONICA M. HENDERSON, JENNIFER PARR-CHRISTMAS, JAMES D. GEYER, AND PAUL R. CARNEY

KEY CONCEPTS/LEARNING OBJECTIVES

The key concepts for this chapter include a discussion of degenerative neurologic diseases, a description of the impact of degenerative neurologic diseases on polysomnography and sleep, and a review of patient management issues in the sleep laboratory.

KEY TERMS

Alzheimer disease
Dementia with Lewy bodies
Multiple system atrophy
Nocturnal stridor
Parkinson disease
Pick disease
Progressive supranuclear palsy
Rapid eye movement (REM) sleep behavior disorder
Restless legs syndrome
Vascular dementia

DEGENERATIVE DISORDERS AND SLEEP

Degenerative neurologic disorders encompass a broad range of diseases. They include common entities such as dementia and rare diseases such as amyotrophic lateral sclerosis (ALS, or Lou Gehrig disease). The incidence of such diseases in the general population increases with advancing age. Given the increasing age of the demographically large baby boom generation, sleep technologists can expect to deal with patients with these degenerative diseases on an increasingly frequent basis.

Neurologic disorders and sleep disorders are linked in a complex fashion. For most of the syndromes, little is known about how the disorders affect normal sleep, because the typical clinical description of patients with degenerative diseases has largely reflected data gathered during wakefulness, paying little attention to the manifestations of these disorders during sleep. There has been even less attention focused on the effects that preexisting sleep disorders have on neurologic function during wakefulness of patients affected with these disorders. This chapter will examine the relationship of sleep and some of the more common neurologic disorders as well as a few rare but more well-known conditions. We have also included practical information to help sleep technologists to establish guidelines to effectively address the physical needs of the patient with neurologic impairment.

GENERAL PATIENT MANAGEMENT ISSUES

The sleep technologist must be aware of the potential cognitive and physical limitations of each patient. A patient with dementia may have difficulty following directions and may not be compliant with standard monitoring protocols. Patients with physically debilitating diseases may need assistance turning or ambulating. It is not uncommon for patients with degenerative neurologic conditions to have previously undiagnosed parasomnias, which may disrupt sleep monitoring. Patient safety is paramount. Once the sleep study has been initiated, the technologist may choose to limit interruptions of monitoring once the patient is asleep, even if electrodes are not making good electrical contact. A recording with the loss of some electrophysiologic signals can still provide clinically important data.

DEGENERATIVE NEUROLOGIC DISORDERS

The relationships between sleep-related breathing disorders, especially obstructive sleep apnea/hypopnea, neurobehavioral and cognitive function, and dementia, are incompletely defined and are the subject of frequent study and debate. The relationships are even less well described for the degenerative movement disorders. We have attempted to present the most current information available, while keeping unproven theories to a minimum.

Dementia

Dementia, including all its subtypes, is one of the most common and debilitating degenerative neurologic disorders. It is frequently undiagnosed in the older adults, with symptoms dismissed as normal aging. There are numerous subtypes that are categorized based on etiology and pathologic findings; however, they often have similar effects on sleep. Dementia is defined as a syndrome characterized by deterioration of baseline mental function in multiple cognitive/intellectual areas, with little or no disturbance of perception or consciousness. Dementia is not necessarily an irreversible condition. Although most common types of dementia are permanent and progressive, some forms are treatable and reversible, such as those caused by thiamine deficiency, hypothyroidism, and long-standing untreated sleep apnea.

Dementia should not be confused with delirium, a transient confusional state that is characterized by an inability to think with proper speed, clarity, and coherence and that is associated with disorientation, reduced attention and concentration, impaired immediate recall, and diminution of all mental activity. Delirium has a variety of causes, the most common of which include infection, medication side effects, alcoholic or other drug intoxication, acute drug withdrawal in a person with substance use disorder, and metabolic abnormalities, which complicate liver failure, renal failure, etc. In comparison, the more common types of dementia arise from primary changes occurring within the brain cells. Although the symptoms of most types of dementia develop over the course of months to years, delirium typically arises over hours to a few days and may last several weeks. The initial signs and symptoms of delirium usually include reduced concentration, irritability, tremulousness, insomnia, and poor appetite. The patient will typically describe vivid and unpleasant dreams, which are further complicated by transient illusions and hallucinations during wakefulness. Seizures are relatively common, occurring in approximately one-third of cases. Later in the course of the condition, patients may experience paranoia, tremor, and autonomic hyperactivity. Unlike dementia, recovery from delirium is usually complete and heralded by increased lucid intervals and sound sleep.

In contrast, dementia is conventionally said to involve impairment in memory and at least one other cognitive sphere (language, praxis or the ability to perform simple tasks, calculation, judgment, visuospatial orientation, abstract thinking, or concentration). There may be behavioral abnormalities and personality changes with little or no disturbance of consciousness or perception. Delirium and dementia may coexist, and because of diminished brain function, patients with dementia are at increased risk of developing delirium from minor infections, changes in medication, etc.

Alzheimer Disease

Alzheimer disease (AD) is the most common cause of degenerative dementia and is estimated to be the etiology in 60% to 80% of patients with dementia. The figures are not exact because a definite diagnosis of AD requires detection of characteristic lesions on postmortem examination of brain tissue. For this reason, clinical trials and studies of AD have likely contained significant numbers of patients with other dementia subtypes.

AD occurs with equal frequency in men and women and usually begins after 60 years of age. Risk factors include advanced age, family history, Down syndrome (essentially all patients with Down syndrome who are over 35 years of age have AD), low educational level, chromosomal mutations on chromosomes 1, 14, and 21, apolipoprotein E ε4 genotype, and a history of brain injury. Regardless of the cause, AD is characterized by decreased levels of the neurotransmitter acetylcholine in the hippocampus and neocortex because of loss of cholinergic projections from the nucleus basalis of Meynert. The clinical features of AD include a gradual decline of intellectual function, poor short-term memory with relative sparing of long-term memory in the early stages of the disease, visuospatial disorientation, language/speech problems, and personality changes. Patients develop difficulty performing simple tasks, including activities of daily living such as eating, drinking, and walking. New-onset seizures occur in approximately 10% of Alzheimer patients.

More recently, obstructive sleep apnea syndrome has been related to AD. The degree of the impact of obstructive sleep apnea syndrome on the development and progression of AD continues to be a topic of research.

Dementia With Lewy Bodies

Dementia with Lewy bodies (DLB) is the second most common cause of degenerative dementia, representing approximately 15% to 20% of cases. It occurs twice as often in men as in women. The onset of symptoms typically begins between 50 and 80 years of age. The hallmark pathologic feature in brain tissue is Lewy bodies, which are inclusions seen within neurons. The clinical features of DLB include dementia, psychosis, and mild extrapyramidal symptoms such as spasticity. The presenting symptoms are usually personality changes and behavioral problems, followed by deterioration of memory over months to years. Hallucinations and delusions are common.

Pick Disease

Pick disease is one of the dementias that are associated with loss of neurons in the frontotemporal region of the brain. It is a rare degenerative dementia occurring in less than 10% of the patients with dementia. Unlike DLB, it occurs more frequently in women than in men. The onset of symptoms is typically in the sixth decade of life.

The hallmark pathologic features of Pick bodies are cytoplasmic inclusion bodies that are present in affected neurons. Similar to DLB, the clinical features of Pick disease include personality changes and behavioral problems usually associated with poor judgment. There is a gradual decline of intellectual function and poor short-term memory. Patients may develop Kluver-Bucy syndrome, which is characterized by hypersexuality, hyperorality, and docile behavior.

Vascular Dementia

Vascular dementia is the cause of approximately 10% of cases of dementia. It occurs in patients with a history of stroke and cerebrovascular disease. As with other types of atherosclerotic vascular disease, it is more common in men. Because stroke and cerebrovascular disease are so common, vascular factors may also complicate other dementia subtypes. Vascular dementia can be caused by ischemic stroke, cerebral hemorrhage, anoxic/ischemic brain injury, or vasculitis. Unlike AD, which has a gradual cognitive decline, there is typically a stepwise progression of symptoms associated with each new vascular event.

Sleep Disorders Associated With Dementias

Patients with dementia have the same risk of developing sleep disorders as the general population. It is speculated that sleep-related breathing disorders may be one of the underlying factors contributing to vascular dementia, but definitive data regarding this relationship are lacking at present. In general, the effect of restful sleep versus unrefreshing sleep on the dementias is poorly understood. Untreated or inadequately treated obstructive sleep apnea/hypopnea in the general population causes excessive daytime somnolence, depressed mood, reduced quality of life, and subsequent cognitive dysfunction. Treatment of obstructive sleep apnea can improve this cognitive dysfunction (1,2). Treatment with positive airway pressure (PAP) in neurologically intact individuals improves attention, speed of thinking, short-term memory, and general cognitive status (3). There are limited data regarding the effect of sleep apnea treatment on the cognitive status of patients with degenerative dementia, yet our experience has been that many patients will receive some benefit. An important consideration is that treatment of sleep disorders improves the bed partner's (and usually the primary caregiver's) quality and amount of sleep (4). Theoretically, improvement in the quality of sleep can result in some improvement in the patient's level of cognitive function, so diagnosis and correction of any underlying sleep disorder is desirable for the benefit of both the patient and their bed partner.

Patients with DLB appear to have a greater risk of rapid eye movement (REM) sleep behavior disorder (RBD), although the prevalence is not yet known (5-7). RBD is so common that it is now regarded as a supportive feature for the diagnosis of DLB (8). RBD typically begins years before the onset of other symptoms of dementia. The differential diagnosis for the abnormal behaviors includes RBD as well as epileptic seizures and wandering, behaviors that commonly occur in the demented population. Episodes of wandering are usually less violent, do not appear to be associated with REM sleep, and are often of longer duration than a typical REM period. Polysomnography with video monitoring, a full electroencephalogram (EEG) montage, and additional electromyography leads on all four extremities can help confirm the diagnosis of RBD. Clonazepam is the drug of choice in treating RBD and is effective in most cases (9). If clonazepam proves ineffective or is not tolerated, alternative treatments include carbamazepine, melatonin (10), and dopamine agonists. Aggressive treatment of any underlying sleep-related breathing disorder is extremely important in the management of RBD.

The epidemiology of restless legs and periodic limb movements (PLMs) in patients with degenerative neurologic disorders is not well understood. Restless legs syndrome (RLS) is quite common, occurring in at least 10% of the population who are generally affected by degenerative cognitive disorders.

Restless legs may occur as a genetic disorder or may be secondary to arthritis, peripheral vascular disease, peripheral neuropathy, or relative iron deficiency. A number of medications have shown efficacy for the treatment of restless legs, including ropinirole, carbidopa/levodopa (L-dopa), pramipexole, benzodiazepines, opiates, pregabalin, and gabapentin enacarbil, but some of these medications should be used cautiously in the population with dementia. L-Dopa has been associated with augmentation of symptoms, a paradoxic worsening of the frequency and severity of symptoms related to the medication itself, as well as an increased risk of psychosis and insomnia. Dopamine agonists (pramipexole and ropinirole) have a lower risk of augmentation but can be associated with an increased risk of psychosis, insomnia, and the possibility of inappropriate sleepiness. As sedatives or central nervous system depressants, benzodiazepines and opiates can help overcome restlessness but may have unacceptable cognitive consequences in patients with dementia. Likewise, the antiepileptic medications can also have adverse cognitive side effects. Patients who have decreased levels of serum ferritin may experience a sufficient reduction in symptoms with iron replacement such that medication may be unnecessary. It is uncommon for patients without RLS to experience PLMs during wakefulness; however, PLMs occur during sleep in about 80% of patients with RLS. PLMs are more common in the normal older population than in younger individuals. PLMs without associated sleep disruption should not be treated, especially in patients with dementia who are more likely to have adverse medication side effects.

Hypersomnolence is also common among patients with degenerative neurologic disorders, although the etiology is unknown. The sleepiness can result from a number of underlying factors, including sleep apnea/hypopnea, nocturnal movement disorders, circadian rhythm disorders, and medication side effects. The patient should be screened for treatable underlying sleep disorders. When all identified instigating factors are remedied, residual sleepiness typically responds to proalerting medications such as armodafinil or modafinil. Traditional stimulants such as amphetamines may also be of some benefit. Behavioral complications caused by these stimulant medications are rare but may occur, and the patient's behavior should be monitored for agitation and worsening of cognitive function.

The origin of insomnia in patients with degenerative neurologic disorders is poorly understood (11,12). The patient with dementia and insomnia should be evaluated for medical causes, including medication side effects, before symptomatic treatment is initiated. Many of the medications traditionally used for treatment of dementia conditions can result in a paradoxic worsening of insomnia, with subsequent decline of cognitive function and a worsening of undesirable behaviors. Circadian dysrhythmia is an abnormal fragmentation of the normal sleep-wake cycle that is common in patients with dementia (3,12) and is often associated with wandering behavior. Degeneration of the suprachiasmatic nucleus of the hypothalamus is most likely the basis for circadian dysrhythmia in this population. Supplemental melatonin and phototherapy are the two primary treatment modalities. Melatonin may improve sleep architecture and continuity with an increase in the total sleep time; however, it should be used with caution. Because melatonin is classified as a supplement rather than a medication, its production is not regulated by the U.S. Food and Drug Administration, and it has not undergone rigorous testing for long-term detrimental side effects. Phototherapy may also be beneficial, but a standardized treatment protocol has not been established.

Patient Management

In the setting of the sleep center, it is useful to keep in mind that patients with degenerative dementias show a broad range of cognitive dysfunction and coexisting psychiatric symptoms, so the approach to each patient should be tailored to their individual needs. Some patients may seem "a little forgetful" and have some degree of confusion on awakening in a strange environment. "Sundowning" is a relatively common phenomenon in which the patient's functional status deteriorates in the late afternoon and evening and may complicate monitoring with increasing confusion or agitation. Other patients may have paranoid tendencies, limiting their ability to cooperate with the sleep technologist. These affected patients have lost the ability to process complex instructions and explanations and, as a result, respond to the actions and tone of the voice of the technologist rather than the content of the explanations that are given. Their confusion may result in combativeness. The technologist should maintain a calm, reassuring demeanor because arguing with a patient with dementia will likely worsen the agitation and aggressive behavior. As an added precaution, the sleep center should establish a policy for dealing with patients who are violent. It is best to limit patient interaction to reduce external stimuli. Benzodiazepines and similar sedative hypnotic medications should be avoided, as these drugs can worsen the degree of confusion. Alternative medications that should be used with combative or difficult patients include antipsychotics, such as quetiapine and risperidone. It is important that home medications be administered routinely, because missed doses may compound cognitive symptoms.

Nocturnal wandering may occur, and patients should be carefully monitored to prevent falls. Patients should be gently redirected back to bed, and medications used as needed. Insomnia, sundowning, and wandering can be extremely disruptive (11), both at home and in the sleep center. Because AD is associated with an increased incidence of seizures, monitoring should be performed with standard seizure precautions in place. Surprisingly, many patients with dementia tolerate continuous positive airway pressure (CPAP) therapy quite well. For those patients who find the mask intolerable, positional treatment of sleep apnea may be an acceptable alternative in the appropriate patient.

Urinary incontinence is commonly seen in patients with degenerative neurologic disorders. Family members should be discreetly asked about the use of adult diapers at home.

Although some patients with dementia may seem quite difficult and unpleasant to the sleep center staff, it is important that the staff understand that this is part of the patient's disease process and cannot be controlled by the patient.

Technical Aspects of Recording

There are no specific technical requirements for recording patients with degenerative neurologic disorders. Degenerative dementias may be associated with slowing of the alpha rhythm. There may be increased delta activity in the EEG even during wakefulness, making sleep staging difficult.

MOVEMENT DISORDERS

Movement disorders are a diverse group of neurologic diseases, which share some symptoms while differing in many other respects. As a group, they have more diverse clinical manifestations than the dementias previously discussed. What the syndromes share is a progressive downhill course that leads in many patients to death from aspiration pneumonia or complications of falls. The more common diseases and those that have a known association with sleep disorders are discussed in the following paragraphs. Given the scope of this textbook, the discussion is not exhaustive, and other less common entities such as Huntington disease, Wilson disease, and tic disorders have been excluded.

Parkinson Disease

Parkinson disease is one of the more common and well-known progressive degenerative movement disorders. Its hallmark features include resting tremor, bradykinesia (slowness of movement), rigidity, and gait disturbance. In contrast, Parkinsonism is a syndrome that occurs in patients without Parkinson disease who develop some but not all the Parkinsonian symptoms, usually consisting of tremor, bradykinesia, and rigidity. It frequently occurs as a side effect of medications such as antipsychotic and antiemetic drugs, although several other neurologic disorders may result in Parkinsonism. As with the dementias, little is known about the interaction between sleep and most movement disorders.

Parkinson disease affects about 1% of the population over 50 years of age and occurs slightly more often in men than in women. The age of onset for Parkinson disease is quite broad, ranging from 20 to 80 years, with a peak in the sixth decade of life. The symptoms typically slowly progress over a course of years, but some sleep abnormalities may arise in the presymptomatic phase.

The pathophysiology of Parkinson disease is dominated by a loss of pigmented neurons in the substantia nigra of the basal ganglia and locus ceruleus, which results in decreased levels of dopamine in the brain. The four characteristic clinical features of Parkinson disease are rigidity with cogwheeling (increases in muscle tone with alternating catches and release), bradykinesia (slowness of movement), resting tremor (often described as a pill-rolling movement), and postural instability (difficulty maintaining standing posture, resulting in a tendency to fall forward). Patients may also have a stooped posture, reduced blinking, an unusually quiet voice, difficulty writing, and drooling. Depression is a common complicating factor. Approximately 30% of afflicted patients will develop dementia.

A number of treatments are available for Parkinson disease and its associated complications. L-dopa or its most common clinical form, Sinemet (carbidopa/L-dopa), crosses the blood-brain barrier and is metabolized to dopamine. Side effects include nausea, vomiting, orthostatic hypotension, dyskinesias (increased involuntary movements), restlessness, and hallucinations. Many of these side effects are dose related and are sometimes reversible. Sleep-related side effects include insomnia, nightmares, and anxiety. Monoamine oxidase inhibitors such as Selegiline are used less often. These drugs have a stimulant effect and must be given early in the day to avoid insomnia at night. Dopamine agonists, drugs that can bind to the cell's dopamine receptor and act in a dopaminergic fashion, include bromocriptine (Parlodel), pergolide (Permax), ropinirole (Requip), and pramipexole (Mirapex). The dopamine agonists can be used to delay the need for L-dopa and can be combined with L-dopa to allow a reduction in the dosage of L-dopa, which reduces medication side effects. The dopamine agonists have side effects similar to those of L-dopa, including orthostatic hypotension, nausea, hallucinations, and dyskinesias. Sleep-related side effects include drowsiness and sleep attacks.

Multiple System Atrophy

Multiple system atrophy (MSA) is present in 10% of the patients with Parkinsonian features. MSA is a neuropathologic term that encompasses several overlapping disorders, which are known as the Parkinson plus syndromes. A Parkinson plus syndrome should be suspected when the patient has Parkinsonism plus one or more of the following non-Parkinsonian symptoms: prominent dysautonomia (abnormal autonomic control of blood pressure and heart rate), ataxia (unstable gait), corticospinal tract findings (including weakness, increased muscle tone, and increased reflexes), bilateral, symmetric onset of symptoms (both arms with the same degree of increased tone), lack of resting tremor, or a poor response to L-dopa treatment.

Progressive Supranuclear Palsy

Progressive supranuclear palsy (Steele-Richardson-Olszewski syndrome) is a Parkinsonian syndrome with typically less tremor and poor response to Parkinson medication. It is commonly misdiagnosed as Parkinson disease. Similarly to Parkinson disease, it occurs more frequently in men, with an onset of symptoms occurring typically after 40 years and with a peak in the sixth decade of life.

The clinical features of progressive supranuclear palsy include reduced balance and falling, typically backward compared with the forward direction of falls usually seen in patients with Parkinson disease, supranuclear gaze palsy (reduced ability to produce voluntary vertical eye movements), and axial dystonia with an erect posture and difficulty bending or stooping. There is minimal tremor, and the dementia usually develops late in the syndrome and is relatively mild.

Corticobasal Ganglionic Degeneration

Corticobasal ganglionic degeneration is a degenerative movement disorder that occurs equally in men and women. The onset of symptoms typically occurs in the seventh decade of life, with the average patient surviving 5 to 10 years. The clinical features include unilateral extrapyramidal rigidity (difficulty moving, with rigidity and stiffness), tremor both at rest and during movement, apraxia (reduced higher mental function, which results in difficulty performing simple tasks), and "alien hand syndrome" of the involved upper extremity. Alien hand syndrome is an interesting phenomenon, where the affected hand or arm not only cannot be voluntarily controlled by the patient but also appears to act in a fashion that actively opposes the goal the patient wishes to achieve. There can also be cortical sensory loss, clumsiness, and supranuclear gaze palsy (difficulty in making voluntary eye movements). The disorder is slowly progressive and eventually involves both sides of the body.

Sleep Disorders Associated With Movement Disorders

Parkinson disease is the most common of the movement disorders and has the most data regarding coexisting sleep disorders. There are virtually no data available for the more obscure degenerative diseases, and the incidence of sleep disorders remains largely unknown. Sleep-disordered breathing, which includes obstructive sleep apnea/hypopnea, central sleep apnea, Cheyne-Stokes breathing, and periodic breathing, is relatively common in Parkinson disease. Although it appears to occur at a frequency above that of the normal population, the exact epidemiology is not known. Many patients tolerate CPAP or bilevel PAP (BPAP) therapy and experience significant functional improvement after the sleep apnea/hypopnea has been adequately treated. The spouse of a patient with Parkinson disease and sleep apnea/hypopnea may also experience improved sleep efficiency and sleep architecture, with less daytime sleepiness when their bed partner with Parkinson disease and sleep apnea is effectively treated.

Insomnia can result from a primary sleep disorder such as RLS, psychophysiologic insomnia, poor sleep hygiene factors, side effects of medications, as well as the Parkinsonism resulting in the difficulty or inability to turn over in bed. Severe sleep maintenance insomnia is common in progressive supranuclear palsy (13).

RLS is one of the most common primary sleep disorders experienced by patients with Parkinson disease. Unfortunately, treatment of the neurologic symptoms with L-dopa commonly results in a worsening of the RLS by producing the daytime augmentation phenomenon in which RLS paradoxically worsens during the afternoons rather than evenings. Often, a change from L-dopa to a dopamine agonist such as pramipexole or ropinirole is needed, but this may result in less optimal control of the neurologic symptoms. Antiepileptic medications such as pregabalin or gabapentin enacarbil can be of benefit in the treatment of RLS. Alternatively, addition of an opioid such as hydrocodone or a benzodiazepine before bedtime may help improve RLS. Patients so treated must be carefully monitored for worsening cognitive status and daytime sleepiness.

RBD is characterized by increased muscle tone during REM sleep and the "acting out of dreams." Limb movements and vocalization during REM sleep are frequently associated with violent behavior consistent with dream content. Injuries to the patient and/or the bed partner are common; however, directed violence is uncommon. The abnormal behavior does not occur with every REM period and may vary in frequency, duration, and the degree of violence. RBD may precede the onset of degenerative neurologic disorders by several years and then tends to reduce in severity as the specific neurologic disorder progresses (1). RBD is the initial manifestation in approximately half of patients with Parkinson disease (9). The frequency is even greater in patients with MSA. Interestingly, RBD in MSA occurs frequently in both males and females, whereas RBD in Parkinson disease occurs predominantly in male patients.

RBD has been reported but is rare in patients with progressive supranuclear palsy. Although most patients with MSA have RBD, REM sleep without atonia occurs in 95% of cases. REM sleep without atonia is also relatively common in corticobasal ganglionic degeneration, but, unlike MSA, RBD is uncommon. Up to 80% of patients with RBD respond to clonazepam. Alternative treatments include carbamazepine, L-dopa, and dopamine agonists such as ropinirole and pramipexole. Management of RBD in MSA is similar to that in the other degenerative neurologic disorders, except that clonazepam should be avoided, if possible, because of its detrimental effect on respiratory stridor, autonomic respiratory instability, and significant gait instability. The use of this medication may, however, be necessary in some patients with MSA. When used, the patient should be monitored carefully for worsening of nocturnal stridor and periodic breathing. Fall precautions should be taken.

As in patients with dementia, excessive daytime sleepiness is very common in Parkinson disease. Potential causes include depression, sleep apnea, restless legs, and intrinsic hypersomnolence. Severe Parkinson disease is associated with excessive somnolence unrelated to any other sleep disorder. "Sleep attacks" or sudden, irresistible, and overwhelming episodes of sleepiness have been reported in a few patients with Parkinson disease, occurring more often in those receiving dopamine agonists (pramipexole, ropinirole, L-dopa, and bromocriptine) (14). The episodes of sleepiness improved following discontinuation of the dopamine agonist. Nocturnal stridor, a high-pitched inspiratory sound that is frequently unrecognized by the patient but commonly reported by the patient's bed partner, occurs in at least 10% to 15% of patients with MSA (15) and may be the presenting feature of the disorder (16). It probably has a central cause that produces abnormally enhanced vocal cord adduction. The stridor can lead to decreased oxygen saturation and severe respiratory compromise.

Tracheostomy has traditionally been the recommended treatment for nocturnal stridor, but the procedure has not been well received by patients. Treatment with CPAP has had mixed results. A number of other respiratory disorders have been associated with MSA, including central sleep apnea, obstructive sleep apnea, central hypoventilation, Cheyne-Stokes breathing, apneustic breathing, and irregular breathing. Brainstem degeneration is thought to be the common etiology for these disorders. Sleep-related breathing disorders are not common in corticobasal ganglionic degeneration but may occur as a concomitant disorder. The exact frequency of sleep-related breathing disorders is not known in the population of patients with corticobasal ganglionic degeneration. CPAP therapy can be problematic for such patients because their lack of motor control sometimes creates difficulty in wearing and adjusting the headgear.

Unilateral PLMs during sleep have been reported in patients with MSA (17) and progressive supranuclear palsy but are not as commonly seen as in Parkinson disease. PLMs can increase fragmented sleep if they cause EEG arousals and complicate the management of the sleep apnea/hypopnea syndrome.

Patient Management

When monitoring patients with known movement disorders, the sleep technologist should be prepared for parasomnias such as RBD, especially because the patient may demonstrate significantly better mobility during an episode of RBD than during wakefulness. Monitoring can be complicated by the patient's lack of motor control. Electrodes, monitors, and CPAP masks are frequently and repeatedly dislodged, and fall precautions should be employed at all times. The patient should be assisted to the restroom, and a bedside toilet should be made available if the patient wishes one. Patients may require assistance with turning during the night. The patient and the caregiver should be asked about these requirements before the sleep study is begun. It is also important to remember that mild dementia is a common component of many movement disorders, so possible cognitive impairment may also be present.

Technical Aspects of Recording

Abnormal sleep architecture may be seen in degenerative movement disorders and is prevalent in patients with progressive supranuclear palsy. Sleep spindles are typically decreased in both number and amplitude. One study in such patients revealed decreased total sleep time, reduced sleep efficiency, increased wake time after sleep onset, and increased stage N1 sleep. REM sleep was reduced with decreased REM period duration (14). Sleep-related breathing disorders are uncommon in progressive supranuclear palsy but may occur as a concomitant disorder.

OTHER DEGENERATIVE NEUROLOGIC DISORDERS

Amyotrophic Lateral Sclerosis (Lou Gehrig Disease)

ALS, or Lou Gehrig disease, causes relentlessly progressive weakness, which leads to death in 3 to 5 years after initial diagnosis. Death is usually secondary to respiratory failure and/or pneumonia. ALS occurs more frequently in men than in women, and the onset of symptoms usually begins after age 50.

The clinical features of ALS include weakness, muscular atrophy, and fasciculations (involuntary muscle twitches). Hyperreflexia, spasticity, and upgoing toes also occur. Initial symptoms may be asymmetric, typically involving only the extremities (eg, foot drop). As the weakness progresses, bulbar muscles of the throat and mouth become affected and result in dysphagia (difficulty swallowing) and dysarthria (difficulty speaking).

Associated Sleep Disorders

Central alveolar hypoventilation is a common component of ALS because of weakness of the respiratory muscles, including the diaphragm and intercostals. As bulbar weakness progresses, the muscle tone of the upper airway is decreased, and obstructive sleep apnea/hypopnea may develop. Obstructive breathing events may be associated with hypoventilation, further complicating treatment. Patients may be intolerant of CPAP because they have difficulty exhaling against the pressure. BPAP or variable PAP may be more appropriate for such patients. Elevation of the head of the bed may alleviate this problem for several months or perhaps longer, and as the disease progresses, these patients typically require BPAP in the spontaneous or S mode. As the condition progresses, BPAP in the spontaneous-timed mode or noninvasive positive pressure ventilation may be necessary. As the disease progresses even further, tracheostomy with nocturnal ventilation may become the only effective treatment. Unfortunately, at this stage, many patients may elect to forgo further treatment because of end-of-life choices.

Patient Management Issues

Patients with ALS may require assistance with turning during the night and with other activities, including using the restroom. Because of bulbar weakness, aspiration is a constant hazard. Hypoventilation is also a concern. Because patients may have trouble exhaling, BPAP may be preferable over CPAP. Elevating the head of the bed, either with a wedge pillow or with a hospital bed, during sleep monitoring may reduce pressure requirement and improve patient comfort.

Technical Aspects of Recording

Patients with ALS are typically weak and may have difficulty cooperating with calibrations.

Fatal Familial Insomnia

Fatal familial insomnia is a rare familial autosomal dominant disorder caused by a mutation in a normal protein, the "prion protein," which causes it to transform into a prion, an infectious, self-reproducing protein structure. The prion subsequently damages the region in the thalamus that regulates normal sleep patterns. There is severe disruption of the sleep-wake cycle, with extremely low sleep efficiency, reduced delta sleep, and reduced or absent REM sleep. Myoclonic jerks are frequent, and RBD or REM sleep without atonia may occur (18). Although insomnia is the most prominent feature of fatal familial insomnia, other features include cognitive decline, bradykinesia, ataxia, dysautonomia, and hallucinations. Hypersomnolence may occur, but the affected patients, although sleepy, are unable to initiate restful sleep. The disease occurs equally in men and women, with a wide age of onset. The disorder progresses to death, usually within 4 years after onset. Death in fatal familial patients with insomnia usually occurs secondary to pneumonia (15).

REFERENCES

1. Shi L, Chen SJ, Ma MY, et al. Sleep disturbances increase the risk of dementia: a systematic review and meta-analysis. *Sleep Med Rev*. 2018;40:4-16. doi:10.1016/j.smrv.2017.06.010
2. Lal C, Weaver TE, Bae CJ, Strohl KP. Excessive daytime sleepiness in obstructive sleep apnea. Mechanisms and clinical management. *Ann Am Thorac Soc*. 2021;18(5):757-768. doi:10.1513/AnnalsATS.202006-696FR
3. Chapman JL, Serinel Y, Marshall NS, Grunstein RR. Residual daytime sleepiness in obstructive sleep apnea after continuous positive airway pressure optimization: causes and management. *Sleep Med Clin*. 2016;11(3):353-363. doi:10.1016/j.jsmc.2016.05.005
4. Fietze I, Rosenblum L, Ossadnik S, et al. Nocturnal positive pressure ventilation improves relationship satisfaction of patients with OSA and their partners. *Sleep Med*. 2023;111:191-198. doi:10.1016/j.sleep.2023.08.023
5. Pacchetti C, Manni R, Zangaglia R, et al. Relationship between hallucinations, delusions, and rapid eye movement sleep behavior disorder in Parkinson's disease. *Mov Disord*. 2005;20(11):1439-1448. doi:10.1002/mds.20582
6. Ferman TJ, Boeve BF, Smith GE, et al. The REM sleep behavior disorder/dementia syndrome: neuropsychological differences when compared to Alzheimer's disease. *Neurology*. 1998;50(suppl 4):A282.
7. Boeve B, Silber M, Ferman T, et al. Association of REM sleep behavior disorder and neurodegenerative disease may reflect an underlying synucleinopathy. *Mov Disord*. 2001;16:622-630.
8. Jiang H, Huang J, Shen Y, et al. RBD and neurodegenerative diseases. *Mol Neurobiol*. 2017;54(4):2997-3006. doi:10.1007/s12035-016-9831-4
9. Hu MT. REM sleep behavior disorder (RBD). *Neurobiol Dis*. 2020;143:104996. doi:10.1016/j.nbd.2020.104996
10. Howell M, Avidan AY, Foldvary-Schaefer N, et al. Management of REM sleep behavior disorder: an

American Academy of Sleep Medicine clinical practice guideline. *J Clin Sleep Med.* 2023;19(4):759-768. doi:10.5664/jcsm.10424

11. Peter-Derex L, Yammine P, Bastuji H, Croisile B. Sleep and Alzheimer's disease. *Sleep Med Rev.* 2015;19: 29-38. doi: 10.1016/j.smrv.2014.03.007
12. Todd WD. Potential pathways for circadian dysfunction and sundowning-related behavioral aggression in Alzheimer's disease and related dementias. *Front Neurosci.* 2020;14:910. doi:10.3389/fnins.2020.00910
13. Montplaisir J, Petit D, Decary A, et al. Sleep and quantitative EEG in patients with progressive supranuclear palsy. *Neurology.* 1997;49:999-1003.
14. Katsuki H, Michinaga S. Anti-Parkinson drugs and orexin neurons. *Vitam Horm.* 2012;89:279-290. doi:10.1016/B978-0-12-394623-2.00015-9
15. Elder GJ, Lazar AS, Alfonso-Miller P, Taylor JP. Sleep disturbances in Lewy body dementia: a systematic review. *Int J Geriatr Psychiatry.* 2022;37(10):10.1002/gps.5814. doi:10.1002/gps.5814
16. Goh YY, Saunders E, Pavey S, et al. Multiple system atrophy. *Pract Neurol.* 2023;23(3):208-221. doi: 10.1136/pn-2020-002797
17. Llorens F, Zarranz JJ, Fischer A, Zerr I, Ferrer I. Fatal familial insomnia: clinical aspects and molecular alterations. *Curr Neurol Neurosci Rep.* 2017;17(4):30. doi: 10.1007/s11910-017-0743-0
18. Baldwin KJ, Correll CM. Prion disease. *Semin Neurol.* 2019;39(4):428-439. doi:10.1055/s-0039-1687841

Chapter 24
Psychiatric Disorders That Affect Sleep

GEORGE P. EVANS AND RITA J. BROOKS

KEY CONCEPTS/LEARNING OBJECTIVES

The key concepts in this chapter include describing the characteristic changes in sleep architecture associated with specific psychiatric illnesses, appreciating changes in sleep structure caused by common psychotropic medications, and anticipating problems in conducting sleep studies on various patients with psychiatric disorders.

KEY TERMS

Anxiety disorder
Bipolar disorder
Major depressive disorder
Posttraumatic stress disorder
Schizophrenia
Seasonal affective disorder

There is an intimate relationship between emotional functioning and sleep. Psychiatric disorders are common in our society, and as a result, patients with psychiatric disorders will be seen frequently in sleep disorder centers. Understanding the symptoms associated with these conditions is critical to evaluating the patient properly, creating the optimal sleep environment, and addressing the challenges that can arise during the polysomnographic (PSG) testing procedure. Psychiatric disorders are often treated with medications, and this usually occurs well before an overnight sleep study is performed. Some of the changes in sleep architecture observed during the study may reflect the effects of medications rather than primary illness. We will try to differentiate between the effects of the illness as opposed to medications.

This chapter will review the sleep characteristics of the major psychiatric disorders, including mood disorders, anxiety disorders, schizophrenia, and alcoholism. In this chapter, we will discuss the major disorders and their effects on sleep, including defining the disorder, discussing presenting symptoms, and determining what challenges the sleep technologist may face.

MOOD DISORDERS

It is normal for people to have changes in their mood or affect. However, when these mood changes are extreme, or when they shift from one extreme to the other, or when their mood is not consistent with their life events, they are said to have a mood disorder (1). The mood disorders include major depressive disorder (MDD), bipolar disorder, and seasonal affective disorder (SAD).

Major Depressive Disorder

MDD requires a minimum symptom duration of 2 weeks with no manic or hypomanic episodes. Symptoms include depressed mood; reduced level of interest in most or all activities; weight loss or gain; difficulty falling asleep or sleeping too much; feelings of inadequacy; feelings of extreme guilt; a reduced ability to think, concentrate, or make decisions; frequent thoughts of death or suicide; fatigue; and behavior that is agitated or slowed (2). MDD occurs at some time in the lives of up to 20% of the North American population, and at any given time about 5% of the population is affected (3). Depression is most likely to begin in adolescence or in the early adult years, but the incidence seems to be increasing in younger populations (4). Between puberty and menopause, women are about 2 times as likely to develop major depression (5). The lifetime prevalence of MDD is 8% to 12% of men and 20% to 26% of women (6). Throughout a lifetime, an individual may experience several episodes of major depression, so it is a recurrent illness. Sleep disturbance is more pronounced during active illness but sleep problems may persist during remission as well.

Sleep disturbance is so common in mood disorders that many individuals are given a diagnosis of depression on the basis of the symptom of insomnia. This may be due to a poor understanding in the general medical community of the variety of sleep disorders, or it may be because of an often erroneous assumption that antidepressant medications are good hypnotics. Although depression is perhaps overdiagnosed in patients with insomnia complaints, sleep disturbance is clearly a common feature of most psychiatric illnesses, including depression. For example, subjective sleep complaints are reported by more than 80% of patients with MDD (7).

Although the specific cause of mood disorders has not been determined, several theories have been proposed that may elucidate the connection between mood disorders and sleep-related changes. First, a number of neurotransmitters have been implicated in mood disorders. Specifically, relative deficiencies of noradrenergic (NE) or serotonergic (5-HT) activity or increased cholinergic activity may be involved in depression (8). Notably, cholinergic activity is responsible for initiating rapid eye movement (REM) sleep, and norepinephrine and serotonin are responsible for terminating REM sleep and making the transition back to non-REM (NREM) sleep. Changes in these neurotransmitters would be expected to influence REM sleep, and, in fact, REM sleep changes are among the most robust findings in depressive disorders. In addition, antidepressant medications typically enhance NE or 5-HT activity (by blocking the neurotransmitter uptake mechanisms), and patients taking these medications usually show characteristic changes in REM sleep (3).

Another theory proposed for depression is that it may be caused by excessive amounts of REM sleep and a resulting decrease in REM sleep pressure. According to this theory, total or partial sleep deprivation can result in significant improvement in depression primarily through the mechanism of REM sleep suppression, and, thereby, increasing the pressure to get into REM. Sleep deprivation studies have shown significant improvement in depressive symptoms in about 40% to 60% of patients, but the effect is only temporary and goes away after the REM sleep deprivation is stopped and that patient is allowed to have REM sleep again. Specifically, the improvement in mood is short-lived, because 50% to 80% of responders have partial or complete relapse after recovery of REM sleep.

A third theory regarding depression involves disruption of circadian and ultradian rhythms that control sleep-wake activity and REM-NREM cycles. It has been suggested that the circadian timing mechanism that controls REM sleep, core body temperature, and the hormone cortisol is phase-advanced. It has been hypothesized that REM sleep is phase-advanced relative to the sleep-wake cycle in patients with depression and that depression occurs because of awakening at sensitive circadian phases. Other circadian models of depression have focused on the flattening (reduction) of the amplitude of circadian rhythms, including the core body temperature rhythm and rest-activity cycles (derived from actigraphy). It has even been hypothesized that this circadian disruption may be linked to an increased susceptibility to having mood disorders across the lifespan.

Subjective Findings

Sleep disturbance can be assessed with subjective measures such as questionnaires, objectively with PSG, or inferentially with actigraphy. As previously noted, 80% of patients with MDD complain about their sleep. These subjective complaints include difficulty falling asleep, frequent awakenings, early morning awakening with difficulty falling back to sleep, nonrestorative sleep, insufficient total sleep time (TST), and disturbing dreams. Some patients report increased daytime fatigue. The word *fatigue* is often used to reflect low energy or lethargy, as opposed to daytime sleepiness or drowsiness (difficulty remaining awake).

Subjective measures correlate well with some, but not all, objective measures. For example, patients are fairly good at reporting time in bed, TST, and sleep latency. They are less accurate when reporting the number of awakenings, sleep quality, sleep depth, and how rested they feel on awakening.

Subjective reports on sleep quality may have clinical utility in managing MDD. Survey data have demonstrated that sleep disturbances can occur *before* the onset of other symptoms of MDD. For example, insomnia occurred as the first symptom in 41% of initial cases of MDD and was the first symptom in 56% of relapses. This association is so strong that some investigators can almost predict that a depressive episode will occur sometime in the future, perhaps even months or years, after insomnia first develops. Furthermore, improvement in sleep-related disturbances has been found to be positively correlated with the remission of depressive symptoms. This is in contrast to anxiety disorder, where the insomnia complaint typically begins with, or after, the onset of anxiety symptoms (4). The astute clinician should anticipate a relapse of depression in a "controlled" patient if such a patient starts complaining about a recurrence of their sleep disturbance.

Objective Findings

Many studies have objectively documented electroencephalographic (EEG) changes associated with MDD. Most studies show changes in the timing or distribution of sleep stages, particularly slow-wave sleep and REM sleep. A symptomatic but unmedicated adult with MDD typically shows a prolonged sleep-onset latency (SOL), bouts of intermittent wakefulness, increased N1 sleep, and reduced N3 sleep. The N3 deficits are greatest in the first NREM sleep period, whereas the amount of N3 sleep is normal or even increased during the second NREM period. Even more profound and more consistent changes are seen in REM sleep parameters. Nonmedicated patients show a substantially shortened latency to the first REM period (REM latency). REM latency in patients with depression is often on the order of 30 to 50 minutes, compared with the typical 90 to 100 minutes seen in nondepressed age- and sex-matched controls. There is also a significant increase in REM density (the number of eye movements per unit of time). Some studies show that the first REM period is longer and may have the highest REM density compared with later REM periods. This is just the opposite of normal sleepers, who have longer duration and more intense REM episodes later on in the sleep period. These sleep changes are not as robust in children and adolescents with depression as they are in nonmedicated adults with MDD. In fact, younger groups with depression are very similar to individuals without depression on most sleep variables.

The severity of the depression may or may not correlate with the severity of the sleep disturbance. There is good evidence that disturbed sleep, particularly a shortened REM latency, may be a trait marker (show a propensity for) rather than a state marker (actively depressed). First-degree relatives of individuals with depression also commonly have short REM latencies. The abnormal REM changes may also be observed during remission of depression. These findings suggest that a shortened REM latency is associated with an increased risk of developing depression, as opposed to actively manifesting the disorder.

As previously noted, most antidepressant medication will influence REM sleep by lengthening the REM latency, decreasing REM density, and decreasing the REM percentage, particularly during the first third of the night. As stated previously, the mechanism for the antidepressant action was thought to be through REM suppression and increased REM sleep pressure. However, a number of effective antidepressant medications (eg, bupropion, nefazodone, and trazodone) do not reduce REM sleep, which suggests another potential mechanism of action.

Cognitive behavioral therapy (CBT) has been shown to decrease REM density but has no effect on REM latency. It is suggested that trait-dependent variables, such as shortened REM latency, decreased N3 sleep ratio, and decreased percentage of N3 sleep, remain stable over time and that state-dependent measures, such as REM density and sleep efficiency, may improve with CBT treatment. However, a small percentage of subjects in remission have persistent sleep state–dependent abnormalities after CBT.

Bipolar Disorder

Bipolar disorder is characterized by the alternating pattern of two emotional extremes: depression and euphoria. An individual with bipolar illness cycles between periods of potentially severe depression and mania, an agitated and often elated emotional state. In addition to the aforementioned symptoms of depression, manic episodes may be characterized by irritable mood, thoughts of grandiosity, rapid or pressured speech, distractibility, and compulsive behavior (eg, shopping sprees, drinking, sexual activity) (2).

Bipolar disorder is much less common than unipolar depression and has a lifetime prevalence rate of 2.8% to 6.5%. However, if the diagnostic criteria stipulate hypomania and not full mania (bipolar II), the incidence could include about one-half of currently diagnosed patients with unipolar depression. There is no gender preference for bipolar disorder I, but bipolar II may affect more women than men. There may be a seasonal pattern for the occurrence of depressive and manic/hypomanic episodes. The onset of depression in bipolar disorder tends to be in the fall to winter, whereas mania tends to peak in the spring or fall.

Subjective Findings

The literature on sleep and bipolar disorder is not as complete as with unipolar depression. Subjective reports indicate that patients with bipolar disorder have concerns about their sleep much like unipolar depressives. In one study, 70% of patient population with bipolar disorder had significant sleep concerns, including impaired sleep efficiency, higher levels of anxiety, fear about poor sleep quality, lowered daytime activity levels, and a tendency to misperceive sleep. One major difference between unipolar and bipolar disorder is a stronger tendency for patients with bipolar disorder to report symptoms of hypersomnia, with extended nocturnal sleep periods, difficulty awakening, and excessive daytime sleepiness, during the depressed phase. However, when the level of hypersomnia was objectively tested using the multiple sleep latency test (MSLT), no increased physiologic sleep propensity was demonstrated in the bipolar group. The authors stated that the reported hypersomnia might reflect lack of interest, social withdrawal, decreased energy, or psychomotor retardation, rather than a true increase in sleep propensity. Another notable subjective difference between bipolar disorder and MDD is that during the manic phase, although sleep may be severely curtailed, the patients have much less concern over their sleep. They feel that they do not need as much sleep. Prodromal episodes of insomnia tend to be more common in mania than depression, and the shift to mania may be exacerbated by periods of sleeplessness.

Objective Findings

Objective data on sleep during mania shows decreased TST, increased time awake in the last 2 hours of the study, a short REM latency, and increased REM density. These findings are similar to the sleep changes seen in MDD.

Manic episodes are often preceded by periods of sleeplessness, and case reports have suggested that mania can be triggered by sleep deprivation. It has been suggested that the curtailed sleep time associated with mania may be potentially self-reinforcing. However, it appears that sleep deprivation may have the same beneficial effects on bipolar disorder as on patients with MDD. There is some concern that sleep deprivation can precipitate a manic episode; however, the rate of switching from depression to mania following sleep deprivation is not more than what is observed in patients using antidepressant medication.

Bipolar type II disorder is characterized by one or more depressive episodes accompanied by at least one hypomanic episode. There are no psychotic features such as delusions or hallucinations that can occur with bipolar I disorder. It should be noted that bipolar II is not a milder form of bipolar disorder. The depressive phase can be as severe in either disorder. As such, the increased sleep time seen in the depressive phase of either disorder can be similar. The manic phase is less pronounced in type II, but there is still a reduced need for sleep in over 80% of patients.

Seasonal Affective Disorder

SAD was first proposed in 1984 and is currently used as a specifier of either bipolar or recurrent MDD. The symptoms usually present during winter and remit during the spring. Symptoms also improve when the patient is exposed to daylight or bright light therapy. Although patients report depression, the other signs of SAD are quite different from those of MDD. Patients with SAD typically report increased appetite and increased need for sleep. The disorder is more common in young adults, particularly in women.

Disturbances of sleep are a primary component of SAD as they are of other mood disorders. However, patients with SAD most often report hypersomnia. Among responses of 293 patients with SAD on a symptom questionnaire, 95% acknowledged sleep concerns. The vast majority (80%) complained of winter hypersomnia, with only 10% reporting insomnia and 5% reporting insomnia and hypersomnia. TST increased by about 2.7 hours during the fall/winter months compared with the spring/summer months. Increasing sleep length by up to 2 hours during the winter months occurs in about one-half of a random sample of the general population, and, thus, this symptom alone is not necessarily indicative of a disorder.

In contrast to the subjective impressions of increased sleep, actual sleep measurement of patients with SAD experiencing depression in winter showed reduced sleep efficiency, decreased N3 sleep percentage, and increased REM density, but normal REM latency. These findings were consistent when the patients were compared with themselves in the summer, compared with themselves following 9 days of bright light therapy, and compared with age- and gender-matched healthy controls. Although there may be a natural tendency to increase TST in the winter months, patients with SAD show sleep architecture changes that are different from normal controls. Bright light therapy, especially morning light administration, appears to be an efficacious and safe treatment for this disorder. Bright light therapy is now being studied in more traditional forms of depression. There is some concern that light therapy can precipitate hypomanic or manic episodes, so caution is advised in using bright light therapy with bipolar patients.

Effect of Antidepressant Medications

A full review of medication and sleep appears elsewhere in this textbook. However, any discussion of psychiatric disorders and sleep must include some comments about the psychotropic medications. Generally, the antidepressant medications are REM-suppressing drugs. They tend to delay the onset of REM sleep and may decrease both the amount and the percentage of REM sleep. The REM suppression is most pronounced early in the treatment and tends to diminish with the long-term treatment (3). However, even in patients using these medications long term, a short REM latency is typically not seen. Although many of the older tricyclic antidepressants (eg, amitriptyline, imipramine, clomipramine) are sedating, most of the selective serotonin reuptake inhibitor (SSRI) antidepressants (eg, fluoxetine, paroxetine, sertraline) and other new agents (eg, venlafaxine, bupropion) tend to be activating or alerting. As such, they may improve sleep by treating depression but probably have little primary hypnotic efficacy, and they may actually worsen sleep. In addition, most antidepressants increase the incidence of periodic limb movements (PLMs) during sleep and may exacerbate restless legs syndrome. However, bupropion seems to be an exception in that the drug does not exacerbate symptoms of restless legs syndrome or suppress REM sleep like most of the other antidepressants. The SSRI fluoxetine can cause REMs in NREM sleep and scoring the record could be challenging if the scorer is unaware of this fact. Most antidepressants improve muscle tone in the upper airway and can slightly reduce snoring and the apnea-hypopnea index (AHI) in patients with obstructive sleep apnea syndrome (OSAS). This effect has been most studied with the antidepressants fluoxetine and protriptyline. In addition to increasing muscle tone, the REM-suppressing aspect of these drugs limits the time during sleep that is most conducive to having obstructive respiratory events.

Sleep Studies in Mood Disorders

In untreated patients with depression, the lengthened SOL, frequent awakenings, or early morning awakening may limit the amount of time available to allow for accurate assessment of other sleep disorders. A shortened REM latency is different from REM onset. Generally, individuals with depression show REM latencies in the 50- to 70-minute range, as opposed to a "sleep-onset" REM period in which the REM latency is 15 minutes or less, sometimes being a true sleep-onset (0-minute latency) REM period.

If a patient with depression is being treated with antidepressant medication, a thorough understanding and documentation of the medications is helpful in completing an accurate interpretation of the results. Owing to the REM-suppressing characteristics of these medications, it may not be possible to diagnose narcolepsy in an individual taking an antidepressant medication if the patient's tendency to have a sleep-onset REM period is weak. The medication may also exacerbate leg movements during sleep and could slightly improve breathing during sleep. Fluoxetine can cause REMs in NREM sleep. All these changes can be misleading without good documentation. Moreover, the time of year that a study is conducted may be important if the patient has SAD. The phase of a bipolar illness that a patient is experiencing at the time of the study could produce drastically different results depending on whether the patient is in the depressed or the manic phase of the disorder. Good technologist observations and documentation are important for all sleep studies, but particularly for the patient with psychiatric/sleep disorder.

ANXIETY DISORDERS

Anxiety is a normal response to various situations that include threat. Dangerous or even important situations can elicit anxiety in almost anyone, and brief episodes of moderate anxiety are a normal part of life for most people. For some people, anxiety is so intense or longstanding that it becomes an anxiety disorder. There are several types of anxiety disorders:

1. Generalized anxiety disorder (GAD): Occurs when the anxiety is excessive and long-standing but is not focused on any particular object or situation. Because the source of the anxiety cannot be specified, it is also called "free-floating" anxiety. This anxiety disorder affects about 5% of the US population at some time in their lives. Anxiety disorder is 2 times more common in women as compared to men.
2. Panic disorder (PD): Individuals experience recurrent extremely intense terrifying panic attacks that may come without warning or without an obvious cause. Symptoms may include heart palpitations, pressure in the chest, dizziness, nausea, sweating, and faintness. Many people with panic attacks feel they are having a heart attack. As many as 30% of the population may experience at least one panic attack within a given year (1).
3. Phobias: An intense, irrational fear of an object or situation that is not likely to be dangerous. Thousands of phobias have been described, but two of the most common are social phobia and agoraphobia. Social phobia is a fear of being negatively evaluated by others. Agoraphobia is a strong fear of being separated from a safe place like a home or from a safe person like a spouse or of being trapped in a place from which escape would be difficult or help would be unavailable (1).
4. Obsessive-compulsive disorder (OCD): Individuals with OCD experience persistent, upsetting, and unwanted thoughts (obsessions) that may motivate them to perform repetitive behaviors (compulsions) that the person believes will prevent the events associated with the obsession (1). Obsessions typically involve thoughts of contamination or harming oneself or others. Compulsions can take the form of incessant cleaning, checking behavior, or counting (1).
5. Posttraumatic stress disorder (PTSD): This is a stress reaction to a severe trauma. Among the characteristic reactions are anxiety, irritability, inability to concentrate, jumpiness, intense startle reactions, and hypervigilance. The most notable feature of PTSD is reexperiencing the trauma through nightmares or vivid memories. Occasionally, the individual will experience flashbacks in which the person behaves as if the trauma was happening again (1).

Anxiety is a state of increased cortical and peripheral arousal and, as such, is a state that makes sleep difficult. Sleep complaints are common in anxiety disorders and are among the diagnostic criteria for many of the anxiety disorders. Anxiety disorders are clearly among the most common causes of insomnia. In a study by the National Institute of Mental Health Epidemiologic Catchment Area, 7,954 respondents were questioned about their sleep complaints. Of these, 10.2% of the 811 respondents reported chronic insomnia. The single most common psychiatric diagnosis was anxiety disorder followed by depression and dysthymia (5).

According to a large European survey of over 14,000 individuals in the general population, insomnia was often a prodromal feature, or a coincident occurrence, in respondents with depression. When anxiety disorders were implicated, insomnia appeared concurrently or after the onset of the anxiety disorder (4).

Generalized Anxiety Disorder

Sleep difficulty is very common in patients with GAD. Between 50% and 70% of these patients have difficulty sleeping (5). The principal cognitive feature associated with GAD is "excessive worry," which goes hand in hand with the development and maintenance of the insomnia complaint (6). Despite the high prevalence of sleep problems in these patients, little research has focused specifically on this disorder. Patients with GAD report having difficulty both falling asleep and staying asleep and feeling that their sleep is unrefreshing. Objectively, PSG studies have shown that, relative to controls, patients with GAD take longer to fall asleep, have lower sleep efficiency, have less N3 and more N1 sleep, and less TST. They have more frequent arousals during the first half of the sleep period and a lower REM density. In contrast to patients with depression, patients with GAD generally have a normal REM latency (of about 90 minutes). In these patients, sleep deprivation does not improve symptoms of anxiety as it does with depression.

Panic Disorder

As with GAD, most patients with PD have significant sleep complaints. Their subjective complaints are similar to those patients with GAD. They report difficulty falling asleep, difficulty remaining asleep, and decreased TST. The exceptional difference with patients with PD is the presence of panic attacks. These attacks occur both during the day and during sleep. One study found 69% of patients with PD had a lifetime occurrence of sleep panic attacks, and 33% reported recurrent sleep panic attacks. Over one-half of the patients indicated that sleep deprivation and relaxation acted as a trigger for panic attacks. Patients with PD can differentiate REM sleep anxiety dreams from panic attacks. The panic attack has no dream content or vivid imagery. Patients have full awakenings from the event; they are not confused at the time of the event and are not amnestic for the events the following day, as is the case with night terrors. These findings help separate panic attacks from both REM-related nightmares and slow-wave sleep night terrors. Even patients with PD who do not experience sleep panic attacks have disturbed sleep.

Objective studies show that sleep panic attacks generally occur from late N2 or early N3 sleep. If the attacks are frequent, some patients with PD may develop a sleep phobia to avoid the panic symptoms. Patients with PD have longer sleep-onset latencies, reduced sleep efficiency, and decreased TST. However, N3 sleep is normal, REM latency is normal or increased, and REM density is normal. In addition, increased motor activity during sleep has been reported in patients with PD, with evidence that they may move less on the nights when there is a sleep-related panic attack.

Phobia

Insomnia or other sleep complaints are rare in phobias unless the phobia is related to sleep itself. For example, individuals with sleep panic attacks may develop a fear of sleep as a way to avoid the panic attack. Other phobias such as fear of the dark can usually be dealt with by providing light or with cognitive therapy. Other than sleep-onset problems that are directly related to the phobia, sleep appears to be normal. However, some studies on social phobia have found subjective reports of poorer sleep quality, longer sleep latency, more frequent sleep disruption, and increased daytime dysfunction compared with control subjects. It has been suggested that sleep problems in social phobia may be associated with comorbid depression in some individuals (6).

Obsessive-Compulsive Disorder

The core features of OCD do not include primary disturbances of sleep (6). Early studies subjectively reported abnormal sleep patterns and objective changes in sleep characteristics (eg, decreased TST, increased number of awakenings, shortened REM latency, reduced N3 sleep, and reduced sleep efficiency). These findings are very similar to patients with MDD, and they could suggest an overlap between OCD and MDD, or they could indicate that many patients with OCD also suffer from depression. In addition, the presence of the obsessions and compulsions may prevent individuals with OCD from going to bed because of the need to check their alarm clock or kitchen stove repeatedly. However, more recent studies on patients with OCD failed to replicate these PSG findings and have concluded that sleep patterns in OCD are basically normal.

The obsessions and compulsions of this disorder may lead to significant sleep disturbances. This can prove a challenge to performing a sleep study. A compulsion such as checking behavior may delay bedtime. Fears of contamination may keep patients from undergoing a sleep study owing to fears about the sleep environment or cleanliness of the electrodes. This may be particularly true with nasal continuous positive airway pressure (CPAP) and wearing a mask worn by previous patients (despite undergoing proper sterilization in between patients).

Posttraumatic Stress Disorder

PTSD is categorized in the *Diagnostic and Statistical Manual of Mental Disorders, 5th edition (DSM-V)* (6) under a new category of Impairing Emotional Outbursts. Disorders in this category include displays of anger or distress that are manifested verbally and/or behaviorally, such as with aggression (eg, physical aggression toward people, property, or self) that leads to significant functional impairment. PTSD is characterized by the recurrent and intrusive distressing recollections of a traumatic event (eg, violent attack with physical injury, sexual assault, death of a loved one) (6). Sleep complaints are varied and typically severe in patients with PTSD. Patients with PTSD may report poor sleep for decades, with corroborating evidence by their bed partners. In fact, insomnia (both sleep initiation and sleep maintenance subtypes) and nightmares (viewed as reexperiencing of the traumatic event) are part of the *DSM-V* criteria for making the diagnosis (2). A survey conducted with male Vietnam War veterans with PTSD confirmed that insomnia complaints were very common, but the presence of recurrent nightmares was more specific for PTSD. In another community survey conducted in Canada, PTSD was frequently associated with violent behavior during sleep, sleep paralysis, sleep talking, and both hypnopompic and hypnagogic hallucinations. It is postulated that these sleep complaints are associated with features of heightened somatic arousal and hypervigilance, which are part of the diagnostic criteria for PTSD.

Some studies have objectively recorded increased awakenings and decreased N3 sleep in patients with PTSD, while other studies have failed to find these changes, and one study found no objective sleep differences at all, with the exception of an increase in brief arousals from REM sleep. The reason for these discrepancies is unknown. However, it is speculated that a number of factors may be responsible. The amount of substance misuse, psychiatric comorbidities, degree or types of trauma, and patient demographics may substantially differ in study populations. It has also been proposed that patients with PTSD may be prone to sleep state misperception or that they find the sleep laboratory a safe environment and, therefore, sleep better there than at home.

Nightmares are commonly reported in PTSD, occurring more frequently in combat veterans with PTSD compared to combat veterans without PTSD. Some studies have found increases in REM density or shortened REM latencies, whereas others have failed to detect these changes. It should be noted that the nightmare or "flashback" experienced during sleep may or may not be REM related; this could account for some of the discrepancies in the findings.

One interesting line of investigation has found a high rate of obstructive sleep apnea (OSA) in both male and female patients with PTSD. There have been reported improvements in insomnia, nightmares, and PTSD symptoms with treatment of the OSA with CPAP, independent of other psychiatric intervention. It is possible that once the REM sleep normalized with the continued use of CPAP, the intensity of the nightmares and sleep fragmentation diminished.

Treatment for sleep disturbances in PTSD has focused on both psychological and pharmacologic approaches. The use of evidence-based psychotherapy is generally a primary or adjuvant therapy for PTSD. Pharmacologic therapy has focused on SSRI medications, mainly sertraline and paroxetine. More recent research has shown that prazosin, through the reduction of norepinephrine synthesis in the brain, may be effective in the reduction of nightmares in PTSD patients (7). This supports the hypothesis that NE stimulation may be contributing to the ongoing sleep disturbances and nightmares in PTSD.

Sleep Studies in the Patient With Anxiety

Stressors may exacerbate anxiety symptoms, and a sleep study can certainly be sufficiently stressful to cause a worsening of symptoms. Preparing the patient with anxiety for a sleep study is very important. Showing the room and fully explaining the procedure to the patient perhaps days before the actual study may be helpful. The interpersonal skills of the technologist are probably most important when working with patient experiencing anxiety. The ability to apply electrodes and to convey to the patient in a calm and reassuring manner that they will be able to complete the study will improve the likelihood of obtaining an accurate sleep study. In addition, anxious patients with sleep apnea may have a particular problem with a CPAP mask, and spending time desensitizing the patient to CPAP therapy well before the study may allow for a more successful CPAP titration study. In particular patients with anxiety, there may be a great deal of muscle tension artifact in the recording during wakefulness. This artifact may persist into stage N1 sleep and reappear with arousals during the study. This artifact can make determining sleep onset challenging and may cause wakefulness to be overscored.

The sleep-related panic attack might include symptoms of heart palpitations, shortness of breath, sweating, chest pain, and nausea (2). These symptoms are similar to the warning signs of a heart attack, and many patients with PD indeed feel that they are having one. It must be remembered that patients with psychiatric issues also have medical problems, and it is important to take these symptoms seriously. If the patient experiences these symptoms during the sleep study, the technician should respond to the symptoms in a medically appropriate manner and not simply assume that they are a manifestation of a psychiatric illness.

Benzodiazepines (BZD) are often used to treat anxiety disorders. These medications will suppress N3 sleep and can slightly worsen the AHI in patients with OSAS, because of increased respiratory suppression. They can also reduce the arousal index related to leg movements but may not actually decrease the number of leg movements. If the patient has an elevated PLM index, a low PLM arousal index, and is taking a BZD, it needs to be understood that the PLM arousal index would almost certainly be higher if the patient were not taking a BZD.

PSYCHOSES

Schizophrenia

Psychoses are defined as mental disorders characterized by the occurrence of delusions, hallucinations, incoherence, catatonic behavior, or inappropriate affect that cause impaired social or work functioning. Schizophrenia is a psychotic disorder and is considered one of the most severe and disabling of all mental disorders (1). It is considered to be a neurodevelopmental disorder that manifests as a result of both hereditary and environmental factors.

The worldwide prevalence of schizophrenia is about 1% of the population; there are no gender differences. The severe symptoms of schizophrenia often dwarf sleep complaints. However, sleep can be severely disrupted in this disorder, and it was once hoped that understanding sleep would help explain the illness.

Severe insomnia is one of the prodromal features of the onset of schizophrenia, or psychotic relapse (8). During episodes of intense psychotic agitation, schizophrenics may display insomnia or a total lack of sleep. Sleep-wake reversals, with daytime sleeping being the predominant pattern, are quite common. This sleep-wake pattern may also reinforce the social isolation that they desire during their psychotic break. Patients with schizophrenia who are considered "clinically stable" with the use of antipsychotic medication may still experience some sleep disturbance, such as early and middle of the night insomnia.

Dreaming associated with REM sleep can be thought of as a model for psychosis. The discovery of REM sleep with its vivid hallucinations and perceptual distortions suggested that abnormalities of REM sleep might be related to the symptoms of schizophrenia. As early as 1955, attempts were made to establish a relationship between REM sleep and schizophrenia (9). These investigations hoped to find intrusion of REM sleep into waking life or at least an unusual distribution or quality of REM sleep during the night. Unfortunately, PSG investigations have failed to find major changes in REM sleep in this group of patients.

A shortened REM latency has been reported in patients with schizophrenia, and it has also been reported that following REM sleep deprivation, patients with schizophrenia do not show a "REM rebound," as would be expected. These findings led to speculation that REM phasic events could be intruding into wakefulness and causing, or at least contributing to, the thought and perceptual problems of the disorder. Studies have failed to find much evidence supporting this hypothesis. There has not been any compelling evidence that REM sleep directly underlies the severe symptoms associated with schizophrenia.

Subjective Findings

Subjectively, patients with schizophrenia report that their sleep is frequently disrupted and that it is more fragmented during psychotic episodes. Although sleep quality may improve during remission, sleep problems can persist. Typically, the sleep complaint is difficulty falling asleep or remaining asleep during the night. These patients are reported to have a higher incidence of nightmares, as do patients without schizophrenia, highly creative individuals.

Objective Findings

The most reliable sleep changes found in schizophrenia occur in NREM sleep, particularly deficits of N3 sleep or delta wave (0.5-2 Hz) activity. Most studies have found a significant reduction in the total number of delta waves and an inverse correlation between delta activity and the severity of negative symptoms, such as affective flattening and impoverishment of speech.

In a review of the major studies on sleep in schizophrenia, findings include an increased SOL of about 36 minutes, increased wake time after sleep onset, an increased number of awakenings, and reduced TST of about 1 hour. Sleep efficiency was found to be reduced by about 15%, delta wave counts were decreased in NREM sleep, and total delta wave counts were decreased. REM latency was moderately decreased or normal. A longitudinal study of sleep in schizophrenia found that between baseline, 4 weeks, and 1 year, there were changes in the REM measures, but no significant changes in N3 parameters. It has been suggested that the stable N3 sleep changes reflect a trait of the patient with schizophrenia, whereas the REM measures may reflect the state of the schizophrenic disorder.

Sleep Studies in the Patient With Psychosis

Sleep studies in active patients with psychosis may have research interest but probably have little clinical utility. Most patients obtaining a clinical sleep evaluation will do so either while in remission or while medicated. As with all patients, the interpersonal skills of the sleep technologist are very important when working with patient with psychosis. It may be difficult to explain the procedures, and there may be concerns that the equipment is doing more than is explained. For example, a patient with schizophrenia may believe that the EEG is reading the mind or inserting thoughts.

Pharmacologic Treatment of Schizophrenia

Many of the antipsychotic medications can improve sleep quality but may also be quite sedating. In addition, older antipsychotics are often associated with movement disorders because of the effect of blockade of the dopaminergic postsynaptic receptors (eg, parkinsonism and dystonia) (8). Some of the newer antipsychotics (eg, olanzapine and risperidone) are also sedating, because they increase slow-wave sleep, promote sleep maintenance, and enhance stage N2 sleep, but they have less effect on REM sleep than the older antipsychotic drugs (8). Flexible scheduling of studies to avoid psychotic exacerbations and approaching the patient in a calm, professional manner should allow for an accurate clinical study.

ALCOHOLISM

Ethyl alcohol (ethanol) is the second most commonly used psychoactive substance in the world, whereas caffeine is the first. It is similar to the sedative hypnotics and can have significant effects on both subjective sleep and the polysomnogram. The effects of alcohol use in normal subjects have been extensively studied. An adult can metabolize about 10 mL (1/3 oz) of 100% alcohol per hour regardless of the blood alcohol concentration. It takes an adult about 1 hour to metabolize a 1-oz glass (29.6 mL) of 80-proof whiskey, a 4-oz glass (118.3 mL) of wine, or a 12-oz (354.9 mL) can of beer.

Although not all studies are consistent, it generally appears that acute alcohol use decreases SOL, suppresses REM sleep in a dose-dependent manner during the first half of the night, and may increase N3 sleep. However, the second half of the night shows increased N1 sleep and more awakenings. The sleep disruption observed in the second half of the night is considered a rebound effect following the metabolism of ethanol. Metabolism may be completed in 4 to 5 hours after consumption, and the drug-induced sleep effects can rebound before the sleep cycle is completed. Studies that show REM suppression during the first half of the night may be followed by REM rebound during the second half of the night. With nightly dosing of alcohol, tolerance to these sleep changes can develop within 3 days, but a REM rebound may still be seen on discontinuation.

The effect of alcohol in alcoholics is different. When they are drinking, they may fall asleep rapidly, but their TST is decreased, and it is composed primarily of light NREM sleep because REM sleep and N3 are largely suppressed. The latter portion of the sleep cycle is fragmented with little REM sleep.

Patients often state that they cannot fall asleep without alcohol. With acute discontinuation of alcohol, there is decreased N3 and more frequent, albeit shorter, REM episodes. Total REM sleep time is not increased. Patients in recovery form alcohol use disorder often show very disturbed sleep. It takes them longer to fall asleep, and they sleep for shorter periods of time. Their sleep can be fragmented with frequent brief arousals, and N3 sleep is decreased.

Insomnia occurs in 36% to 72% of patients with alcohol use disorder and may persist for months after beginning abstinence. Confounding factors with alcoholic patients and sleep are increased anxiety, depression, and tobacco use. Sober alcoholics may have more sleep-disordered breathing and more PLMs during sleep. Insomnia in alcoholism is important because it has been associated with relapse, possibly using alcohol to initiate sleep. It is not known if treatment of insomnia can reduce relapse.

Ethanol also selectively decreases muscle tone in the upper airway and can lead to the development or worsening of the degree of both snoring and obstructed breathing during sleep. This effect is more pronounced in men than in women, and older men are more vulnerable than younger men. Normal women are resistant to the development of sleep apnea after alcohol consumption regardless of menopausal status. In addition, ethanol may blunt the arousal response so that obstructive apnea and hypopnea events become much longer in duration. The negative effects of alcohol on breathing are most pronounced during the first 1 to 2 hours following consumption, when alcohol concentrations are the highest. Therefore, proximity of alcohol consumption to bedtime is important. A single glass of wine several hours before bedtime would likely have little effect on sleep or breathing during sleep. An individual who routinely drinks alcohol in the evenings may not snore in the sleep center or may not have expected apnea if they happen to be studied without alcohol. Controlled use of alcohol in a sleep center or the use of a recording pulse oximeter at home may help clarify this issue. The use of alcohol may also bring into question the accuracy of a CPAP titration study if the pressure of a habitual drinker is set on an alcohol-free night. However, one study suggests that moderate alcohol consumption does not cause more apneas when the optimal pressure has been previously titrated (10).

CONCLUSION

Patients with psychiatric disorder often present a special challenge for the sleep technologist. Psychiatric illnesses generally have negative effects on sleep. The medications used to treat these illnesses also affect sleep architecture and may exacerbate other primary sleep disorders. This group of patients requires the utmost patience and interpersonal skills on the part of the sleep technologist, more than other patient groups. It is incumbent on the technologist to provide a calm, reassuring environment for conducting the sleep study. Explanation regarding the process of hooking up and conducting the study will help relax the patient before the study. Understanding the impact that psychiatric illnesses and medications have on sleep will allow an accurate interpretation of the sleep study and may provide some information on the patient's prognosis as well.

REFERENCES

1. Bernstein DA, Clarke-Stewart A, Roy EJ, et al. *Psychology*. 4th ed. Houghton Mifflin Company; 1997.
2. American Psychiatric Association. *Diagnostic and Statistical Manual of Mental Disorders*. 4th ed. American Psychiatric Association; 1995.
3. Wilson S, Argyropoulous S. Antidepressants and sleep: a qualitative review of the literature. *Drugs*. 2005;65(7):927-947.
4. Ohayon MM, Roth T. Place of chronic insomnia in the course of depressive and anxiety disorders. *J Psychiatr Res*. 2003;37(1):9-15.
5. Anderson DJ, Noyes R, Crowe RR. A comparison of panic disorder and generalized anxiety disorder. *Am J Psychiatry*. 1984;141:572-575.
6. Benca RM. Anxiety disorders. In: Kryger MH, Roth T, Dement WC, eds. *Principles and Practice of Sleep Medicine*. 4th ed. Elsevier Saunders; 2005:1311-1326.
7. Raskind MA, Peskind ER, Kanter ED. Reduction of nightmares and other PTSD symptoms in combat veterans by prazosin: a placebo-controlled study. *Am J Psychiatry*. 2003;160:371-373.
8. Benson KL, Zarcone VP Jr. Schizophrenia. In: Kryger MH, Roth T, Dement WC, eds. *Principles and Practice of Sleep Medicine*. 4th ed. Elsevier Saunders; 2005:1327-1336.
9. Dement WC. Dream recall and eye movements in schizophrenics and normals. *J Nerv Ment Dis*. 1955;122(3):263-269.
10. Berry RB, Desa MM, Light RW. Effect of ethanol on the efficacy of nasal continuous positive airway pressure as a treatment for obstructive sleep apnea. *Chest*. 1991;99(2):339-343.

SECTION III

Patient Care and Assessment

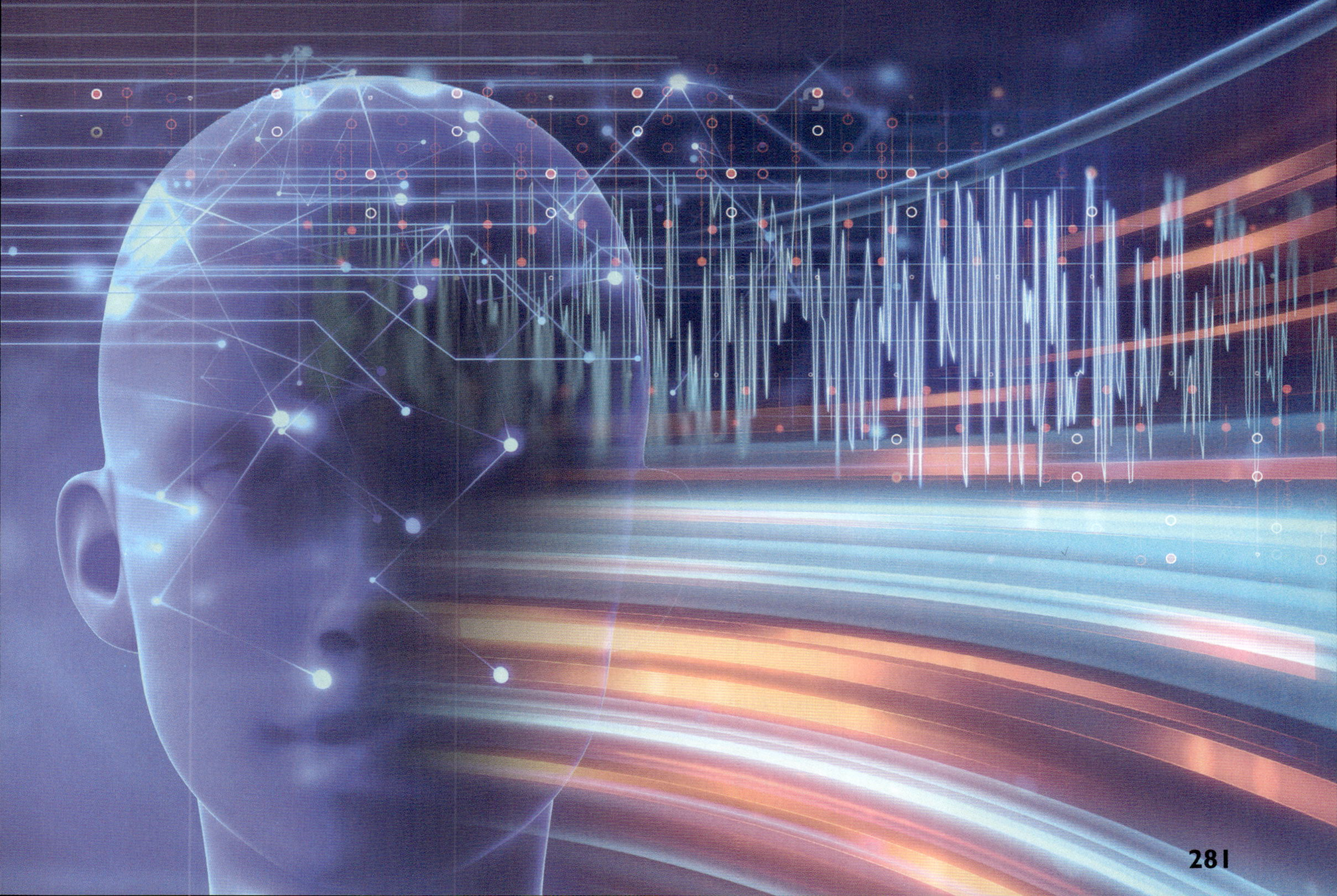

Chapter 25 Patient Rights and the Provision of Sleep Medicine

JAYME R. MATCHINSKI

KEY CONCEPTS/LEARNING OBJECTIVES

The key concepts for this chapter include a review of how to construct a Patient Bill of Rights for a sleep center, health care regulations, the risks and benefits of health care professionals ensuring patient privacy, and how to maintain privacy of protected health information in the electronic health record.

KEY TERMS

Advance directive
Anti-Kickback Statute (AKS)
Breach notification
Business associate
Covered entity
Electronic health record (EHR)
False Claims Act
HIPAA
HITECH Act
HIPAA Omnibus Rule
Notice of privacy practices (NPP)
Office for Civil Rights (OCR)
Office of the Inspector General (OIG)
Protected health information (PHI)
Safe harbor
Stark Law

The provision of sleep medicine to patients by sleep centers, sleep medicine professionals, and durable medical equipment (DME) companies requires compliance with applicable state and federal regulations. Patients have certain rights pursuant to state and federal regulations that govern the provision of patient care, maintenance and retention of the patient's medical records, and transfer of patient medical records to other entities and individuals.

Patient rights include the right to make decisions regarding medical care, the right to accept or refuse treatment, and the right to formulate advance directives, which may include written instructions, such as a living will or durable power of attorney for health care, as recognized by the state where the patient resides. This chapter focuses on patient rights during the provision of sleep medicine.

PATIENT BILL OF RIGHTS

Many states have promulgated a Patient Bill of Rights to ensure the basic rights of patients for independence of expression, decision and action, personal dignity, and to define the responsibilities of patients who receive care from health care providers and facilities. Health care providers, including sleep centers, sleep medicine professionals, and DME companies, must comply with the applicable state law related to Patient Bill of Rights. Sleep centers, sleep medicine professionals, and DME suppliers should consider drafting a Patient Bill of Rights and posting the Patient Bill of Rights in the sleep center and on its websites. The Patient Bill of Rights should also be printed and included in the patient's orientation packet prior to the provision of a sleep study.

Outline of a Patient Bill of Rights for the Sleep center

Sleep centers will need to determine how to structure, draft, and implement a Patient Bill of Rights and related policies and procedures. State laws often require that certain provisions be included in a health care facility's Patient Bill of Rights. For example, the State of Illinois has promulgated a Medical Patient Rights Act, which sets forth certain rights that patients in Illinois have regarding the provision of health care by a health care provider, which is defined as any public or private facility that provides, on an inpatient or outpatient basis, preventative, diagnostic, therapeutic, convalescent, rehabilitation, mental health, or intellectual disability services, including general or special hospitals, skilled nursing homes, extended care facilities, intermediate care facilities, and mental health centers (1,2).

The Illinois Medical Patient Rights Act requires that health care providers notify patients that they have the following rights regarding the provision of their health care:

- The right of each patient to care consistent with sound nursing and medical practices, to be informed of the name of the physician responsible for coordinating their care, to receive information concerning their condition and proposed treatment, to refuse any treatment to the extent permitted by law, and to privacy and confidentiality of records except as otherwise provided by law (3).
- The right of each patient, regardless of source of payment, to examine and receive a reasonable explanation of their total bill for services rendered by the physician or health care provider, including the itemized charges for specific services received (3). In the event an insurance company or health services corporation cancels or refuses to renew an individual policy or plan, the insured patient shall be entitled to timely, prior notice of the termination of such policy or plan (3). An insurance company or health services corporation that requires any insured patient or applicant for new or continued insurance or coverage to be tested for infection with human immunodeficiency virus or any other identified causative agent of acquired immunodeficiency syndrome shall (1) give the patient or applicant prior written notice of such requirement, (2) proceed with such testing only upon the written authorization of the applicant or patient, and (3) keep the results of such testing confidential. Notice of an adverse underwriting or coverage decision may be given to any appropriately interested party, but the insurer may disclose the test result itself only to a physician designated by the applicant or patient, and any such disclosure shall be in a manner that assures confidentiality (3). The right of each patient to privacy and confidentiality in health care. Each physician, health care provider, health services corporation, and insurance company shall refrain from disclosing the nature or details of services provided to patients, except that such information may be disclosed: (1) to the patient; (2) to the party making treatment decisions if the patient is incapable of making decisions regarding the health services provided; (3) for treatment in accordance with state law; (4) for payment in accordance with state law; (5) to those parties responsible for peer review, utilization review, and quality assurance; (6) for health care operations in accordance with state law; (7) to those parties required to be notified under the Abused and Neglected Child Reporting Act or the Illinois Sexually Transmissible Disease Control Act; or (8) as otherwise permitted, authorized, or required by state or federal law. This right may be waived in writing by the patient or the patient's guardian or legal representative, but a physician or other health care provider may not condition the provision of services on the patient's, guardian's, or legal representative's agreement to sign such a waiver (3). Any patient who is the subject of a research program or an experimental procedure, as defined under the rules and regulations of the Hospital Licensing Act, shall have, at a minimum, the right to receive an explanation of the nature and possible consequences of such research or experiment before the research or experiment is conducted, and to consent to or reject it (4).
- Every health care facility in this state shall permit visitation by any person or persons designated by a patient who is 18 years of age or older and who is allowed rights of visitation unless (1) the facility does not allow any visitation for a patient or patients, or (2) the facility or the patient's physician determines that visitation would endanger the physical health or safety of a patient or visitor, or would interfere with the operations of the facility (5).

Most states have penalties and fines that will be assessed against a health care provider, including a sleep center, that violates a patient's rights pursuant to the state's Patient Bill of Rights regulations (6).

Sleep centers and other health care providers are often required by state law to post a statement of the Patient Bill of Rights and provide a written statement of all the rights to the patient on admission to the facility. The statement shall also include the right not to be discriminated against by the sleep center on the basis of the patient's race, color, or national origin, where such characteristics are not relevant to the patient's medical diagnosis and treatment. The statement shall further provide each admitted patient or the patient's representative or guardian with notice of how to initiate a grievance regarding improper discrimination with the facility and how the patient may lodge a grievance with the relevant government agencies, as applicable (7,8).

In certain jurisdictions, a health care facility, including a sleep center, that provides treatment or care to a patient requires each employee of or volunteer for the facility, including a student, who examines or treats a patient to wear an identification badge that readily discloses the first name, licensure status, if any, and staff position of the person examining or treating the patient (10).

SAMPLE PATIENT BILL OF RIGHTS

Although sleep centers will need to comply with the applicable state law regarding the regulatory requirements for Patient Bill of Rights, sleep centers and sleep medicine professionals should also consider patient care issues and the delivery of patient care related to the screening, evaluation, testing, diagnosis, and treatment of sleep disorders when drafting a Patient Bill of Rights. The following is a sample Patient Bill of Rights Policy:

Patient Bill of Rights Policy

It is the policy of the sleep center to respect the individual rights of all persons that come to this sleep center for care. Patient rights include the following: the right to make decisions regarding medical care, the right to accept or refuse treatment, and the right to formulate advance directives, including written instructions, such as a living will or durable power of attorney for health care as recognized under state law, relating to the provision of such, when an individual is incapacitated.

Patient responsibilities include those actions on the part of patients that are needed so that sleep center and health care professionals can provide appropriate care, make accurate and responsible care decisions, address patient needs, and maintain a sound and viable health care sleep center.

The implementation of a comprehensive Patient Bill of Rights is essential for sleep centers not only to ensure ethical patient care but also to maintain compliance with federal reimbursement programs. As sleep centers rely heavily on Medicare and Medicaid reimbursements for diagnostic polysomnography, continuous positive airway pressure (CPAP) titration studies, and DME provisions, understanding the intersection of patient rights and federal health care regulations becomes critical for operational sustainability and legal compliance.

Access to Care

Patients shall be afforded impartial access to treatment that is available and medically indicated, regardless of race, creed, sex, national origin, religion, sexual orientation, disability, or source of payment. Free translation services are available if needed.

The patient has the right to considerate, respectful care at all times, under all circumstances, with recognition of their personal dignity and worth.

Privacy and Confidentiality

The patient has the right, pursuant to applicable state and federal law, to personal privacy and information privacy, as demonstrated by the right to the following:

- Be interviewed and examined in surroundings designed to assure reasonable audiovisual privacy.
- Expect that any discussion or consultation involving the patient's care will be conducted discreetly and that individuals not involved in direct care will not be present without permission of the patient.
- Have the patient's medical record read only by individuals directly involved in treatment or monitoring of quality and by other individuals only on written authorization by the patient or their legally authorized representatives.
- Refuse to talk with or see anyone not officially connected with the sleep center, including visitors and persons officially connected with the sleep center but who are not directly involved in the patient's care.
- Wear appropriate personal clothing and religious or other symbolic items, as long as such clothing and religious or other symbolic items do not jeopardize safety or interfere with diagnostic procedures or treatment provided by the sleep center and its professionals.
- Expect that all communications and other records pertaining to the patient's care, including the sleep study and source of payment for treatment, be treated as confidential.
- Expect that information provided to family members or significant other legally qualified person be delivered in privacy and with consideration of confidentiality.

Personal Safety and Security

The patient has the right to expect reasonable safety in the sleep center, including compliance with the sleep center's policies and procedures, practices, and environment regarding patient safety and security. Other safety and security measures include: limited access to the sleep center through the use of electronic access cards and readers on exterior entrances, video monitoring in numerous areas of the sleep center, including the patient's treatment area, and the use of employee identification badges that are to be displayed by health care professionals providing services to the patient.

Identity

The patient has the right to know the identity and professional status of individuals providing service and which physician or other practitioner is primarily responsible for their care. This includes the patient's right to know of the existence of any professional relationship among individuals who are treating them, as well as the relationship to any health care or other institution, facility, or professional involved in their care. Participation by patients in research programs, or in the gathering of data for research purposes, shall be voluntary with a signed informed consent.

Communication

The patient has the right of access to people outside the sleep center by means of oral and written communication. When the patient does not speak or understand the predominant language of the community, or is hearing impaired, the patient shall have access to an interpreter, if at all possible.

Information

The patient has the right to obtain from the health care professional responsible for coordinating their care complete and current information concerning their diagnosis, treatment, and any known prognosis. This information should be communicated in terms the patient can reasonably be expected to understand. When it is not medically advisable to give such information to the patient, the information shall be made available to a legally authorized representative.

The patient has the right to access their medical records. The patient shall complete the Authorization to Disclose Protected Health Information (PHI) form and submit it to the sleep center.

The patient may access, request an amendment to, and/or receive an accounting of disclosures of their own PHI as permitted under applicable law, including the Health Insurance Portability and Accountability Act (HIPAA) regulations and standards.

Consent

The patient has the right to reasonably informed participation in decisions involving their health care. To the degree possible, this shall be based on a clear, concise explanation of their condition and of all proposed technical procedures, including the possibilities of any risk of mortality or serious side effects, issues related to the patient's diagnosis and treatment, and probability of success and outcomes. The patient shall not be subjected to any procedure without their voluntary, competent, and informed consent or that of their legally authorized representative. Where medically significant alternatives for care or treatment exist, the patient shall be so informed. The patient has the right to know who is responsible for authorizing and performing the diagnostic testing and/or treatment.

Sleep Study–Specific Informed Consent

For sleep studies, informed consent should also address the following issues:

- The nature of overnight monitoring, including electroencephalogram (EEG), electrooculogram (EOG), electromyogram (EMG), electrocardiogram (ECG), respiratory effort, and oxygen saturation measurements
- Video and audio recording procedures, retention periods, and access limitations
- The presence of sleep technologists throughout the night and their role in patient care
- Circumstances under which a study may be terminated (eg, medical emergencies, patient request, technical failures)
- Patient rights to request cessation of recording at any time
- Procedures for CPAP or bilevel positive airway pressure (BiPAP) trials during titration studies
- Poststudy data retention, analysis, and sharing protocols

The patient shall be informed if the health care professional proposes to engage in or perform human experimentation or other research/educational projects affecting their care or treatment, and the patient shall sign an informed consent if participation is desired and maintains the right to refuse to participate or withdraw from any such activity at any time.

The patient may refuse treatment to the extent permitted by law. When refusal of treatment by the patient or their legally authorized representative prevents the provision of appropriate care in accordance with ethical and professional standards, the relationship with the patient may be terminated upon reasonable notice by the sleep center.

If a patient is unconscious or is determined to be mentally incompetent and no consent can be obtained from an appropriate family member, legal action may be taken to obtain a court order for diagnostic testing procedures. In life-threatening emergencies, where the patient is incompetent or unconscious, appropriate treatment may be administered without consent.

Consultation

The patient, at their own request and expense, has the right to consult with a specialist.

Transfer and Continuity of Care

A patient may not be transferred to another facility unless they have received a complete explanation of the need for the transfer and the alternatives to such a transfer and unless the transfer is acceptable to the other facility. The patient has the right to be informed by the responsible health care professional or their delegate of any continuing health care requirements following discharge from the sleep center.

Regardless of the source of payment for their care, the patient has the right to request and receive an itemized and detailed explanation of their total finalized bill for services rendered in the sleep center. The patient shall be informed of eligibility for reimbursement by any third-party coverage during the admission or preadmission financial investigation.

Sleep Center Rules and Regulations

The patient shall be informed of the sleep center's rules and regulations applicable to their conduct as a patient. The sleep center's notice of privacy practices (NPP) is available from the administrator and can be found on the sleep center's website.

Complaint Process

The patient has the right to file a complaint regarding services and is entitled to information regarding the sleep center's mechanism for the initiation, review, and resolution of such complaints.

Patient Responsibilities

Patients have the responsibility for:

- providing complete and accurate information about medical complaints and issues, past illnesses, hospitalizations, medications, pain, and other matters relating to the patient's health;
- keeping appointments, arriving on time, and contacting the sleep center if the appointment cannot be kept;
- following the treatment plan recommended by those responsible for the patient's care;
- the patient's actions if they refuse treatment or do not follow the sleep center's instructions;
- providing complete and accurate information about the patient's health insurance coverage and promptly paying bills in a timely manner;
- following the sleep center's policies and procedures and applicable rules and regulations;
- being considerate of the rights of other patients and the sleep center's health care professionals; and
- seeking information and, in the event the patient has any questions, asking such questions.

HEALTH CARE REFORM

The Patient Protection and Affordable Care Act ("ACA") was enacted in March 2010. As a result of the ACA, substantial changes have occurred, and continued changes are anticipated in the US health care system. The ACA is impacting the delivery of health care services, the financing of health care costs, reimbursement of health care providers, and the legal obligations of health insurers, providers, employers, and consumers, including regulatory compliance and enforcement activities. These provisions are slated to take effect at specified times over approximately the next decade from adoption, and, therefore, the full consequences of the ACA on the health care industry will not be immediately realized. The ramifications of the ACA may also become apparent only following implementation or through later regulatory and judicial interpretations. Thus, the health care industry is the subject of significant new statutory and regulatory requirements and consequently structural and operational changes and challenges for a substantial period of time. Portions of the ACA have already been limited and nullified as a result of legislative amendments and judicial interpretations, and future actions and amendments may further change its impact. In addition, the uncertainties regarding the implementation of the ACA create unpredictability for the strategic and business planning efforts of health care providers, and this in itself constitutes a risk.

The ACA addresses almost all aspects of health care delivery and has changed, and is changing, how health care services are covered, delivered, and reimbursed. These changes will result in new payment models with the risk of lower health care provider reimbursement from Medicare, utilization changes, increased government enforcement, and the necessity for health care providers to assess, and potentially alter, their business strategy and practices, among other consequences. Although many providers will receive reduced payments for care, millions of previously uninsured Americans may have coverage. Requirements for state "health insurance exchanges" could fundamentally alter the health insurance market and negatively impact health care providers, enabling insurers to aggressively negotiate rates (9-13).

HEALTH CARE REGULATION

Federal Issues

A wide array of regulatory issues impact sleep medicine and the provision of care to patients by sleep centers and DME companies as related to the health care industry. Various levels of government agencies are involved with health care oversight, not only in the role of regulators but also as significant third-party payors.

Medicare, a federal health insurance program for the older adults and certain disabled persons, and Medicaid, a jointly administered federal and state program for certain indigent persons, are very important payors for most health care providers, including sleep centers. There are numerous complex rules governing payments and methodology, documentation, claim forms, cost reporting forms, as well as certification processes for participation and conditions of participation in the Medicare and Medicaid programs.

The sleep center must be approved for participation in the Medicare and Medicaid programs in order to become enrolled in the programs, receive provider numbers, and be permitted to bill Medicare and Medicaid for services rendered to patients who are Medicare and Medicaid beneficiaries. Failure to maintain certification by Medicare could have a materially adverse effect on the sleep center's business. The sleep center will also be required to revalidate its compliance with the Medicare regulations, including the conditions of participation, and such Medicare revalidation requirements have increased since the implementation of the ACA. Given the current regulatory environment, sleep centers and DME companies will continue to be subject to intensive regulation, including increased audits and investigations to enforce regulatory compliance, at the state and federal levels.

"Fraud" and "False Claims"

Health care "fraud and abuse" laws have been enacted at the federal and state levels to broadly regulate the provision of services to government program beneficiaries and the methods and requirements for submitting claims for services rendered to the beneficiaries (14). Under these fraud and abuse laws, health care providers and suppliers who submit claims for services provided to government program beneficiaries can be penalized for a wide variety of conduct, including submitting claims for services that are not provided, billing in a manner that does not comply with government requirements or including inaccurate billing information, billing for services deemed to be medically unnecessary, and/or billings accompanied by an illegal inducement to utilize or refrain from utilizing a service or product.

Federal and state governments have a broad range of criminal, civil, and administrative sanctions available to penalize and remediate health care fraud, including the exclusion of the provider or supplier from participation in the Medicare or Medicaid programs, recoupment of previous payments, civil monetary penalties, suspension of Medicare or Medicaid payments, and criminal sanctions and imprisonment. Fraud and abuse cases may be prosecuted by one or more government entities and/or private individuals, and more than one of the available sanctions and penalties may be, and often is, imposed for each violation. The ACA authorizes the Secretary of the U.S. Department of Health and Human Services (DHHS) to exclude a provider's participation in Medicare and Medicaid, as well as suspend payments to a provider pending an investigation or prosecution of a credible allegation of fraud against the provider.

Laws governing fraud and abuse may apply to nearly all individuals and entities with which a health care provider does business. Fraud investigations, settlements, prosecutions, and related publicity can have a material adverse effect on health care providers. Major elements of these often highly technical laws and regulations are generally summarized in what follows.

False Claims Act

The federal False Claims Act ("FCA") makes it illegal to knowingly submit or present a false, fictitious, or fraudulent claim to the federal government. Because the term "knowingly" is defined broadly under the law to include not only actual knowledge but also deliberate ignorance or reckless disregard of the facts, the FCA can be used to regulate and oversee a wide range of conduct. Centers for Medicare and Medicaid Services (CMS) adopted a new 60-day overpayment rule at 42 CFR § 401.305 (effective January 1, 2025). An overpayment is now "identified" when the provider has—or should have—actual knowledge, deliberate ignorance, or reckless disregard of the facts, mirroring the FCA "knowing" standard. A one-time 180-day investigation grace period suspends the 60-day clock while a good-faith probe is underway.

Federal Anti-Kickback Statute

The federal "Anti-Kickback Statute" (AKS) prohibits anyone from soliciting, receiving, offering, or paying any remuneration, directly or indirectly, overtly or covertly, in cash or in kind, in return for a referral (or to induce a referral) for any item or service that is paid by any federal or state health care program. The ACA amended the AKS to provide that a claim that includes items or services resulting from a violation of the AKS now constitutes a false or fraudulent claim for purposes of the FCA. Another amendment provides that an AKS violation may be established without showing that an individual knew of the statute's proscriptions or acted with specific intent to violate the AKS but only that the conduct was generally unlawful. The new standards have significantly expanded criminal and civil fraud exposure for transactions and arrangements where there is no intent to violate the AKS, and these new standards have also led to increased enforcement activities by federal agencies, including audits and investigations of providers and suppliers (13).

Violation or alleged violation of the AKS often results in settlements that require significant dollar payments and the imposition of formal, government-monitored compliance programs. The AKS can be prosecuted criminally or civilly. Violation of the AKS is a felony, subject to potentially substantial fines for each act (which may be each item or each bill sent to a federal program), imprisonment, and/or exclusion from the Medicare and Medicaid programs, any of which would have a significant detrimental effect on the financial stability of most providers. In addition, significant civil monetary penalties may be imposed. Increasingly, the federal government and qui tam relators are prosecuting violations of the AKS under the FCA, on the basis of the argument that claims resulting from an illegal kickback arrangement are also the submission of false claims for FCA purposes. In 2023, the First Circuit held that "but-for causation" is required to attach automatic FCA liability to AKS violations, raising the evidentiary bar for whistleblower actions.

The AKS applies to many common health care transactions between individuals and entities involved in the ownership and operation of a health care facility, including the ownership interests of physicians who refer patients to such health care facilities center, medical director agreements, and other related arrangements and agreements. Because the provisions of the AKS are so broad, the DHHS, Office of the Inspector General has published regulations, including "safe harbors," advisory opinions, and fraud alerts, outlining certain categories of activities that are deemed *not* to violate the AKS, provided all required elements of the safe harbor are met. The preambles to the safe harbor regulations state that the failure to comply with a safe harbor does not mean that the arrangement violates the AKS and that many legitimate ventures do not fall within one. If the statute is violated, the preambles state that the degree of the risk of prosecution depends on an evaluation of the many factors that are part of the decision-making process regarding case selection for investigation and prosecution.

Stark Law

The federal Stark Law and implementing regulation prohibits the referral of Medicare and Medicaid patients for certain designated health services ("DHS") (including inpatient and outpatient hospital services, clinical laboratory services, and radiation and other imaging services) to entities ("DHS Entities") with which the referring physician has a financial relationship unless the relationship fits within a stated exception. The Stark Law also prohibits a DHS Entity from furnishing the DHS and subsequently from billing Medicare for services performed pursuant to a prohibited referral. The government does not need to prove that the DHS Entity knew that the referral was prohibited to establish a Stark violation. Unless certain technical requirements are met, many ordinary business practices and economically desirable arrangements between hospitals and physicians arguably constitute improper "financial relationships" within the meaning of the Stark statute, thus implicating the prohibition on referrals and billing. Most providers of the DHS with physician relationships have some exposure to liability under the Stark Law (13).

Changes to the regulations issued under the Stark Law have rendered illegal a number of common arrangements under which physician-owned entities provide services and/or equipment to hospitals and may increase risk of violation because of lack of clarity of the technical requirements necessary to satisfy exceptions.

Medicare may deny payment for all services related to a prohibited referral, and a DHS Entity that has billed for prohibited services may be obligated to refund the amounts collected from the Medicare program. For example, if a medical director agreement between a DHS Entity and a physician is found to violate the Stark Law, the DHS Entity could be obligated to repay CMS for the payments received from Medicare for all of the Medicare-covered services performed by the physicians during the time the arrangement was out of compliance, a potentially significant amount, and the physician and DHS may be excluded from the Medicare program. The government may also seek substantial civil monetary penalties, and in some cases, a DHS Entity may be liable for fines up to 3 times the amount of any monetary penalty and/or be excluded from the Medicare and Medicaid programs. Potential repayments to CMS, settlements, fines, or exclusion for a Stark violation or alleged violation could have a material adverse impact on a health care provider. Increasingly, the federal government is prosecuting violations of the Stark Law under the FCA, on the basis of the government's position that claims resulting from an illegal referral arrangement are also false claims for FCA purposes. The federal government is also increasingly attempting to recover the federal portion of Medicaid claims referred to DHS Entities by physicians with whom they have a prohibited financial relationship.

State Issues

In addition to federal issues, compliance with state law by a sleep center and a DME company is very important in the ongoing operation of the facilities and provision of sleep medicine. Most states regulate licensure, certificate of need, and other matters relative to medical practice and the operation of a health care facility, including sleep centers and DME companies.

MAINTAINING PATIENT PRIVACY

HIPAA and Privacy Requirements

Health Insurance Portability and Accountability Act

HIPAA of 1996 adds additional civil penalties and criminal sanctions for health care fraud and applies to all health care benefit programs, whether public or private. HIPAA also provides for penalties and sanctions on a health care provider for knowingly and willfully embezzling, stealing, converting, or intentionally misapplying any money, funds, or other assets of a health care benefit program. A health care provider convicted of health care fraud could be subject to mandatory exclusion from Medicare.

HIPAA also addresses the confidentiality of individuals' health information, including privacy and security aspects of confidential health information. Disclosure of certain broadly defined PHI is prohibited unless expressly permitted under the provisions of the HIPAA statute and regulations, authorized by the patient, and meets exceptions related to the patient's treatment, payment, and health care operations. HIPAA's confidentiality provisions extend not only to patient medical records but also to a wide variety of health care clinical and financial information. These patient privacy restrictions impose communication, operational, accounting, and billing restrictions that add costs and create potentially unanticipated sources of liability. HIPAA imposes civil monetary penalties for violations and criminal penalties for knowingly obtaining or using individually identifiable health information.

Special Considerations for Sleep Medicine Data Privacy

Due to the continuous monitoring of data, sleep centers face unique privacy challenges. Polysomnography generates extensive physiologic data over 6 to 8 hour periods, creating large datasets that require secure storage and transmission protocols. Centers must implement encryption for both stored data and data in transit.

CPAP compliance monitoring is utilized to ascertain compliance with PAP therapy. PAP devices transmit usage data through cellular or Wi-Fi connections. Sleep centers must (1) establish business associate agreements with CPAP manufacturers; (2) inform patients about remote monitoring capabilities; (3) obtain specific consent for compliance data sharing with insurers; (4) ensure secure data transmission protocols are in place.

Sleep studies often include video monitoring to assess sleep behaviors and movements. Centers should post clear notices about video recording areas, limit access to video recordings to authorized clinical staff, establish retention and deletion schedules for video data, prohibit use of personal recording devices by staff, and address patient requests to opt out of video recording when clinically appropriate.

The HITECH Act

Provisions in the 2009 Health Information Technology for Economic and Clinical Health Act (the "HITECH Act"), enacted as part of the American Recovery and Reinvestment Act ("ARRA"), increase the minimum and maximum civil monetary penalties for violations of HIPAA and grant enforcement authority of HIPAA to state attorneys general. The HITECH Act also (1) extends the reach of HIPAA beyond "covered entities," (2) imposes a breach notification requirement on HIPAA-covered entities, (3) limits certain uses and disclosures of individually identifiable health information, (4) restricts covered entities' marketing communications, and (5) permits imposition of civil monetary penalties for a HIPAA violation even if an entity did not know and would not, by exercising reasonable diligence, have known of a violation (15).

The breach notification obligation, in particular, may expose covered entities such as sleep centers and DME companies to heightened liability. Under the HITECH Act, in the event of a data privacy breach, covered entities are required to notify affected individuals and the federal government. If more than 500 individuals in any one state are affected by the breach, (1) the covered entity must also notify the media, and (2) the federal government posts a description of the breach on its website. Although HIPAA does not provide for a private right of action, these reporting obligations increase the risk of government enforcement as well as class action lawsuits filed under state privacy or consumer protection laws, especially if large numbers of individuals are affected by a breach.

On January 25, 2013, DHHS issued comprehensive modifications to the existing HIPAA regulations to implement the requirements of the HITECH Act, commonly known as the "HIPAA Omnibus Rule." The HIPAA Omnibus Rule became effective on March 26, 2013, and covered entities were required to be in compliance by September 23, 2013 (although certain requirements had a longer time frame). Key aspects of the HIPAA Omnibus Rule include, but are not limited to: (1) a new standard for what constitutes a breach of private health information, (2) establishing four levels of culpability with respect to civil monetary penalties assessed for HIPAA violations, (3) direct liability of business associates for certain violations of HIPAA, (4) modifications to the rules governing research, (5) stricter requirements regarding nonexempt marketing practices, (6) modification and redistribution of notices of privacy practices, and (7) stricter requirements regarding the protection of genetic information. Although the effects of the HIPAA Omnibus Rule cannot be predicted at this time, the obligations imposed thereunder could have a material adverse effect on the financial condition of the Credit Group.

The HITECH Act revises the civil monetary penalties associated with violations of HIPAA as well as provides state attorneys general with authority to enforce the HIPAA privacy and security regulations in some cases through a damages assessment of $100 per violation or an injunction against the violator.

Criminal penalties will be enforced against persons who obtain or disclose personal health information without authorization. DHHS is also beginning to perform periodic audits of health care providers and group health plans to ensure that required policies under the HITECH Act are in place. Finally, individuals harmed by violations will be able to recover a percentage of monetary penalties or a monetary settlement based on methods to be established by DHHS for this private recovery.

The Office for Civil Rights ("OCR") is the administrative office that is tasked with enforcing HIPAA. The OCR has stated that it has now moved from education to enforcement in its implementation of the law, and in March 2016, the OCR began its Phase 2 HIPAA Privacy, Security, and Breach Notification Audit Program, which requires providers to submit certain data to the OCR. Recent settlements of HIPAA violations for breaches involving lost data have reached millions of dollars. Any breach of HIPAA, regardless of intent or scope, may result in penalties or settlement amounts that are material to a covered health care provider or health plan.

Business Associates

Under existing HIPAA regulations, covered entities must include certain required provisions in their contractual relationships with organizations that perform functions on their behalf that involve use or disclosure of PHI. These organizations are called business associates and have been indirectly regulated by HIPAA through contractual obligations. The HITECH Act and the final rules promulgated thereunder provide that all of the HIPAA security administrative, physical, and technical safeguards, as well as security policies, procedures, and documentation requirements now apply directly to all business associates. In addition, the HITECH Act makes certain privacy provisions directly applicable to business associates. These changes are significant because business associates will now be directly regulated by DHHS for those requirements and, as a result, will be subject to penalties imposed by DHHS and/or state attorneys general. Likewise, to the extent a business associate is deemed to be an agent of the covered entity under the federal common law, the covered entity will be liable for the breaches of the business associate. Importantly, all telehealth technology vendors used by sleep centers are now considered business associates and must have proper business associate agreements in place.

Security Breaches and Unauthorized Releases of Personal Information

State and local authorities are increasingly focused on the importance of protecting the confidentiality of individuals' personal information, including patient health information. Many states have enacted laws requiring businesses to notify individuals of security breaches that result in the unauthorized release of personal information. These notification requirements may be triggered even where information has not been used or disclosed but rather has been inappropriately accessed. Violations can lead to individual or class action lawsuits and increased enforcement by state consumer protection agencies.

Notable 2024 actions include California's $49 million settlement with Kaiser for improper PHI disposal and New York's enforcement actions against health care providers using website tracking pixels without proper patient consent.

Sleep centers qualify as a "covered entity" under the Administrative Simplification Provisions of HIPAA, and as a covered entity, sleep centers are required to comply with these regulations, including privacy and security standards. Failure to comply would expose the sleep center to civil and criminal penalties. Also, failure to submit claims electronically in compliance with the electronic data interchange (EDI) regulation may result in denial of claims and possible exclusion from participation in federal health care programs.

How to Maintain Privacy of PHI in Electronic Health Records

The HIPAA regulations and security standards address how a patient's PHI must be protected from unauthorized disclosure to other entities and individuals. Many sleep centers and DME companies utilize electronic health record (EHR) to document, retain, and transmit a patient's PHI. Given the utilization of EHR and potential for data breaches and unauthorized disclosure of patients' PHI, it is imperative that sleep centers and DME companies comply with the HIPAA regulations and set up safeguards and security measures pursuant to the HIPAA security standards. The following is an overview of how a sleep center and its sleep medicine professionals can maintain privacy of patients' PHI in an EHR pursuant to the HIPAA regulations and security standards.

Patients have the right to receive a notice explaining how a provider, including a sleep center or health plan, uses and discloses their health information. Health care providers usually give patients this notice on their first visit to the sleep center and post it in the center where patients may see it. Health plans typically send their notices by mail after patient enrollment (15).

An NPP will often contain jargon that can be difficult for patients to understand.

The HIPAA regulations require that an NPP (15):

- include how the HIPAA Privacy Rule allows the covered entity to use and share PHI and state that it will obtain the patient's permission for any other reason;
- tell patients about their rights under the HIPAA Privacy Rule;
- tell patients how to file a complaint with the covered entity;
- tell patients how to file a complaint with the DHHS OCR;
- provide information about a patient's rights to restrict fund-raising solicitations; and
- explain the need to obtain a patient's written authorization for marketing or the sale of the patient's PHI.

For more information about notices of privacy practices, see the DHHS website at: www.hhs.gov or 45 CFR §164.520.

Health care providers, including sleep centers, should ask patients to sign a form saying that they received a copy of the NPP. The law does not require patients to sign this. However, signing does not waive a patient's rights under HIPAA and does not mean that the patient agrees with the privacy policy. If a patient refuses to sign, it does not prevent a health care provider from using or disclosing information in ways already permitted under HIPAA. A provider may not deny treatment if a patient refuses to sign an acknowledgment of having received an NPP (16).

The NPP will provide information about whom to contact with privacy questions and how to complain. If a patient does not have a copy of the notice, there may be one on the provider's or health plan's website. If there is not an NPP on the health care provider's website, a covered entity's administrative office will be able to provide the information and a copy of the notice.

HIPAA gives patients the right to see and receive a copy of their medical records but not the original medical records. To find out how to request access to a medical record, the patient should review the sleep center's NPP. Patients can always request a copy of the notice, which should provide instructions for requesting records as well as contact information for asking questions or filing complaints (17).

Patients have the right to access both paper and electronic records. An individual may request information in a specific format, and the covered entity must comply with the request if the data are readily producible. If the data are not readily producible in the patient's specified format, the covered entity and the individual can agree on another format. If the sleep center and the patient cannot reach an agreement, the covered entity will produce a hard copy (17).

For example, a patient might ask the sleep center to provide their records on an external portable storage device such as a USB drive. If the sleep center does not agree to use the USB drive because it believes it is a security risk, the sleep center and the patient may reach agreement about another format. If they do not reach an agreement, the sleep center may provide a hard copy to the patient.

Often, patients want providers to send their health information, including PHI, to third parties such as another doctor, a relative, or an attorney. To authorize this transfer and disclosure of PHI, the patient should sign a request that clearly identifies which medical records need to be sent, who has been designated to receive the medical records, and where the patient's medical records need to be sent. HIPAA allows covered entities, including sleep centers, to charge a "reasonable, cost-based fee." The covered entity can charge for supplies, staff time for copying and processing, and mailing, if applicable (17).

The covered entity may charge for the time staff spends copying and processing the record. However, the sleep center may not charge for the time a staff member spends searching for the record. In addition, the covered entity should not adopt a policy of charging a flat fee or charging a patient to view a record. Many states have laws that limit a covered entity's ability to charge for medical records. Sleep centers should check the applicable state laws to ensure that its charges for patient medical records comply with the applicable state regulations (17).

A covered entity, including a sleep center, must produce a patient's medical records 30 days from the date of request. HIPAA allows a covered entity one 30-day extension if the sleep center provides written notice to the patient stating the reason for the delay and the expected date. This applies to both paper and electronic records (17).

A sleep center, as the covered entity, may deny a patient's request for access under certain circumstances. Typically, the covered entity must issue a written denial letter, and in some cases, an individual may be able to appeal a denial. As a general rule, patients do not have the right to access their own psychotherapy notes or information a covered entity compiled for legal proceedings. Patients may be denied access to their PHI without the right to review the denial in the following situations: (17)

- Correctional institutions may deny an inmate's request for a copy of PHI if it jeopardizes the health, safety, security, custody, or rehabilitation of the individual or other inmates. It may also deny a request that jeopardizes the safety of any person at the correctional institution or those responsible for transporting the inmate.
- If a covered health care provider obtains or creates PHI in the course of research, it may temporarily suspend access while the research is in process. This applies if the individual agreed to the denial when they decided to participate in a study and understands that the right will be reinstated when the research is complete.
- If a record that contains PHI is subject to the HIPAA privacy standards, there are certain circumstances where an individual may not be able to access the record.
- If the PHI was obtained from someone other than a health care provider under a promise of confidentiality and the access requested would likely reveal the source of the information, an individual may not be able to access the information.

Sometimes, patients have the right to have denials of access reviewed by a licensed health care professional. If so, the patient should receive instructions telling them how to appeal the denial. The covered entity will designate a reviewing official who did not participate in the original decision to deny access.

When patients access a medical record and find information they believe is inaccurate, they may file a written request that the record be corrected. The covered entity, including sleep centers, must respond to the request within 60 days. The sleep center may decide to take an additional 30 days but must provide the patient with a written explanation for the delay and a date by which it will complete the action (18).

If the covered entity denies the request, it must provide the patient with the following information in writing:

- The basis for the denial. For example, the covered entity did not create the medical record, the information is not part of the designated record set, the patient is not allowed to access the medical record under another HIPAA provision, or the medical record is accurate and complete;
- That the patient has a right to submit a written statement disagreeing with the denial;
- That the patient may request that the covered entity provide the request for amendment and the denial with any future disclosures that pertain to the request; and
- How the patient may complain.

Under the HIPAA regulations and privacy and security standards, covered entities, including sleep centers, must allow a patient to make specific privacy requests. Although a patient has the right to make a request, in most situations, the covered entity is not required to agree (19).

If a covered entity agrees to honor an individual's privacy request, it must comply unless the individual needs emergency treatment and the restricted PHI is necessary to provide the treatment. In an emergency situation where the covered entity must disclose information it agreed to restrict, it must request that the information not be further disclosed.

HIPAA enables patients to learn to whom the covered entity has disclosed their PHI. This is called an "accounting of disclosures." The accounting will cover up to 6 years prior to the patient's request date and will include disclosures to or by business associates of the covered entity. For each disclosure, the accounting must state: (20)

- the date of the disclosure;
- the name of the entity or person who received the PHI, and, if known, the address;
- a brief description of the PHI disclosed; and
- a brief statement of the purpose of the disclosure.

The accounting does not include information about disclosures the covered entity made:

- to carry out treatment, payment, or health care operations;
- to the individual for information about them;
- incident to a use or disclosure that HIPAA permits or requires;
- that the patient authorized;
- for a sleep center's directory or persons involved in the patient's care;
- for national security or intelligence purposes;
- to correctional institutions or law enforcement officials;
- as part of a limited data set that excludes a number of identifiers and is disclosed for research, public health, or health care operations; or
- that occurred prior to the date by which the covered entity had to comply.

Within 60 days of receiving a request for an accounting, a covered entity, including sleep centers, must: (20)

- provide the accounting; or
- extend the time by no more than 30 days as long as it provides the individual with a written statement of the reasons for the delay and date by which it will provide the accounting.

A covered entity must provide the first accounting, during any 12-month period, free of charge. If an individual requests more than one accounting during a year, the covered entity may impose a cost-based fee on subsequent requests. However, if it is going to charge, the covered entity must inform the individual of the fee in advance and give them an opportunity to withdraw or modify the request (20).

Under the HIPAA Privacy Rule, a covered entity can disclose a minor child's PHI to a parent acting as a child's "personal representative" as long as it is consistent with state and other law. DHHS provides the following examples of situations where a parent may not access a minor's medical record (21):

- a minor consents to care, and law does not require parental consent; (21)
- a court or person appointed by the court directs a minor to obtain care; and (21)
- a parent agrees that the minor and health care provider may have a confidential relationship (21).

Sleep centers and DME companies should carefully review their policies and procedures and patient forms related to the provision of patient care, administration, and operational functions to ensure compliance with the applicable state and federal regulations, specifically, regulations that address Patient Bill of Rights requirements, protection of patient's PHI, maintenance of privacy of patient's PHI in an EHR, and identify risks and benefits of health care professionals who provide sleep medicine services to patients to ensure patient privacy and protection of PHI.

The provision of sleep medicine services requires careful navigation of complex patient rights regulations at both state and federal levels. Sleep centers must balance clinical excellence with regulatory compliance, ensuring that patients' rights to privacy, informed consent, and quality care are protected while meeting the technical requirements of Medicare, Medicaid, and commercial insurance programs.

Key compliance priorities for sleep centers include:

- Implementing and posting a comprehensive Patient Bill of Rights
- Maintaining HIPAA-compliant procedures for all patient data, including polysomnography recordings and CPAP compliance data
- Ensuring proper documentation and billing practices to avoid FCA violations
- Structuring physician relationships to comply with Stark Law and AKS requirements
- Providing appropriate training to all staff on patient rights and privacy requirements

Regular review and updates of policies and procedures, combined with ongoing staff education, will help sleep centers maintain compliance while delivering high-quality patient care in this evolving regulatory landscape.

REFERENCES

1. Illinois General Assembly. Medical Patient Rights Act, 410 ILCS 50/0.01. 2024.
2. Illinois General Assembly. Medical Patient Rights Act, 410 ILCS 50/2.03. 2024.
3. Illinois General Assembly. Medical Patient Rights Act, 410 ILCS 50/3. 2024.
4. Illinois General Assembly. Medical Patient Rights Act, 410 ILCS 50/3.1. 2024.
5. Illinois General Assembly. Medical Patient Rights Act, 410 ILCS 50/3.2. 2024.
6. Illinois General Assembly. Medical Patient Rights Act, 410 ILCS 50/4. 2024.
7. U.S. Government Publishing Office. Rights to request privacy protection for protected health information. 45 CFR §164.522. Electronic Code of Federal Regulations. 2023.
8. Illinois General Assembly. Medical Patient Rights Act, 410 ILCS 50/5. 2024.
9. Illinois General Assembly. Medical Patient Rights Act, 410 ILCS 50/6. 2022.
10. Centers for Medicare & Medicaid Services. Medicare Access and CHIP Reauthorization Act of 2015 (MACRA): quality payment program overview. 2024.
11. Legal Information Institute. National Federation of Independent Business v. Sebelius: Wex Summary. Cornell Law School. 2012.
12. American Medical Association Journal of Ethics. King v. Burwell: U.S. Supreme Court upholds ACA subsidies. 2015.
13. U.S. Government Publishing Office. 42 U.S.C. § 1396d(y)—Medicaid-Expansion FMAP. 2010.
14. Office of Inspector General. Fraud & abuse laws for physicians. 2024.
15. U.S. Department of Health and Human Services. Summary of the HITECH Act enforcement interim final rule. 2009.
16. U.S. Government Publishing Office. Notice of privacy practices for protected health information. 45 CFR. §164.520. Electronic Code of Federal Regulations. 2023.
17. U.S. Department of Health and Human Services. Notice of privacy practices for protected health information. 2024.
18. U.S. Department of Health and Human Services. Individuals' Right Under HIPAA to access their health information. 2025.
19. U.S. Government Publishing Office. Amendment of protected health information. 45 CFR §164.526. Electronic Code of Federal Regulations. 2023.
20. U.S. Government Publishing Office. Accounting of disclosures of protected health information. 45 CFR §164.528. Electronic Code of Federal Regulations. 2023.
21. U.S. Department of Health and Human Services. Guidance: Personal representatives. 2024.

Chapter 26
Patient and Employee Safety

SHANNA STEVEN

KEY CONCEPTS/LEARNING OBJECTIVES

The key concepts for this chapter include recognizing unsafe situations within the work environment, expressing that personal and patient safety involves each employee, participating in safe practices, describing how to prevent accidents or injury in the sleep center and react appropriately to an unsafe environment or situation and the importance of infection control standards.

KEY TERMS

Cardiopulmonary resuscitation (CPR)
Chemical spills
Electrical grounding
Medical waste

The importance of effective workplace safety cannot be overstated. The safety of employees affects morale, attendance, and workmen's compensation. Well-written policies and procedures are imperative in patient and employee safety. Policies help clarify and reinforce the standards expected of employees. Federal, state, and local organizations and agency guidelines assure the occupational health and safety of the technologist and patients who visit the sleep center. The Occupational Safety and Health Administration (OSHA) is a division of the US Department of Labor. OSHA provides regulatory standards for workplace safety. These standards are intended to protect employers, employees, and patients in and around the work environment. Personal and environmental hazards that the sleep technologist may be subjected to should be addressed in the department policy and procedures manual. A Quality Improvement (QI) plan is a formal documented action plan that targets areas of practice within an organization that will be the focus of safety and outcomes to obtain the highest quality of patient care. Quality assurance measures are then evaluated quarterly to track the effectiveness of the plan. The plan is adjusted appropriately to ensure that quality goals are being met. The American Academy of Sleep Medicine requires sleep centers to perform a safety risk analysis at least every 5 years to identify and make a plan to lessen the risk of events such as falls, medical emergencies, or harassment allegations (1).

PERSONAL SAFETY/CHEMICALS

An aspect of personal safety in the sleep disorder clinic that may be neglected is frequent exposure to fumes/odors from cleaning solutions and adhesive materials. Chemical exposure for health care workers is a possible threat at any sleep center. Causes may include improperly used or maintained disinfectant solutions or sterilizing agents. OSHA requires manufacturers to provide safety information on chemical products in a uniform format to ensure safety and proper handling of the chemical products that are utilized in the workplace (2). Staff meetings discussing the hazards of chemicals and solutions used and quick and easy access to safety data sheets (SDS) are ways to educate workers about the potential dangers surrounding these compounds.

The SDS is not meant for consumers but for employees who may be occupationally exposed to hazardous products or chemicals while in the working environment. The SDS is designed to provide workers with the proper procedures for handling, storing, and working with a particular substance. Basic supplies used by the sleep technologist during patient hookup procedures or cleaning equipment that require an SDS include the following:

- Electroencephalography (EEG) conductive paste or cream
- Disinfectant/cleaner concentrate
- Germicidal deodorizing cleaner
- Abrasive skin prep gel
- Adhesive to secure electrodes
- Alcohol prep pads
- Diaphoretic skin prep

The OSHA Quick Card identifies the required format for the SDS (3).

Section 1, Identification includes product identifier; manufacturer or distributor name, address, phone number; emergency phone number; recommended use; and restrictions on use.

Section 2, Hazard(s) identification includes all hazards regarding the chemical's intrinsic properties, including a change in the chemical's physical form and chemical reaction products associated with known or reasonably anticipated uses or applications and required label elements.

Section 3, Composition/information on ingredients includes information on chemical ingredients such as names; Chemical Abstracters Service (CAS) numbers or other unique identifiers; and prescribed concentration ranges and trade secret claims.

Section 4, First aid measures include important symptoms/effects (acute, delayed) and required treatment.

Section 5, Firefighting measures comprise suitable extinguishing techniques and equipment and chemical hazards from fire.

Section 6, Accidental release measures comprise emergency procedures, protective equipment, and proper methods of containment and cleanup.

Section 7, Handling and storage provides precautions for safe handling and storage, including incompatibilities.

Section 8, Exposure controls/personal protection lists OSHA's Permissible Exposure Limits (PELs); ACGIH Threshold Limit Values (TLVs); and any other exposure limit or range used or recommended by the chemical manufacturer, importer, or employer for chemicals listed in Section 3, appropriate engineering controls, and personal protective equipment (PPE).

Section 9, Physical and chemical properties list the chemical's characteristics, including particle size.

Section 10, SFIGility and reactivity lists chemical stability and the possibility of hazardous reactions, including those associated with any foreseeable emergencies.

Section 11, Toxicologic information includes routes of exposure; related symptoms, acute and chronic effects; numerical measures of toxicity and interactive effects.

Section 12, Ecologic information

Section 13, Disposal considerations

Section 14, Transport information

Section 15, Regulatory information

Section 16, Other information includes the date of preparation or last revision.

It is crucial to the safety of sleep technologists to have access to an SDS manual containing information for each chemical used in the sleep center. This reference should be available for employees at all times.

INFECTION CONTROL

Infection control should be an integral part of the health care facility's objectives. It is the responsibility of each member of the health care team to ensure the use of proper techniques to eliminate the spread of infection (2). Cooperation from the organization's administration, medical staff, and other health care personnel is necessary to maintain infection control standards. The following elements are necessary to attain appropriate infection control:

- Coordination with other departments
- Employee medical evaluations
- Health and safety education
- Employee immunization programs
- Management of job-related illnesses and exposure to infectious diseases, including policies for work restrictions for infected or exposed personnel
- Counseling services for personnel on infection risks related to employment
- Guidelines for COVID-9 (6)
- Maintenance and confidentiality of personnel health records

According to the Centers for Disease Control and Prevention and OSHA, the use of "universal precautions" or "standard precautions" refers to an infection control system that assumes any direct contact with a patient, particularly with body fluids, has the potential for transmitting disease (4). Health care personnel are at risk for occupational exposure to blood-borne pathogens, including hepatitis B virus, hepatitis C virus, and HIV. Standard precautions are designed to reduce the risk of transmission of blood-borne pathogens and to reduce the risk of transmission of pathogens from moist body substances. Standard precautions apply to blood, secretions, excretions except sweat, and all other body fluids of patients receiving care in hospitals or other medical settings, regardless of their diagnosis or presumed infection status. It is important to note that bodily fluids can be considered contaminated, whether or not they contain visible blood, nonintact skin, or mucous membranes. Exposures may occur through needle sticks or abrasions caused by contaminated sharp objects. Infection may occur through contact with mucous membranes of the eyes and mouth, skin, or the patient's blood. Contact with any bodily fluid, regardless of quantity, is considered to be a potential source of infectious agents (5). Using appropriate barriers such as gloves, goggles, or gowns when contact with blood is expected can prevent many exposures. Remove gloves promptly after use and wash hands immediately to avoid the transfer of microorganisms. If exposure occurs, wash needlestick injuries and cuts with soap and water; flush splashes to the nose, mouth, or skin with water; and irrigate the eyes (2). Prompt reporting of exposures to the department that handles such situations is essential so that proper treatment can be initiated.

Handwashing must occur after touching blood, body fluids, secretions, excretions, and contaminated items, whether or not gloves are worn. Wash hands immediately after gloves are removed, between patient contacts, and any time contamination has occurred, to avoid transfer of microorganisms to other patients or environments (2). Handwashing is also essential before eating and after using the bathroom.

It is important for technologists to handle used patient care equipment in a manner that prevents skin and mucous membrane exposure, contamination of clothing, and transfer of microorganisms to other patients and environments. Adequate procedures should be in place and followed for routine care, cleaning, and disinfection of environmental surfaces, beds, bedrails, bedside equipment, and other frequently touched surfaces.

Cleaning and disinfecting reusable equipment in the sleep center is a safety standard that cannot be compromised. It is the responsibility of *every* staff member to prevent the spread of infection with proper handwashing and effective cleaning of reusable equipment. Consider utilizing central processing for sterilizing reusable patient care equipment. Some facilities opt for disposable equipment and supplies (ie, individual use Nuprep and Ten20) to minimize contamination risk, as well as the cost of disinfecting agents and staff time. Some supplies, electrodes, masks, and even respiratory inductance plethysmography belts come in a disposable variety. Facilities using full tubs and tubes of conductive pastes and prep products must ensure that they are not cross contaminating the product between patients; recommended practice is to utilize individual use containers when available.

OSHA defines decontamination as the use of physical or chemical means to remove, inactivate, or destroy blood-borne pathogens on a surface or item to the point where they are no longer capable of transmitting infectious particles and the surface or item is rendered safe for handling, use, or disposal. Sterilization is the use of a physical or chemical procedure to destroy all microbial life, including highly resistant bacterial endospores (8).

In 1968, Spaulding devised an approach to disinfect and sterilize patient care items or equipment that is still used today. This approach classifies medical equipment into categories according to degree of risk of infection involved in the use of the items. Spaulding describes these categories as critical, semicritical, and noncritical. Positive airway pressure (PAP) masks, airflow sensors, and EEG cup electrodes fall into the category of semicritical, meaning that they come in contact with mucous membranes or skin that may not be intact. Semicritical items require high-level disinfection, in a separate cleaning area, with wet pasteurization or a chemical disinfectant. Today, most accrediting bodies recommend single-use EEG electrodes, PAP masks, tubing, humidifiers, and headgear. If PAP items are cleaned, there must be a method in place to track the number of times each item has been disinfected, and they must be discarded after they have been cleaned the maximum number of times indicated by the manufacturer. Reprocessing guidelines differ by manufacturer, by specific interface within manufacturers, and sometimes even for different parts of a continuous positive airway pressure (CPAP) mask—so this can be daunting to track and manage.

Electromyogram (EMG) and body sensor electrodes generally fall into the noncritical category. These items may come in contact with skin but not with mucous membranes. Most noncritical reusable items may be disinfected where they are used and do not need to be transported to a central processing area. There is generally little risk of transmitting infectious agents to patients by means of noncritical items. A high-level disinfectant wipe should be used to clean most noncritical items (Table 26-1).

PAP Mask Cleaning

According to the Spaulding criteria for medical device classification, PAP masks are considered semicritical medical equipment. Semicritical items contact mucous membranes or nonintact skin. It is recommended that centers utilize a single-use mask program. The sleep center may have a maintenance agreement with a mask manufacturer that allows the patient to take home the mask that was used in the sleep center during the titration study. The manufacturer then replaces that mask for the sleep center, although small replacement fees may apply.

Cleaning and disinfection requirements should adhere to those approved by the Food and Drug Administration (FDA) for each individual mask in order to ensure elimination of tuberculosis spores. Semicritical items minimally require high-level disinfection containing a tuberculocidal disinfectant. Glutaraldehyde, hydrogen peroxide, *ortho*-phthalaldehyde, and peracetic acid with hydrogen peroxide are FDA-approved semicritical

Table 26-1 Disinfecting Chart

	Noncritical Spaulding Category	Semicritical Spaulding Category	Cleaning
CPAP masks		X	Single-patient use CPAP masks are preferred. If re-used, soak in a high-level disinfectant according to disinfectant manufacturer's guidelines or pasteurize. Rinse and dry thoroughly.
EEG electrodes		X	Due to the abrading preparation of the skin, single-use disposable EEG electrodes are preferred. Reusable electrodes: Rinse with warm water. Soak in a high-level disinfectant or sterilize according to manufacturer's directions after each patient use. Wipe lead wires using a cloth soaked in a solution of low-level disinfectant, or wipe with a disinfectant towelette. Air dry prior to plugging into head box.
Snap electrodes	X		Wipe using a cloth soaked in a solution of low-level disinfectant, or wipe with a disinfectant towelette.
Airflow sensors		X	Disposable airflow sensors are preferred. Wipe using a cloth with a high-level disinfecting agent or towelette that is not corrosive to metal or plastic. Air dry.
Belts	X		Disposable belts are preferred. Straps may be safely soaked in low-level disinfectant solution. Air dry.
			The wire-set may be wiped with disinfecting cloth or towelette. Do not immerse in liquid.
Body position sensor	X		Wipe using a cloth with a low-level disinfecting agent or towelette that is not corrosive to metal or plastic. Do not immerse in liquid. Air dry.
Snore microphone	X		Wipe using a cloth with a disinfecting agent or towelette that is not corrosive to metal or plastic. Do not immerse in liquid. Air dry.
Spo_2 sensor	X		Disposable sensors are preferred. Remove disposable adhesive from permanent sensors and discard; wipe with a low-level disinfecting agent or towelette that is not corrosive to metal or plastic. Do not immerse in liquid. Air dry.
Headgear	X		Single-patient use headgear is preferred. Follow manufacturer's guidelines.
Linen	X		Blanket, sheets, and pillowcases must be washed between patients. Contaminated linens should be placed in impermeable bags.

CPAP, continuous positive airway pressure; EEG, electroencephalogram.
Retrieved from Rutala WA, Weber DJ; Healthcare Infection Control Practices Advisory Committee. Guideline for disinfection and sterilization in healthcare facilities, 2008. Centers for Disease Control and Prevention. Published 2024. Updated June 2024. https://www.cdc.gov/infection-control/media/pdfs/Guideline-Disinfection-H.pdf

method(s) of disinfection (ie, Control III, Cavicide, Sanizide Plus, and CIDEX OPA). Follow each specific manufacturers' recommendations. Consider using a timer to remind you when the equipment can be removed from the disinfecting agent to avoid excessive wear.

Sleep centers have also found pasteurizing to be a cost-effective way to clean and disinfect equipment. Pasteurization is a form of cleaning/high-level disinfecting of health care equipment using water temperatures of 160 °F to 170 °F (71 °C-77 °C). This eliminates or reduces the use of expensive toxic chemicals and saves labor costs of staff handwashing supplies. Guidelines on sterilization processes vary from state to state and, in some cases, from facility to facility.

Patient Room, Electrode, and Sensor Cleaning

Work surfaces, bed rails, EMG electrodes, thermal airflow sensors, head straps, snore microphones, and belts are considered noncritical medical equipment. Noncritical items come in contact with intact skin but not mucous membranes. In addition, the surfaces in patient rooms and work surfaces must be decontaminated to avoid transmission of infection. A low-level disinfectant such as isopropyl alcohol (70%-90%), sodium hypochlorite (5.25%-6.15%) diluted with water at 1:500, or a germicidal (ie, Control III, Sani-Cloth HB wipe, Super Sani-Cloth wipe, and Sani-Cloth Plus) wipe may be used to decontaminate noncritical items.

Proper handling and cleaning of sensors will prolong their durability and longevity. All equipment and sensors, masks, and belts coming into contact with the patient are considered contaminated. The sleep center must maintain a separation of "clean" and "dirty" equipment by keeping clean and dirty equipment in distinct areas designated as clean and dirty, respectively. All dirty equipment must be cleaned and disinfected after each use according to manufacturer guidelines. Single-use items must be discarded after each use.

Reusable equipment must be completely disassembled and thoroughly washed using an approved cleaning solution. OSHA requires staff to wear PPE such as gloves and goggles while cleaning equipment to reduce exposure to hazardous chemicals. Ensure that reusable equipment is not used for the care of another patient until it has been cleaned and processed appropriately. Personnel are more likely to comply with an infection control program if they understand the rules and the importance of such rules. Personnel education is the key element of an effective infection control program.

MEDICAL WASTE

Medical waste generated by health care providers can pose a risk of disease transmission if not managed properly. Hazardous waste and discarded chemicals that are toxic, flammable, or corrosive can cause fires, explosions, and pollution of air, water, and land. Knowing how to identify and properly dispose of medical and other hazardous waste is critical. Hazardous waste is a serious safety and health problem that continues to endanger human and animal life and environmental quality (7). Unless hazardous waste is properly treated, stored, or disposed, it will continue to do great harm to all living things that have contact with it now or in the future.

Because of the seriousness of the safety and health hazards related to hazardous waste operations, OSHA has issued regulations to protect workers and help them handle hazardous waste safely and effectively (8).

Medical "sharps" is the term used to describe any needle or sharp object, including glass. If not cared for properly, sharps can cause puncture wounds and/or lacerations that may create a point of entry for infectious agents. Infectious agents are any organisms that cause disease to or an adverse health impact on humans (2). Take care to prevent injuries when using needles and other sharp devices before, during, and after procedures, when cleaning used devices, and when disposing of used needles. Never recap used needles. Place used disposable syringes and needles and other sharp items in appropriate puncture-resistant containers and dispose of as regulated medical waste. Patient disposal of syringes, such as syringes used for insulin injections, should be monitored to prevent needles in the patient room. Sharps or products contaminated with blood or body fluids that are disposed of in the health care setting should be placed in properly identified and labeled sharps containers to be sent to the waste treatment center for decontamination.

PROPER LIFTING TECHNIQUES

Back injuries account for nearly 25% of occupational injuries. Not only are these injuries costly to the Worker's Compensation program, but they also leave the worker prone to recurrent injury. Attention to posture, conditioning, and body mechanics are essential to maintaining a healthy back while on the job. Body mechanics refers to the way we use our body to accomplish a task (Table 26-2). Eighty percent of Americans will experience back pain some time in their lives. Of these, 90% are due to strain of back muscles, ligaments, or soft tissue. These conditions generally heal completely but often recur if prevention strategies are not used. The National Institute of Occupational Safety and Health (NIOSH) has researched and developed a lifting equation taking into account such things as weight of the object lifted, distance of the hands above the floor, angle of the distance of the object from the core of the body at the beginning or end of the lift, and twisting of the legs, shoulders, or torso in assessing physical stress with unassisted two-handed lifting.

Injury may occur when using poor posture, awkward positioning, or overreaching. When preparing to lift, stand close to the object or individual being moved or lifted, position your feet a comfortable distance apart, bend at the knee, keep the back straight, and grip the

Table 26-2 Body Mechanics to Promote Back Injury Prevention

	Do	Do Not
Bending	Stoop with bent knees	Bend at the back
Reaching	Use step stool	Stretch overhead
Pulling or pushing	Use entire body	Use arms only
Lifting	Stand close to object	Reach
	Bend at knees and hips	Bend or twist at the waist

item firmly. While lifting, slowly straighten your legs, keep the object close to your body, bring your back to a full upright position, and move your feet; never twist your shoulders or torso. Ask for help when necessary.

According to the NIOSH, back injuries cost American industry $10 to $14 billion in workers' compensation costs and about 100 million workdays annually. Lifting/pushing supplies and equipment; lifting, positioning, and/or transporting patients; and reaching, stooping, bending, kneeling, and crouching are physical abilities required of the sleep lab technologist to perform essential job functions. Care must be taken to maneuver correctly to avoid injury.

EMERGENCY PLAN

A workplace emergency is an unforeseen situation that threatens your employees or patients. It may even disrupt your business because of physical or environmental damage to your facility. Nobody expects an emergency or disaster. Yet the simple truth is that emergencies and disasters can strike anyone, anytime, anywhere, and at any sleep center. The best way to protect yourself, your workers, and your patients is to expect the unexpected and develop a well-thought-out emergency action plan (EAP) to guide you when immediate action is necessary. An EAP is a written document required by OSHA standards and is often part of the sleep center's policy and procedure manual. Facilities must conduct and document emergency drills annually (1).

Emergencies may be natural or man-made and include the following:

- Floods
- Hurricanes
- Tornadoes
- Fires
- Toxic gas releases
- Chemical spills
- Radiologic accidents
- Explosions
- Civil disturbances
- Workplace violence resulting in bodily harm and trauma
- Active shooter

It is best to prepare to respond to an emergency before it happens. Few people can think clearly and logically in a crisis, so it is important to do so in advance when you have time to be thorough.

An EAP covers designated actions that employers and employees must take to ensure employee safety from fire and other emergencies. Even if you are not specifically required to do so, compiling an EAP is a good way to protect yourself, your employees, and your patients as well as your business during an emergency. An EAP should consist of the following:

- A preferred method for reporting fires and other emergencies
- An evacuation policy and procedure
- Emergency escape procedures and route assignments, such as floor plans, workplace maps, and safe or refuge areas
- Proper use of firefighting equipment such as extinguishers
- Contact list of names, titles, departments, and telephone numbers of individuals both within and outside your organization to contact for additional information or explanation of duties and responsibilities under the emergency plan (9)
- Procedures for employees who will perform critical tasks, such as shutting down critical plant operations, operating fire extinguishers, or carrying out other essential services before evacuating
- Rescue and medical duties for any workers designated to perform them. Designate an assembly location and procedures to account for all employees after an evacuation (9).

When developing your EAP, it is important to determine the following:

- Conditions under which an evacuation would be necessary
- A clear chain of command and designation of the individual in your facility authorized to order an evacuation or shutdown. Consider designating an evacuation warden to assist others in an evacuation and to account for patients and personnel.
- Specific evacuation procedures, including routes and exits. Post these procedures where they are easily accessible to all employees.
- Procedures for assisting people with disabilities or those who may have difficulty understanding verbal direction
- A designated group of people who will shut down critical operations during an evacuation
- A system for accounting for personnel and patients following an evacuation. Consider employees' transportation needs for community-wide evacuations.

Accounting for all employees and patients following an evacuation is critical. Confusion in the assembly areas can lead to delays in rescuing anyone trapped in the building, or unnecessary and dangerous search-and-rescue operations. To ensure the fastest, most accurate accountability of your employees and patients, you may want to consider including these steps in your EAP:

- Designate assembly areas where employees and patients should gather after evacuating.

- Take a head count after the evacuation. Identify the names and last-known locations of anyone not accounted for, and pass them to the official in charge.
- Establish procedures for further evacuation in case the incident turns into a major one. This may consist of sending employees and patients home by normal means or providing them with transportation to an off-site location.

Protecting the health and safety of everyone in the facility should be the first priority. In the event of a fire, an immediate evacuation to a predetermined area away from the facility is the best way to protect employees and patients.

When preparing your EAP, designate primary and secondary evacuation routes and exits. To the extent possible, ensure that evacuation routes and emergency exits meet the following conditions:

- Clearly marked and well lit
- Wide enough to accommodate the number of evacuating personnel
- Unobstructed and clear of debris at all times
- Unlikely to expose evacuating personnel to additional hazards

If drawings are prepared to show evacuation routes and exits, post them prominently for all employees to see.

The best EAP includes employees in the planning process. Specify employee procedures during an emergency, and ensure that employees receive proper training for emergencies. Encourage employees to offer suggestions about potential hazards, worst-case scenarios, and proper emergency responses. After developing the plan, allow employees to review procedures that take place before, during, and after the emergent event. Keep a copy of the EAP in a convenient location where employees can access it readily. With 10 or fewer employees, plans may be communicated orally (9). A review of the EAP should be performed and documented annually.

SECURITY THREATS

Terrorist threats both inside and outside of hospitals and clinics have grown steadily over the years. But security has often remained unchanged. Facilities lack electronic lockdown capability, creating vulnerability of patient data and making it difficult to defend against cyberattacks. Insider threats against hospitals from fired or disgruntled employees, physicians, patients, or relatives of patients who may find reason for revenge are growing. Physician terrorist "suicide/homicide" bombers were and are a continuing threat. Intensive international background checks of physician groups found potential bombers. Extensive background checks revealed misrepresentation of certifications and education, which exposes trusting patient populations to unqualified practitioners or other dangers.

In the event of a bomb threat, it is imperative for employees to maintain a calm environment and gather as much information as possible from the caller.

1. Ask the caller specific questions relating to the type, location, and time of detonation of the bomb.
2. Listen carefully to assess the voice quality of the caller. Are they calm? Excited? Angry? Do they speak fast? Slow? Loud? Slurred? With an accent? Note any background sounds such as traffic, airplanes, machinery, animals, music, or other details, which may assist in locating the caller.
3. Once the call has been terminated, immediately call 911 and give the operator specific details. This should be done as confidentially as possible so as not to incite panic.
4. Notify management that a bomb threat has been received.
5. Employees should awaken all patients and disconnect the head box from the amplifier. Evacuate and wait at a safe distance from the building for the authorities to arrive.
6. During the evacuation, employees should make a visual sweep for any unusual or suspicious items. If such an item is found, make a mental note of its description and location and report it once the authorities are on the scene. Do not touch or attempt to move the item.

With many sleep facilities located off-site, physical separation of workers from patients or the general public through the use of bullet-resistant barriers or enclosures has been proposed. The height and depth of counters are important considerations in protecting workers because they introduce physical distance between employees and potential attackers. Consideration must be given to the continued ease of conducting business; a safety device that increases frustration for workers or patients may be self-defeating.

Sleep technologists often find themselves alone at night in an office complex awaiting patient arrival for sleep testing. Visibility and lighting of parking areas and entrances are environmental design considerations that can be implemented to discourage workplace assaults. There should be safeguards to prevent patients from entering the building through unlocked doors, particularly at night. Consider minimal use of landscaping near entrances where attackers could hide. Security devices such as entry buzzers, closed-circuit cameras, alarms, card key access, and an intercom system in the entryway may deter potential perpetrators and improve staff safety. Advantages of providing panic buttons worn by technologists to immediately alert a facility security team or emergency services should be considered in the event the technologist is unable to reach a phone or is at immediate risk of injury or harm.

FIRE SAFETY

All employees should be educated on fire hazards in the workplace and trained for what to do in case of fire (9,10). A popular acronym used to remember the best approach to fire safety is RACE (rescue, alarm, contain, and evacuate).

- **Rescue:** Assistance to the patient is priority. Remove all patients from immediate danger.
- **Alarm:** Alert coworkers to a fire emergency. This may be accomplished using an alarm system, voice communication, or sound signals such as bells, whistles, or horns. Alert emergency personnel using an alarm system such as a fire alarm pull box or by dialing 911.
- **Contain:** Close doors, if possible, to contain a fire. Facilities may have an automatic door release when a fire alarm is activated. Attempts should be made to extinguish the flame by using an appropriate fire extinguisher for the classification of fire (Table 26-3). Many facilities have multipurpose extinguishers available. Multipurpose or "combination" extinguishers can be used for more than one classification of fire (10).
- **Evacuate:** Exit the building. The workplace must have exits suitably located and well-marked. Exits must be clearly visible and marked as an EXIT (9). Fire doors must not be blocked or locked. Exit routes must be kept clear of obstruction. No materials or equipment may be placed, either permanently or temporarily, within the exit route (10).

Correct use of a fire extinguisher should be revisited with staff during annual fire safety drills (10).

The acronym **PASS (pull, aim, squeeze, sweep)** reminds how to use the extinguisher:

- **Pull** the pin
- **Aim** the nozzle
- **Squeeze** the trigger
- **Sweep** at the base of the flame

Emergency evacuation plans must also be implemented for other environmental disasters that may be common to your geographic area. All employees should understand evacuation plans, be familiar with how to alert emergency personnel, and always be prepared to respond to disasters, such as fire, or severe weather, be it tornadoes, earthquakes, or hurricanes.

Table 26-3 Fire Classifications
Class A Fires
Fires of this type consist of ordinary combustibles, such as wood, paper, or cloth, and can be put out with water. Approach the fire and aim the nozzle toward the base of the flames, sweeping the extinguisher nozzle from side to side across the base of the flame. Continue spraying until all smoldering material is saturated.
A multipurpose dry-chemical extinguisher can also be used on class A fires. Attack at the edge of the fire, directing the nozzle in a sweeping motion. The powdered chemical becomes sticky when heated, allowing it to form a film that clings to the heated material and smothers the fire.
Class B Fires
Fires that burn flammable liquids, such as oil, gasoline, solvents, and paints, as their primary fuel are class B.
Dry-chemical extinguishers are the type usually used—starting about 8 ft (2.1 m) away from the fire and slowly moving closer, applying the substance from side to side near the fire's base.
Carbon dioxide extinguishers are also effective on flammable liquid fires. You must use this type near the edge of the fire at close range in an enclosed area where no wind or draft exists. Fires can spread with the presence of oxygen, but carbon dioxide decreases the amount of oxygen surrounding the fire until the air can no longer support the combustion.
Class C Fires
These fires involve electrical equipment. Water cannot be safely used to extinguish this type of fire because of the electrical conduction properties of water, which may deliver a shock to the firefighter. If the equipment can be deenergized, extinguishers for class A or B fires may be safely used. Otherwise, carbon dioxide and dry-chemical extinguishers are the best. Carbon dioxide is nonconductive and noncorrosive and leaves no sticky film, making cleanup easy.
Class D Fires
Class D fires involve combustible metals, such as magnesium, titanium, zirconium, sodium, lithium, and potassium. Special dry-compound powders, such as powdered graphite and sodium chloride, powdered talc, soda ash, and limestone, are made to extinguish these fires. In case of emergency, dry sand can be used.

ELECTRICAL SAFETY

OSHA's electrical standards address electricity as a serious workplace hazard, exposing employees or patients to such dangers as electric shock, electrocution, burns, fires, and explosions. OSHA electrical standards help minimize these potential hazards by specifying safety aspects in the design and use of electrical equipment and systems. Almost every electrical accident is preventable. To avoid accidents and potential injuries, some basic precautions can be taken.

Computers, fans, PAP devices, home sleep apnea testing devices, televisions, and any other electrical equipment should be tracked, inspected, and monitored annually. Reports of failures of such equipment must be logged.

Volts, watts, and amps measure electricity. Volts measure the "pressure" under which electricity flows. Amps measure the amount of electric current. Watts measure the amount of work done by a certain amount of current at a certain pressure or voltage. To understand this relationship, think of water in a hose. Turning on the faucet supplies the force that is comparable to the voltage. The amount of water moving through the hose is like the amperage. A lot of water (more wattage) is needed to wash a muddy car. Less water (lower wattage) is needed to fill a glass.

Resistance to the flow of electricity is measured in ohms. Some substances, such as metals, offer very little resistance to the flow of electric current and are called conductors. Other substances, such as porcelain, pottery, and dry wood, offer such a high resistance that they can be used to prevent the flow of electric current and are called insulators. Dry wood has a high resistance, but when saturated with water, its resistance drops to the point where it will readily conduct electricity. This is also true of human skin. When it is dry, the skin has a fairly high resistance to electric current, but when it is moist there is a radical drop in resistance. Pure water is a poor conductor, but small amounts of impurities, such as salt and acid (both of which are contained in perspiration), make it a ready conductor. When water is present either in the environment or on the skin, anyone working with electricity should exercise even more caution than they normally would.

Electricity travels in closed circuits, and its normal route is through a conductor. Ideally, current enters a device, flows through the electronics, and exits. Electric shock occurs when the body becomes a part of the electric circuit. The current must enter the body at one point and leave at another. If a person touches a bare conductor carrying current, this current will flow through the person to the ground. The effects of electric shock are variable depending on the amount of voltage, current, and duration of the contact. Effects can range from a barely perceptible tingle to immediate cardiac arrest. A severe shock can cause considerably more damage to the body than is visible. One may suffer internal hemorrhages and destruction of tissues, nerves, and muscles. In addition, shock is often only the beginning in a chain of events. The final injury may be from a fall, cuts, burns, or broken bones associated with the shock (Table 26-4).

Table 26-4 Effects of Electric Current in the Human Body

Current (mA)	Reaction
1	Perception level. Just a faint tingle.
5	Slight shock felt; not painful but disturbing. Average individual can let go. However, strong involuntary reactions to shocks in this range can lead to injuries.
6–25 (women)	Painful shock, muscular control is lost.
9–30 (men)	This is called the "freezing current" or "let-go" range.
50–150	Extreme pain, respiratory arrest, severe muscular contractions.[a] The individual cannot let go. Death is possible.
1,000–4,300	Ventricular fibrillation. (The rhythmic pumping action of the heart ceases.) Muscular contraction and nerve damage occur. Death is most likely.
10,000	Cardiac arrest, severe burns.

[a]If the extensor muscles are excited by the electric shock, the person may be thrown away from the circuit.

Electrical accidents are typically caused by a combination of three possible factors:

- Unsafe equipment and/or installation
- Workplaces made unsafe by the environment
- Unsafe work practices

Ways of protecting people from the hazards caused by electricity include proper insulation, proper electrical grounding, and safe work practices. The power cord is a conductor that is insulated by the rubber cording. This prevents accidental exposure to electrical current. The integrity of all power cords must be checked routinely. Equipment with a damaged cord should be taken out of use (Table 26-5).

Grounding is another method for protecting employees from electric shock. The term "ground" refers to a connecting circuit from the equipment to the earth. By grounding a tool or electrical system, a low-resistance path to the earth is intentionally created. Electrical current will follow the path of least resistance. This does not guarantee that no one will receive a shock, be injured,

Table 26-5 Safety Tips for Power Cords

Replace, do not attempt to fix, cords that have been cut or damaged. Exposed strands of wire can cause shock or burns.
Never unplug a power cord by pulling the cord.
If a cord or plug is warm or hot to the touch, unplug it immediately.
Check wires, cords, and electrical equipment for signs of wear.
Never place electric cords across traffic areas or under a carpet.
Never bend or remove the ground (third prong on a plug). It is designed to help prevent shock.

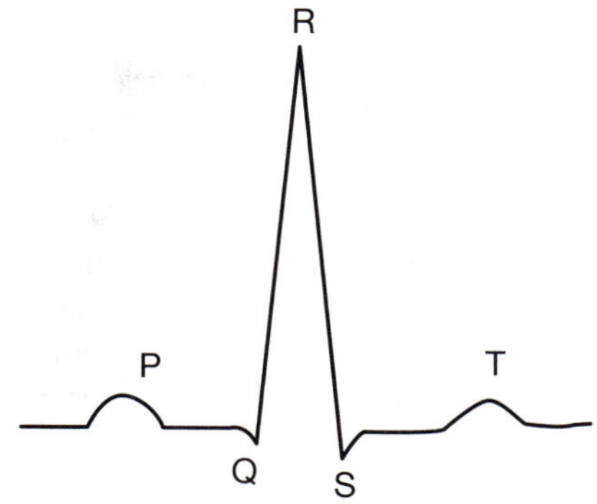

Figure 26-1 The electrocardiogram complex represents the electrical impulse traveling through the cardiac conductive pathway.

or be killed. It will, however, substantially reduce the possibility of such accidents.

Equipment grounding for safety should not be confused with the patient-ground connection. A patient-ground connection is used to help prevent line-frequency interference (50 or 60 Hz) by providing a conductive pathway from the patient to the ground through the recording system. In this case, the ground connection actually becomes a potential hazard because it may also become a pathway for a stray current. To prevent this possibility, a patient-ground connection must be isolated and equipped with a circuit breaker. Technologists must also be aware that all wires connected to the patient pose a potential electrical hazard to the patient. Care must be taken to prevent the electrode from coming in contact with any electrical equipment or any conductive or wet surfaces.

Employees and others working with electric equipment need to use safe work practices. This includes unplugging electric equipment before inspecting or making repairs, using electric tools that are in good repair, and using appropriate protective equipment. To ensure that they use safe work practices, employees must be aware of the electrical hazards to which they will be exposed. Through cooperative efforts, employers and employees can learn to identify and eliminate or control electrical hazards.

PATIENT EMERGENCIES

Cardiovascular Events

Patients with comorbid conditions such as underlying cardiac or pulmonary disease, coupled with hypoxia due to sleep-disordered breathing, are susceptible to cardiac arrhythmias. Early detection of, and response to, cardiac arrhythmia can save lives. Each heartbeat is the result of an electrical impulse traveling through the heart, causing depolarization of the atria and ventricles (Figure 26-1). Viewing the electrocardiogram (ECG) complex allows us to distinguish normal electrical conduction from cardiac ectopy, or abnormal electrical conduction. The P wave of the ECG complex represents atrial contraction. The P-R interval represents the hold time of the atrioventricular node. The QRS represents ventricular contraction. Knowing this helps us determine where in the electrical pathway the disruption occurs, thus better identifying the type of arrhythmia.

During sleep, heart rates of greater than 90 bpm indicate tachycardia, whereas a heart rate of less than 40 bpm indicates bradycardia (11). P waves of variable morphology indicate an atrial arrhythmia such as premature atrial contraction, atrial flutter, or atrial fibrillation. Atrial, or narrow complex, arrhythmia are generally not life-threatening. The technologist should document any occurrence in the technologist notes or study summary. The medical director must be notified if the patient becomes symptomatic, experiencing dizziness, light-headedness, syncope, cyanosis, or dyspnea.

A normal P-R interval has a duration of 0.12 to 0.20 seconds. An elongated P-R interval indicates a heart block. Varying degrees of heart blocks may be present. The normal duration of the QRS complex is 0.04 to 0.12 seconds. A longer, or wider, QRS segment indicates ventricular ectopy. Ventricular arrhythmias include premature ventricular contractions (PVCs), ventricular tachycardia, and ventricular fibrillation. Occasional PVCs are not uncommon and should be noted. Ventricular tachycardia and ventricular fibrillation are life-threatening. Technologists must activate the emergency medical system (EMS) and initiate cardiopulmonary resuscitation (CPR).

A pause of 3 seconds or more between beats is considered an episode of asystole (11). In the event of a cardiac or respiratory arrest, the patient care staff is responsible for activating the EMS and administering CPR until the emergency medical personnel arrive

(Table 26-6). Use mouthpieces, resuscitation bags, or other ventilation devices as an alternative to mouth-to-mouth resuscitation methods (12,13). Refer to Chapter 37 for more detail on arrhythmia.

The association between sleep apnea and systemic hypertension, stroke, congestive heart failure, and myocardial infarction has become more evident. Sudden cardiac arrest is the major complication of cardiovascular

Table 26-6 Medical Emergency Response

Emergency Situation	Response
• Chest pain, neck, jaw, or arm pain	• Initiate 2 L/min O_2 through nasal cannula. • Call the medical director. • Monitor the patient.
• Mild-to-moderate difficulty breathing	• Call the medical director. • Monitor the patient.
• Severe difficulty breathing	• Activate EMS. • Monitor the patient.
• Seizures without cardiac arrest	• Turn the patient on the side in case of vomiting. • Call the medical director. • Remain at the bedside to monitor and protect the patient.
• Symptoms of stroke, that is, paralysis, weakness of limbs, difficulty speaking, difficulty comprehending (F.A.S.T)	• Activate EMS. • Monitor the patient.
• Nausea/vomiting	• Provide emesis basin for patient. • Call the medical director.
• Fall/injury	• Call the lead technologist. • Complete the incident report.
• Spo_2 below 80% on 4 L/min of oxygen	• Awaken the patient. • Call the medical director. • Monitor the patient.
• Ventricular tachycardia for 10 s or more	• Awaken the patient. • Call the medical director. • Monitor the patient.
• Runs of premature ventricular contractions (six or more) occurring 3 or more times	• Awaken the patient. • Call the medical director. • Monitor the patient.
• Tachycardia 120 bpm or more over a minute or more or not associated with periods of apnea	• Awaken the patient. • Call the medical director. • Monitor the patient.
• Bradycardia <40 bpm over a minute or longer or not associated with periods of apnea	• Awaken the patient. • Call the medical director. • Monitor the patient.
• No electrocardiographic activity	• Assess the patient. • Activate EMS—first tech. • Begin cardiopulmonary resuscitation—additional staff.
• Parasomnia mobility (sleepwalking, active night terrors)	• Maintain patient safety. • Call security for assistance if applicable.
• Psychiatric emergency	• Maintain patient safety—remain with the patient. • Call security for assistance if applicable. • Visually monitor the suicidal patient until the situation is resolved.
• Grand mal seizures	• Activate EMS. • Go to the bedside to maintain patient safety. • Avoid placing anything in or near the patient's mouth. • Roll the patient on the side to prevent aspiration. • Document clinical observations.

EMS, emergency medical system.

disease. The American Heart Association (AHA) has defined separate *chains of survival* for in-hospital and out-of-hospital events to summarize the present understanding of the best approach to the treatment of persons with sudden cardiac arrest (12). The chain of survival consists of five links:

1. *Surveillance and Prevention*
   - Recognize patients at risk and have the necessary equipment available to resuscitate if needed.
2. *Call for help*
   - Recognize the warning signs of heart attack or stroke, and activate the EMS by calling 911 or code blue where available.
3. *Initiate CPR*
   - Immediate high-quality CPR increases positive outcomes. Compress the chest 2 in (5 cm) at a rate of 100 to 120 per minute. Allow for full recoil of the chest between compressions. Deliver 2 breaths after 30 compressions. Repeat as needed.
4. *Provide defibrillation*
   - The interval between collapse and defibrillation is critical for successful conversion from ventricular fibrillation to a normal heart rhythm. Every minute that passes reduces the chance of survival. Without CPR and defibrillation, few attempts at resuscitation are successful. Automatic external defibrillators (AEDs) are easy to use and provide automatic recognition of a shockable cardiac arrhythmia. Voice commands warn before a shock is administered.
5. *Advanced life support and post arrest care*
   - Advanced cardiac life support provides equipment to support ventilation, establishes intravenous access, administers drugs, and controls arrhythmias.

These links are interdependent and must all be strong to increase the patient's chance of survival.

Warning signs of heart attack include lingering chest discomfort; discomfort in other areas of the upper body such as arms, back, neck, or stomach; sweating; nausea/vomiting; shortness of breath; and light-headedness. These signs may develop in persons of any age or sex, at any time or place.

Signs and symptoms of acute stroke include alterations in consciousness (seizures, confusion, delirium, stupor, or coma), intense or unusually severe headache, incoherent speech, facial weakness, poor balance/clumsiness, visual loss, intense vertigo, double vision, unilateral hearing loss, and nausea or vomiting. The American Stroke Association recommends utilizing F.A.S.T warning signs as a tool to spot a stroke (14).

- F = Face Drooping—One-sided facial drooping. Ask the patient to smile; is it uneven?
- A = Arm Weakness—One arm with weakness or numbness; can the patient raise both arms? Does one arm fall to the side?
- S = Speech difficulty—Slurred speech?
- T = Time to call 911 immediately, every minute matters. Document time of first symptom and report.

Sleep center personnel are first responders for medical emergencies. It is imperative that technologists are certified in CPR and trained to recognize a change in a patient's condition that may be life-threatening. American Heart Association's Guidelines for CPR and ECC are the recommended guidelines to follow.

In 2010, the AHA changed the emphasis of CPR away from assessment and more toward action, changing the A-B-Cs (airway, breathing, and circulation) to C-A-Bs (circulation, airway, and breathing). The survivability rate is 40% to 70% when CPR is performed, and an AED is utilized in the first 3 to 5 minutes post arrest (13). Compress the victim's chest at least 100 times per minute with enough force to circulate blood to the brain (Table 26-6). Every interruption in chest compressions stops blood flow to the brain, which can lead to brain death. Cease compressions only long enough to allow the AED to analyze a cardiac rhythm or to deliver two breaths. Immediately resume compressions. It takes several compressions to get the blood moving again. Consider "hands-only CPR" if protective or airway equipment is not available. Reassess the victim every 2 minutes to evaluate the need for continued efforts.

Attach a defibrillator to the bare chest of anyone needing CPR, ensuring the pads do not touch. If the victim has an implantable pacemaker or port where the pads should reside, place the pad 1 inch (2.5 cm) below the device. Dry shave a hairy chest before placing the pads. Follow the AED voice prompts. The AED shocks for ventricular fibrillation only.

Pediatric adaptable AEDs are available. These use either pediatric pads or a dose attenuator adapter. If you are in a situation where a child requires CPR and no pediatric AED pads are available, use adult pads, but be sure that the pads do not touch. For a small child, place one pad on the sternum and the second pad on the victim's back between the shoulder blades.

Seizures

A seizure is a sudden discharge of electrical activity in the brain. There are two broad categories of seizures: generalized and partial (also called local or focal). Generalized seizures broadcast across the entire brain, while a small area of the brain produces partial seizures. Symptoms may include a brief loss of consciousness, lip smacking, chewing, muscle rigidity, spasms, or convulsions. The duration of a seizure may be several seconds to several minutes.

The technologist's response to patient seizure activity will vary according to the type of seizure occurring. The technologist's responsibility is to keep the patient safe. Knowing the patient history and the manifestation of the seizure will help with preparedness. Pad the headboard and use padded side rails as necessary. During grand mal seizures, also known as generalized tonic-clonic seizures, go to the patient's bedside to keep the patient safe by turning them on the side to prevent aspiration, loosen tight clothing around the neck, and put something soft under the head. Never attempt to restrain a patient or to stop their movement, and never place any object or fingers in or near the patient's mouth.

Document clinical observations such as the duration of the seizure, cyanosis, diaphoresis, movement type, and involvement. Speak calmly and reassuringly to the patient during and after the event. Give nothing by mouth until the patient is fully alert.

Activate EMS if the Following Occur

- The seizure lasts 5 minutes or longer or if one seizure occurs right after another without the person regaining consciousness between seizures.
- Seizures occur closer together than usual for the patient.
- This is a first-time seizure.
- The patient is injured or pregnant.
- Breathing becomes difficult, or the person appears to be choking.

Psychiatric Emergency (Suicidal Ideation)

According to the National Institute of Mental Health (NIHM), people of all backgrounds can be at risk of suicide, which has become the leading cause of death in the US. Emergency policies must address psychiatric emergencies specifically relating to suicidal ideation. Technologists must be prepared should a psychiatric emergency arise in the sleep lab setting (1,15).

If a Patient Threatens Harm to Themselves

1. Assess the situation; are staff or the patient in immediate danger?
2. Activate emergency personnel; call 911 immediately.
3. Contact facility director or call physician if patient threatened suicide.
4. Remain calm, listen attentively to the patient, do not offer advice.
5. Keep the patient within view at all times.
6. Document all information in the medical record.
7. Include facility director's and clinical managers' contact information in the policy.

PATIENT SAFETY EVENT REPORTING

The American Academy of Sleep Medicine (AASM) has formalized standards and policy for risk management in sleep facilities. These include Patient Safety Risk Analysis, Significant Adverse and Unusual Event Reporting. Sleep facilities must have formal written policies in place outlining the risk management processes of the facility. This should include reporting patient safety risks, documentation, and analysis of adverse events. Risk analysis must be reviewed and documented on an annual basis (1).

VIOLENT PATIENTS

Although uncommon, the sleep technologist may encounter an aggressive or violent patient in the sleep center setting. The best way to reduce the chances of such an encounter is through careful screening of patients before a sleep study. However, to ensure the safety of the patient and the staff, it is important for sleep technologists to understand how to handle inappropriate behavior. Sleep facilities and organizations should provide formal de-escalation training for staff.

Aggression may take the form of angry shouting or accusing others of wrongdoing. Aggression may also involve physical violence such as breaking objects or harming others. When working with patients who have a history of mental illness or dementia, it is recommended that a familiar caregiver stays with the patient. Some individuals may be easily confused and suspicious that others are trying to do harm to them. A recognizable caregiver may ward off such suspicions. Other causes of violence include delusions or hallucinations, reactions to drugs, and pain. Medication may reduce aggression and violence. On the contrary, medications that calm the patient may produce sleepiness or increase confusion.

Many patients who become violent are not violent from the moment they come through the door. A patient should be provided with alternatives to correct inappropriate behavior to enable them to maintain a good working relationship with the technologist while maintaining dignity. There are several important things to keep in mind to avoid escalating a potentially violent situation. Some suggested methods of working with potentially violent patients include the following:

1. Avoid eye contact with the patient.
2. Do not block exits, and leave the door to the room open.
3. Maintain distance from a potentially violent patient; do not invade the patient's "space."
4. Adopt a passive, nonconfrontational posture and attitude, and allow the patient to ventilate feelings.
5. Develop a therapeutic alliance with the patient.
6. Treat the patient as you expect them to behave.

7. Offer food or drink.
8. Do not make challenging, provocative, or belligerent remarks.
9. If the patient acts out, tell them directly, "Your behavior is frightening others, and we cannot allow such behavior."
10. Do not turn your back on a potentially violent patient.
11. Never underestimate the potential for violence.

If a situation arises in which the technologist feels uncomfortable with the patient, the former should call security and/or send the patient home.

Policies and procedures should be in place for training staff to recognize escalating behavior that might lead to violence and to assess and report threats and allow employers to track and follow up on threats and violent incidents in the workplace. Training employees in nonviolent conflict resolution, de-escalation techniques, cultural/ethical diversity training, and how to handle complaints will help alleviate behavior that could escalate to physical violence.

SUMMARY

Federal, state, and local agencies and accrediting bodies have developed guidelines to ensure the safety of all individuals visiting or working in the health care setting. A written emergency and safety plan will ensure that each employee understands the practices required to maintain the highest level of safety. It is the responsibility of each member of the health care team to understand and implement safety standards to prevent accident, injury, or illness from occurring.

REFERENCES

1. American Academy of Sleep Medicine. Standards for accreditation. Published 2025. Accessed April 1, 2025. https://aasm.org/wp-content/uploads/2024/05/Standards-for-Accreditation-1.1.2025-New-Model_Final.pdf
2. Centers for Disease Control and Prevention. Infection control: infection control in healthcare personnel: infrastructure and routine practices. 2024. https://www.cdc.gov/infection-control/hcp/healthcare-personnel-infrastructure-routine-practices/
3. United States Department of Labor. OSHA quick card. Published 2024. Accessed March 10, 2024. http://www.osha.gov/sites/default/files/publications/OSHA3493QuickCardSafetyDataSheet.pdf
4. OSHA Bloodborne Pathogen Standard. Title 29 Code of Federal Regulation, Part 1910.1030. US Department of Labor.
5. Rutala WA, Weber DJ; Healthcare Infection Control Practices Advisory Committee. Guideline for disinfection and sterilization in healthcare facilities, 2008. Centers for Disease Control and Prevention. Published 2024. Updated June 2024. https://www.cdc.gov/infection-control/media/pdfs/Guideline-Disinfection-H.pdf
6. American Academy of Sleep Technologists. *Covid-19 sleep lab guideline*. Published 2020. Accessed April 8, 2025. http://aastweb.org
7. United States Environmental Protection Agency. Learn the basics of hazardous waste. Accessed April 1, 2025. https://www.epa.gov/hw/learn-basics-hazardous-waste
8. Occupational Safety and Health Administration. Hazardous waste operations and emergency response (Standard 1910.120). United States Department of Labor. 2025. https://www.osha.gov/emergency-preparedness/hazardous-waste-operations/standards
9. Occupational Safety and Health Administration. Exit routes and emergency planning. Subpart E, part 1910. Accessed April 1, 2025. https://www.osha.gov/laws-regs/regulations/standardnumber/1910/1910.38
10. Fire Extinguisher: 101. Fire hazards (fire prevention tips). Accessed April 1, 2025. http://www.fire-extinguisher101.com/hazards.html
11. Troester MM, Quan SF, Berry RB, et al; for the American Academy of Sleep Medicine. *The AASM Manual for the Scoring of Sleep and Associated Events: Rules, Terminology and Technical Specifications: Version 3*. American Academy of Sleep Medicine; 2023.
12. American Heart Association. *Basic Life Support for Healthcare Providers*. American Heart Association; 2020.
13. American Heart Association. *CPR Guidelines*. American Heart Association; 2020.
14. American Stroke Association. *Stroke symptoms*. Published 2025. Accessed April 8, 2025. http://stroke.org
15. National Institute of Mental Health. *Suicide prevention*. Published 2024. Accessed April 1, 2025. https://www.nimh.nih.gov/health/topics/suicide-prevention

SUGGESTED READING

The Joint Commission. *Sentinel Event Alert issue 59: physician and verbal violence against health care workers*. June 18, 2021. https://www.jointcommission.org/en-us/knowledge-library/newsletters/sentinel-event-alert/issue-59

Chapter 27 Patient Interviewing and Assessment

KIMBERLY A. TROTTER

KEY CONCEPTS/LEARNING OBJECTIVES

On completion of this chapter, the reader should be able to:

1. Review patient chart documentation, including physician order, history, and physical examination; review protocols; and analyze and respond to unclear, inappropriate, or contradictory orders.
2. Interview and observe the patient to assess special physical, cognitive, or emotional needs, recognize patients with special needs (mental age, physical, or emotional discomfort) and assess patients' readiness to learn and their ability to cooperate, orient the patient to the facility and testing procedure utilizing appropriate technologist-patient interaction, and determine the need for any special precautions or special testing considerations (prosthetic devices, electromechanical devices, etc).
3. Identify the patient's current sleep schedule, recent caffeine or alcohol intake, and current medications, and interview the patient during the setup to clarify any gaps in history or symptoms identified during chart review, documenting any special needs identified or pertinent clinical information in the patient's chart.
4. Discuss positive airway pressure and other therapeutic modalities with the patient and assist with pre- and postprocedure questionnaires and follow-up processes.

KEY TERMS

Emotional needs
Forensic patients
Patient assessment
Physical limitations
Prosthetic devices
Readiness to learn
Safe Patient Handling
Sundowning
Universal precautions

It is a unique encounter every night when the sleep technologist performs a polysomnogram (PSG) and reviews a patient's chart for the first time. The technologist may not know anything about the patient they are about to see. Perhaps a sleep consultation was performed before the PSG; however, the needs of the patient have to be evaluated during the initial meeting in the sleep center by the sleep technologist. Sometimes, clinical notes are not as exact as we would like them to be. If the sleep consultation was performed by the referring physician, it may be vague and general. This is why patient interviewing and assessment are so important in making the most of the sleep study and, most importantly, ensuring that the patient's accommodations are met.

CHART REVIEW

It is important for a daytime sleep technologist or other clinical staff to review all charts before the night shift, because there may be special testing or equipment that needs to be set up before the night shift arrives. Once the nighttime sleep technologist arrives, they should thoroughly review the chart as well.

The chart should contain a recent history and physical (H&P). This is a report of the patient's general health status, regular medications, past surgeries, and family history. The H&P can come from the primary care physician or referring physician. Reviewing this information is helpful to understand the patient's general status. If the patient is a "direct referral," meaning they bypassed the sleep consultation and workup with the sleep specialist, and is referred directly for a sleep study, then a comprehensive H&P with sleep-specific information is very important and is a required American Academy of Sleep Medicine (AASM) accreditation standard.

The sleep consultation is an integral part of the chart. It should be reviewed by the sleep technologist. Information such as sleep medications, sleep schedule, chief complaint, and family sleep history should all be addressed in the sleep consultation. During the consultation, a sleep questionnaire, sleepiness scale, and a sleep diary that typically consists of 2 weeks of data are usually obtained.

If the patient was referred directly to the sleep disorders center by the referring physician, the sleep questionnaire may be administered to the patient on their arrival at the sleep center. The technologist will need to assess whether the patient is able to read, understand, and answer the questions. The technologist may need to assist the patient by asking the questions. Once the sleep questionnaire is filled out, then the technologist will have information needed to determine what degree of special or accommodating treatment the patient may need. The technologist must make certain that the patient is able to fill out the pre- and postsleep questionnaires as well and assist if necessary.

The physician order form must be included in each PSG patient chart. It must give clear instructions regarding what type of procedures are to be performed. It must also be clear if the patient has any special needs or considerations for their care. This documentation is very important to the technologist and, consequently, to the patient.

MEETING AND ASSESSING THE PATIENT

As mentioned, the sleep technologist is at a disadvantage before they first meet the patient, unless they have had prior information that can be reviewed. Meeting and assessing the patient may be the only information the technologist gets regarding special needs or other considerations.

Visual Assessment

Visual assessment occurs when the sleep technologist first meets the patient. How does the patient look, in terms of appearance, attire, demeanor, and general health? Is the patient alert or sleeping in the chair? Does the patient seem nervous or relaxed? Are there any visible challenges?

Readiness to Learn

Once the formal introductions are made, and the technologist escorts the patient to the sleep room, it is time to check their readiness to learn. Readiness to learn is based on the perceived need, attitude, and beliefs (1). It is a phrase used to determine by casual interview of the patient if they are ready to learn. Obstacles to readiness to learn include emotional factors, such as anxiety, distraction, or inattention; knowledge or experiential, such as not understanding the language or not understanding the reason for the sleep study; and physical conditions, such as hearing loss or excessive sleepiness.

Mental and Developmental Age

Mental age is defined as cognitive abilities compared to the typical abilities of individuals at various chronologic ages. Similarly, developmental age encompasses a broader concept of physical, emotional, and social development alongside cognitive abilities (2). Do they seem to understand simple words and phrases? Does the patient act as though they are 13 years old, although they are really 35? This is important information, so the sleep technologist can simplify their presentation to the patient if necessary, assuring the patient that they will be able to understand the process and cooperate better.

Physical Limitations

Often, physical limitations will be obvious when the sleep technologist first greets the patient. This valuable information may also be found in the patient's chart, the physician order form, sleep questionnaire, or consultation notes. If the patient was referred directly to the sleep center and the referring physician conducted the sleep consultation, this information may not be present because the referring physician was familiar with the patient and may not have considered it an issue for the sleep study. This can result in a challenge for the technologist.

Emotional Needs

Emotional needs may be the most difficult to determine. If the patient seems withdrawn or distant, it will be a difficult night for both the sleep technologist and the patient, unless the technologist is able to break through and reach the patient, making them feel more comfortable and assured. Sometimes, emotional needs are related to mental or developmental age; the patient may need more reassuring and attention. It is important to note that patients will sometimes act out in order to receive this added attention. In cases like this, the sleep technologist needs to set boundaries with the amount of attention and service they can give the patient. This is important when the sleep technologist is monitoring two patients because if they are overly busy with one, then the other patient suffers.

PATIENT ORIENTATION PROCESSES

Facility Orientation

When the patient arrives, the sleep technologist will escort them to the sleep room and show them other pertinent areas of the facility that they may need to use, such as the bathroom, showers, and areas to store food. The technologist should allow them the opportunity to ask questions.

Patient Confidentiality, Patient Rights, and Other Forms

The Health Insurance Portability and Accountability Act of 1996 requires each patient to sign an acknowledgment of receipt of patient confidentiality regulations. If this is the patient's first visit to the center and they have not previously signed this form, this must be collected by the technologist. Many facilities, particularly hospitals, also make a copy of information pertaining to patient rights and responsibilities available to the patient.

Procedure Consent

In many sleep centers, the technologist may have the patient review and sign a consent form, which describes the procedure. If the patient is to be videotaped, the technologist may obtain consent for this as well.

Recognizing and Accommodating Patients With Special Emotional Needs

Once the sleep technologist has had time to assess the patient's emotional needs, it is time to work with the patient to obtain a quality sleep study.

What Are Special Emotional Needs?

Special emotional needs are related to patients with disorders that include posttraumatic stress disorder (PTSD), depression, panic attacks, claustrophobia, and more serious mental illnesses. As stated previously, mental and developmental age can play a part in relation to special emotional needs.

The sleep technologist must develop strategies for dealing with these types of patients. For patients with PTSD, it is important to find out the best way to communicate with them during the night and, more importantly, the best way to wake them up should the technologist need to adjust sensors or apply positive airway pressure (PAP). Waking a patient with PTSD the wrong way can result in injury to the technologist! Ask the patient before lights out how they should be awakened. Some patients may prefer being awakened using the intercom, and others may need the light on and to be called from the doorway. A night light may also be appropriate.

PAP titration for these patients, as well as patients with claustrophobia, can be tricky, and these patients should be treated with caution and great care. Always allow the patient to be in control of the mask on the face. If the patient starts feeling panicky (a common symptom of PTSD), then they can take the mask off the face and try again later. Always remind the patient to breathe slowly, focusing on breathing out. A full-face mask, which equalizes the positive pressure delivered between the nose and the mouth allowing the patient to breathe with the mouth open, may be helpful. Sometimes, a nasal mask or nasal pillows can make the patient feel less claustrophobic. Nasal pillows or other types of small masks that do not touch the patient's face can be less restrictive and more comfortable. The technologist's impressions should always be documented in the patient's chart.

Depression is not evident in all patients, but in those who seem down or disengaged, it is important to identify possible depression. It is important to note that the technologist is not licensed to diagnose the patient but to merely document their impressions. Dealing with depressed patients can be challenging, and the technologist should try to be sensitive to the patient's needs. Spending extra time with the depressed patient is important, especially if they seem withdrawn about the procedure.

Some patients may tell the technologist that they have panic attacks at night. These panic attacks may be related to obstructive sleep apnea (OSA) or PTSD. Assure such patients that you are nearby should they feel anxious.

The best way to handle the patient with a mental disorder is to be calm and not argumentative. Ideally, the medical director or sleep physician would have screened out unstable patients, and you will not see them in the sleep center until they are stable. If the technologist feels threatened in any way, they should immediately leave the room and contact security, if available, or the medical director or call 9-1-1. A technologist should never allow a patient to stand between them and the exit of the room. A sleep center policy for these types of situations should be available.

Recognizing and Accommodating Patients With Special Physical Needs

Patients who come to the sleep center with physical disabilities can be a challenge for the technologist. The referring physician should mention these disabilities in the H&P or consultation notes. If the patient is severely disabled, then it may be helpful for a caregiver to be present for the entire sleep study to assist with lifting and other personal needs. Sleep technologists should also be trained in Safe Patient Handling (SPH) and get practical annual training and competency in assistive devices such as lifting equipment and transfer sheets (3).

If the patient has a prosthetic device or some other type of device necessary for mobility, the technologist must be aware of such devices and work around the device during the setup. If the patient has a prosthetic leg, the electromyographic electrodes must be placed on the leg above the prosthetic device or on the forearms for the detection of periodic limb movement disorder, and the alternative placement must be documented. If a patient has a prosthetic eye, it is important to document this information in the patient's chart, the technologist notes, and on the record. Some prosthetic eyes do generate some eye movements if attached to the muscle, while others do not. The sleep technologist should pay close attention to the movements during biocalibrations.

If the patient has an unusually shaped head or has a plate or cover over a part of the skull, the technologist must modify the 10-20 system of electrode placement and document in the patient chart and in the technologist notes.

Infection control is another important area for using precautions with patients. If the patient is incontinent, then the technologist must know how to deal with body fluids properly. An in-service on infection control techniques by the hospital's infection control nurse is important so that the technologist knows how to protect themself and the patient. The same is true if the patient has a severe productive cough. Universal precautions (gloves, masks, and protective wear) must be strictly followed for all patients but are particularly important for patients requiring special precautions. Droplet or airborne precautions may need to be instituted to prevent the spread of certain respiratory pathogens.

If the patient complains of pain, discomfort, or anxiety, immediate interventions are needed. The technologist must check on the patient, assess the situation, and determine a solution. The solution might be calling the on-call sleep physician to get input or to have the physician talk to the patient over the phone to calm and reassure them. If the sleep center is in a hospital, it may involve paging the on-call physician or nursing supervisor so they can evaluate the patient and determine if there is any risk in continuing the study. Some patients may need to end the study and go to the emergency department for further evaluation and treatment.

OTHER CHALLENGES

Sundowning

Sometimes, older patients can present as normal and fully functional during the daytime for the sleep consultation, but at night, they may exhibit "sundowning." Patients showing signs of sundowning become confused and agitated during the early evening. Patients with sundowning can be a challenge to work with. These patients may already be diagnosed with Alzheimer disease or other forms of dementia. Sleep disorders can make the symptoms worse (4). If a patient is known to have sundowning, then they should be required to bring a loved one or attendant for the sleep study. Bringing familiar items from home can be helpful too, such as bedding and photos. If the sundowning comes as a "surprise" to the technologist, then the technologist should calmly talk to the patient, with the lights on, so the patient can become accustomed to the surroundings and remember that they are at the sleep center. If the patient continues to fight the testing procedure and becomes aggressive and agitated, then the technologist will have no other choice but to call a family member or caregiver to pick up the patient. This situation can be dangerous to the technologist who is not trained to deal with sundowning.

Violent/Inappropriate Behaviors

If a patient becomes violent or abusive to the technologist, be it verbal abuse, sexual innuendo, or physical movements or action, the technologist should immediately address the situation. Does the technologist feel physically threatened? If so, the technologist should leave the patient's room immediately and follow the sleep center security policy, which may include calling security or the local police. If the technologist feels that the patient is being inappropriate but believes the sleep study could still be performed, a technologist switch (if there is more than one technologist working) is usually the best first step and is usually successful in stopping such behavior. Simply have another technologist (same sex as the patient if possible) come in and assume care of the patient. If the patient is reminded that they are being videotaped, inappropriate behavior usually stops as well.

Forensic Patients

Another situation that appears to be dangerous, but that is actually the safest of all patient interactions, is dealing with the forensic patient. Incarcerated patients, or forensic patients, are those who are brought in from prison for a sleep study. These patients are secured in shackles and are accompanied by two guards who remain in the sleep center for the entire night. Other than the shackles getting in the way of the hookup, and the space needed for two guards and a patient in one room, there is little threat. If the sleep center is in a hospital setting, then the hospital will have its own policy on forensic patients. Most policies involve contacting security on the day of the study and having the forensic patient and guards check in and out with security on arrival and after the sleep study. It is important to be sensitive to the other patients by rooming the forensic patient, if possible, before others arrive.

Diabetes

Some medical disorders, such as diabetes, may involve the patient requiring medications and food during the night. Simply allow the patient to do what they need to do, as if they were at home. It is, however, important that the patient be reminded to bring their regular medication, supplies, and snacks for their sleep study because most sleep centers are outpatient based, with no readily available sources of food or medications. If the patient uses injections, the syringes will need to be disposed of properly, preferably in a sharps container.

Language Barriers

The technologist may see patients who do not speak English. If the sleep center is stand-alone and not supported by a hospital or does not have translation technology available, the patient should bring an interpreter or family member who speaks English, and that person should remain with the patient for the entire sleep study to ensure that the technologist can communicate with the patient. Another option is using a language line service with a live phone or video interpreter. Many of these services offer most of the spoken languages. If the patient requires PAP during the night, the patient will most likely not understand the equipment or process being initiated without an interpreter.

REVIEW PHYSICIAN ORDERS

When reviewing the chart, the physician orders need to make sense to the technologist. After assessing the patient, the technologist should ask themselves the question, are the orders appropriate? If the orders are unclear or inappropriate or contradictory, it is important to contact the referring physician or the medical director to confirm the order or discuss a change in procedure. It is important to note that when a revised order is taken over the phone it must be documented, dated, and timed and that the sleep physician must sign the revised order the next day. This is easily completed if the sleep center uses an electronic health record (EHR), which is accessible securely and remotely.

ORIENT PATIENT TO TEST PROCEDURE

Explain PSG Protocol to Patient

Education begins with the patient instructions given to the patient when they are scheduled for their sleep study. Sometimes, these instructions are electronic, allowing for an embedded video that can describe the process ahead of time. Educating the patient about the setup and monitoring process will help the patient feel more at ease with the procedure. Explain that a PSG is a test that records various physiologic signals during sleep and that testing may vary on the basis of individual patient needs and physician's orders. Describe what the PSG measures and the sensors as you apply them. A common concern voiced by patients is that they may be unable to sleep with all the monitoring leads attached. A reassuring response to this concern may be, "surprisingly, most people sleep very well. After a period of adjustment, you easily forget about the electrodes. All the attachments are made in such a way as to provide easy movement during sleep." Document how the patient feels about undergoing the PSG and their level of cooperation with the procedure.

Discuss Therapeutic Modalities

The most common therapeutic procedure technologists perform during PSG is PAP titration for sleep-related breathing disorders. The technologist has an important role in the orientation of the patient to the PAP device because the patient's first impression and experience with the device is likely to strongly influence their compliance. The patient should be shown and allowed to handle the equipment. Many centers utilize educational videos, which are readily available through PAP equipment manufacturers. It is best to fit the patient and let the patient apply the PAP mask and experience PAP at a low level for a short trial period before the beginning of the study, especially if the order is for a split-night sleep study. This will avoid having to wake the patient to fit the mask and get acclimated for PAP therapy in the middle of the night.

The patient may display poor sleep hygiene, such as watching late night TV, scrolling on their tablet or phone, or eating or drinking throughout the night. This should be documented in the chart, and good sleep hygiene education can be performed by the sleep technologist at the beginning or following the sleep study. Sleep hygiene education can also be made available to the patient during the follow-up, provided the technologist documented the behavior.

PATIENT INTERVIEW

Patient Questionnaire

Most sleep centers require the patient to complete a sleep-focused questionnaire that is reviewed by the technologist. The technologist should discuss key information in the questionnaire with the patient and clarify any incomplete or missing information. Ask for a brief history of medical illnesses and compare the patient's response with the physician's consult notes. Patients often forget to discuss certain problems with their physician. A review of medications is also necessary, keeping in mind that many medications affect electroencephalographic patterns. The questionnaire should have a section for additional technologist notes from the patient interview. The questionnaire may be the primary tool for the technologist to understand their patient's needs, especially if they were a direct referral with an abbreviated H&P.

Presleep Questionnaire

After the technologist asks the patient to complete a presleep questionnaire (Figure 27-1), the technologist will review the patient's responses and ask for missing information. This questionnaire generally reviews caffeine or alcohol intake, medications, physical complaints, sleep within the previous 24 hours, and unusual aspects of the day's activities. It may also include a sleepiness scale (Tables 27-1 and 27-2). For patients returning for a subsequent sleep study, further information should be obtained regarding interim treatments, change in medications, or changes in sleep patterns. Questions and sleepiness scale numbers can also be compared from previous studies and visits.

Verbal Interview

In addition to the patient questionnaire, there are a number of verbal questions (Figure 27-2) the technologist may ask the patient in order to get a clearer picture of their sleep habits and sleep problems. If the bed partner is present, obtain their input during the written or verbal interview. Many sleep problems, such as snoring

Name: ____________________ Date: __________

How many hours of sleep did you have last night? __________

How many hours do you normally have? __________

Did you take any naps today? Yes No

If yes, how long did you nap? __________ minutes

Did you get your normal amount of exercise today? Yes No

If no, why not? __________

Has today been an unusual day in any respect? Yes No

If yes, please explain: ____________________

Do you have any physical discomfort now? Yes No

If yes, what? ____________________

If you had alcohol, coffee, tea, or soft drinks today, specify amounts and times:

Type	Amount	Time

List all medications you took today:

Medications	Amount	Time

Figure 27-1 Presleep questionnaire.

Table 27-1 Stanford Sleepiness Scale

Degree of Sleepiness	Scale Rating
Feeling active, vital, alert, or wide awake	1
Functioning at high levels but not at peak; able to concentrate	2
Awake but relaxed; responsive but not fully alert	3
Somewhat foggy, let down	4
Foggy; losing interest in remaining awake; slowed down	5
Sleepy, woozy, fighting sleep; prefer to lie down	6
No longer fighting sleep, sleep onset soon; having dream-like thoughts	7
Asleep	X

From Hoddes E, Zarcone V, Smythe H, Phillips R, Dement WC. Quantification of sleepiness: A new approach. *Psychophysiology*. 1973; 10(4):431-436. Reprinted by permission of John Wiley & Sons, Inc.

or cessation of breathing, are not evident to the patient, and the bed partner is able to give a more objective assessment of these symptoms.

The best way for a technologist to begin the verbal interview is to discuss the patient's nighttime routine before bedtime. Assess whether the patient may have special needs. Ask if there are any specific physical or psychological discomforts that may prevent a patient from achieving a normal night's sleep. If a PAP titration is ordered, ask if the patient has nasal congestion or blockage.

Table 27-2 Epworth Sleepiness Scale

0 = Would *never* doze or sleep	
1 = *Slight* chance of dozing or sleeping	
2 = *Moderate* chance of dozing or sleeping	
3 = *High* chance of dozing or sleeping	
Situation	**Chance of Dozing or Sleeping**
Sitting and reading	_______
Watching TV	_______
Sitting inactive in a public place	_______
Being a passenger in a motor vehicle for an hour or more	_______
Lying down in the afternoon	_______
Sitting and talking to someone	_______
Stopped for a few minutes in traffic while driving	_______
Total score	_______
Score results	
1–6	Within normal limits
4–8	Moderately sleepy
9 and over	Excessively sleepy

From Johns MW. A new method for measuring daytime sleepiness: The Epworth sleepiness scale. *Sleep*. 1991;14(6):540-545. Reproduced by permission of American Sleep Disorders Association and Sleep Research Society.

Patient Interaction/Interview During Testing

The technologist should reassure the patient that they can contact the technologist at any time during the night using the intercom system. If a patient is restless and not sleeping, check to see if they need something to make them more comfortable.

If the patient has difficulty tolerating initiation of PAP therapy, take the time to determine if there is a physical barrier such as nasal blockage or if the patient simply cannot or does not want to use the device.

If the technologist notices a significant physiologic event, such as a possible seizure or cardiac event, the technologist must immediately go to the patient and assess their vital signs and cognitive status through verbal questioning. Utilize the sleep lab's medical emergency protocols and document.

Medications

The technologist must also confirm the patient's medications and document the medications taken on the day of the study, including over-the-counter medicines, vitamins, supplements, caffeine, and alcohol intake. In most states, medications cannot be administered by a sleep technologist. Medications can be brought in by the patient and self-administered. The technologist must document what medications were taken, dosage, and time. Medications, especially sleeping medications that the patient may take before the testing, must be closely monitored. If a patient takes a sleeping medication and then wants to discontinue the study, the sleep center and technologist might be liable if the patient drove home incapacitated from the medication. If a patient takes sleeping medication, then wakes up during the night and wants to discontinue the sleep study, the technologist must ensure that the patient is driven home or stays until it is safe for them to drive (typically, until morning). It is important for the sleep technologist to understand the half-life (how long a medication stays in the patient's system) of the most common sleeping medications, so they can determine when it may be safe for a patient to drive themselves home.

Sleep Schedule

The sleep questionnaire should have a section dedicated to documentation of the patient's normal sleep schedule. The technologist should make sure that all sections

What activities does the patient undergo before bedtime?
Does the patient bath, brush teeth, or perform other grooming activities before bedtime?
Does the patient watch TV in bed?
Does the patient perform rigorous mental work just before bedtime?
Does the patient perform rigorous physical exercise in the 3 to 4 hours before bedtime?
What time does the patient usually retire/begin sleeping?
How long does it take the patient to fall asleep?
What time does the patient usually awaken in the morning?
How does the patient feel after awakening? Is he or she still sleepy?
Is the patient a restless sleeper?
Does the patient snore, choke, gasp, or breathe noisily at night?
Is the snoring/noisy breathing intermittent or continuous?
Has the patient been told that he or she stops breathing at night?
Does the patient typically arise to use the bathroom during the night?
Does the patient typically awaken during the evening? Why? How often?
Does the bed partner have complaints about the patient's sleep symptoms?
How many pillows do you sleep with?
Can you lie on your back?
Do you keep the TV on at night?
Are you tired during the day?
Do you nap during the day? How much?
Is the bed partner complaining of abnormal movements or sounds at night?
Does the patient kick his or her legs at night?
Does the patient suffer from insomnia?
Does the patient have nasal congestion?
Does the patient frequently have headaches in the morning?
Does the patient have a dry mouth in the morning?
Does the patient fall asleep at inappropriate times?
What time of day is it the hardest to stay awake?
Does the patient smoke?
What time does he or she get home from work?
What does the patient do after dinner?
Does the patient fall asleep watching TV or reading?

Figure 27-2 Interview questions.

of sleep questionnaire and logs are filled out completely. If the patient normally goes to bed at 2 AM and the night technologist's shift ends at 7 AM, then this is a problem. The patient should not feel obligated to fall asleep unusually early or be awakened earlier than their normal wake time. Accommodations should always be made for the patient's sleep schedule. This can be accomplished by having a daytime technologist take over monitoring in the morning. Alternatively, if no daytime technologist is available, slowly shifting the patient's sleep schedule earlier prior to testing may work.

Postsleep Questionnaire and Follow-Up Process

A postsleep questionnaire (Figure 27-3) will assess pertinent details of the patient's sleep period. Before the patient leaves the facility, answer any of their questions,

Name: ______________________________ Date: ____________

How long did it take you to fall asleep last night? ____________

How long does it usually take you to fall asleep? ____________

How many times do you remember waking up last night? ____________

How many times do you usually wake up? ____________

How long were you awake during the night? ____________

How long do you feel you slept last night? ____________

How long do you usually sleep every night? ____________

How would you say your sleep last night compares with your typical night?

Better ______ Same ______ Worse ______

Were you bothered by sleeping in the lab? Yes No

If yes, please explain ______________________________

____

Did you get enough sleep? Too little Just right Too much

Do you have any physical discomfort at the present time? Yes No

If yes, please explain ______________________________

____

Please add any additional comments you might have: ______________________________

____

____

____

Figure 27-3 Postsleep questionnaire.

being careful to avoid discussing detailed diagnostic results with the patient. Ensure the patient is aware of the follow-up process they will undergo with the physician.

Chart Documentation

If special needs were identified during the sleep study that are not already documented in the patient chart, then the technologist should document these needs.

Postprocedure Documentation and Follow-Up Processes

After the procedure, the technologist will need to verify that all the PSG forms have been completed and signed, including any consent forms. The technologist will want to administer a postsleep questionnaire in the morning to get a sense of how the patient felt while they slept. This is a subjective measure. A technologist's preliminary assessment is also completed in the morning that the sleep physician will review while interpreting the sleep study. Most sleep centers use an EHR; therefore, the technologist's documentation can be reviewed immediately by the medical director. Remote access to sleep studies is common.

There is a fine line related to what the technologist should tell the patient after sleep testing. The patient wants to know if they have a sleep disorder or not. If the diagnosis was OSA and the patient tried PAP during a split-night study, it is most likely that they have OSA; however, it is important to leave the diagnosis to the sleep physician. It is inappropriate for the technologist to diagnose the patient. The technologist can simply tell the patient that the sleep physician will review the sleep study and discuss the diagnosis and treatment options with them.

After the study is over and before the patient has left, it is important to make sure that the patient has a follow-up scheduled with the sleep physician to go over results, initiate treatment, and track their treatment success. A follow-up visit and compliance documentation are required by Medicare and many other insurance providers. Follow-ups may be scheduled through the sleep center office staff once the patient has completed testing. These may be video or phone follow-ups, and if PAP was utilized, may be accompanied by compliance data obtained from the Durable Medical Equipment company (DME), or PAP manufacturer.

SUMMARY

It is beneficial to the sleep testing and patient treatment process for the sleep technologist to gather as much pertinent information about the patient as possible. This information gathering begins before the patient's arrival through chart review and continues until the patient has completed their sleep study and left the sleep center. The process begins with a thorough review of the patient's chart, where the technologist will review the patient's H&P and physician orders for the sleep study. When the patient arrives, the technologist must orient the patient to the sleep facility and testing process. The patient questionnaire must be reviewed by the technologist and clarified with the patient. The technologist can ask additional clarifying questions pertaining to the patient's sleep complaints and document any additional information obtained. Observation and interviewing the patient to assess for special needs is important for obtaining a high-quality sleep study.

The patient entrusts the sleep center, sleep physician, and the sleep technologist with their care. The technologist's duty is to screen patients and determine they are well enough to obtain a safe and valid sleep study. The first screening step rests with the physician. If the technologist has any doubt or discomfort related to testing a patient with special needs and there is no documentation in the patient's chart, a call to the ordering physician may be in order. If a patient's special needs are beyond the scope of practice of the technologist, such as requirements for lifting (if no SPH equipment is available or the technologist is not trained), personal care, or assisting the patient in the bathroom, then a decision needs to be made as to whether it is safe and in the best interest of the patient to perform the study. An acceptance policy that outlines the types of patients accepted for a sleep study can be beneficial (Figure 27-4). A well-trained, competent technologist is the expectation of every patient.

PATIENT ACCEPTANCE CRITERIA

Section I: Purpose

A. Outlines the acceptance criteria for the safety and appropriateness of patients referred for a sleep study in an outpatient setting.

POLICY:	All patients scheduled for sleep studies will either be seen in consultation by a sleep physician of the center and have a history and physical (H&P) placed in the patient chart, or the case will be discussed by the sleep physician and the referring physician, with the H&P in the chart. Patients with certain limitations will not be seen at the center for a polysomnography (PSG), until their condition changes.
PROCEDURE:	Any patients who need a PSG must first be either seen by the sleep physician or the sleep physician must discuss the case with the referring physician before the PSG is done. If the patient has certain limitations, then the PSG will not be done until his or her condition changes. These limitations include the following:
	24-hour nursing care, including catheters, intravenous medication, glucose checks, severe incontinence, or anything that requires a nurse or orderly (lifting, bed pan, and diaper changes).
	Mentally diminished capacity that could interfere with the PSG, such as dementia, severe developmental delay, or other disorders.
	Patients who may need additional care, and the sleep physician knows will benefit from a PSG, may be studied only if attended by a nurse or attendant, who will be able to perform nursing or patient care duties, and not interfere with the PSG testing, or the technologist performing the testing.
	Patients who require an attendant, but do not have one present will be sent home after the sleep physician has been notified. Sleep technologists are not licensed or trained in nursing care.

Figure 27-4 Acceptance policy.

Section II: Procedure

A. Before all sleep studies, the sleep physicians review the medical chart and write the orders.

1. Acceptance criteria:
   a. Age newborn and up
   b. Patients can be seen in the sleep lab provided:
      i. They do not have an intercurrent or viral illness.
      ii. They have a guardian present if they are a minor.
      iii. A caregiver is present if needed, regardless of age.
2. Evidence-based exclusion criteria:
   a. Age premature to newborn
   b. Patient has an intercurrent or viral illness.
   c. Patient needs 24/7 nursing care.
   d. Caregiver not available to stay the night with patient

REFERENCES

1. Harding MM, Kwong J, Roberts D, Hagler D, Reinisch C. *Lewis's Medical-Surgical Nursing: Assessment and Management of Clinical Problems*. 11th ed. Elsevier; 2020.
2. NeuroLaunch. Mental age in psychology: definition, measurement and impact. Published September 14, 2024. Accessed February 23, 2025. https://neurolaunch.com/mental-age-psychology-definition/#google_vignette
3. Occupational Safety and Health Administration. Worker safety in hospitals: caring for our caregivers: safe patient handling. Accessed February 23, 2025. https://www.osha.gov/hospitals/patient-handling
4. Cleveland Clinic. Sundown syndrome. Published April 26, 2022. Accessed February 23, 2025. https://my.clevelandclinic.org/health/articles/22840-sundown-syndrome

SUGGESTED READINGS

Chokroverty S. Approach to the patient with sleep complaints. In: Chokroverty S, ed. *Sleep Disorders Medicine: Basic Science, Technical Considerations, and Clinical Aspects*. 3rd ed. Saunders/Elsevier; 2009.

Kryger MH, Roth T, Dement WC. *Principles and Practice of Sleep Medicine*. 7th ed. W.B. Saunders; 2021.

Chapter 28
Caring for the Patient With Disability in the Sleep Center

JOHNATHAN SIMPSON

KEY CONCEPTS/LEARNING OBJECTIVES

The key concepts for this chapter include a review of the practices and challenges in caring for the patient with disability within the sleep center setting and a variety of methods for providing safe, effective and high-quality care based on education and training surrounding common disabilities and methods for managing them.

KEY TERMS

Physical
Sensory
Cognitive
Neurologic
Quadriplegic

This chapter explores current practices and challenges in caring for patients with disability within the sleep center setting. Disabilities can impact diagnostic procedures and patient comfort and thus call for adapted protocols to ensure safe, effective, and patient-centered care. Patient-centered adaptations are based on a synthesis of multiple peer-reviewed sources and clinical practice standards. This chapter reviews the literature on best practices, discusses methodologic considerations for adapting sleep center environments, and offers a framework for staff training and facility modifications. Emphasis is placed on communication adaptations, accessibility, equipment calibration, and the physical environment. Figure 28-1 illustrates a sample patient assessment flowchart used to streamline these adaptations. Evidence suggests that a systematic approach to adapting protocols improves both patient outcomes and the operational efficiency of sleep center.

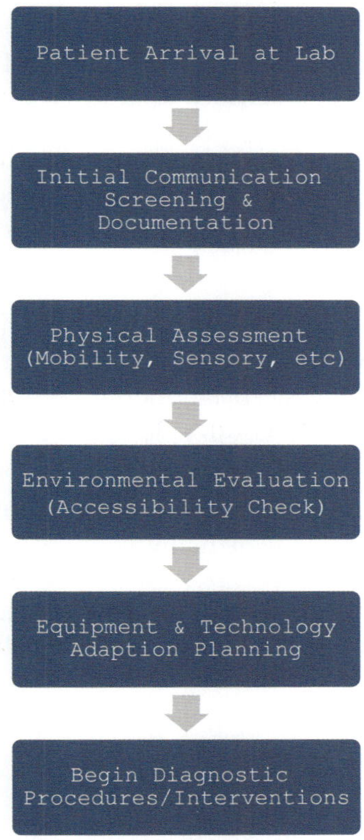

Figure 28-1 Patient assessment flowchart. Figure 28-1 outlines the systematic process for evaluating the care needs of patients with disabilities upon arrival at the sleep center. The flowchart includes steps for initial communication screening, physical assessment, environment evaluation, and planning for equipment adaptation. This tool is integral to ensuring that each patient's unique requirements are identified and met promptly.

PRACTICES AND CHALLENGES IN CARING FOR THE PATIENT WITH DISABILITY

Patients with disabilities often present unique challenges in clinical settings. In the sleep center, factors such as impaired mobility, communication difficulties, and sensory sensitivities can influence diagnostic accuracy and patient comfort. As the incidence of sleep disorders in diverse populations increases, sleep center protocols must evolve to meet the needs of patients with disabilities. This chapter outlines the rationale for specialized care, highlights gaps in existing literature, and sets forth recommendations based on both clinical experience and published guidelines (1). The guidelines provided by the American Academy of Sleep Medicine have been instrumental in shaping the framework discussed in this chapter.

Understanding Disability in Sleep Medicine

Disability encompasses a wide range of conditions, including physical, sensory, cognitive, and neurologic impairments. Patients with disabilities may experience unique challenges in sleep studies, such as difficulty positioning for polysomnography (PSG), heightened sensitivity to stimuli, or the need for specialized equipment.

Physical Accessibility in the Sleep Center

Ensuring that the sleep laboratory complies with the Americans with Disabilities Act (ADA) is crucial. Key considerations include the following:

- **Entrance and facility accessibility:** Ramps, automatic doors, and wide hallways allow for ease of movement.
- **Adjustable equipment:** Beds with adjustable heights and accessible control interfaces aid in patient comfort.
- **Restroom accommodations:** Wheelchair-accessible restrooms should be available and clearly marked.

Communication Strategies

Effective communication is essential in providing care for patients with disabilities. Strategies include the following:

- **Verbal and nonverbal communication:** Using clear, concise language, and visual aids where necessary
- **Assistive technology:** Providing text-to-speech devices or sign language interpreters for patients with hearing impairments
- **Patient-centered care:** Encouraging patients to express their needs and preferences for optimal study conditions

Adaptive Testing Methods

Patients with disabilities may require modifications to traditional sleep study protocols:

- **Alternative electrode placement:** Patients with mobility limitations may benefit from flexible electrode configurations.
- **Sensory accommodations:** Reducing ambient noise and minimizing bright lighting for sensory-sensitive individuals
- **Extended setup time:** Allowing additional time for preparation ensures patient comfort and cooperation

Special Considerations for Common Disabilities

1. **Patients with mobility impairments**
   - Use of hoists or transfer boards for bed positioning
   - Ensuring emergency procedures account for mobility limitations
2. **Patients with cognitive impairments**
   - Simplified explanations and step-by-step guidance
   - Presence of a caregiver to provide reassurance and assistance
3. **Patients with sensory impairments**
   - Adjustments in auditory or visual communication methods
   - Tactile cues or written instructions for patients with hearing impairments

CASE STUDY: ADAPTING SLEEP STUDIES FOR A PATIENT WITH QUADRIPLEGIA

A patient with quadriplegia requiring overnight PSG presented challenges in positioning, communication, and monitoring. Modifications included the use of specialized pillows, Hoyer style lift, continuous monitoring with adaptive equipment, two team-member assistance, and real-time feedback from caregivers. This approach ensured successful data collection without compromising patient safety or comfort.

Literature Review

An increasing body of literature addresses the integration of disability accommodations in clinical settings. Studies have highlighted the importance of environmental modifications, adapted communication techniques, and specialized staff training to improve patient safety and satisfaction. For instance, recent reviews have underscored the necessity of physical accessibility enhancements in sleep laboratories as well as the integration of assistive communication technologies (2,3). Figure 28-1 presents an example of a patient assessment flowchart designed to identify specific needs upon the arrival of a patient with disability at the sleep laboratory.

Methods

This chapter synthesizes data from current peer-reviewed journals, policy statements from professional organizations, and practice guidelines from leading sleep medicine centers. The methodologic approach encompasses a narrative review, followed by an analysis of case studies that discuss modifications in sleep center settings. Key areas of focus include the following:

- **Communication techniques:** Utilization of alternative and augmentative communication (AAC) devices
- **Physical accessibility:** Modifications to the sleep center infrastructure to ensure ease of access
- **Equipment adaptation:** Calibrating sleep diagnostic equipment to accommodate patients with unique anatomic or physical considerations
- **Staff training:** Implementing regular disability-awareness training modules

Results

The review of the literature and analysis of case studies show that systematic adaptations in sleep laboratories result in improved patient adherence to protocols and higher overall satisfaction. For example, centers that implemented specialized training and facility adjustments reported fewer diagnostic interruptions and a more streamlined patient workflow. Additionally, patient feedback emphasizes the benefits of dedicated communication aids and a physically accessible environment (4,5). See Figure 28-1 for an overview of the patient assessment process that integrates these findings.

DISCUSSION

Implementing a framework to accommodate patients with disabilities in the sleep center involves a multidimensional approach. This includes ergonomic modifications, adjustments in communication strategies, and ongoing staff education. The proposed strategies offer a cohesive protocol that can be tailored to the needs of individual patients, thereby reducing anxiety and enhancing the diagnostic process. Moreover, Table 28-1 summarizes key adaptation strategies across several domains, and Table 28-2 provides suggestions for adaptive modifications to the sleep study for different disabilities. It is imperative for administrative leadership to invest in periodic staff training and facility upgrades to ensure sustained improvements in care delivery for this vulnerable population.

Table 28-2 Adaptive Sleep Study Modifications for Different Disabilities

Disability Type	Modification
Mobility impairment	Hoists, transfer boards, extended setup time
Cognitive impairment	Simplified instructions, caregiver presence
Sensory impairment	Auditory/visual adjustments, tactile cues

CONCLUSION

The evolving demographics of patients requiring sleep diagnostic services necessitate that sleep laboratories adopt adaptive practices to ensure comprehensive care. Integrating accessibility measures, specialized communication tools, and environmental modifications into standard protocols can significantly enhance patient outcomes. Future studies should aim to quantify the benefits

Table 28-1 Summary of Special Considerations and Adaptations in the Sleep Center for Patients With Disabilities

Area of Concern	Adaptation Strategy	Implementation Details
Communication	Utilization of AAC devices	Provide access to communication boards, speech-generating devices, etc.
Accessibility	Wheelchair and mobility adaptations	Ensure wide passageways, ramps, and accessible restrooms are available.
Equipment adaptation	Customized sensor placement	Adjust sensor positions to account for physical limitations or positioning.
Staff training	Disability awareness programs	Regular workshops and competency training for handling diverse needs
Entrance accessibility	Ramps, automatic doors, wide hallways	Use sound-dampening materials and adjustable lighting to enhance comfort.
Adjustable equipment	Beds with adjustable height and control access	Ensure beds have the capability to adjust by the head, feet, and height.

ACC, augmentative and alternative communication.

of these interventions using controlled clinical trials and extend the findings to diverse patient populations.

REFERENCES

1. American Academy of Sleep Medicine. *The International Classification of Sleep Disorders*. 3rd ed. American Academy of Sleep Medicine; 2014.
2. Aurora RN, Kristo D, Bista SR, et al. The management of patients with sleep disorders. *Journal of Clinical Sleep Medicine*. 2016;12(3):323–329.
3. Oliven A, Munson D. Approaches for healthcare professionals caring for disabled individuals in sleep laboratories. *Sleep Medicine Reviews*. 2018;37:79–85.
4. Jackson C, Huang X, Kim J, et al. Improving the sleep laboratory environment for disabled patients. *Sleep Health*. 2019;5(4):376–383.
5. Williams T, Smith J. Disability, sleep disorders, and care strategies in clinical settings. *Journal of the Neurolological Sciences*. 2020;417:117–123.

Chapter 29

Preoperative Assessment and Perioperative Monitoring

DANIELIZA JUNIIS-JOHNSON AND KRISTINA WEAVER

KEY CONCEPTS/LEARNING OBJECTIVES

The key concepts for this chapter include a review of perioperative morbidity in patients with obstructive sleep apnea (OSA), comorbid conditions that may affect perioperative management, evaluating known and patients with suspected OSA preoperatively, perioperative risks associated with sleep-disordered breathing, minimizing the risk posed by OSA intraoperatively, and determining postoperative disposition of a *suspected* and known patient with OSA after general anesthesia.

KEY TERMS

Diabetes
Hypertension
Intraoperative
Multimodal analgesia
Opioids
Pain-sedation mismatch
Perioperative

The global prevalence of obstructive sleep apnea (OSA) is utterly astounding. Recent research has estimated that worldwide, nearly 1 billion adults between the ages of 30 and 69 years old have OSA (1). Moderate OSA with an apnea-hypopnea index (AHI) greater than 15 is estimated to be present in 425 million (45%) of these individuals (1). In the surgical population, a significant number of patients present for procedures that may have undiagnosed OSA and need effective screening tools to enhance surgical patient outcomes. In a 1-year cross-sectional study, researchers found that the Berlin Questionnaire and STOP-Bang screening tool were the most sensitive and accurate OSA screening tools (2, 3).

Identification of patients at risk for OSA is important to optimize perioperative outcomes. Patients with OSA may be more likely to have increased airway compromise with administration of sedative and anesthetic medications. These medications may decrease arousal responses that prevent collapse of the upper airway, leading to worsening of obstructive symptoms.

Perioperative morbidity in patients with OSA (diagnosed and undiagnosed) is still a major concern, and the American Academy of Sleep Medicine (AASM) continues to defer to the American Society of Anesthesiologists (ASA) to assist with the most updated research.

The ASA addressed the issue of perioperative management by creating a task force to develop guidelines regarding management of patients with OSA who may be at risk for perioperative morbidity (4). In October 2012, the ASA Committee on Standards and Practice Parameters elected to collect new evidence to determine if recommendations in the 2006 version of the ASA Practice Guidelines were supported by current evidence (4). Although the research is still limited, on October 16, 2013, the ASA Task Force updated their recommendations to include the following items: preoperative evaluation, inpatient versus outpatient surgery, preoperative preparation, intraoperative management, postoperative management and criteria for discharge to unmonitored settings (4). The purpose of these guidelines is to improve perioperative care and reduce the risk of adverse outcomes in patients with confirmed or suspected OSA who receive sedation, analgesia, or anesthesia for diagnostic or therapeutic procedures under the care of an anesthesiologist (4).

Sleep technologists involved in perioperative assessment of patients require an understanding of the problems encountered by patients with OSA who are facing upcoming surgical procedures.

PERIOPERATIVE RISKS ASSOCIATED WITH SLEEP-DISORDERED BREATHING

Sleep in the Hospitalized Patient

Sleep for the hospitalized patient leaves much to be desired, for it is often disrupted, fragmented, and/or minimally obtained. This disruption of sleep is often caused by environmental factors (noise, light, medical devices), patient characteristics (sex, age, pain intensity), or primary sleep disorders like OSA (5). Sleep deprivation or interruption decreases immune system function, slows healing, impairs cognitive function, and increases stress levels, stroke risk, and cardiovascular events, which can impact the overall health outcome of the patient, including length of stay (5). Medications also play a significant role in the disruption of sleep as well as in the increased incidence of OSA. Clinicians quite often fail to document sleep disturbances and are often unaware of best practices to improve sleep quality in the hospitals, despite the myriad of both intrinsic and extrinsic factors presenting the perioperative patient (6).

Perioperative Medications

Medications administered during the perioperative period can induce and exacerbate OSA. Medications such as intravenous (IV) analgesics, opioids, pentothal, muscle relaxants, benzodiazepines, nitrous oxide, and propofol reduce the tone of the pharyngeal musculature, which maintains airway patency, thus increasing airway collapsibility (7). The primary site of occlusion is at the level of the soft palate; however, multiple sites of airway collapse incidents of hypoxemia and compete airway obstruction are more common in patients with OSA (7). Thus, perioperative patients with known or unknown OSA are at an even higher risk for complications. The ASA and its consultant members strongly agree that regional analgesic techniques should be considered to eliminate or reduce the requirement for systemic opioids in patients at increased perioperative risk from OSA (4). Studies show that the incident rate of complications among patients with OSA was an astounding 48.9% compared to 31.4% of patients without OSA (7). Respiratory complications accounted for 40.4% of patients versus the 23.2% of control patients (7). A systematic review and meta-analysis study revealed the effectiveness of perioperative positive airway pressure (PAP) therapy. Patients with OSA undergoing noncardiac surgery had a 28% decreased risk of postoperative respiratory complication, and a 56% reduction rate in unplanned ICU admissions (7). PAP applications in cardiac and thoracoabdominal surgeries have been associated with decreased pulmonary complications to include reintubation and reduction in hypoxemia (7). The ASA advises patients treated for OSA to continue to use PAP therapy before surgery and during their entire hospitalization, while serious consideration of initiating PAP therapy should be given to untreated individuals who exhibit severe OSA or episodes of desaturation postoperatively (4).

Comorbid Conditions

It is imperative that health care providers involved in the care of the surgical patient be aware of comorbidities associated with OSA to provide the best possible health care outcome.

OSA is associated with multiple medical conditions that can affect management in the perioperative and postoperative period of surgical patients. Comorbidities associated with OSA include cardiovascular disease (CVD), arrhythmias, heart failure, hypertension, encephalic and behavioral alterations, metabolic syndrome, and obesity (8). These comorbidities increase the mortality rate of patients with OSA compared to the general population (8).

Sleep Apnea and Its Link to Cardiac Disease

OSA is characterized by the partial or complete recurrent upper airway obstruction during sleep, which if left untreated, can cause many adverse consequences (Pinto). These consequences can include hypertension, obesity, diabetes mellitus, cardiac and encephalic alterations, including behavioral alterations that result in a significant source of public health care by generating a high financial and social impact (Pinto).

In 2021 in the United States, coronary heart disease (CHD) was the leading cause of deaths (40.3%) attributable to CVD, followed by stroke (17.5%), other CVD (17.1%), high blood pressure (13.4%), heart failure (9.1%), and diseases of the arteries (2.6%) (9). CVD accounted for approximately 19.91 million global deaths in 2021 (9). CVD is a class of prevalent diseases including heart failure, myocardial infarction, coronary revascularization procedure, angina pectoris and stroke (12). In the United States, CVD is the cause of 655,000 deaths each year, and OSA frequently coexists with CVD (12). Between 2017 and 2020, 127.9 million US adults (48.6%) had some form of CVD (9). The financial health care expenditure continues to climb. CVD accounted for 12% of total US health expenditures from 2019 to 2020, more than any major diagnostic group (9). Between 2019 and 2020, direct and indirect costs of CVD totaled \$422.3 billion (\$254.3 billion in direct costs and \$168.0 billion in lost productivity/mortality) (9). The identification and treatment of OSA can significantly reduce these CVD instances.

Sleep Apnea and Its Link to Obesity and Diabetes

Many Americans continue to choose to maintain an unhealthy diet of fast food, and the increasing use of technology contributes to a reduction in physical activity. Food choices and reduction in physical activity can ultimately lead to a more sedentary lifestyle, which, in turn, can lead to obesity. The rates of obesity in the United States continue to rise. According to the American Heart Association, the prevalence of obesity in the United States among adults from 2017 to 2020 was 41.8% in males and 41.8% in females (9). Severe obesity in adults in the United States in 2017 to 2020 was 6.6% in males and 11.7% in females (9). OSA pathogenesis is multifactorial, yet in patients with obesity, excess weight may contribute to OSA pathogenesis through several mechanisms (10). Upper airway crowding is arguably the most thoroughly investigated factor of OSA, as it directly induces airway obstruction at the pharynx (10). The presence of more adipose tissue around this segment or in the tongue contributes to an elevated extra-luminal pressure, thereby precipitating collapse (10). Increasing values of BMI progressively worsens upper airway collapsibility (10).

Those individuals suffering from OSA are more likely to be overweight, and they are also more likely to develop type 2 diabetes (T2D) and glucose metabolism dysregulation (4). The alarming increase in overweight and obesity has played a pivotal role in the rise of prediabetes and type 2 diabetes (4). In the past 30 years, the number of American adults with diabetes nearly quadrupled, with an estimated 29 million people, or 9.3% of the US population, estimated to have diagnosed or undiagnosed diabetes (4). Type 2 diabetes represents 90% to 95% of all cases of diabetes, and the number of American adults that have prediabetes is estimated at 86 million (4). The role of sleep fragmentation and intermittent hypoxemia on glucose metabolism has been demonstrated in multiple human experiments that indicate an independent association between the severity of OSA and insulin resistance even in individuals without T2D (4). In a cross-sectional study of healthy volunteers, exposure to 5 hours of intermittent hypoxia during wakefulness, inducing an average of 24 desaturation events per hour, led to a 17% reduction in insulin sensitivity without a simultaneous increase in insulin secretion (4).

Hospitalized inpatients and inpatients awaiting surgery who have OSA are at an increased risk for complications that can include longer hospitalization, higher reintubation rates, oxygen desaturations, hypercapnia, cardiac arrhythmias, myocardial injury, delirium, unplanned ICU transfers, and sudden unexpected death (11). The role of sleep in regard to health and well-being, continues to be an underestimated concern, and OSA still remains a highly undiagnosed disease. However, developing an inpatient assessment and monitoring program can assist when it comes to diagnosis, prognosis, patient care, interaction, and education for patients in the hospital setting.

INDICATIONS FOR PREOPERATIVE SLEEP ASSESSMENT

Early identification of sleep apnea helps to reduce risk, coordinate care, and facilitate perioperative management strategies such as postsurgical PAP needs or perioperative monitoring. Preoperative sleep assessment is indicated for patients showing signs of sleep-disordered breathing (eg, loud snoring, daytime sleepiness); those with high-risk factors like obesity, CVD, or difficult airway history; and for surgeries involving general anesthesia or high postoperative respiratory risk. Screening is also warranted if the patient has a known but untreated or poorly managed diagnosis of OSA. ASA guidelines highlight the importance of perioperative diagnosis and management of OSA, in which the "gold standard" screening tool continues to be the nocturnal polysomnogram (6). However, because of time constraints, cost, and personnel requirements, it can be an impractical screening tool for the perioperative patient (6). Thus, the use of other OSA screening tools that are less time-consuming and more cost-effective should be considered in perioperative management. Common screening tools include the Epworth Sleepiness Scale (ESS), STOP Questionnaire, STOP-BANG Questionnaire (SBQ), BQ, and the Wisconsin Sleep Questionnaire. These assessment tools are time efficient and have evidence-based reliability and validity.

METHODS FOR PREOPERATIVE SLEEP ASSESSMENT

Preoperative sleep apnea assessment is most effective when conducted early in the surgical planning process, ideally, during the initial surgical consult in the surgeon's office or at the preadmission testing (PAT) clinic. At the time of surgical consultation, patients can be screened using validated tools such as the STOP-Bang often completed by nursing staff or via digital intake. Patients who score high or report concerning symptoms are flagged for further evaluation during their PAT. In the PAT clinic, a more detailed review is conducted by a nurse, advanced practice provider, or anesthesiologist to assess sleep history, continuous positive airway pressure (CPAP) use, and comorbidities. This information is used to guide anesthesia planning, determine the need for postoperative respiratory monitoring, and assess the appropriateness of same-day surgery. If OSA is suspected or confirmed, EMR alerts are added to ensure care teams are aware and prepared. Early assessment allows for safe, tailored perioperative management; helps avoid unexpected complications; and improves coordination among surgical, anesthesia, nursing, and respiratory teams. The ASA guidelines were created by a task force to optimize care for patients with diagnosed or undiagnosed OSA who may have increased risk in the perioperative period (12). This group recommended the development of protocols to screen patients suspected of having OSA preoperatively for the identification of high-risk patients.

There are several screening tools that have been utilized in the preoperative assessment of patients suspected of having OSA. In addition, on initial physical examination, some physical findings may increase suspicion. These include obesity and craniofacial abnormalities, such as retrognathia and macroglossia. Questions regarding signs and symptoms of OSA should be asked, such as loud snoring, observed apnea, and daytime hypersomnolence. Several of the screening tools utilize these assessments as well.

Protocols have also been established at numerous medical centers on the basis of specific management of high-risk patients.

Sleep apnea screening tools vary in complexity and purpose, each offering unique value in clinical practice. STOP-Bang is the most widely used and validated, combining eight factors such as snoring, tiredness, BMI, and neck circumference to identify patients at high risk for OSA, particularly in preoperative and inpatient settings. STOP is a shorter, four-question version that is quicker to administer but less accurate, making it more suitable for basic screening. The Berlin Questionnaire assesses risk based on snoring, fatigue, and comorbidities, offering more detail but requiring more time, and is often used in outpatient or research settings. The ESS measures daytime sleepiness and is helpful for symptom tracking, although it is not diagnostic on its own.

A study published in *BMC Anesthesiology* evaluated the effectiveness of the STOP-Bang questionnaire for preoperative screening of OSA, in which it demonstrated a high sensitivity, correctly identifying 85% of all cases, 88% of moderate cases, and 90% of severe cases, making it a reliable tool for identifying risk. A STOP-Bang score of less than 3 was associated with effectively ruling out severe OSA in 93% of surgical patients. In clinical practice, STOP-Bang remains the preferred first-line screening tool for OSA due to its high sensitivity and ease of use (13).

Diagnostic Testing

Polysomnography (PSG), as a preoperative diagnostic tool, is not feasible for all high-risk patients because it is expensive, requires a significant time commitment for the study and preoperative initiation of therapy (if indicated), and would burden already busy sleep centers. PSG is typically limited to patients with severe comorbidities, such as decompensated heart failure, uncontrolled hypertension, or pulmonary hypertension.

Overnight oximetry is an option in patients who are considered at risk for postoperative complications related to undiagnosed OSA. Figure 29-1 is an example

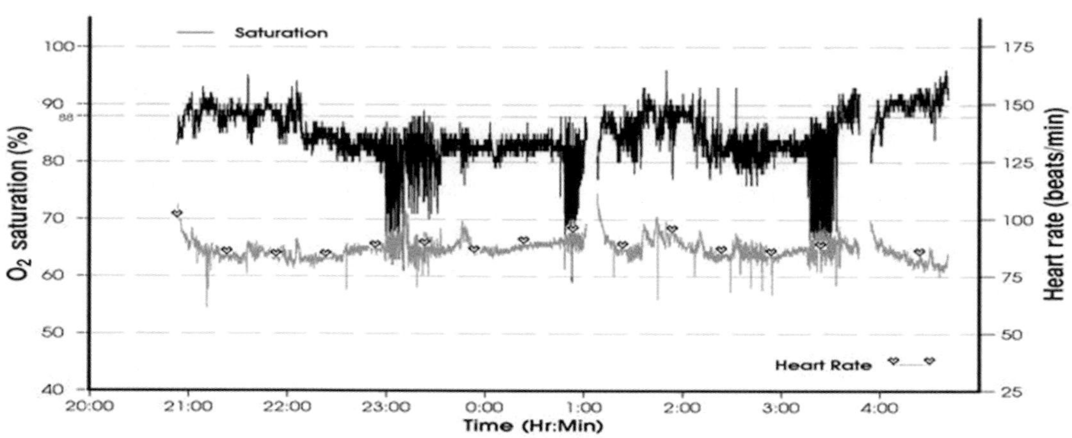

Figure 29-1 Oximetry result of a patient with severe obstructive sleep apnea (OSA) and chronic obstructive pulmonary disease with obesity hypoventilation. The reduced mean saturation is an indication that there is coexisting cardiopulmonary disease, and the prolonged time at low oxygen saturation suggests that pulmonary hypertension is also present. The frequency of 4% oxygen desaturations (4% oxygen desaturation index) per hour of 47 supports the diagnosis of severe OSA and corresponds with the patient's AHI from a polysomnogram showing an AHI of 40/h. Lastly, the clustered desaturations (icicles from the rooftop) to 59% identify the severe rapid eye movement desaturations typically occurring in this type of patient.

of overnight oximetry in a patient with severe chronic obstructive pulmonary disease, obesity hypoventilation syndrome, and OSA. Review of this study indicates co-existing cardiopulmonary disease with reduced mean saturation. A prolonged time at low oxygen saturation may suggest that pulmonary hypertension is also present.

Recent studies continue to support the use of overnight oximetry—particularly the oxygen desaturation index (ODI)—as a valuable, low-cost tool for screening patients at risk for OSA prior to surgery. ODI has been shown to closely correlate with the AHI from polysomnography (PSG), making it a reliable surrogate when full PSG is not feasible. In a study of 172 surgical patients, those with a 4% ODI greater than or equal to 5 events per hour experienced a significantly higher rate of postoperative complications (15.3%) compared to those with ODI less than 5 (2.7%). Complication rates increased further for patients with ODI greater than or equal to 15. Most complications involved increased respiratory support, such as supplemental oxygen. ODI values greater than 10 have demonstrated a sensitivity of 71% to 85% and a specificity of 90% to 95% for detecting mild-to-moderate OSA, reinforcing its utility in preoperative risk stratification. When PSG is unavailable or delayed, overnight oximetry can help identify high-risk patients and inform perioperative planning to reduce complications (14).

Recent evidence supports the use of portable monitoring and home sleep apnea testing (HSAT) as reliable and cost-effective alternatives to in-lab polysomnography (PSG) for identifying OSA in preoperative patients. A 2024 study found HSAT identified OSA in up to 82% of surgical patients when combined with clinical tools like the STOP-Bang questionnaire, while another study showed that 47% of patients had undiagnosed moderate-to-severe OSA not recognized until HSAT was performed. Patients with a STOP-Bang score indicating high risk and an ODI greater than 10 were significantly more likely to have OSA confirmed. A 2023 systematic review further confirmed the validity of HSAT and Type III monitors for surgical screening, particularly when PSG is not available. HSAT is increasingly accepted by payers for confirming diagnosis and initiating CPAP therapy preoperatively, although patients with complex cardiopulmonary or neurologic conditions should still undergo in-lab testing when appropriate.

Preoperative Positive Airway Pressure

Recent studies underscore the importance of PAP therapy adherence in patients with OSA undergoing surgery. A systematic review and meta-analysis found that in patients with OSA undergoing noncardiac surgery, PAP therapy was associated with a 28% reduction in the risk of postoperative respiratory complications and a 56% reduction in unplanned ICU admissions. In cardiac surgery patients, PAP therapy decreased the risk of postoperative cardiac complications and atrial fibrillation by 37% and 41%, respectively (15). Despite these benefits, adherence to PAP therapy remains a challenge. To mitigate perioperative risks, it is recommended that patients with known OSA resume PAP therapy preoperatively. When patients cannot recall their PAP settings, the use of auto-titrating PAP devices during hospitalization can be considered. Documentation of PAP usage in the preoperative evaluation is crucial to inform perioperative care providers and optimize patient outcomes. There is still no definitive guidance specifying the optimal preoperative PAP therapy duration. However, expert opinion and observational data suggest that a period of 4 to 6 weeks of PAP therapy may be beneficial prior to surgery. This timeline is based on the physiologic benefits that accrue over several weeks of therapy, including reduction of upper airway edema, improved oxygenation, decreased sympathetic nervous system activation, and stabilization of blood pressure and cardiovascular function. While shorter durations of therapy such as one night preoperatively and several nights postoperatively have shown some benefit, they may not allow enough time for these physiologic improvements to take full effect. Therefore, when feasible, 4 to 6 weeks of PAP therapy is often recommended to optimize patient outcomes. The duration should still be tailored based on the urgency of surgery and individual clinical factors, with close monitoring of adherence and therapeutic effectiveness (16).

INTRAOPERATIVE MANAGEMENT

Patients with diagnosed or suspected sleep apnea face a heightened risk of perioperative complications, particularly respiratory depression and airway obstruction. Due to this risk, the Society of Anesthesia and Sleep Medicine (SASM), recommend a set of key safety principles: avoid sedation in unsupervised areas, minimize the use of opioids and sedatives, and maintain heightened vigilance for airway management challenges, such as difficult intubation or upper airway collapse. Anesthetic plans should prioritize short-acting agents (eg, desflurane over sevoflurane) to support faster emergence and reduce postoperative hypoventilation. Regional anesthesia techniques—such as neuraxial or peripheral nerve blocks—are strongly encouraged when feasible as they reduce or eliminate the need for general anesthesia and systemic opioids, both of which contribute to respiratory compromise. Multimodal analgesia strategies should be used to reduce opioid burden. Propofol, while commonly used, is known to increase upper airway collapsibility and should be administered cautiously. For patients receiving moderate or deep sedation, securing the airway with a supraglottic device or endotracheal tube is preferable to leaving the airway unprotected. Importantly, capnography is recommended intraoperatively for real-time detection of hypoventilation, particularly during sedation. By following these principles, anesthesia teams can proactively reduce the risk of postoperative complications, including oxygen desaturation, respiratory failure, and unplanned ICU admissions (17).

Monitored Anesthesia Care

Monitored anesthesia care (MAC) is a form of anesthesia in which patients receive intravenous sedation for procedures that do not require general anesthesia but still demand vigilant monitoring and the ability to convert to general anesthesia if needed. In patients with sleep apnea, MAC carries increased risk due to the respiratory depressant effects of commonly used sedatives such as benzodiazepines, opioids, and propofol, which can worsen upper airway obstruction and blunt responses to hypoxia and hypercapnia. Updated guidance from the ASA and the SASM recommends enhanced intraoperative monitoring—particularly capnography—to promptly detect hypoventilation. When appropriate, alternative techniques such as regional anesthesia without sedation should be considered to reduce airway and respiratory risks in patients at high risk for sleep apnea (17).

Airway Management

Anatomic changes can be associated with OSA that may affect airway management intraoperatively. Patients may have increased neck circumference, macroglossia, retrognathia, and maxillary constriction. These anatomic features can be associated with difficult mask ventilation and intubation. A 2021 study reported that patients with OSA had a higher incidence of difficult intubation compared to patients without OSA (14.5% vs 7.7%). Additionally, studies show that patients with OSA were more likely to experience difficult intubation, with an incidence of 20% compared to 10% in patients without OSA. Given these findings, the ASA Practice Guidelines for Management of the Difficult Airway emphasize the importance of preoperative airway assessment in patients with OSA. The guidelines recommend strategies such as preoxygenation with 100% oxygen, utilization of video laryngoscopy, and having alternative airway devices readily available. Because of these issues, preparation for the induction of anesthesia and intubation should follow the ASA difficult airway guidelines. Preparations should be made for unanticipated difficulty in these patients. Sedatives should be administered slowly to avoid sudden loss of consciousness and resultant unanticipated obstructions. Patients with obesity should be placed in a ramped or sitting position. This involves elevation of the torso and head tilt with chin upward to optimize airway visualization and should be combined with approximately 30° head-up position. Preoxygenation with 100% oxygen given by tight-fitting mask for 3 minutes should be performed. This can increase time of tolerance to apnea in case of intubation difficulties.

Alternate airway devices, such as laryngeal mask airway, video laryngoscope, or fiberoptic scope, should be readily available. If awake intubation is planned, topical anesthetics are utilized for the upper airway and oropharynx. If the surgical procedure is short in duration, care providers should be vigilant about residual topical anesthesia causing impaired upper airway reflexes at the end of the surgery.

Extubation following surgical procedure should be carefully planned, because residual anesthetics may increase the risk of obstruction. Often, nondepolarizing muscle relaxants are administered during surgery to optimize performance of the surgical procedure. It is important to ensure that the muscle relaxant is fully reversed to avoid increased risk of upper airway obstruction. A nerve stimulation device should be utilized to assess appropriate reversal of muscle relaxant. Patients should be fully awake, breathing with adequate respiratory rate and tidal volume before extubation. Immediately after extubation, careful monitoring for evidence of obstruction and asynchrony of respiratory efforts should be performed (18).

MANAGEMENT OF SLEEP-DISORDERED BREATHING IN THE RECOVERY PERIOD

Postanesthesia Care Unit

Patients routinely recover in the postanesthesia care unit (PACU) following surgical procedures, where continuous cardiopulmonary monitoring is standard. During this time, patients may still experience residual effects from anesthetic and analgesic agents, placing them at increased risk for respiratory complications. Vigilant recovery care is provided by PACU nurses, with close monitoring for signs of respiratory depression, apnea, desaturation, and pain-sedation mismatch. The PACU is a critical period because patients often receive their highest doses of postoperative opioids during this time, compounding the effects of residual sedation. Studies have shown that combining a high preoperative sleep apnea risk score with recurrent PACU respiratory events—such as apnea, bradypnea, or oxygen desaturation—strongly predicts postoperative complications, with odds ratios exceeding 20 in some studies (19).

Patients at risk for sleep apnea should be positioned sitting upright or in a lateral decubitus position during recovery, both of which promote better airway patency. For patients with known sleep apnea and prescribed

PAP therapy, continuation of CPAP or auto-PAP in the PACU is strongly recommended. This enables careful observation while resuming their preoperative airway support settings. Patients with known sleep apnea who are noncompliant with PAP therapy should be monitored even more closely, as they are at highest risk for postoperative complications. For patients suspected of having undiagnosed sleep apnea, careful consideration should be given to the use of PAP therapy in a monitored setting.

Postoperative Analgesia

IV analgesics and opioids (common analgesic) not only increase airway collapsibility but suppress REM sleep (6). REM sleep allows the body to heal and restore itself for optimal function. The reduction of REM sleep has a higher occurrence after major surgery in which recovery REM (or REM rebound) is usually observed on the second or third postoperative day (6). During REM sleep, the neural drive to the pharyngeal muscles is minimized, causing hypotonia of the muscles, thus increasing severity of OSA during REM rebound (6). REM rebound can contribute to myocardial ischemia and infarction, stroke, hemodynamic instability, mental confusion, and wound breakdown (6). Patients with OSA are at higher risk for these effects.

Anesthetic and sedative drugs are central nervous system depressants that also inhibit respiration, causing oxygen desaturations, hypoxemia, and hypercapnia. In a case study of 23 patients with unrecognized sleep apnea, undergoing an outpatient procedure with conscious sedation, 17 (74%) patients developed OSA.

Postoperative Location

Patients with OSA or at high risk for OSA may require a higher level of care than that provided on a routine hospital unit after surgery. The ASA guidelines recommend a monitored setting or pulse oximetry that is continuously observed for high-risk patients (12). Perioperative risk is dependent on the severity of OSA, whether PAP is being utilized, invasiveness of the surgery, and requirement for postoperative opioids.

Using this algorithm (Figure 29-2), patients are at high risk if they have OSA (left) or high suspicion by preoperative screening. On the left-hand side of Figure 29-2, patients are at high risk when noncompliant with CPAP, AHI greater than 30, or recurrent PACU events. The PACU events are assessed at 30-minute intervals and are positive if they have events at two of the three periods. These events are as follows:

1. Apnea greater than or equal to 10 seconds
2. Bradypnea less than or equal to eight breaths per minute (three episodes needed)
3. Desaturations less than 90% (three episodes needed)
4. Pain-sedation mismatch, high pain score with a high level of sedation. These patients may need a higher level of care, and possibly PAP.

The right-hand side of the algorithm guides the management of patients suspected of OSA, identified as high risk by screening tools. They are also considered high risk if they have recurrent PACU events in addition to high risk by screening and should be considered for a higher level of care postoperatively as well. If a patient requires initiation of PAP postoperatively, including someone with known OSA noncompliant with therapy, the patient should go to a step-down or monitored setting. Initiation of PAP on the unit without close observation will be difficult, and the acceptance of a new PAP is often difficult.

MONITORING

Oximetry

Pulse oximetry is an external diagnostic tool that is used to indirectly measure the percentage of oxygenated hemoglobin in the blood. The pulse oximeter probe, which can be placed on the finger or earlobe, uses a red-infrared light source that measures the light absorption properties of hemoglobin that produces a reading called the Spo_2. It is widely used in the perioperative and intensive care settings and in pediatric patients to identify hypoxemia or an indication of respiratory complication that may require clinical intervention. Pulse oximetry contributes to maintaining patient safety and reducing the risk of complications for the perioperative and postoperative patient, especially someone with a higher risk of OSA.

Capnograph

Capnography is the measure of concentration of partial pressure of carbon dioxide (CO_2) in respiratory gases, which provide important information about a patient's ventilatory status.

End-tidal CO_2 ($Etco_2$) provides a noninvasive means of measuring CO_2 levels through a patient's exhaled breath, normal values ranging between 35 and 45 mm Hg (Figure 29-3). Higher than normal $Etco_2$ values (hypoventilation) indicate ventilation is not effective at eliminating CO_2 and can be associated with obesity, pulmonary disease, or respiratory distress. Lower than normal $Etco_2$ values (hyperventilation) can be seen in diabetic complications or anxiety. Transcutaneous CO_2 ($Tcco_2$) provides a reading of CO_2 levels in the blood by a heated sensor placed on the skin.

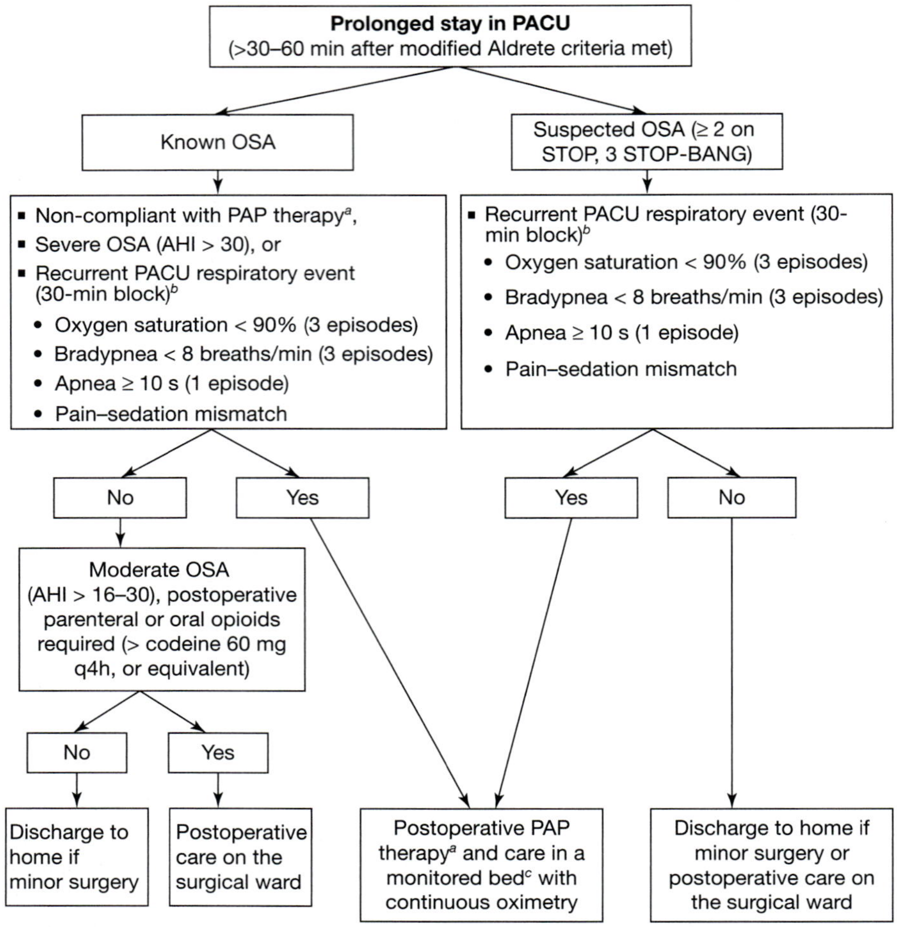

Figure 29-2 Postoperative management of the known or suspected patient with obstructive sleep apnea (OSA) after general anesthesia. [a]Recurrent postanesthesia care unit (PACU) respiratory event—any event occurring more than once in each 30-minute evaluation period (not necessary to be the same event). [b]Positive airway pressure (PAP) therapy—including continuous PAP, bilevel PAP, or auto-titrating PAP. [c]Monitored bed—environment with continuous oximetry and the possibility of early nursing intervention (eg, intensive care unit, step-down unit, or remote pulse oximetry with telemetry in surgical ward). Pain-sedation mismatch, simultaneous occurrence of high pain scores and high sedation levels. AHI, apnea-hypopnea index. (Reprinted by permission from Springer: Seet E, Chung F. Management of sleep apnea in adults—functional algorithms for the perioperative period: Continuing Professional Development. *Can J Anaesth*. 2010;57(9):849-864. Copyright © 2010 Canadian Anesthesiologists' Society.)

The ASA updated practice guidelines for perioperative management of patients with OSA indicate that if moderate sedation is used, ventilation should be continuously monitored by capnography or another automated method if feasible because there is an increased risk of undetected airway obstruction (4).

Protocols

Continued use of sedative agents in the postoperative period can contribute to obstructions and apneas in patients with OSA. Many institutions have initiated protocols to limit sedative agents given to high-risk patients also receiving analgesic medications. These include limitation of sleep-enhancing medications and benzodiazepines to minimize pharmacologic sedative effects that could worsen OSA symptoms. Often, these protocols include recommendations about patient positioning. The ASA guidelines recommend the use of nonsupine positions, if possible, during the recovery period (4).

The ASA updated practice guidelines for perioperative management of patients with OSA suggest CPAP or noninvasive positive pressure ventilation should be continuously administered to patients who were using these modalities preoperatively (4). Initiation of nasal CPAP or noninvasive positive pressure ventilation

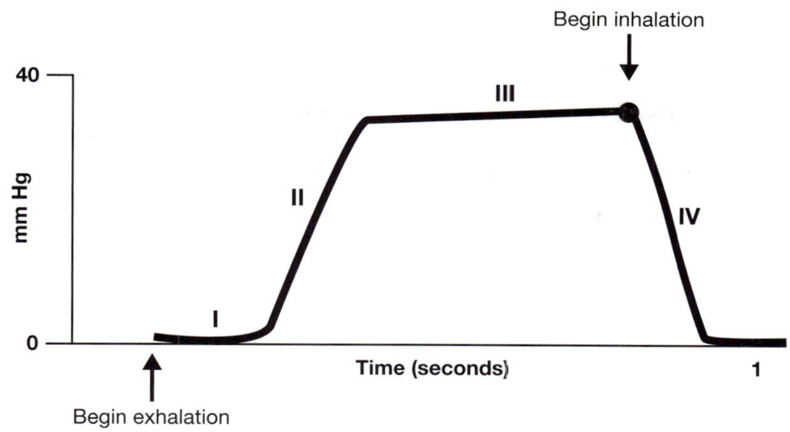

Figure 29-3 The "normal" capnogram is a waveform that represents the varying carbon dioxide level throughout the breath cycle. Phase 1: Beginning of exhalation. Dead space is cleared from the upper airway. Phase II: Rapid rise in CO_2 concentration as alveolar CO_2 reaches the upper airway. Phase III: Plateau. Entire exhaled breath stream is alveolar gas. Maximum value for that tidal breath is the end-tidal CO_2 Phase IV: Beginning of inhalation. Atmospheric air replaces alveolar CO_2 (Reprinted with permission from Fleisher GR, Ludwig S. *Textbook of Pediatric Emergency Medicine*. 6th ed. Wolters Kluwer Health/Lippincott Williams & Wilkins; 2011. Figure 1 [Appendix].)

should be considered in patients showing severe or frequent airway obstruction during postoperative monitoring (4). If possible, patients should bring in their own equipment, unless contraindicated by the surgical procedure (4).

Multiple studies in controlled and randomized settings with non-OSA diagnosed and patients with OSA who were compliant with their CPAP or where CPAP was used as a prophylactic measure had a decreased hospital length of stay and reduced rate of pulmonary complications (11).

SUMMARY

Patients with known and suspected OSA are at risk for complications in the perioperative period. Both the AASM and the ASA have addressed this issue and provided recommendations to assist in management. Both intraoperative and postoperative management can be challenging. Regional analgesic techniques are considered more ideal than systemic opioids. Regional analgesic techniques may reduce difficult airway management; however, airway management remains a concern for the intraoperative medical team. Postoperatively, OSA may be linked to multiple complications. Identification of patients with undiagnosed OSA may allow increased vigilance during their perioperative period. Careful history and physical examination and the use of clinical screening tools to identify patients at high risk for OSA should be carried out.

Patients with suspected OSA with comorbidities thought to be associated with OSA, such as heart failure and uncontrolled hypertension, should undergo further evaluation before proceeding with elective surgery. This will require evaluation by both sleep medicine and other subspecialists to optimize their medical condition. Patients with known OSA and those identified as high risk should be managed similarly in the perioperative period. Attention to the severity of OSA, invasiveness of the surgical procedure, postoperative opioid requirements, and positioning should be considered for the determination of requirements for postoperative monitoring.

Information regarding optimal management continues to be a work in progress. Current AASM and ASA guidelines should be reviewed in the development of institutional approaches to management of this high-risk group. Further work in this area is necessary to better understand the risks and optimal management strategies.

REFERENCES

1. Benjafield AV, Ayas NT, Eastwood PR, et al. Estimation of the global prevalence and burden of obstructive sleep apnoea: a literature-based analysis. *Lancet Respir Med*. 2019;7(8):687-698. doi:10.1016/S2213-2600(19)30198-5
2. Amra B, Javani M, Soltaninejad F, et al. Comparison of Berlin questionnaire, STOP-Bang, and Epworth Sleepiness Scale for diagnosing obstructive sleep

apnea in Persian patients. *Int J Prev Med*. 2018;9:28. doi:10.4103/ijpvm.IJPVM_131_17

3. Bixler EO, Vgontzas AN, Ten Have T, et al. Effects of age on sleep apnea in men: I. Prevalence and severity. *Am J Respir Crit Care Med*. 1998;157:144-148.
4. Practice guidelines for the perioperative management of patients with obstructive sleep apnea: an updated report by the American Society of Anesthesiologists Task Force on Perioperative Management of Patients with Obstructive Sleep Apnea. *Anesthesiology*. 2014;120(2):268-286. doi:10.1097/ALN.0000000000000053
5. Vincensi B. Sleep in the hospitalized patient: nurse and patient perceptions. *Medsurg Nursing*. 2016;25(5):351-356.
6. Morse AM, Bender E. Sleep in hospitalized patients. *Clocks Sleep*. 2019;1(1):151-165. doi:10.3390/clockssleep1010014
7. Chaudhry RA, Zarmer L, West K, Chung F. Obstructive sleep apnea and risk of postoperative complications after non-cardiac surgery. *J Clin Med*. 2024;13(9):2538. doi:10.3390/jcm13092538
8. Pinto JA, Ribeiro DK, Cavallini AF, Duarte C, Freitas GS. Comorbidities associated with obstructive sleep apnea: a retrospective study. *Int Arch Otorhinolaryngol*. 2016;20(2):145-150. doi:10.1055/s-0036-1579546.
9. Martin SS, Aday AW, Almarzooq ZI, et al; on behalf of the American Heart Association Council on Epidemiology and Prevention Statistics Committee and Stroke Statistics Subcommittee. 2024 Heart disease and stroke statistics: a report of US and global data from the American Heart Association. *Circulation*. 2024;149(8):e347-e913. doi:10.1161/CIR.0000000000001209
10. Messineo L, Bakker JP, Cronin J, Yee J, White DP. Obstructive sleep apnea and obesity: a review of epidemiology, pathophysiology and the effect of weight-loss treatments. *Sleep Med Rev*. 2024;78:101996. doi:10.1016/j.smrv.2024.101996
11. Vasu TS, Grewal R, Doghramji K. Obstructive sleep apnea syndrome and perioperative complications: a systematic review of the literature. *J Clin Sleep Med*. 2012;8(2):199-207. doi:10.5664/jcsm.1784
12. Li A, Roveda JM, Powers LS, Quan SF. Obstructive sleep apnea predicts 10-year cardiovascular disease-related mortality in the Sleep Heart Health Study: a machine learning approach. *J Clin Sleep Med*. 2022;18(2):497-504. doi:10.5664/jcsm.9630 PMID: 34437053; PMCID: PMC8805009.
13. Hwang M, Nagappa M, Guluzade N, et al. Validation of the STOP-Bang questionnaire as a preoperative screening tool for obstructive sleep apnea: a systematic review and meta-analysis. *BMC Anesthesiol*. 2022;22:366. doi:10.1186/s12871-022-01912-1
14. Hwang D, Shakir N, Limann B, et al. Sleep study and oximetry parameters for predicting postoperative complications in patients with obstructive sleep apnea. *Chest*. 2020;157(5):1210-1220. doi:10.1016/j.chest.2019.11.010
15. Chaudhry, R. A., Zarmer, L., West, K., & Chung, F. Obstructive sleep apnea and risk of postoperative complications after non-cardiac surgery. *J Clin Med*. 2024;13(9), 2538. doi:10.3390/jcm13092538
16. Bae E. Preoperative risk evaluation and perioperative management of patients with obstructive sleep apnea: a narrative review. *J Dent Anesth Pain Med*. 2023;23(4):179-188. doi:10.17245/jdapm.2023.23.4.179
17. Memtsoudis SG, Cozowicz C, Nagappa M, et al. Society of Anesthesia and Sleep Medicine guideline on intraoperative management of adult patients with obstructive sleep apnea. *Anesth Analg*. 2018;127(4):967-987. doi:10.1213/ANE.0000000000003434
18. Apfelbaum JL, Hagberg CA, Connis RT, et al. Practice guidelines for management of the difficult airway: an updated report by the American Society of Anesthesiologists Task Force on Management of the Difficult Airway. *Anesthesiology*. 2022;136(1):31-81. doi:10.1097/ALN.0000000000004002
19. Fernandez-Bustamante A, Bartels K, Clavijo C, Golisch W. Preoperative screening and postoperative respiratory outcomes in patients at risk for obstructive sleep apnea. *Anesth Analg*. 2020;130(4):976-985. doi:10.1213/ANE.0000000000004543

Chapter 30

Developing an Inpatient Assessment and Monitoring Program

KELLY W. GLADDEN AND KEIR MORRISON NOE

KEY CONCEPTS/LEARNING OBJECTIVES

The key concepts in this chapter include identifying hospitalized patients at risk for sleep disorders, developing an assessment plan appropriate to hospitalized patients with an increased risk of sleep disorders, reviewing the patient's comorbid disorders that contribute to multiple hospitalizations and readmissions, and developing a program for hospitalized patients identified with sleep disorders.

KEY TERMS

Case management
Certified Clinical Sleep Health Educator (CCSH)
Chronic obstructive pulmonary disease (COPD)
Congestive heart failure (CHF)
Obstructive sleep apnea (OSA)
Sleep disorders (SD)

INTRODUCTION

This chapter aims to provide sleep programs with a fundamental approach to developing a program for identifying, assessing, and managing hospital inpatients at an increased risk for sleep disorders. The complex interaction between untreated sleep issues and other common disorders such as treatment-resistant hypertension, chronic obstructive pulmonary disease (COPD), type 2 diabetes, atrial fibrillation, stroke, and congestive heart failure (CHF) is associated with multiple hospitalizations and readmissions. Many patients, including inpatients and outpatients undergoing surgery, are also at an increased risk of sedation complications and medication interactions.

RATIONALE

Despite widely available information about the clinical importance of screening for sleep-disordered breathing (SDB) and The Joint Commission's citation of SDB (1) as a patient safety issue, the majority of patients with SDB remain unrecognized and undiagnosed. There may be a variety of reasons for this. The symptoms and risk factors for SDB are neither sensitive nor specific for SDB and overlap with many other important medical conditions, some of which may be the conditions driving admission to the hospital.

The recent declaration by the U.S. Preventive Services Task Force that "the current evidence is insufficient to assess the balance of benefits and harms of screening for obstructive sleep apnea (OSA) in asymptomatic adults" has led to some unfortunate confusion. Health care professionals may mistakenly apply this recommendation to the acute care setting, where symptoms are often present, and where the balance of risk and benefit favors screening for SDB.

Adult and pediatric patients with SDB are at risk of complications during hospitalization or surgery. These patients may experience complications when receiving sedatives, opioid analgesics, or general anesthesia, increasing the risk of prolonged apnea and respiratory arrest.

Evidence suggests an association between SDB and COPD and CHF readmissions, conditions monitored closely by Medicare's Hospital Readmission Reduction Program. Untreated obesity hypoventilation syndrome increases the risk of acute and chronic hypercapnic episodes, as well as having a significant impact on long-term survival. SDB screening programs are an important way to identify these patient populations. Implementation of treatment in these patients has been shown to convey benefits. Studies have shown that patients hospitalized with CHF and/or COPD who also have SDB, and who are adherent to treatment, have a lower 30-day readmission rate than patients with SDB who are untreated.

Sleep technology professionals, especially sleep health educators with established core competencies, have an opportunity to participate in implementing procedures that help reduce readmission by establishing screening solutions. These strategies include building processes that identify, screen, and facilitate testing and initiate treatment of patients with SDB.

The Joint Commission issued an advisory on safety and quality issues relating to patients with OSA in June 2015. The advisory cites sentinel events in which patients were diagnosed or suspected to have OSA, which may have been a contributing factor in some of the cases.

In this advisory, staff from The Joint Commission's Division of Healthcare Improvement cite the following concerns regarding OSA:

- Lack of training for health care professionals to screen for and recognize OSA
- Failure to assess patients for OSA
- Lack of guidelines for the care and treatment of individuals at risk for, and those diagnosed with, OSA
- Failure to implement appropriate monitoring of patients with risk factors associated with OSA
- Lack of communication among health care providers regarding patients with OSA or potential risk factors associated with OSA
- Lack of pre-/postoperative evaluation and treatment for OSA

These concerns should be kept in mind as you develop your program to ensure that they are addressed.

THE PURPOSE OF SCREENING

Screening of inpatients for sleep disorders is intended to prevent related complications, protect patients from potential harm, reduce readmissions, and provide exceptional patient-centered care by improving overall patient wellness. The role of the registered polysomnographic technologist (RPSGT) or certified clinical sleep health (CCSH) educator is to collect and summarize patient health information including vital signs and questionnaires necessary for evaluation of risk for sleep disorders. There should be set protocols in place to alert appropriate health care providers when patients meet the criteria for an elevated risk of SDB. The RPSGT or CCSH can manage the process of monitoring patients during hospitalization and work with the patient care team to coordinate an appropriate sleep care follow-up plan.

BUILDING THE TEAM

Development and implementation of a sleep disorders screening program require working with a variety of members of the patient care team and creating policies and procedures to guide team members.

The composition of this team will vary from hospital to hospital and may require the involvement of a variety of stakeholders to implement and manage the process. Some of the key players may include the following:

a. **Physician advocate:** One of the biggest assets to starting any hospital program is having a physician advocate. This physician should be well versed in hospital politics, know about the medical community, and understand the positive impact the program will have on patient care. This person does not have to be a sleep physician; a current referring physician such as a surgeon, cardiologist, or hospitalist may be a good option.

b. **Members of the sleep care team:** The medical director and other sleep physicians, hospitalists, nurse practitioners, physician assistants, and all other staff need to be on board and well informed about the program. An inpatient program may require your sleep physicians and practitioners to see inpatients in consultation, and order sleep studies or consultations while the patient is in-house. A staff of RPSGT and CCSH educators is essential to the program. These professionals will require sufficient time for chart review, patient education, and requesting consults and/or sleep studies for follow-up postdischarge.

c. **Administrators:** When a plan has been developed and you have a physician and staff buy-in, the next step is to present the plan to administration. Hospital administrators are responsible for the financial well-being of the hospital, and a program that is focused on improving patient outcomes and reducing readmissions is one way of achieving that. Administrators will be interested in the effect the screening program will have on the quality of patient care, meeting Joint Commission recommendations, and achieving good outcomes. You may also note increased referrals to the sleep center. The presentation should be short, factual, and include a financial analysis for the program.

d. **Nursing administrators:** Determine if the nursing staff is already using a STOP-Bang or modified sleep questionnaire about symptoms of OSA on admission. It will be important to develop an ongoing relationship with nursing staff as well as develop training for the nurses.

e. **Risk management or patient safety officers:** Risk management involvement will guide you through the risks, safety precautions, and policies needed for the program.

f. **Surgical team members:** Preoperative screening can be beneficial in setting up appropriate monitoring during postoperative patient recovery for those at risk for OSA. Some of these teams should include members from programs for bariatric surgery, anesthesiology, general surgery, and cardiology.
g. **Case managers and discharge planners:** It is important to educate this group because they are typically the last to see the patient before discharge. They can make a significant difference in ensuring appropriate ongoing care for the patient after discharge.

PROCEDURAL STEPS

Identify Hospitalized Patients With Sleep Disorders

Identifying at-risk patients is the first step. It would be prudent to check to see if or how the admitting nursing staff is collecting sleep-related information. If the hospital utilizes an electronic medical record (EMR), established sleep screening tools such as the Epworth Sleepiness Scale (ESS), Apnea Risk Evaluation System, the Berlin questionnaire, or the STOP-Bang should be implemented in the admitting process. One method to obtain a referral to the program could be triggering the referral based on a specific score on the screening questionnaire. If the admitting nursing staff completes the sleep questionnaire during admission, the Informational Technology (IT) team can develop a report to flag all new admissions that scored positive on the questionnaire. Additionally, further parameters collected such as previous OSA diagnosis or a body mass index (BMI) of more than 35 could trigger a referral.

Established risk factors that can be used to identify populations at risk for sleep disorders and OSA include:

- BMI more than 35 kg/m^2.
- Comorbid conditions with SDB such as resistant hypertension, COPD, type 2 diabetes, atrial fibrillation, stroke, and CHF.
- Known symptoms of SDB such as complaints of witnessed apneas, snoring, gasping/choking at night, nonrestorative sleep, excessive daytime sleepiness.
- Clinical symptoms such as nocturnal hypoxemia, nocturnal shortness of breath, waking with angina.
- Previous diagnosis of sleep apnea and nonadherence to treatment.
- Using medications that (a) might increase the risk of SDB (eg, opiates, muscle relaxants), (b) address common symptoms of SDB (eg, hypnotics, stimulants/wake promoting agents), or (c) treat common comorbidities of SDB (eg, antiarrhythmics, antiobesity drugs, diabetes agents).

Safeguard and Monitor At-Risk Patients

It is important to recognize that inpatients are acutely ill and, if suspected of having OSA or diagnosed but noncompliant with therapy, need to be monitored continuously upon admission. An automated alert system when a patient scores positive for OSA on admission to the following departments can help create a well-informed and active patient care team.

Some important team members include:

- Respiratory therapists and/or educators, who may initiate or request continuous telemetry, pulse oximetry monitoring, or even continuous positive airway pressure (CPAP) therapy.
- Pharmacy staff, who review the patient's medications and effects on SDB.
- Attending physicians and care team partners, who should be notified of patient risk.
- A sleep consult, which can be offered, if appropriate, or a referral to the sleep physician after discharge.
- Case managers/discharge planners, who should be informed to make appointments for the patient or arrange for home setup of CPAP therapy.

Educate At-Risk Patients, Families, and Staff

In some hospitals, it may be possible to automatically initiate a consult with the sleep physician who assesses the condition of the patients and the appropriateness for an inpatient home sleep apnea test (HSAT). Another option is an EMR alert for the attending physician who will discuss the risk with the patient and/or family and initiate a sleep physician consult if appropriate at that time. In all cases, the sleep center should provide an educational visit to the patient's room. Provide personalized patient information on sleep health and hygiene, sleep disorders, SDB and comorbidities, and therapeutic options. A discussion regarding possible OSA, screening, and testing, and, if applicable, therapy adherence with the patient and family members may be appropriate. Always be respectful, because most patients will not be in a proper frame of mind to talk about snoring or how they are sleeping as a result of their condition. In such a scenario, leave them with an educational sheet that includes a phone number to call when they feel better. Approach them later if an opportunity arises.

Tips to Remember

- Determine the appropriate literacy level and educate the patient and family.
- Follow the American Association of Sleep Technologists (AAST) standardized Patient Education Curriculum guidelines.

- Document education provided in patients' medical records.
- Consider using the hospital patient education TV channel, if available.

Educate the Health Care Team

In general, the education plan for the program should include the following:

- Outlining the program and educating hospitalists, nursing staff, cardiologists, pulmonologists, risk management, case management, and the respiratory therapy team (with special attention to night shift care teams) about the risk of SDB for inpatients and available resources
- Referencing the AAST OSA Care Plan and the AAST Patient Education Curriculum
- Providing Continuing Education Credits (CEC)/ Continuing Education Units (CEU) in-service programs for staff
- Providing a method to contact the sleep health educator and other members of the sleep care team for support

Coordinate Diagnostic Testing

Work with the patient care team to assess the benefits of immediate testing. Inpatients with chronically poor health may not return after discharge, and therefore, inpatient testing may be warranted.

- Triage patients based on the risk assessment.
- Obtain an order for additional screening tests as needed (consider overnight oximetry or HSAT).
- Schedule postdischarge in-lab studies, if appropriate.
- Report the outcome of testing to the attending physician and patient care team.
- Obtain an order for treatment from a sleep specialist or another physician if appropriate.

Ensure Treatment Implementation

Identify any barriers to treatment and work with the health care team to resolve them. The hospital case manager and discharge planner will be assisting before discharge. There are many choices they must provide the patient to maintain compliance with state and federal regulations. Be sure to include them in the treatment planning process.

The sleep team should be prepared to do the following:

- Assist with the implementation of positive airway pressure (PAP) therapy.
- Ensure appropriate documentation to support the durable medical equipment (DME) order.
- Document the DME supplier, the interface type and size, and treatment settings.
- Coordinate with the DME supplier to ensure appropriate equipment is in place upon discharge.

Monitor Patient Adherence and Outcomes

Implement a follow-up monitoring plan that may include the following:

- Monitor adherence data, beginning with the first week and continuing until adherence to therapy is established.
- Technologist or educator telephone support for patients on PAP therapy. Follow policies and procedures to determine and document the need for intervention.
- Ensure timely and appropriate physician follow-up.
- Utilize digital patient engagement tools to support therapy adherence.
- Track and report patient outcomes and establish metrics and reporting process (data collection tool or EMR). Track and report previous history of readmission and adherence to therapy.
- Track and report overall program outcomes.
- Maintain a database for outcomes tracking (readmission rates, adherence to therapy, improvement in quality of life, or other appropriate measures).

HOW TO START AN INPATIENT SLEEP PROGRAM

There are many different ways one can start an inpatient sleep program. The person has to be driven, expect to hear no, and if no occurs, find a workaround until one achieves their goal. The person has to be a good public speaker and interact well with different teams. Since several programs are using some form of inpatient screening for sleep apnea, there is more data available that can be presented to your hospital administration team to show the value of creating a sleep navigator role to help reduce readmissions and improve patient outcomes.

If a CCSH educator advocate can present data showing how an inpatient sleep screening program can save hospital money by reducing readmissions or increase revenue by increasing sleep center in-lab or home testing referrals along with increasing sleep outpatient office consult and follow-up referrals, your chances for being approved should have improved. The bonus of having such a program is improving patient outcomes. If the patient is compliant with sleep apnea treatment, that will help reduce their yearly out-of-pocket expenses and modify the individual's health for the better.

As you begin your thought process in creating such a program, start simply. Depending on the personality of your hospital system, sometimes starting small is better than going broad. Once your program is up and running successfully, expand out because you will then have more contacts, and your previous contacts will help introduce you to other departments in the hospital system. Always helpful if the sleep center has a Head of Department (HOD) hospital leader, who takes the time to listen to the ideas of their team members. The HOD leader may be an asset to help grow your program.

The best way to understand how to start a program by combining the information summarized in this chapter is by laying out an example of how one hospital system started a successful sleep navigation program.

1. Need an advocate such as your direct manager and your medical sleep director to start the process of discussing the idea of having a new role using a CCSH to start a sleep navigation program at their team management organizational meetings.
2. If the above was not already occurring, then the CCSH should gather the data to present to their direct manager and medical sleep director as to why a sleep navigator would benefit the sleep center.
3. The CCSH needs to have a plan in place because once you have permission, the meetings will begin with various department leaders approving or denying your proposal.
4. This one hospital sleep center system goal was to screen every patient admitted to the hospital, which required many meetings with different leaders/teams such as the hospitalist team, emergency department team, and cardiac teams. Depending on your request, your teams may differ.
5. Once the sleep navigator role is approved amongst the hospital teams, the CCSH will need to have a plan in mind to build what is needed in the hospital's EMR system.
6. The CCSH will need to create a ticket for such a build to occur with the hospital IT team. Do not expect the IT team to know how to build what you need. The navigator needs to talk with the IT team about what is needed. One advantage is with other hospital systems having some form of sleep apnea screening in their EMR system, there may be a build that can be copied.
7. Think about who is going to ask the screener and to which population. Do you screen the entire hospital, or do you screen specific comorbid individual floors?
8. What is the sleep navigator staffing going to look like?
9. What happens if there is one sleep navigator, but that person wants to take off? Is there another CCSH that can cover?
10. What other forms do you want to have in the EMR besides the screener?
11. What forms do you want to leave with the patient?
12. How are you going to document that the sleep health education was completed?
13. How are you going to track your time with each patient?
14. How are you going to track the patients you see?
15. How are you going to know when the patient is discharged?
16. What is your progress note going to look like?
17. Are you going to be able to order the sleep study or outpatient sleep consult while the patient is in the hospital?
18. If you are not able to order a consultation or sleep study, what is your plan to get the patient scheduled after discharge? Once the patient leaves, it is hard to get them to respond to calls or messages because they are feeling better.
19. How are you going to track readmissions?
20. What is your plan going to be to move the patient quickly through the sleep center for testing, office visits, and treatment to help reduce 30-day readmissions?
21. After the Go-Live date, think about how to expand the program either within the hospital system or outside of the hospital system.

There are many ways to move a patient through the hospital system. One example of a successful inpatient sleep navigation consultation to help reduce readmission and improve the patient's outcomes would be the following case study.

- 48-year-old male
- History of obstructive sleep apnea, hypertension, anxiety, and depression
- Admitted 10/28/24 for a new CHF
- STOP-Bang score = 7 by the nurse and Cardiology Nurse Practitioner sent a sleep navigator education order to speak with the patient
- The patient was stable, and the sleep navigator spoke with the patient and wife on 10/28/24 in the Intensive Care Unit (ICU).
- Home bilevel positive airway pressure (BiPAP) device was 10 years old. The patient stated he could not sleep without it.
- The patient never followed up with a sleep physician since obtaining BiPAP.
- 50 lb heavier since tested

- The BiPAP machine had a warning message that motor was declining.
- He wanted the sleep study first and then follow up with the sleep physician for results to obtain a new home device.
- He was willing to drive anywhere if he could not get into the lab near his home quickly.
- The sleep navigator ordered the sleep study, and the hospitalist signed the order.
- The sleep navigator expedited sleep referral to sleep center insurance authorization team.
- Insurance approved in-lab sleep study on 10/29/24.
- The patient accepted the insurance estimate on 10/30/24.
- The patient called the sleep navigator on 10/30/24 stating that 12/12/24 first available appointment near his home was too long to wait. Can he get in quicker?
- The sleep navigator reached out to sleep scheduling.
- Scheduled at another lab location on 11/4/24
- On 11/1/24, the sleep navigator emailed the sleep day support team to expedite him.
- He showed up for an in-lab study, and he was Split with an Apnea Hypopnea Index (AHI) = 132.6, 79% low saturation, and with severe periodic leg movement disorder (PLMD).
- Auto BiPAP was suggested in the sleep interpretation report.
- On 11/7/24, he called the sleep navigator stating he saw the results in his medical record. What are the next steps?
- On 11/12/24, the sleep navigator called him because the navigator did not see an appointment and the supervisor of the sleep office said he was not returning her calls.
- On 11/13/24, he scheduled a video call with pulmonary sleep on 11/22/24 in a different office to get in quicker.
- On 11/22/24, he called in for the telehealth visit.
- An Auto BiPAP was ordered.
- All done in less than 1 month.

The above case study is an excellent example showing the need for an inpatient sleep navigator. If not for this hospital system having such a role, this patient would not have moved through the large health care system as quickly to help reduce readmissions and improve the patient's outcome.

SUMMARY

Developing a program for identifying, assessing, and managing inpatients at increased risk for sleep disorders is a significant undertaking. In the inpatient arena, there are many overlapping priorities. Making the identification of hospitalized patients at risk for sleep disorders that may extend or complicate their hospital stay is no small undertaking.

An organized plan that includes all facets of the organization from administration and physicians to the nursing and ancillary staff is essential. Policies and procedures must be a part of the plan, and education for staff in all areas is key to the success of an inpatient program. Screening tools, diagnostic tools, discharge and follow-up care, as well as measurement of outcomes and success of the program are each important pieces of the overall plan.

The success of an inpatient screening program depends on the cooperation and coordination of a multitude of people and services, but if done well, it can result in improved care and better outcomes for all patients who are at risk for sleep disorders. It is definitely worth the effort!

REFERENCES

1. AAST Technical Guidelines. *Best Practice for Inpatient Sleep Disordered Breathing Screening and Management.* American Association of Sleep Technologists; February 2018. Accessed July 2, 2018. https://aastweb.org/wp-content/uploads/2025/03/Best-Practice-for-Inpatient-Sleep-Disordered-Breathing.pdf

SUGGESTED READINGS

Gladden KW. *A Diary Build and Grow a Hospital Navigation Program.* 1st ed. Book Patch; 2023.

Quick Safety: An Advisory on Safety and Quality Issues. *At Risk: Obstructive Sleep Apnea Patients* (Issue 14). Joint Commission; June 2015.

Chapter 31
Medications and Their Effect on Sleep and Sleep Disorders

DEBBIE AKERS AND TIFFANY NEALY

KEY CONCEPTS/LEARNING OBJECTIVES

On completion of this chapter, the reader should be able to identify the major classes of drugs that may alter the polysomnogram, detect sleep disturbances that may occur because of specific medications, discuss the relationship between sleep and medications and intervene on behalf of patient safety.

KEY TERMS

ACE inhibitor
Antidepressant
Gamma-aminobutyric acid (GABA)
Hypnotics
Oxybates
Polysomnography (PSG)
Respiratory drugs
Sedative
Selective serotonin reuptake inhibitors (SSRI)
Tricyclic antidepressants

The Centers for Disease Control and Prevention (CDC) reported in 2020 that 47% of the US population used at least one prescription drug within the past 30 days, 21% used three or more prescription drugs, whereas 12% used five or more prescription drugs (1). Chances are that three out of four of the 84% using a prescription drug within the past 30 days are being seen in the sleep laboratory tonight. The purpose of this chapter is to assist the technologist to provide better patient care by understanding how daily medications can affect sleep and sleep disorders.

MEDICATIONS AND HOW THEY AFFECT SLEEP

About 89% of patients rely on some sort of prescribed medications. Most of these medications are for chronic conditions, whereas some are used for acute ailments. Medications for high blood pressure, heart disease, respiratory issues (asthma, chronic obstructive pulmonary disease), headaches, smoking cessation, colds, and allergies, to name a few, can affect sleep by either depriving the patient of sleep or causing daytime sleepiness.

Some of the more commonly prescribed medications are antiarrhythmic drugs used to treat heart rhythm issues, which can cause difficulty initiating and maintaining sleep or insomnia. Beta-blockers are used to treat hypertension, arrhythmias, and angina. Beta-blockers increase the likelihood of awakenings during the night, nightmares, and/or insomnia. Cholesterol medications are associated with poor sleep. Asthma medications can cause insomnia because the chemicals in theophylline are related to caffeine and can make the patient feel fidgety. Thyroid conditions can cause tremendous sleepiness (specifically, hypothyroidism), whereas the medication used to treat this disorder causes insomnia. These are a few of the common prescription medications often seen on the patient's medication list. This chapter will review medications that can affect a patient's sleep and the effects of medications on the polysomnography (PSG).

Hypnotics

Barbiturates

Barbiturates, sometimes called "downers," are medications that act on the central nervous system (CNS) by depressing or inhibiting nerve signals in the brain. They work by depressing the reticular formation, a comprehensive network of nerves found in the central area of the brainstem, thus promoting sleep. Other uses include, but are not limited to, anesthesia during surgery, an anticonvulsant, and for anxiety attacks. Barbiturates are derived from barbituric acid (2) that scientists have synthesized and are grouped according to how fast they produce an effect and how long that effect lasts and are classified as sedative hypnotics that lead to the slowing down of the body's functions. This slowing down of the body's functions can include physical signs such as lethargy, slurred speech, shallow breathing, fatigue, drowsiness, and difficulty in concentrating.

Expected and possible effects on PSG (acute):

Decrease: Sleep latency (SL), wake after sleep onset (WASO), N1, rapid eye movement (REM), N3, arousals, and body movement.
Increase: Sleep efficiency (SE), total sleep time (TST), N2, spindles, N3, REM latency (RL), sleep apnea, and daytime sleepiness.
Withdrawal: Decrease TST and increase REM (REM rebound).

Barbiturates are now rarely used most likely because of the numerous adverse side effects and high incidence of tolerance and dependence. They used to be the "go-to drug" for insomnia but have lessened in popularity with the advent of benzodiazepines (BZDs).

Benzodiazepines

BZD is a psychoactive medication used as a sedative or muscle relaxant. When one suffers from anxiety or panic attacks, the brain becomes overactive, and BZDs are chemicals that will help it to slow down. Although it is not clear how BZDs work, they are believed to affect the GABA receptors of the brain. GABA, or gamma-aminobutyric acid, is a major inhibitory brain chemical that blocks the transmission of a signal from one brain cell to another. Although GABA is an amino acid, it is classified as a neurotransmitter; it inhibits and relaxes, therefore inducing relaxation and sleep.

Expected and possible effects on PSG (acute):

Decrease: SL, WASO, REM, N3 (for most agents), periodic limb movements (PLMs), and arousals.
Increase: SE, TST, N1, N2, spindles, N3 (for some agents), RL, sleep apnea, and daytime sleepiness.
Withdrawal: Increase WASO, decrease TST, increase REM (REM rebound), increase SL, and arousals.

Although BZDs contain chemicals like those found in the body to induce calming, adding them to what is already in the body helps GABA receptors send out a greater number of these signals to the brain, resulting in sedation or relaxation. BZDs are also used for general anesthesia, sedation before medical procedures, alcohol withdrawal, nausea, and vomiting. Although BZDs are used for various reasons, some are more commonly prescribed for certain conditions (3):

Alcohol withdrawal: Chlordiazepoxide (Librium)
Anesthesia: Diazepam (Valium), lorazepam (Ativan), and midazolam (Versed)
Anxiety: Alprazolam (Xanax), chlordiazepoxide (Librium), clorazepate (Tranxene), diazepam (Valium), lorazepam (Ativan), and midazolam (Versed)
Insomnia: Estazolam (Prosom), flurazepam (Dalmane), quazepam (Doral), temazepam (Restoril), and triazolam (Halcion)
Irritable bowel syndrome: Chlordiazepoxide/clidinium (Librax)
Muscle relaxant: Diazepam (Valium)
Seizure: Clonazepam (Klonopin), clorazepate (Tranxene), and diazepam (Valium)
Reduce PLMs: Clonazepam (Klonopin)

Keeping in mind that some BZDs have been used for a multitude of medical conditions, one should then not assume that a patient who, for illustration purposes, takes diazepam suffers from seizures. The sleep technologist should always take the time to read each patient's medical history (Table 31-1).

Nonbenzodiazepine (Z-Drugs and Gamma-Aminobutyric Acid Receptor Agonists)

Nonbenzodiazepine (NBZD), a relatively newer class of drugs, is also used for surgical anesthesia but is more widely advertised as a short-term treatment for insomnia. These drugs work in the same area of the brain as BZDs do but tend to be more specific for inducing sleep.

NBZDs are generally known to have a shorter half-life, so it is rare to wake up with a "hangover" feeling the following day. Newer controlled-release formulations may extend the half-life of the medication as in the case of zolpidem. Information released by the Food and Drug Administration (FDA), however, states that the termination half-life for controlled-release zolpidem (12.5 mg) is no different from that of the immediate release formula (10 mg).

The use of NBZDs is less likely to cause addiction but may cause amnesia and erratic behavior (as parasomnia). One should keep in mind, however, that these medications would not address any underlying medical problems that may cause insomnia and should therefore not be seen as a cure (Table 31-2).

Dual Orexinergic Antagonists

Orexin neuropeptides A and B, also known as hypocretin 1 and 2, are known to play a part in sleep/wake regulation. Dual OX1R/OX2R antagonists (dual orexinergic antagonists [DORAs]) and selective OX2R antagonists (2-SORAs) have been studied for their potential as sleep aids. There are formulations currently registered as a treatment for insomnia (suvorexant, lemborexant, and

Table 31-1 Benzodiazepines

Generic Name	Popularly Known as/ Brand Name	Time to Peak (Onset of Action [h])	Elimination Half-life (h) (Active Metabolite)
Alprazolam	Xanax	1-2	6-12
Chlordiazepoxide	Librium	1.5-4	5-30 (36-200 h)
Clonazepam	Klonopin	1-4	18-50
Clorazepate	Tranxene	Varies	(36-100 h)
Diazepam	Valium	1-2	20-100 (36-200 h)
Estazolam	Prosom	0.5-5	10-24
Flunitrazepam	Rohypnol	0.5-3	18-26 (36-200 h)
Flurazepam	Dalmane	1-1.5	(40-250 h)
Halazepam	Paxipam	1-3	(30-100 h)
Lorazepam	Ativan	2-4	10-20
Midazolam	Versed	0.5-1	3 (1.8-6 h)
Oxazepam	Serax	3-4	4-15
Quazepam	Doral	1-5	25-120
Temazepam	Restoril	0.5-3	8-22
Triazolam	Halcion	0.5-2	2
Expected Effects of Benzodiazepines on Polysomnography			
<	SL		
>	SE		
>	TST		
<	WASO		
>	NREM 1		
>	NREM 2 > Spindles		
<<	SWS		
>	RL		
<	REM		
<	Arousals		
<,>	PLMs		
≥	Sleep apnea		
>	Daytime sleepiness		
	Withdrawal		
<	TST		
>	REM (REM rebound)		
>	Arousals		
>	SL		
Expected Effect on Polysomnography			
<	SL		
>	SE		
>	TST		
<	WASO		
<	NREM 1		

(continued)

Table 31-1 Benzodiazepines (*continued*

Expected Effect on Polysomnography	
>	NREM 2 (spindles)
≤	SWS
>	RL
≤	REM
<,>	Arousals
=	PLMs
=	Sleep apnea
	Withdrawal
≥	WASO

NREM, nonrapid eye movement; PLM, periodic limb movement; REM, rapid eye movement; RL, REM latency; SE, sleep efficiency; SL, sleep latency; SWS, slow-wave sleep; TST, total sleep time; WASO, wake after sleep onset.

daridorexant), and many more are being studied across the world. Many studies show that there is an improvement in TST as well as a subjective improvement in reported sleep quality and insomnia scale scores (https://pubmed.ncbi.nlm.nih.gov/35065036/). Upon review of the current up-to-date evidence, these medications appear to increase REM pressure and overall reduce RL (https://pubmed.ncbi.nlm.nih.gov/32505969/)

Oxybates

Oxybates (sodium oxybate or mixed oxybate salts) are CNS depressant drugs with both hypnotic and sedative properties used for the treatment of cataplexy and excessive daytime sleepiness in patients with narcolepsy. Patients with narcolepsy have dysregulated nighttime sleep, disordered sleep/wake stages, and overall

Table 31-2 Nonbenzodiazepines

Generic Name	Popularly Known as/ Brand Name	Onset of Action (min)	Half-life (h)
Eszopiclone	Lunesta	60	4-6
Zaleplon	Sonata	15-30	1
Zolpidem	Ambien	15-30	2-3
Expected Effects of Nonbenzodiazepines on Polysomnography			
<,>	SL		
<,>	SE		
>	TST		
<	WASO		
>	NREM 2 (spindles)		
≥	SWS		
>	RL		
<<	REM		
>	PLMs		
≥	Daytime sleepiness		
	Withdrawal		
>	WASO		
>	REM		

NREM, nonrapid eye movement; PLM, periodic limb movement; REM, rapid eye movement; RL, REM latency; SE, sleep efficiency; SL, sleep latency; SWS, slow-wave sleep; TST, total sleep time; WASO, wake after sleep onset.

sleep state instabilities (https://pubmed.ncbi.nlm.nih.gov/20082240/). Sodium oxybate is the sodium salt of gamma hydroxybutyrate (GHB), which is a metabolite of GABA. Oxybate acts as a GABA-B and GHB receptor agonist, which helps stabilize sleep in patients with narcolepsy.

Prior studies show that oxybates help decrease the number of shifts per hour from Stages N2, N3, and REM to Stage N1 and Wake, which results in improved continuity and decreased disruptions https://pubmed.ncbi.nlm.nih.gov/27807903/. Overall, oxybates improve sleep architecture in patients with narcolepsy. The expected effects include decreased N1 sleep, increased Slow-wave sleep (SWS) (N3), decreased REM sleep, and a decrease in overall arousals (https://pubmed.ncbi.nlm.nih.gov/37755650/)

Other Hypnotic Agents

Two examples of hypnotic agents are ramelteon and chloral hydrate. Ramelteon is considered a melatonin receptor agonist, thus inhibiting the wake-promoting activity of the suprachiasmatic nucleus. It also helps reduce SL and increase TST, while having no effect on sleep architecture. Chloral hydrate, an alcohol-type hypnotic, is occasionally used in the older adults. It has a short half-life (4-6 hours) and will decrease SL and arousals. SWS is also slightly depressed, but overall REM sleep is unchanged (4).

Antidepressants

There are occasions when doctors prescribe antidepressants to promote sleep even though none of these are specifically approved as sleep medications.

Antidepressants, the third most prescribed drug in this country, were first developed in the 1950s to help relieve the symptoms of depression. Tricyclic antidepressants (TCAs) and selective serotonin reuptake inhibitors (SSRIs) are the two most popular on the market today (5).

Tricyclic Antidepressants

TCAs are considered a first-generation antidepressant medication and are named for the molecular structure of most of the drugs in this class. They are one of the oldest classes of antidepressants and continue to be prescribed today. They are thought to act by blocking the reuptake or reabsorption of two critical brain hormones, the neurotransmitters serotonin and norepinephrine. Some block one, some the other, and some block both.

Neurotransmitters are different types of chemical messengers that the brain contains, which act as communication agents between various brain cells. Two of these transmitters are serotonin, also known as 5-hydroxytryptamine, and norepinephrine. Serotonin's effects are normally inhibitory. It diminishes appetite and sexual behavior and suppresses pain perception and has also been correlated with eating and sleep disorders (6). Norepinephrine plays a significant role in how the body responds to stress. It is more involved in maintaining normal body functions such as heart rate, blood pressure, and blood sugar levels and in regulating attention, emotions, and sleep (7).

TCAs will also block the reuptake of histamine and acetylcholine (ACh) activity. Histamine helps control the sleep-wake cycle and promotes the release of epinephrine and norepinephrine, whereas ACh is a neurotransmitter with an important role in the enhancement of sensory perceptions when we are awake and in sustaining attention. ACh is known to be the most important inducer of REM sleep (8) (Table 31-3).

A low-dose doxepin formulation is approved by the FDA for the treatment of insomnia. Studies have shown

Table 31-3 Tricyclics

Generic Name	Popularly Known as/Brand Name	Half-life (h)
Amitriptyline	Elavil	10-50
Amoxapine	Asendin	8
Clomipramine	Anafranil	21
Doxepin	Silenor, Sinequan	8-24
Desipramine	Norpramin	12-24
Imipramine	Tofranil	11-25
Maprotiline	Ludiomil	8-16
Nortriptyline	Pamelor	18-44
Protriptyline	Vivactil	16-90
Trimipramine	Surmontil	14-46

(*continued*)

Table 31-3 Tricyclics (*continued*)

Expected/Effects of Tricyclics on Polysomnography	
<	SL
<	SE
<	TST
≥	WASO
</>	NREM 1
≤	SWS
>	RL
<	REM
>	Arousals
≥	PLMs
≥	Daytime sleepiness
>	NREM eye movement
>	RBD

NREM, nonrapid eye movement; PLM, periodic limb movement; RBD, REM behavior disorder; REM, rapid eye movement; RL, REM latency; SE, sleep efficiency; SL, sleep latency; SWS, slow-wave sleep; TST, total sleep time; WASO, wake after sleep onset.

that low-dose doxepin (3 and 6 mg) may be an alternative to hypnotics such as Ambien for primary insomnia. Doxepin decreases WASO and SL, increasing TST. These results were the same for patients with chronic or transient insomnia.

Selective Serotonin Reuptake Inhibitors

SSRIs were developed in response to the need for better tolerated, if not safer, antidepressants than TCAs. They were developed to inhibit the reuptake of only serotonin and not other neurotransmitters, which were also affected by TCAs. Because of this desired result, plus the benefit of improved tolerability and safety if taken in excess, SSRIs now replace TCAs as the drug of choice to treat depression. It should be noted, however, that there remain clinical situations where TCAs are still deemed more appropriate (eg, severe depression).

SSRIs are stimulants and are more likely to produce insomnia. Several patients have reported sleeping better, and the remaining issues of insomnia are expected to improve with continued use. Although they may encourage better sleep, they have also been linked to REM behavior disorder (RBD). SSRIs' effect on sleep architecture includes a decrease in SL, SE, TST, and REM sleep and an increase in WASO, N1, and PLMs (Table 31-4).

Serotonin and Norepinephrine (Noradrenaline) Reuptake Inhibitors

Serotonin and norepinephrine (noradrenaline) reuptake inhibitors (SNRIs) are also known as "dual reuptake inhibitors" because they act on both serotonin and norepinephrine. The former regulates a variety of bodily functions and feelings, whereas the latter is a chemical messenger in the brain that influences sleep and alertness. Duloxetine (Cymbalta), venlafaxine (Effexor), and desvenlafaxine (Pristiq) are SNRIs. Aside from being antidepressants, duloxetine and venlafaxine are also indicated for the treatment of generalized anxiety and social anxiety disorders. Duloxetine may also be prescribed for painful diabetic neuropathy and may soon be used for stress urinary incontinence (9). Newly diagnosed with RBD? Effexor may be the culprit (Table 31-5).

Monoamine Oxidase Inhibitors

Monoamine oxidase inhibitors (MAOIs) are a class of antidepressants that affect serotonin, norepinephrine, and dopamine levels in the brain. Dopamine is responsible for motivation, interest, and drive and is also involved in muscle control and function. It is associated with positive stress states such as being in love, exercising, listening to music, and sex.

MAOIs are mostly effective in major depression and are typically prescribed for those who do not respond well to other antidepressants and as a last resort because of numerous side effects. They are effective for some forms of depression when other medications have failed (5).

Expected and possible effects on PSG:

Decrease: SE, TST, SWS, and REM.
Increase: SL, WASO, PLMs, and daytime sleepiness.

Atypical Antidepressants

There are some antidepressants that are both non-SSRI and non-TCA. An example of this is buspirone (Buspar).

Table 31-4 Selective Serotonin Reuptake Inhibitors

Generic Name	Popularly Known as/Brand Name	Half-life (h)
Citalopram	Celexa	35
Escitalopram	Lexapro	27-32
Fluoxetine	Prozac	48-96
Paroxetine	Paxil	20
Sertraline	Zoloft	26
Expected Effects of SSRIs on Polysomnography		
>	SL	
<	SE	
<	TST	
>	WASO	
>	NREM 1	
>	RL	
<<	REM	
>	PLMs	
≥	Daytime sleepiness	

NREM, nonrapid eye movement; PLM, periodic limb movement; REM, rapid eye movement; RL, REM latency; SE, sleep efficiency; SL, sleep latency; SWS, slow-wave sleep; TST, total sleep time; WASO, wake after sleep onset.

Table 31-5 Serotonin and Noradrenaline Reuptake Inhibitors

Generic Name	Popularly Known as/Brand Name	Duration of Effect/Elimination Half-life (h)
Desvenlafaxine	Pristiq	11
Duloxetine	Cymbalta	12
Venlafaxine	Effexor	5-7
Expected/Possible Effects of H1 Blockers on PSG		
<	SL	
>	TST	
>	NREM 1	
>	NREM 2	
>	SWS	
<	REM	
Expected/Possible Effects of H2 Blockers on PSG		
>	SWS (for cimetidine)	
=	Usually have no effect on sleep stages or sleep continuity	
+	Somnolence and lethargy for older patients	

NREM, nonrapid eye movement; PSG, polysomnography; REM, rapid eye movement; SL, sleep latency; SWS, slow-wave sleep; TST, total sleep time.

Because it lacks the anticonvulsant, sedative, and muscle relaxant properties associated with other anxiolytics, buspirone has been termed "anxioselective" (10). It is nonsedating and shows no effect on SL, sleep continuity, SWS, or REM sleep and does not increase incidence of PLMs.

Cardiovascular Drugs

Antihypertensive Drugs

There are many different types of antihypertensive drugs, some of which affect how the heart pumps blood, whereas others cause vasodilation. The types that are most commonly used are beta-blocker drugs, angiotensin-converting enzyme (ACE) inhibitor drugs, angiotensin II blocker drugs, calcium-channel blocker drugs, and diuretic drugs.

Angiotensin-Converting Enzyme Inhibitors

ACE inhibitors are drugs used to treat heart failure and high blood pressure and to treat diabetic kidney disease. ACE inhibitors help prevent, although not completely, the normal formation in the body of angiotensin II, which is a hormone that causes constriction (narrowing) of blood vessels. By reducing the amount of hormone present in the blood, ACE inhibitors allow blood vessels to dilate. This dilation or widening of blood vessels throughout the body reduces blood pressure, making it easier for the heart to pump blood, and results in alleviating heart failure (11). Although these drugs help improve quality of life and cognitive performance, there is some question as to whether they may cause insomnia.

Angiotensin II Blockers

Like ACE inhibitors, angiotensin II drugs are used to treat heart failure and high blood pressure and to prevent kidney failure. They are an alternative to ACE inhibitors and work by blocking the action of angiotensin II that is produced naturally by the body and causes blood vessels to constrict (11).

Beta-Blockers

Beta-blocker drugs, or beta-adrenergic blocking agents, are most often prescribed to treat high blood pressure. They work by blocking the action of epinephrine (adrenaline) and norepinephrine (noradrenaline), two chemicals produced by the body that increase heart rate and raise blood pressure (11).

Expected and possible effects on PSG:

Decrease: TST, SWS, and REM.
Increase: SL, WASO, N1, REM, total wake time, and daytime sleepiness (after daytime administration).

The effects on sleep quality and staging seem to be limited to lipophilic as opposed to hydrophilic beta-blockers (12). Lipophilic agents include propranolol, pindolol, and metoprolol, whereas hydrophilic agents include atenolol and sotalol. Beta-blockers have also been associated with complaints of insomnia, fatigue, hallucinations, and nightmares.

Calcium-Channel Blockers

Calcium-channel blockers reduce the amount of calcium entering the muscle cells in blood vessel walls. Muscle cells need calcium to contract, and reducing the amount of calcium induces the muscle cells to relax and the blood vessels to widen (11).

Calcium-channel blockers are not known to affect sleep, sleep continuity, or sleep stages. However, they are associated with insomnia and nightmares (13).

Diuretic Drugs

Diuretics work by reducing the amount of liquid and salts reabsorbed into the blood, thereby increasing the volume of urine that is produced. The reduced blood volume helps reduce blood pressure (11). Impact on sleep is secondary because of increased nocturia.

Centrally Acting Alpha-Adrenergic Agonists: Clonidine

Several studies have demonstrated that clonidine disrupted the quality of nighttime sleep by inducing more shifts to N1 or wakefulness (13,14). Clonidine increases sedation and has also been known to suppress or reduce REM sleep.

Hypolipidemic Drugs

Cholesterol is a waxy, fat-like substance that is made by the liver. It forms part of every cell in the body, helps maintain healthy cell walls, and produces hormones, bile acids for the digestion of fat, and vitamin D. Excess cholesterol clogs blood vessels and increases the risk of heart disease and stroke.

Although cholesterol medications are often prescribed, there are no supporting data showing the relationship between the use of cholesterol medication and sleep architecture. Some reports, however, show that atorvastatin, lovastatin, and simvastatin may lead to insomnia or disrupt sleep, whereas Gemfibrozil and clofibrate are reported to cause sleepiness (15).

Stimulants

Stimulants are a class of drugs that work by increasing the dopamine levels in the brain. They include, among others, amphetamines, methylphenidate, modafinil, pemoline, and xanthene derivatives (namely, caffeine and theophylline) (16). Xanthene derivatives, including caffeine, are also considered CNS stimulants. The exact mechanism of modafinil (Provigil) is not known. It is primarily used in the management of narcolepsy and is approved for persistent daytime sleepiness in patients on continuous positive airway pressure, circadian rhythm sleep disorder, and shift work. It is a wakefulness-promoting agent and decreases TST and REM sleep (16).

Stimulants, as a rule, affect wakefulness. They are known to increase SL and reduce both SE and SWS. Discontinuing their use may result in sleepiness as a rebound effect (except for modafinil) (16).

Caffeine users are more readily aroused by sudden noises and exhibit an increase in body movements during sleep and a reduction in the reported quality of sleep. When caffeine is used, REM sleep tends to occur earlier, but researchers have not yet determined whether the duration of REM sleep is increased or decreased (17).

Respiratory Drugs

As previously noted, theophylline is a methylxanthine that acts as a respiratory stimulant medication that is used to treat obstructive airway disease. There is consideration for use in treatment of central sleep apnea syndromes (CSAS) related to chronic heart failure (CHF), although it is not routinely prescribed for the aforementioned (https://aasm.org/wp-content/uploads/2017/07/CSA.pdf).

Theophylline has an affinity to adenosine receptors, which can alter sleep architecture similar to caffeine and other xanthene derivatives. In healthy individuals, sleep onset is typically delayed, and patients tend to have increases in WASO (https://pubmed.ncbi.nlm.nih.gov/8417877/). Limited studies have been conducted on the effects theophylline has on sleep architecture, some of which have shown limited differences in architecture and others an increased Stage N1 sleep. It is still being studied as a potential treatment option for OSA (https://pubmed.ncbi.nlm.nih.gov/10939035/).

Antihistamines

Histamine agonist or antihistamines are a class of medications used to treat millions who suffer from allergies and their symptoms. It is a pharmaceutical drug that inhibits the action of histamine by blocking it from attaching to histamine receptors. With the increase in the number of people suffering from allergy today, more and more people take antihistamines (Table 31-6).

Antihistamines are classified as either H1 receptor blockers (further grouped into first generation and second generation) or H2 receptor agonists. First-generation H1 blockers are sedating and the second generation, mild or nonsedating. The first-generation H1 blockers may decrease SL and REM and increase TST, N1, N2, and SWS. Cimetidine, an H2 receptor, is known to increase SWS. Other drugs in its class, including ranitidine and famotidine, have no documented effect on sleep stages or sleep continuity.

Anticonvulsants

Anticonvulsant or antiepileptic drugs can have either detrimental or beneficial effects on sleep. Most anticonvulsants appear to improve and stabilize sleep as a direct consequence of seizure suppression. Effect on sleep architecture is dependent on which anticonvulsant is prescribed (18).

Table 31-6 Antihistamines

Generic Name	Popularly Known as/ Brand Name	Agent Type	Sedating	Nonsedating
Cetirizine[a]	Zyrtec	H1	☐	√
Chlorpheniramine	Chlor-Trimeton		√	☐
Cimetidine	Tagamet	H2	☐	☐
Cyproheptadine	Periactin	H1	√	☐
Desloratadine[a]	Clarinex	H1	☐	√
Diphenhydramine	Benadryl		√	☐
Fexofenadine[a]	Allegra	H1	☐	√
Levocetirizine	Xyzal		☐	√
Loratadine[a]	Claritin	H1	☐	√
Levocetirizine	Xyzal		☐	√
Montelukast	Singulair		☐	√

H1, effective in the symptomatic treatment of acute allergies; H2, effective in the control of gastric secretions, often used in the treatment of gastroesophageal reflux.

[a]Second-generation H1 blockers considered less sedating. Cetirizine, however, may be (more sedating) in higher doses.

Gabapentin (Neurontin): Increase TST, SE, N1, SWS, REM, PLMs, and arousals.

Clonazepam (Klonopin): Increase TST, N1, N2, and arousals while also decreasing SE, SWS, and REM.

Some anticonvulsants have been prescribed for other medical conditions. Gabapentin is also prescribed for neuropathic pain and hot flashes, and clonazepam for panic attacks.

Opioids/Opiates

Opiates are drugs derived from opium, whereas opioids refer to synthetic opiates, created to emulate opium; however, they are chemically different (19). Opioids refer to the entire family of opiates, including natural, synthetic, and semisynthetic.

An opioid is any agent that activates the opioid receptors, the protein molecules located on the membranes of some nerve cells. These receptors are found principally in the CNS and gastrointestinal tract. Opiates activate the receptors once they reach the brain, facilitate pain relief, and stimulate pleasure centers in the brain that then signal reward. They suppress perception of pain and calm an individual's emotional response to pain by reducing the number of pain signals sent by the nervous system. Drugs under this class include methadone, morphine, and oxycodone.

Opiates can cause sedation with acute use and insomnia with chronic use. They can increase wakefulness, thereby decreasing TST and SE. They are also known to increase N1 sleep. The limited data from sleep studies show a decrease in REM sleep and SWS. Subjective sleep has been reported as improved, possibly resulting from improved pain control (20). Withdrawal leads to sleep disturbances, affecting SL, SWS, and REM sleep (21).

Antipsychotics

Antipsychotic drugs are a class of medications used to treat a serious mental disorder characterized by defective or lost contact with reality (psychosis) and other mental and emotional conditions. They are also known as tranquilizers used to treat conditions when a calming effect is desired.

Tranquilizers can be divided into different groups, called "major tranquilizers" and "minor tranquilizers." Although they are both groups of CNS depressants, their mechanisms of action, medical uses, and misuse potential are very different. Major tranquilizers (antipsychotics) are used to treat mental illnesses, whereas minor tranquilizers (BZDs) have therapeutic uses including the treatment of anxiety, insomnia, seizures, muscle spasms, and alcohol withdrawal. BZDs can be highly addictive, whereas antipsychotics are nonaddictive and have very little potential for misuse (22).

Reports on studies conducted on patients diagnosed with schizophrenia limit the drugs used to haloperidol, olanzapine, and clozapine. There is virtually no change in sleep architecture with haloperidol use except for an increase in RL. An increase or no change has been seen in N3, whereas a decrease, or no change, has been noted in REM density. The use of either olanzapine or clozapine shows an increase in N2 sleep. An increase in SWS is seen in the former but a decrease in the latter. The drug affects neither RL nor the duration of REM sleep (23).

Mood Stabilizers

Mood stabilizer drug types include antimania, anticonvulsant, antipsychotic, and antihypertensive medications. They are used to treat acute mania defined as an abnormally elevated mood state characterized by symptoms as inappropriate elation, increased irritability, severe insomnia, grandiose notions, increased speed and/or volume of speech, disconnected and racing thoughts, increased sexual desire, markedly increased energy and activity level, poor judgment, and inappropriate social behavior. They are also used to treat hypomania (a mild form of mania), depression, and mania + depression episodes. Regular use of mood stabilizers can help reduce the risk of suicide, prevent relapse, and improve the emotional well-being of any individual.

The use of an anticonvulsant, such as carbamazepine, has been an accepted treatment for mood disorders for some time. Studies in healthy volunteers have shown that carbamazepine and lithium carbonate, another mood-stabilizing drug, will increase SWS but will suppress REM sleep. Lithium carbonate also increases RL (24).

Other Sleep Aids

Over-the-counter (OTC) sleep aids and herbal supplements fall in this category. Most OTC products do contain antihistamines (diphenhydramine) and will cause drowsiness, so they can be effective for occasional use. Side effects include dry mouth, nausea, a hangover effect, blurred vision, and constipation.

Examples of herbal sleep aids include melatonin, valerian root, and chamomile tea. Melatonin is a natural hormone that regulates sleep cycles. It decreases SL and may help normalize irregular sleep-wake patterns without affecting sleep architecture. It lost popularity when the side effects, depression, weepiness, and headaches, became known.

Some patients have found the use of valerian root calming and beneficial in treating mild cases of insomnia. It is somewhat like chamomile tea because it produces a soothing feeling of relaxation. Side effects of valerian root include headaches, indigestion, and restlessness, whereas chamomile tea can cause dermatitis or other allergic reactions. The use of chamomile tea with antiepileptic medications can increase their sedative effects. It can increase the risk of bleeding for individuals who are already taking aspirin or other blood-thinning medications (as in warfarin, etc) (25).

This section will not be complete if two other popular OTC sleep aids go unmentioned: alcohol and nicotine (cigarettes).

The decision on when to consume alcohol appears to influence sleep. Taken too early (about 6 hours before bedtime), alcohol increases wakefulness by the second half of the night and when taken at bedtime (about an hour before), causes fitful sleep by the second half of the night (26). Taken at bedtime, alcohol shortens SL, increases NREM, and reduces REM sleep. Whatever the timing, alcohol's depressant effects can increase the duration of periods of apnea or worsen any preexisting obstructive sleep apnea (27).

Nicotine can have a biphasic effect because it initially relaxes and then stimulates. It can raise blood pressure, speed up the heartbeat, stimulate brain wave activity, and can even make breathing shallower and faster (28). By stimulating the release of aminergic neurotransmitters (such as dopamine and serotonin), nicotine in cigarette smoke may disturb the normal regulation of NREM sleep and shift the distribution of sleep architecture toward lighter stages of sleep (29,30). Use can decrease SL and increase frequency of arousals, resulting in reduced TST.

SUMMARY

The vast array of substances currently available to patients will always challenge the ability to interpret the PSG data. Many of these substances will alter sleep in some form. Sleep technologists need to be aware of the latest trends in the use and misuse of drugs, as well as the literature linking drugs to altered sleep. Technologists should ask themselves if and how each PSG might be affected by medications, whether taken on the day of the study or earlier. Close attention to patients' medications will significantly aid in the interpretation of the PSG and increase the number of correct diagnoses (29,30).

REFERENCES

1. National Center for Health Statistics. Health, United States, 2016: with chartbook on long-term trends in health. 2020. Accessed May 24, 2025. https://www.cdc.gov/nchs/hus/topics/rx-drug-use.htm
2. Korsmeyer P, Kranzler HR, eds. Barbiturates. In: *Encyclopedia of Drugs, Alcohol, and Addictive Behavior*. 3rd ed. Gale Cengage Learning; 2008.
3. RXList. Benzodiazepine drug information. Accessed November 1, 2025. https://www.rxlist.com/benzodiazepines/drugs-condition.htm
4. Schatzberg AF, Nemeroff CB. *Textbook of Psychopharmacology*. American Psychiatric Publishing; 2009.
5. Mayo Foundation for Medical Education and Research. *Antidepressants*. Author; 1998-2001.
6. Carlson N. What is serotonin and what does it do? 2001. https://my.clevelandclinic.org/health/articles/22572-serotonin
7. New World Encyclopedia. Norepinephrine. 2007. http://www.newworldencyclopedia.org/entry/Norepinephrine
8. PediaView.com. Acetylcholine. https://my.clevelandclinic.org/health/articles/24568-acetylcholine-ach
9. Kaplan HI, Saddock BJ. *Synopsis of Psychiatry: Behavioural Sciences/Clinical Psychiatry*. Lippincott Williams & Wilkins; 2007.
10. Taylor DP, Eison MS, Riblet LA, Vandermaelen CP. Pharmacological and clinical effects of buspirone. *Pharmacol Biochem Behav*, 1985;23(4):687-694. https://www.sciencedirect.com/science/article/pii/0091305785904381
11. Patel J, Swierzewski SJ. High blood pressure medication. 2011. https://my.clevelandclinic.org/health/treatments/21811-antihypertensives
12. Rosen RC, Kostis JB. Biobehavioural sequelae associated with adrenergic-inhibiting antihypertensive agents: a critical review. *Health Psychol*. 1985;4(6):579-604.
13. Schweitzer PK. Drugs that disturb sleep and wakefulness. In: Kryger M, Roth T, Dement W, eds. *Principles and Practice of Sleep Medicine.* 4th ed. Elsevier Saunders; 2005.
14. Spiegel R, DeVos JE. Central effects of guanfacine and clonidine during wakefulness and sleep in healthy subjects. *Br J Clin Pharmacol*. 1980;10(suppl. 1):165S-168S.
15. Roman F. Medication effects on sleep. *Focus J*. 2008;52-53.
16. Qureshi A, Lee-Chiong T Jr. Medications and their effect on sleep. *Med Clin North Am*. 2004;88(33):751-766.
17. Schneerson JM, ed. Drugs and sleep. In: *Handbook of Sleep Medicine*. Blackwell Science; 2000.
18. Bazil CW, Malow BA, Sammaritano MR. *Sleep and Epilepsy: The Clinical Spectrum*. Elsevier Health Sciences; 2002.
19. National Alliance of Advocates for Bupren-orphine Treatment. Common buprenorphine side effects: headache, constipation, dry mouth. https://www.nhs.uk/medicines/buprenorphine-for-pain/side-effects-of-buprenorphine/
20. Overeem S, Reading P. *Sleep Disorders in Neurology: A Practical Approach*. Wiley-Blackwell; 2010.
21. Dimsdale JE, Norman D, DeJardin J, et al. The effect of opioids on sleep architecture. *J Clin Sleep Med*. 2007;3(1):33-36.

22. Addiction Technology Transfer Center. Psychotherapeutic medications. https://archive.org/details/pstr-meds-2011
23. Lader MH, Cardinali D, Pandi-Perumal SR. *Sleep and Sleep Disorders: A Neuropsychopharmacological Approach*. Springer; 2006.
24. Eisen J, MacFarlane J, Shapiro CM. ABC of sleep disorders: psychotropic drugs and sleep. *Br Med J*. 1993;306:1331-1334.
25. Hirshkowitz M, Smith P, eds. I can't sleep a wink: examining insomnia. In: *Sleep Disorders for Dummies*. Wiley Publishing, Inc; 2004.
26. Landolt, HP, Roth C, Dijk DJ, et al. Late-afternoon ethanol intake affects nocturnal sleep and the sleep EEG in middle-aged men. *J Clin Psychopharmacol*. 1996;16(6):428-436.
27. Dawson A, Lehr P, Bigby BG, et al. Effect of bedtime ethanol on total inspiratory resistance and respiratory drive in normal non-snoring men. *Alcohol Clin Exp Res*. 1993;17(2):256-262.
28. Hirshkowitz M, Smith P, eds. Adopting a sleep-well life-style. In: *Sleep Disorders for Dummies*. Wiley Publishing, Inc; 2004.
29. Zhang, L., Samet, J., Caffo, B., et al. Cigarette smoking and nocturnal sleep architecture. *Am J Epidemiol*. 2006;164(6):529-537.
30. Wettach GR., Ware IC, Vorona RD, et al. Pharmacologic effects on the polysomnogram. In: Butkov N, Lee-Chiong T, eds. *Fundamentals of Sleep Technology*. Lippincott Williams & Wilkins.

Chapter 32

Consumer Sleep-Tracking Technologies and Sleep-Promoting Devices

KEVIN ASP

KEY CONCEPTS/LEARNING OBJECTIVES

The key concepts for this chapter include a review of the technologies available for monitoring and improving sleep and the effects of recovery tools, supplements, and biohacking strategies available to provide new streams of data and extend care beyond the sleep laboratory.

KEY TERMS

Sleep trackers
Wearables
Contactless sensors
Thermal regulation
Noise modulation
Circadian lighting
Smart thermostats

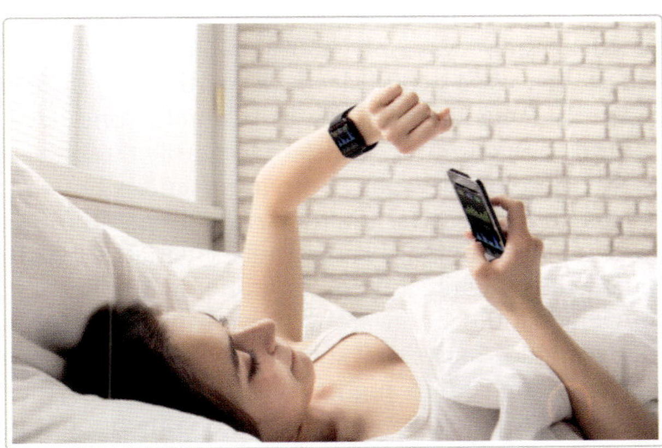

INTRODUCTION

Public awareness of the importance of healthy sleep has surged in recent years (1). Alongside this trend, consumer sleep technologies have rapidly advanced and gained widespread adoption. Modern sleep-tracking devices empower individuals to monitor their own sleep patterns conveniently at home, using minimal sensors compared to traditional polysomnography (PSG) (1,2). Recent estimates indicate that approximately one in three Americans has used an electronic sleep tracker, with most finding the data helpful and many even changing their sleep behavior as a result. As technology companies like Apple, Samsung, Google, and Oura integrate sophisticated algorithms and biosensors into consumer devices, sleep tracking is becoming a mainstream wellness tool.

Despite their popularity, it is essential to critically assess what these tools can and cannot do. Consumer sleep trackers are not medical devices—they generally lack the Food and Drug Administration (FDA) approval for diagnosing or treating sleep disorders and are marketed as wellness products (3). The purpose of this chapter is to provide an evidence-based overview of current consumer sleep-tracking technologies (wearables and nonwearables) and sleep-promoting smart devices, including their capabilities, accuracy, and potential uses in both general populations and clinical settings. We will review the latest promising wearable trackers (such as smartwatches and smart rings) and nonwearable systems (undermattress sensors and smart home integrations), as well as environmental technologies designed to enhance sleep (cooling bedding, sound machines, circadian lighting, climate and air quality controls). Throughout, we highlight supporting scientific studies, discuss benefits and limitations, and consider how these technologies might interface with clinical practice for patients with sleep disorders. The goal is to help clinicians and researchers understand the state of consumer sleep technology in 2025, enabling informed guidance to patients and integration of useful tools while maintaining a critical perspective on their validity and appropriate application.

CATEGORIES OF CONSUMER SLEEP-TRACKING TECHNOLOGY

Consumer sleep trackers can be classified into three broad categories based on how they collect data: (7)

- Wearables: Devices worn on the body (wristbands, smartwatches, rings, etc) that track sleep via movement and physiologic signals.
- Nearables (Nonwearable Sensors): Contact-free devices placed near the sleeper (under the mattress or bedside) that detect motion, respiration, or other signals without being worn.
- Airables (Smartphone Apps and Environmental Sensors): Systems that utilize microphones, speakers, or other ambient sensors in the bedroom environment (often via a smartphone or smart home device) to infer sleep metrics (3).

Each category has distinct advantages and limitations. Here, we examine the most prominent examples and recent developments in each group.

Wearable Sleep Trackers: Smartwatches and Smart Rings

Wearable sleep trackers are among the most popular consumer devices for monitoring sleep. These include fitness tracker bands, multifunctional smartwatches, and dedicated ring or wrist devices. Modern wearables are typically equipped with accelerometers to sense movement and photoplethysmography (PPG) sensors to measure heart rate and blood flow signals (3). Using these inputs (movement, heart rate, heart rate variability, etc), proprietary algorithms estimate sleep parameters such as total sleep time, sleep stages (light, deep, rapid eye movement [REM]), and awakenings.

Smartwatches and Fitness Bands: Leading brands like Fitbit, Apple Watch, Garmin, and Samsung Galaxy Watch have integrated sleep-tracking features (3). Fitbit, for example, uses accelerometer and heart rate data to estimate sleep stages and durations, providing users with nightly breakdowns of light, deep, REM sleep and comparative "sleep scores." Newer Fitbit models (eg, Sense 2) also include oxygen saturation sensors and can detect variations that might signal breathing disruptions during sleep. The Apple Watch, which introduced native sleep tracking in 2020, similarly records motion and heart signals; newer versions add blood oxygen monitoring that can be relevant to sleep breathing issues. These wrist-worn devices aim to improve sleep habits by giving users feedback on their sleep duration, consistency, and even bedtime routines (eg, schedule reminders).

Smart Rings: A notable innovation in wearables is the emergence of ring-based trackers. The Oura Ring is a prominent example—a small ring worn on the finger that contains sensors for motion, pulse, and body temperature. By measuring subtle pulse waveform changes and skin temperature, smart rings like Oura claim to track sleep stages and even offer insights into circadian alignment and recovery. Another example is the less common Thim ring (introduced around 2017), which was designed not only to track sleep but also to train sleep patterns by delivering gentle vibrations to nudge the user toward sleep at specific intervals (1). In general, rings provide an alternative form factor for those who dislike wristbands, and their inclusion of skin temperature sensing is a unique feature potentially aiding sleep phase estimation.

Scientific Validation of Wearables: Early validation studies of wearables in the mid-2010s found that while devices could fairly detect sleep versus wake (comparable to actigraphs), their staging accuracy was limited (4).

However, recent evidence suggests significant improvements. In a comprehensive 2023 multicenter study, researchers tested five modern wearables (including Apple Watch Series 8, Fitbit Sense 2, Oura Ring Gen3, Google Pixel Watch, and Samsung Galaxy Watch 5) against lab PSG. The results showed that some of the latest wearables achieved substantial agreement with PSG on certain measures (4).

In particular, devices like the Oura Ring 3 and Fitbit Sense 2 demonstrated improved accuracy in sleep stage detection compared to their earlier versions (1). The top-performing wearables had overall sleep/wake accuracy in the mid-80% range (similar to medical-grade actigraphy) and showed better concordance for deep sleep detection (4). For example, one study found the Oura Ring's estimates of total sleep time differed by less than 12 minutes on average from PSG recordings (4). That said, sleep stage classification remains imperfect—in the ring validation, overall per-epoch agreement on the exact sleep stage was only ~50% to 55% (vs PSG) for the best devices (4). REM sleep was particularly difficult to identify (sensitivity as low as ~14% for one device in a study). In summary, modern wearable trackers can closely approximate total sleep time and sleep/wake patterns for many users, and their stage differentiation is improving, but they still cannot reliably match PSG for detailed sleep architecture on an individual night basis. Clinicians should be aware that even the most promising wearables may show substantial errors for certain individuals or certain nights, underscoring that these gadgets are trending toward research-quality but not yet diagnostic-grade.

Benefits and Uses of Wearables: For the general consumer, wearable trackers offer a convenient "mirror" of their sleep habits. Many users report that tracking data increases their awareness of sleep duration and encourages healthier behaviors (like setting earlier bedtimes) (3,4). Some programs use wearable data to motivate improvements in sleep hygiene, and researchers note that long-term data from consumer wearables can enable large-scale sleep studies that were previously impractical. From a clinical standpoint, wearables might serve as a form of objective sleep diary—patients can bring longitudinal data on bedtimes, total sleep, and variability to supplement their history. For example, a patient's smartwatch data showing chronically short sleep or irregular sleep-wake times could help identify behaviors contributing to insomnia or circadian rhythm disorders. Importantly, wearables today also incorporate wellness monitoring that can intersect with sleep medicine: some track heart rate and heart rate variability trends, which might reflect sleep quality or stress; others measure overnight Spo_2 or even listen for snoring, which can hint at possible sleep apnea (although not conclusively diagnose it). This additional data can prompt users to seek medical evaluation if, say, a device consistently flags low oxygen or excessive awakenings.

Limitations of Wearables: Despite their convenience, wearable trackers have well-recognized limitations (4). Accuracy varies between devices and between individuals—validation studies show that devices may be reasonably accurate on average, yet for a given person on a given night, the error can be large. Quiet wake periods (lying still in bed awake) are often mis-scored as sleep, meaning trackers tend to overestimate total sleep time and sleep efficiency in those with insomnia or fragmented sleep. They also often misclassify light versus REM versus deep stages, since movements and heart rate are only rough proxies for brain states. Another concern is user compliance and comfort—some people forget to wear the device to bed or find it uncomfortable to wear nightly, limiting data continuity. Battery life and charging schedules present practical issues; for instance, a smartwatch used heavily in daytime may need charging at night, interfering with sleep tracking. Additionally, there are data privacy considerations as wearables often upload sensitive health data to cloud servers, something clinicians should mention when patients use these tools (5). Finally, an emerging phenomenon termed "orthosomnia" has been described, in which individuals become overly obsessed with achieving "perfect" sleep metrics from their tracker and develop anxiety that paradoxically worsens their sleep (3). Reports have documented patients with insomnia who, driven by tracker data, spend excessive time in bed or develop maladaptive routines in pursuit of better sleep scores. Clinicians should counsel patients that tracker data is an estimate and that chasing ideal numbers can be counterproductive. In summary, wearable sleep trackers are useful for raising awareness and tracking trends, but their data should be interpreted with caution and never in isolation for clinical decision-making.

Contactless and Nonwearable Sleep Trackers

Not everyone is willing or able to wear a device to bed each night. Nonwearable sleep trackers offer a more passive approach by embedding sensors in the sleep environment (1). These systems include undermattress pads, bedside radar devices, and mobile apps that use a phone's sensors. They are sometimes called "nearables" or contact-free trackers, since they work without direct attachment to the body.

Undermattress and Bedside Sensors: A number of products use pressure or radar sensors to detect sleep. For example, the Withings Sleep mat (a thin pad placed under the mattress) measures subtle pressure changes from cardiac contractions, breathing, and movement. It can log heart rate, snoring episodes, and breathing disturbances in addition to sleep cycles. Another example is the Sleep Number 360 smart bed, which has built-in mattress sensors to track movement and respiration for each sleeper, automatically adjusting mattress firmness and providing sleep metrics each morning. Bedside radar devices have also emerged: the Google Nest Hub (2nd Gen) uses a low-power motion-sensing radar (Soli) to monitor the rise and fall of the sleeper's chest and overall movements from the nightstand. Similarly, Amazon's Halo Rise is a standalone bedside gadget with environmental sensors and a contactless radar that tracks sleep phases. These devices appeal to consumers who want "invisible" monitoring—nothing to wear or remember to charge—making the process frictionless.

Smartphone Sleep-Tracking Apps: Many people already have the necessary hardware in their smartphones to do basic sleep tracking. Apps like SleepCycle, SleepScore, or Pillow use the phone's accelerometer and microphone to monitor movement and sound during the night. Typically, the user places the phone on the mattress or nightstand close to the bed, and the app analyzes vibrations or noises (such as snoring or bed squeaks) to infer sleep/wake cycles (1). Some apps emit barely audible sound pulses (sonar) from the phone's speaker and use the reflections to detect respiration and motion (eg, SleepScore app). These "air-based" sensors essentially turn the bedroom into part of the device's sensing system. Many apps include smart alarm features that attempt to wake the user during a lighter sleep stage (based on detected movements) within a set window, aiming for a more refreshed awakening. While basic versions of such apps are often free or low cost, they may offer premium upgrades with more detailed analytics or coaching.

Accuracy and Evidence for Nonwearables: The performance of contactless trackers varies widely and has been less extensively validated than wearables. A 2020 study by Chinoy et al., for instance, tested a bed sensor (EarlySense Live) and a smartphone sonar app (SleepScore Max) alongside several wearables and found that their sleep/wake detection was in a similar range as the wearables but that sleep stage accuracy was limited (1). More recently, the 2023 validation study mentioned earlier also evaluated three nonwearables (Withings mat, Nest Hub 2, and Halo Rise) and three smartphone-based solutions (including SleepScore and Pillow apps) (1). The findings indicated that *certain contactless devices achieved only "fair" or "slight" agreement with PSG on sleep stage classification*—for example, the Google Nest Hub and a popular phone app showed very low concordance with PSG-defined sleep stages (2). On the other hand, some undermattress sensors like the Withings mat performed comparably to actigraphy for estimating total sleep time and sleep efficiency (within ~90% agreement range). The sleep/wake sensitivity of the best contactless devices can be high (they catch most of the sleep periods), but specificity for detecting awakenings is often lower, meaning they tend to overcount sleep. In plain terms, nonwearables can usually tell when you have been in bed and generally still, but they might miss brief wake episodes or restlessness.

It is worth noting that contactless devices that measure respiratory signals (like bed sensors or radar) have an edge in potentially detecting sleep-disordered breathing or snoring. Some have companion apps giving a "snore score" or even an apnea likelihood index based on detected breathing pauses. For example, the Withings Sleep Analyzer pad claims to detect signs of sleep apnea by analyzing breathing patterns and sound; one validation study showed it could detect moderate-to-severe sleep apnea with reasonable sensitivity, although with some false positives, leading to its CE-marking as a medical device in Europe. These developments hint that in the near future, contactless monitors might aid in screening for conditions like obstructive sleep apnea (OSA) at home—but as of 2025, they are not yet replacements for formal diagnosis. They may, however, prompt users to seek professional evaluation if the device consistently reports heavy snoring or possible apneic events.

Practical Considerations: Nonwearable trackers offer improved comfort and compliance, since they require no action from the user beyond setup. This makes them attractive for long-term nightly monitoring or for populations like children or older adults who might not keep a device on. They can seamlessly integrate with the bedroom environment—for instance, the Nest Hub's sleep sensing can tie into a smart home system (dimming lights, adjusting alarms, etc). The tradeoff is that these devices can be sensitive to placement and environment. A mattress sensor must be positioned correctly to pick up signals; thick memory foam or two people in bed can interfere with accuracy. Radar-based devices might pick up movements from a partner or even a pet if they are in range. Phone apps depend on the user remembering to start the app and place the phone properly each night, and they can drain battery or be disrupted by notifications (which is why some apps prompt airplane mode usage). Data privacy is also a consideration—for example, bedside devices by big tech companies may send data to cloud services for analysis. Users should be informed about what is recorded (audio snippets of snoring?) and how it is used.

Overall, contactless sleep trackers provide a comfortable, low-effort way to monitor sleep patterns, and some have demonstrated accuracy approaching wearables for basic metrics. But like wearables, their data should be viewed as approximate. They are best used for observing trends over time (eg, "your average sleep duration this month vs last month"), rather than exact nightly metrics. In clinical contexts, they might be useful when continuous long-term monitoring is needed without burden—for instance, tracking sleep continuity in an older patient at home to gauge response to insomnia treatment, where wearing a device is impractical. Still, clinicians must validate any unusual or concerning readings (eg, possible apneas) with proper medical evaluation.

ENVIRONMENTAL SLEEP-PROMOTING TECHNOLOGIES

Beyond tracking sleep, a growing market of sleep-promoting devices aims to optimize the bedroom environment for better sleep. These technologies address key environmental factors known to influence sleep quality: temperature, sound, light, and air quality. By intelligently controlling or modulating these factors, the goal is to create an ideal sleep setting or even to therapeutically enhance certain aspects of sleep (like deep sleep). In what follows, we explore several categories of these devices and the evidence behind them.

Thermal Regulation: Cooling Mattresses and Climate Control

Sleep is tightly linked to body temperature regulation—a slight drop in core body temperature is part of normal sleep onset, and thermal environment can influence sleep stages (6). Recognizing this, companies have introduced cooling/warming mattress systems and smart thermostats to optimize sleep temperature. For example, the Eight Sleep Pod is a mattress cover with built-in water-based cooling and heating controlled by algorithms. It can cool one's bed during the first part of the night and warm it near morning, in line with circadian body temperature patterns (6). A 2024 manufacturer-sponsored study (Eight Sleep) tested 1 week of sleep with the active cooling/heating mattress cover versus 1 week without it, in 54 adults. The results showed measurable improvements in sleep architecture: when the bed was cooled during the first half of the night, participants gained on average +14 minutes of deep sleep (a 22% increase) and +9 minutes of REM sleep (+25%) compared to nights without cooling. In the latter half of the night, warming the bed slightly was associated with more light sleep in men (which could potentially ease awakening). Additionally, the study found cardiovascular benefits—overall nightly heart rate was ~2% lower and heart rate variability ~7% higher (indicating better recovery) with the thermal regulation system (6). These findings suggest that dynamically adjusting bed temperature can positively impact sleep depth and autonomic recovery, although the study's funding by the device maker warrants interpreting results cautiously.

Apart from specialized bedding, smart thermostats (like Google Nest or Ecobee) can be programmed to adjust the bedroom ambient temperature through the night. Many sleep experts recommend a slightly cool room (around 65 °F or ~18 °C) for optimal sleep. A thermostat could be set to lower temperature at bedtime and ease up by morning. While this is more about comfort and following good sleep hygiene practices, it is now often integrated into "smart home" sleep routines (for instance, a user can set a bedtime mode that cools the house, dims lights, and turns on a fan) (7). There is general consensus and some research evidence that cooler environments facilitate falling asleep and increase slow-wave sleep, up to a point. Overly hot conditions reliably cause sleep fragmentation. Some studies have explored even more targeted thermal tricks: for example, warming the feet or hands (vasodilating extremities to shed heat) or cooling the head. These have had mixed but interesting results in small trials.

Overall, thermal sleep technologies—whether active cooling mattresses or climate control—are grounded in solid physiology: a comfortable, well-regulated temperature can improve sleep quality. Individuals who sleep hot or experience night sweats might particularly benefit from cooling devices, whereas those with poor circulation might appreciate timed bed warming. Clinically, such devices might be considered in patients with insomnia linked to thermal discomfort or in certain conditions like menopause-related night sweats. However, cost can be high, and simpler interventions (like breathable bedding; fans; or adjusting existing heating, ventilation, and air conditioning [HVAC]) should be tried first. If used, these devices should be paired with guidance, since improper use (excess cooling or heating) could also disturb sleep.

Sound Machines and Noise Modulation

Noise in the sleeping environment can significantly impact sleep continuity. Sound machines that produce constant soothing noise (white noise, pink noise, nature sounds, etc) have become popular tools to mask disruptive sounds and lull the brain into a more stable auditory environment. White noise machines emit a steady broad-spectrum sound (resembling radio static or a humming fan) that can drown out sudden environmental noises (like traffic or a neighbor's music) that might otherwise wake the sleeper (8). The theory is that a consistent noise floor reduces the difference between background sound and a jarring noise, thereby reducing sleep interruptions. Many people subjectively report better sleep with a fan or white noise, and these devices are commonly recommended for adults and infants alike. But what does research say?

A 2021 systematic review examined 38 studies on noise as a sleep aid and found the overall evidence to be of very low quality (8). The studies were heterogeneous and often small. Some reported improved sleep onset or maintenance with continuous noise, while others found no benefit or even potential harm. Notably, one included study suggested that introducing white noise might increase sleep fragmentation in certain cases (8). The review's authors cautioned that despite the ubiquity of white noise machines, we lack high-quality data proving their efficacy. They also raised concerns about possible downsides: *masking important sounds* (like alarms or a baby's cries) and potential long-term effects on hearing or auditory processing from constant noise exposure. In summary, white noise can subjectively help some individuals sleep better, especially in noisy environments, but it is not a universally proven solution. Clinicians should ensure that patients are using these machines safely (moderate volume, not completely eliminating critical sounds like smoke alarms). If a patient finds white noise helpful and it causes no harm, it can be a useful adjunct for insomnia or for sleeping in new environments. However, they should not expect miraculous improvements, and any significant sleep issues should still be evaluated for underlying causes rather than simply masked with noise.

Beyond white noise, research has explored "pink noise" and other frequency-tuned sounds. *Pink noise* is a deeper sound with more power in lower frequencies (think of rainfall sounds)—it is often perceived as more soothing than the higher-pitched hiss of white noise (9,10). Intriguingly, small trials have experimented with timed pink noise bursts synchronized to slow-wave sleep, aiming to enhance deep sleep (10). In older adults, this approach showed increased slow-wave electroencephalogram (EEG) activity and some memory consolidation benefits in initial studies. For instance, a 2017 study and a 2019 pilot in people with mild cognitive impairment found that playing brief pink noise pulses during deep sleep (detected in real time by EEG) led to deeper slow waves and was correlated with improved memory recall the next day. Although this is a promising avenue, it requires controlled lab setups or advanced home EEG headbands to time the stimulation—not yet a typical consumer scenario. Some high-end consumer devices (like certain sleep headbands or smartphone apps paired with wearable EEG) have started to include "deep sleep stimulation" sound modes, but their real-world efficacy is still under investigation.

Lastly, adaptive soundscapes are being introduced in some smart bedroom systems. These use microphones to detect environmental noise and then augment the output sound to mask it. For example, if loud cars pass by occasionally, the device might raise the volume or change the frequency profile momentarily to cover the intruding noise. Smartphone apps also offer sound environments that can be tailored (mixing rain with gentle music, etc) as part of wind-down routines. While pleasant sound environments can certainly aid relaxation and sleep onset for many, it is essential to personalize it—some people sleep best in complete quiet. If a patient suffers from insomnia and is bothered by every little noise, a white noise machine or app might be recommended as a trial, but with the understanding that evidence for benefit is mixed (8).

Circadian Lighting and Smart Light Systems

Light is the most powerful regulator of our circadian rhythms. Exposure to bright, blue-enriched light in the morning helps signal the body to wake up and suppresses melatonin, while dim, warm light in the evening allows melatonin to rise and promotes sleepiness. Traditional advice for good sleep hygiene includes getting natural daylight and avoiding bright screens or bulbs at night. Now, technology offers ways to automate and enhance these lighting patterns through circadian lighting systems.

Smart bulbs and fixtures (Philips Hue, LIFX, and others) can adjust their color temperature and intensity on a schedule. For instance, bulbs can be cool-white (~6,500 K, high blue content) during daytime and gradually shift to warm amber (~2,700 K, low blue) in the evening, simulating sunset. They can also be set to very low levels or off overnight and then slowly brighten in the morning as a simulated dawn. Devices like the Philips Somneo or Casper Glow are consumer "sunrise alarm" lights that brighten over 30 minutes to wake a person more naturally than a sound alarm. The question is, does circadian-tuned lighting tangibly improve sleep or health?

Emerging research suggests it can have benefits, especially for those with irregular schedules or in low natural light environments. A 2024 study on circadian-informed lighting for night shift workers found that providing tailored light exposure (bright blue in the evening/night for night shifters and blocking blue light in daytime when they slept) accelerated circadian adjustment and improved sleepiness and performance during shifts (11-13). In home settings, a small pilot study using smart bulbs that turned red at night and bright in the morning showed improved subjective sleep quality in participants compared to a control condition. In that 3-week crossover trial, those who experienced the true light intervention (fading lights at bedtime and brightening at wake time) reported significantly better sleep quality on the PROMIS sleep scale than when they had a sham (normal lighting). This suggests that gradually dimming lights in the evening and simulating sunrise can make people feel like they slept better. The effect was modest but statistically significant, and, importantly, all participants improved somewhat just by adhering to a consistent schedule and bedtime routine (highlighting that routine itself is beneficial).

From a practical standpoint, smart lighting is an easy intervention to recommend: many LED bulbs are available with app or voice control, and users can set up "bedtime" and "wake-up" scenes. In a clinical context, patients with circadian rhythm disorders (like delayed sleep phase syndrome) might benefit from strict light schedules—for example, bright light exposure soon after their desired wake time to help shift their clock earlier and avoiding blue light at night. Smart lights and automated window blinds could facilitate these regimens. There is also interest in using dynamic lighting in elder care or hospitals to support circadian rhythms for better sleep and mood. A case study in a nursing home found that 1 hour of circadian lighting (bright bluish light) in the morning helped regulate sleep and improve mood in residents (14).

Overall, circadian lighting technology is a tool to implement well-established chronobiologic principles. While not a substitute for medical treatment of, say, insomnia or depression, it can be a helpful environmental modification. Key caveat: if not used correctly (for instance, exposing oneself to stimulating light at the wrong times), it could be counterproductive (eg, bright light late at night will worsen insomnia). Therefore, education on timing is crucial when patients use these tools.

Smart Thermostats and Air Quality Monitors

A comfortable bedroom environment extends beyond temperature and light to include air quality. Poor ventilation leading to high carbon dioxide (CO_2) levels or excessive humidity can degrade sleep quality. New devices and monitors allow users to keep an eye on these parameters. Smart thermostats often integrate not only temperature control but also humidity sensors and sometimes even CO_2 or volatile organic compound (VOC) sensors (or they can tie in separate air quality monitors). Maintaining an ideal temperature (cool) and humidity (around 40%-50% RH) is generally recommended for sleep; too dry can irritate airways, too humid can cause stuffiness.

CO_2 and Ventilation: Humans breathe out CO_2, and in an unventilated bedroom (doors/windows closed), levels can rise overnight to concentrations high enough to cause stuffy air and microawakenings (15,16). Research has shown that when bedroom CO_2 levels climb above about 1,000 parts per million (ppm) (indicating poor ventilation), sleepers experience poorer sleep depth and next-day cognitive performance. One study found that reducing CO_2 from ~2,500 ppm to ~900 ppm by opening a window or using a fan led to significantly better objectively measured sleep quality and higher reported freshness in the morning (17,18).

In another intervention, increasing ventilation (with a fan or open door) improved sleep efficiency and reduced awakenings, correlating with lower CO_2 levels overnight (17,18). These findings highlight that fresh air and ventilation are important for good sleep. In response, some smart home systems will automatically turn on an exhaust fan or crack a window via a smart window opener when CO_2 gets high. Devices like air quality monitors (eg, Awair, Airthings) can be placed in the bedroom to display CO_2, temperature, and humidity, often giving a simple "air quality score." While these monitors do not directly improve sleep, they raise awareness—a patient who sees their CO_2 is routinely 1,500+ ppm at night might decide to keep a door ajar or get an air purifier with a fresh air inlet. Clinically, for patients complaining of morning headache or poor sleep in a small bedroom, checking air quality could provide insight (eg, high CO_2 could be a factor).

Noise and Air Purifiers/Fans: Interestingly, air purifiers and fans serve dual roles—they can improve air freshness and provide white noise. A high-efficiency particulate air (HEPA) purifier can remove allergens that might cause nighttime congestion, indirectly aiding sleep for allergy sufferers, and simultaneously the hum of the device can mask noise. Smart purifiers can auto-adjust speed based on air quality or schedule. If a patient has environmental allergies affecting sleep (dust mites, etc), recommending a HEPA filter and monitoring particulate levels might be worthwhile.

In summary, environment-focused sleep technologies like smart thermostats, ventilators, humidifiers, and air quality monitors all aim to create an optimal bedroom atmosphere. These devices are particularly useful when specific issues are identified: for example, a hot sleeper can use a cooling bed; an urban apartment dweller with noisy streets can use a white noise machine and double-paned smart windows; a person in a stuffy dorm can use a CO_2 monitor and window fan. The general principle for clinicians is to ensure patients cover the basics of sleep hygiene—a dark, quiet, cool, and comfortable environment—and then consider high-tech solutions if standard measures fall short or if the patient is enthusiastic about tech-based self-improvement.

ACCURACY AND EFFICACY: WHAT THE EVIDENCE SHOWS

With the proliferation of consumer sleep devices, researchers have been rigorously evaluating their accuracy and efficacy. It is important for an academic and clinical audience to understand how these technologies stack up against gold-standard measurements and whether they truly benefit sleep outcomes.

Accuracy of Sleep-Tracking Devices: As discussed in the previous sections, wearable and contactless trackers have variable accuracy. On the whole, *they are reasonably good at measuring total sleep time and sleep interruptions but less reliable at distinguishing sleep stages or detecting specific sleep disorders* (2). A 2024 review concluded that consumer sleep-tracking devices now perform "as well, or even better, than actigraphy" for basic sleep measurements (2). Actigraphy, the medical-grade wrist movement sensor used in sleep medicine for decades, typically has accuracy in the 80% range for sleep/wake; modern consumer devices meet or exceed that level for many populations. Moreover, the same review suggested these trackers could *overtake actigraphy in research* soon, due to their low cost and ability to collect long-term data unobtrusively. This sentiment is echoed by other experts who note that millions of nights of sleep data can now be gathered via wearables, enabling large-scale studies that were not possible before. For example, anonymized data from users worldwide has been used to map sleep patterns by age and country, offering epidemiologic insights.

However, limitations persist, especially in fine-grained accuracy. Consumer devices tend to overestimate sleep duration because they have trouble detecting quiet wakefulness (2). They also often misidentify light sleep and REM. In one comparative study of seven popular trackers (including Fitbit and Garmin models), researchers found that while devices could fairly accurately pinpoint sleep versus wake periods, *none* were highly sensitive in correctly classifying REM sleep and that all had room for improvement in stage tracking (3). In plain terms, if a device app says "you got 25% REM last night," that should be taken with caution (3). It might have mis-scored some of that time. Breathing and oxygen measurements on some devices (like detecting snoring or SpO_2 dips) also need validation—while promising, they are not diagnostic. The American Academy of Sleep Medicine (AASM) emphasized, in a 2018 position statement, that *consumer sleep technology is no substitute for a medical evaluation* and that data from such devices should be considered adjunctive information only. That stance remains essentially true in 2025: use the data as a conversation starter or to monitor trends, but do not treat or diagnose a patient based solely on a Fitbit or app report.

Efficacy of Sleep-Promoting Devices: For the various sleep-enhancement gadgets (cooling systems, noise machines, lights, etc), evidence is often device specific or anecdotal, with a need for more independent trials (6). We saw that the Eight Sleep cooling cover did show improved sleep in a study (17,18), but that was industry funded. Other independent studies have demonstrated that simply optimizing temperature or ventilation improves sleep (eg, lowering CO_2 levels improved sleep depth, and cooler room improves slow-wave sleep) (8). So the core concepts of these environmental technologies are backed by science, even if each brand's proprietary solution has not been individually vetted in peer-reviewed trials (13). White noise and pink noise have mixed outcomes in studies—some individuals clearly benefit (especially if baseline environment is noisy), while others may see no change or even slight disruption. The placebo effect and individual preference play a big role; if a person believes a sound machine helps, it may relax them enough to fall asleep faster, regardless of objective changes. Light-based interventions are strongly supported by chronobiologic research (bright light therapy is an accepted treatment for circadian disorders), but using consumer smart lights to improve general sleep quality is still a relatively new practice with limited but encouraging data.

In sum, when advising on these gadgets, clinicians should ground recommendations in basic sleep science and personalize it to the patient's issues. For example, if a patient struggles with racing thoughts at night (anxiety insomnia), a soothing sound machine or guided meditation app might be suggested, while for someone who cannot wake up on dark winter mornings, a dawn-simulator lamp could be effective. Always check if the patient has tried low-tech solutions first (earplugs, fans, keeping a window open, getting morning sun), as these often achieve the same effects without cost.

INTEGRATING CONSUMER SLEEP TECHNOLOGY INTO CLINICAL PRACTICE

As patients become more engaged with tracking their sleep, many are now bringing their device data or questions about gadgets to their health care providers. This presents both an opportunity and a challenge for sleep clinicians.

Uses for General Sleep Coaching: Personal sleep trackers can serve as an objective record of a patient's sleep patterns over weeks or months (3). This can complement traditional sleep diaries. For instance, instead of relying purely on self-reported bed and wake times (which are often inaccurate), a clinician can look at a printout from a tracker that shows the patient was inactive (likely in bed) from 11:30 PM to 6:30 AM on most nights, with frequent awakenings between 3 and 4 AM. This objective data may reveal consistency or inconsistency that the patient was not aware of (3). In a literature review, combining subjective reports with objective measures like wearables yielded the most accurate insight into sleep habits. Thus, clinicians can use tracker data as a supplemental "electronic sleep log." It can help identify patterns (eg, "On nights you exercised in the evening, your tracker shows it took longer to fall asleep") and facilitate conversations about sleep hygiene (eg, showing the cumulative effect of variable bedtimes). Importantly, providers should validate the data's plausibility (sometimes devices log "sleep" when the person was just lying still watching TV). If something looks off, it is okay to trust clinical judgment or get further information.

Applications for Sleep Disorders: Different sleep disorders intersect with consumer tech in specific ways:

- Insomnia: Sleep trackers can both help and hurt. On the one hand, they give insomniacs some external feedback, which can counteract the tendency to misestimate sleep (many insomniacs *underestimate* their sleep time). Seeing that they did sleep, say, 5 hours when they felt it was 3 might provide reassurance. Trackers can also be used to monitor progress during cognitive-behavioral therapy for insomnia (CBT-I)—for example, tracking if total sleep time increases after sleep restriction therapy. On the other hand, as noted, some patients become overly fixated on the numbers (orthosomnia), which can perpetuate insomnia. Clinicians should gauge whether a given patient finds the tracker calming (objective evidence) or anxiety-provoking. If the latter, a therapeutic recommendation might be to take a break from the tracker. In research, there is interest in integrating tracker data into CBT-I apps or clinician dashboards, but standard practice has not caught up yet.
  OSA: Most consumer devices cannot diagnose OSA, but some provide clues. A number of wearables now record blood oxygen variation or use the microphone for snoring detection (3). If a patient's watch or ring is frequently flagging low oxygen saturation drops or heavy snoring, a clinician should take that as a sign to screen for sleep apnea (using questionnaires or moving to a home sleep apnea test).

Wearables that measure heart rate might also show an elevated resting heart rate or bursts of heart rate spikes at night, which can correlate with apneic arousals. However, normal readings on a tracker *do not rule out* OSA. The AASM has been clear that normal consumer tracker data should not create false reassurance in someone at risk for a sleep disorder (3) For patients with apnea on continuous positive airway pressure (CPAP) therapy, the relevant "gadgets" are actually the CPAP machines themselves—virtually all modern CPAP devices are internet-connected and come with apps (ResMed's myAir or React Health Connect, for example) that show nightly usage, mask fit, and residual apneas. These apps empower patients to track their therapy and often motivate better adherence (some give a daily score out of 100, which appeals to those who like gamification). Clinicians can capitalize on this by encouraging patients to review their positive airway pressure (PAP) data and troubleshoot issues (many will know their nightly usage or have questions ready via the app). Moreover, clinicians can remotely monitor this data through secure portals, allowing outreach if a patient's usage drops. This integration of consumer-style data from medical devices has measurably improved compliance and outcomes in sleep apnea care. It represents a successful model of technology interfacing with clinical practice—one that perhaps personal sleep trackers might emulate in the future for other conditions.

- Circadian Rhythm Disorders: Patients with irregular sleep schedules or circadian misalignment (eg, teenagers with delayed sleep phase or shift workers) can benefit from using tracking and environmental tech. A simple actigraph or wearable can objectively demonstrate a patient's sleep times and variability, which is useful for diagnosis (eg, documenting a delayed phase). Light therapy devices and apps that schedule exposure can then be used as part of treatment. For instance, a patient with delayed sleep phase syndrome might use a combination of a smart light that mimics sunrise at 6 AM and a pair of blue-blocking glasses at 9 PM to help shift their rhythm earlier. The adherence to these can be logged (some apps ask if you used the light or glasses). Clinicians can encourage the use of reminders and automation—for example, "Have your smart lighting system gradually dim the lights at 10 PM each night to cue wind-down." Over weeks, the wearable data might show if the patient's sleep onset is indeed moving earlier. In more complex circadian cases (like non–24-hour sleep-wake disorder), continuous tracking via wearables provides invaluable data since these patients may not keep reliable diaries.
- Movement Disorders (Restless Legs Syndrome (RLS)/Periodic Limb Movements): Consumer trackers are generally not adept at capturing leg movements specifically (especially if worn on the wrist). They might detect that sleep is fragmented but not know why. Bed sensors could potentially pick up periodic limb movement vibrations, but this is not a common feature yet. One indirect use is to see if sleep improves once RLS is treated (eg, less fragmentation on the tracker). But for diagnosis, we still rely on patient history and PSG for periodic leg movement (PLM) index.

Patient Education and Expectations: It is important for clinicians to educate patients on what their devices can tell them and what they *cannot*. For example, if a patient says "My smartwatch says I only get 10 minutes of deep sleep—is something wrong with me?" the clinician should explain that the device's staging is not perfect and that there's huge night-to-night variability in deep sleep. Focus instead on whether the patient feels refreshed and is getting adequate total sleep. Similarly, if a tracker indicates a high "sleep score" but the patient feels terrible, the clinical evaluation should prioritize the patient's subjective experience and look for underlying issues (the tracker might be missing microawakenings or an undiagnosed sleep disorder).

When used appropriately, consumer sleep technologies can enhance patient engagement. Some sleep physicians encourage patients to use trackers as part of therapy—for instance, during CBT-I, a patient might enjoy seeing their sleep efficiency percentage improve over weeks of training, which can reinforce the positive behavior changes. The key is to ensure the data is accurate enough and interpreted correctly. In cases of discrepancy, trust the medical-grade evaluation. The ultimate message to patients is that these devices provide estimates and trends, not definitive judgments about one's sleep health.

Future Directions: The landscape of sleep technology is evolving rapidly. There is active work on integrating multisensor arrays (combining movement, heart, respiration, oxygen, and even EEG in unobtrusive ways) to get closer to PSG-level detail at home. Some headband and earbud devices already provide single-channel EEG to track sleep stages; their accuracy is better for sleep stages but comfort and user adoption are lower than wrist wearables. We may see FDA-cleared sleep trackers in the coming years for specific uses, such as screening for apnea or tracking circadian rhythms for therapeutic monitoring. Big data and AI are being applied to the troves of consumer sleep data—one can imagine predictive algorithms that warn a user "you are heading toward sleep deprivation" or that detect early signs of disorders (like subtle elevation in heart rate and limb movement patterns that correlate with developing neuropathy or RLS). In clinical trials, wearables are starting to be used to gather endpoints on sleep (eg, measuring how a new drug affects patients' daily sleep at home). The AASM and other bodies are watching these developments; guidelines will likely adapt as validation studies accumulate.

CONCLUSION

Consumer sleep-tracking devices and sleep-promoting technologies have become ingrained in the public's approach to sleep health. These tools—from smartwatches and rings to smart beds, noise machines, and adaptive lighting—offer exciting possibilities for monitoring and improving sleep outside of the traditional clinical setting (3). They empower individuals to engage with their sleep patterns and make environment changes conducive to better rest. For clinicians and researchers, they provide new streams of data and opportunities to extend care beyond the sleep lab. However, it is critical to maintain an evidence-based perspective. Consumer devices, while improving, do not replace formal medical evaluation or proven therapies. Their readings should be used as supplemental information and interpreted in context. When utilized thoughtfully, personal sleep technologies can enhance patient education, aid in tracking treatment progress, and possibly improve adherence and lifestyle behaviors. But over-reliance or misinterpretation can mislead or even exacerbate anxiety about sleep.

In the current state (circa 2025), the consensus is that personal sleep trackers are best for raising awareness and monitoring trends, not for diagnosing sleep disorders (3). Environmental devices can certainly improve comfort and potentially sleep quality, but one should ensure they are addressing a real need (eg, noisy neighborhood, hot bedroom) and not simply adding more gadgets into the mix of potential sleep distractions. Clinicians are encouraged to stay updated on validation studies and to ask patients about any sleep tech they use. Dismissing a patient's tracker data outright can alienate them; instead, discuss it and put it into proper context. Likewise, recommending a helpful tech adjunct (like a light therapy lamp for a patient with circadian issues or a white noise machine for an insomniac with a noisy apartment) can be a compassionate and practical addition to a treatment plan.

Good sleep will always rest on the fundamentals—behavior, environment, and in some cases medical intervention—but technology is steadily weaving its way into each of those domains. As further research and development occur, we may see consumer devices validated for clinical use and new innovations that blur the line between medical device and wellness gadget. Until then, the prudent path is to embrace the useful aspects of consumer sleep technology (engagement, data collection, comfort) while clearly understanding its limits. By doing so, sleep professionals can harness these tools to supplement care, all in the service of helping patients achieve healthier sleep. Future advancements hold promise for more robust integration, and it will be exciting to see if upcoming personal sleep devices can attain the accuracy and reliability needed to become true extensions of clinical practice (3). For now, they remain allies in concept—bringing sleep awareness to the masses—but still junior partners in the clinical management of sleep health.

REFERENCES

1. Lee T, Cho Y, Cha KS, et al. Accuracy of 11 wearable, nearable, and airable consumer sleep trackers: prospective multicenter validation study. *JMIR Mhealth Uhealth*. 2023;11:e50983.
2. Glazier G. New Research Evaluates Accuracy of Sleep Trackers. Accessed November 1, 2025. https://www.sleepfoundation.org/sleep-news/new-research-evaluates-accuracy-of-sleep-trackers
3. Tribau L. Sleep apps and personal tracking devices. In: Lee-Chiong TL Jr, Mattice C, Brooks R, eds. *Fundamentals of Sleep Technology*. 3rd ed. Philadelphia, PA: Wolters Kluwer Health/Lippincott Williams & Wilkins; 2019:379-384.
4. Herberger S, Aurnhammer C, Bauerfeind S, Bothe T, Penzel T, Fietze I. Performance of wearable finger ring trackers for diagnostic sleep measurement in the clinical context. *Sci Rep*. 2025;15(1):9461.
5. Summer JV, Rehman, A. What is Orthosomnia? Sleep Foundation. Accessed November 1, 2025. https://www.sleepfoundation.org/orthosomnia
6. Moyen NE, Ediger TR, Taylor KM, et al. Sleeping for one week on a temperature-controlled mattress cover improves sleep and cardiovascular recovery. *Bioengineering (Basel)*. 2024;11(4):352.
7. Herberger S, Penzel T, Fietze I, et al. Enhanced conductive body heat loss during sleep increases slow-wave sleep and calms the heart. *Sci Rep*. 2024;14(1):4669.
8. Neurology Learning Network. Systematic review cautions promoting white noise machines as a viable sleep aid. Accessed November 1, 2025. https://www.hmpgloballearningnetwork.com/site/neurology/qas/systematic-review-cautions-promoting-white-noise-machines-viable-sleep-aid
9. Min R. Scientists hope to find out if pink noise can enhance sleep and memory. Accessed November 1, 2025. https://www.euronews.com/health/2024/05/21/scientists-hope-to-find-out-if-pink-noise-can-enhance-sleep-and-memory

10. Paul M. Pink noise boosts deep sleep in mild cognitive impairment patients. News Center. Accessed November 1, 2025. https://news.feinberg.northwestern.edu/2019/07/05/pink-noise-boosts-deep-sleep-in-mild-cognitive-impairment-patients/
11. Guyett A, Lovato N, Manners J, et al. A circadian-informed lighting intervention accelerates circadian adjustment to a night work schedule in a submarine lighting environment. *Sleep*. 2024;47(11):zsae146.
12. Flinders University. Circadian lighting boosts sleep and performance for night shift workers. Accessed November 1, 2025. https://medicalxpress.com/news/2024-09-circadian-boosts-night-shift-workers.html
13. Gartenberg D. Can Smart Lights Improve Your Sleep Quality? Accessed November 1, 2025. https://sleepspace.com/smart-lights-improve-perceived-sleep-quality/
14. Sanders M, Barnaba S, Bowerman L, et al. The impact of a circadian lighting intervention on sleep, mood, & engagement: two case studies. *Am J Occup Ther*. 2023;77(suppl 2):7711510305p1.
15. Kang M, Yan Y, Guo C, et al. Ventilation causing an average CO2 concentration of 1,000 ppm negatively affects sleep: A field-lab study on healthy young people. *Build Environ*. 2023;249:111118.
16. American Association for the Advancement of Science. Ventilate your bedroom at night. You perform better the next day. Accessed November 1, 2025. https://www.eurekalert.org/news-releases/988687
17. Fan X, Liao C, Matsuo K, et al. A single-blind field intervention study of whether increased bedroom ventilation improves sleep quality. *Sci Total Environ*. 2023;884:163805.
18. Strøm-Tejsen P, Zukowska D, Wargocki P, Wyon DP. The effects of bedroom air quality on sleep and next-day performance. *Indoor Air*. 2016;26(5):679-686.

SECTION IV
Polysomnography

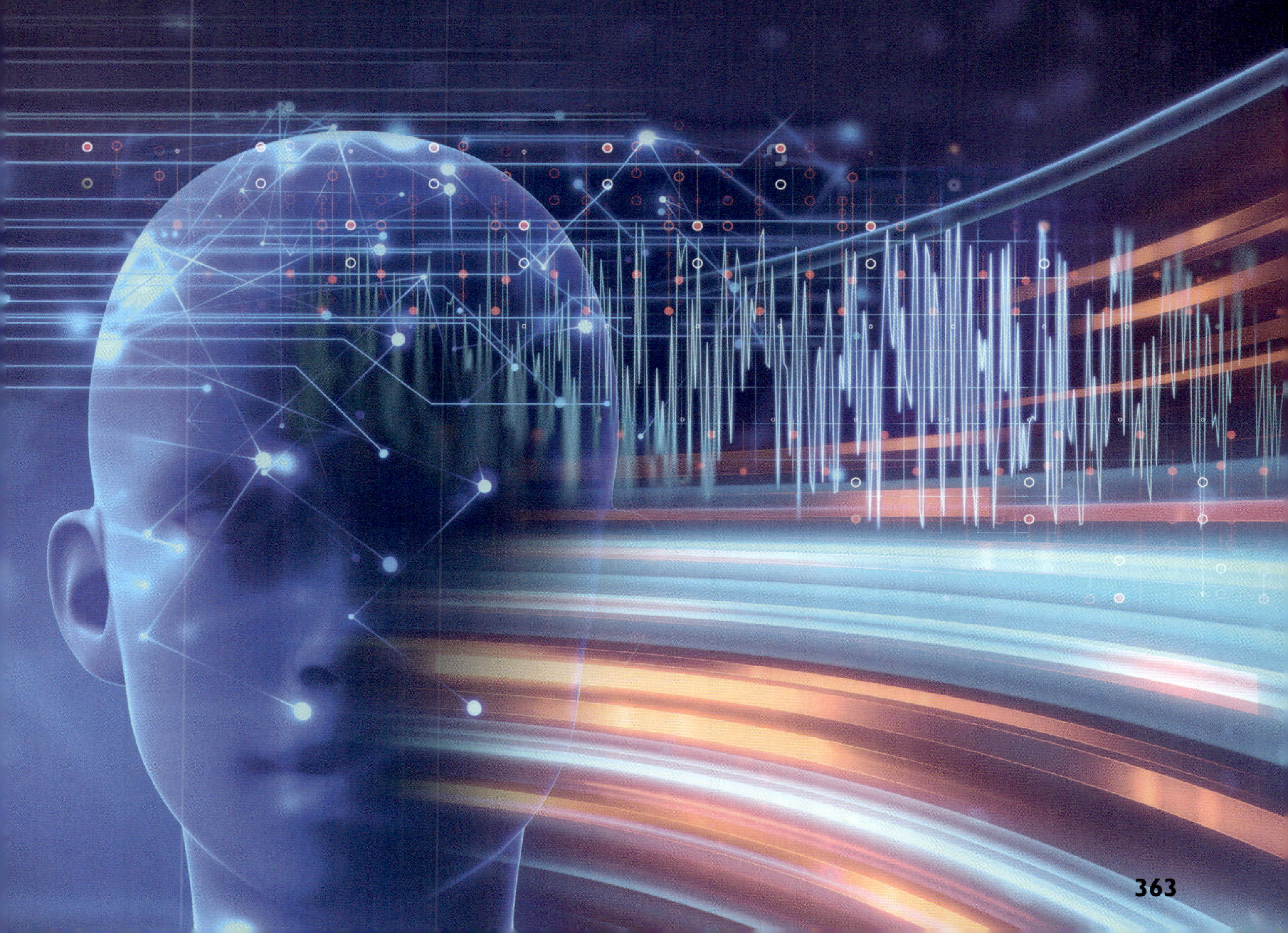

Chapter 33
Digital Polysomnography

JATIN TEKCHANDANI

KEY CONCEPTS/LEARNING OBJECTIVES

The key concepts in this chapter include identification and differentiation of the three main sources of signals in digital polysomnography (PSG): bioelectric potentials, transduced sensors, and ancillary equipment, and a review of how differential amplification affects signal voltage and polarity through the subtraction of electrode inputs. In addition, a discussion of how the summation of neuronal electrical activity is detected and localized through scalp electrodes according to the 10–20 system, how Ohm's law and Nyquist's sampling theory are applied to digital PSG, the complete signal pathway in digital PSG systems from electrode detection through amplification, filtering, and analog-to-digital conversion, the purpose and function of low-frequency, high-frequency, and notch filters in optimizing PSG signal quality and reducing artifacts, and a review of the differences between system calibrations, impedance checks, biocalibrations, and other calibration procedures essential for ensuring PSG recording accuracy are discussed.

KEY TERMS

Amplitude
Analog-to-digital converter
Biocalibrations
Bioelectric signals
Common mode rejection ratio
Conductivity
Fall time constant
Frequency
Frequency response curve
High-frequency filter
Impedance
Low-frequency filter
Notch filter
Nyquist sampling theory
Ohm's law
Polarity
Rise time constant
Sensitivity
Time constant

The word *polysomnography* in its root derivation means many (*poly*) sleep (*somno*) writings (*graphy*). A polysomnogram is produced by a multiple-channel recording instrument comprised of a hardware device (often called an "amplifier") that interfaces with software to produce a digital record of multiple biophysical variables during a sleep session.

Historically, polysomnographic (PSG) recordings were conducted with analog equipment that traced this physiologic activity by mechanical means to paper. Although these paper-based systems performed admirably, the machines were large and resource intensive. They required replenishment of paper and ink and ongoing maintenance of all the mechanical parts, not to mention extraordinary storage requirements. Because the activity was converted by mechanical means, each study required precise mechanical baseline calibrations. Scoring required a page-by-page examination of each epoch, and event marking was done by hand. Present-day digital systems offer sleep professionals all the benefits of software programming and networking. Studies can be viewed on multiple screens, allowing for simultaneous acquisition and scoring. Montages can be adjusted across all parameters during and after the recording, video can be collected and synchronized with the recording, and indices can be estimated or tabulated in real time. Physicians can view studies remotely in real time and in review mode. Reports can be tailored to suit the needs of the health care provider.

The quality and validity of signal processing remain intact in modern digital PSG as long as adequate PSG system specifications and good PSG skills are observed. The American Academy of Sleep Medicine (AASM) Scoring Manual (1) has defined standards and best practices sampling rates, bit rates, screen resolution, etc) for the recording process to ensure that all studies accurately reflect the patient condition.

PRINCIPLES OF ELECTRICAL CONDUCTION

Signal Sources

The basic function of a PSG system is to record signals associated with specific physiologic parameters and convert this activity into visible tracings that can be measured and analyzed. In PSG, there are three sources for these signals:

- Bioelectric potentials
- Transduced signals from sensors attached to the patient
- Signals derived from ancillary equipment

Bioelectric potentials are voltages generated by living tissue. Examples of bioelectric potential recordings include the electroencephalogram (EEG), electrooculogram, electromyogram, and electrocardiogram (ECG). Bioelectric signals are recorded using surface electrodes attached directly to the patient's skin over the area of interest. For the purposes of a discussion regarding the general pathway of these source signals, we concentrate on EEG recordings of the brain.

The brain's electrical charge is the result or summation of the electrical activity of billions of neurons. Neurons are electrically charged (or polarized) by transport proteins that pump ions across their cell membranes. When a neuron receives a signal from its neighbor, an action potential is triggered; it responds by releasing ions into the synaptic space outside the cell. Ions of like charge repel each other, and when many ions are pushed out of many neurons at the same time, they can push their neighbors, who push their neighbors, and so on, in a wave. When the wave of ions reaches the electrodes on the scalp, they can push electrons through the measuring circuit comprising the electrodes and a sensitive amplifier. Thus, the measuring circuit can measure the difference in this electron "push," or voltage, between any two electrodes. Recording these voltage differences over time gives us the EEG (2). Note that the EEG does not directly measure electrical impulses in the cells, but instead the EEG arises from changing ionic concentrations and the resulting charge in the extracellular space.

The electric potentials generated by a single neuron are far too small to be picked by the EEG (3), because the skull and skin act as capacitors and dampen the signal. EEG activity, therefore, always reflects the summation of the synchronous activity of thousands or millions of neurons that have similar spatial orientation (4).

Transduced signals are voltages usually supplied as DC voltages by sensors that are attached to the patient as opposed to voltages that are produced by the body. This can include position sensors, snore sensors, and respiratory sensors.

Table 33-1 Conductivity

Metal	Conductivity σ (1/Ωm) at 20 °C
Silver	6.29×10^7
Copper	5.95×10^7
Gold	4.52×10^7

Ancillary equipment, such as continuous positive airway pressure devices, pulse oximeters, and end-tidal CO_2 ($EtCO_2$) monitors, can be interfaced with the PSG system by using one of many available DC inputs. The industry trend is to integrate pulse oximetry with the amplifier unit.

Electrodes

The first step of the signal pathway external to the body is the electrode. The electrodes, secured using a conductive paste, are the conduits for electron push and, as such, must have, as one of their properties, high electric conductivity. As seen in Table 33-1, the conductivities of copper, silver, and gold are all comparable.

These elements are all from group 12 of the periodic chart and are heavy, dense, malleable metals with high electric conductivity. This high conductivity is due to an atomic makeup of having free outer shell electrons in relation to a dense nucleus. The electrode cups commonly used in PSG are typically silver or gold plated. Those two metals have the additional desirable property of being resistant to the corrosive effects of oxygen, H_2O, and bodily fluids such as sweat. Gold is seen as superior because it optimizes contact impedance over the long duration of a sleep study. Silver–silver chloride and disposable electrodes made of these metals or plastic can also be used.

SIGNAL PATHWAY TO THE DIGITAL POLYSOMNOGRAPHY

The signals previously discussed, whether they originate from the patient or are transduced or ascribed to the patient, follow a pathway that we shall refer to as a "channel." These input signals are amplified and processed so that they are strong enough and clean enough to be converted into a digital signal that is ready for visual display, storage, and analysis.

Bioelectric signals are amplified with differential amplifiers, which reduce recording artifacts by subtracting voltages that are common to an electrode pair. The electrodes are usually routed to the amplifier through a small portable junction box, sometimes referred to as the "headbox." The industry trend is to integrate these

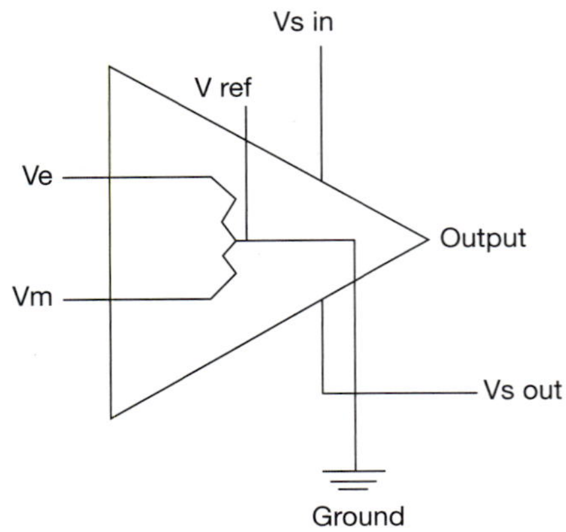

Figure 33-1 Differential amplifier.

functions even further by placing the headbox, amplifier, and digitizer all in the same enclosure. A differential amplifier schematic is shown in Figure 33-1.

OHM'S LAW

The three electric properties that are the variables in the equation known as Ohm's law are voltage, current, and resistance. Ohm's law is commonly represented as

$$I = V/R \text{ or voltage} = \text{current} \times \text{resistance}$$

Ohm's law can be rearranged to show current as a function of voltage and resistance according to the formula $I = V/R$, and from this formula, one can deduce that under conditions of constant voltage, if resistance is increased, current or flow of electrons will be decreased. This concept has practical implications when we consider the fact that in our signal pathway, several factors contribute to higher resistance. This means that the technologist must be vigilant in reducing these effects. Examples of things that could contribute to higher resistance are electrode cups inadequately filled with conductive paste, electrode damage, electrode wire damage, poor patient skin preparation, and incomplete removal of lotions or other skin products.

Notice that what is being measured is the difference in voltage of the two input electrodes as determined by their relation to the reference electrode (Figure 33-1). The first input electrode is the exploring electrode. In PSG, we commonly refer to the mastoid electrodes as the reference electrodes because we have placed them on distant bony electrically neutral sites (M1 and M2). The M1 and M2 electrodes are considered the second input electrodes. The referential electrode is labeled "V_{ref}." Common ground is an additional connection (usually separate from the reference) and is necessary for equalizing electric potentials of the patient and the input circuits of the amplifier. Also, notice the power supply voltage, represented in the diagram by V_s in and V_s out. The power supply is necessary to carry out the function of amplifying the faint biopotential signals.

An essential function of the differential amplifier is that of common mode rejection, or, in plain words, the cancellation of unwanted voltages that are common to both input electrodes. The ability of the differential amplifier to perform this vital function is expressed as the common mode rejection ratio (CMRR). This is the ratio of the differential voltage gain to the common mode voltage gain. If the differential amplifier were perfectly symmetric, the common mode gain would be zero because both voltages would effectively cancel each other out, and the CMRR would be infinite. However, in reality, there is a slight amount of common voltage gain, resulting in industry standard CMRRs of 10,000 to 1 or even as high as 100,000 to 1.

SIGNAL PROCESSING

Signal Polarity and Summation

The processing of bioelectric signals includes conversion from analog-to-digital signal format. Electrodes on the surface of the scalp measure signals of constantly changing voltage, or amplitude, as a function of time. Differential amplifiers process the signals from two electrodes, an exploring electrode and a reference. Because the electrodes are positioned at various locations (according to the 10-20 system), the resulting tracing will vary according to the position of the electrodes and their distance and proximity to the source of voltage (Figure 33-2).

In EEG, it is conventional to represent a negative voltage from a single input in relation to a reference as an upward deflection and, conversely, a positive voltage as a downward deflection. This relationship of the tracing to the electric zero above or below the baseline is referred to as "polarity," as illustrated in Figure 33-3.

With differential amplifiers, signal tracings shown on screen are the result of subtracting the voltage

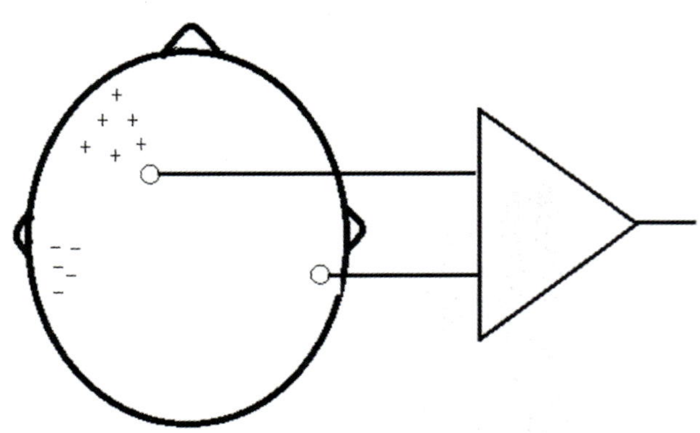

Figure 33-2 Differential amplification of exploring and reference electrodes.

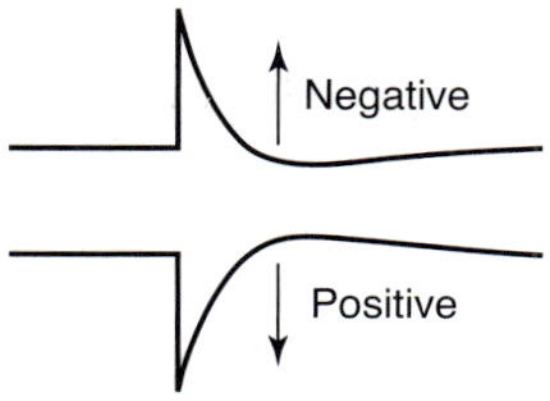

Figure 33-3 Polarity.

contributions from two input electrodes. This is accomplished by inverting the signal from the reference electrode. The formula for combining the signals is exploring electrode (V_1) voltage minus reference electrode (V_2) voltage ($V_1 - V_2$), which we refer to as voltage drop.

In summation, under ideal conditions, the variables that determine bioelectric tracings are as follows:

1. Polarity
2. Voltage
3. Source
4. Electrode proximity
5. Time

Please examine the simple case of two electrodes detecting equal polarity and voltage (50 µV) at the same point in time, at the same distance from the source, in Figure 33-4. We apply the formula for voltage drop 50 – (50) = 0 and see by visual examination the result is no signal.

Now follow along with the case of simultaneous charges of equal polarity and equal proximity but differing voltages. 50 – (25) = 25. In this case, we see the resulting tracing having the same polarity (Figure 33-5), but if the reference electrode is higher in voltage than the input voltage, then the polarity flips. Now take the case of simultaneous charges of opposite polarity, equal proximity, and same voltages: 50 – (–50) = 100, as illustrated in Figure 33-6.

The number of possible combinations is infinite, but we will discuss one more example. That is the combination of two similar polarities, similar signal amplitudes but making their contributions at differing times.

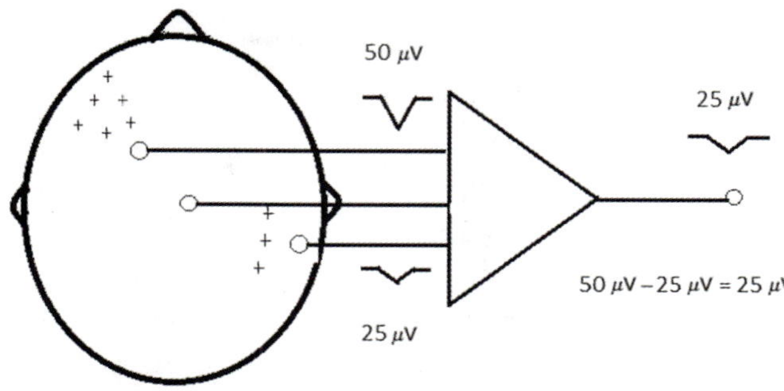

Figure 33-5 Two electrodes with equal polarity and different voltage inputs.

By using our formula, $V_1 - V_2$, as we go along the axis of time, we see the resulting (and recognizable) signal in Figure 33-7.

To a major extent, resulting signal tracings are dependent on time, location of electrodes, source, and signal strength. Additional variables affect the resulting bioelectric tracings in practical applications. They are:

1. Contact impedance
2. Common reference electrode(s)
3. Patient ground electrode

For optimal signal quality, it is necessary to match the input impedance of all electrode pairs as closely as possible. Impedance mismatching allows current to pass through to the amplifier and can lead to artifact (3). If two electrode sites produce a signal with the same amplitude and frequency but one amplifier input receives less voltage because of a higher electrode impedance, then the signals are not perfectly canceling each other, and the effect of common mode rejection is reduced. As a result, synchronized ambient signals can manifest as artifacts in the record. The most common example of this is the noise from the 50 or 60 Hz alternating current of the power grid. To avoid this kind of artifact, the technologist should strive for a uniform approach to site preparation and electrode application. By keeping impedances under 5 kΩ, wide variation in impedances are less likely.

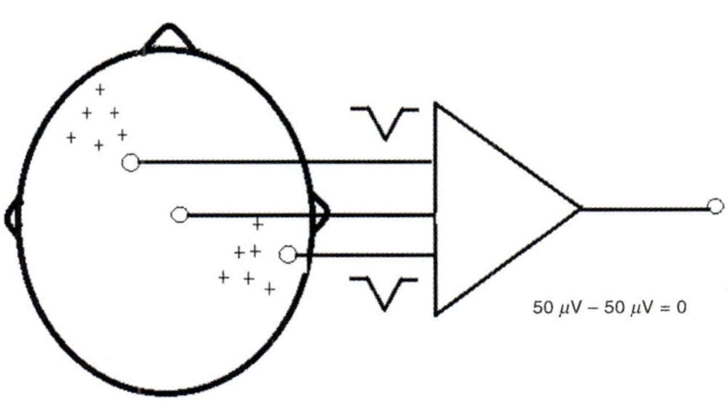

Figure 33-4 Two electrodes with equal polarity and voltage input.

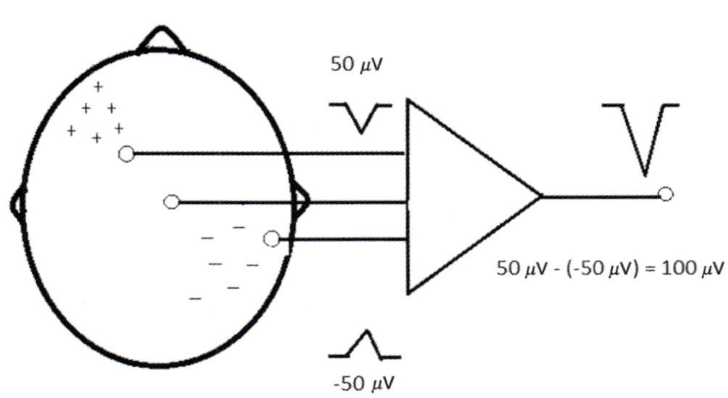

Figure 33-6 Two electrodes with opposite polarity and voltage.

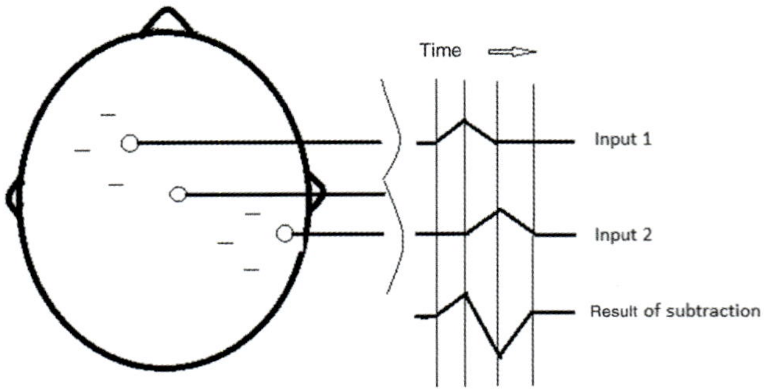

Figure 33-7 Two electrodes with equal polarity and voltage input at dissimilar times.

Many amplifiers utilize a common referential electrode. This electrode allows for re-referencing after the recording has ended and is most effective when placed at a site on the skull that is equidistant to all exploring electrodes and has a low impedance. For this reason, C_z is a good 10/20 site choice for this electrode if it is not required in a custom montage. Some systems have inputs for two common referential inputs, allowing for the use of the best signal. In addition to this, some modern systems also allow the user to assign a common reference electrode, thus alleviating dependence on referential signals that may go bad during the recording.

The patient ground electrode, as previously discussed, provides electrical zero. Without a good stable ground electrode, the electrode pairs will not have a respective electric zero and will, therefore, wander with respect to equal inputs, thus picking up signals that would otherwise be canceled out. Even worse, this wandering common potential may cause amplifier saturation.

SIGNAL MEASUREMENT

Signal tracings are viewed on the display according to two variables, time and amplitude. Time is followed on the horizontal or *x* axis and is the basis for determining the frequency at which a signal intersects the *x* axis. The timescale used in sleep staging is 1 cm per second (Figure 33-8).

Frequency, expressed as cycles per second, is referred to in the unit of measurement known as Hertz (Hz). Frequency describes the period or width of the wave, whereas amplitude describes the height or voltage of the wave. In EEG, actual voltage from the electrodes is in microvolts, or millionth of a volt, and is represented as μV. This abbreviation is often spelled as uV on systems that cannot display Greek characters. Amplitude is followed on the vertical or *y* axis. The typical scale used in PSG to represent voltage amplitude is 50 μV/mm (see Figure 33-9).

The two scales, frequency (time) and amplitude (voltage), can be combined into a useful waveform scale legend or key that can be displayed over the tracings and is available in many PSG systems (Figure 33-10).

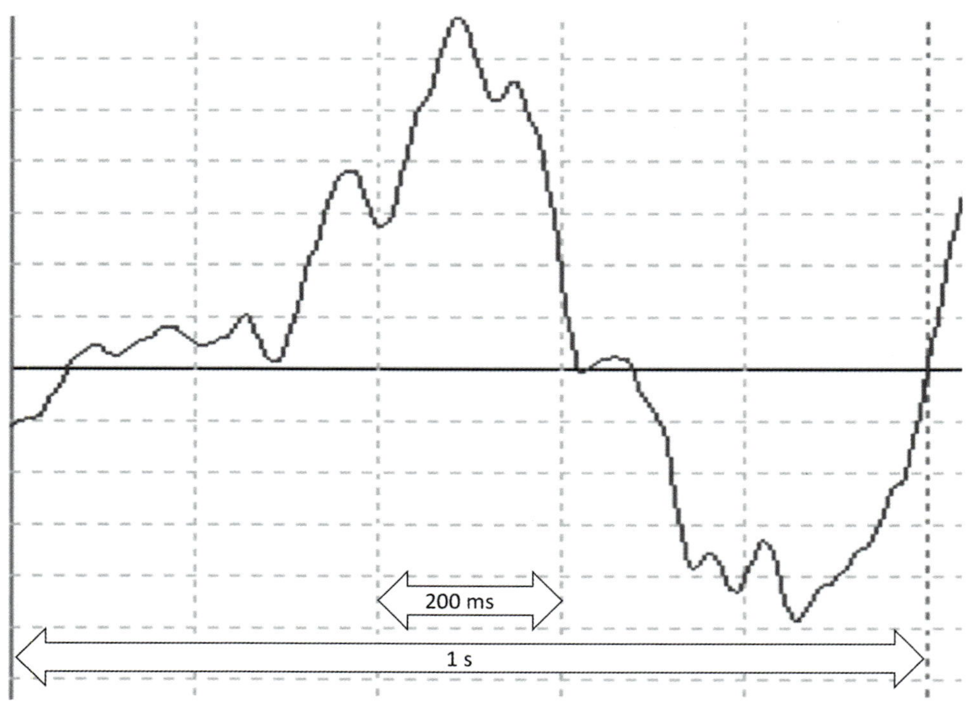

Figure 33-8 The *x* axis—signal frequency.

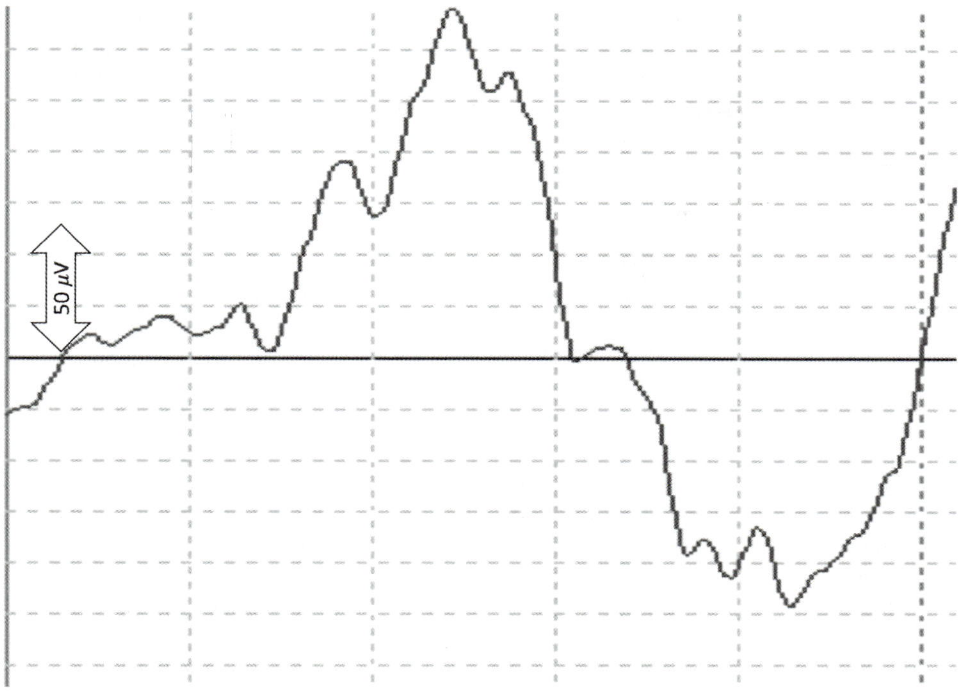

Figure 33-9 The *y* axis—signal amplitude.

This is helpful when screens are resized to fit desktop workspaces and different monitor configurations so that the observer will always be able to relate waveforms to a known scale. Another useful software tool commonly available allows the user to measure voltage and frequency by moving the mouse cursor over the tracing.

The ability to change the amplitude scale is referred to as "sensitivity setting." Sensitivity is determined by the formula

$$S = V/A,$$

where S = sensitivity, V = voltage drop (expressed in μV), A = amplitude (expressed in mm or cm).

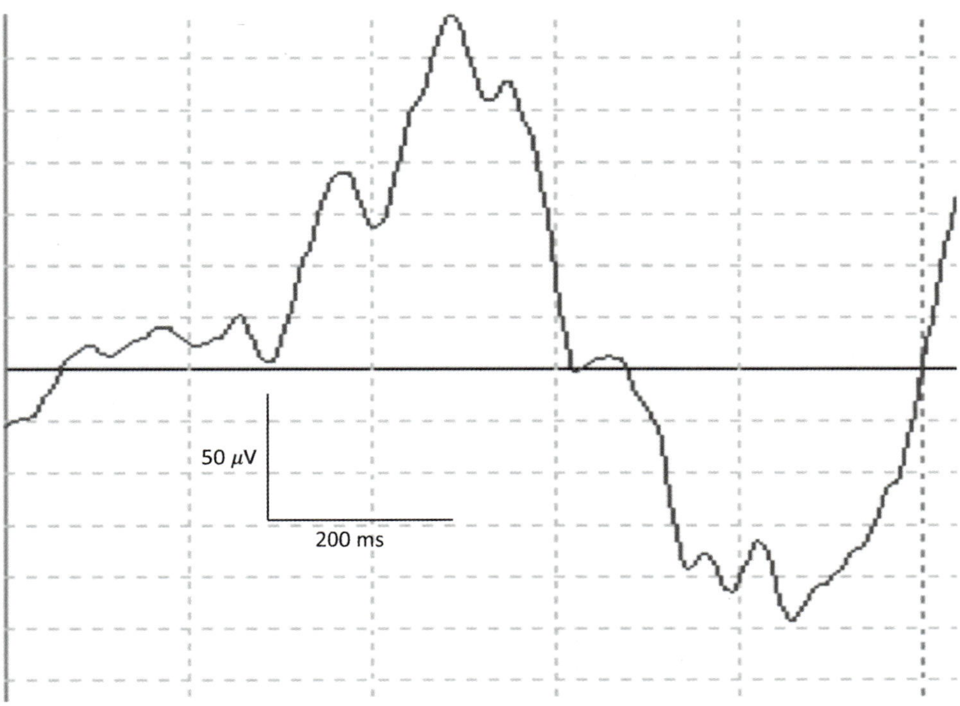

Figure 33-10 Waveform scale.

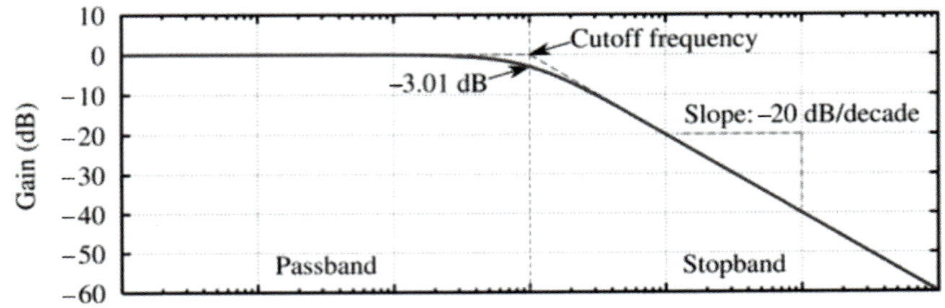

Figure 33-11 Frequency response curve. Image courtesy of Natus Medical Incorporated, natus.com.

We see by our formula that increasing the sensitivity means that higher voltages are represented in the same amount of space, so increasing the sensitivity will decrease the size (amplitude) of the signal on screen. According to the AASM recommended settings, sensitivities for EEG channels are 7 µV/mm.

LOW- AND HIGH-FREQUENCY FILTERS

In any practical setting, amplifier output contains not only physiologic biopotential signals but also noise from various sources, both external (environmental) and internal (inherent in electronic circuit design). High-frequency muscle artifact and slow-frequency respiration or "sweat artifact" are examples of signals that are undesirable in PSG recording, even though they are physiologic in nature. Because there are so many competing signals of varying amplitude and frequency that can obscure the record, we need some way of filtering as much of this undesirable activity as possible. Using low-frequency filters (LFF) and high-frequency filters (HFF), we can limit a "window" of desirable frequency spectrum that is let through to the record. When we set an LFF, we are setting a lower limit of frequencies that are let into the recording. Only signals with frequencies above that limit, called the "cutoff frequency," are allowed to pass. For this reason, an LFF is also referred to as a "high-pass" filter (HPF).

Conversely, when we choose an HFF setting, we are setting an upper limit of allowed signal frequencies. This is also called the "low-pass" filter. By setting the LFF and the HFF cutoff frequencies, we choose the "window" or frequency band that we are interested in viewing.

The extent to which the LFFs and HFFs are successful at filtering out unwanted frequencies is determined by the filter's frequency response. The amount of attenuation of a signal outside the pass band depends on the filter design. Digital filters do not affect the source data, and digital filters of high orders can be easily implemented in software. Digital filters used in PSG systems are usually limited to fourth or lower order to better preserve the signal shape (phase). Filter response can be visualized as a frequency response curve (see Figure 33-11).

TIME CONSTANTS

To understand more fully what we see when we perform a digital machine calibration, it is necessary to understand the concept of time constants. A machine calibration is performed so that there is documentation of the validity of our filter settings. The term "calibrate" in this case is not strictly true because the calibration is actually done once at the factory. The machine calibration shows the effect that amplification and filter settings have on a DC signal oscillating between +50 and −50 μV. This input signal is illustrated in Figure 33-12.

How quickly a signal falls back to the baseline (0 μV) as a function of the filters is known as the signal's time constant.

When a DC voltage is quickly turned on, the signal at the filter output changes almost as quickly (but not immediately because the highest frequencies are filtered out by the HFF). After the signal reaches the peak, it immediately starts to decay back to the baseline (0) because the DC signal (0 Hz frequency) is filtered out by the LFF. As a result, the output after the effects of the filter settings will look as illustrated in Figure 33-13.

Depending on the filter settings, we would see the signal decay at a faster or slower rate. The time it takes for the signal to decay to 37% of its original voltage is known as the "fall time constant." Conversely, the time

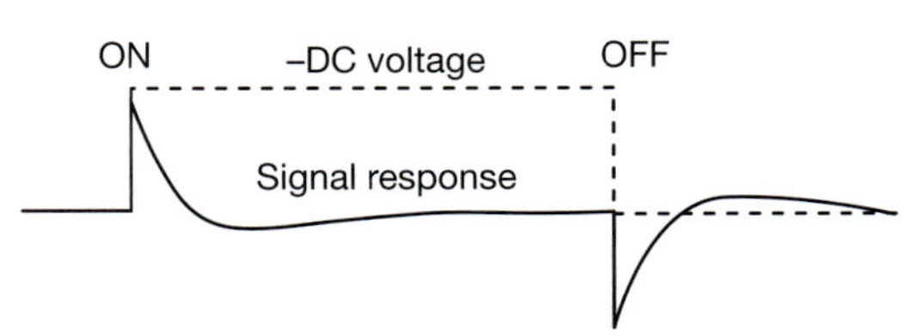

Figure 33-12 Square wave calibration signal.

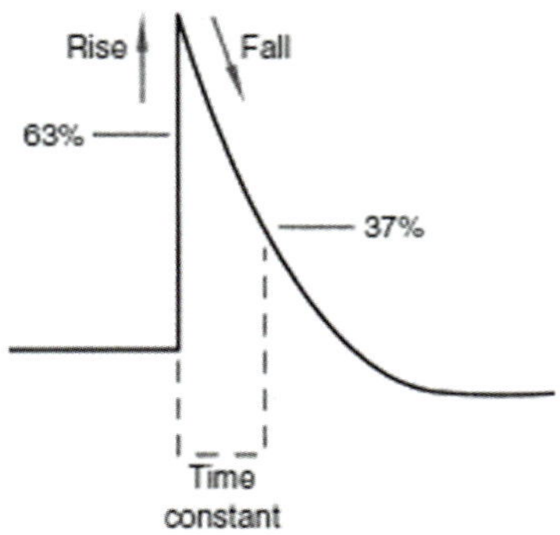

Figure 33-13 Effect of high-frequency filter and low-frequency filter settings on time constant.

it takes for the signal to reach 63% of its peak voltage is the "rise time constant." Now let us compare the effect of varying filter strengths on time constants as we look at Figure 33-14.

Notice that higher filter cutoff frequency settings result in lower fall time constants. This is important because it allows us to illustrate to all who inspect our recorded studies that we were collecting data with verified correct filter settings, as shown in Figure 33-15.

60-HZ OR 50-HZ (NOTCH) FILTERS

Otherwise known as the "notch filter," the purpose of the 60-Hz filter is to eliminate noise caused by power line interference from the record. Many countries use a 50-Hz power grid AC current; therefore, PSG systems often incorporate a 50-Hz notch filter as well. The notch filter allows strong suppression of unwanted electrical noise from the environment.

It is important to make sure that the record is as free of 60-Hz noise as possible without using a notch filter because very strong 60-Hz interference may result in artifacts or amplifier saturation that is not completely eliminated by a notch filter (Figure 33-16).

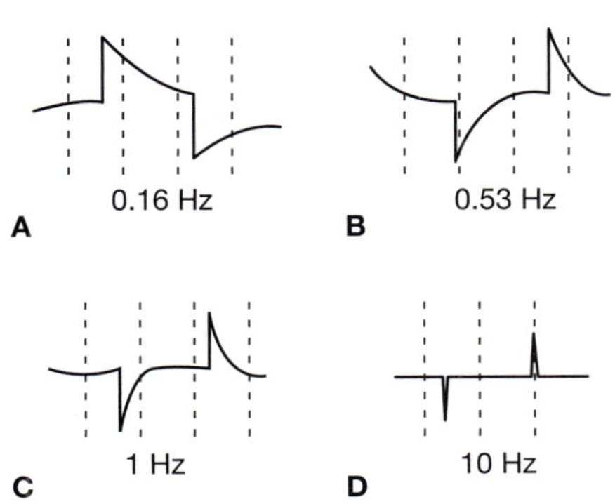

Figure 33-14 Effect of various filter settings on time constant.

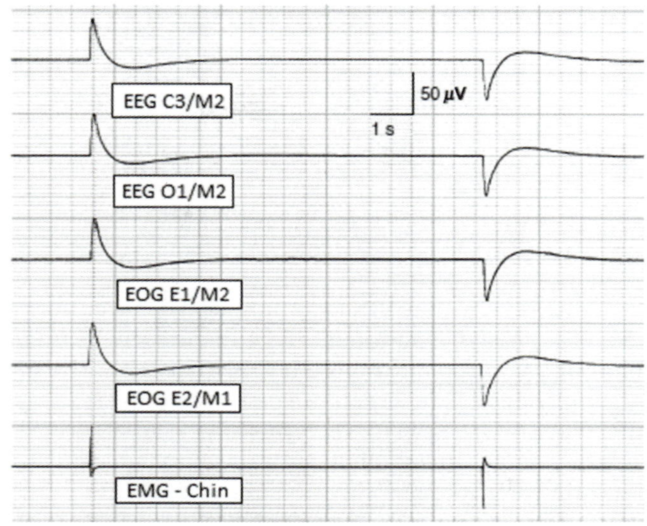

Figure 33-15 Calibration signals.

ANALOG-TO-DIGITAL CONVERTERS

The purpose of analog-to-digital conversion is to translate continuous (analog) bioelectric, transduced, and ancillary device signals into discrete numerical values (Figure 33-17). The analog-to-digital converter (ADC) captures analog signal periodically (at a sampling rate) and creates discrete numeric data points or samples. In order to properly reproduce the analog signal waveform, the sampling frequency needs to be sufficiently high. Specifically, it needs to be at least 2 times higher than the highest frequency that is being measured. This is known as "Nyquist theorem" (5). If this criterion is not followed, then incoming signals that are more than half the frequency of the sampling rate will be "aliased" or replaced with frequencies that are different from the original signal when the waveform is reconstructed for viewing.

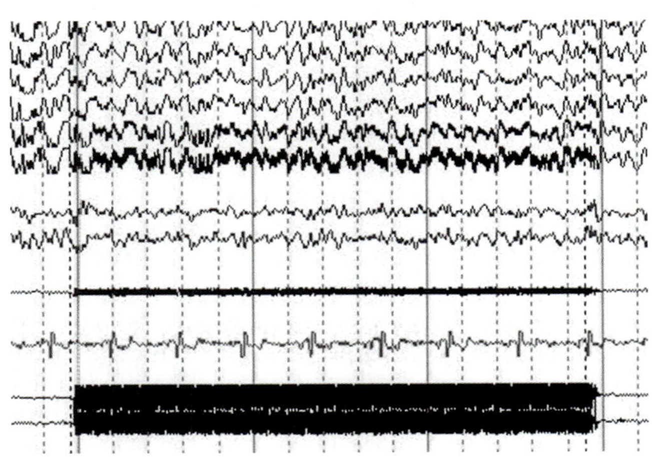

Figure 33-16 A 60-Hz artifact.

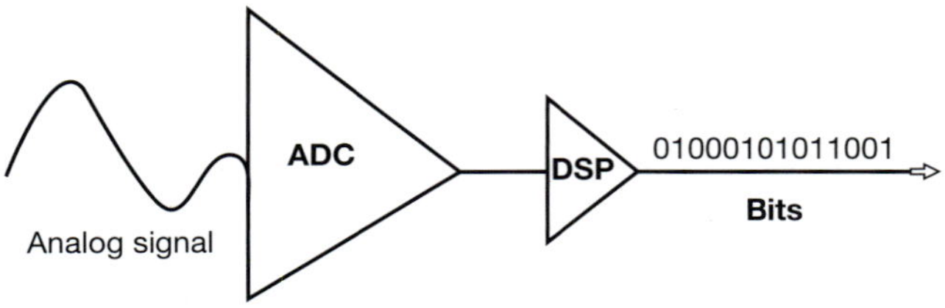

Figure 33-17 Analog-to-digital converter (ADC). DSP, digital signal processing.

This means that the incoming signal needs to be low-pass filtered to eliminate all frequencies higher than half the sampling rate before it gets to an ADC. This is accomplished by an antialiasing filter. In older systems, this type of filter had to be designed as a hardware circuit, making it potentially large, expensive, and suitable for only one fixed sampling frequency.

One of the most important advancements in system design is the shift in importance from hardware to software. The use of digital signal processing allows fewer circuitry components to accomplish the task. As a result, hardware can be miniaturized and costs reduced.

The sampling rate of a modern ADC can exceed 32,000 Hz, and by Nyquist sampling theory, this results in a reliable frequency spectrum of up to 16,000 Hz. This intermediate data stream can be then filtered in software before secondary sampling, which creates an output data stream typically at a sampling frequency of 200 to 4,096 Hz. This technique, called "oversampling," allows a high degree of flexibility in selecting output data rate and aliasing elimination without the use of large and expensive electronic components for LFFs.

Recent AASM technical specifications recommend sampling rates of 500 Hz or higher for polysomnography to ensure accurate signal capture across multiple physiologic parameters. These higher sampling rates provide specific benefits for different recording channels. For EEG signals, sampling at greater than or equal to 500 Hz improves resolution of neurologic spikes and preserves critical waveform details. For ECG recordings, greater than or equal to 500 Hz sampling better defines pacemaker spikes and cardiac waveforms, with HFF set to greater than or equal to 150 Hz to optimize pacemaker detection. Respiratory monitoring also benefits significantly: nasal pressure transducers recorded at higher rates show improved definition of vibration and snoring patterns, while respiratory effort channels display clearer cardiogenic oscillations, allowing better artifact identification. Similar advantages extend to electromyogram (EMG) channels, where higher sampling rates prevent amplitude attenuation in rapidly oscillating signals. Snoring sound analysis at 500 Hz provides more accurate amplitude determination and clearer waveforms. These enhanced sampling specifications ensure that sleep recordings capture the subtle physiologic events necessary for accurate diagnosis and treatment planning.

Multiplexing is the combination of multiple signals into one stream to allow digital conversion to be performed by fewer ADC components (albeit requiring components that work reliably at higher frequencies). Alternatively, multiple independent ADCs may be employed—a dedicated ADC for each recorded channel. With proper design and modern components, adequate signal quality can be achieved with either approach, and it is usually considerations such as size and cost that impact this choice.

The next parameter that we need to consider in the digitization process is voltage or amplitude resolution. To accurately display the EEG signal waveform, a minimum of 12 bits or 2^{12} = 4,096 voltage points has been mandated by the AASM. Some advanced systems use 24-bit ADCs, allowing larger dynamic range and smoother signals.

The number of data points may be further reduced by hardware or software depending on relevant physiologic characteristics. This allows storage constraints to be met. The final result is accurate and noise-free representation of the original exceedingly weak signal at the desired electrode pairings, sensitivity, and filter settings, as exemplified in Figure 33-18.

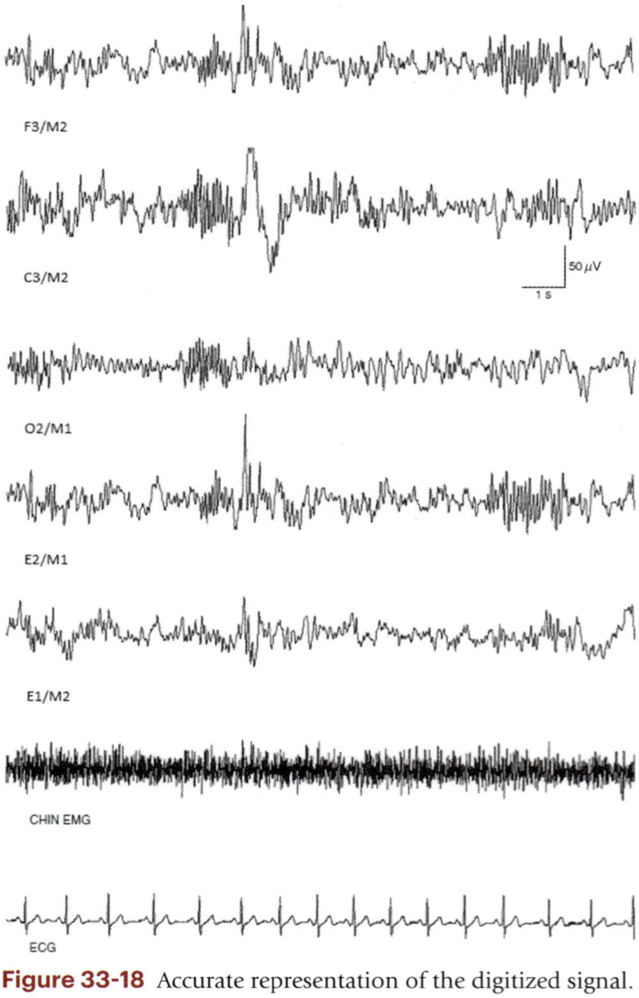

Figure 33-18 Accurate representation of the digitized signal.

CALIBRATIONS

In our discussion of calibrations, we must first be sure that we understand what the term "calibration" means. In its literal sense, calibration is the determination and documentation of the accuracy of a measurement or an observation. In PSG, there are several realms in which calibration comes into play.

Historically, machine calibration was necessary daily to ensure that the writing pens inked out tracings that accurately reflected recording parameters. This was due to the susceptibility of mechanical parts to a gradual loss of their position. In today's PSG systems, everything is digital, and true machine calibrations are no longer performed by the technologist. Rather, the conversion is innate to the amplifier circuitry, thus providing security in the knowledge that what you see is what you get. This does not mean that a well-run study does not attempt to document the scale used when viewing the recording. Therefore, at any time during a study, the technologist can usually initiate a software command that will produce several calibrations useful in the documentation process, including:

1. Square wave—Many systems will produce a channel-by-channel scroll of a square wave that will trace a DC 50 μV/cm on/off signal.
2. Time constant—All PSG systems will record a channel-by-channel tracing that shows the time constant as a function of time and filter settings.
3. Impedance check—Although not a calibration, the impedance check will produce an electronic stamp that shows the contact impedance values of all electrodes. This varies among vendors in the way it is illustrated but usually documents the actual value in kΩ. While running the impedance check, it is possible to see whether the values are acceptable, and the technologist is alerted to any poor electrode connections. It is good practice to aim for similar values below 5kΩ and to make sure that common and reference electrode impedance values are low.
4. Biocalibrations—These are physiologic maneuvers used to assess the integrity of the recording of various parameters. This is discussed in detail in other chapters, but we mention it here only to make sure that technologists do not confuse these patient calibrations with system calibrations.
5. External and integrated pulse oximetry calibrations—Most PSG systems have integrated pulse oximetry that conforms to AASM standards for accuracy and sampling rate. Because the readout of integrated oximetry is what the technologist views on the PSG monitor, the method for obtaining a calibration in this case would be to attach a separate clip from an independent oximeter to another finger and compare the readouts. In the case of using an ancillary oximeter that is plugged into a DC input, the technologist compares the readout on the bedside oximeter with what is being displayed on the PSG monitor and calibrates accordingly.
6. $EtCO_2$ and transcutaneous CO_2 involve the use of ancillary CO_2 monitoring devices that interface with the PSG system through one of the available DC inputs on the bedside amplifier. In either case, calibration involves the assigning of a voltage range to the minimum and maximum measurement values according to the example in Table 33-2.
7. Positive airway pressure (PAP) flow generators—Most manufacturers have developed flow generators capable of multiple measurements, including pressure, flow, leak rate, etc. Calibration of PAP to the PSG system involves the assigning of a voltage range to the desired minimum and maximum values according to the example in Table 33-3.

Table 33-2 Voltage Ranges for Direct Current Signals

Parameter	0 V	1 V
End-tidal CO_2 (mm Hg)	0	100
Transcutaneous CO_2 (mm Hg)	0	100

THE RECORDING MONTAGE

When the minimum criteria for channel recording, as determined in the AASM scoring manual are met, a standard montage can be developed, as shown in Table 33-4.

Digital PSG allows the technologist to re-reference during and after the recording as necessary to maintain signal clarity. This includes the ability to choose an arithmetic average of the left and right mastoid references when ECG artifact contaminates the recording. This has been referred to as "linked ears," and the digital benefit is that because the re-referencing is done using software, the technologist no longer needs to enter the room and combine M1 and M2 with jumper cables.

Table 33-3 Calibration Ranges for Positive Airway Pressure Outputs

Parameter	−1 V	0 V	1 V
Pressure (cm H_2O)		0	30
Flow (L/min)	−60	0	60
Leak (L/min)		0	60

Table 33-4 Sample Montage

Channel	Derivation	Sensitivity (mV/mm)	High Filter (Hz)	Low Filter (Hz)	Sample Rate (Hz)
L outer canthus	E1–M2	5-7	35	0.3	512
R outer canthus	E2–M1	5-7	35	0.3	512
Chin EMG	EMG1–EMG2–EMG3	10	100	10	512
Central EEG	C3–M2 or C4–M1	5-7	35	0.3	512
Occipital EEG	O1–M2 or O2–M1	5-7	35	0.3	512
Frontal EEG	F3–M2 or F4–M1	5-7	35	0.3	512
Left anterior tibialis	LAT1 LAT2	10	100	10	512
Right anterior tibialis	RAT1 RAT2	10	100	10	512
ECG	ECG1 ECG2	20	70	0.3	1,024
Snore		20	100	10	512
P flow AC[a]		20	15	0.1	100
P flow DC[a]	DCx	20	15	N/A	100
Thermo flow[a]		20	15	0.1	100
Thoracic effort belt		10-100	15	0.1	100
Abdominal effort belt		10-100	15	0.1	100
CPAP[a]	DCx	–	5	–	100
SpO_2	DCx	–	5	–	25

[a]flow channel options.
CPAP, continuous positive airway pressure; ECG, electrocardiogram; EEG, electroencephalogram; EMG, electromyogram; SpO_2, pulse oximetry.

Sophisticated digital PSG platforms can digitally subtract ECG artifact contamination from EEG and other physiologic channels through advanced signal processing algorithms, effectively removing cardiac electrical activity that would otherwise contaminate cerebral recordings. The technologist can change many additional recording variables in order to examine more closely those aspects of the recording that warrant documentation. For example, any number of montages can be selected to satisfy the requirements of the ordering physician and aid in diagnosis.

DIGITAL SCREEN RESOLUTION

For the sleep professional to interpret signals accurately, high-quality visual display of waveforms is essential. The AASM specifies a minimum digital screen resolution of 1,600 × 1,050 pixels (horizontal × vertical), which supports the standard visual analysis of sleep in 30-second epochs. Modern displays now offer resolutions up to 3,840 × 2,160 pixels, commonly referred to as 4K or UHD (Ultra High Definition). These enhanced resolutions, paired with larger screen sizes, significantly improve multitasking capabilities and simultaneous visualization of multiple physiologic parameters.

The appropriate display technology facilitates better detection of subtle abnormal waveforms such as EEG spikes and enhances workflow efficiency by allowing technologists to view more channels or longer time periods without sacrificing detail. When combined with the recommended higher sampling rates, high-resolution displays ensure that the detailed information captured in the recording is fully accessible during visual analysis, supporting accurate identification of clinically significant events across all recording channels.

VIDEO AND AUDIO RECORDING IN POLYSOMNOGRAPHY SYSTEMS

The ability to synchronize digital video to the PSG recording introduces an additional valuable diagnostic tool to digital PSG. By converting the analog signal from a high-resolution camera into a digital format, such as MPEG4, video can be streamed into the collection computer, and using various software programs, the video can be time-synchronized with the raw PSG data stream. Modern systems no longer require cumbersome add-on hardware to process the video stream but utilize conversion algorithms such as software compression and available USB ports. On most systems, the video capture bit rate can be adjusted to decrease the video file size. Reviewing physicians can quickly navigate to desired epochs to view video synchronized with the recording. Large video files can also be deleted or clipped to desired epoch ranges or be copied to separate data storage locations to suit the facilities' retention requirements. During the collection process, technologists can pan, tilt, and even zoom to capture the most articulate and fine aspects of patient movement and behavior during the recording.

In the same regard, refined directional and omnidirectional microphone configurations also make it possible to capture even the faintest sounds emanating from the recording bedroom. The end result is a truly detailed composite of all recording parameters of the patient's sleep experience.

PRESENT AND FUTURE CONSIDERATIONS FOR DIGITAL POLYSOMNOGRAPHY

The needs of health care providers and testing facilities demand that present-day diagnostic and treatment platforms are cost-efficient. Owing to software developments and hardware miniaturization, sleep facilities are now able to incorporate improvements in such areas as database customization, storage, networking, portability/mobility, and interfacing with other facility information platforms. Digital PSG has also become more reliable with the inclusion of such technologies as automatic disaster recovery, which, in the case of interruptions to the recording such as power outages, automatically restarts and appends to the existing record.

In the area of patient data and information, there is the issue of ever-expanding storage requirements. Smaller facilities can archive studies to various media. Larger networked facilities can leverage existing infrastructure to make use of more elegant solutions. Study data can be backed up over networks to storage servers that automate periodic redundant backups. Depending on regulatory requirements, data can be archived for the requisite period before they are deleted, if they are deleted at all. Some facilities may also print study reports and interpretations for inclusion in paper files.

With the advent of sophisticated database programming, it is now possible to keep track of patient records using any number of variables, including demographic data and information clinically specific to the patient. Physicians and other users can easily sort patients they are interested in viewing, and management and retrieval of salient information is now as quick as a click of the pointing device.

There is also concurrent application or "multitasking" technology, allowing technologists to simultaneously acquire and review patient data, making it possible to view live recording on one monitor while scoring the same record on a different monitor, or by splitting the screen. Virtualization technology makes it possible to serve multiple instances of the application. Larger facilities may find this technology prudent and actually dedicate servers of this type so that all stakeholders can access patient information regardless of time or place.

Users can also make use of autoscoring algorithms, although these outcomes require review for clinical confirmation. Another valuable addition is the capability of multiuser comparison scoring. This is known as "Interscorer reliability." All these advancements necessitate increased vigilance and protection of sensitive personal health information. This is accomplished using encryption protocols, password-protected user logins, and other administrative forms of data protection.

In other areas of data exchange, most PSG systems now integrate with the facility's electronic medical record. This initiative is known as HL7. Integration of the PSG system with the facility information system means that patient demographics and personal health care information can be imported from existing databases so that valuable clinical history is not overlooked by the sleep specialists. This is important because sleep medicine is particularly concerned with differential diagnosis and comorbid conditions. Along those same lines, most modern PSG systems will also export study files in European Data Format (EDF) and other standard file formats so that patient records can be viewed across varying platforms. Modern PSG systems also integrate with spreadsheets and word processing programs so that reports can be tailored to show data in every way imaginable.

Portable or remote PSG occurs when the technologist is not in the same physical location as the patient is. Digital PSG has also made possible portable monitoring or home sleep apnea testing (HSAT). Most PSG vendors now offer portable amplifiers that do not sacrifice any channels typically included in normal facility–based PSG. These devices can be set up in the facility and taken home with the patient. The technology is quite similar to full PSG with the option of audio and video capture. These devices usually record information to flash storage on the order of 2 GB to as high as 32 GB. This technology is categorized as a type II device. Type III and type IV devices are simpler devices that record fewer channels, and they comprise the devices that are used for HSAT. The next area of improvement in portable diagnostics may well be streaming data from the home to the facility for remote viewing and "real-time" observation and processing. All these improvements will be governed by data integrity, data security, and Health Insurance Portability and Accountability Act (HIPAA) concerns. With the ever-changing landscape of sleep medicine, one thing is certain: PSG will forever be inextricably linked to digital technology.

Technical consulting guidance was provided by Valery Arkhangorodsky (Natus Medical Incorporated; Google) and Michael Tamayo (Natus Medical Incorporated).

REFERENCES

1. Troester MM, Quan SF, Berry RB, et al. *The AASM Manual for the Scoring of Sleep and Associated Events: Rules, Terminology and Technical Specifications* [Version 3]. American Academy of Sleep Medicine; 2023.
2. Tatum WO, Husain AM, Benbadis SR. *Handbook of EEG Interpretation*. Demos Medical Publishing; 2008.
3. Nunez PL, Srinivasan R. *Electric Fields of the Brain: The Neurophysics of EEG*. Oxford University Press; 1981.
4. Klein S, Thorne BM. *Biological Psychology*. Worth; 2006.
5. Forouzan BA, Fegan SC. *Data Communications and Networking*. 2nd ed. McGraw-Hill; 2001.

Chapter 34
Recording the Biopotentials of Sleep

REGINA PATRICK

KEY CONCEPTS/LEARNING OBJECTIVES

The key concepts for this chapter include explaining the frequency and voltage characteristics of the primary biopotentials recorded during polysomnography, recognizing and correcting problems with biopotential signals, explaining the purpose and procedures for pre- and post-physiologic calibrations, recognizing common artifacts and determining the appropriate action or monitoring required to identify and respond to physiologic data, clinical events, patient needs, and medical emergencies.

KEY TERMS

Artifact
Biopotential
Clinical event
Electrocardiogram
Electroencephalogram
Electromyogram
Electrooculogram
High-frequency filter
Low-frequency filter
Physiologic calibration

The desired signals of brainwaves on an electroencephalogram (EEG), eye movements on an electrooculogram (EOG), heartbeats on an electrocardiogram (ECG), and thoracic and abdominal movements on the respiration channels occur in association with signals that are stronger. The stronger signals may obscure the desired signals. On a polysomnograph (PSG), low-frequency filters and high-frequency filters allow for the recording of desired signals while excluding undesired signals. The low-frequency filter setting will not allow any frequency less than that setting to be recorded, and the high-frequency filter setting will not allow any frequency above the setting to be recorded. Thus, any frequency falling between the high- and low-frequency filters will be detected and recorded.

The low- and high-frequency filters are set just below and above, respectively, the desired signal frequency. To optimize signal quality, the American Academy of Sleep Medicine (AASM; Darien, IL) (1,2) recommends specific high- and low-frequency filter settings for the EEG, EOG, electromyogram (EMG), ECG, and respiratory channels. By applying the recommended filter settings, a polysomnographic recording should, ideally, be free of interference from stronger undesired signals.

RECORDING THE BIOPOTENTIALS OF SLEEP

Electroencephalogram

The EEG frequencies of interest range from less than 1 cycle per second (ie, <1 Hz) to 14 Hz. Therefore, a low-frequency filter setting of 0.3 Hz (which allows the detection of slow waves) and a high-frequency filter setting of 35 to 50 Hz (usually, 35 Hz, which allows the detection of alpha waves), are typically used for the EEG channels.

Electrooculogram

A low-frequency filter setting of 0.3 Hz allows the detection of the slow-rolling eye movements that occur with sleep onset, and a high-frequency filter setting of 35 Hz allows the detection of rapid eye movements (REMs) and the fast, low-amplitude EOG activity occurring throughout sleep.

Electromyogram

A low-frequency filter setting of 10 to 20 Hz and a high-frequency filter setting of 100 to 150 Hz are used to detect EMG frequencies of the skeletal muscles (eg, legs and chin). This range is sufficient to record the faster firing rate of the muscles (ie, increased muscle tone) during arousals, wake, or nonrapid eye movement

(NREM) sleep and the decreased firing rate of the muscles (ie, atonia [lack of muscle tone]) during REM sleep.

Electrocardiogram

A low-frequency filter setting of 0.3 Hz and a high-frequency filter setting of 100 Hz are used to detect ECG frequencies. The low-frequency filter setting of 0.3 Hz (ie, 0.3 cycles per second = 1 cycle per 3.33 seconds) allows the recording of each heartbeat, which normally takes about 0.8 seconds. The high-frequency filter setting of 100 Hz (ie, 100 cycles per second = 1 cycle per 0.014 second) allows the recording of a heartbeat's individual waves (ie, P, QRS complex, and T wave; the duration of these waves ranges from <0.10-0.25 seconds). It also allows the detection of pacer spikes (ie, a pacer spike appears as a small vertical line before a heartbeat and represents the electrical pulse generated by the pacemaker to induce a heartbeat) (1,2). To record an ECG, one electrode (negative [ECG2]) is placed below the right clavicle at the midclavicular line, and a second electrode (positive [ECG1]) is placed on the left lower chest at the anterior axillary line in the sixth or seventh intercostal space (1,2). An alternative is to place one electrode each below the right clavicle and left clavicle at the midclavicular line (1,2).

Respiratory Effort

The low-frequency filter setting is 0.1 Hz, and the high-frequency filter setting is 15 Hz for the respiratory effort sensors, usually respiratory inductance plethysmography belts. (In previous guidelines, the AASM considered piezoelectric belts as "acceptable" for recording thoracic and abdominal respiratory effort; however, as of December 31, 2023, this device is no longer allowed) (2). The low-frequency setting allows the motions related to inhalation and exhalation to be presented as sinusoidal waves, whereas the high-frequency setting excludes frequencies (eg, snoring noise, movement artifact, muscle contractions) that could obscure these waves.

Respiratory Airflow

For the airflow sensors (eg, thermistor or thermocouple, pressure transducer), the low-frequency filter setting is 0.1 Hz and the high-frequency filter setting is 15 Hz for thermocouple and thermistor, and the low-frequency filter setting is less than 0.03 Hz and the high-frequency filter setting is 70 to 100 Hz for the pressure transducer (1). As with the respiratory effort channel, these settings allow the sinusoidal waves of inhalation and exhalation to be recorded while excluding higher frequencies that would obscure these waves.

PROBLEMS RECORDING BIOPOTENTIAL SIGNALS

Even when using the correct filter settings, undesired signals (ie, artifacts) can appear in a channel and interfere with the recording of a desired signal. The following sections discuss common problems that can lead to artifact in a channel.

Skin/Electrode Issues

Some skin problems (eg, rash) can affect the electrical properties of the skin by altering normal cellular interactions. This alteration may result in a high impedance reading. If the skin problem is localized, a technologist may need to place the electrode in a slightly different position to avoid the problem area and make a note of this alteration in the patient's chart. If the problem is more widespread, a technologist may need to forgo placing an electrode on that area of the skin. In this instance, the technologist should thoroughly notate in the patient's chart why the electrode was not placed on the patient.

Problems Recording Electroencephalogram Signals

Sweat Artifact

Sweat may cause low-frequency artifact to appear in the EEG, resulting in rolling in the EEG channels. Cooling the patient by increasing air circulation (eg, turning on a fan or air conditioner, opening the door) may eliminate rolling by ameliorating sweating. However, sweat contains salt, and the salt that remains on the skin after the skin cools can cause chemical changes in the electrolyte gel used in the electrode. This factor can cause continued problems with a poor signal. If a poor signal persists, the poorly recording electrode(s) should be replaced.

Movement Artifact

Muscle activity during movement can obscure underlying EOG and EEG signals. During movement, the technologist should describe in the patient's chart and/or on the PSG exactly what is happening—especially if a patient is being monitored for nocturnal seizures or REM sleep behavior disorder (RBD) (ie, a sleep disorder in which muscle atonia does not occur during REM sleep, thereby allowing the person to act out dreams).

Problems Recording Electrooculogram Signals

The retina has a negative charge (reflected by an upward deflection on the EOG channel), and the cornea has a

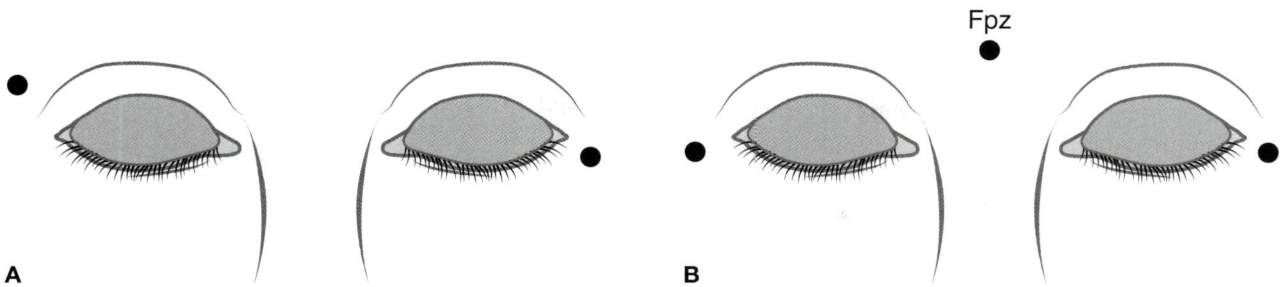

Figure 34-1 The recommended (A) and alternate (B) electrode placement for the electrooculogram channels.

positive charge (reflected by a downward deflection on an EOG channel). The difference in charge between the cornea and retina, called the "corneoretinal potential," is approximately −60 mV. The corneoretinal potential allows eye movements to be recorded from sensors placed on the outer canthus of each eye. When the eyes move in the same direction, one electrode will be close to the retina and record a negative charge, whereas the other electrode will be close to the cornea and record a positive charge.

To ensure equal amplitude of conjugate eye movements (ie, the eyes move in the same direction), the AASM recommends placing one EOG electrode 1 cm above and 1 cm lateral to the midline of the outer canthus of one eye (typically the right eye [ie, E2 electrode]) and one EOG electrode below and 1 cm lateral to the midline of the outer canthus of the other eye (typically, the left eye [ie, E1 electrode]). In general, both EOG electrodes are referenced to the same mastoid site (typically, E1-M2 and E2-M2). When using the recommended placement, the out-of-phase deflections of the EOG signals are greater for horizontal eye movements than for vertical eye movements.

An alternate placement allowed by the AASM for the EOG electrodes is to place each electrode 1 cm below and lateral to the midline of the outer canthus of its respective eye (1,2). Both electrodes are referenced to Fpz. In this configuration, vertical eye movements are in phase, and horizontal eye movements are out of phase (Figures 34-1 and 34-2).

An advantage of using the AASM's recommended eye placement is that all conjugate eye movements produce out-of-phase deflections. However, when using the AASM-recommended eye placement, the deflections of vertical eye movements will be greater than those of horizontal eye movements and eye blinks. As a result,

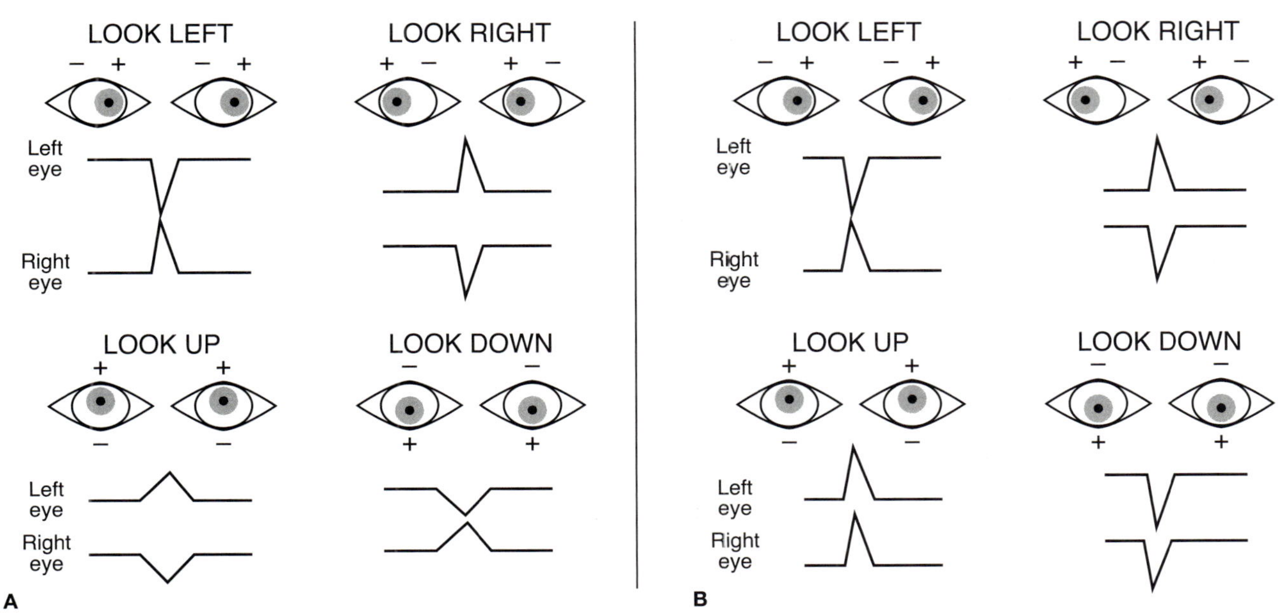

Figure 34-2 Eye deflections with the American Academy of Sleep Medicine (AASM)–recommended electrode placement (A) and the AASM alternate electrode placement (B). The deflections with alternate placement are larger for the vertical movements, compared with those of the recommended placement.

determining the direction of all eye movements can be difficult, and eye movements with low amplitude may be missed. When using the alternate AASM eye placement, the vertical and horizontal eye movement deflections are more pronounced than those of the recommended placement, and the signals for eye blinking are more readily detected (as in-phase deflections). However, with the alternate placement, the Fpz electrode may allow some EEG signals in the EOG recording, which can make distinguishing EEG activity from EOG activity difficult, particularly during vertical eye movements. Even if electrodes are correctly placed using the recommended or alternate EOG electrode placement, several physiologic conditions can affect the recording of biopotential changes in an EOG channel.

An Artificial Eye

An artificial eye does not generate the electrical potential changes as would a natural eye. Therefore, an electrode placed by the artificial eye does not reflect eye movements of the affected eye. However, recording eye movements during REM sleep is still possible. Rather than placing an electrode on the outer canthus of each eye, the technologist can place both electrodes on the unaffected eye. The first electrode should be placed 1 cm from the edge and 1 cm above the midline of the outer canthus, and the second electrode (which would have normally been used on the channel of the affected eye) should be placed 1 cm below the midline of the outer canthus of the same eye. Thus, the electrodes will still pick up the deflections needed to record REMs.

If a technologist were to place an electrode on the outer canthus of the affected eye, the EOG signals on that channel would appear dampened or distorted because the electrode continues to record frontal EEG activity. The technologist should make a note in the patient's chart that the patient has an artificial eye and indicate whether the EOG electrodes are placed on one eye or on both eyes. If the technologist places an electrode by the affected eye, they need to describe in the patient's chart how the signal is affected (eg, "the patient has an artificial right eye; the right EOG signal is dampened").

Eye Diseases That Affect the Retina

Damage to or destruction of the rods or cones in the retina alters these cells' ability to undergo the photochemical reactions that are necessary for visual perception. The retina's electrical potential consequently decreases, and this factor can affect the corneoretinal potential. A diminished corneoretinal potential may dampen the EOG signal of one or both eyes in people who have diseases that affect the retina, such as Best disease (ie, congenital macular dystrophy) (Figure 34-3). The technologist may need to increase the sensitivity of the channels to record the EOG signal. The technologist should make a note in the patient's chart if sensitivity was increased for the affected eye.

Eye Muscle Problems

Six muscles in the eye, which are arranged as three sets of opposing muscles, allow a person to move the eyes in all four directions (up, down, left, and right) and obliquely (ie, at an angle rather than vertically or horizontally). If a problem such as a stroke affects how these muscles move, one or both eyes will not move correctly.

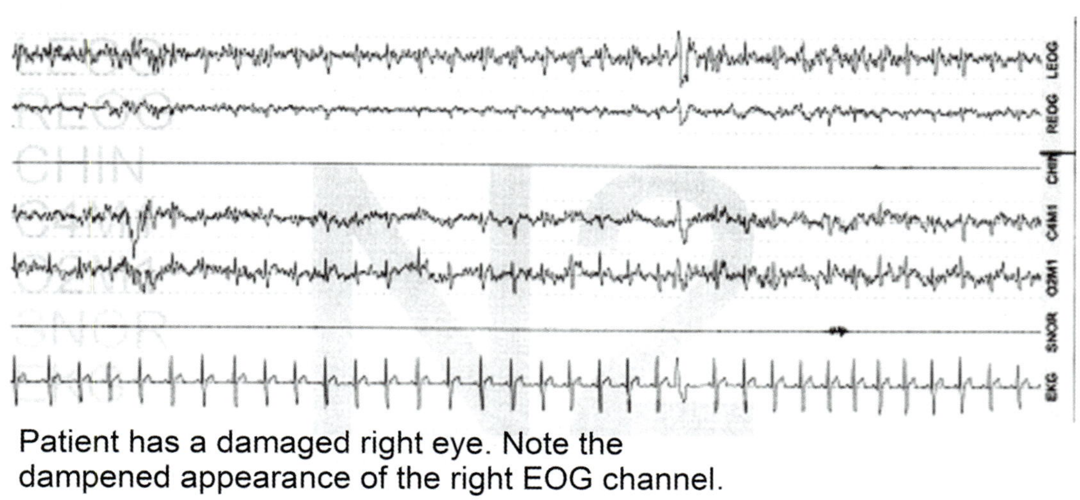

Figure 34-3 Electrooculogram (EOG) recording of a patient who had a right eye injury. (Image used with permission of Regina Patrick, RPSGT, RST, and obtained on the SomnoStar system, version 9 [2008; Cardinal Health Respiratory Technologies].)

As a result of impaired muscle movement, EOG signals may be altered (ie, nonexistent or dampened). The technologist may need to increase the sensitivity of the EOG channels to record the signal. The technologist should make a note in the patient's chart if sensitivity was increased for the affected eye.

Problems Recording Electromyogram Signals

Problems recording biopotential changes on the chin or leg EMG channels usually result from improper electrode placement, from high impedances (eg, the skin is insufficiently cleaned), or from electrodes becoming dislodged during sleep. To reduce the likelihood of poor signal quality in the EMG channels, the technologist must show the same care in preparing the electrode sites as when applying EEG and EOG electrodes. For EEG, EOG, and chin EMG, an impedance should ideally be less than or equal to 5 kilo-ohms (kΩ) and, for the leg EMG, the impedance should be less than or equal to10 kΩ (1). The electrodes must also be securely attached to the chin or legs to prevent their being easily dislodged during the night. For example, an extra piece of tape may be placed on the leg sensors to ensure that they remain on the patient during the night. However, vigorous movement by a patient may dislodge an electrode, no matter how well secured. If the PSG recording system provides re-referencing capabilities, the EMG channel can be re-referenced to a backup electrode. If necessary, electrodes may need to be reapplied.

Problems Recording Electrocardiogram Signals

Problems with the ECG recording are generally caused by poorly attached or dislodged ECG electrodes. If an ECG electrode becomes dislodged during the study (Figure 34-4), an ECG tracing may be temporarily obtained from alternate electrode derivations, provided that the PSG recording system offers re-referencing capabilities. For example, a leg electrode can be used as a temporary substitute for the affected ECG electrode. If re-referencing is not possible, the electrode will need to be reapplied.

Problems Recording Respiratory Effort

People with certain neurologic problems that affect the abdominal and thoracic muscles or who have chest deformities such as kyphosis (commonly called "hunchback") may be unable to fully expand and contract the chest wall. This insufficient movement may reduce respiratory signals, even if the abdominal and thoracic sensors are properly placed on the patient. The technologist may therefore need to increase the sensitivity of a respiratory channel to record respiratory signals.

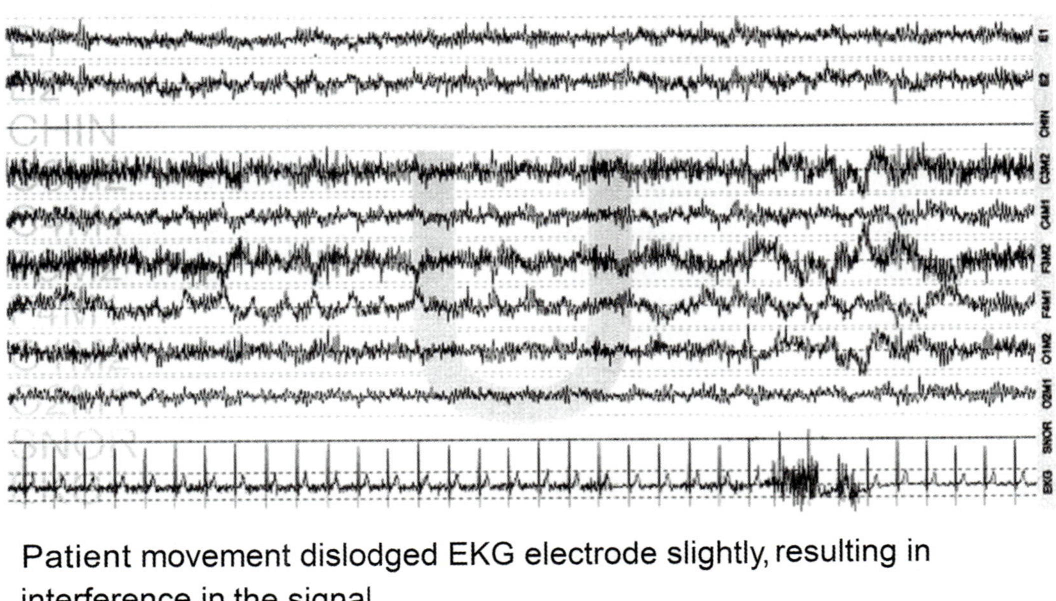

Figure 34-4 Poor electrocardiogram (ECG) signal. (Image used with permission of Regina Patrick, RPSGT, RST, and obtained on the SomnoStar system, version 9 [2008; Cardinal Health Respiratory Technologies].)

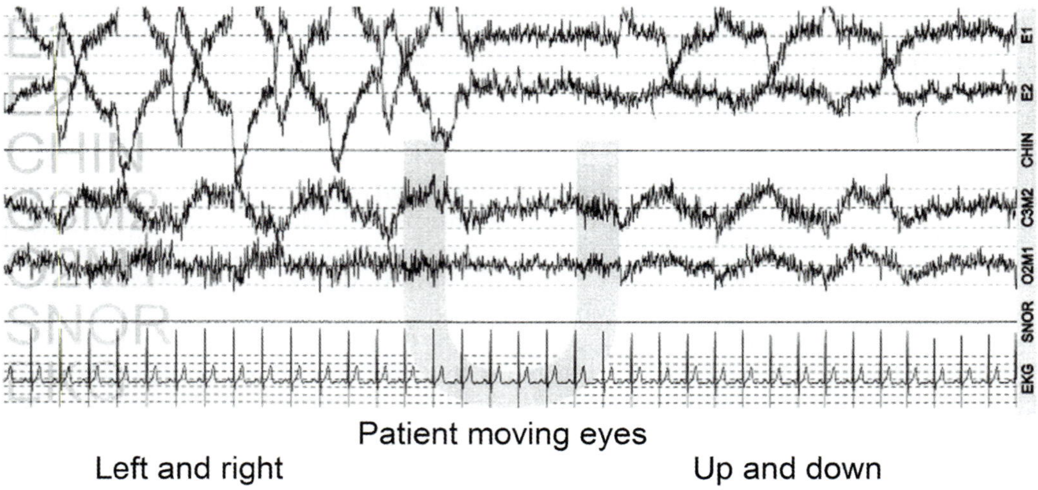

Figure 34-5 Eye deflections with the AASM-recommended electrode placement. (Image used with permission of Regina Patrick, RPSGT, RST, and obtained on the SomnoStar system, version 9 [2008; Cardinal Health Respiratory Technologies].)

Problems Recording Respiratory Airflow

A common problem with recording airflow pressure changes is that the pressure transducer sensor may become plugged by excessive mucus, especially in a person with an upper respiratory infection or sinus infection. This obstruction will interfere with the proper recording of the signal. The technologist may need to clean or replace the sensor during the study to obtain a clear airflow signal. Another common problem with the airflow transducer sensor is that the air tube may become kinked with patient movement or the patient may lie on the air tube. The technologist may need to enter the patient's room to unkink the air tube or dislodge it from under the patient.

PROCEDURES FOR PRE- AND POSTPHYSIOLOGIC CALIBRATIONS

Physiologic calibrations (sometimes called "biocalibrations" or "patient calibrations") are performed before and after a sleep study. The physiologic calibrations are a series of instructions that are designed to determine that the sensors are correctly recording signals from a patient, the polarity of the signals is correct, the strength of the signal is sufficient for recording, and no unwanted interference exists. The following are features that should appear for each channel during the physiologic calibration procedure.

The Electrooculogram Channels

For these channels, the eye signals of each channel must deflect in opposite directions when the person's eyes move conjunctively (ie, in the same direction). To mimic the conjunctive eye movements of REM sleep, ask the patient to look left and right 5 times, then up and down 5 times (Figure 34-5). As a result of the corneoretinal potential, the signal on one eye channel should deflect upward, and the signal on the other eye channel should deflect downward with each movement. (However, if one uses the alternate EOG electrode placement, horizontal eye movements produce deflections in the opposite direction, and vertical eye movements produce deflections in the same direction.)

The next physiologic calibration that involves the eyes elicits alpha waves. To do this, ask the patient to close the eyes for 30 seconds and then open the eyes for 30 seconds. In most people, when the eyes are closed, alpha waves become prominent in the EEG, especially in the occipital channels. When the eyes are opened, the EEG resumes its original waking activity, which consists of a mixture of fast, low-frequency waves, primarily alpha and beta waves (the latter of which have a frequency of 18-30 Hz) (Figure 34-6).

The third physiologic calibration involving the eyes involves having the patient blink 5 times rapidly (Figure 34-7). During wake, a patient may blink at a rate of 0.5 to 2.0 Hz. As drowsiness develops, the blinking rate begins to slow and may be replaced by slow oscillating eye movements.

The Chin Electromyogram Channel

For this channel, sufficiently detecting muscle tone when the person is in NREM sleep is important. To ensure muscle tone is being recorded appropriately, ask the patient to grit the teeth together or chew

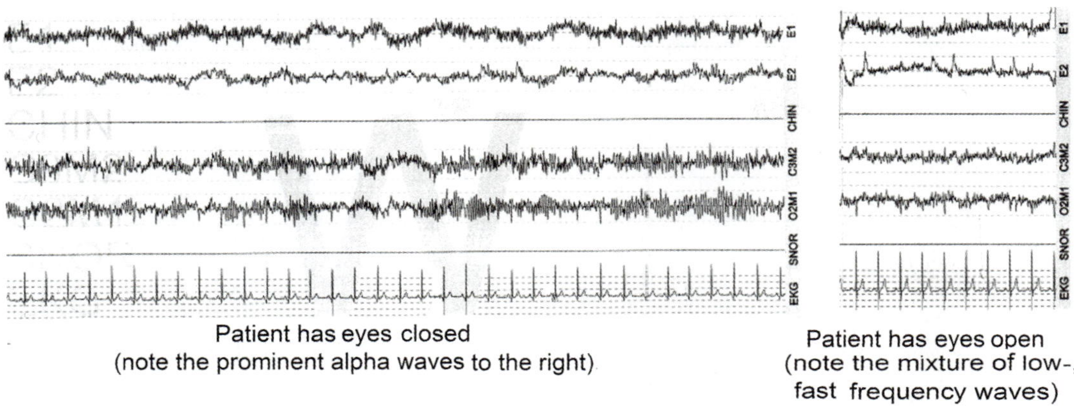

Figure 34-6 Electroencephalogram changes with eyes closed (left) and open (right). (Image used with permission of Regina Patrick, RPSGT, RST, and obtained on the SomnoStar system, version 9 [2008; Cardinal Health Respiratory Technologies].)

(for 5 seconds), and then relax (Figure 34-8). The amplitude of the signal should increase by at least 0.5 cm. This increase reflects an increase in muscle tone. For patients who have no teeth, ask them to open the mouth or yawn instead.

The Snore Channel

For this channel, the sensor must detect the increased vibration of the upper airway muscles that occurs with snoring. Ask the patient to make a snoring noise or hum

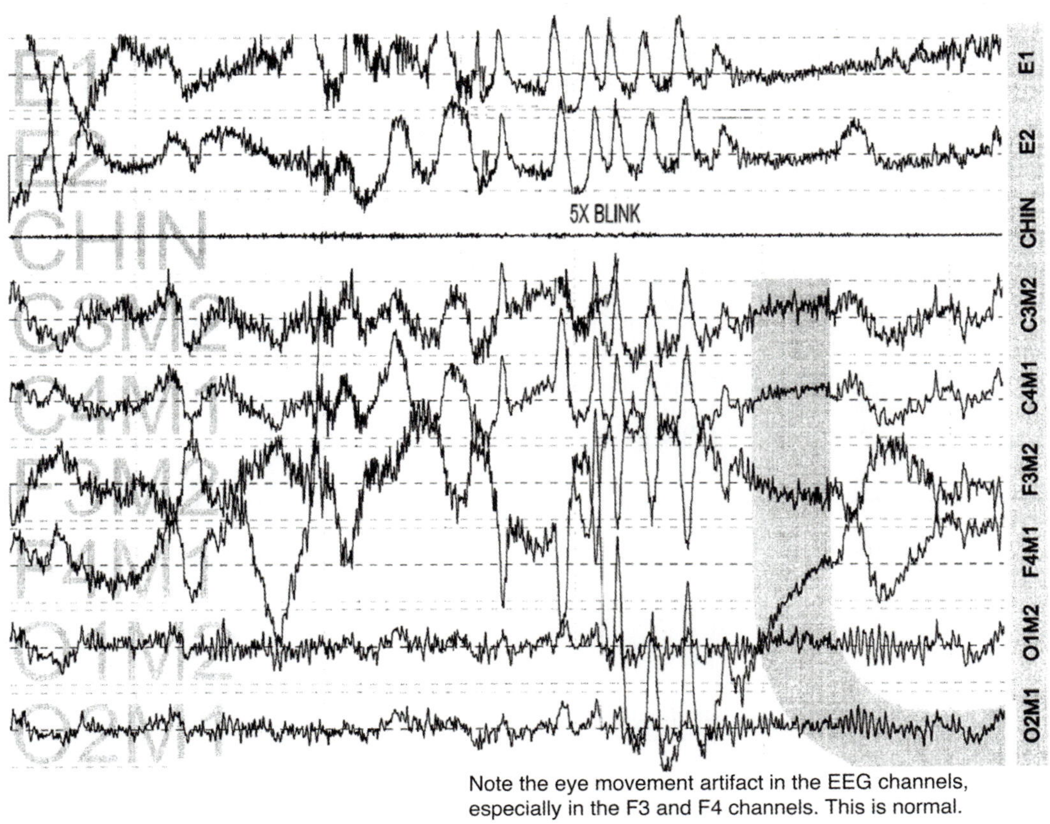

Figure 34-7 The appearance of the electrooculogram channels with eye blinking. EEG, electroencephalogram. (Image used with permission of Regina Patrick, RPSGT, RST, and obtained on the SomnoStar system, version 9 [2008; Cardinal Health Respiratory Technologies].)

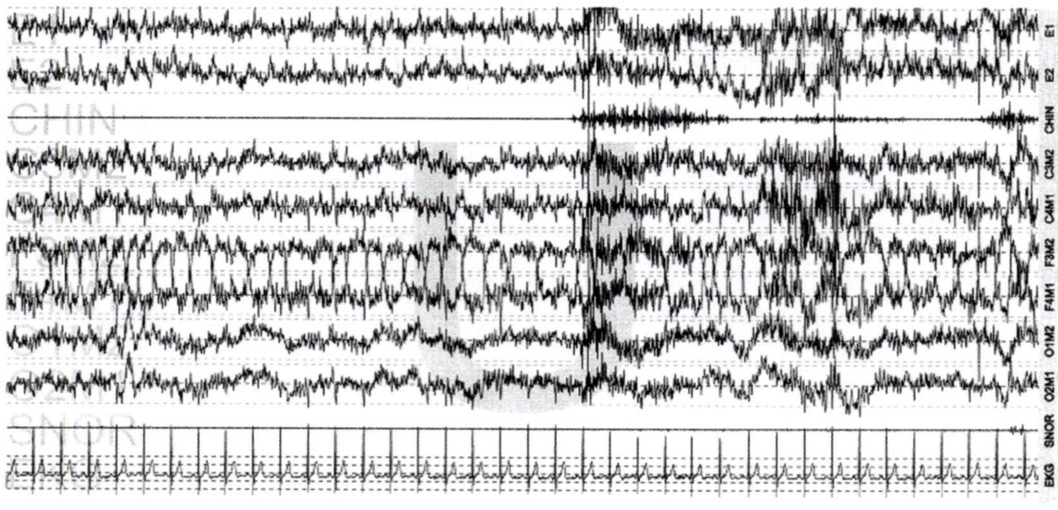

Patient gritting teeth

Figure 34-8 Change in chin electromyogram activity with gritting. (Image used with permission of Regina Patrick, RPSGT, RST, and obtained on the SomnoStar system, version 9 [2008; Cardinal Health Respiratory Technologies].)

for 5 seconds (Figure 34-9). If the patient is unable to make a sufficient snoring noise, an alternative is to ask the patient to make a vocalization such as counting "1, 2, 3" or saying "A, B, C." The signal should increase briefly with each vocalization.

The Leg Electromyogram Channels

For these channels, detecting the leg movements that occur with periodic leg movement (PLM) disorder or restless legs syndrome is important. Some patients with PLM disorder may bend the legs at the knee or hip level; however, more often, a person with PLM disorder may flex the ankle or toes. Therefore, leg sensors must be able to detect the slightest leg movements (eg, flexing of the toes) that occur during a sleep study. To mimic PLMs, ask the patient to flex the foot or raise the toes of the right (or left) foot 5 times and then to flex the foot or raise the toes of the opposite foot 5 times (Figure 34-10). A burst of activity should occur with each flex.

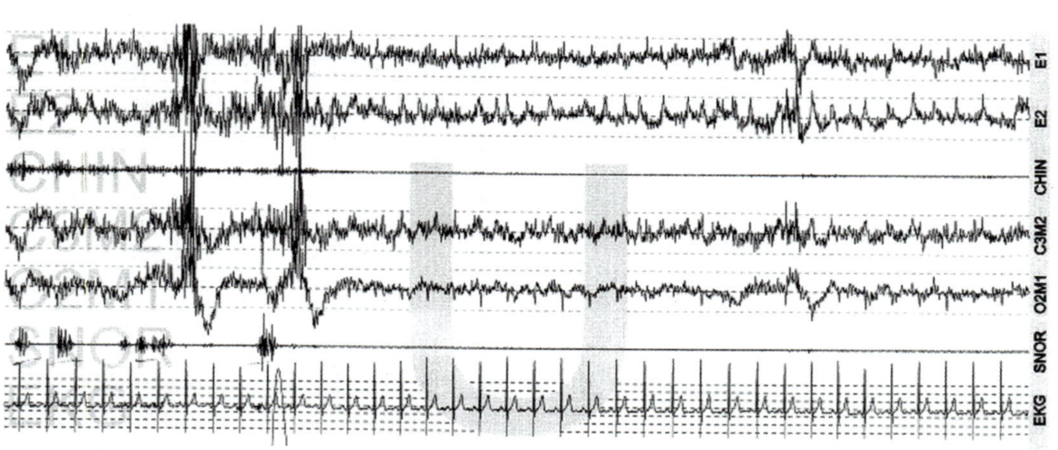

Patient making snoring noises

Figure 34-9 Simulation of snoring. (Image used with permission of Regina Patrick, RPSGT, RST, and obtained on the SomnoStar system, version 9 [2008; Cardinal Health Respiratory Technologies].)

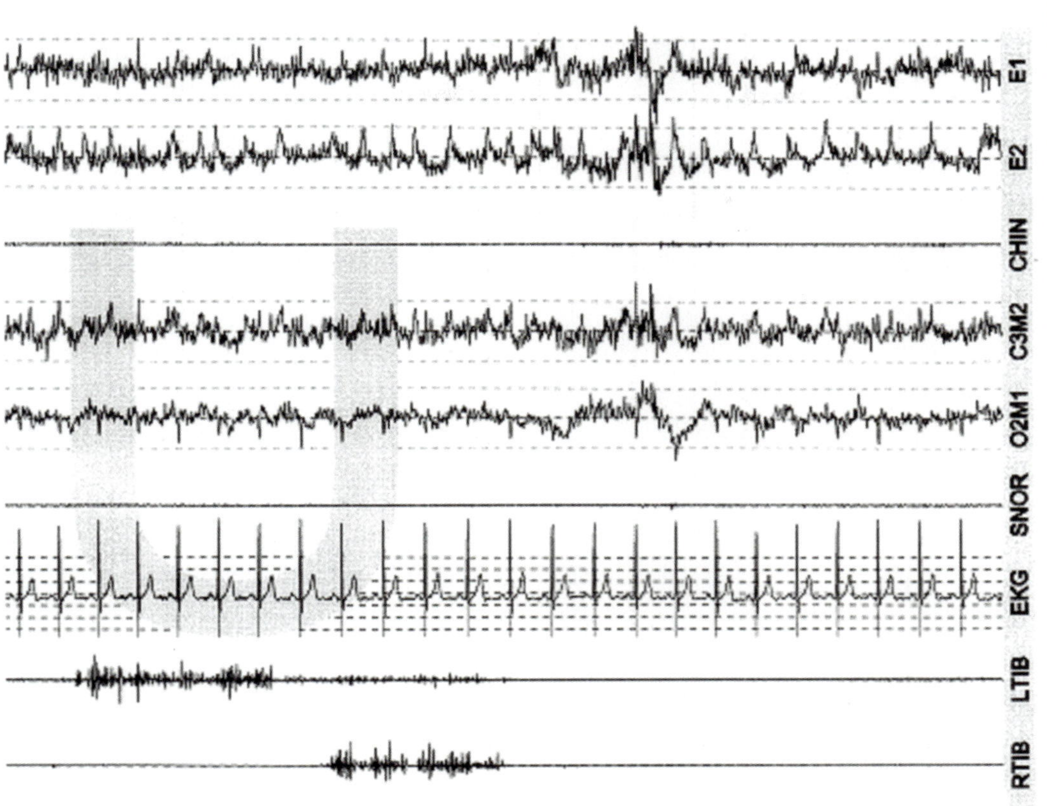

Figure 34-10 Change in leg electromyogram activity with toe flexes. (Image used with permission of Regina Patrick, RPSGT, RST, and obtained on the SomnoStar system, version 9 [2008; Cardinal Health Respiratory Technologies].)

The Airflow Channels

For these channels, the airflow sensor (ie, thermistor or thermocouple, both of which indirectly reflect airflow by detecting temperature changes that occur with inhalation and exhalation) and a pressure transducer sensor, which detects air pressure changes that occur with inhalation and exhalation, should be used. Also important to ensure is that these sensors detect the lack of airflow during an apnea episode. To verify that the airflow sensors are detecting nasal breaths and oral breaths, ask the patient to breathe through the nose only for 10 seconds and then to breathe through the mouth alone for 10 seconds (Figure 34-11). As the person inhales and exhales, the thermistor or thermocouple should generate sinusoidal signals on the airflow channel. Nasal pressure transducers typically only measure nasal airflow; therefore, the signal in this channel should be flat during oral breathing maneuvers.

To mimic apnea, ask the patient to take a deep breath and hold it for 10 seconds. The airflow and air pressure signals should be flat because no air is passing through the nose or mouth (Figure 34-12).

The Abdominal and Thoracic Effort Channels

For these channels, the sensors should detect the movements of the abdomen and chest during normal respiration and during an apnea. During the airflow tests, the abdominal and thoracic effort channels should have a sinusoidal signal moving in correlation with the airflow signal for inhalation and exhalation. When the patient is holding the breath to mimic apnea, the abdominal and thoracic channel signals should be flat (Figure 34-12).

Another respiratory feature usually tested during physiologic calibrations is paradoxic breathing—the movement of the abdomen and thorax in opposite directions. It can occur when the upper airway is fully blocked but the person continues to make respiratory efforts to breathe during an obstructive sleep apnea (OSA) episode. To mimic paradoxic breathing, ask the person to hold their breath while making breathing movements. An alternative is to ask the person to pant. Either of these actions will cause the thoracic and abdominal channel signals to move in opposite directions (Figure 34-13).

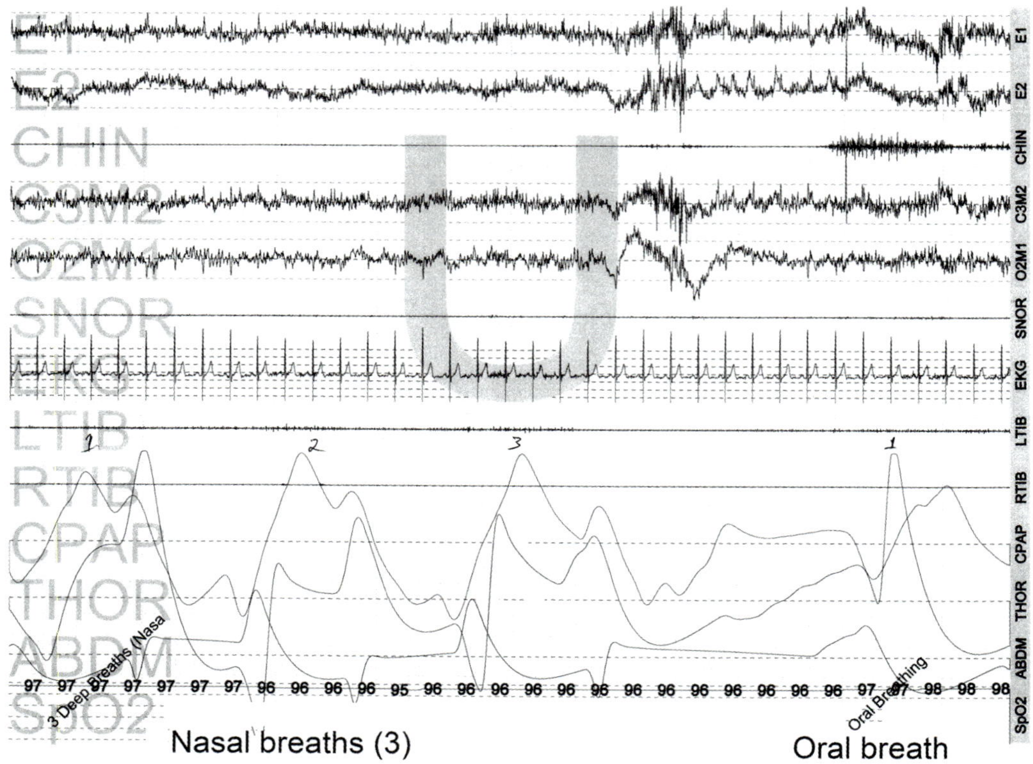

Figure 34-11 Oral/nasal airflow tests. (Image used with permission of Regina Patrick, RPSGT, RST, and obtained on the SomnoStar system, version 9 [2008; Cardinal Health Respiratory Technologies].)

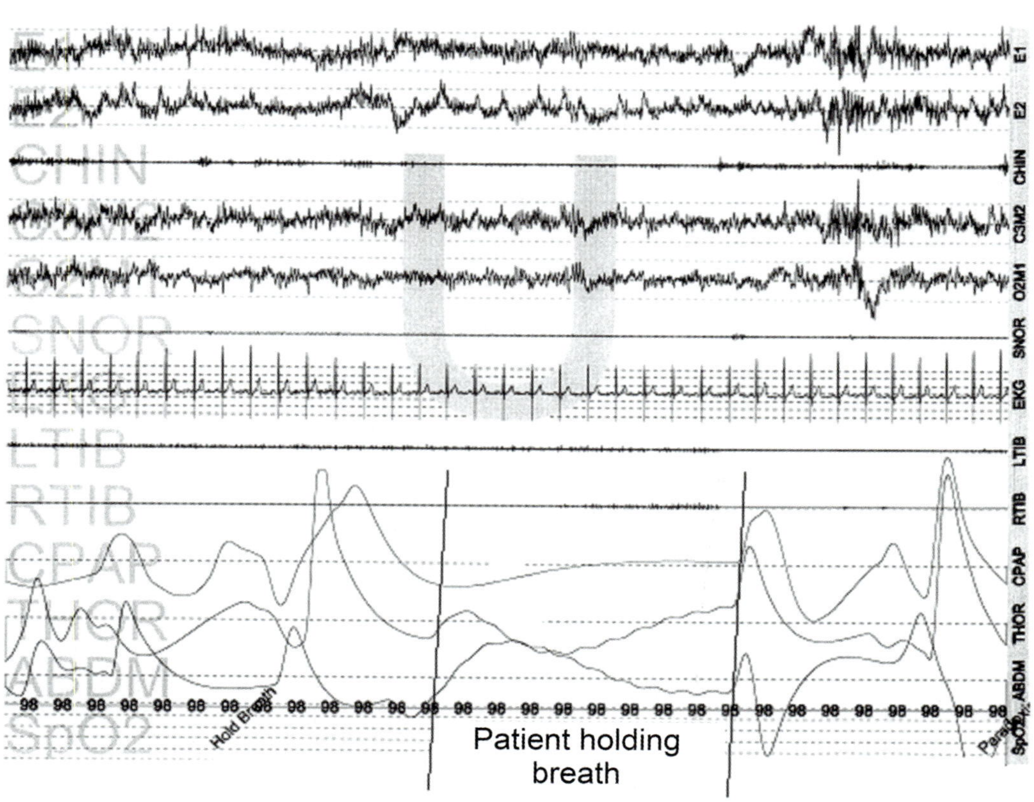

Figure 34-12 Simulation of apnea. (Image used with permission of Regina Patrick, RPSGT, RST, and obtained on the SomnoStar system, version 9 [2008; Cardinal Health Respiratory Technologies].)

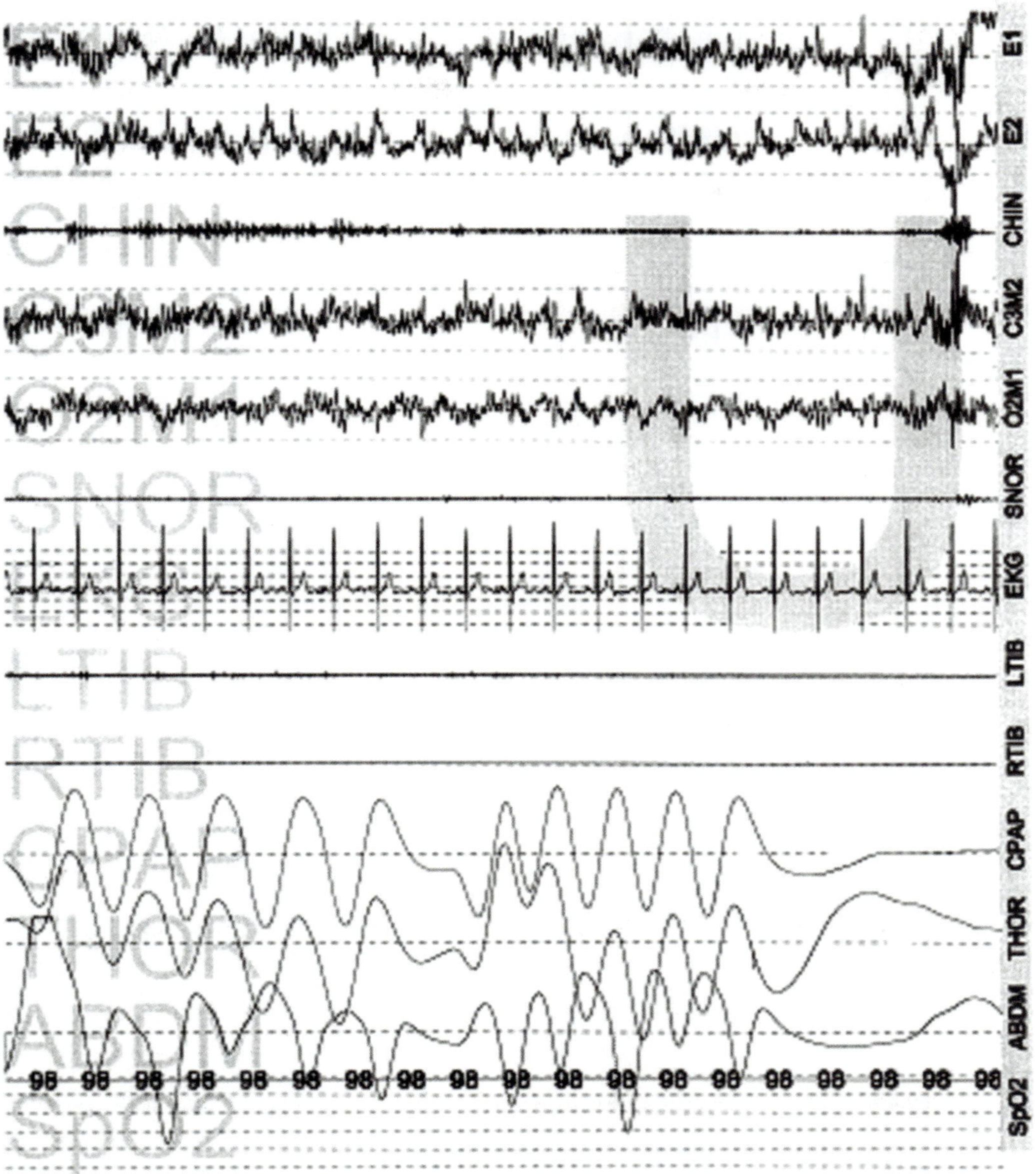

Paradoxic breathing (note that the thoracic and abdominal channels deflect in opposite directiions)

Figure 34-13 Simulation of paradoxic breathing. (Image used with permission of Regina Patrick, RPSGT, RST, and obtained on the SomnoStar system, version 9 [2008; Cardinal Health Respiratory Technologies].)

The Electrocardiogram Signal

The ECG signal is not tested as part of the physiologic calibrations procedure. However, the technologist should confirm that the ECG signal has the correct polarity. The P wave should deflect upward, the QRS complex should have a down-up-down deflection, and the T wave should deflect upward. If the waves are in the wrong directions, the polarity should be corrected before lights out (Figures 34-14 and 34-15).

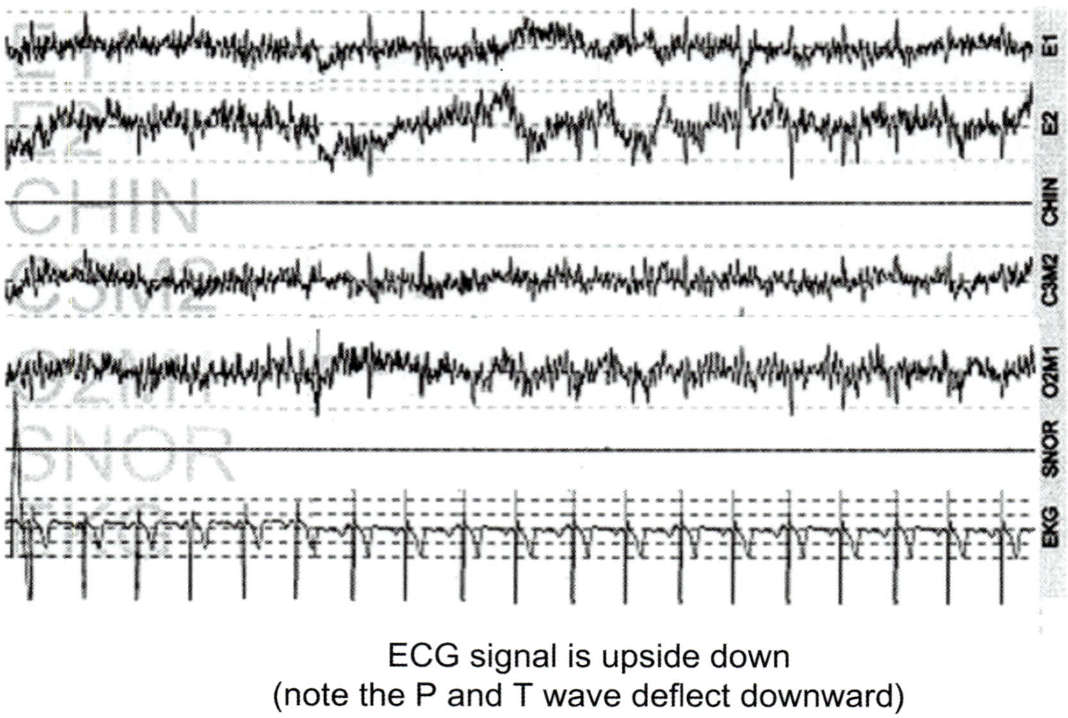

Figure 34-14 Electrocardiogram (ECG) before correction. (Image used with permission of Regina Patrick, RPSGT, RST, and obtained on the SomnoStar system, version 9 [2008; Cardinal Health Respiratory Technologies].)

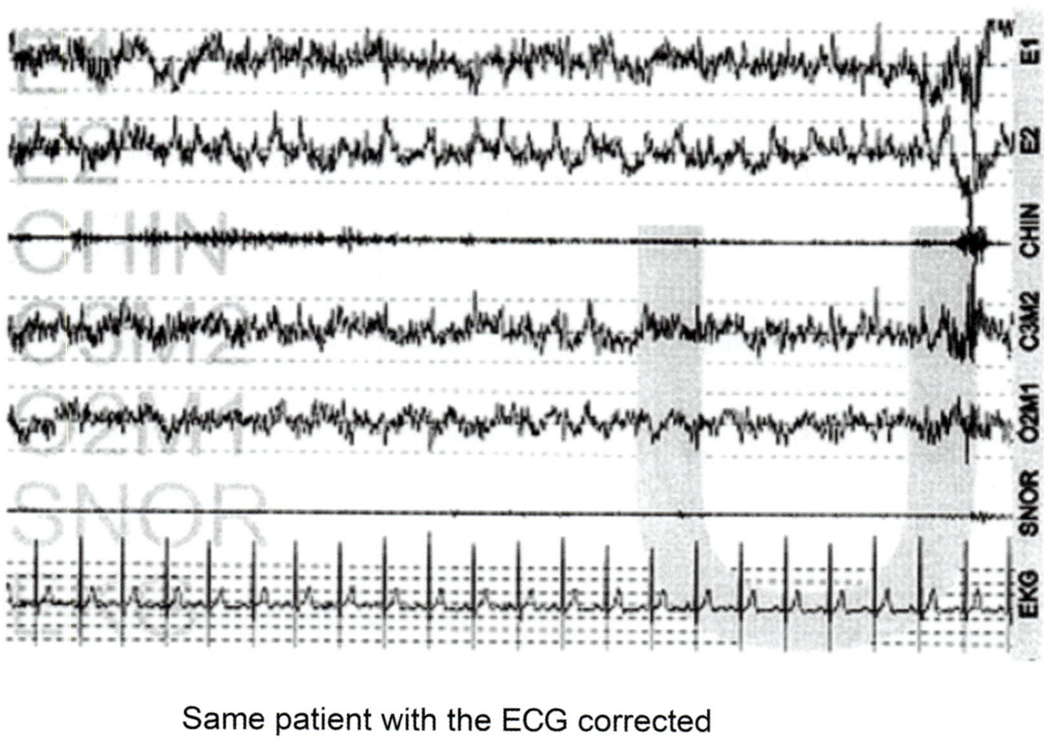

Figure 34-15 Electrocardiogram (ECG) after correction. (Image used with permission of Regina Patrick, RPSGT, RST, and obtained on the SomnoStar system, version 9 [2008; Cardinal Health Respiratory Technologies].)

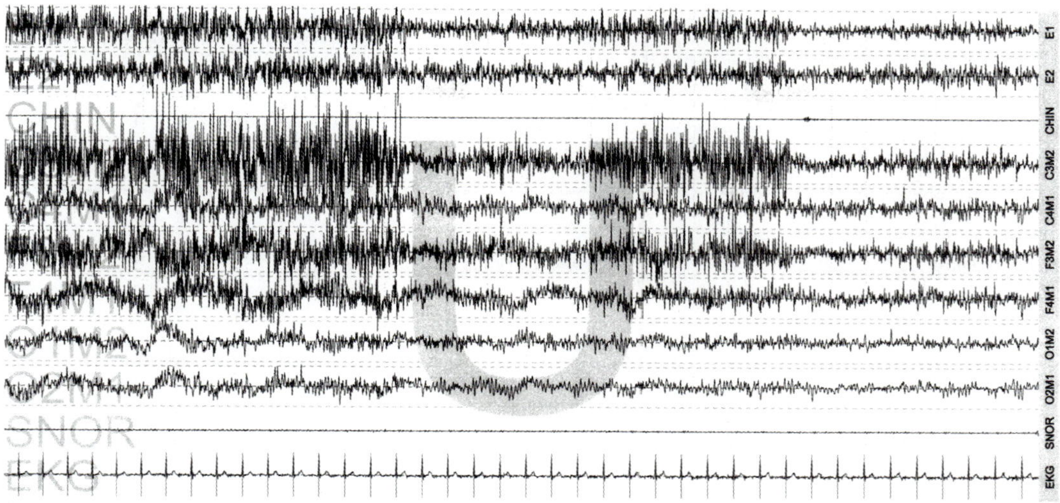

Muscle artifact (note it obscures the underlying EEG and EOG signals)

Figure 34-16 Patient movement resulting in muscle artifact. EEG, electroencephalogram; EOG, electrooculogram. (Image used with permission of Regina Patrick, RPSGT, RST, and obtained on the SomnoStar system, version 9 [2008; Cardinal Health Respiratory Technologies].)

ARTIFACT RECOGNITION AND RESPONSE DURING POLYSOMNOGRAPHY

The biggest contributor to artifact on a PSG during a study is patient movement. Patient movement increases muscle activity to the point that the activity obscures the EEG and EOG signals as artifact (Figure 34-16).

The muscle artifact in these channels cannot be filtered out. A patient's movement is usually short, lasting less than 30 seconds, which would normally not interfere with the scoring of the record. However, if the movement is prolonged (eg, patient is tossing and turning in bed), the technologist needs to make a notation of this on the PSG.

Muscle artifact can also result from fast rhythmic muscle contractions induced by a seizure. During a seizure, a technologist needs to record on the PSG and in the patient's chart what activity occurred (eg, flailed arms; jerked leg) *and* in what order (eg, "Patient had rhythmic jerking of the left leg, followed by rapid flailing of both arms."). This description may later help a neurologist or physician determine the origin and progression of the seizure in the patient's brain.

Patient movement may also dislodge electrodes. If a ground electrode, system electrode, or reference electrode (eg, M1 or M2) becomes dislodged, all channels referenced to that electrode will contain artifact. The solution is to switch to the other reference or to a second ground or system reference electrode, if it is available, or to replace the electrode.

Another source of artifact is 60-Hz interference from external sources such as electronic equipment, television, and radios. This artifact appears as a somewhat thick line that may overlay the EEG, ECG, or EOG signals (Figures 34-17 and 34-18). If the patient has any electronic devices operating near the electrode headbox, turning off the device should clear up the signal. At times, accessory equipment (such as a continuous positive airway pressure machine) near the electrode headbox may emit 60-Hz interference. If possible, moving the equipment away from the headbox may reduce the interference. If the interference remains, the technologist may need to look for other sources of 60-Hz interference or, as a last resort, apply the 60-Hz notch filter.

IDENTIFYING AND RESPONDING TO CLINICAL EVENTS AND MEDICAL EMERGENCIES

Some clinical events that can occur during a study are seizures, ECG arrhythmias, and parasomnias. The advent of these events during a study may require technologist and/or clinical intervention.

CLINICAL EVENTS

Seizures

A seizure is the sudden transient disturbance of brain activity that may result in sensory disturbances, loss of

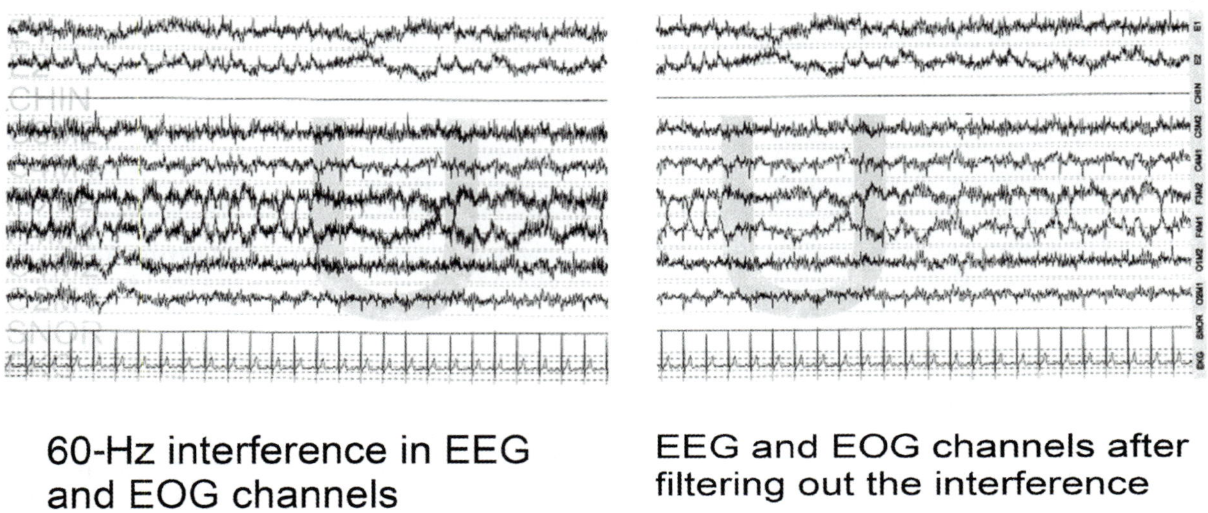

Figure 34-17 60-Hz interference in the EEG and EOG channels. EEG, electroencephalogram; EOG, electrooculogram. (Image used with permission of Regina Patrick, RPSGT, RST, and obtained on the SomnoStar system, version 9 [2008; Cardinal Health Respiratory Technologies].)

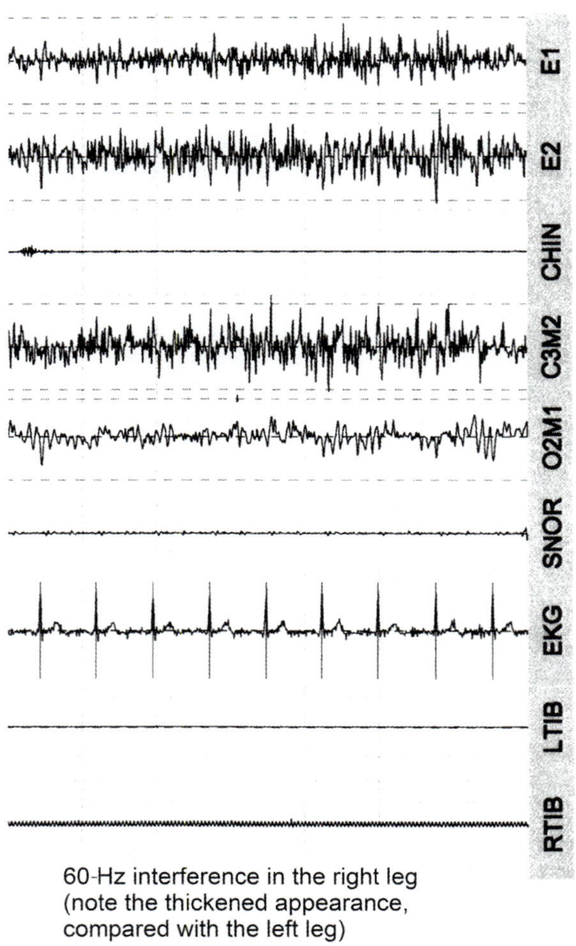

Figure 34-18 Sixty-hertz interference in the right leg EMG channel, which has a thickened appearance, compared with the normal signal of the left leg channel. (Image used with permission of Regina Patrick, RPSGT, RST, and obtained on the SomnoStar system, version 9 [2008; Cardinal Health Respiratory Technologies, Palm Springs, CA].)

consciousness, abnormal motor activity, or disturbance of the autonomic nervous system. A seizure can be partial or generalized. A partial seizure occurs if the origin of the dysfunctional activity is limited to a discrete area (ie, the focus) in the brain. A generalized seizure occurs if the dysfunctional activity involves a large area of the brain (eg, one hemisphere) or if the dysfunctional activity involves the whole brain.

The two types of partial seizures are simple and complex. During a simple partial seizure, a person maintains consciousness throughout the episode; however, impaired neuronal firing may manifest in a variety of ways, depending on the location of the focus and the pathway the dysfunctional signals travel. The person may have uncontrolled motor phenomenon (eg, muscle twitching); sensory dysfunction (eg, olfactory hallucination such as smelling rotten meat); autonomic symptoms (eg, urinary urgency); or psychic signs (eg, sense of *déjà vu* [ie, the sense of having experienced something before]). During a complex partial seizure, an episode may begin with an "aura"—a preliminary sign of an impending seizure. (An aura is actually the manifestation of a simple partial seizure.) For example, an aura may involve muscular twitching in one arm. As the complex partial seizure continues, the person may exhibit altered consciousness or may lose consciousness. For example, during a complex partial seizure, the person may have automatisms (ie, involuntary aimless behavior such as lip smacking or picking at clothing) but later have no memory of the activity.

Simple and complex partial seizures can progress to a generalized seizure. A generalized seizure involves a loss of consciousness. At its simplest, a generalized seizure may involve a 1- to 10-second lapse of awareness (ie, absence seizure), after which the person may continue the pre-seizure activity, unaware of the passage of time. However, during the seizure, onlookers may note the person staring unresponsively or blinking or rolling the eyes.

A tonic-clonic seizure is a generalized seizure at its worst. This type of generalized seizure begins with a sudden rigid extension of muscles (ie, tonic phase), which is soon followed by violent shaking, the result of extremely fast, rhythmic muscular contractions (ie, clonic phase). A tonic-clonic seizure may last from 2 to 5 minutes. Afterward, a person may be confused, be extremely sleepy, or may complain of headache, muscle aches, or muscle weakness.

The violent muscle contractions occurring during a tonic-clonic seizure obscure the signals in all channels on a PSG. The technologist needs to immediately go into the patient's room to ensure that they do not harm themself as a result of the violent jerking. The patient should be turned to the side to prevent aspiration of fluids (eg, saliva), and the sleep center's emergency protocol should be followed.

Other types of generalized seizures are tonic seizures, which involve muscle rigidity but are not followed by a clonic phase; clonic seizures, which involve violent rhythmic contractions but are not preceded by a tonic phase; myoclonic seizures, in which a person has brief involuntary jerking of the torso or extremities; and atonic seizures, in which the skeletal muscles lose all tone, causing the person to suddenly drop to the floor.

A person with epilepsy (ie, recurrent episodes of seizures) may have spikes or spike-and-slow wave complexes in the EEG channels on a PSG. On observing this activity in the EEG channel, a technologist should make a notation of it in the patient's chart.

Cardiac Arrhythmias

Cardiac arrhythmias may appear on the ECG channel during a sleep study, even in a person who does not have a diagnosed heart problem. Some common arrhythmias that may be seen on the ECG channel during a sleep study are sinus tachycardia (ie, a fast heart rhythm), atrial tachycardia, sinus bradycardia (ie, a slow heart rhythm), bradytachycardia (ie, slowing of the heart rhythm, followed by a sudden increase in the heart rhythm), premature atrial contraction (PAC), premature ventricular contraction (PVC), atrioventricular (AV) branch block (more commonly called an "AV block"), premature junctional contraction (PJC), junctional tachycardia, and bundle branch block (BBB). Some arrhythmias require immediate emergency intervention.

Sinus tachycardia is a heart rhythm of 100 bpm or greater in adults. This rate is initiated by the sinoatrial (SA) node. Sinus tachycardia can occur in association with other illnesses such as hyperthyroidism, chronic obstructive pulmonary disease, and congestive heart failure.

Atrial tachycardia is a heart rhythm of 150 to 250 bpm. This rate is initiated by an atrial focus outside the SA node. Atrial tachycardia usually occurs in association with heart problems such as Wolff-Parkinson-White syndrome, but it can occur with excessive use of stimulants (eg, caffeine), use of certain drugs (eg, marijuana), electrolyte imbalances, hypoxia, and psychological or physical stress.

Sinus bradycardia has a heart rhythm of less than or equal to 60 bpm. This rate is initiated by the SA node. Sinus bradycardia can occur as a result of a drug effect (eg, β-blocker drugs) or in association with other disorders such as hypothyroidism. However, bradycardia can be a normal finding in athletes.

Bradytachycardia most often occurs during an OSA episode, although it can occur in association with heart problems (eg, sick sinus syndrome in which SA node dysfunction causes episodes of tachycardia, bradycardia, sinus arrest or pause, or bradytachycardia). In bradytachycardia occurring in association with an OSA episode, the heart rhythm progressively slows to less than or equal to 60 bpm during the cessation in breathing (ie, apnea) and as the blood oxygen level falls. When a person briefly arouses to take deep breaths, the heart rate suddenly speeds up to greater than or equal to 100 bpm. Soon after taking deep breaths, the heart rate returns to normal as the blood oxygen level is restored to normal.

A PAC is an atrial contraction that occurs too soon after the preceding beat because a focus in an atrium but outside of the SA node (which would normally induce an atrial contraction) instead triggers the contraction of the atria. A PAC may or may not be followed by a ventricular contraction. The P wave appears different from one that originates in the SA node. If the premature signal travels the normal pathway through the SA node, through the AV node, and down the bundle of His, the heartbeat will appear normal. PACs can occur in association with heart disease (eg, heart failure), respiratory failure, hypoxia, electrolyte imbalances (ie, improper levels of minerals such as calcium and potassium or molecules such as phosphate [HPO_4^-] and bicarbonate [HCO_3^-]), as an adverse drug effect (eg, digitalis toxicity), or with the use of certain substances (eg, alcohol, cigarettes). An occasional PAC in some people may be normal and present no danger. However, in people with heart disease, the presence of PACs can lead to more serious arrhythmias (eg, atrial flutter, atrial fibrillation).

A PVC occurs when a focus in the ventricle triggers a ventricular contraction before the atria contract. The result is a deformed and wide QRS complex because the signal has not passed through the normal route (ie, SA node to AV node, and through the bundle of His). PVCs can occur in people without heart problems; however, they often occur in association with heart disease and can be a prelude to a lethal ventricular arrhythmia (eg, ventricular tachycardia, ventricular fibrillation). PVCs can

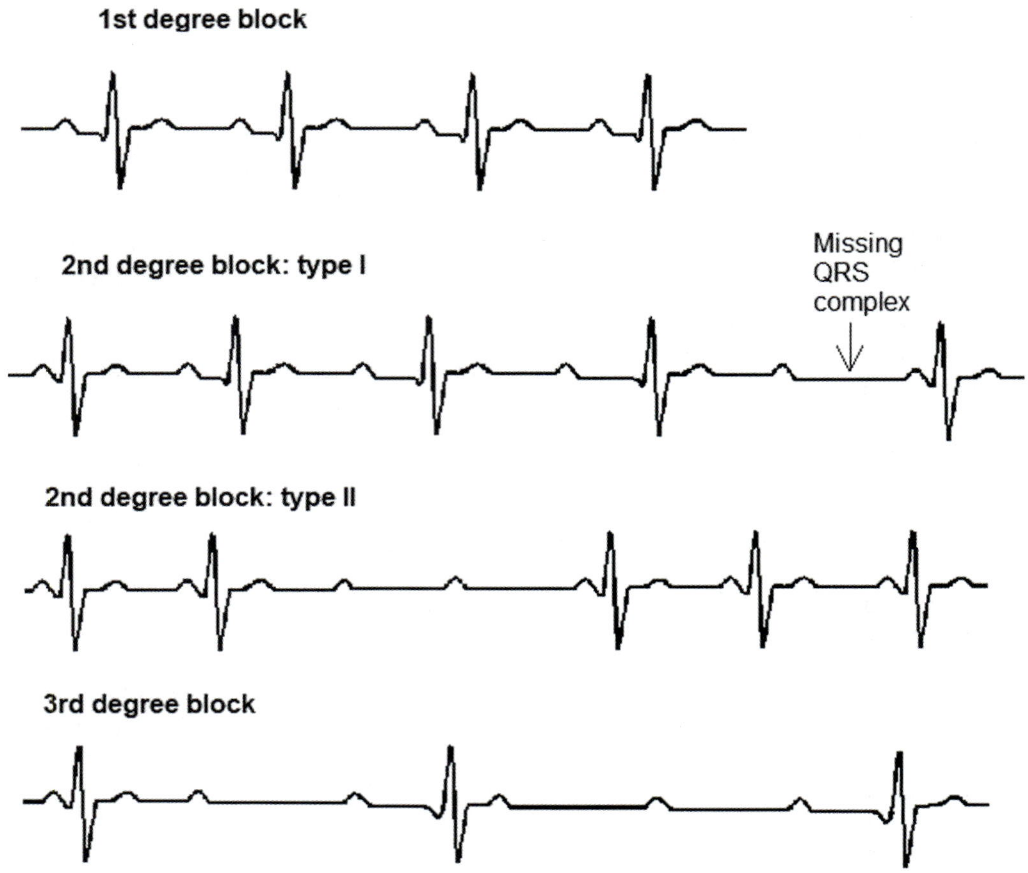

Figure 34-19 Schematic of first-degree, second-degree (type I [Mobitz I] and type II [Mobitz II]), and third-degree atrioventricular blocks.

occur because of metabolic acidosis (ie, an acidic state in the body resulting from an improper acid-base balance), hypoxia, a drug effect (eg, tricyclic antidepressants, amphetamines), a heart defect, or damage to the ventricles.

An AV block occurs when the conduction of a signal from the atria to the ventricles is impeded (ie, blocked). A problem at the level of the AV node, bundle of His, or the right or left branches of the bundle of His can result in an AV block. An AV block can be first-degree (ie, delayed conduction of signals from the atria to the ventricles), second-degree (ie, partial disconnection between atrial contractions and ventricular contractions so that not every atrial contraction results in a ventricular contraction), or third-degree (ie, complete disconnection between atrial contractions and ventricular contractions so that the atria and ventricles contract independently). An AV block can occur because of ischemia (ie, low blood flow) or infarction (ie, dead tissue caused by blocked blood flow) of the heart muscle, an adverse drug effect, structural defect in the ventricles, or damage to the AV node.

In a first-degree block, each P wave is followed by a QRS complex, and the P wave and the QRS complex appear normal. However, after the P wave, a delay occurs that lasts greater than 0.2 seconds before the QRS complex appears. (The normal interval between the end of the P wave and the beginning of the QRS complex is 0.12-0.20 seconds.) The delay occurs because the signal from the SA node cannot be conducted quickly through the AV node because of a problem at the level of the AV node (Figure 34-19—first-degree block).

A second-degree block consists of two types: type I block (also called Mobitz I block or Wenckebach phenomenon) and type II block (also called Mobitz II block). In a type I block, P waves appear rhythmically. However, the interval between each P wave and the following QRS complex progressively lengthens until a QRS complex does not appear after a P wave. Therefore, the ventricular contractions are irregular, but the atrial contractions are regular (Figure 34-19—second-degree block: type I and type II).

In a type II block, a signal is occasionally not conducted from the AV node. The type II block can result from a problem at the level of the bundle of His or bundle of His branches. Atrial contractions are regular, whereas ventricular contractions may or may not be regular in a type II block.

In a third-degree block, the atria and the ventricles contract regularly but independently of each other. The atrial contractions do not induce ventricular contractions. For example, the atria may contract at a rate of 90 bpm, whereas the ventricles contract at a rate of 30 bpm (Figure 34-19—third-degree block).

A PJC occurs before a normal sinus contraction can occur. The origin of the junctional signal is the area around the AV node and bundle of His (collectively called the "AV junction"). A junctional signal travels simultaneously toward the atria and through the bundle of His. The result is an inverted P wave but normal QRS and T waves. PJCs can occur with excessive use of caffeine, digoxin toxicity, and heart problems affecting the heart wall (eg, inferior wall infarction, swelling of the AV junction after heart surgery).

Junctional tachycardia is when three or more successive PJCs occur. The rate of the contractions is 100 to 200 bpm.

Atrial arrhythmias, ventricular arrhythmias, and BBBs may require emergency intervention. When to intervene will be discussed later in the Medical Emergencies section.

Parasomnias

RBD, night terrors (also called "sleep terrors"), nightmares, sleepwalking, and enuresis are parasomnias for which a technologist may need to intervene to protect a patient from hurting themself. RBD typically occurs in older men, although it can occur in women. The other parasomnias—night terrors, nightmares, sleepwalking, and enuresis—typically occur in children, although they can also occur in adults. Each of these parasomnias is associated with a specific sleep stage. Therefore, a technologist needs to be vigilant when a patient enters the stage during which a particular parasomnia is likely to occur.

Rapid Eye Movement Sleep Behavior Disorder

RBD is often a prodrome (ie, an early symptom indicating the onset of a disease or illness) of Parkinson disease. Symptoms of RBD manifest during REM sleep. In a person with RBD, REM sleep muscle atonia does not occur, leaving the person free to act out dreams. Dreams reported by people with RBD are usually violent, with themes of being chased or attacked. As a result, people with RBD may strike out against an attacker, unaware that they are actually striking a bed partner or a wall or other hard object. During REM sleep, the technologist monitoring a patient with RBD needs to record in the PSG and in the patient's chart exactly what the patient does. Such documentation can aid a sleep physician's diagnosis and treatment planning. If the patient is hurt during an episode, the technologist may need to initiate the sleep center's emergency protocol.

Night Terrors (Pavor Nocturnus)

Night terrors (also called pavor nocturnus) most commonly occur in children during slow-wave sleep in the early part of the night. Night terrors are more common in boys but can occur in girls. A child with night terrors awakens screaming and apparently in distress. Parents often note the child looks dazed. Attempts to calm the child agitate the child more, and the child is unable to respond or explain what scared them. After a few minutes, the episode is usually over, and the child goes back to sleep as if nothing has happened. In the morning, the child has no awareness of having awakened with a night terror. Because night terrors tend to occur during slow-wave sleep, the technologist needs to be vigilant for the onset of slow-wave sleep during a sleep study to anticipate the occurrence of a night terror and to note in the patient's chart everything a child does during an episode.

Sleepwalking (Somnambulism)

A sleepwalking episode (also called "somnambulism") occurs most often during slow-wave sleep and in children. A child who sleepwalks gets out of bed and begins to walk in a somewhat haphazard fashion. The child appears dazed and may or may not respond to questions put to them by onlookers. The child may settle back in bed or settle in another setting. During a sleep study, the technologist needs to be vigilant to note the onset of slow-wave sleep and to note everything a child does during an episode of sleepwalking. If the child gets out of bed and appears to be in danger of hurting themself, the technologist may need to enter the room to intervene.

Enuresis

Enuresis is bed-wetting. It occurs in children who are beyond the age by which urinary control is normally accomplished. It generally occurs during slow-wave sleep. During a sleep study, the technologist needs to be vigilant to note the onset and the end of slow-wave sleep. Enuresis alarms can be used to signal an episode of bed-wetting. If an alarm is unavailable, then at the end of the slow-wave sleep episode, the technologist needs to enter the child's room to assess whether the child has urinated. If so, the bedding should be changed. Afterward, the child can return to bed.

MEDICAL EMERGENCIES

A medical emergency is an acute injury or illness that results in an immediate risk to a person's life or long-term health. Medical emergencies in a sleep center are rare but can occur. To effectively manage a medical emergency and potentially reduce the risk of injury or death to a patient, a technologist should be aware of the medical emergency protocols of their sleep center and when to implement them. Cardiorespiratory arrest and falls are the most common events that may occur in a sleep center and would require a technologist to initiate the center's medical emergency protocol. Other events that would require a technologist to initiate a center's medical emergency protocol are certain cardiac arrhythmias, stroke, asthma attack, and diabetic ketoacidosis. A technologist's awareness of the impending signs of an adverse event or implementation of steps to prevent an adverse event from occurring could potentially save a patient's life or mitigate injury to a patient. Patients experiencing a medical emergency may need to be transported to an emergency room. Depending on the severity of the emergency, the patient may then be admitted to a hospital.

Cardiorespiratory Arrest

Cardiorespiratory arrest is a cessation in the heartbeat and in breathing. A patient who goes into cardiac arrest, respiratory arrest, or both (ie, cardiorespiratory arrest) during a sleep study can die within minutes and therefore requires immediate medical attention. A delayed response by a technologist could jeopardize the patient's life and health. For a patient in cardiac and/or respiratory arrest, a technologist should utilize an automated external defibrillator (AED), initiate cardiorespiratory resuscitation, alert the emergency medical service (EMS), and follow the emergency protocol of the sleep center.

Heart Attack

A heart attack (ie, myocardial infarction) is a sudden episode in which blood flow in one or more vessels supplying the heart becomes blocked and thereby damages or results in the death of a part of the heart muscle. As a heart attack progresses, the heart rhythm may become unstable and ultimately stop, which may result in a person's death. Some warning signs that a person may be having a heart attack are shortness of breath; complaint of squeezing or crushing chest pain originating below the breast bone, which may radiate to the left arm, jaw, neck, or shoulder blades; cool extremities (a sign that the heart is not pumping efficiently); sweating; or complaint of indigestion (individuals often mistake a heart attack for indigestion). If a technologist suspects a heart attack in a patient who is alert but manifesting these symptoms, the technologist should initiate the center's emergency protocol.

Cardiac Arrhythmias

A normal heartbeat will contain a P wave, which represents atrial contraction, a QRS complex, which represents ventricular contraction, and a T wave, which represents repolarization of the ventricles (Figure 34-20). Atrial repolarization occurs during ventricular contraction; however, the much stronger signals produced by a ventricular contraction obscure the atrial repolarization signal. The normal heart rhythm is typically 60 to 100 bpm. Cardiac arrhythmia is a change from the normal rhythm and results from changes in the heart rate, regularity of signals, pathway of signals, or sequence in the activation of the heart. Cardiac arrhythmias may originate from the atria, ventricles, AV junction, and bundle of His branches.

Atrial Arrhythmias

Atrial arrhythmias that may be of concern during a sleep study are sinus tachycardia and atrial tachycardia, sinus bradycardia, PACs, atrial flutter, and atrial fibrillation. Atrial tachycardia, atrial bradycardia, and PACs may not be problematic in healthy people without heart disease. However, in people with an underlying heart condition, these atrial arrhythmias can lead to serious

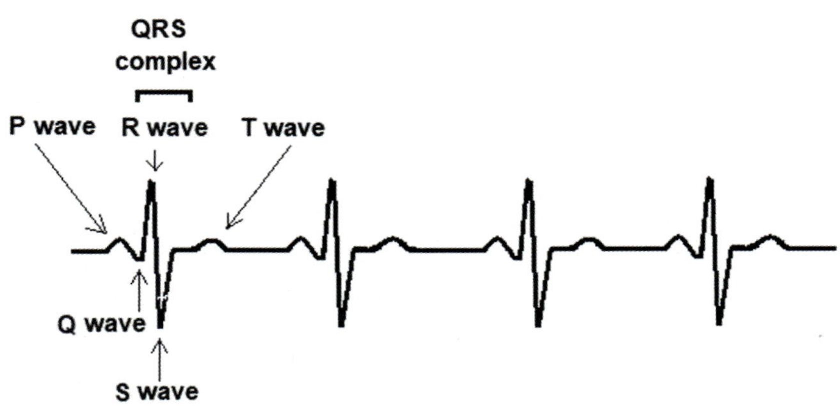

Figure 34-20 Schematic of a normal heart rhythm.

life-threatening arrhythmias. Atrial fibrillation is a serious life-threatening rhythm that requires implementing a center's emergency protocol.

Sinus Tachycardia and Atrial Tachycardia

Sinus tachycardia is a heart rhythm greater than 100 bpm. The origin of the signals is the SA node. Sinus tachycardia can be nonclinical (eg, a person's heart rate can rise to more than 100 bpm with exercise), an adverse drug effect (eg, amphetamine use), or the effect of using stimulants (eg, caffeine, nicotine, alcohol). In a healthy person with no known heart problems, a technologist should make a notation of the rhythm in the patient's chart and follow the center's protocol regarding arrhythmias (eg, contacting the center's medical director to make the director aware of the situation or ending a study, if necessary). However, if a patient with sinus tachycardia but no known heart problems complains of symptoms such as heart pain and palpitations, or faints, the technologist should implement the center's emergency protocol (eg, initiating the AED and cardiopulmonary resuscitation, contacting EMS, transferring the patient to an emergency room, and calling a staff physician [if the center is located in a hospital]).

Sinus tachycardia can be problematic in people with heart problems. The increased rate of contractions increases the heart's requirement for oxygen. If the heart muscle cannot meet this demand, a person with heart trouble and tachycardia may complain of chest pain, palpitations, a pounding chest, or skipped beats. The patient may also have blurred vision and hypotension (ie, low blood pressure), or may faint. The center's emergency protocol should be implemented for a patient with heart problems and tachycardia who is experiencing these symptoms. Sinus tachycardia can progress to heart failure (ie, inability of the heart to pump blood efficiently throughout the body), stroke, sudden cardiac arrest, and death. Features of sinus tachycardia are (1) a regular but fast rhythm; (2) normal P wave, QRS complex, and T wave; and (3) the P wave is close to the T wave (Figure 34-21).

Atrial tachycardia is the abrupt appearance of three or more atrial contractions that originate from a focus other than the SA node. The sinus rhythm resumes after the episode. These atrial contractions have a rate of 150 to 250 bpm. At this rate, the ventricles cannot properly fill with blood. Therefore, the amount of blood the heart pumps in a minute (ie, cardiac output) throughout the circulatory system is reduced. In a healthy person without heart disease, episodes of atrial tachycardia may be benign. It can occur in people who ingest excessive amounts of stimulants such as caffeine, who use marijuana, who have electrolyte imbalances, or who are undergoing psychological or physical stress. Atrial tachycardia can also occur with hypoxia or as an adverse effect of digitalis toxicity. A technologist should make a notation of atrial tachycardia in the patient's chart and follow the center's protocol regarding cardiac arrhythmias. If the person complains of palpitations, angina, blurred vision, dizziness, trouble breathing (ie, dyspnea); has syncope (ie, faints); or has hypotension, a technologist should implement the center's emergency protocol.

In a person with a heart problem, atrial tachycardia can precede serious ventricular arrhythmias. Therefore, on noting this rhythm, a technologist should follow the center's protocol regarding cardiac arrhythmias and carefully monitor the person. If the ECG pattern changes to a life-threatening rhythm (eg, atrial fibrillation) or a patient complains of palpitations or angina, faints, or has hypotension, the center's emergency protocol should be initiated. Features of atrial tachycardia are (1) each P wave induces a QRS complex; however, the P wave may be indiscernible because of the rapid rate of 150 to 250 bpm, and (2) the QRS complex appears normal (Figure 34-22).

Sinus Bradycardia

Bradycardia is a heart rhythm initiated by the SA node at a rate of less than or equal to 60 bpm. Bradycardia is problematic when the rhythm falls to less than 45 bpm. In a healthy person without heart disease, sinus bradycardia may be benign. For example, a slow heart rhythm can be a normal finding in athletes. It can also be a drug effect (eg, β-blocker drugs such as propranolol). A technologist should make a notation of bradycardia in the patient's chart and follow the center's protocol regarding cardiac arrhythmias.

Patients with known heart problems and bradycardia should be monitored carefully because bradycardia can lead to more serious arrhythmias such as ventricular

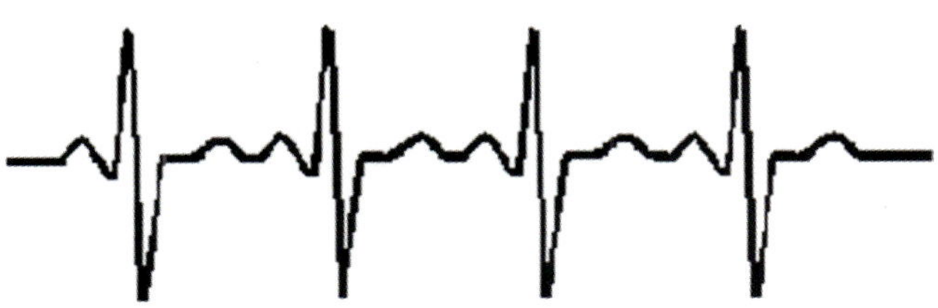

Figure 34-21 Schematic of sinus tachycardia.

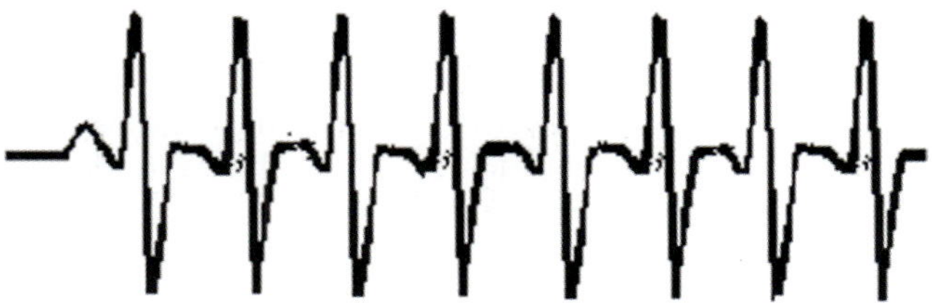

Figure 34-22 Schematic of atrial tachycardia.

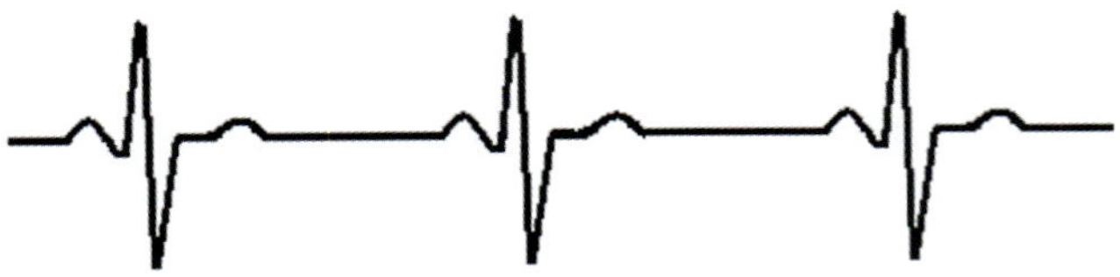

Figure 34-23 Schematic of sinus bradycardia.

tachycardia and ventricular fibrillation. A patient who is experiencing symptoms of bradycardia may complain of dizziness, faint, or have hypotension. If a patient has these complaints, the technologist should implement the center's emergency protocol. Features of sinus bradycardia are (1) the P waves and QRS complex are normal, and (2) each P wave is followed by a QRS complex (Figure 34-23).

Premature Atrial Contraction

A PAC occurs because a focus outside the SA node initiates one or more beats independently of the SA node. A PAC may or may not trigger a ventricular contraction.

In a person without heart problems, a PAC is rarely dangerous. PACs can be associated with pain, anxiety, use of alcohol or cigarettes, fever, and infectious diseases. A patient may experience them as palpitations or as a skipped beat. However, if PACs are frequent, a technologist should follow the center's protocol regarding cardiac arrhythmias.

PACs are problematic in people with coronary heart disease, hypoxia, respiratory failure, pulmonary disease, electrolyte imbalances, or digitalis toxicity because they can lead to more serious arrhythmias such as atrial flutter and atrial fibrillation. If a patient with PACs complains of heart palpitations, skipped beats, or a fluttering sensation, a technologist should initiate the center's emergency protocol. Features of a PAC are (1) the P wave occurs prematurely and may or may not be followed by a QRS complex, (2) the P wave may appear abnormal because the signal does not arise from the SA node, and (3) PACs may occur every other beat (ie, bigeminy), every third beat (ie, trigeminy), or in couplets (ie, two sequential PACs) (Figure 34-24).

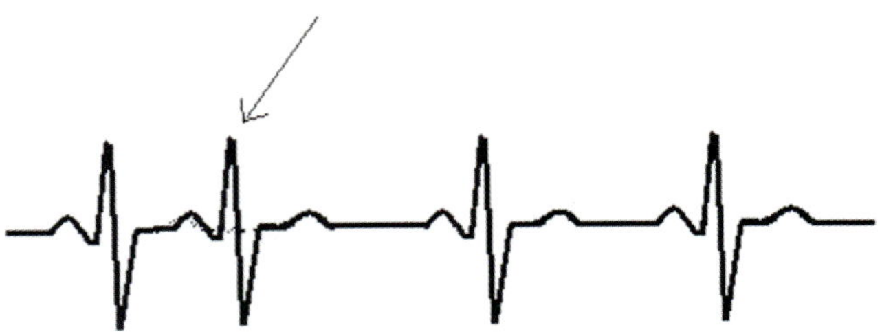

Figure 34-24 Schematic of premature atrial contraction.

Atrial Flutter

Atrial flutter is a form of atrial tachycardia in which atrial contractions occur at a rate of 250 to 400 bpm (typically 300 beats). At this rate, not every atrial contraction will induce a ventricular contraction. Instead, every second, third, or fourth atrial signal may be conducted through the ventricles because the AV node can only respond to signals up to 180 bpm. The number of atrial contractions that occur with each ventricular contraction is called the "conduction ratio" (eg, four atrial contractions per one ventricular contraction is a 4:1 conduction ratio; the normal conduction ratio is 1:1). If the ventricular rate that occurs with atrial flutter is too slow (<40 bpm) or too fast (>150 bpm), the cardiac output is reduced. In general, the faster the ventricular rate that is occurring with atrial flutter, the more dangerous is the rhythm.

Atrial flutter rarely occurs in healthy people. It tends to occur in people with heart problems (eg, mitral valve disease) and can occur in people with chronic obstructive pulmonary disease or systemic arterial hypoxia. People with atrial flutter may experience symptoms of low cardiac output, complain of dizziness and lightheadedness, or faint. Technologists should implement the center's emergency protocol for patients complaining of these symptoms. Atrial flutter can lead to the life-threatening arrhythmia, atrial fibrillation. Features of atrial flutter are (1) not every P wave is followed by a ventricular contraction, (2) the P waves that appear between ventricular contractions occur so rapidly that they have a sawtooth appearance, and (3) the QRS complex appears normal (Figure 34-25).

Atrial Fibrillation

In atrial fibrillation, many foci in the atria fire rapidly at a rate of 400 to 600 times per minute. This phenomenon may occur in association with heart problems such as severe mitral valve stenosis and coronary artery disease, hyperthyroidism, the use of stimulants (eg, coffee, alcohol, nicotine), or the use of medications (eg, digitalis, aminophylline). The result of signals from multiple foci in the atria is that the atria cannot contract but instead quivers. Some atrial signals are conducted from the atria to the AV node, allowing the ventricles to contract. However, because of the lack of coordinated contractions from the atria, the ventricles cannot properly fill with blood, and the cardiac output is reduced.

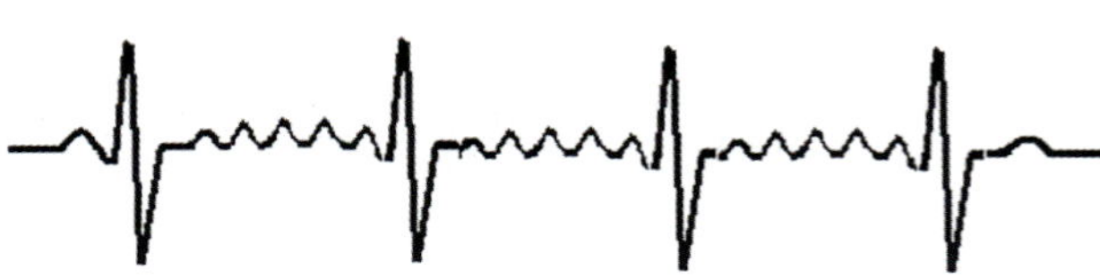

Figure 34-25 Schematic of atrial flutter.

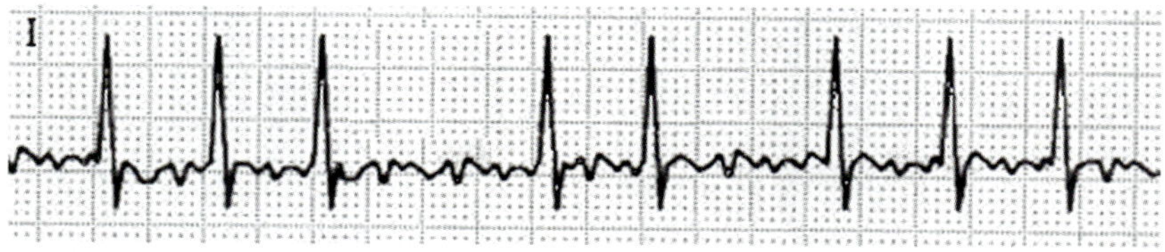

Figure 34-26 Electrocardiograph of atrial fibrillation.

A patient with atrial fibrillation may complain of symptoms such as lightheadedness, dizziness, mild shortness of breath, pain, and blurred vision, or the patient may faint or be unresponsive. Atrial fibrillation is a dire emergency because it can lead to sudden death. On noting this rhythm, a technologist should immediately implement the center's emergency protocol. Features of atrial fibrillation are (1) P waves are lost and appear as a thin narrow wavy line, and (2) QRS complexes typically occur at a rate of 100 to 150 bpm (but the rate can be lower) (Figure 34-26).

Ventricular Arrhythmias

Ventricular arrhythmias that may be of concern during a sleep study are PVCs, ventricular tachycardia, and ventricular fibrillation. PVCs may not be problematic in healthy people with no known heart problems but may be serious in people with heart problems. Ventricular tachycardia and ventricular fibrillation are serious life-threatening rhythms in people with and without heart problems and require medical intervention.

Premature Ventricular Contraction

A PVC occurs when a focus located below the level of the bundle of His fires a signal before a P wave can be conducted. The subsequent QRS complex has a widened appearance because the ventricular signal is not conducted through the normal path. In addition, because the ventricles contract before the atria contract, cardiac output is decreased. Patients with PVCs may complain of symptoms associated with low cardiac output such as hypotension, angina, syncope, and respiratory distress.

PVCs can be benign in healthy people with no heart problems. However, if PVCs are frequent (ie, six or more PVCs per minute), a technologist should make a notation of the arrhythmia in the patient's chart, follow the center's protocol regarding cardiac arrhythmias, and monitor the patient.

A technologist should carefully monitor a person with heart problems who has PVCs because such a person is at greater risk of PVCs progressing to ventricular tachycardia or ventricular fibrillation. If a patient with a heart problem is known to have PVCs, a technologist should carefully monitor the patient for an increase in frequency or a change from the baseline pattern. On noting an increase in the number of PVCs from the baseline or on noting a change from the baseline pattern such as the appearance of paired PVCs, bigeminy or trigeminy, or PVCs that look different from each other (ie, multifocal PVCs, which indicates they have different foci), a technologist should immediately implement the emergency protocol of the sleep center. Paired PVCs, bigeminy or trigeminy, and multifocal PVCs are dangerous patterns that can induce ventricular tachycardia or ventricular fibrillation, either of which can lead to death. Features of a PVC are (1) it is not preceded by a P wave, (2) the QRS complex is wide and distorted, (3) it can regularly alternate with normal beats (eg, bigeminy [Figure 34-27] or trigeminy [Figure 34-28]), (4) two PVCs can occur in succession (ie, PVC couplet [Figure 34-29]), and (5) PVCs may have multiple foci (Figure 34-30).

Ventricular Tachycardia

Ventricular tachycardia is when three or more PVCs occur successively and the ventricular rate is greater than or equal to 100 bpm. The rapid ventricular contractions prevent the ventricles from properly filling with blood, which can quickly lead to ventricular fibrillation, followed by cardiac arrest and death. Ventricular tachycardia can be associated with the use of certain drugs (eg, digitalis, cocaine, procainamide), heart disease (eg, myocardial infarction, coronary heart disease),

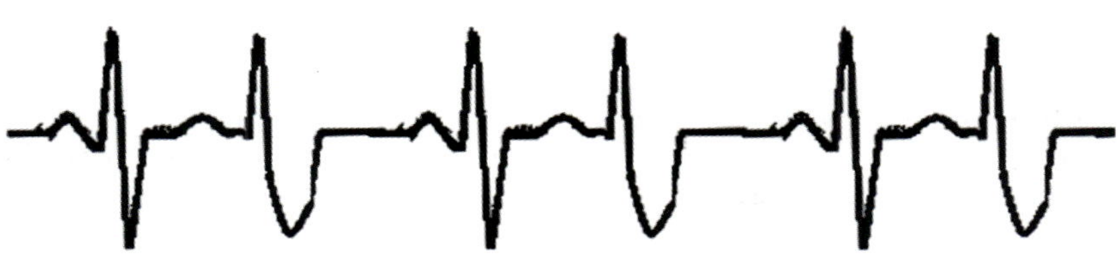

Figure 34-27 Schematic of bigeminy (every second beat is irregular).

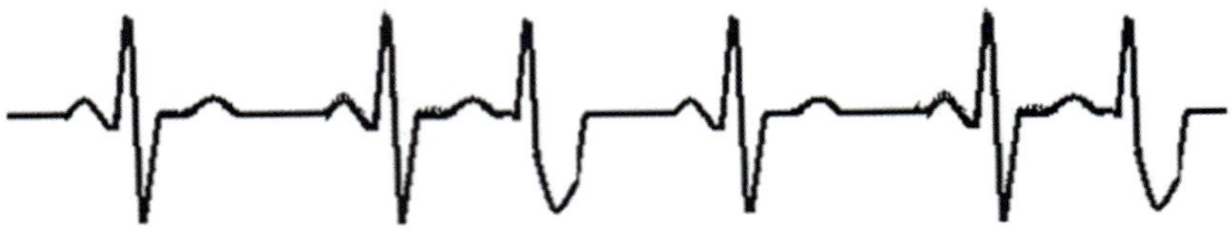

Figure 34-28 Schematic of trigeminy (every third beat is irregular).

and electrolyte imbalances. A patient experiencing ventricular tachycardia may complain of angina, will have hypotension, and may have a decreased level of consciousness that may progress to unresponsiveness.

Ventricular tachycardia can occur in short bursts lasting less than 30 seconds and cause few to no problems. However, sustained ventricular tachycardia is a serious rhythm that requires the immediate implementation of a center's emergency protocol, which may include the use of an AED. Ventricular tachycardia appears as a somewhat sinuous pattern, which represents successive and uniformly distorted QRS complexes (Figure 34-31).

Ventricular Fibrillation

As with atrial fibrillation, ventricular fibrillation occurs because many foci in the ventricles but outside the AV node fire rapidly, causing the ventricles to quiver, rather than to contract. No cardiac output occurs during ventricular fibrillation. As ventricular fibrillation progresses, the ventricles ultimately come to a standstill and death occurs. On noting this pattern, a technologist should immediately initiate a center's emergency protocol, which may include the use of an AED device. Features of ventricular fibrillation are as follows: (1) no discernible P waves, (2) lack of QRS complexes, and (3) lack of T waves. On an ECG, ventricular fibrillation appears as a fine squiggly line (ie, fine ventricular fibrillation) or a coarse line (ie, coarse ventricular fibrillation); on a PSG, because of its slower recording speed, ventricular fibrillation appears as a low thick somewhat flat line or as a compact angular zigzag line, respectively (Figure 34-32).

Junctional Arrhythmias

Junctional arrhythmias arise from improper signals from the AV junction. Junctional arrhythmias that may be of concern during a sleep study are PJC and junctional tachycardia.

Premature Junctional Contraction

A PJC occurs when a focus in the area of the AV node and bundle of His (collectively called the "AV junction") initiates a heart contraction before the SA node can initiate an atrial contraction. When a signal originates from the AV junction, a wave of depolarization simultaneously travels upward toward the SA node and downward through the bundle of His branches. A PJC is usually not dangerous, although patients should be monitored for symptoms (eg, light-headedness). PJCs can occur in people with certain heart conditions (eg, Wolf-Parkinson-White syndrome, rheumatic heart disease, myocardial infarction), with the use of certain drugs (eg, digitalis), and with excessive use of caffeine.

A technologist should make a notation of this arrhythmia in a patient's chart and follow the center's protocol regarding cardiac arrhythmias. If a patient complains of palpitations or feeling a "quickening" in the chest, a technologist should implement the sleep center's emergency protocol. Features of a PJC are (1) an upside-down P wave (the result of retrograde depolarization) and (2) a normal QRS complex; however, the P wave may precede the QRS complex, come after the QRS complex, or be embedded within the QRS complex (Figure 34-33).

Junctional Tachycardia

In junctional tachycardia, three or more successive junctional contractions occur. This phenomenon occurs because a focus in the AV junction takes over as the heart's pacemaker at a rate of approximately 100 to 200 bpm. Junctional tachycardia typically occurs in people who have heart problems that affect the heart's wall such as congenital heart disease, infarction in the inferior or posterior wall, or trauma-induced swelling of the

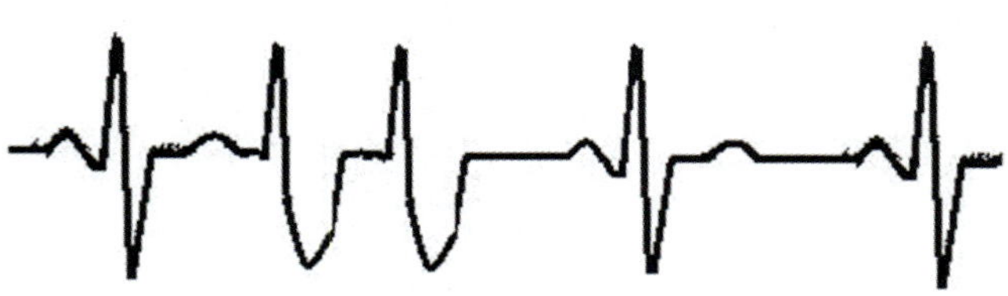

Figure 34-29 Schematic of a premature ventricular contraction couplet.

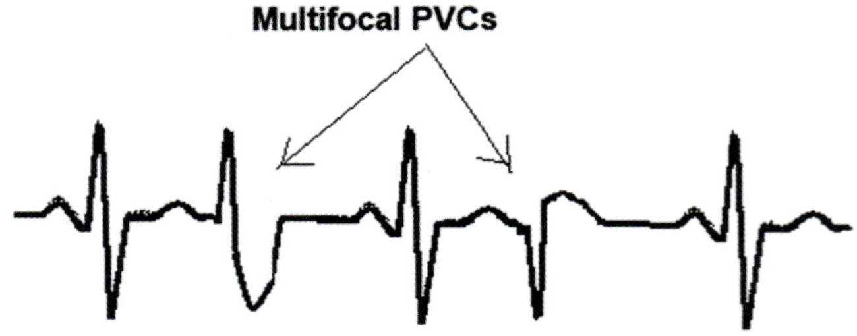

Figure 34-30 Schematic of multifocal premature ventricular contraction (PVC).

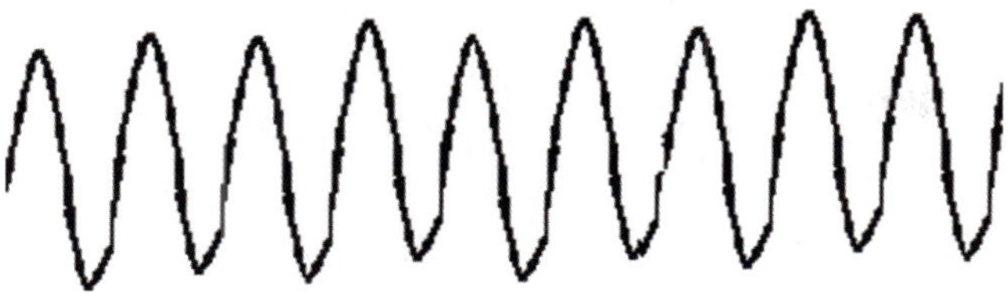

Figure 34-31 Electrocardiograph of ventricular tachycardia.

AV junction after heart surgery. It can also occur with digitalis toxicity. The rapid ventricular contractions can reduce cardiac output and decrease blood flow into the ventricles. As a result, a patient may complain of palpitations or feeling a "quickening" in the chest or may show signs of low cardiac output (eg, light-headedness, fainting, dizziness). For a patient experiencing symptoms, a technologist should implement the center's emergency protocol. Features of junctional tachycardia are (1) a regular but fast ventricular rhythm (100-200 bpm), (2) an inverted P wave, which may appear just before, within, or after the QRS complex, (3) a normal QRS complex, and (4) a normal T wave (unless the rate is so rapid the T wave cannot be detected) (Figure 34-34).

Branch Bundle Block

In the upper portion of the interventricular septum, the bundle of His fibers divide into two branches, the left bundle branch and the right bundle branch. Each branch travels down its respective side of the interventricular septum and then spreads throughout the myocardium (ie, muscle tissue) of its respective ventricle. When stimulated, the bundle branch fibers allow the simultaneous contraction of ventricles. Injury to the heart (eg, heart attack) can impede the conduction of a signal through the left bundle branch or right bundle branch; this impedance is called a "left bundle branch block" (LBBB) or "right bundle branch block" (RBBB), respectively. Both types of blocks can occur with heart disease or injury. An RBBB can occur in people without heart disease, whereas an LBBB never occurs in a healthy person. If a signal is impeded in one branch, the P wave and T wave will be normal because the SA node and AV node are functioning correctly, but the QRS complex will be wider than normal and may appear doubled (reflecting the slower contraction of the ventricle affected by the BBB).

Many people with a BBB do not experience symptoms. However, some people with a BBB may have a slow heart rate, which may cause fainting. In addition, people with a BBB are at greater risk of sudden cardiac death because of the faulty conduction in the heart. On noting a BBB, a technologist should make a notation of the arrhythmia and follow the center's protocol for cardiac arrhythmias. If the ECG pattern changes to a life-threatening rhythm (eg, severe bradycardia) or a patient with a BBB faints, or complains of feeling as if they will faint, the technologist should implement the center's emergency protocol. Features of a BBB are (1) the QRS complex will be wider than normal (ie, >0.12 seconds), (2) the QRS complex is wider than normal and

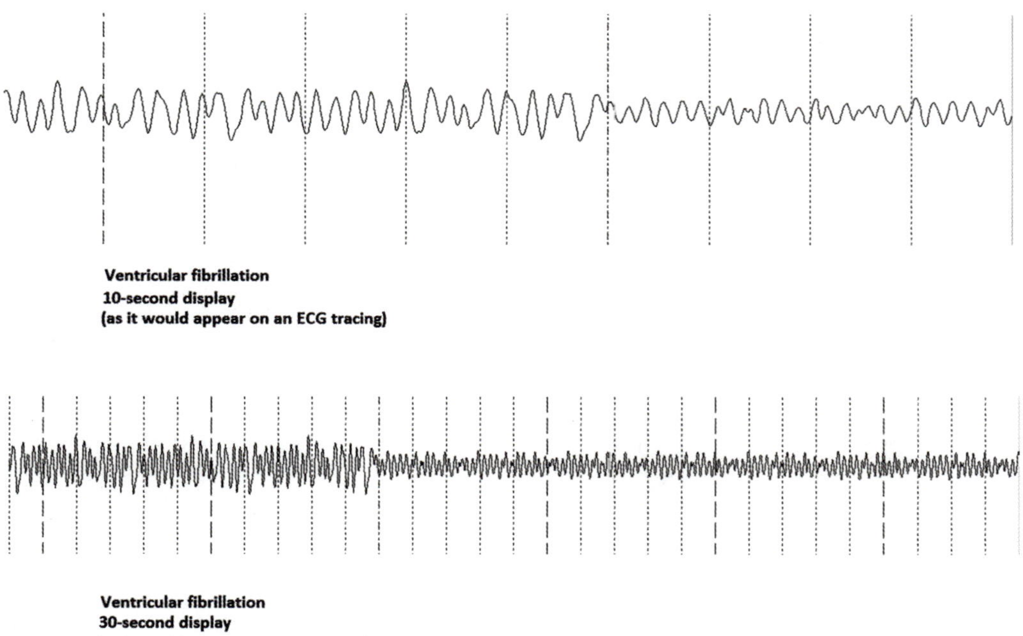

Figure 34-32 Ventricular fibrillation (coarse, seconds 1-6 [left]; fine, seconds 7-10 [right]) as it would appear on an ECG (top) and on a PSG (bottom). ECG, electrocardiogram; PSG, polysomnograph. (Courtesy of Jon Atkinson.)

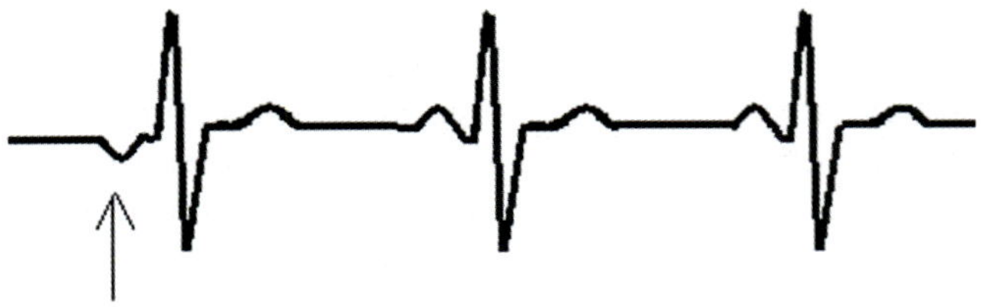

Figure 34-33 Schematic of premature junctional contraction.

may appear doubled, (3) the QRS complex has an "M" pattern in LBBB and a "rabbit ear" pattern in RBBB, and (4) the heart rhythm may be normal (approximately 60-100 bpm) but can be slower or faster (Figure 34-35).

Falls

A fall is a sudden unexpected descent to the floor from standing, sitting, or other positions (eg, rolling out of a bed) with or without injury to the patient. Neurologic conditions such as Alzheimer disease and Parkinson disease, stroke, cerebral palsy; musculoskeletal disorders such as scoliosis; and the use of ambulatory devices such as wheelchairs and walkers can increase a patient's risk of falling. Fall precautions involve practices with the goal of preventing a patient from falling. Examples of precautions that a technologist may need to take to reduce the likelihood of a fall in patients with a fall risk are assisting the patient with ambulation to and from the toilet or during walks to various areas in the sleep center (eg, to and from the hookup room, lounge, office); allowing the patient to use a bedpan, portable toilet placed by the bedside, or urinal (male patients); and removing items from the floor such as area rugs that could become caught on a patient's foot or on an ambulatory device and cause a fall.

In older patients, in particular, the risk of falls can be increased by the use of certain types of medications

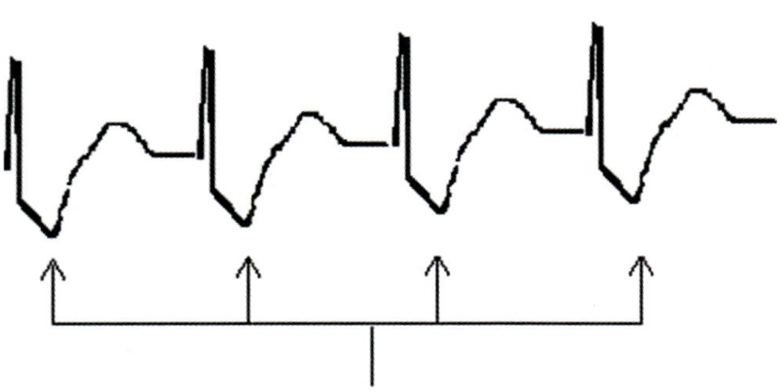

Figure 34-34 Schematic of junctional tachycardia.

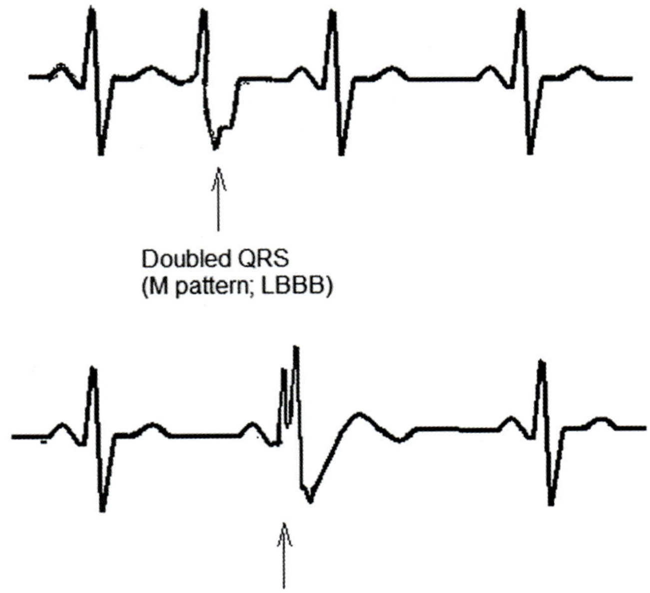

Figure 34-35 Schematic of bundle branch block: left bundle branch block (LBBB) (top) and right bundle branch block (RBBB) (bottom).

such as hypnosedatives (eg, zolpidem, ramelteon) and benzodiazepines (eg, lorazepam, diazepam), antidepressants (eg, tricyclic drugs such as amitriptyline and imipramine; selective serotonin reuptake inhibitors [SSRIs] such as fluoxetine and paroxetine; non-SSRIs such as mirtazapine), neuroleptic drugs (eg, risperidone), and antipsychotic drugs (eg, thioridazine), or by the use of four or more medications that are known to increase the risk of falls. Therefore, a technologist's awareness of the medications a patient is taking allows the technologist to be more diligent in following the fall prevention protocols of a sleep center.

Once a patient is in the center, some methods that can help prevent falls include the following:

- Increase the lighting level. In some patients, reduced vision can increase the risk of falls. Increasing the light level could help a patient see objects more readily and thereby reduce the risk of falling.
- Keep floors free of clutter and remove area rugs or other objects that can become entangled on a patient's feet or in walking assistance devices.
- Provide a nonskid bath mat in a shower or tub.
- Administer a questionnaire to assess a patient's fall risk. The following are some examples of questions that can assess fall risk:
  1. "Have you fallen in the last year?"
  2. "Are you taking four or more medications?"
  3. "Do you have any vision problems such as blurry vision, cataracts, glaucoma, macular

degeneration, diabetic retinopathy, poor depth perception, or tunnel vision?" (Peripheral vision loss [ie, "tunnel vision"] may prevent a person from seeing objects on the floor and consequently tripping over them.)

4. "Have you ever had a stroke?"
5. "Have you been diagnosed with Parkinson disease or other neurologic disorder (eg, cerebral palsy, multiple sclerosis, amyotrophic lateral sclerosis [also called "Lou Gehrig's disease"]), or do you have numbness or tingling in your feet or legs?"
6. "Do you have any problems with balance or walking?"
7. "Do you have difficulty getting up from a chair?" (Difficulty arising from a chair can be caused by leg weakness or poor balance, which increases fall risk.)
8. "Do you have any inner ear problem (eg, Meniere disease, vertigo) or hearing loss?" (Hearing loss, particularly in older individuals, has recently been associated with an increased risk of falls; however, the extent to which correcting hearing loss, eg, with hearing aids, reduces the risk of falling has not been determined) (3,4).

If a patient falls despite these efforts and is injured, the technologist should initiate the center's emergency protocol. Depending on the severity of the injury, the patient may need to be transported to a hospital for assessment and treatment.

Stroke

Recognizing the warning signs of a stroke in a patient is important for a technologist. As with a heart attack, a delayed response could jeopardize the patient's life and health. Some warning signs of a stroke are slurred speech or incoherent speech (eg, a person may speak "gibberish" or use the wrong words for an object); uncoordinated gait; weakness or numbness in part of the body such as the face; altered consciousness; drowsiness; and patient complaints of dizziness, headache, and double vision or unilateral blindness (ie, blindness in only one eye). If a technologist suspects a stroke in a patient who is alert but manifesting these symptoms, the technologist should initiate the center's emergency protocol and record symptoms in the patient's chart.

Asthma Attack

Asthma is an overactive immune response to an allergen. After exposure to the allergen, the air passages in the lungs contract, thereby causing difficulty in breathing, which is manifested by wheezing, coughing, and a sense of chest tightness. The sudden appearance of these symptoms is called an "asthma attack." An asthma attack can be a life-threatening condition. During such an attack, the bronchial airway passages suddenly narrow after exposure to the allergen. As the narrowing in the air passages worsens, wheezing may become louder, the person may begin to use neck muscles (ie, accessory muscles) to raise the rib cage in an effort to get air into the lungs, or the person may begin to breathe fast (ie, "pant"; the Greek word *asthma* means "to pant"). As an asthma attack continues, airway inflammation and narrowing prevent oxygenation, and a person may become cyanotic (ie, has a blue tinge to the skin, especially the lips, face, and fingers). Continued reduction in oxygenation can result in unconsciousness and death.

For some patients with asthma, positive airway pressure (PAP) treatment can trigger an asthma attack. The force of the air into the lungs and/or the plastic particles from the PAP mask and hose may induce an asthma attack. Depending on the severity of the symptoms, a patient may be able to continue PAP treatment by using an inhaler to open the airway. However, the technologist should immediately stop PAP treatment and implement the center's emergency protocol if symptoms worsen, for example, wheezing becomes substantially worse, the person begins using accessory muscles to breathe, or the person becomes cyanotic.

Diabetic Ketoacidosis

Diabetic ketoacidosis is a complication of diabetes, a disease involving improper blood glucose levels. Diabetic ketoacidosis occurs when insulin insufficiency (ie, lower-than-normal insulin production) or insulin resistance (ie, inability to use insulin correctly) causes the body to sense a "starvation" state. (Insulin is a hormone that removes glucose from the blood so that body tissues can utilize glucose.) In a starvation state, stores of carbohydrates (ie, sugars, starches) from which glucose can be synthesized are typically depleted. To restore glucose levels, the body produces glucose from noncarbohydrate sources such as fat. This process is called "gluconeogenesis." However, a by-product of gluconeogenesis is ketone bodies (ie, acetone, acetoacetic acid, and beta-hydroxybutyric acid). These molecules are acidic and raise the acidity of the blood, which can alter consciousness, cause coma, and, ultimately, death, if left untreated.

Ketoacidosis can result from insulin insufficiency, severe infection or other illness, prolonged fasting, severe dehydration, or a combination of these factors. Ketoacidosis typically occurs in people with type 1 (ie, insulin-dependent) diabetes. People with this type of diabetes produce little or no insulin. However, ketoacidosis can occur in people with type 2 (ie, noninsulin-dependent) diabetes when blood sugar levels are high because of poor blood sugar control or poor treatment compliance. In people with type 2 diabetes, insulin resistance allows excessive amounts of glucose to remain in the blood and not enter the body's tissues; thus, the body erroneously senses a starvation state and initiates gluconeogenesis.

Signs and symptoms of diabetic ketoacidosis develop quickly—sometimes within 24 hours—as the levels of ketone bodies increase. At the onset of ketoacidosis, a person may have excessive thirst, dry mouth, frequent urination, and dry or flushed skin. As ketoacidosis progresses, the patient may experience nausea and vomiting, abdominal pain, weakness or fatigue, and shortness of breath. In the later stages of ketoacidosis, the person develops a fruity or nail polish remover–like smell to the breath because of the excessive production of acetone and other ketone bodies; rapid deep breathing; confusion; coma; and, at worst, death.

The treatment for ketoacidosis involves correcting a person's blood glucose and insulin levels. Some patients may recognize early symptoms of improper blood glucose or insulin levels and attempt to take precautions. For example, a patient may state "My blood sugar feels like its high, I better take my insulin" or "My sugar feels like its low, I better eat something." To confirm whether blood glucose levels need to be decreased (eg, taking insulin) or increased (eg, ingesting a meal or candy), a patient may use test strips to test the blood for a high glucose level or test the urine for high ketone level and act accordingly. The sleep technologist should record this information in the patient's chart. If a patient does not improve or appears to be getting worse within 20 to 30 minutes after attempting to correct blood glucose or insulin levels, a sleep technologist should initiate the sleep center's emergency protocol or contact EMS.

SUMMARY

Recording biopotentials accurately during a sleep study and recording factors or events that affect the recording of biopotentials are very important aspects of a sleep technologist's job. The quality of a record produced by a technologist can affect the quality of care a patient receives. If a sleep physician is unable to read a record because of uncorrected artifacts or improper signals (eg, low-amplitude respiratory signals), the physician may be unable to accurately diagnose a patient's sleep problem and effectively treat it. Factors (eg, blindness) and events (eg, the onset of a seizure, parasomnias) that affect a recording need to be recognized, addressed (if necessary), and recorded in a patient's chart by the technologist. Recording these factors and events gives a sleep physician a clearer picture of what is occurring with a patient during sleep. This information may then impact how a physician diagnoses and treats a sleep disorder in a patient.

In addition to recording a PSG, recognizing when a patient may be in danger of injury or experiencing a life-threatening event during the sleep center visit is important for technologists. A technologist's quick and appropriate actions in managing medical emergencies could lessen injury to a patient, avoid the long-term consequences of an injury to a patient, or avoid the death of a patient in a sleep center.

REFERENCES

1. Berry RB, Wagner MH, Ryals SM. *Fundamentals of Sleep Medicine*. 2nd ed. Elsevier Health Sciences; 2025.
2. Troester M, Quan S, Berry R, Plante DT, Abreu AR, Alzoubaidi M. *The AASM Manual for the Scoring of Sleep and Associated Events. Rules, Terminology and Technical Specifications Version 3*. American Academy of Sleep Medicine; 2023.
3. Riska KM, Peskoe SB, Gordee A, Kuchibhatla M, Smith SL. Erratum to "Preliminary evidence on the impact of hearing aid use on falls risk in individuals with self-reported hearing loss". *Am J Audiol*. 2021;30:1150. doi:10.1044/2021_AJA-21-00143
4. Riska KM, Peskoe SB, Gordee A, Kuchibhatla M, Smith SL. Preliminary evidence on the impact of hearing aid use on falls risk in individuals with self-reported hearing loss. *Am J Audiol* 2021;30: 376-384. doi:10.1044/2021_AJA-20-00179

Chapter 35
Preparing the Patient for Polysomnography

CYNTHIA D. MATTICE AND RITA J. BROOKS

KEY CONCEPTS/LEARNING OBJECTIVES

The key concepts in this chapter include applying the standard electrodes and sensors used in polysomnography, performing measurements for electroencephalogram using the International 10/20 System of Electrode Placement, developing techniques for electrode and sensor application, and troubleshooting poor quality signals.

KEY TERMS

Biocalibration
Electroencephalogram
Electromyogram
Electrooculogram
Inion
Nasion
Preauricular points
Respiratory inductance plethysmography
Thermistor
Thermocouple

The application of electrodes and sensors to the patient is one of the most important parts of a sleep study. If done poorly, the quality of the data will be compromised, and a significant part of the night will be spent troubleshooting and problem-solving. Filters should not be used to compensate for poor-quality electrode application. Excessive use of filtration can significantly alter the integrity of the data and impact how the study is analyzed.

There are many different approaches to preparing a patient for a sleep study. This chapter will focus on the standard or classic methods. In addition to the varied techniques utilized by different sleep centers, each sleep technologist will develop their own method of performing electrode and sensor application. Exchanging ideas with other technologists is an excellent way to continue to improve and refine one's technique.

BASIC SUPPLIES AND EQUIPMENT

To expedite the hookup process, it is helpful to have all your supplies close at hand while preparing the patient (Table 35-1). Applying electrodes takes dexterity and care, so being well organized is essential.

BEFORE THE PATIENT ARRIVES

It is critical to allow time at the beginning of the shift before the patient arrives to prepare for the night ahead. The technologist should use this time to review the practitioner's orders, set up and calibrate the recording equipment, prepare the necessary supplies, and assess and respond to any special needs the patient may have.

Undergoing a sleep study can be stressful for a patient. An informed and knowledgeable technologist helps reduce that anxiety and creates a positive patient experience. Become familiar with the patient's medical history by reviewing the chart before the patient arrives. Be sure to label any questionnaires or forms that require completion, and check the physician's order to determine which type of study has been prescribed (positive airway pressure [PAP] titration, diagnostic study, split-night study, or extended channel montage). If an order is unclear, contact the sleep center manager, on-call physician, or the practitioner who wrote the order for clarification.

The hookup procedure will be faster and more efficient if the supplies are prepared and organized in advance. For example, you can precut the tape and gauze, lay out gold cup electrodes, check for broken or damaged sensors, and stock the supply tray before the patient arrives. Ensure all reusable items that will come into contact with a patient have been cleaned and disinfected according to infection control standards before use.

Table 35-1 Basic Supplies

General Supplies
Nonlatex gloves
Scissors
Towels
Various types of medical tape (Transpore, Hypafix, or Medipore, and Scanpor) Impedance meter
For Applying Scalp and Face Electrodes (To Record EEG, EOG, and Chin EMG)
Air compressor (if using collodion)
Tape measure
Grease pencil
Hair pins/clips
Hair comb
Electrodes (gold cup with center hole)
Alcohol swabs
Abrasive skin preparation (NuPrep or Lemon Prep)
Cotton-tip applicators
EEG conductive paste
Electrolyte gel or cream
Collodion/EC2 paste
Collodion remover/acetone
Gauze (4 × 4 squares and/or roll of single-ply gauze)
Medical tape (Micropore, Transpore, and fabric tape)
Double-sided electrode collars
For Applying ECG Electrodes (To Record the ECG)
Disposable ECG snap pads
ECG electrodes
For Applying Leg EMG Electrodes (To Record Leg Movements)
Gold cup electrodes with extra long leads (72 in [182.9 cm])
Small ECG patches (optional)
For Applying Respiratory Belts (To Record Respiratory Effort)
Thoracic/abdominal belts in various sizes
Inductive plethysmography belts
For Applying Airflow Sensor (To Record Respiratory Airflow)
Nasal cannula with pressure transducer and thermocouple, or thermistor
For Applying Snore Sensor
Snore sensor
For Applying Oximeter Probe (To Record Spo_2)
Oximeter probe (disposable or reusable)
Oximeter calibration tool (may have autocalibration)

ECG, electrocardiogram; EEG, electroencephalogram; EMG, electromyogram; EOG, electrooculogram.

APPLYING THE ELECTRODES AND SENSORS

Proper electrode and sensor placement is essential for recording a quality polysomnogram. Every technologist should be familiar with all electrodes and sensors, what they measure, where they are placed, and how they plug into the headbox (also called a jackbox). All electrodes and sensor leads should be easily identifiable to avoid confusion when connecting them to the headbox. Some technologists prefer to use labeled gold cup electrodes, whereas others plug each electrode into the headbox immediately after it is attached.

Suggested Routine for Electrode and Sensor Application

This chapter provides a suggested sequence for applying electrodes and sensors, but all technologists develop their own routine. Do not be afraid to experiment and develop a system that suits your individual style.

1. Scalp and face electrodes
2. Snore sensor
3. Electrocardiogram (ECG) electrodes
4. Leg electrodes
5. Respiratory bands
6. Airflow sensor(s)
7. Oximeter probe

The airflow sensor and oximeter probe are typically applied shortly before bedtime as these sensors are more cumbersome to the patient. However, for some patients, it may be helpful to have a longer assessment of the individual's waking oxygen levels. In those cases, the oximeter should be attached upon arrival to allow oxygen levels to be monitored throughout the hookup procedure.

General Suggestions to Optimize Electrode Application

- During the application procedure, the technologist should explain the procedure to the patient. This is an ideal time to provide education on sleep hygiene, obstructive sleep apnea, and/or whatever sleep topic seems appropriate for the patient.
- The patient's skin and hair should be clean and dry. Electrodes applied to oily skin or hair will likely have high impedance levels, resulting in poor signal quality, and are more susceptible to becoming detached during the night. Patients should be instructed by the daytime staff to shower or bathe before arriving. If necessary and if shower facilities are available, ask the patient to shower at the sleep center before beginning the hookup. If the patient has

very dirty or oily hair and a shower is not possible, use alcohol or acetone wipes to remove the excess oil. Alcohol dries quickly, so the site can be prepped and the electrode attached almost immediately.

- When using tape or gauze to adhere an electrode, scrub only the small area where the electrode will be placed. If excess prep material remains in the vicinity of the electrode, gently cleanse the area with rubbing alcohol because tape will not stick to the gritty prep.
- Facilitate tape removal in the morning by using small pieces of tape and making tabs by folding down one end. The tape should be just large enough to secure the sensor and wire throughout the study (Figure 35-1).
- Point the wires toward the crown of the head or nape of the neck to make them more manageable. Consider where the headbox will be placed during the night when selecting how to bundle the wires.
- Provide extra slack in the wires to avoid putting stress on the electrodes.

Attaching Gold Cup Electrodes

Before starting the application process, all electroencephalogram (EEG) electrode sites should be measured and marked using the International 10/20 System (1) described later in the chapter. Scalp electrodes can be attached using paste or collodion. When deciding which method to use, signal quality, stability of sensor, convenience of application, and removal as well as cleanup should be considered. Collodion requires an air compressor to dry the glue, has a strong odor, is highly combustible, and requires storage in fireproof safe and a solvent to remove in the morning. Paste is removed with water, but electrodes may move slightly or loosen during the night, particularly if the patient sweats. Although collodion is more secure, most labs use paste because it is more convenient and less caustic.

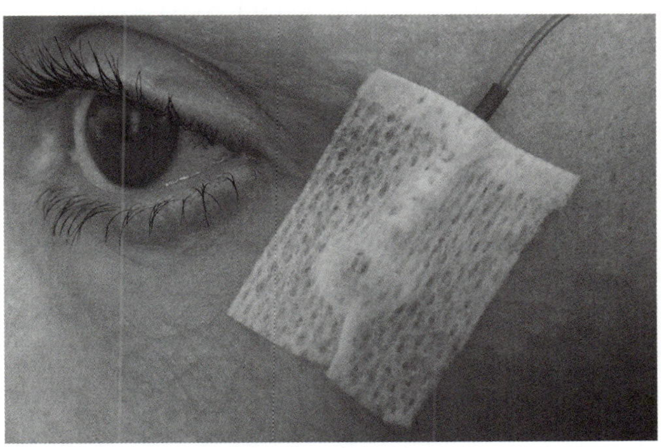

Figure 35-1 Suggested approach to tabbing tape. Note the small crease at the bottom center of the tape.

Preparing the Electrode Sites

Preparing the skin before attaching the electrode is essential for reducing impedance levels and ensuring signal quality. Be sure to discuss the procedure with the patient so that they are not surprised by the process. First, clean the area with an alcohol swab to remove any makeup or oil on the skin. Then, using a small cotton-tipped applicator, gently scrub the area where the sensor will be placed with an abrasive skin preparation, such as NuPrep or Lemon Prep, for 5 to 10 seconds, applying moderate pressure. The skin may redden slightly from the procedure.

To prevent signal contamination and possible bridging with other electrode sites, be sure to only scrub the area covered by the electrode cup. Likewise, avoid using excessive amounts of prep material, because it has conductive properties and electrodes attached with tape will not stick to the prep. If there is excess prep material, the area can be cleaned again with rubbing alcohol. Be sure to wipe away from the electrode site to avoid transferring skin oils from the surrounding area.

Attaching Gold Cup Electrodes With Electrode Paste

Fill the electrode disk with conductive paste, so the surface is slightly rounded, making sure that there are no air pockets. Using the wooden side of the cotton-tipped applicator or a comb, part the hair in the same direction in which the lead wire will be positioned. Hair clips can be used to keep the site clear. Spread a small amount of electrode paste evenly on one side of a 3-cm square of gauze. Position the electrode in the center of the prepped site so the paste is against the skin. Cover the electrode with the gauze square, paste side down. Distribute the electrode paste around the head of the electrode, keeping it firmly in place until the paste begins to set. Check for a secure application by gently tugging on the electrode wire.

Attaching Gold Cup Electrodes With Collodion

When using collodion, the hookup process should be performed in a well-ventilated area as the glue is very pungent and flammable. If there is limited space available, an air filtration or exhaust system can be used to reduce the fumes. For safety purposes, collodion and acetone should always be handled carefully and stored in a fireproof safe. Collodion and acetone spills pose a safety risk; consequently, all sleep centers should have a protocol for handling and properly disposing of these materials.

A towel should be placed around the patient's shoulders to protect their clothing from the glue. Separate the hair using a comb or the wooden side of the cotton-tipped applicator so that the skin is visible. Hair clips can be used to help hold the hair in place and keep the electrode site in view. Once the site is prepped, position a clean gold-cupped electrode on the scalp, and place a small square of single-ply gauze on top (~2-3 cm). Insert the air compressor stylus through the gauze into the hole at the top of the electrode to hold it in place against the scalp. Using a syringe or another disposable applicator, apply just enough glue to saturate the gauze. If the electrode is moved after the glue is applied, the collodion may seep between the scalp and the electrode, which will raise the impedance level and compromise signal quality. Smooth the gauze tightly over the scalp while the glue is dried with the air compressor, taking care not to adhere your gloves to the electrode. If long enough, the patient's hair can be used to help anchor the electrode to the scalp. Before removing the stylus, twist the end to break any seal that may have formed from the glue. The collodion bottle should be kept tightly closed when not in use to avoid spills and maintain the liquid nature of the glue. When collodion is exposed to air for an extended time, it becomes viscous and difficult to apply in moderation.

When all electrodes are glued in place, use a blunt-tipped needle syringe to fill the electrodes with electrolyte gel or cream. Be careful not to overfill the electrode cup, or the gel may leak out the side and break the collodion seal, causing electrode popping artifact during the recording.

Attaching Gold Cup Electrodes With Tape

Fill the electrode cup with conductive paste or electrolyte gel so it is slightly rounded, making sure there are no air pockets. To help ensure a solid connection with the skin, center a double-sided electrode collar over the cup and remove the paper backing. Place the electrode onto the prepped site, paste side down, with the wire pointed toward the crown of the head, and cover with a piece of tape. Press firmly around the rim of the cup to obtain a good seal. To facilitate removal in the morning, fold one end of the tape, creating a small tab; this makes it easier to pull the tape off at the end of the study (Figure 35-1).

Managing the Electrode Leads

Organizing and securing the wires during the electrode application procedure will reduce the likelihood of electrodes being inadvertently pulled off during the night. After attaching the electrodes to the face and scalp, gather all the wires together into a ponytail at the crown of the head or nape of neck, making sure no wire is pulled taut. Bundle the wires together with pieces of tape or Velcro strips. If tape is used, both ends should be folded over for easy removal. The wires should be secured every 4 to 6 inches (10.2-15.2 cm) to reduce tangling. The leads from the other sensors can also be grouped separately and taped together to make the wires more manageable.

If using tape to bundle the electrodes becomes problematic because of the sticky tape residue, try using Coban tape. This tape sticks to itself, comes in many colors, and is disposable. Posey straps can also be used.

Experienced sleep technologists usually develop their own approach for arranging and managing the wires, which helps facilitate easy removal in the morning. A neatly organized application also makes it easier to troubleshoot recording problems and replace sensors when necessary.

Electroencephalography Scalp Electrodes

According to the standard practice, EEG electrodes are applied using the International 10/20 System of Electrode Placement (1). When applying the electrodes, there are three key elements that are vital to collecting quality data:

1. Electrodes must be placed in the correct location.
2. Electrode sites must be properly prepared.
3. Electrodes must be securely attached.

The current American Academy of Sleep Medicine Scoring Manual (2) recommends six EEG scalp electrodes for polysomnography (PSG): two frontal electrodes (F3 and F4), two central electrodes (C3 and C4), and two occipital electrodes (O1 and O2). In addition, two mastoid electrodes, M1 and M2, are placed on the mastoid processes, the bony protrusion located behind each ear.

The primary recording derivations are F4-M1, C4-M1, and O2-M1. Backup electrodes should be placed in order to record the backup derivations F3-M2, C3-M2, and O1-M2 in the event an electrode signal becomes compromised during the study. Most sleep centers include both the recommended and the backup electrode derivations in a standard PSG recording montage to ensure all EEG channels are visible during data collection and allow for troubleshooting.

Determining the Electroencephalogram Electrode Placements: The International 10/20 System

The International 10/20 System of Electrode Placement (1) is a standardized method for identifying equally spaced electrode positions on the scalp on the basis of four identifiable skull landmarks. This method was developed in 1958 to provide a consistent procedure for collecting EEG data and to develop common terminology. The system is termed 10/20 because the measurements are spaced either 10% or 20% of the distance between a given pair of skull landmarks. Percentages are used rather than absolute distances to allow for normal variations in head shape and size.

Each location is named with a letter indicating the corresponding lobe of the brain and a number or letter identifying the exact site. The locations on the left side of the head are odd numbered, those on the right side are even numbered, and the midline is represented by the letter "z." From front to back, the lobes are: prefrontal (Fp), frontal (F), temporal (T), central (C), parietal (p), and occipital (O).

Before starting the measuring process, have the patient sit in a chair that is low enough to allow you to see the top of the head. Ensure that all reusable equipment (grease pencil, hair clips, measuring tape) has been cleaned and disinfected according to facility protocols for infection control. When using a paper measuring tape, be sure to fold the end down at the zero line to avoid computation errors.

Identifying the Landmarks

The four standard landmarks used in the 10/20 system are the nasion, inion, and left and right preauricular points (Figure 35-2). If the landmarks are not correctly identified, electrode placement will not be accurate. Each site should be marked to facilitate the measuring process, keeping in mind that these sites are used as landmarks only and are not electrode positions.

Preauricular Points

The opening of the ear canal is protected by a small piece of cartilage called the "tragus." The preauricular points are the indentations just above this cartilage. If you are unsure of the location, place a finger on the patient's cheek, touching the tragus, and ask the patient to open and close their jaw. The indentation will become more pronounced with this movement.

Nasion

The nasion is the indentation between the forehead and the nose formed by the intersection of the frontal bone and two nasal bones of the skull. While facing the patient, find the small dip at the bridge of the nose between the eyes and lightly mark the point with a grease pencil.

Inion

The inion is the ridge or knob at the back of the head. When running your finger up the back of the neck to the skull, you should feel a depression with the ridge of the protruding inion just above it. This landmark may be difficult to find on some individuals, so ask the patient to tilt their head all the way back, or forward, while you try to feel the ridge. If you are unable to locate the inion, mark it at the same level as the preauricular points. A common mistake is to use the underside of the protrusion instead of the tip, which will impact the accuracy of electrode placement.

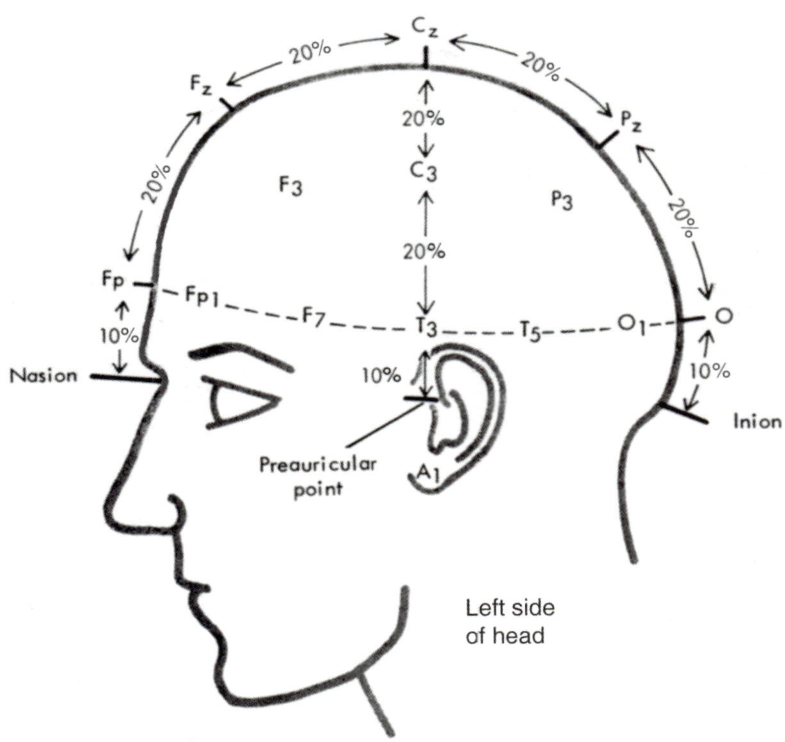

Figure 35-2 Identifying the landmarks. (From Harner PF, Sannit T. *A Review of the International Ten–Twenty System of Electrode Placement*. Grass Instrument Co.; 1974. Image courtesy of Natus Medical Incorporated, natus.com)

Measuring the Scalp Electrode Sites

Each electrode site is determined by the intersection of two lines created by calculating distances, measured in centimeters, stemming from the four main landmarks (Figure 35-3). Start the measuring process by marking each of these landmarks with the grease pencil.

Step 1 in Determining Cz

Many PSG software systems use Cz for the system reference electrode, which is not the same as the patient ground. Even if an electrode is not attached at Cz, it should be marked as a reference point for identifying other electrode sites.

While standing to one side of the patient, place the zero line of the measuring tape on the marked inion. Stretch the tape measure upward, over the crown of the head, until it reaches the marked nasion. Determine the total distance between the inion and the nasion in centimeters. Using your grease pencil, mark the values for 10%, 50%, and 90% of that total distance. The marks at 10% and 90% will be used for identifying other electrode sites. Next, measure the distance between the marks made at 10% (will become Fpz) and 50% (will become Cz) and draw a line halfway between the two for Fz. Be sure to mark these sites with straight horizontal lines that are prominent enough to be easily located later.

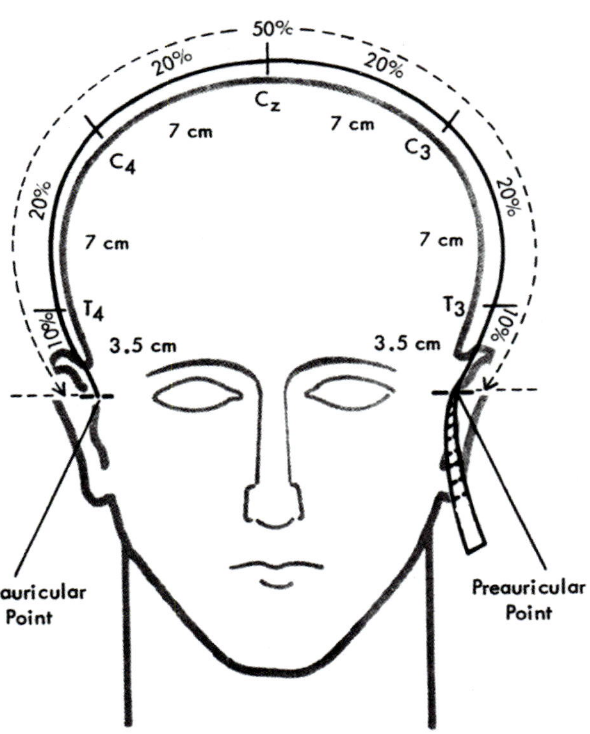

Figure 35-3 Measuring the scalp between the two preauricular points. The measured distances in centimeters are provided as an example; actual distances will vary depending on the size and shape of the scalp. (From Harner PF, Sannit T. *A Review of the International Ten–Twenty System of Electrode Placement.* Grass Instrument Co.; 1974. Image courtesy of Natus Medical Incorporated, natus.com)

Step 2 in Determining Cz

Standing behind the subject, reposition the zero end of the tape measure on one of the preauricular marks. Stretch the measuring tape over the top of the head through the 50% mark that was made during step 1, until it reaches the opposite preauricular mark. Determine the total distance from preauricular to preauricular point. Calculate 10%, 50%, and 90% of the total distance and mark each location. The point where the 50% mark intersects with the line drawn indicating 50% of the distance between nasion and inion is the site for Cz.

Step 1 in Determining C3 and C4

Standing to one side of the patient, place the zero line of the measuring tape on Cz and measure the distance to the mark made at 10% above one of the preauricular points (T3 or T4). Calculate 50% of this distance and mark the location. Repeat the process standing on the other side of the patient. These are the first set of marks necessary in determining C3 and C4. The second set of marks will be established after O1 and O2 have been identified.

Step 1 in Determining O1, O2, Fp1, and Fp2

Standing in front of the patient, draw a vertical line in the middle of the forehead (lining up with the bridge of the nose), intersecting the line drawn 10% up from the nasion. This location is Fpz. Standing to the side of the patient, place the zero end of the measuring tape at Fpz and wrap the tape around the entire circumference of the head, until it meets the zero end at Fpz. Calculate 50% of the head circumference and make a vertical mark at the back of the head, intersecting the 10% mark above the inion. This location is Oz. Next, calculate 5% of the circumference and make a vertical mark 5% to each side of Oz. Repeat the same procedure at the front of the head, drawing vertical marks 5% to each side of Fpz.

Step 2 in Determining O1, O2, Fp1, and Fp2

Extend the horizontal lines marked at Oz and Fpz during step 1 in determining Cz until they intersect with these new lines. At the back of the head, the points at which the lines intersect are O1 and O2, with O1 being on the patient's left side and O2 on the right. At the front of the head, the intersecting lines identify Fp1 and Fp2.

To double-check these locations, measure the distance between the two new vertical lines drawn on the back of the head. This distance should equal 10% of the total head circumference, with the original 50% line (Oz) in the center. Fp1 and Fp2 should be verified similarly on the forehead.

Step 1 in Determining F3 and F4

Place the zero line of the measuring tape on the newly marked Fp1 and stretch the tape to the line you made 10% up from the left preauricular point (T3), and mark 10% of the total head circumference to create F7, which will be used later to calculate F3. Repeat the process on the right side to identify F8. The total distance between F7 and F8, passing through Fpz, should be 30% of the total head circumference, and all measurements should be in the same plane.

Step 2 in Determining C3 and C4 and F3 and F4

Standing to the left of the patient, place the zero end of the measuring tape at O1 and extend the tape over the left side of the head to Fp1. Calculate 50% of the distance between O1 and Fp1 and make a vertical mark, intersecting the line drawn during step 1 in determining C3 and C4. The intersection of these two lines determines the location for C3.

Once C3 has been identified, measure the distance between Fp1 on the forehead and C3, and mark the halfway point. This will be the first line for F3.

Repeat the process standing on the right side of the patient, measuring the distance between O2 and Fp2 to determine the location for C4 (Figure 35-4). Then mark 50% between Fp2 and C4 to identify the first mark for F4.

Step 3 in Determining F3 and F4

To complete the process of locating F3 and F4, measure the distance between F7 and F8, passing through the line marked earlier for Fz. Determine 50% of this distance to identify the second mark for Fz. Locate the final mark for F3 halfway between Fz and F7. Repeat the process to identify the second mark for F4 between Fz and F8.

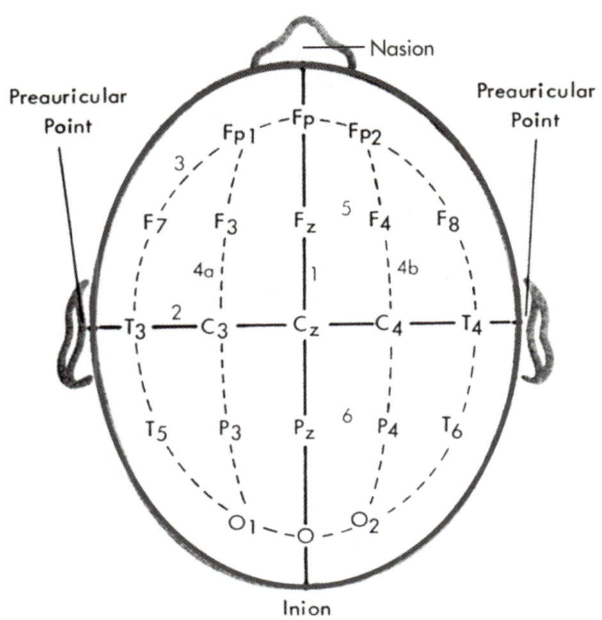

Figure 35-4 Overview of electrode locations. (From Harner PF, Sannit T. *A Review of the International Ten–Twenty System of Electrode Placement*. Grass Instrument Co.; 1974. Image courtesy of Natus Medical Incorporated, natus.com)

Preparing the Electrode Site

The EEG electrode sites must be prepared using the procedure described earlier. Perform a visual check as the sites are prepped to ensure that the sites are correctly aligned. If the pattern does not match Figure 35-4, the measurements should be checked before attaching electrodes.

Attaching the Electrode

The EEG electrodes are generally attached using paste, although collodion or taping using double-sided electrode collars and paper tape may also be used.

Reference Electrodes

Determining the Reference Electrode Placement (M1 and M2)

The reference electrodes M1 and M2 are placed over the mastoid process (bone behind the earlobe). The electrodes should be placed on the skin between the crease of the earlobe and where the hairline begins. To reduce artifacts, the sensors should be placed over the flattest and boniest area. M1 is placed behind the left ear and M2 behind the right ear.

Preparing the Electrode Site

The reference electrode sites should be prepared using the same procedure described earlier for attaching gold cup electrodes.

Attaching the Electrode

The reference electrodes can be attached with tape if there is enough space between the ear and the hairline to secure the tape. Paste or collodion application can also be used.

Ground Electrode

Determining the Ground Electrode Placement

The ground electrode is typically placed in the middle of the forehead between the nasion and the start of the hairline at the site that was identified as Fpz during the measurement process. However, the exact location for the ground electrode is not critical. It is more important to ensure a good connection, so avoid areas with deep creases or wrinkles. A flat area just below the hairline also works well for this application.

Preparing the Electrode Site and Attaching the Electrode

The ground electrode site should be prepared using the procedure described earlier. The ground electrode may be attached with either conductive paste or electrolyte gel, using tape or a double-sided electrode collar and tape.

Electrooculogram Electrodes

Two electrodes, E1 and E2, are used to measure eye movements. Both electrooculogram (EOG) electrodes are referenced to the M2 electrode. In keeping with the International 10/20 System's naming convention, E1 is near the patient's left eye and E2 near the right eye.

Determining Electrooculogram Electrode Placements (E1 and E2)

The standard placement for EOG electrodes (2) is designed to record both vertical and horizontal eye movements. To accomplish this, the left eye electrode (E1) is attached 1 cm below and 1 cm lateral to the left outer canthus (outside corner of the eye), whereas the right eye electrode (E2) is secured 1 cm above and 1 cm lateral to the outer canthus of the right eye. Use caution when prepping and placing these electrodes because the skin near the eye tends to be very thin and sensitive.

The AASM alternate placement is to position both electrodes 1 cm lateral and 1 cm below the outer canthus of each eye (2). When using the alternate derivation, both electrodes are referenced to Fpz.

Preparing the Electrode Sites and Attaching the Electrodes

The sites should be prepared using the procedure described earlier. Use caution with prepping and attaching electrodes close to the eye to prevent discomfort and skin irritation. The EOG electrodes are attached using paste and tape or a combination of double-sided electrode collars and tape. It is important to remember that the skin around the eye is very sensitive, particularly in older patients, so use tape sparingly. There are specialty tapes and skin barrier products commercially available to make removal of tape more comfortable for sensitive patients.

Chin Electromyogram Electrodes

The AASM recommends using three electrodes: two primary electrodes referenced to each other to create a bipolar signal and one backup electrode in the event that one of the primary sensors fails. Obtaining an adequate signal can be challenging with subjects with obesity, so a third electrode can be particularly helpful in this population. The muscle tone information relayed through this channel is essential for determining rapid eye movement (REM) onset and bruxism. It can also help identify sleep onset and arousals. For an extended bruxism montage, two additional electrodes can be placed on the masseter muscles when clinically indicated. The masseter muscles are located just below the cheekbone and can be easily felt by having the patient grit their teeth.

Determining the Chin Electromyogram Electrode Placements

Three electrodes are placed for recording chin electromyogram (EMG) (2). The third chin EMG electrode is useful as a backup, in case one of the EMG electrodes becomes loose or detached during the night. The first electrode, ChinZ, is placed at the midline of the chin, 1 cm above the inferior edge of the mandible.

The other two electrodes, Chin1 (lower left lateral) and Chin2 (lower right lateral), are placed on the submentalis, which is the large muscle located below the chin. It is important to place the electrodes over the muscle. The submental electrodes are placed 2 cm below the inferior edge of the mandible and 2 cm to the right and left of the midline so they are 4 cm apart. As with any pair of electrodes, it is imperative that they are sufficiently far apart to avoid electrode bridging; not even the tape should touch.

Preparing the Electrode Sites and Attaching the Electrodes

The sites should be prepared using the procedure described earlier. Chin EMG electrodes typically need extra security to guarantee they will stay in place through the night. Using a paste and tape or a double-sided electrode collar and gauze tape reduces the chance of these electrodes coming off during the study. For patients with facial hair, collodion or EC2 paste is recommended.

Electrocardiogram Electrodes

The ECG data collected during a polysomnogram is an abbreviated ECG generally using only one ECG channel instead of twelve. Therefore, the ECG is not typically used as a definitive test to diagnose subtle arrhythmias. However, signal quality must be sufficiently clear to allow recognition of significant arrhythmias, which should be reported to the clinician. Standard ECG electrodes should be used to record the ECG to minimize artifact and assure signal quality. Additional ECG leads can be ordered by the physician and added to the montage if clinically indicated.

Locating the Electrocardiogram Sites

To record a modified lead II ECG using the recommended torso electrode placement (2), one ECG electrode is placed approximately 3 to 5 cm (two finger widths) below the right clavicle. The other ECG electrode is placed on the left lower rib cage. The electrodes should be aligned in parallel to the right shoulder and left hip.

An alternate (modified lead I) placement is sometimes used on very obese patients, whereby the second electrode is positioned below the left clavicle.

Preparing the Electrode Sites and Attaching the Electrodes

Standard ECG electrodes with snap leads should be used to record the ECG. The electrode sites should be cleaned with rubbing alcohol to remove skin oils. The area should be lightly scrubbed with a prep material to reduce impedance before the electrode is attached. For male patients, it may be necessary to shave the area before applying the electrodes. This will reduce artifact and make it easier to remove the sensors in the morning.

Snap the electrode to the lead wire before applying it to the patient's skin. Remove the backing from the electrode and place the gel side down. Feed the connector end of the wire up through the patient's bedclothes.

Be sensitive to the patient's modesty when attaching ECG electrodes; lift only as much of the garment as necessary. It is important to put your patients at ease and make them as comfortable as possible during the electrode application process. Communication is key; understanding what to expect will make patients feel more relaxed.

If the polarity of the ECG derivation is reversed, the ECG recording will be inverted, so ensure the leads are plugged into the headbox correctly to avoid confusion. Polarity can also be corrected using the PSG software to invert the signal.

Anterior Tibialis (Leg) Electromyogram Electrodes

Movement activity from both legs should be monitored during a PSG on two separate channels. The recommended approach for collecting this data is to use surface electrodes. Gold cup electrodes are the most sensitive for recording EMG activity. Because the leg electrodes have the longest wires, they are more likely to have 50/60-Hz interference and can be difficult to manage. Taking time during the application to ensure that the electrodes and lead wires are securely in place and protected will improve the signal and reduce the likelihood that an electrode will be pulled off during the night. An extended EMG montage (2) can be used to monitor arm movements or another specific type of EMG activity if clinically indicated.

Locating the Electrode Sites

To monitor lower limb movements, two electrodes are attached to the anterior tibialis muscle that runs along the outside edge of the tibia (shin bone). The electrodes should be placed vertically along the muscle ridge 2 to 3 cm apart or one-third of the length of the anterior tibialis muscle, whichever is shorter.

It is essential to position the sensors on the muscle rather than the tibia bone. To ensure you have the correct placement, ask the patient to flex the foot back and forth to see the muscle move. Once you have correctly identified the location, mark the sites with a pencil. Figure 35-5 illustrates the correct electrode placement.

To monitor upper limb movements, two electrodes should be placed 2 cm apart on the anterior of the forearm along the flexor digitorum superficialis muscle and/or the extensor digitorum communis muscle that is located on the posterior of the forearm. To ensure correct placement on the flexor digitorum superficialis muscle, ask the patient to flex the hand at the base of the fingers (where fingers attach to the hand, not at the finger joints) to see the muscle move, and mark the site. To identify extensor digitorum communis muscle electrode placement, ask the patient to extend the fingers back without moving the wrist and mark the site.

Preparing the Electrode Sites and Attaching the Electrodes

Standard prepping procedure should be used. In male patients, it may be necessary to shave the area where tape will be applied. This will improve impedance and reduce discomfort when the tape is removed after the study.

Each electrode is attached to the leg, arm, or other EMG recording site with paste and tape or double-sided electrode collars and about 2 inch (5.1 cm) of tape to ensure that the sensor will remain in place throughout the night. A stress loop should be used after both electrodes are attached to reduce the likelihood of the electrodes being pulled off during the study (Figure 35-5). Using a 2 inch (5.1 cm) piece of tape, secure the loop between or above the two electrodes. With this method,

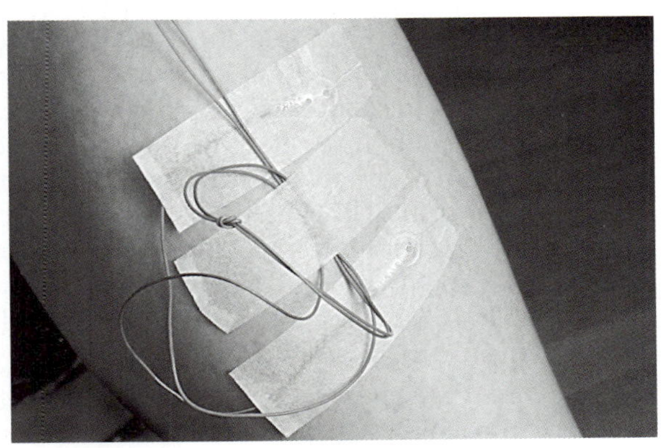

Figure 35-5 Stress loop used to avoid tension on leg electrodes.

if the wires are inadvertently tugged, the tape from the stress loop will be pulled off, not the electrodes.

Managing the Electrode Leads

The limb EMG lead wires should be threaded up through the patient's night clothes to keep them from becoming tangled and unmanageable. Ask the patient to reach down from the waist and pull the sensors up through the pajamas. You can help by passing the ends up from the bottom of the bedclothes. Be sure that the leads are not pulled too tightly; there should be enough slack in the lines so the patient can stand up and move around comfortably. If the patient is wearing shorts or a nightgown, tape the wires to the thigh, again making sure to leave enough slack for movement. Use similar techniques to secure upper limb electrode lead wires.

Respiratory Effort Sensors

Accurately assessing ventilatory effort and the differentiation between abdominal and thoracic movement is critical for distinguishing between obstructive, central, and mixed breathing events. The 2023 AASM Scoring Manual Version 3.0 (2) specifies that either esophageal manometry or inductance plethysmography (calibrated or uncalibrated) may be used to classify abnormal breathing events.

Esophageal manometry is considered the gold standard because it is a calibrated signal that can measure subtle changes in breathing effort. However, it is an invasive measure and is therefore employed judiciously. Although esophageal pressure manometry is recommended for scoring respiratory effort-related arousals, nasal pressure and inductance plethysmography are acceptable alternatives.

Most sleep centers use respiratory inductance plethysmography (RIP) bands to meet the AASM criteria for monitoring respiratory effort. The bands are placed around the chest and abdomen and generate a respiratory effort signal on the basis of changes in body circumference associated with breathing. The RIP bands are embedded with wires, woven in a sinusoidal pattern, that encircle the body. An electrical current is applied to the wires, generating an oscillating signal in response to variations in resistance associated with changes in body circumference.

Dual thoracoabdominal polyvinylidene fluoride (PVDF) belts are an acceptable alternate method to detect breathing effort. PVDF belts produce an electrical signal when subjected to force, sound, acceleration, pressure, or heat and do not require an external battery. Piezo-sensor bands do not meet AASM recommendations for monitoring respiratory effort.

Selecting the Band Size

Selecting the correct RIP band or PVDF belt size will simplify the process of fitting the effort sensors and reduce the need to make adjustments during the night. Bands and belts are available in both pediatric and adult sizes and should be chosen according to the size of the subject. If the bands are too small, they will cause patient discomfort, and the band will be stretched too tight, distorting the signal. If the bands are too long, they may be loose and difficult to adjust properly.

Determining the Position of the Bands

The bands are placed around the thorax and abdomen. The thoracic band is positioned just below the armpits. The abdominal band is secured around the waist, below the lower edge of the rib cage. For patients with obesity, find the location that will provide a snug fit, and allow the bands to stay in place throughout the night. Have the subject stand and move around to ascertain whether the bands are likely to shift during the night.

Fitting the Bands

A buckle may be used to fasten the bands, or they may be self-adhering where the ends of the bands overlap. Fit the bands so they are snug, but not too tight or too loose, with the lead wires pointing upward toward the headbox. Bands may need to be taped in place to ensure that they will stay in place for the entire night. Incorrect placement can cause poor signals and restrict the patient's comfort.

Snore Sensor

There are multiple AASM-approved devices to detect snoring, including an acoustic sensor, a piezoelectric sensor, and a nasal pressure transducer (cannula). The acoustic sensor is thought to detect snore events with lower volume and higher fundamental frequency than both the nasal pressure transducer and the piezoelectric sensor (3). However, the piezoelectric sensor is more commonly used and works by measuring vibration at the skin surface. The cannula measures snoring by pressure vibration in the nares.

Locating the Appropriate Site

To locate the ideal position, place two fingers on the anterior side of the patient's neck above the larynx and ask them to hum. The sensor should be secured over the area with the strongest vibration.

Preparing the Site and Attaching the Sensor

Clean the area with rubbing alcohol to remove any oil from the skin, because tape will adhere better to clean skin; no site preparation is required.

Attach the sensor using tape. The tape should be applied in such a way as to ensure a solid connection between the sensor and the skin, as well as to secure the wire. To be sure that the tape will not restrict movement, ask the patient to hold the head naturally, looking straight ahead while attaching the sensor. Avoid placing the sensor or tape along the slope of the jaw or on the jawbone.

Airflow Sensors

Airflow is monitored using an oronasal thermal sensor and nasal cannula pressure transducer. AASM standards require both types of sensors for scoring breathing events (2). The thermal sensor is used to identify apneas, and a thermistor, thermocouple, or PVDF sum signal can be used. Many sleep centers use oronasal PVDF sensors in place of a thermal sensor; however, these are not currently AASM approved (2).

Thermistors generate their signal by changes in temperature. When a patient breathes out, the heat that is applied to the thermistor produces a signal. An oronasal thermocouple measures change in temperature and does not require a power source. The oronasal thermistor creates a signal by passing a constant current through the thermistor junction of two dissimilar metals and requires a voltage source. The PVDF sum signal is a derived flow signal from the PVDF belts. PVDF airflow sensors use a specially treated plastic film that is flexible and lightweight to generate a voltage when exposed to temperature changes, pressure changes, force changes, vibration, and sound, so it is responsive to changes in both air temperature and pressure and does not require an external voltage source.

The nasal air pressure transducer (with or without square root transformation of the signal) is used to identify hypopneas. It measures qualitative change in air pressure with inspiration and expiration but does not measure oral breathing. Although each system uses a different technology, the sensor placement at the nares and in front of the oral airway is similar.

Securing the Sensors

Thermal sensors are typically designed to monitor both nasal and oral airflow. A three-pronged sensor is placed under the patient's nose, with the two nasal prongs positioned directly in the flow of nasal air, whereas the third prong is situated in front of the mouth. Most oronasal sensors are secured by looping the wires around the ears and connecting them under the chin. Additionally, small pieces of tape can be used to fasten the wires to the cheeks to prevent the sensor from becoming dislodged. The tips of the sensors should not touch the lips, skin, or nasal membranes.

Pressure transducers use nasal cannula–type sensors that fit into the nares to record nasal pressure. These cannulas also loop around the patient's ears and can be taped to the cheeks if necessary. When both a pressure transducer and a thermal sensor are used, the thermal transducer is generally placed over the nasal cannula.

Oximeter Probe

The finger oximeter indirectly records pulse and blood oxygen levels using a small light that shines through the finger to a photodetector on the other side. The maximum acceptable signal averaging time for pulse oximetry during PSG is 3 seconds.

Determining the Appropriate Recording Site

If possible, the sensor should be placed on the index finger of the hand nearest to the oximeter. If the index finger does not yield an accurate reading, the ring or pinkie finger can be used as an alternate placement. There are alternate sensors available for most pulse oximeters that can record from the bridge of the nose and pediatric sensors that can be used to record from the base of the foot in infants.

Preparing the Recording Site

The fingernail should be free of nail polish and cleaned with rubbing alcohol before the sensor is attached. Artificial fingernails may prevent the probe from accurately measuring the oxygen saturation. Ideally, nail polish and artificial nails should be removed before the study, but, in reality, that is not always possible. If the patient has artificial fingernails, try applying the sensor to one of the patient's toes.

Applying a Disposable Oximeter Probe

To gauge accurate placement of a disposable probe and to ensure that the light-emitting diode (LED) aligns with the receptor diode, bend the probe in half before removing the tape so the two diodes line up, and place it over the patient's finger. Once the correct fit is assured, peel off the paper backing, place the LED above the nail, fold the sensor over the top of the finger so that the receptor diode is positioned opposite the LED against the pad of the fingertip. Wrap the tape around the finger, making sure the two sides are vertically aligned, and the diodes face each other directly. Then, to secure the finger sensor, tape the sensor wire to the wrist.

Take care to assure that the probe is not taped too tightly around the finger. After securing the sensor, ask the patient if any discomfort is felt. If the finger throbs, loosen and reapply the sensor.

Applying a Reusable Oximeter Probe

Place a flexible fingertip sensor over the tip of the finger, with the LED positioned above the nail and the receptor diode opposite the LED against the pad of the fingertip. Secure the sensor with tape and tape the sensor wire to the wrist. After securing the sensor, check to be sure that the tape is not too tight. Ask the patient if any discomfort is felt. If there is throbbing, loosen the tape and reapply the sensor.

A clip-type finger sensor fits over the tip of the finger. This type of sensor is typically placed on an index finger but in some patients, may be placed on another finger. Check for an acceptable signal, and then tape the wire to secure it to the wrist.

Position Sensor

The AASM recommends a position sensor to monitor the patient's sleeping position (2). However, some sleep centers still require the technologist to document any changes in body position in technologist notes to ensure that accurate information is available to the physician reviewing the study. Most position sensors are attached to one of the respiratory effort bands and recognize five different patient positions (standing/sitting, supine, prone, left side, and right side).

SETTING UP AND CALIBRATING THE EQUIPMENT

Enter the patient information into the computer, select the correct montage, test the equipment, and document the performance of the equipment. Equipment calibrations are essential for accurate signal measurement and data interpretation, so a 30-second machine calibration must be performed and stored as part of the record before and after every sleep study. More detailed information about technical settings can be found in other chapters in this textbook.

The mechanism to perform the calibration process will vary depending on the type of equipment and software used. The industry standard is to apply a negative 50-µV DC voltage to all channels to evaluate individual channel signal responses. This will document the correct signal polarity, amplitude, and time constant for each channel. During the calibration, the following features should be assessed:

- Correct signal polarity (confirm that there is an upward deflection in response to the negative voltage)
- Appropriate sensitivity settings for each channel (gauge the amplitude or height of the calibration wave in relation to the applied voltage)
- Correct filter settings for each channel (inspect the time constant or duration of the calibration wave)

If one of the channels does not give the expected response to the 50-µV DC voltage input, check the filter settings to be sure they are correct. For all channels, sensitivity (also called gain) should be adjusted at the beginning of the recording. Although in digital PSG changes made during the acquisition process are not permanent alterations to the incoming signal, the technologist should avoid unnecessary changes unless an adjustment is required to preserve the quality of the signals. Any changes to settings should be documented in the technologist notes.

CHECKING ELECTRODE IMPEDANCES AND SIGNAL QUALITY

After the machine calibrations are completed, the impedance levels of each electrode, including the ground and reference electrodes, must be checked. The impedance readings should be stored as part of the recording to document the quality and accuracy of the recorded signals. This is followed by a series of patient calibrations, also called "biocalibrations." AASM standards require repeat impedance checks and biocalibrations in the morning to document that signals did not deteriorate during the night (2).

Low-individual impedance levels ensure accurate signal transmission from each electrode and minimize the possibility of external signal interference by providing a clean pathway for the signal. High impedances defeat the passage of signals between the subject and the electrode, resulting in a poor signal. Most PSG recording systems use an internal impedance meter, although older software packages may still require the use of an external meter.

It is critical to understand the system you are using because some of the internal meters do not read individual impedance levels; instead, they measure the imbalance between selected pairs of electrodes. Therefore, to achieve accurate impedance readings, it is necessary to identify problematic electrodes or use an external meter such as a handheld AC impedance meter to check electrode impedances.

Ideally, the *individual* impedance level of all electrodes on the face and scalp should not exceed 5 kΩ. The impedance *differences* between paired EEG electrodes are also critical for preventing undesirable artifacts. Maintaining low-individual impedance readings (below 5 kΩ) assures that the difference in impedance levels between paired electrodes will be minimal. On some systems, the ground electrode connection may yield an artificially elevated reading because of the safety circuit breaker in the headbox, sometimes reporting as much as 5 kΩ more than the true impedance. Move this electrode to another position in the headbox or use a handheld meter to evaluate the true impedance level.

It is not always possible to obtain ideal impedance readings, particularly for the leg EMG channels. If the electrode impedance at a particular site remains high despite troubleshooting, the efforts to resolve the problem should be documented in the technologist notes.

TROUBLESHOOTING TECHNIQUES

Troubleshooting equipment issues begins with the basics; always start by checking that the system is plugged in properly, turned on, and that all cables and wires are securely connected.

- If an electrode has a high impedance level (>5 kΩ), it should be removed and the site re-prepped before the electrode is reattached. Care should be taken not to overscrub an area, because patient discomfort, bruising, or, in extreme situations, skin injury can result from too much scrubbing.
- If electrical noise is seen in all channels, check the patient ground and/or system reference connection.
- If the impedance reading is still high after reprepping and reattaching an electrode, there are two possible problems. The lead wire or electrode may be damaged, or the area of skin has unusually high impedance. A faulty electrode should be removed and replaced. If necessary, the electrode may be reattached immediately adjacent to the previous site.

BIOCALIBRATIONS

Biocalibrations are a series of exercises performed before initiating a study to verify correct input derivations, signal quality, and accurate signal response. It is essential to record the AASM-recommended biocalibrations at the beginning and end of each study to facilitate scoring and interpretation of the study (2). Additional calibrations must be performed if additional signals, such as upper limb EMG, are recorded. During biocalibrations, be sure to allow enough time between each set of instructions to make the corresponding signal response distinct and easily identifiable. Record each step of the process in the technologist notes.

If a signal does not respond in the expected fashion, always repeat the instruction and watch the video monitor to ensure that the patient correctly carried out the procedure. It may be helpful to explain the exercise in a different way or go into the bedroom to demonstrate the action. See Table 35-2 for an example set of biocalibrations.

Table 35-2 Example Set of Biocalibrations

Instruction	Channel	Expected Response	Possible Fixes
None	ECG	Correct signal polarity, R wave should deflect upward.	Change headbox or invert signal.
None	EEG, EOG, EMG	Impedances within acceptable range	Check electrode, reattach if necessary.
Eyes open (30 s)	EEG	Mixed-frequency EEG	Check electrode placements.
Eyes closed (30 s)	EEG	EEG should change from mixed frequency to alpha rhythm.	Check electrode placements.
Look left and right (5 times each direction)	EOG	Distinct, opposite deflections that are somewhat blunt or squared. Looking left should bring the signals together; looking right should take the signals apart.	Check derivations, filter settings, and electrode placements.
Look up and down (5 times each direction)	EOG	Distinct, opposite deflections that come together in a peak. Looking down should bring the signals together; looking up should take the signals apart.	Check derivations, filter settings, and electrode placements.
Blink (5 times)	EOG	Distinct, opposite deflections going first apart and then coming together before returning to baseline	Check derivations, filter settings, and electrode placements.
Grit teeth or chew (5 s)	Chin EMG	Bursts of activity on chin EMG channel	Check derivations, filter settings, and electrode placements, or try re-referencing to backup electrode.
Simulate a snore or hum (5 s)	Snore	Bursts of activity on snore channel, which may bleed over to the chin EMG	Check filter settings and position of sensor or replace sensor.
Breathe normally (10 s)	Respiratory	Clean sine wave, without spikes or electrical noise with all respiratory channels in phase (move together). Check polarity and note IN vs OUT.	Adjust sensitivity or gain levels, or invert signal if appropriate.

(*continued*)

Table 35-2 Example Set of Biocalibrations (*continued*)

Instruction	Channel	Expected Response	Possible Fixes
Hold breath (10 s)	Respiratory	Simulates a central apnea. Respiratory effort and flow channels should be flat.	Reposition or replace bands or flow sensors.
Breathe through nose only (10 s)		Clean sine wave, without spikes or electrical noise on nasal cannula.	Reposition or replace bands or flow sensors.
Breathe through mouth only (10 s)		Clean sine wave, without spikes or electrical noise on oral thermal sensor.	Reposition or replace bands or flow sensors.
Transfer breath	Respiratory	Simulates paradoxic breathing. Respiratory effort deflections should be out of phase (opposite movements), and flow channels should be flat.	Reposition or replace bands or flow sensors.
Flex right foot (5 times)	Leg EMG	Bursts of activity on right leg EMG channel	Check electrode placements.
Flex left foot (5 times)	Leg EMG	Bursts of activity on left leg EMG channel	Check electrode placements.

This table includes an example of instructions to give the patient at both the beginning and the end of the study, which electrode should be impacted, how the recording should change during the task, and suggested corrections. If a signal does not show the anticipated response, always confirm if the patient correctly performed the exercise before making any adjustments.
ECG, electrocardiogram; EEG, electroencephalogram; EMG, electromyogram; EOG, electrooculogram.

Electrocardiogram Channel

Take a moment to verify that the polarity of the ECG signal is correct. If it is reversed, the ECG leads should be switched in the headbox. If changing the leads in the headbox is not possible or does not correct the problem, the ECG signal can be inverted using the PSG software, and the alteration should be documented.

Electroencephalogram Channels

Ask the patient to relax with their eyes open for at least 30 seconds and then with the eyes closed for 30 seconds. Alpha waves are typically prominent and should be seen in the occipital channels when the eyes are closed.

If no alpha waves are present and the patient definitely has their eyes closed, check the electrode placement of O1 and O2 to be sure that the electrodes are in the correct location. If the measurements are confirmed, it is possible that the individual is not an alpha producer, which should be documented in the technologist's notes along with all troubleshooting efforts.

Electrooculogram Channels

Instruct the patient to keep the head still and move just the eyes left and right several times. Then instruct them to look up and down several times. Next, ask the patient to blink the eyes slowly and distinctly 5 times. The tracings should show prominent deflections in the EOG channels, with a significant difference between the three types of movements.

If no movement is detected on the EOG channels, it may be necessary to demonstrate the exercise to the patient to confirm whether they understood the instructions. If the patient is following the instructions correctly but the waveforms are still not responding, the derivations and filter settings should be confirmed. Finally, the placement of the two eye electrodes (E1 and E2) should be verified.

Chin Electromyogram Channel

Ask the patient to grit the teeth or chew for 5 seconds. The EMG tracing should show a burst of activity when the teeth are clenched or the patient is chewing. Next, instruct the patient to relax, to be sure the EMG tracing shows an adequate level of baseline muscle tone (at least 0.5 cm in amplitude).

If the chin EMG does not pick up the muscle activity and you are sure the patient is gritting their teeth, confirm whether the derivation and filter settings are correct and whether the EMG electrodes are correctly placed. Try re-referencing the EMG channel to the backup electrode in an effort to improve the signal and identify which electrode is the source of the problem.

Snore Channel

Ask the patient to simulate a snore or hum for 5 seconds. The snore channel tracing should show a high degree of deflection during this maneuver. If the snore channel does not show a response, the filter settings should be checked and, if necessary, the sensor should be repositioned. If moving the sensor does not rectify the problem, replace the sensor.

Respiratory Channels

With normal breathing, the airflow and respiratory effort channels should show a clean sine wave, without spikes or electrical noise. All channels should be in phase. The sensitivity or gain levels of the respiratory channels should be adjusted to obtain adequate deflections and to avoid signal blocking.

During the night, as the subject moves or changes body positions, the respiratory bands may shift and cause changes in signal amplitude, requiring channel sensitivity adjustments. If the bands become too loose, or the airflow sensor becomes displaced, manual readjustment of the sensors may be necessary to maintain a quality signal. Any changes to the bands or to the settings made after lights out should be well documented in the technologist notes.

To test the signals, instruct the patient to lie still and breathe normally for 15 to 20 seconds and then hold their breath for 10 seconds. During the breath hold, the respiratory channels should show a flat line. Next, ask the patient to breathe through the nose for only 10 seconds and then through the mouth only for 10 seconds. To simulate paradoxic breathing effort, you may ask the patient to make breathing efforts during a breath hold. This instruction can be relayed as trying to sip a very thick milkshake through a clogged straw. This should result in out-of-phase (opposite) deflections in the respiratory effort channels while the airflow channels remain flat.

Leg Electromyogram

Ask the patient to flex or extend the big toe of each foot several times to see a burst of activity in the recording. Each leg should be tested separately. If there is no change in recorded muscle activity, it may be necessary to demonstrate the exercise to the patient to confirm if they understood the instructions. If the patient is correctly performing the task and there is still no change in signal, the derivation and filter settings should be checked. If the problem persists, verify that the leg EMG electrodes are in the proper position over the anterior tibialis muscle. If upper limb EMG is recorded, the appropriate maneuvers to verify correct operation of these sensors must also be completed.

CONCLUDING A POLYSOMNOGRAM STUDY

Overnight polysomnograms are typically run for at least 6 hours to ensure sufficient data are collected to adequately assess the patient's sleep. PAP titrations should continue for at least 3 hours after initiating treatment in order to allow adequate time for the patient to progress through all the sleep stages and body positions at the optimal PAP level.

Because of the higher percentage of REM sleep in the last third of the night, it is not unusual for a patient to be in REM when it is time to end the study. If time permits, allow patients to complete the REM period before calling lights on and waking the patient up.

After the patient is awake but before being disconnected, check and document impedance levels, and repeat biocalibrations and machine calibrations before stopping the recording. If a polysomnogram is terminated early at the specific request of the patient, the technologist may need to complete an against medical advice form, and the technologist must document the circumstances.

Procedure for Waking a Patient

1. Enter "lights on" in the technologist notes, and record the time in the study log.
2. Enter the patient's room and explain that the test is over and that calibrations will be performed. If conducting a PAP study, remove the mask and turn off the PAP machine.
3. Repeat the impedance check and biocalibrations performed at the beginning of the night. Note any equipment that is malfunctioning in the technical summary.
4. End the acquisition according to system software instructions.
5. Ask if the patient needs to use the bathroom. When the patient is comfortable, remove all the electrodes and sensors from the patient.
   a. Remove electrode paste from the scalp and face with warm water.
   b. Remove electrodes attached with collodion using acetone or collodion remover, taking care to avoid the patient's eyes. A syringe with collodion remover or small cotton balls or pieces of gauze are best used for this procedure. Carefully soak each electrode site until the electrode loosens, and then wipe away any excess collodion residue. Ask the patient to tilt the head backward, to prevent any acetone or remover from dripping toward the face.
   c. Loosen tape by moistening with water, alcohol, or adhesive remover as needed for patient comfort.

Documentation

Documentation protocols vary by sleep center; however, the key information to be relayed is usually fairly standard. It is standard in most sleep centers to include the following information in the technical summary report at the end of a shift:

- "Lights off" and "lights on" times
- Patient's overall sleep quality
- Degree of snoring, if any
- Positions in which the patient slept, positional effects on respiratory events, oxygen saturation levels, and sleep quality
- Presence, frequency, and severity of respiratory disturbances
- Presence, frequency, and severity of ECG abnormalities
- Presence, frequency, and severity of periodic limb movements
- Lowest oxygen saturation recorded
- Any cardiac, respiratory, seizure, or other medical conditions that may require follow-up or medical attention
- Any other pertinent patient observations (unusual sleep patterns or unusual behaviors)
- Optimal PAP setting(s), if used
- Equipment problems or persistent recording artifacts, if any

Before signing off on a patient chart, confirm whether all the necessary patient and technologist paperwork has been completed, and then place all patient records in locked storage, following standard procedures of the Health Insurance Portability and Accountability Act (HIPAA). In case of medical conditions that require immediate attention, contact the attending or on-call physician before allowing the patient to leave the sleep center.

Discharging the Patient

Be sure to allow adequate time in the morning for the patient to complete any morning paperwork required by the sleep center protocol and get ready for the patient's day. It may be helpful to ask the patient the night before how long they will need to shower and get dressed once disconnected from the electrodes. After a long, overnight shift it may be tempting to rush the patient out in the morning, but customer service is an important part of the job. Taking a few extra minutes to attend to the patient's needs will significantly improve their experience. After the patient has been discharged from the sleep center or while they are getting ready to leave, clean all the equipment and the work area.

SUGGESTED READINGS

American Association of Sleep Technologists. *Standard polysomnography: technical guideline.* 2021. Retrieved March 9, 2025. https://www.aastweb.org/Portals/0/Docs/Resources/Guidelines/AAST%20PSG%20Guideline%20Final.pdf

Harner PF, Sannit T. *A Review of the International Ten–Twenty System of Electrode Placement.* Grass Instrument; 1974.

Kapur VK, Auckley DH, Chowdhuri S, et al. Clinical practice guideline for diagnostic testing for adult obstructive sleep apnea: an American Academy of Sleep Medicine clinical practice guideline. *J Clin Sleep Med.* 2017;13(3):479-504.

Kushida CA, Littner MR, Morgenthaler T, et al. Practice parameters for the indications for polysomnography and related procedures: an update for 2005. *Sleep.* 2005;28:499-521.

REFERENCES

1. Harner PF, Sannit T. *A Review of the International Ten–Twenty System of Electrode Placement.* Grass Instrument; 1974.
2. American Academy of Sleep Medicine. The AASM manual for the scoring of sleep and associated events: rules, terminology and technical specifications, version 3. 2023. Accessed November 8, 2025. https://aasm.org/clinical-resources/scoring-manual/
3. Arnardottir ES, Isleifsson B, Agustsson JS, et al. How to measure snoring? A comparison of the microphone, cannula and piezoelectric sensor. *J Sleep Res.* 2016;25(2):158-168.

Chapter 36
Polysomnographic Recording Procedures

RACHEL FORDYCE

KEY CONCEPTS/LEARNING OBJECTIVES

The key concepts of this chapter include identifying the key prerequisites for obtaining quality artifact-free data, describing appropriate patient monitoring and documentation procedures, recognizing clinical and technical issues that require a technologist response. The recording technologist must recognize common causes of recording artifacts, identify and correct common artifacts in various recording parameters, and utilize principles of system referencing, re-referencing techniques, and other strategies to maintain recording quality as well as describe the processes related to ending the study and discharging the patient.

KEY TERMS

50/60-Hz artifact
Artifacts
Montage
Signal derivations
System referencing
Re-referencing

The basic concepts of obtaining high-quality, artifact-free recordings have not changed despite considerable technologic advancements over the years that have impacted how we collect, process, and view polysomnographic (PSG) data. The three major factors include the following:

- Proper electrode and sensor application
- Accurate signal processing
- Conscientious maintenance of the recording

This chapter focuses on how to utilize the available tools offered by today's digital sleep recording systems to obtain a high-quality, artifact-free sleep study.

ELECTRODE APPLICATION

The first step toward obtaining an artifact-free polysomnogram is the proper application and correct placement of the electrodes and sensors. Although all data collection systems have mechanisms to filter data, they are meant to fine-tune the signal being collected, not disguise or repair a nonexistent or bad signal related to poor electrode application. Poor electrode application cannot be fixed through aggressive filtration and signal manipulation because excessive signal filtering will obscure or alter the data.

Careful attention should be paid to each of the following steps during the hookup process to attain a quality recording:

- Precise head measurements for the electroencephalogram (EEG) electrodes
- Careful site preparation, scrubbing an area no larger than the size of the electrode cup
- Utilization of high-quality electrodes (typically, gold cup electrodes)
- Secure adhesion of the electrodes to the skin
- Low and relatively equal electrode impedances (<5 kΩ as measured by an AC impedance meter)
- Proper management of the electrode wires

For a more detailed explanation of electrode application techniques, see Chapter 35, *Preparing the Patient for Polysomnography*.

SIGNAL PROCESSING

Once the electrodes and sensors are in place, the resulting signal must be processed in a standardized manner to ensure consistent output across individuals as well as sleep centers. Signal processing includes amplification of the signal, filtration, analog-to-digital conversion, and signal display.

Basic considerations for proper signal processing include the following:

- The use of high-quality amplifiers
- Sturdy electrical connections

- Adequate electrical shielding
- Proper electrical grounding of equipment
- Appropriate filter settings for each recorded parameter
- Adequate sampling rates for each recorded parameter
- Correct signal polarity
- Adequate computer screen resolution (digital screen and video card must be at least 1,600 × 1,200)
- Documentation of all signal manipulations

The American Academy of Sleep Medicine (AASM) updates its guidelines (1) regularly. Every technologist is responsible for reviewing the current standards, including requirements for digital PSG recording, because they represent the essential requirements for performing and scoring polysomnograms.

Today, it is recommended that a digital PSG system include the following features:

- A mechanism to perform visual (on-screen) electrical calibrations for all channels by applying a negative 50 mV DC voltage to document correct signal polarity, amplitude, and time constant
- A separate 50/60-Hz notch filter for every channel
- The ability to program sampling rates for each channel
- The capacity to measure individual impedance levels for each electrode against a common reference (may be the sum of all other applied electrodes)
- The capability to retain and display all settings used by the attending technologist, including adjustments to derivations, sensitivity, filters, and temporal resolution
- A filter design that mimics conventional, analog-style frequency response curves

The AASM also suggests as an optional feature that all systems have the flexibility to choose and/or change the electrode input signal derivations without relying on a common reference electrode.

SELECTING THE APPROPRIATE MONTAGE

Today, virtually all digital sleep systems allow you to select which channels to monitor during a study by allowing customizable settings for the electrode derivation, sensitivity, filter settings, label, color, and analysis properties for each channel. The arrangement of the recording channel selections and their settings is called a montage. Multiple montages can be developed and saved. The proper montage will be developed and chosen based on the study type and requirements specified by the sleep physician. An example of a sleep apnea diagnostic montage using the AASM-recommended specifications is shown in (1,2). The technologist must ensure that the correct montage is chosen during the setup process because the montage cannot be changed once the recording is initiated.

Examples of common montages include the following:

- Sleep apnea diagnostic evaluation
- Positive airway pressure (PAP) titration
- Seizure
- Multiple sleep latency test (MSLT)/maintenance of wakefulness test (MWT)
- Specialty equipment (transcutaneous CO_2, end-tidal CO_2)

Before choosing a montage, carefully review the physician's order to be sure you select the montage that will record the appropriate physiologic data. A quality hookup is a wasted effort if the appropriate information is not recorded, and the study has to be repeated.

INITIATING THE RECORDING

It is time to initiate the recording when the montage has been selected, patient demographics have been entered in the system, and the patient is properly hooked up. Once the study is recording, electrical calibrations are performed for at least 30 seconds to ensure that the equipment is functioning properly and the correct filter settings and sampling rates have been selected.

The next step is to start the system to test the impedance levels of each electrode to confirm a secure attachment. Most sleep systems have an impedance meter built into the software, but an external AC impedance meter can be used if necessary. Ideally, all electrodes should have relatively equal and low (<5 kΩ) impedance readings. If any channel reports a high level of impedance, the electrode should be reapplied or replaced before starting the recording.

After verifying that each electrode provides an optimal signal, perform biocalibrations to assess whether the sensors are in the correct location and record appropriate physiologic information. The patient should be walked through a series of exercises known as biocalibrations designed to provide a baseline signal for each channel. It is important to document each of these instructions in the technologist's notes and allow several seconds between successive exercises to allow time for the signals to return to baseline.

Once all these items have been completed, the patient is ready for bed. Turn the lights off in the bedroom, and document the "lights out" information in the technologist's notes. It is common to record details such as the bedtime, body position, and oxygen saturation at the beginning of a study.

MONITORING THE PATIENT AND DOCUMENTING DURING THE RECORDING

Once the patient is in bed for the night, the pace of the night usually changes significantly, but that does not mean the work is done. Every patient must be carefully monitored over the course of the night to ensure the patient is safe, the necessary information is collected, and there are no disruptions to data collection.

Q30 Documentation

One element of cohesive data collection is the detailed and professional documentation, throughout the night. Some sleep centers require Q30 documentation, which is a structured technologist note entered every 30 minutes. It is possible to program some of the digital systems to prompt for a technologist note at preselected intervals with a pop-up dialog box. The content of these notes varies depending on sleep center policy. Standard comments include information such as body position, PAP setting (if applicable), heart rate, Sao_2, CO_2 levels (if available), and any other relevant patient updates like sleep stage, snoring, or unresolved artifact. Keep in mind that the technologist notes are part of the official medical record, so they should contain facts rather than opinions or speculations about a diagnosis.

Waveform Recognition

A sleep technologist must be able to read and interpret the data being collected to effectively run a sleep study. A basic knowledge of sleep stages is necessary to differentiate wake from sleep and assess the quality of sleep throughout the night. However, monitoring a patient is more than just identifying sleep spindles or rapid eye movements. A sleep technologist must also be able to understand how the various channels of data impact one another to truly understand whether the data being viewed are a true physiologic event or artifact requiring correction.

Sleep apnea, in particular, is a complex phenomenon that impacts multiple biologic systems. Abnormal breathing events impact not only respiration and oxygen saturation but also cardiac function, muscle tone, and, of course, sleep consolidation. Therefore, the data should be interpreted as a whole in addition to assessing each channel independently.

Assessment of Sleep Disorders

The most common reason patients undergo overnight PSG is for evaluation of sleep-related breathing disorders (SRBDs), which is an umbrella term for disorders related to abnormal breathing during sleep with repeated interruption of breathing. There are several different types of sleep-disordered breathing, including obstructive sleep apnea (OSA), central sleep apnea (CSA), mixed sleep apnea (MSA), and upper airway resistance syndrome (UARS). During sleep, apneas can be caused by a physical obstruction, such as that seen in OSA, the most common type of SRBD. Breathing pauses can also be caused by a disruption of the central nervous system, as is seen in CSA. Each disorder has a spectrum of severity levels ranging from mild to severe.

Each type of sleep apnea has a different approach to treatment; therefore, it is imperative that every sleep technologist understands the differences between the disorders and is able to correctly identify which type of event is being witnessed. The technologist must also be able to differentiate between different types of obstructive events (respiratory effort-related arousal [RERA], hypopnea, and apnea).

Although sleep apnea is the most prevalent disorder seen in the sleep center, other disorders should not be overlooked. Understanding the physiologic data that is seen during the recording is key to the correct diagnosis and treatment for any patient. Most sleep centers have a copy of the *International Classification of Sleep Disorders*, third edition (*ICSD-3*), which can be consulted when necessary.

RESPONDING TO PATIENT NEEDS

For many patients, a night in the sleep center is uneventful. However, the technologist must be vigilant throughout the night to ensure the patient is safe and comfortable at all times.

Responding to Physiologic Data

There are a number of factors, ranging from a medical emergency to a restroom break, that require the technologist to intervene during a sleep study. The technologist must be alert and attentive to identify a potential issue, assess the situation, and, if appropriate, take action.

Signal Issues

There are numerous opportunities for signal failure during a sleep study. The key is to identify a compromised signal as soon as possible and take the appropriate corrective action based on the situation.

Medical Emergencies

Medical emergencies are fairly uncommon; however, the unexpected can occur at any time, so it is imperative that every sleep technologist is certified in cardiopulmonary resuscitation (CPR) and basic life support, is able to use an automated external defibrillator (AED), and is familiar with the sleep center's emergency protocol.

Cardiac issues are the most likely to be encountered in patients with sleep-disordered breathing, so a basic knowledge of cardiac arrhythmias is essential to distinguish life-threatening issues such as ventricular tachycardia from benign irregularities.

Medication Needs

Today, many sleep centers are not located in a hospital, so there is no convenient way to distribute medications. Therefore, patients are typically instructed by the daytime staff to bring with them any medications they need to take while at the sleep center on the night of the sleep study. Even if the sleep center is situated in a hospital with access to medications, most sleep centers avoid dispensing medications because sleep technologists are not generally authorized to administer medications. In most sleep centers, the patient will bring and self-administer the medication. If a patient arrives for the sleep study without the necessary medications, the on-call physician or medical director should be contacted to ensure that the study may proceed nonetheless.

Treatment Interventions

When a split-night study is indicated, it is imperative to clearly understand when the study should transition from diagnostic to PAP titration. Criteria for starting PAP are typically based on Medicare guidelines, although the exact policy may vary from one sleep center to another. The key is to obtain sufficient diagnostic data to document the presence of sleep apnea to both the clinician and the insurance company while leaving enough time to identify a therapeutic PAP pressure.

Early Termination of the Study

On occasion, a patient may ask to end the study early and leave the sleep center in the middle of the night. In this situation, the technologist should make a reasonable effort to convince the patient to stay and complete the study. However, if the patient insists on leaving, the technologist should document the situation and terminate the study. Early termination may result in patient safety and possible billing issues. Depending on the sleep center protocol, it may be necessary to have the patient sign an against medical advice form.

MAINTAINING THE RECORDING

A quality sleep recording requires vigilance to ensure the data recorded at the end of a study is just as accurate as the data collected at the beginning. Patients, especially children, often move, perspire, change body position, and pull at the electrode wires in their sleep. The sleep technologist is responsible for monitoring the data as it is recorded and making appropriate adjustments and corrections to the signals or replacing electrodes that have been inadvertently dislodged during the study. See Figure 36-1 for an example of a high-quality, artifact-free sleep tracing.

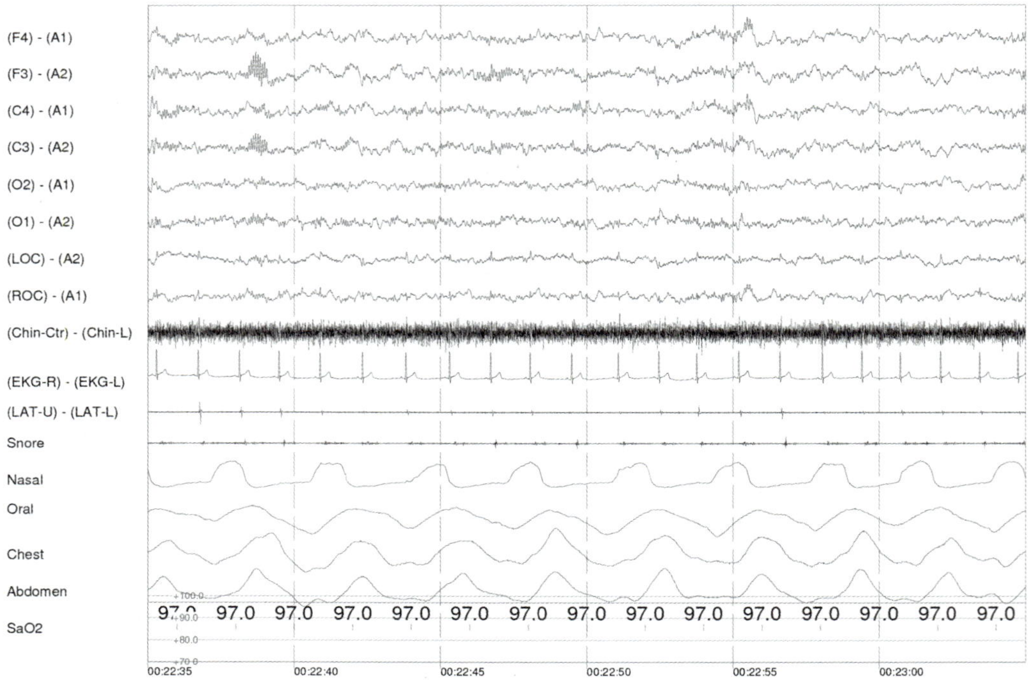

Figure 36-1 Artifact-free tracing. Example of a high-quality, artifact-free sleep tracing using the 2018 AASM-recommended derivations.

Selecting Display Features

The viewing resolution of each signal is dependent on the size and resolution of the computer monitor as well as the number of channels being displayed. When too many channels are viewed simultaneously, the subtle nuances of the waveform become lost due to their small size. Therefore, an overcrowded display can alter the recording technologist's perception as well as the scorer's or interpreter's perception of the data. In essence, viewing a limited number of flawlessly acquired channels may be more clinically relevant than viewing a large number of poorly recorded ones.

The 2023 AASM criteria (1) for scoring and review of sleep study data must meet or exceed the following standards:

- A 15-in screen size with a minimum of 1,600 pixels horizontal and 1,050 pixels vertical
- A minimum digital resolution of 12 bits per sample
- Histograms with stage, respiratory events, leg movement events, O_2 saturation, and arousals to be displayed
- Ability to position the cursor on the histogram and jump to the page selected
- Ability to view a screen on a timescale ranging from 5 seconds to the entire night
- Ability to synchronize the recorded video data with the PSG data and have an accuracy of at least one video frame per second
- Ability to display whether sleep staging scoring was performed visually or computed automatically by the software

The AASM also suggests the following optional criteria:

- Ability to turn pages automatically or scroll through the study
- Control key or toggle to turn off or invert a channel
- Ability to click and drag a channel to change display order
- Display setup profiles (including colors) that may be activated at any time
- Analysis options such as fast Fourier transformation or spectral analysis on specifiable intervals, including omission of data tagged as artifact
- Ability to turn on and off highlighting of EEG patterns used to make sleep stage decisions (eg, sleep spindles, K complexes, alpha activity)
- Ability to turn on and off highlighting of respiratory patterns used to make sleep stage decisions

Utilizing System References

The original analog amplifiers that processed sleep study data included an electrode selector panel used to specify the electrode derivations for each channel. During the night, the technologist could easily re-reference the signal by changing the selector panel to avoid waking the patient if an electrode became dislodged. Although this technique was very convenient, all changes to the data were permanent and, therefore, impossible to reverse once recorded. Today, digital recording systems are designed to collect and store each signal separately. The most common method references all EEG signals to a common electrode, typically placed on the midline of the scalp (Cz). This approach is known as system referencing. It has the advantage of allowing the viewer to change the electrode derivations at any time through software functions without permanently altering the raw data. Any desired derivation can then be viewed by digitally subtracting the common reference from any pair of EEG electrodes. For example, the signal for C3-M2 is created by simultaneously subtracting Cz from C3 and M2.

Despite this technique's advantages, such as preserving data integrity, system referencing does create risks for error because any electrode, including the system reference, may potentially become the source of artifacts. If the system reference signal becomes degraded, the entire recording is affected, and no amount of re-referencing will resolve the issue. Therefore, sleep technologists, as operators of digital recording equipment featuring system referencing, must be especially aware of the possibility of reference-generated artifacts and be cognizant of how signals should be combined to produce reliable, accurate waveforms.

Most software systems use a common reference to record and store data. Including systems with the flexibility to choose and/or change the electrode input signal derivations without relying on a common reference electrode, as suggested by the AASM, is currently an optional feature on most digital systems. It is essential that the recording software allows the capability of storing all derivation changes or any other signal manipulations performed by the technologist during the study so that the scorer/interpreter does not have to duplicate this process.

Utilizing Multiple Channel Recordings

An alternative solution to using a common system reference is to program the montage to include multiple derivations for each parameter. For example, both C3/M2 and C4/M1 can be recorded, which gives the viewer the option to change from C3/M2 to C4/M1 if the M2 channel should fail. The rationale is that if an electrode becomes dislodged, another derivation will be able to produce a readable alternative signal. The drawback to this approach is that preselecting derivations limits the options for re-referencing during the night. This is especially important if multiple electrodes go bad and creativity is needed to correct the issue. For example, if the C3 and M1 signals are both degraded, neither the C3-M2 nor the C4-M1 derivation will be acceptable. With re-referencing capabilities, a derivation of C4-M2 may be selected, at least temporarily, until the problem can be corrected without unduly disturbing the patient.

Utilizing Filters and Filtering

Filters are used in PSG to isolate and record specific frequency bandwidths relevant to each recording parameter while eliminating surplus signal information. The AASM has set standard filter configurations for each channel to minimize the presence of unwanted signal frequencies while preserving the signals of interest (1,2). As a general rule, the filter settings should be changed only when all other efforts to eliminate unwanted artifact have failed. There are three different types of filters that can be employed to correct artifact: low-frequency filter (LFF), high-frequency filter (HFF), and 50/60-Hz notch filter.

Low-Frequency Filter

The LFF (high-pass filter) allows high-frequency signals through while reducing signals with frequencies lower than the cutoff value, which is determined by the time constant. The LFF can be increased to diminish or eliminate the presence of slow-wave artifact resulting from sweat or respiratory artifact (see section Common Recording Artifacts). The standard LFF setting for EEG and electrooculogram (EOG) is 0.3 Hz.

High-Frequency Filter

The HFF (low-pass filter) does the exact opposite of the LFF by attenuating high-frequency signals while preserving low-frequency signals. It is unusual to alter the HFF during the night. The HFF is generally set at 35 Hz for EEG and EOG channels.

50/60-Hz Notch Filter

The 50/60-Hz notch filter reduces interference caused by outside electrical interference from outlets, power cords, and electrical ancillary equipment. Common mode rejection should eliminate most 50/60-Hz artifact if the electrodes have been properly attached and the surrounding equipment is functioning correctly; therefore, additional filtration should not be needed. However, the 50/60-Hz notch filter can be used to temporarily resolve artifacts until the problem can be identified and corrected.

Overfiltering affects the integrity of the recording by hiding problems that should be corrected at the source rather than filtered. Care must be taken, therefore, not to overprocess the input signals. Using filters to reduce artifacts is only appropriate when the underlying physiologic signals are intact, which means the electrode impedances are in an acceptable range and the connections are sound. Filters can be used to temporarily correct an artifact that is caused by body movements, sweat, or direct pressure against one of the electrodes. If the underlying physiologic signals from the patient are lost or distorted, filtering the signal will not solve the problem.

RECORDING ARTIFACTS

Even when careful attention is devoted to the hookup process, some degree of artifact can be expected to occur in virtually every sleep study. By definition, artifacts are extraneous signals appearing within any of the recorded parameters of the polysomnogram. These signals can originate from the patient's body, from recording instruments and devices used on the patient, or from the surrounding environment. The task of the sleep technologist includes recognizing the artifact, determining its origin, and deciding on the most appropriate way to address the problem.

It is important to keep in mind that not all artifacts are considered undesirable. For example, the "snoring artifact," often seen in the chin electromyogram (EMG) channel, is useful for confirming the accuracy of the snore channel (Figure 36-2). Muscle-generated artifacts seen during patient movement help identify arousals. These and certain other physiologic artifacts can be quite useful in the interpretation of the polysomnogram and should not be removed from the recording.

However, many types of artifacts are undesirable and can severely impede the scoring and interpretation process. These include 50- or 60-Hz power line frequencies; slow-frequency artifacts caused by sweat; electrode "popping" artifacts; electrocardiogram (ECG) artifacts recorded in the EEG, EOG, or EMG channels; and various other interfering signals recorded within any of the channels.

Artifact Recognition

Most recording artifacts can be recognized by their exaggerated appearance. However, in some cases, it may be difficult to discern artifacts and physiologic signals of interest. For example, sweat artifact in the EEG is usually identified by excessively slow frequency, but sometimes, the intruding waves may appear similar to high-amplitude delta waves. An advantage offered by multichannel PSG is the ability to cross-examine the recording to see whether the signals in question correlate with other recorded parameters. For example, if questionable slow waves are seen in the central EEG channel but are not appropriately reflected in the occipital or eye movement channels, they are likely artifact. For this reason, EEG frequencies are not filtered from the eye

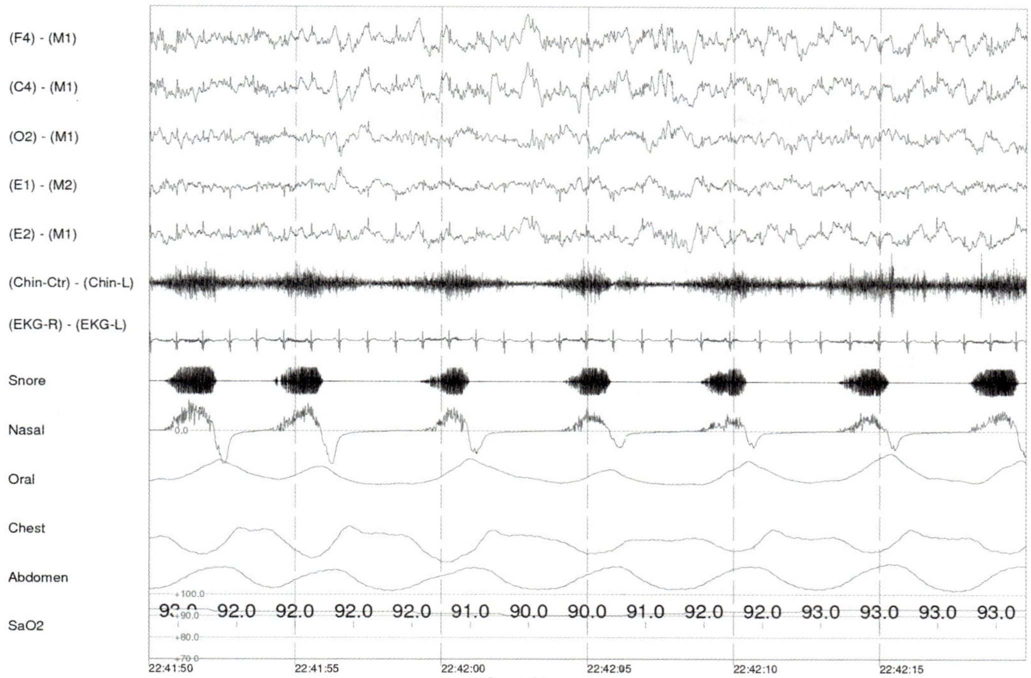

Figure 36-2 Snoring artifact in the chin electromyogram, electrocardiogram, and nasal airflow channels. Notice that the respiratory effort bands are out of phase, which may suggest paradoxic breathing.

channels. In addition to detecting eye movements, EOG channels record frontal EEG activity. The combined tracings from the central, occipital, and eye movement channels allow for cross-examination of these signals to confirm normal voltage distribution (higher voltages in the frontal region and lower voltages in the occipital region) and identify exaggerated, stray voltages that do not correlate with adjoining channels.

Cross-examining channels can also help identify the source of the artifact by comparing adjacent channel tracings. For example, if an identical artifact is seen in two or more channels sharing the same reference (eg, C3-M2 and O1-M2), it can be assumed that the artifact originates from the reference electrode. Alternatively, if an artifact appears in only one channel (sharing a common reference with other channels), the problem can be attributed to the exploring electrode.

Artifact Correction

When an unwanted artifact is detected, whether environmental or biologic in nature, it should be documented and corrected as soon as possible. As a general rule, when an artifact is localized to just one channel, it typically indicates that the problem lies with just one electrode. Unfortunately, there is no hard and fast rule for how to correct artifact, because there are many different causes of signal interference and often multiple solutions. In some scenarios, like muscle artifact, no corrective action is required because the situation will resolve itself. Other circumstances require immediate intervention to correct the problem, such as a displaced airflow sensor or an oximeter.

If a problem is detected during the impedance check or biocalibrations, every effort should be made to resolve the issue before starting the study, even if it requires reattaching electrodes or replacing sensors. However, if an artifact develops after the patient has fallen asleep, replacing the electrode may not be the best course of action. Often, it is possible to eliminate undesirable artifacts by re-referencing the input signal derivation to an alternate exploring or reference site, with proper documentation. For example, if an artifact contaminates the C4 channel, the signal input can be changed to C3. If the artifact originates from a reference site, such as M2, then the reference input may be changed to the opposite side (M1). However, if the patient awakens to use the restroom, the problematic electrode should always be fixed at the source, and the system should be returned to the standard derivations.

Artifacts often originate from the side of the head or face on which the patient is lying, usually due to sweat or direct pressure against the electrode. Because the patient changes body position during a sleep study, several derivation changes may be necessary. To perform signal derivation changes, the recording equipment must provide a method for making these changes. Essentially, all digital systems have this functionality through either system referencing or the ability to simultaneously record multiple electrode derivations.

Although a sleep center may have a policy regarding re-referencing or artifact tolerance, the sleep technologist must often use judgment to assess whether the problem warrants waking the patient. For instance, if the recording is compromised to the point where the sleep stage cannot be determined, the patient should be disturbed to correct the issue. However, if there is still sufficient readable data being recorded to adequately monitor the patient, the best course of action may be to wait until the patient awakens naturally to repair the problem.

COMMON RECORDING ARTIFACTS

50/60-Hz Artifact

The most pervasive interfering signal is the 50- or 60-Hz power line frequency (60 Hz in the United States and 50 Hz in many other countries). Artifact caused by 50/60-Hz interference appears as a regular, sinusoidal wave, which completely obscures the physiologic signal, turning it into a thick, dark tracing. To qualify as 60-Hz interference, there must be exactly 60 oscillations (if recorded in the United States) per second. The oscillations should be counted on a 1-second display. If there are not exactly 60 oscillations, there is another cause for the artifact such as increased muscle tone. Figure 36-3A shows how 50/60-Hz artifact can obscure an EEG channel, and Figure 36-3B presents the same channel at a slower speed to demonstrate the regular appearance of the 60-Hz artifact. With the signal expanded from 30 seconds to 1 second, the 60-Hz artifact on the O1/M2 channel is easily distinguished from muscle artifact by the uniformed sinusoidal pattern (Figure 36-3C).

Normal levels of 50/60-Hz interference are minimized or eliminated with common mode rejection, provided the impedance levels among the electrodes are low (<5 kΩ) and relatively equal. The patient-ground electrode, which is not the same as the electrical ground, also helps dissipate 50/60-Hz interference. Despite these routine measures to combat 50/60-Hz interference, abnormally high levels of interference may still impact a recording. Excessive 50/60-Hz artifact is usually caused by high-electrode impedance levels or a poor electrical connection.

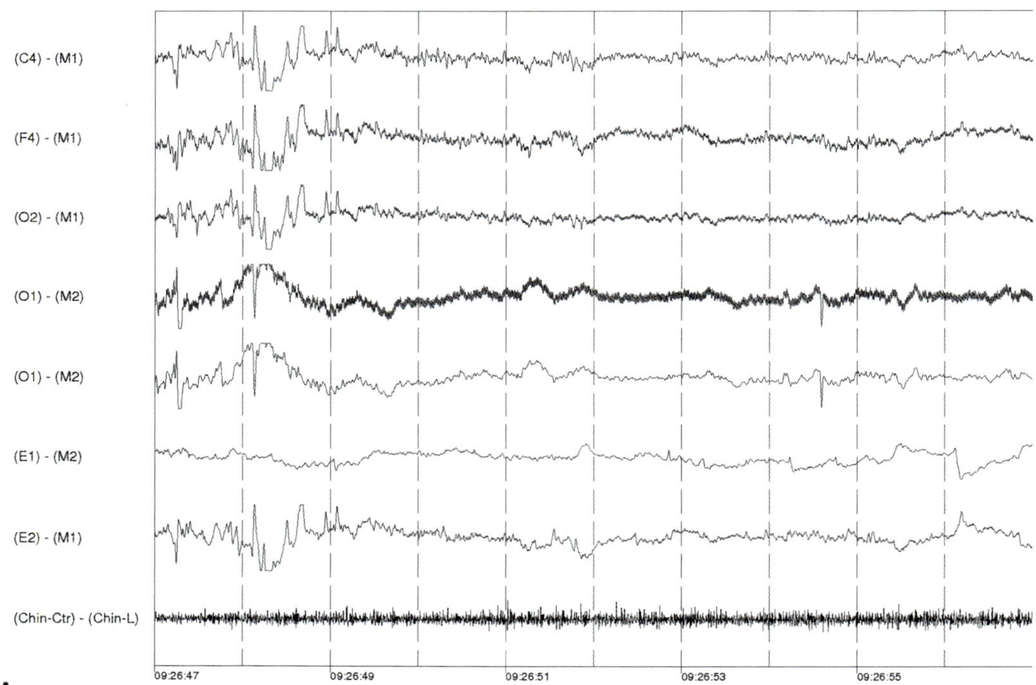

A

Figure 36-3 A: A 30-second epoch with 50/60-Hz artifact in the occipital channel. In this example, the O2/M1 channel appears twice. The top display shows the channel with the 60-Hz interference. The second instance uses the 60-Hz notch filter to correct the display and confirm the cause of the problem. In this scenario, the electrode should be reattached at the next available opportunity. B: 50/60-Hz artifact in occipital channel with a 1-second epoch. C: With the signal expanded from 30 seconds to 1 second, the 60-Hz artifact on the O1/M2 channel is easily distinguished from muscle artifact by the uniformed sinusoidal pattern.

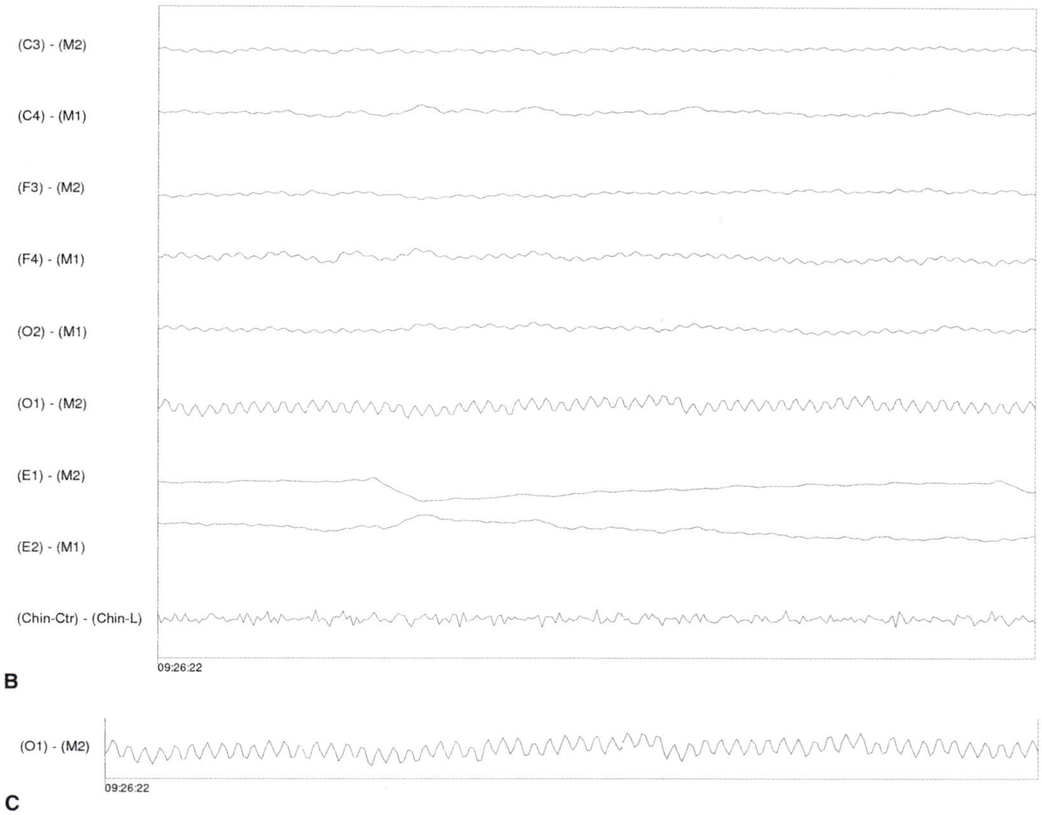

Figure 36-3 *(continued)*

Another cause of 50/60-Hz artifact is an excessive amount of current leakage originating from electrical ancillary equipment, extension cords, lamps, televisions, electric beds, fans, and so on. When the artifact originates from poorly shielded electrical equipment, it will impact all channels that include the 50/60-Hz frequency bandwidth.

The source of the artifact and the electrode in question dictate which technique should be used to resolve the problem. For example, the leg EMG recordings require extra-long leads and are therefore more likely to absorb 50/60-Hz interference from the surrounding environment. When minor line frequency interference appears in a leg EMG channel (which includes the 50/60-Hz frequency bandwidth), a 50/60-Hz notch filter can be used to remove the artifact. However, 50/60-Hz notch filters should not be used in the EEG or EOG channels, which are typically set below the 50/60-Hz bandwidth. The appearance of a 50/60-Hz artifact in any of these channels invariably indicates high impedances, a poor connection, a broken lead wire, or an unplugged lead. In these cases, the use of 50/60-Hz filters merely conceals the problem. To eliminate 50/60-Hz interference in EEG or EOG channels, the electrode connection causing the artifact must be identified and corrected.

Muscle Artifact

Muscle artifact is another form of fast or high-frequency artifact routinely encountered in the EEG, EOG, and, occasionally, the ECG tracings. Although the thick, dark tracing can look similar in appearance to 50/60-Hz interference, muscle artifact is distinguished by its irregular high frequency, as seen in Figure 36-4.

Muscle artifact is caused by localized muscle activity in the vicinity of an exploring or reference electrode and is commonly seen in tense or anxious patients. Muscle artifact usually disappears when the patient relaxes or falls asleep. If the artifact does not resolve on its own and the source of the artifact (usually a reference electrode) can be identified, the electrode derivation should be changed to a backup configuration. Then, at the next opportunity, correct the issue by repositioning the M1 and M2 electrodes to decrease extraneous muscle signals.

Cell Phone Artifact

A new variation of electrical interference comes from the use of cell phones and tablets in the sleep center. If a patient places a device near the headbox, intermittent communication with the service provider and incoming

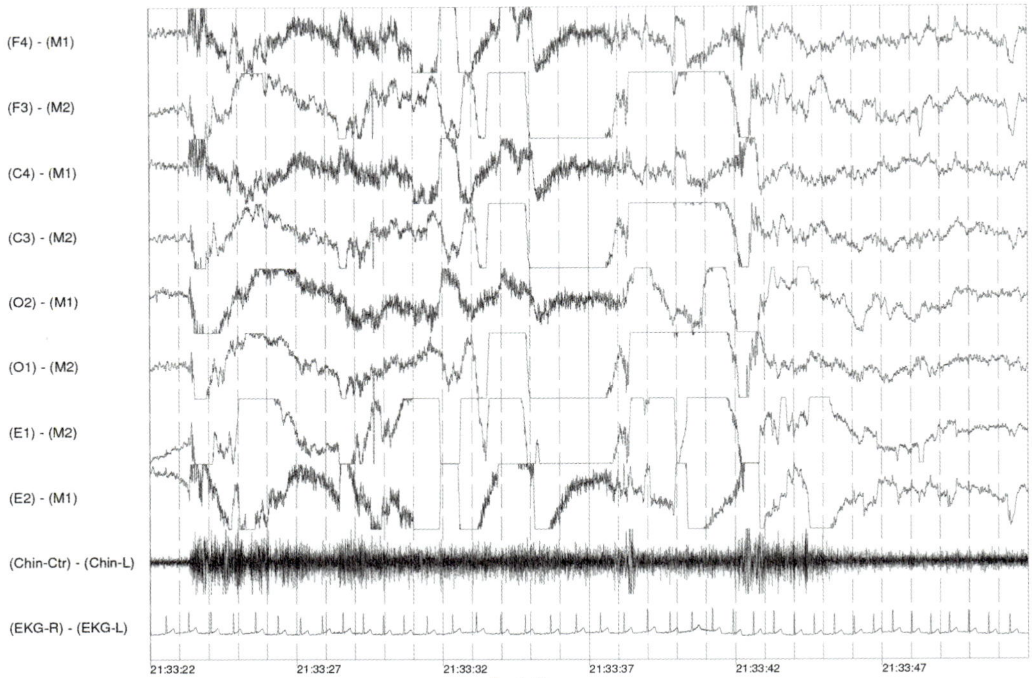

Figure 36-4 Muscle artifact in the electroencephalogram and electrooculogram channels. In this example, note how the artifact coincides with the increase in muscle activity measured by the chin electromyogram at the start of the epoch. As the muscle tone decreases, the artifact disappears, and the waveforms are once again readable.

messages or alerts may result in 100-μV low-frequency (5-9 Hz) sharply contoured waveforms with intermittent high-frequency (20-50 Hz) sinusoidal waves (2). This can be particularly problematic because EEG interference at this frequency can mimic spindles (11-16 Hz) and cause confusion with sleep staging. To mitigate this type of interference, mobile devices should be kept at least 32 inches away from recording equipment.

Electrocardiogram Artifact

ECG artifact consists of a visible intrusion of the ECG signal on the EEG, EOG, and/or EMG channels. ECG artifact is easily recognizable by the spike-like waves that coincide with each QRS complex of the ECG channel. Refer to Figure 36-5 for an example of ECG artifact.

Extraneous ECG signals are normally canceled by common mode rejection. However, due to the relatively long interelectrode distances used in standard PSG derivations (such as C3 referenced to M2), it is sometimes impossible to eliminate a small amount of ECG artifact in the EEG and EOG channels. This is particularly true when studying obese patients.

When an ECG artifact is found in just one channel, it is usually caused by impedance imbalances between the exploring and the reference electrodes. As with any form of undesirable artifact, utilizing proper electrode application techniques minimizes ECG interference. If an excessive ECG artifact originates in one of the reference electrodes, multiple channels will be affected. The electrodes should be reattached slightly above the mastoid process, over the firm bony area behind the ear (taking care not to place them too high). In order to reduce the possibility of ECG artifacts, avoid soft, fatty tissue behind the ears when applying the reference EEG electrodes M1 and M2 during the initial hookup procedure. If altering the placement of the reference electrodes does not correct the problem, the interference can be minimized or eliminated by linking the two reference electrodes M1 and M2. Double referencing an EEG or EOG channel essentially creates three divergent ECG signals that cancel each other out, thereby reducing the artifact. Using analog equipment, this was accomplished by double referencing the EEG and EOG channels through the electrode selector panel. Digital systems have provisions for double referencing using the system reference approach described earlier.

There are drawbacks to double referencing electrodes, so this technique should not be used routinely. Once the channels are double referenced, any other signal interference (such as sweat or muscle artifact) originating from either of the cross-linked reference electrodes will contaminate all the linked channels. In addition, if the artifact originates from one of the reference electrodes, cross-linking the reference electrodes

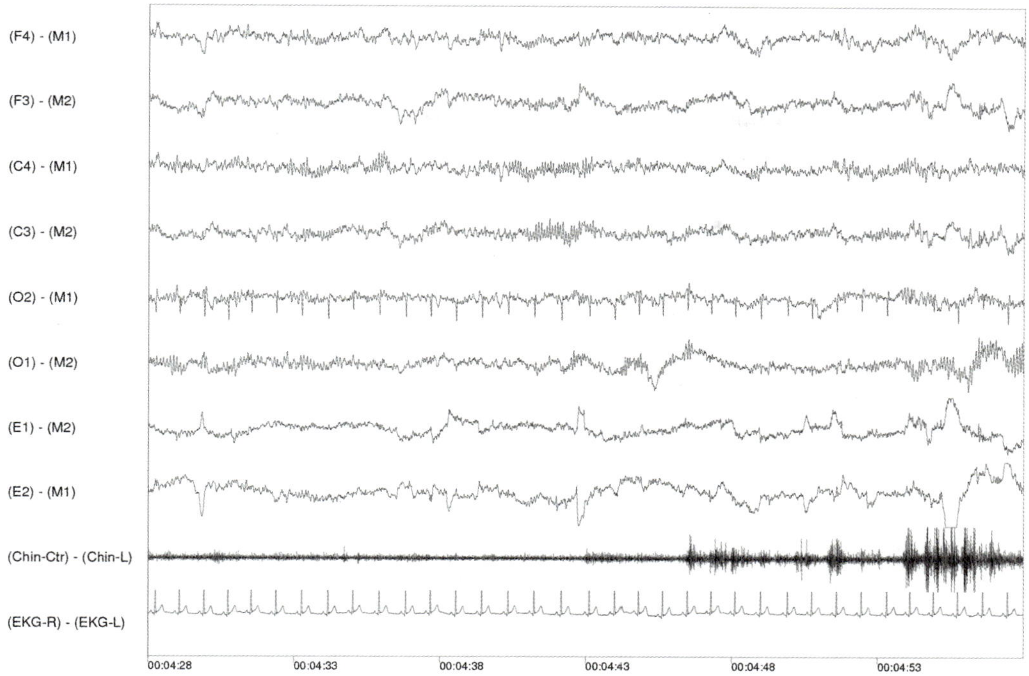

Figure 36-5 Electrocardiogram (ECG) artifact in the O2 channel. In this example, a prominent ECG signal can be clearly detected in the O2/M1 channel, but not in the other electroencephalogram or electrooculogram channels. Because the artifact is localized to just one channel, double referencing M1 and M2 is unlikely to resolve the problem.

will increase the artifact rather than reducing it. Furthermore, the use of additional reference electrodes on any channel may attenuate the signal of interest.

Slow-Frequency Artifacts

There are three main categories of slow-wave frequency artifacts routinely seen in PSG: sweat artifact, respiratory artifact, and electrode popping. These artifacts are occasionally confused with slow-wave sleep because of their slow frequency.

Sweat Artifact

Perspiration induces chemical changes in the electrolyte interface between the electrode and the patient's skin, causing the slow-oscillating wave patterns, commonly referred to as "sweat artifact." The huge, slow sways and wandering baseline differentiate sweat artifact from slow-wave sleep. See Figure 36-6 for an example of sweat artifact in the EEG and EOG channels.

If a patient perspires enough to cause sweat artifact in multiple channels, the technologist should attempt to cool the room with a fan or air-conditioning. If the artifact is affecting one side of the head, changing the derivation or re-referencing the electrodes is appropriate while waiting for the temperature in the room to decrease. As a last resort, the LFF in the EEG and/or EOG channel(s) can be raised from 0.3 to 1 Hz to reduce the amount of slow-wave activity in that channel. Any changes to the electrode derivation or filters must be properly documented.

Respiratory Artifact

Slow-frequency artifacts often appear synchronous with the patient's breathing patterns, as shown in Figure 36-6. However, "respiratory artifact" is a misleading term because it is unlikely that respiration alone is responsible for the problem. Although the slight movement of the head associated with breathing is often a contributing factor to slow artifacts, the underlying cause of these artifacts can usually be attributed to either a chemical or mechanical instability of the electrode/patient interface. Body movements associated with respiration may aggravate slow-frequency artifacts but, again, are rarely the direct cause of the problem.

It is very difficult to eliminate artifact caused solely by the slight head or body movements associated with respiration. If the artifact is excessive, the LFF in the EEG and/or EOG channel(s) can be raised from 0.3 to 1 Hz to decrease the slow-wave artifact. Modifications to the filter settings must be documented in the technologist's notes. If another type of slow-frequency artifact is being exacerbated by respiration, the primary cause of the artifact should be addressed.

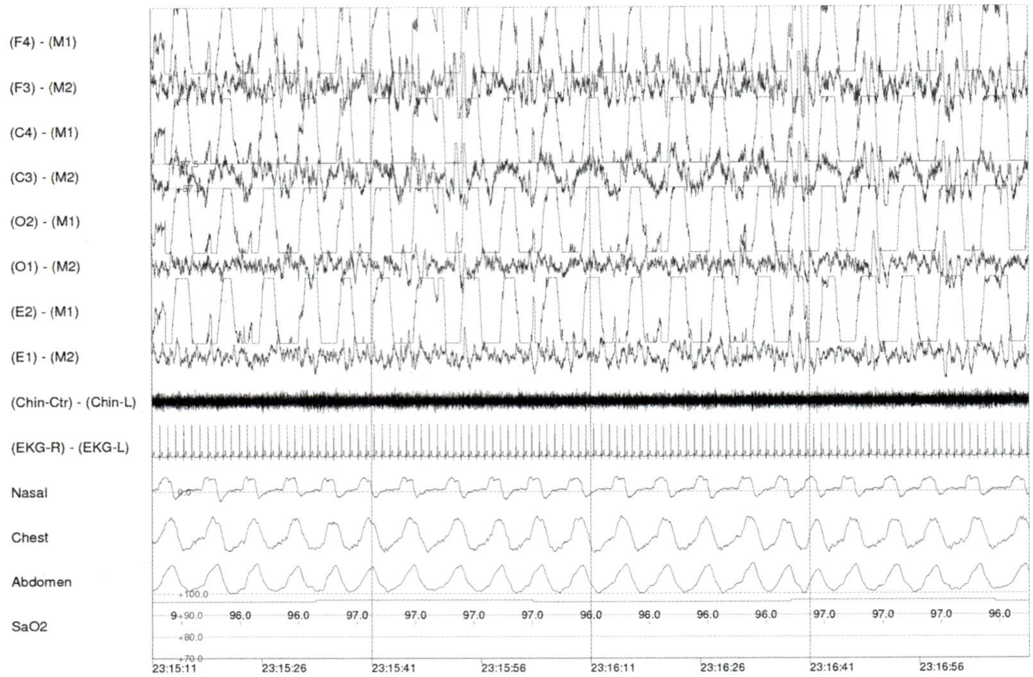

Figure 36-6 Slow-frequency artifact. The slow-frequency artifact originating in the M2 lead has caused multiple channels to block. Notice how the sway of the electroencephalogram (EEG) coincides with the respiration. In this situation, the technologist should re-reference the EEG and electrooculogram to M1 until the room cools.

Electrode Popping

The difference between sweat and popping artifacts may not always be readily apparent. In general, electrode popping produces sharper, higher amplitude waves, causing a signal-blocking effect in the EEG or EOG channels, which is illustrated in Figure 36-7. Popping artifacts in the EMG channels will produce a sharper, spiky wave due to the higher filter settings of these channels.

Electrode popping can be generated by applying pressure against an electrode or by creating tension on an electrode wire. Dirty or faulty electrodes can also cause electrode popping. Maintaining a tight seal between the electrodes and the patient's skin will minimize electrode popping artifact. When direct pressure against one of the electrodes causes an artifact, a solution (other than repositioning the patient) is to temporarily raise the channel's LFF. This strategy is effective only if the electrode is well attached and the underlying physiologic signal remains intact. An alternative technique when the artifact is limited to the side of the head on which the patient is lying is to change the input derivation to the opposite side of the head.

In many cases, a combination of all three scenarios described (sweat, pressure against an electrode, and slight body movements associated with breathing) contributes to slow-frequency artifacts. As with most signal interference, slow-frequency artifacts can be minimized by paying close attention to the quality of the electrode application. This prevents the electrode from "floating" over the electrode site, which can cause a disruption of the input signal with even the slightest movement.

Movement Artifacts

The term "movement artifact" is a general expression that describes a mixture of artifacts caused by body movement, which obscure multiple channels. When major body movements occur, as seen in Figure 36-8, different types of artifacts, such as muscle, electrode popping, and generalized signal blocking, may overlap. Although artifacts related to movement are unavoidable, they can be exacerbated by poor-quality electrode application. The only way to minimize movement artifacts is to practice proper electrode application techniques and to reduce strain or tension on the electrode leads.

Artifacts in the Respiratory Channels

Unlike bioelectric recordings, such as the EEG, inaccurate respiratory recordings do not always demonstrate obvious signs of signal distortion, like 50/60-Hz artifact. Instead, artifacts appearing in the respiratory channels tend to be more subtle and usually consist of conflicting information being displayed. Therefore, it is essential to examine all available respiratory channels and

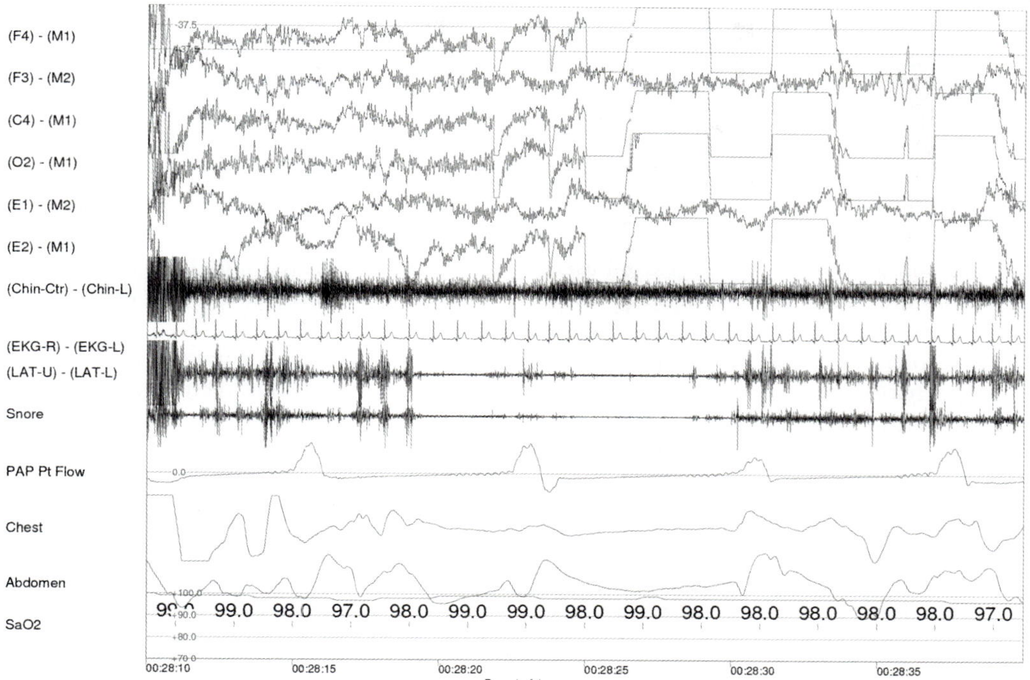

Figure 36-7 Electrode popping artifact in the electroencephalogram and electrooculogram channels. This sample shows popping in the M1 lead, which has caused a significant disruption to multiple signals, causing them to block out of range.

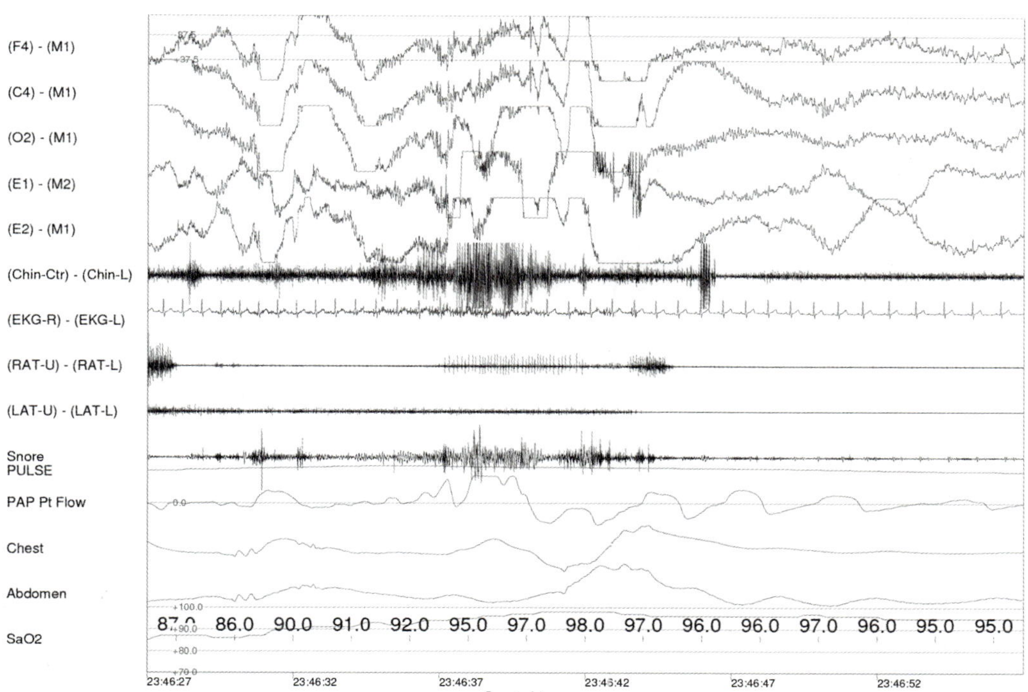

Figure 36-8 Movement artifact. In this sample, the recording is significantly distorted due to patient movement. Note the electrode popping in the electroencephalogram and the artifact on the channel monitoring the right leg (RAT).

view them within the context of other PSG parameters to avoid treating signal inaccuracies caused by patient movement or transducer displacements as factual data.

Most forms of respiratory monitoring in clinical PSG are based on external, noncalibrated, indirect representations of the patient's breathing patterns. These representations are generally imprecise and susceptible to signal distortion. For example, respiratory airflow sensors are typically either temperature-based or pressure-based. Both types of sensors are susceptible to signal loss or distortion due to sensor displacement. In addition, each type of sensor has its own peculiarities and limitations. Temperature-based sensors are less responsive to minor changes in airflow than pressure transducers. They are also more susceptible to drift caused by air currents or contact with the patient's skin. Cannula-based pressure transducers are more sensitive to minor changes in airflow but are more susceptible to signal loss due to mouth breathing or cannula occlusion.

Respiratory effort tracings are most commonly obtained with inductive plethysmography belts, which are susceptible to signal distortion caused by body movements, body position changes, shifting or twisting of the belts, or belts that are either too loose or overtightened.

Oximetry Channel Artifacts

As with respiratory artifact, inaccuracies of the oximetry channel can be identified when the oximetry output varies with no apparent correlation to respiratory pattern (Figure 36-9 for an illustration). Oximetry artifact may be caused by improper probe attachment, probe displacement, poor perfusion, motion artifact, or imprecise equipment calibrations, and/or faulty oximeter/computer interface. All these factors must be considered when evaluating the oximetry tracing. To ensure signal accuracy, sleep technologists must know how to recognize a potentially false signal and be adequately trained in the proper use and calibration of the oximeter. Typically, replacing the probe or recalibrating the system will correct the issue.

Most present-day recording systems provide some form of oximetry signal verification and/or method of deleting "bad" data. However, no signal detection system is foolproof; therefore, a visual inspection of the entire oximetry channel tracing should be conducted for every study. False oximetry readings may significantly alter the interpretation of the recording; therefore, any false readings must be tagged or deleted so they do not appear as factual data in the sleep study report.

Artifacts Specific to Digital Recording Systems

There are numerous digital recording systems, each of which uses a different technology; as a result, the appearance of recording artifacts may vary across systems. Some systems may overprocess signals, minimizing the

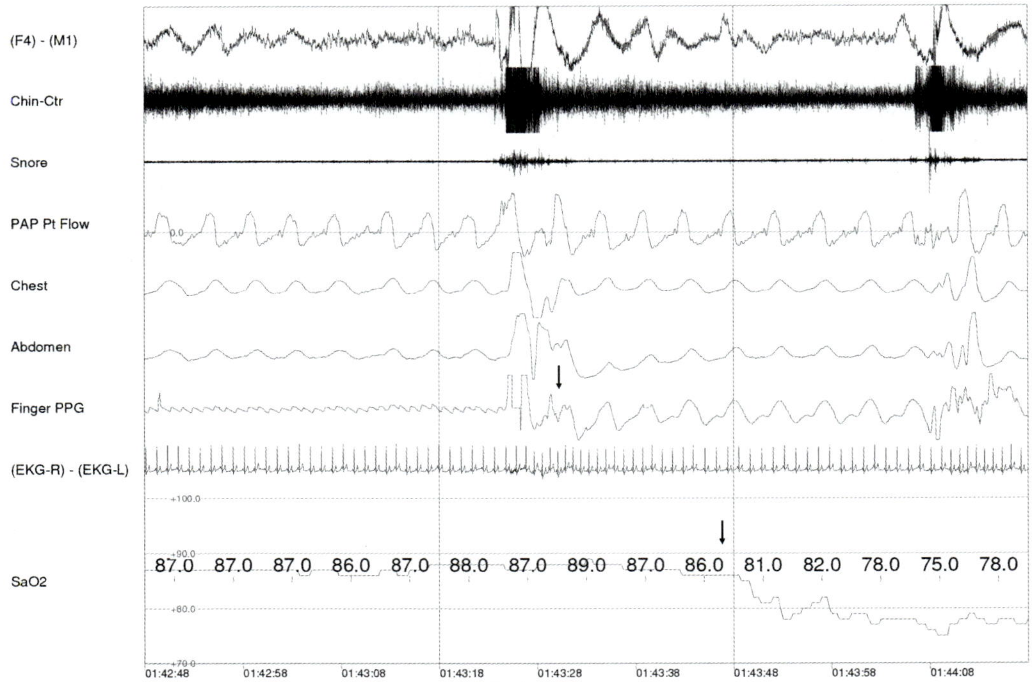

Figure 36-9 Oximetry channel artifact. The oximetry signal in the second half of this epoch is erroneous. The sharp drop in Sao_2 does not correspond with the breathing pattern, and the finger photoplethysmography (PPG) signal confirms the tracing is invalid.

appearance of artifacts, at the cost of losing essential detail. Other systems generate tracings that resemble conventional paper recordings, preserving all the necessary detail and allowing the presence of artifacts to alert the technologist to a potential problem.

Using an analog recording system, when a connection to the patient deteriorates or is lost, the technologist is immediately alerted by the obvious presence of artifact, usually in the form of 50/60-Hz artifact. Some digital systems generate a flat line when a signal is lost. This is equally problematic because a brief or intermittent loss of signal could be misinterpreted as a physiologic event, such as an asystole in the ECG channel.

Miscellaneous Artifacts

In addition to the commonly recognized recording artifacts, many other atypical or unique artifacts may be encountered during PSG. Some may have physiologic origins, whereas others may be related to the equipment or to external signal interference. The task of the sleep technologist involves a careful evaluation of any unusual patterns that do not seem to be related to the signal of interest. As noted previously, care must be exercised not to remove all suspicious patterns arbitrarily. Instead, the technologist should develop strategies to identify the cause of the pattern, decide whether its presence is useful or detrimental to the evaluation of the sleep study, and then proceed accordingly.

ENDING THE STUDY

When morning arrives and it is time to wake your patient(s), do your best to put behind you whatever technical issues you may have struggled with during the night to ensure you are polite, cheerful, and courteous to your patient. This is a key time to exercise good customer service. For additional details about ending a sleep study, see Chapter 35.

Morning Calibrations

After marking "lights on" and waking the patient, perform and record an impedance check and repeat biocalibrations to confirm that all the electrodes are still collecting relevant data. When the calibrations have been completed, the patient can be disconnected from the equipment and allowed to get out of bed.

Removing and Cleaning Sensors, Electrodes, and Equipment

Unhooking a patient is much faster and easier than applying the electrodes, but it should still be performed with care. Acetone or collodion remover should be used if the EEG electrodes were attached with collodion. If paste was used, warm water can be used to soften the paste for removal. If it is difficult to remove tape, moisten it with alcohol or adhesive remover to avoid causing the patient discomfort.

Documentation

At the end of your shift, review the documentation completed during the night to ensure all relevant information has been relayed according to sleep center policy. Typically, in addition to technologist notes, most sleep centers have the patient complete a morning questionnaire to gather subjective information about the night.

Patient Discharge Procedures

Once the patient has completed all the necessary paperwork and is ready to leave the sleep center, be sure to explain what they can expect to happen next. Typically, that will include a follow-up phone call or appointment with the clinician to discuss the test results. Providing a time frame for when that contact is likely to happen will facilitate the process and keep the individual's expectations in line with what the sleep center can provide. Be careful not to predict what the doctor may say about the sleep study results. Conflicting information will complicate the process and undermine the reputation of the facility.

SUMMARY

The sleep technologist has a very complex role that requires a unique range of skills in addition to a strong understanding of sleep and sleep disorders. A good technologist must be able to interact well with patients, be dexterous enough to apply the electrodes and sensors, and be adept at troubleshooting equipment and software issues. The technologist must be able to identify medical emergencies and know when to intervene as well as identify and correct different types of artifacts quickly and effectively. By properly maintaining the sleep recording, the attending sleep technologist assures the safety of the patient and records a polysomnogram with minimal signal distortion caused by artifacts.

SUGGESTED READINGS

Barkoukis TJ, Avidan AY. *Review of Sleep Medicine*. 2nd ed. Butterworth-Heinemann; 2007.

Butkov N. *The All-Night Sleep Recording Manual*. Synapse Media; 1994.

Butkov N. *Atlas of Clinical Polysomnography*. Vols I & II. Synapse Media; 1996.

REFERENCES

1. Troester MM, Quan SF, Berry RB, et al; for the American Academy of Sleep Medicine. *The AASM Manual for the Scoring of Sleep and Associated Events: Rules, Terminology and Technical Specifications* [Version 3.0]. American Academy of Sleep Medicine; 2023.
2. Rasquinha RJ, Moszczynski AJ, Murray BJ. A modern artifact in the sleep laboratory. *J Clin Sleep Med.* 2012;8(2):225-226.

Chapter 37
Understanding Cardiac Arrhythmias

JON W. ATKINSON

KEY CONCEPTS/LEARNING OBJECTIVES

The key concepts for this chapter include polysomnographic cardiac monitoring and recording techniques and normal electrocardiogram parameters. These key concepts also include using the American Academy of Sleep Medicine (AASM) algorithm to identify cardiac arrhythmias using systematic analysis steps and the rule of differing morphology.

KEY TERMS

Accelerated junctional and ventricular rhythms
Atrial and ventricular fibrillation
Atrial flutter
Atrial, junctional, and ventricular tachycardias
First-, second-, and third-degree AV block
Normal sinus rhythm
Sinus bradycardia

THE AMERICAN ACADEMY OF SLEEP MEDICINE MONITORING AND REPORTING GUIDELINES

In 2007, shortly after the first edition of *Fundamentals of Sleep Technology* was published, the American Academy of Sleep Medicine (AASM) published *The AASM Manual for the Scoring of Sleep and Associated Events: Rules, Terminology and Technical Specifications* (1). This manual contains information about the technical aspects of recording the electrocardiogram (ECG) as well as recommendations for reporting abnormal cardiac events. Little change in the cardiac section of the scoring manual has occurred through the subsequent versions of the manual, except in the latest version 3.0 (2), which includes a slight revision of the definition of atrial fibrillation.

Technical Considerations

The AASM manual provides the following technical specifications for the recording of ECG during polysomnography:

1. The sampling rate should be greater than or equal to 500 Hz desirable, 200 Hz minimum, with a digital resolution of 12 bits per sample.
2. The maximum electrode impedance for ECG is not specifically stated; however, 5 kΩ is appropriate.
3. Recommended low-frequency filter is 0.3 Hz and high-frequency filter 100 Hz.
4. The recommended recording derivation is a modified lead II with the right shoulder (typically subclavian) negative and the left lower torso (typically at the bottom of the rib cage) positive. A modified lead I derivation with right subclavian negative and left subclavian positive may also be employed.

Notes provided suggest that the recommended filters may be prone to various artifacts such as movement, perspiration, and muscle. Employing standard ECG electrodes instead of electroencephalogram (EEG) electrodes may make these problems less likely to occur. Additional ECG electrodes may be placed at the discretion of the practitioner.

Scoring Rules

The AASM manual recommends indicating the presence of the arrhythmias listed here, which should be acknowledged by responding "yes" if they occur and providing the heart rate (HR) or the duration of the pause.

1. Sinus tachycardia (ST) during sleep for sustained (>30 seconds duration) sinus HR greater than 90 bpm for adults.
   - Report (yes/no); report highest HR observed
2. Bradycardia during sleep for sustained (>30 seconds duration) HR of less than 40, ages 6 through adult.
   - Report (yes/no); report lowest HR observed (defined as HR <40 bpm)
3. Asystole for pauses greater than 3 seconds' duration for ages 6 through adult.
   - Report (yes/no); report longest event

4. Wide complex tachycardia for a rhythm of 3 or more consecutive beats at a rate greater than 100 bpm with a QRS duration of more than or equal to 0.12 seconds.
   - Report (yes/no); report highest HR observed
5. Narrow complex tachycardia for a rhythm of 3 or more consecutive beats at a rate greater than 100 bpm with a QRS duration of less than 0.12 seconds.
   - Report (yes/no); report highest HR observed
6. Atrial fibrillation for an irregularly irregular ventricular rhythm where the normal, consistent P waves have been replaced by rapid oscillations of varying timing, size, and shape.
   - Report (yes/no); report highest HR observed
7. Score AV (atrioventricular) heart blocks. This would include type II (distinguish between Mobitz I and Mobitz II blocks, described later in this document) and type III atrioventricular (AV) blocks.
   - Report (yes/no); report type(s) of blocks observed
8. Score cardiac pacer rhythms with pacer spikes occurring before the P wave, before the QRS complex or both.
   - Report (yes/no)

The notes in the cardiac scoring section of the manual state that significant arrhythmias should be reported if the single lead recorded is sufficient for accurate scoring. This could include escape rhythms, atrial flutter, and so on. Ectopic beats should also be reported if deemed clinically significant. Included in this group are frequent premature ventricular contractions (PVCs), patterned PVCs, ventricular couplets, and frequent atrial or junctional extrasystoles. These events may be reported similarly to the aforementioned as other arrhythmias (yes/no); report the arrhythmia.

ANATOMY AND PATHWAYS

This portion of the chapter is reproduced with modification from Atkinson JW, with permission (3). There are numerous other excellent resources for arrhythmia interpretation (4-6).

Arrhythmia recognition and identification is a fairly logical process that is based on a good working knowledge of the anatomy and pathways of the conduction system of the heart. Within the myocardium, there are areas of specialized tissue that have the primary function of generating electrical impulses or transmitting these impulses to other areas of the conduction system and, finally, to the cardiac muscle mass. The main areas of interest are the sinoatrial (SA) node, the AV node, the AV bundle or bundle of His, the left and right bundle branches, and the Purkinje system (fibers).

The normal sequence of events is as follows:

1. The cycle begins with a discharge of the SA node, which causes the atria to depolarize.
2. The AV node receives input through the internodal pathways and holds the signal for a brief period (a brief pause between atrial and ventricular depolarization that facilitates ventricular filling).
3. The impulse is passed from the AV node to the AV bundle.
4. The signal is then sent down the right and left bundles (the left bundle divides into an anterior and a posterior fascicle).
5. The left and right bundles distribute the impulse through the Purkinje system to the ventricular myocardium such that all the cardiac muscles contract simultaneously as a unit.

See Figure 37-1 for a graphic illustration of the conducting system.

CARDIAC CYCLE

The cardiac cycle is the repetitive sequence of atrial depolarization, atrial repolarization, ventricular depolarization, and ventricular repolarization. The corresponding electrophysiologic events appear as the main components of the ECG. These are identified as the P wave, the QRS complex, and the T wave. Furthermore, there is a relationship between the physiology of the cardiac cycle and the waveforms and intervals of the ECG. Table 37-1 shows the physiologic event and related ECG component. Figure 37-2 shows a graphic representation of the events in Table 37-1.

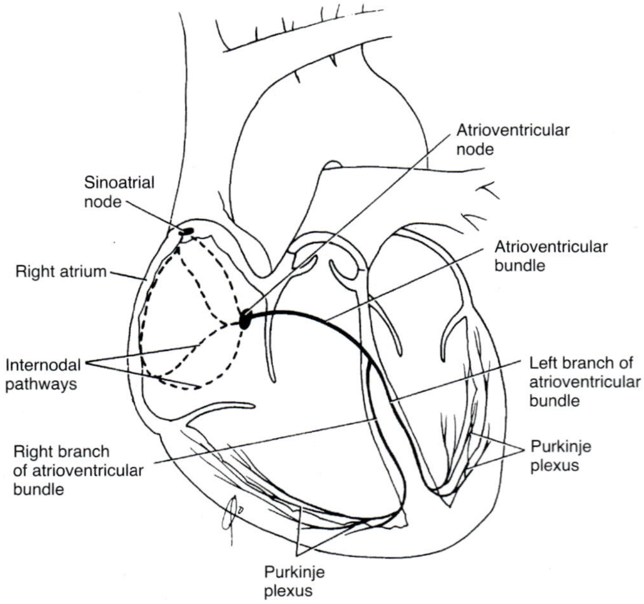

Figure 37-1 The conducting system.

Table 37-1 Physiologic Event and Related Electrocardiogram Component

Physiologic Event	Electrocardiogram Waveform
Atrial depolarization	P wave
Atrial repolarization	None seen (hidden by the timing and magnitude of the QRS complex)
Pause between atrial depolarization and ventricular depolarization	PR interval (the last portion following the P wave, PR segment)
Ventricular depolarization	QRS complex
Ventricular repolarization	T wave

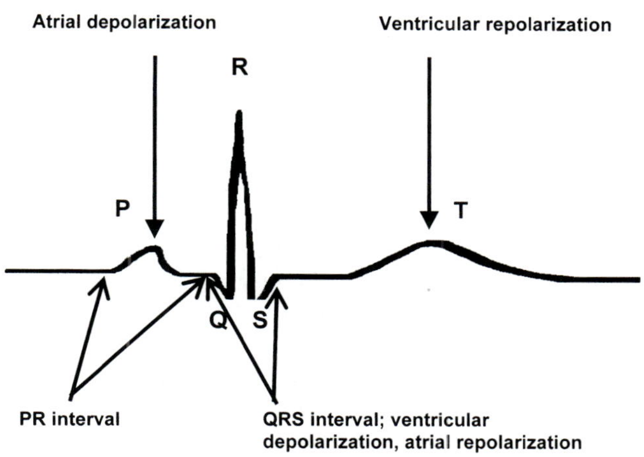

Figure 37-2 Graphic representation of the events in Table 37-1.

NORMAL PARAMETERS

Any presentation of arrhythmias requires an understanding of the ECG in its normal state. The normal ranges for key parameters needed to diagnose arrhythmias are shown in Table 37-2.

The basis for observing and identifying arrhythmias is the normal sinus rhythm (NSR). The following samples are presented in both a 30-second window and a 10-second window for comparison.

One of the better features of digital recordings is the ability to change timescales without changing how the recording is saved. For the purpose of arrhythmia analysis, it is frequently beneficial to view the ECG utilizing a 10-second screen (Figure 37-3[1]) rather than the usual 30-second window (epoch; Figure 37-4) used for sleep staging. This functionality demonstrates a basic concept: If you want to view rapidly occurring activities (ECG, EEG, etc), spread the display out; if you want to view slowly occurring events (apneas, hypopneas, limb movements, etc), compress the display.

[1]Record samples have been reduced to fit the format of this book. The actual appearance of the ECG on a computer screen or printout will vary according to the selected timescale, as well as the size of the active screen display.

Table 37-2 The Normal Adult Ranges for Key Electrocardiogram Parameters Needed to Diagnose Arrhythmias

Key Parameter	Value Range
Heart rate	60-100 bpm, awake 40-90 bpm, during sleep
Rhythm	Regular
PR interval	0.12-0.20 s
QRS interval	0.04-0.11 s
Sinoatrial node discharge rate	60-100/min
Atrioventricular node discharge rate	40-60/min
Ventricular discharge rate	20-40/min

Features of the Normal Sinus Rhythm

P wave: Present, each appears the same
QRS complex: Present, each appears the same
PR interval (start of P wave to start of QRS complex). See Figure 37-2: 0.12 to 0.20 seconds
QRS interval (start of Q wave to end of S wave). See Figure 37-2: 0.04 to 0.11 seconds
P to QRS ratio: 1:1
Rhythm: Regular
Rate: 60 to 100

ARRHYTHMIA BASICS

An ECG arrhythmia occurs if there is a difference from NSR in impulse formation, impulse conduction, or both. Heartbeats that originate outside of the SA node, such as other areas in the atrium, the AV node, or the ventricle, are some examples of impulse formation abnormalities. These abnormal beats will not have a sinus P wave. Abnormal beats with only conduction abnormalities will exhibit a sinus P wave but then show prolonged conduction across the AV node or through the ventricular conduction pathway. The AV blocks and bundle branch blocks are good examples of impulse conduction abnormalities. When both impulse formation and impulse conduction are affected, neither a normal sinus P wave nor a normal QRS complex is present.

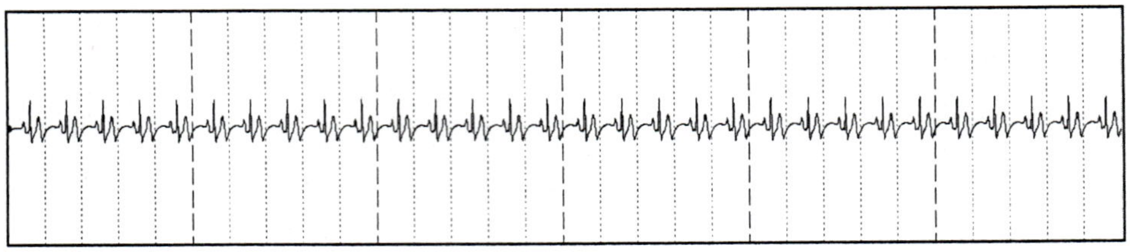

Figure 37-3 Normal sinus rhythm, 30-second display.

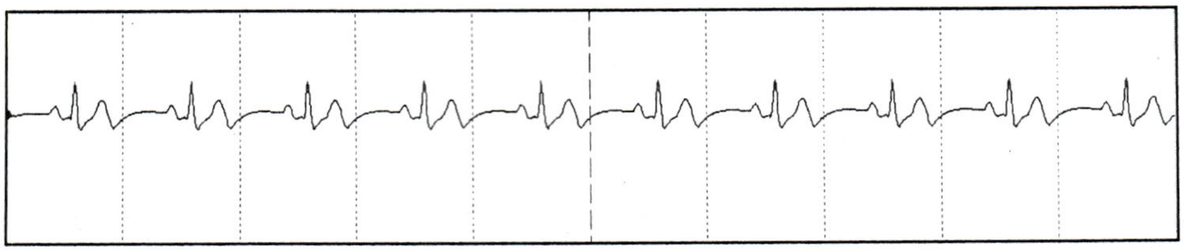

Figure 37-4 Normal sinus rhythm, 10-second display.

Any of the ventricular arrhythmias demonstrate both impulse formation and impulse conduction abnormalities. Essentially, an arrhythmia is present if the rate is too fast or too slow, the rhythm is irregular, the site of origin is abnormal, or the movement of the impulse through the conductive system is abnormal.

ARRHYTHMIA ANALYSIS

Far too often, there is the temptation to "guess" the type of arrhythmia that is presented on the polysomnogram. This section presents a systematic method to accurately analyze cardiac rhythm disturbances. If possible, a second ECG derivation should be added to the montage. This is easily accomplished unless the equipment manufacturer has only a dedicated, two-input amplifier for recording the ECG. Utilizing a second ECG channel may reveal changes in P wave or QRS complex configuration that are difficult to ascertain with a single-channel recording. When examining the ECG for detail, use a 10- or 6-second window to examine the intervals or subtle changes in morphology.

Routine use of the following methodical evaluation system will improve the accuracy of identifying arrhythmias.

Step 1. Examine the P wave.

Is the P wave absent or present? Absence of a distinct P wave would indicate that the arrhythmia is not of atrial origin (except atrial fibrillation or atrial flutter). Do the P waves all look the same (have the same morphology)? A basic concept that should be remembered is as follows: If an ECG complex starts from the same location and takes the same pathway, it will always look the same. This is the *rule of identical morphology*. The corollary to the rule of identical morphology is as follows: If the complex originates from a different location or takes a different pathway, the appearance will be different. This is the *rule of differing morphology*.

Step 2. Examine the QRS complex.

Check for absence or presence and similar appearance of the QRS complex. Absence of the QRS indicates some type of second- or third-degree AV block or severe ventricular disturbance such as ventricular fibrillation or asystole. Differing morphologies of the QRS indicate a shift from a supraventricular origin of the abnormal beat(s) or a different pathway in the ventricle, such as bundle branch block or multifocal ventricular origin.

Step 3. Examine the P and QRS relationship.

Ask the following questions. Is there a P wave for every QRS complex? Is there a QRS complex for every P wave? Is there a 1:1 P to QRS ratio? A P to QRS ratio of more than 1 (more P waves than QRS complexes) indicates some sort of AV block. A P to QRS ratio of less than 1 (more QRS complexes than P waves) indicates a junctional or ventricular arrhythmia.

Step 4. Measure the intervals.

Is the PR interval normal, or is it too long or too short? An abbreviated PR interval may indicate a junctional beat (retrograde P wave) or an accessory pathway (such as in Wolff-Parkinson-White syndrome). A prolonged PR interval indicates that some type of AV block is occurring. Is the QRS interval normal or too long? (Seldom, if ever, will it be too short.) A widened QRS complex likely indicates bundle branch block, a beat of ventricular origin, or, in some cases, an aberrantly conducted beat of supraventricular origin (the beat originates before the ventricular conductive pathway is repolarized during the relative refractory period).

Step 5. Regular or irregular rhythm

Examine the P-P and the R-R intervals. If the intervals are constant, the rhythm is regular. If they vary, the rhythm is irregular. Using calipers on a computer monitor is not advised, so either print the screen image and measure the intervals with calipers on paper or use something like a 3 × 5 index card. Make pencil marks corresponding to a succession of two or more P waves, while holding the card against a stationary screen display. Move the card from one set of P-P intervals to the next and see if they fall on the marks. Do the same for the R waves.

Step 6. Determine the rate.

An accurate determination of HR is obtained from the ECG. Do not rely on the readout from a pulse oximeter. Using the ECG display, HR can be determined in a variety of fashions:

Times two method: Count the number of beats in a 30-second screen display and multiply by two. This can be a bit cumbersome but is quite accurate. Make sure you do this in a frozen screen view.

Times four method: Count the number of beats in a 15-second display and multiply by four. Again, use a stationary screen.

Times six method: Count the number of beats in a 10-second display and multiply by six.

Interval method: Measure the active screen width in millimeters. If you have a 30-second window, multiply this number by two to get the number of millimeters in 60 seconds. If you are using a 10-second window, multiply the active screen width by six to obtain the number of millimeters in 60 seconds. Measure the R-R interval with a ruler and divide into the number of millimeters in 60 seconds.

COMMON ATRIAL ARRHYTHMIAS

- Premature atrial contractions (PACs)
- Sinus bradycardia (SB)
- Atrial tachycardia (AT); ST; supraventricular tachycardia (SVT)
- Sinus arrhythmia
- Sinus pause
- Paroxysmal atrial tachycardia
- Atrial fibrillation
- Atrial flutter

PREMATURE ATRIAL CONTRACTION

Features of Premature Atrial Contractions

P wave: Present, the appearance of the P wave of the abnormal beat will be different (it arises from a different location)

QRS complex: Present, each appears the same

PR interval: 0.12 to 0.20 seconds, may vary slightly with the abnormal beat

QRS interval: 0.04 to 0.11 seconds

P to QRS ratio: 1:1

Rhythm: Irregular because of the premature beat; P-P will be different, so will be the R-R

Rate: 60 to 100

Comments: Note the different appearance of the P wave (origin is from a different source and travels a different pathway) at the arrows in Figures 37-5 and 37-6. There may also be subtle PR interval changes. The QRS and the T wave are normal in appearance, unless the ectopic atrial focus fires so early that it captures the ventricle, whereas the bundle branches or the Purkinje system is still relatively refractory to conduction (PAC with aberrancy).

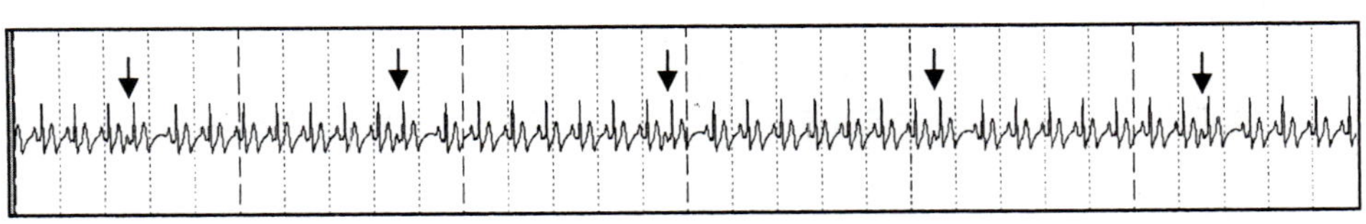

Figure 37-5 Premature atrial contraction, 30-second display.

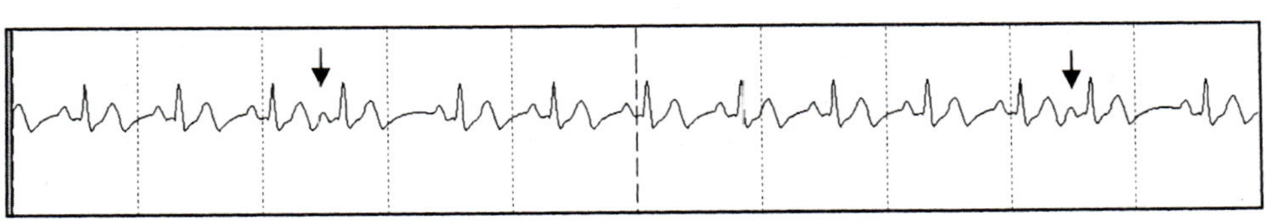

Figure 37-6 Premature atrial contraction, 10-second display.

SINUS BRADYCARDIA

Features of Sinus Bradycardia

P wave: Present, each appears the same
QRS complex: Present, each appears the same
PR interval: 0.12 to 0.20 seconds
QRS interval: 0.04 to 0.11 seconds
P to QRS ratio: 1:1
Rhythm: Regular
Rate: Less than 50, some authors say less than 60 awake. Bradycardia during sleep is regarded as a sustained HR of less than 37 bpm (1,2).

Comments: Sinus bradycardia (Figures 37-7 and 37-8) looks like NSR except the rate is slower. This is not uncommon in athletic individuals and patients on β-blockers.

ATRIAL TACHYCARDIA; SINUS TACHYCARDIA; SUPRAVENTRICULAR TACHYCARDIA

Features of Supraventricular Tachyarrhythmias

P wave: Present, each appears the same, may not be well defined in SVT
QRS complex: Present, each appears the same
PR interval: 0.12 to 0.20 seconds
QRS interval: 0.04 to 0.11 seconds
P to QRS ratio: 1:1
Rhythm: Regular
Rate: Greater than 100 bpm. ST during sleep is regarded as a sustained sinus rhythm of more than 90 bpm (1,2).

Comments: Supraventricular tachyarrhythmias are rapid, regular rhythms with normal-appearing QRS complexes. ST will have a normal sinus P wave. In AT, the P wave will have a morphology different from that of the sinus P wave (Figures 37-9 and 37-10). SVT will not have a clearly defined P wave. It is difficult to distinguish one from the other on the surface ECG. Electrophysiologic studies may be necessary to determine the precise focus. *Sustained tachyarrhythmias will decrease cardiac output. The patient should be assessed for the level of consciousness, chest pain, and blood pressure and the physician notified.* The AASM recommends reporting ST during sleep if sustained. Otherwise, brief runs of these arrhythmias are reported as narrow complex tachycardia.

SINUS ARRHYTHMIA

Features of Sinus Arrhythmia

P wave: Present, each appears the same
QRS complex: Present, each appears the same
PR interval: 0.12 to 0.20 seconds
QRS interval: 0.04 to 0.11 seconds
P to QRS ratio: 1:1
Rhythm: Irregular
Rate: 60 to 100

Comments: Sinus arrhythmia (Figures 37-11 and 37-12) is frequently seen in infants and children. It is

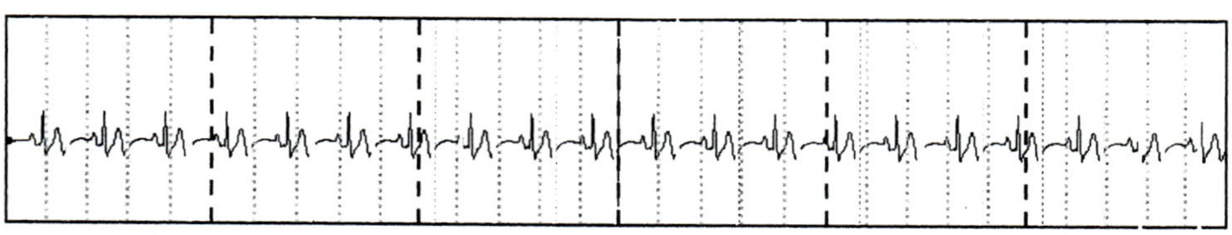

Figure 37-7 Sinus bradycardia, 30-second display.

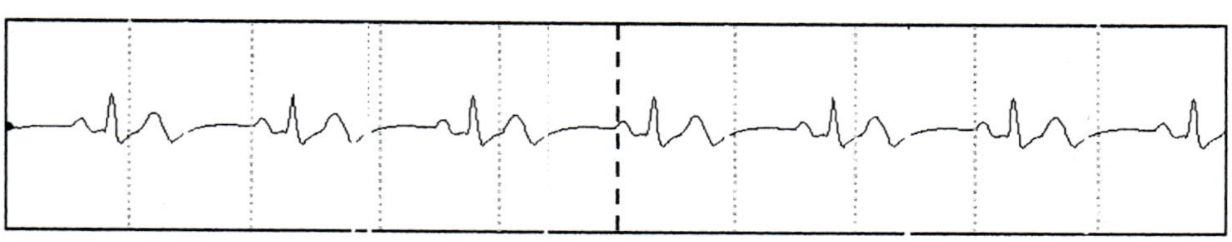

Figure 37-8 Sinus bradycardia, 10-second display.

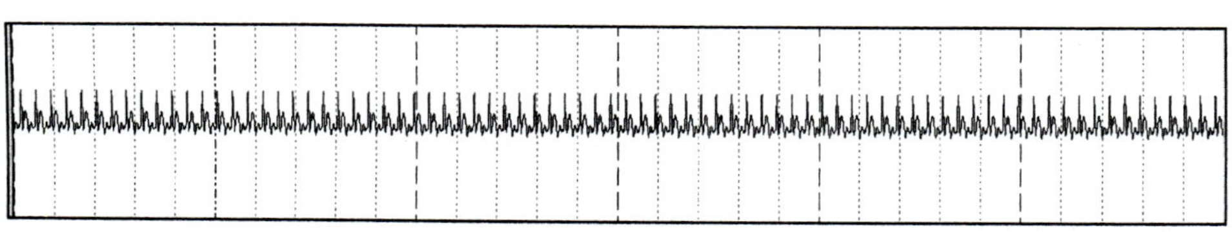

Figure 37-9 Atrial tachycardia, 30-second display.

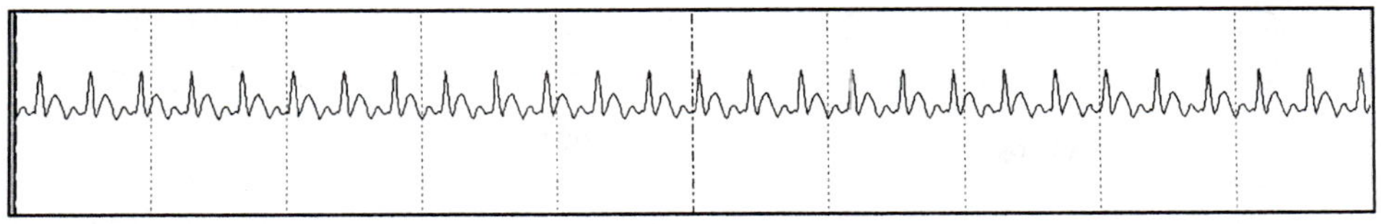

Figure 37-10 Atrial tachycardia, 10-second display.

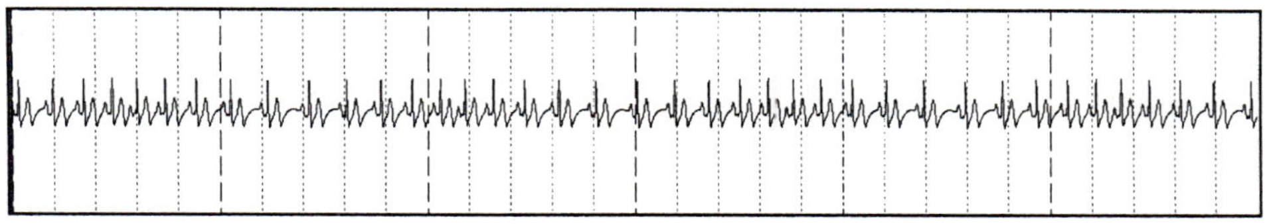

Figure 37-11 Sinus arrhythmia, 30-second display.

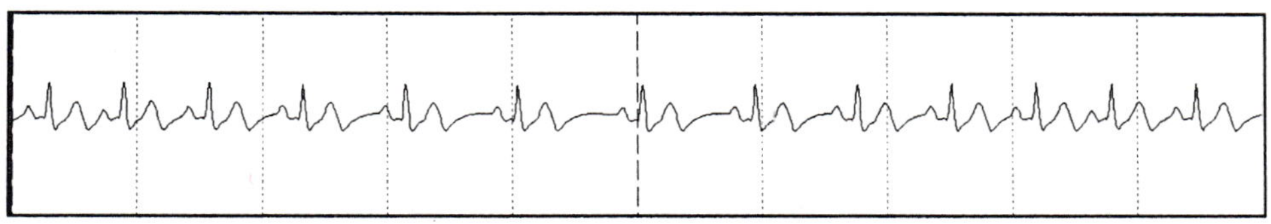

Figure 37-12 Sinus arrhythmia, 10-second display.

often seen in obstructive sleep apnea as a result of the vagal effect of intrathoracic pressure fluctuations. Minor fluctuations of HR associated with inspiration and expiration are quite normal and indicate a "healthy" autonomic control of HR. Lack of HR fluctuation may indicate an underlying pathologic condition such as diabetes mellitus.

SINUS PAUSE

Features of Sinus Pause

P wave: Absent during pause
QRS complex: Absent during pause
PR interval: Absent during pause
QRS interval: Absent during pause
P to QRS ratio: 1:1
Rhythm: Irregular
Rate: 60 to 100, but can occur at any rate

Comments: One cannot distinguish sinus arrest from sinus exit block on surface ECG. This requires electrophysiologic studies of the heart. *If a sinus pause is prolonged, notify appropriate medical personnel according to protocol.* The arrows in Figures 37-13 and 37-14 indicate the areas of absence of the P waves. The AASM recommendation is to report HR pauses of more than 3 seconds' duration as asystole.

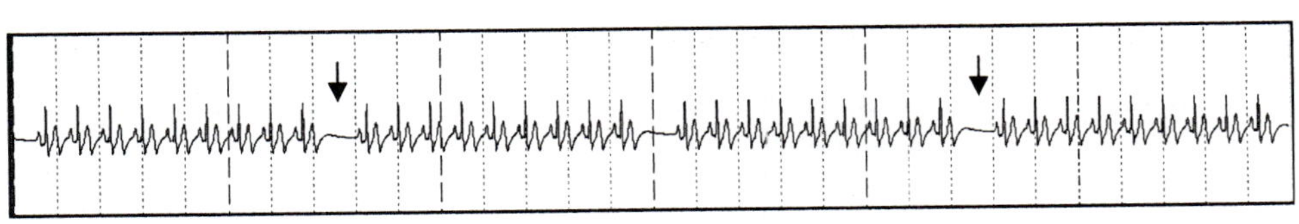

Figure 37-13 Sinus pause, 30-second display.

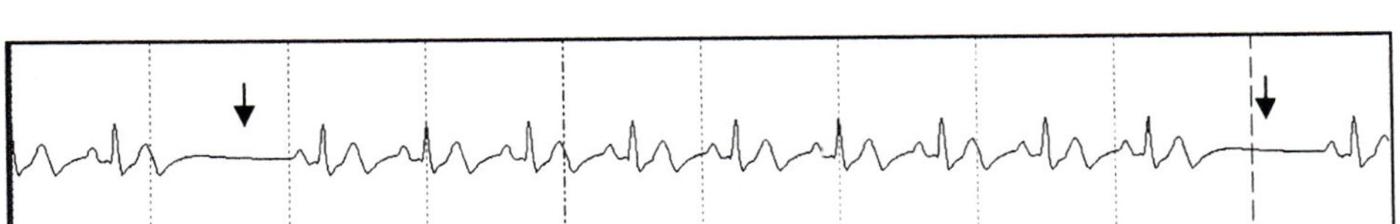

Figure 37-14 Sinus pause, 10-second display.

PAROXYSMAL ATRIAL TACHYCARDIA, PAROXYSMAL SUPRAVENTRICULAR TACHYCARDIA

Features of Paroxysmal Supraventricular Tachyarrhythmias

P wave: Present, aberrant, often hidden
QRS complex: Present, appearance is the same, may be aberrant
PR interval: Not measurable
QRS interval: 0.04 to 0.11 seconds
P to QRS ratio: 1:1
Rhythm: Regular during paroxysm
Rate: 150 to 250

Comments: Supraventricular tachyarrhythmias often occur with reentry phenomena from an accessory pathway. The term *paroxysmal* describes a phenomenon that arises abruptly from the background and abruptly returns to that background. Generally, these arrhythmias are self-limiting, but *if sustained, cardiac output is decreased. Hence, assess the patient and notify appropriate medical personnel according to protocol.* Report these arrhythmias as narrow complex tachycardia. The arrows in Figures 37-15 and 37-16 indicate the onset of the paroxysm.

ATRIAL FIBRILLATION

Features of Atrial Fibrillation

P wave: None, per se; chaotic deflections called "fibrillatory waves"
QRS complex: Present, appearance is the same
PR interval: Not measurable
QRS interval: 0.04 to 0.11 seconds
P to QRS ratio: Not applicable
Rhythm: Irregularly irregular
Rate: Ventricular rate is highly variable.

Comments: Central sleep apnea, Cheyne-Stokes respirations, and mixed apneas (often with a long central component) are frequently seen with atrial fibrillation. This is likely due to decreased cardiac output and a prolonged circulation time, rendering the breathing control centers ineffective. *If sustained or previously undocumented, notify appropriate medical personnel according to protocol.* Indicate in the polysomnographic report as atrial fibrillation. Note the absence of true P waves and the replacement by chaotic fibrillatory waves in the preceding examples (Figures 37-17 and 37-18).

ATRIAL FLUTTER

Features of Atrial Flutter

P wave: None, per se; sawtooth deflections called "flutter waves"
QRS complex: Present, appearance is the same
PR interval: Not measurable
QRS interval: 0.04 to 0.11 seconds
P to QRS ratio: Variable 2:1, 3:1, 4:1, and so on.
Rhythm: Regular or irregular depending on the variability of the block
Rate: Atrial: 250 to 400; ventricular rate depends on the degree of the block and atrial rate

Comments: Atrial flutter often occurs with reentry phenomena from accessory pathway. *If sustained or previously undocumented, notify appropriate medical personnel according to protocol.* Note under Other Arrhythmias on the polysomnographic report. Note the "sawtooth" flutter wave indicated by the arrows in Figures 37-19 and 37-20.

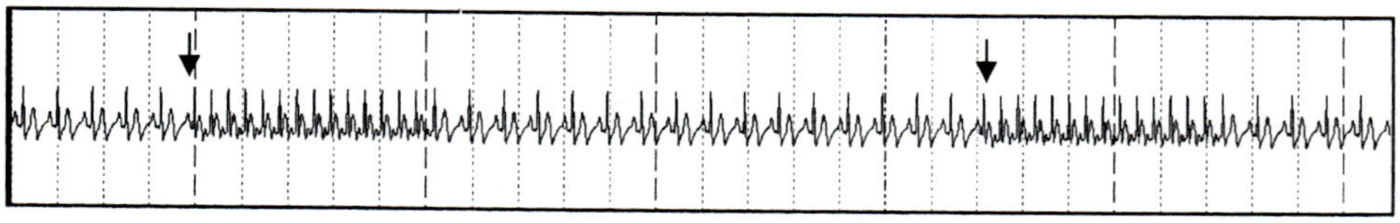

Figure 37-15 Paroxysmal atrial tachycardia, paroxysmal supraventricular tachycardia, 30-second display.

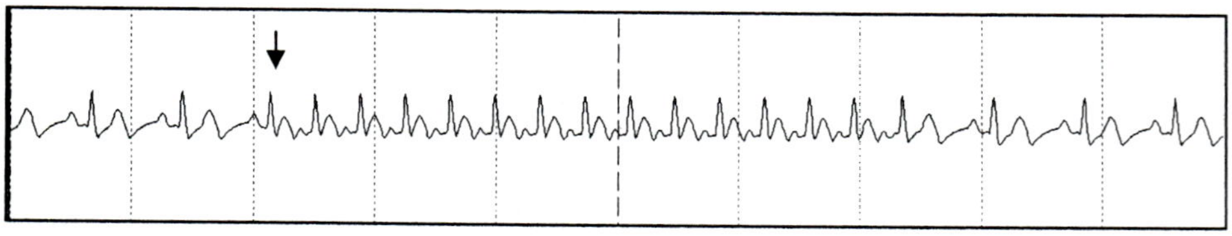

Figure 37-16 Paroxysmal atrial tachycardia, paroxysmal supraventricular tachycardia, 10-second display.

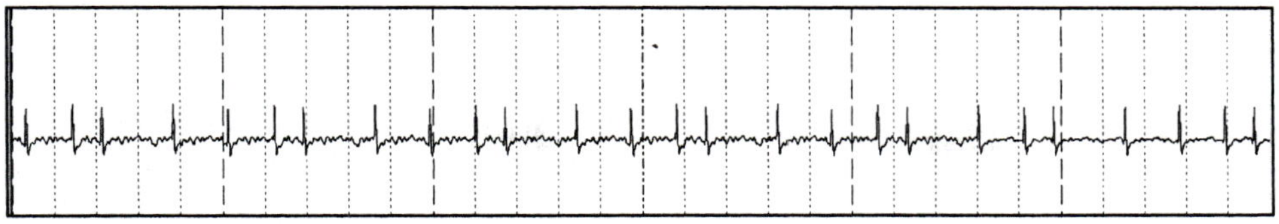

Figure 37-17 Atrial fibrillation, 30-second display.

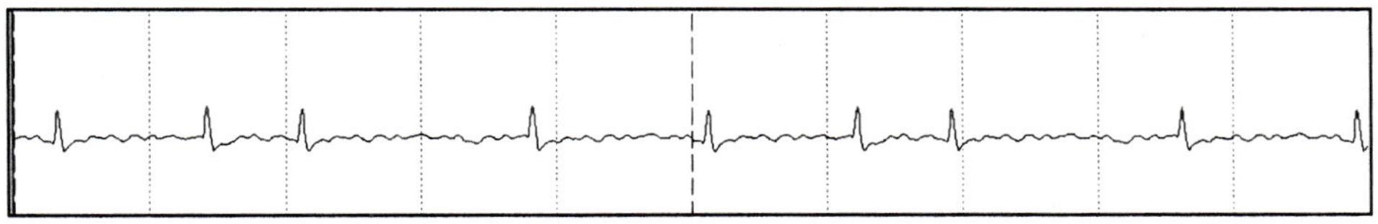

Figure 37-18 Atrial fibrillation, 10-second display.

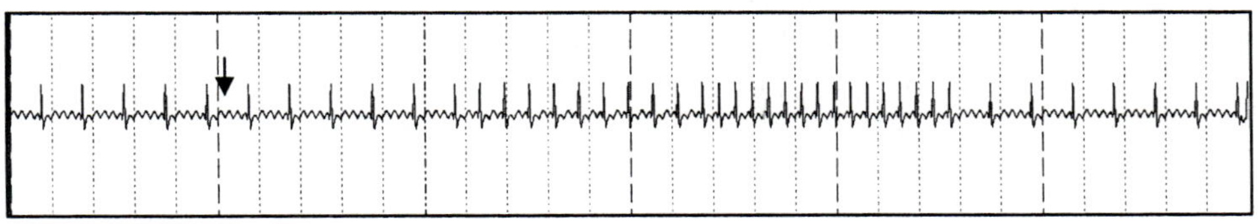

Figure 37-19 Atrial flutter, variable block, 30-second display.

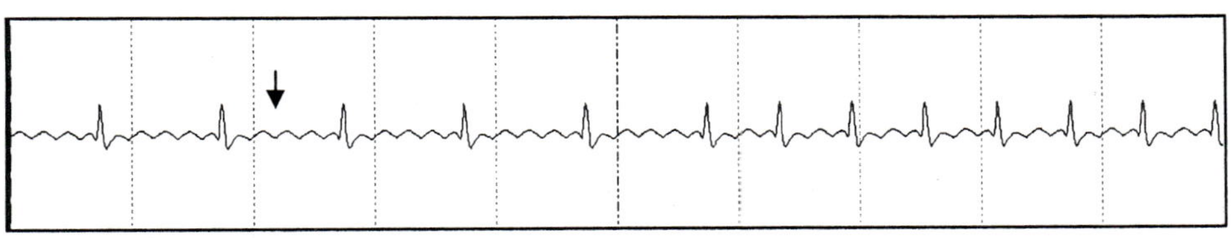

Figure 37-20 Atrial flutter, variable block, 10-second display.

JUNCTIONAL ARRHYTHMIAS

- Premature junctional contraction (PJC)
- Junctional rhythm
- Accelerated junctional rhythm
- Junctional tachycardia

Junctional arrhythmias can occur if the AV nodal tissue fires prematurely or if the atrial mechanism for initiating the cardiac cycle fails. Key features of the junctional arrhythmias are normal-appearing QRS complexes (the pathway distally from the AV bundle is intact). P waves may or may not be seen. If the P waves are seen, they will be inverted (a reverse from the normal P wave vector) and can occur before or after the QRS complex. If they occur before the QRS, the PR interval will be shorter than normal in contrast to the preceding ECG samples.

PREMATURE JUNCTIONAL CONTRACTION

Features of Premature Junctional Contractions

P wave: Premature and abnormal configuration, will be inverted; can be before (with shortened PR interval), after, or hidden in the QRS
QRS complex: Present, appearance is the same
PR interval: Shorter than normal
QRS interval: 0.04 to 0.11 seconds
P to QRS ratio: Less than 1:1 if hidden; 1:1 if inverted P is seen
Rhythm: Irregular
Rate: Usually normal, but can occur in ST or SB

Comments: The premature beats with normal-appearing QRS complexes and absent or hidden P waves are seen at the arrows in Figures 37-21 and 37-22.

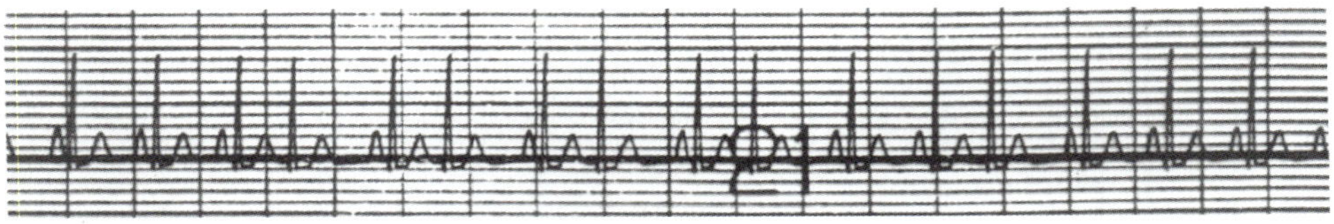

Figure 37-21 Premature junctional (nodal) contraction, 30-second timescale; uncompressed, partial epoch display.

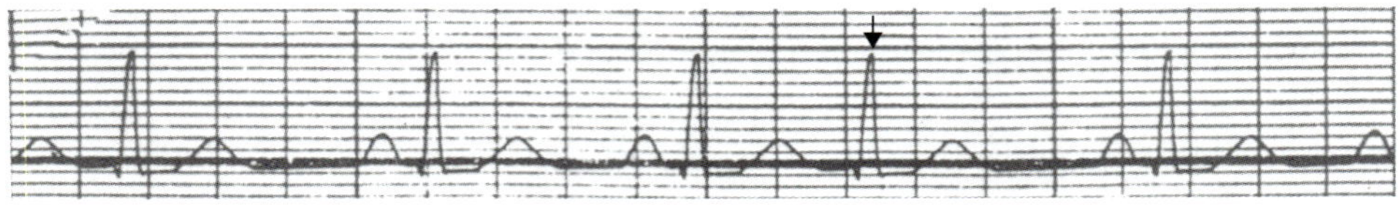

Figure 37-22 Premature junctional (nodal) contraction, 10-second timescale; uncompressed, partial epoch display.

JUNCTIONAL RHYTHM

Features of Junctional Rhythms

P wave: Premature and abnormal configuration, will be inverted; can be before (with shortened PR interval), after, or hidden in the QRS
QRS complex: Present, appearance is the same
PR interval: Shorter than normal; less than 0.12 seconds
QRS interval: 0.04 to 0.11 seconds
P to QRS ratio: Less than 1:1 if hidden; 1:1 if inverted P is seen
Rhythm: Regular
Rate: 37 to 60

Comments: Junctional rhythms are often seen as an escape rhythm with sinus node dysfunction. This type of rhythm should be listed under Other Arrhythmias in the report. Note the inverted P wave and short PR interval in Figures 37-23 and 37-24 at the arrows.

ACCELERATED JUNCTIONAL RHYTHM

Features of Accelerated Junctional Rhythm

P wave: Premature and abnormal configuration, will be inverted; can be before (with shortened PR interval), after, or hidden in the QRS
QRS complex: Present, appearance is the same
PR interval: Shorter than normal; less than 0.12 seconds
QRS interval: 0.04 to 0.11 seconds
P to QRS ratio: Either less than 1:1 if hidden; or 1:1 if inverted P is seen
Rhythm: Regular
Rate: 60 to 100

Comments: Accelerated junctional rhythm is often seen as escape rhythm with sinus node dysfunction. This type of rhythm should be listed under Other Arrhythmias in the report (Figures 37-25 and 37-26).

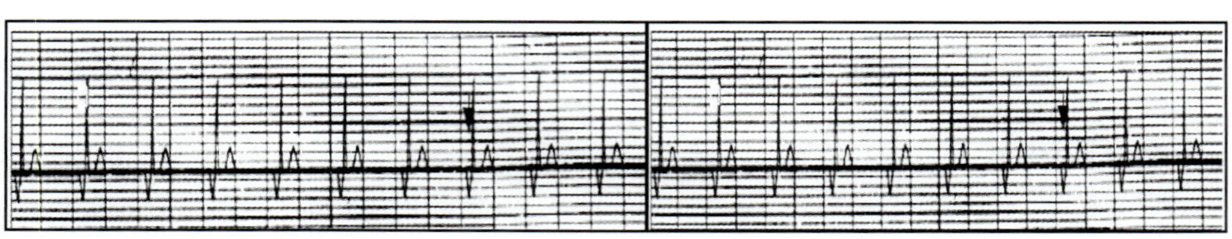

Figure 37-23 Junctional rhythm, 30-second display.

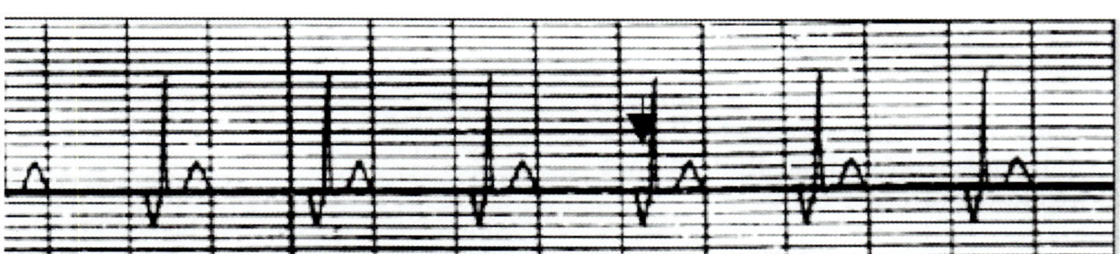

Figure 37-24 Junctional rhythm, 10-second window.

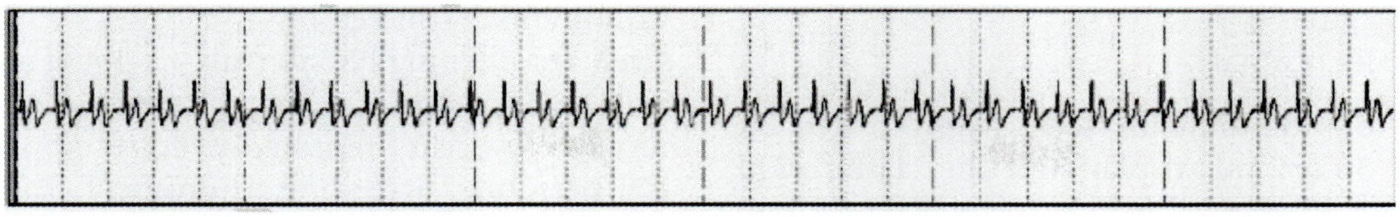

Figure 37-25 Accelerated junctional rhythm, 30-second window.

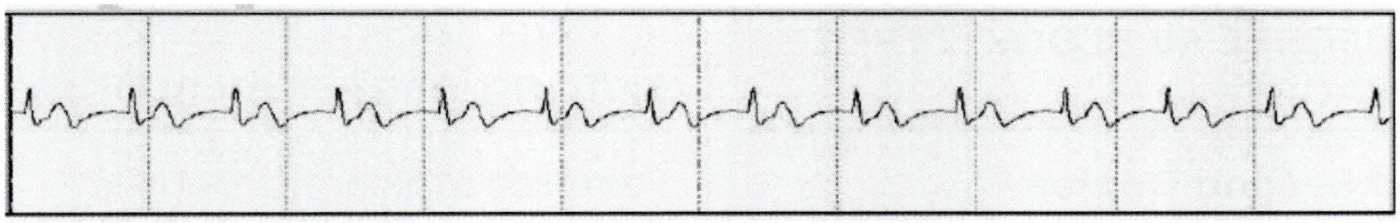

Figure 37-26 Accelerated junctional rhythm, 10-second window.

JUNCTIONAL TACHYCARDIA

Features of Junctional Tachycardia

P wave: Premature and abnormal configuration, will be inverted; can be before (with shortened PR interval), after, or hidden in the QRS
QRS complex: Present, appearance is the same
PR interval: Shorter than normal; less than 0.12 seconds
QRS interval: 0.04 to 0.11 seconds
P to QRS ratio: Less than 1:1 if hidden; 1:1 if inverted P is seen
Rhythm: Regular
Rate: Greater than 100

Comments: Note the inverted P wave following the QRS at the arrows in Figures 37-27 and 37-28. Assess the patient if sustained (due to decreased cardiac output) and notify appropriate medical personnel according to protocol. This type of rhythm should be listed under Narrow Complex Tachycardia in the report.

BLOCKS

- First-degree AV block
- Second-degree AV block, type 1
- Second-degree AV block, type 2
- Third-degree AV block
- Left bundle branch block (LBBB)
- Right bundle branch block (RBBB)

FIRST-DEGREE AV BLOCK

Features of First-Degree Atrioventricular Block

P wave: Present, appearance is the same
QRS complex: Present, appearance is the same
PR interval: Longer than normal; more than 0.20 seconds
QRS interval: 0.04 to 0.11 seconds
P to QRS ratio: 1:1

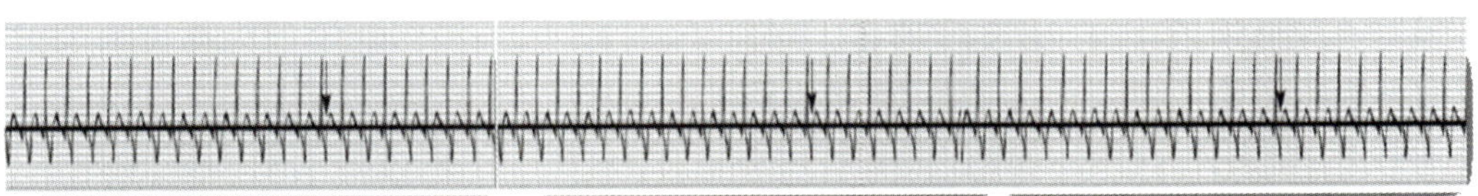

Figure 37-27 Junctional tachycardia, 30-second window.

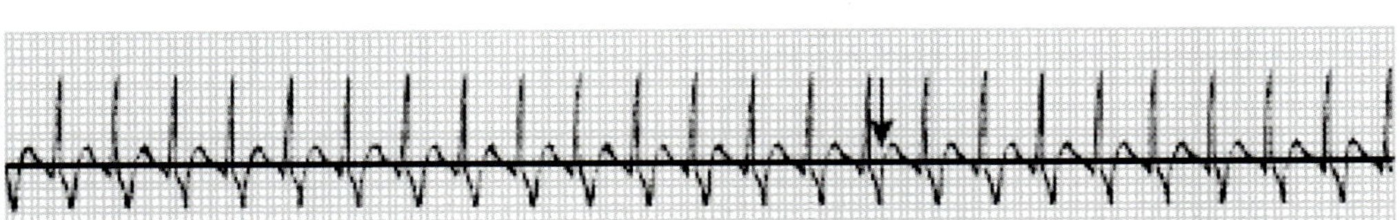

Figure 37-28 Junctional tachycardia, 10-second window.

Rhythm: Regular
Rate: Usually normal

Comments: Note the difficulty seeing a prolonged PR interval on a 30-second display and the clarification provided with a 10-second display (Figures 37-29 and 37-30).

SECOND-DEGREE AV BLOCK, TYPE 1 (WENCKEBACH)

Features of Second-Degree Atrioventricular Block, Type 1

P wave: Present, normal sinus P, some not followed by QRS
QRS complex: Present, appearance is the same
PR interval: Progressively lengthening
QRS interval: 0.04 to 0.11 seconds
P to QRS ratio: More than 1:1, may be 1:1 if the nonconducted P wave is hidden
Rhythm: Irregular
Rate: Usually slow but can be normal

Comments: As in Figures 37-29 and 37-30, the progressively lengthening PR intervals are better appreciated on a 10-second display. This type of block is not uncommon. If it occurs repeatedly, notify appropriate medical personnel according to protocol. The P waves are indicated by the arrows in Figures 37-31 and 37-32. This type of rhythm should be listed under second-degree AV Block (Mobitz I) in the report.

SECOND-DEGREE AV BLOCK, TYPE 2

Features of Second-Degree Atrioventricular Block, Type 2

P wave: Present, normal sinus P wave, 2, 3, or more P waves before QRS
QRS complex: Present, appearance is the same
PR interval: Constant PR interval before dropped QRS, PR interval may be normal or prolonged.
QRS interval: 0.04 to 0.11 seconds
P to QRS ratio: More than 1:1
Rhythm: Irregular
Rate: Usually slow but can be normal

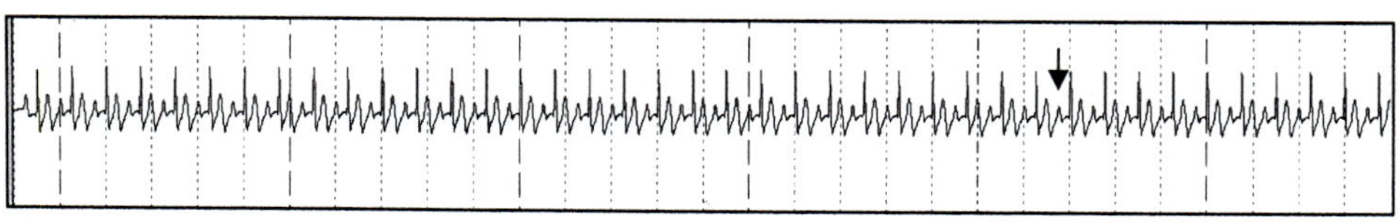

Figure 37-29 First-degree atrioventricular block, 30-second display.

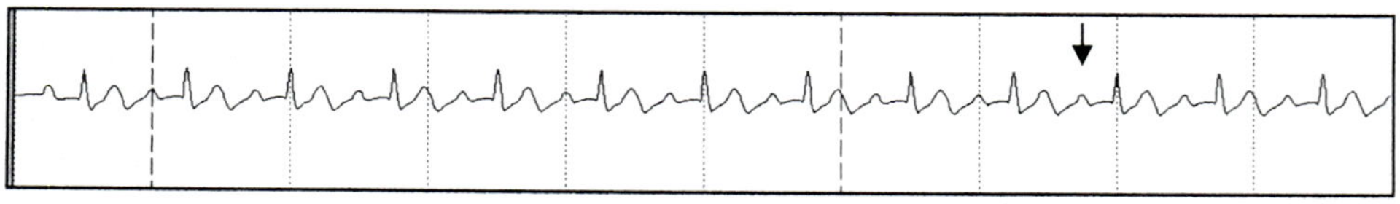

Figure 37-30 First-degree atrioventricular block, 10-second display.

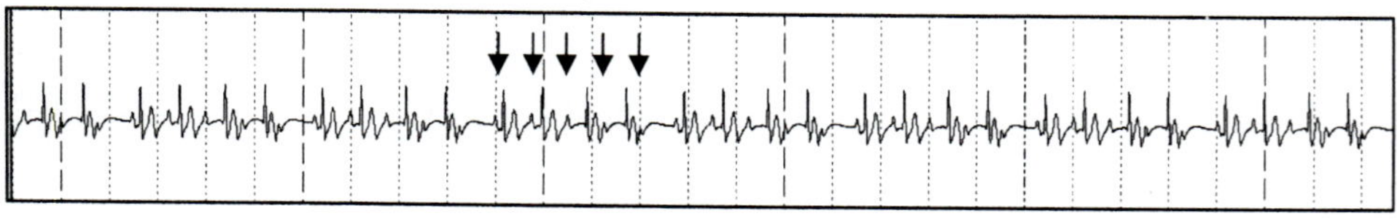

Figure 37-31 Second-degree atrioventricular block, type 1, 30-second display.

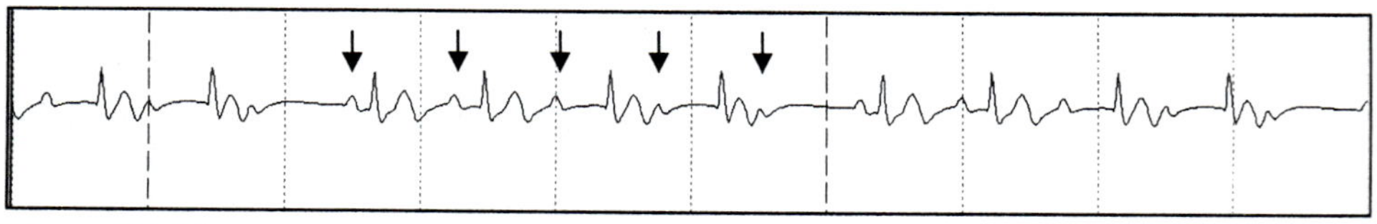

Figure 37-32 Second-degree atrioventricular block, type 1, 10-second display.

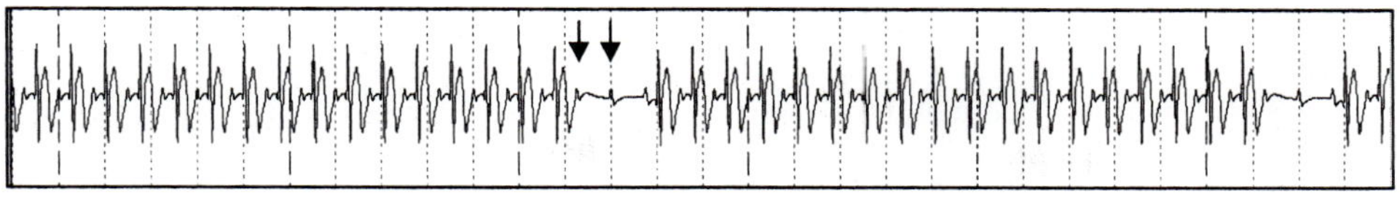

Figure 37-33 Second-degree atrioventricular block, type 2, 30-second display.

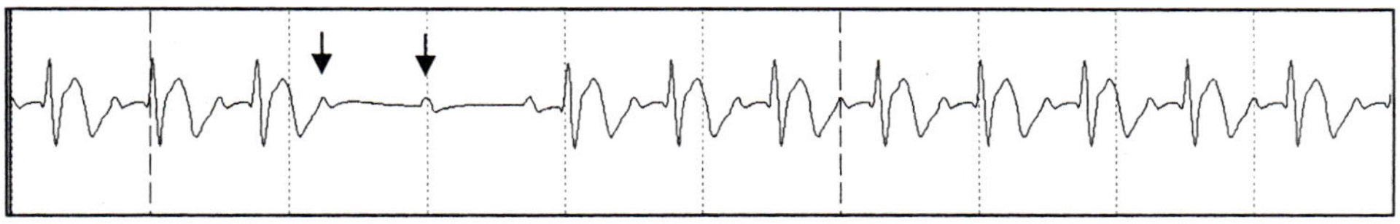

Figure 37-34 Second-degree atrioventricular block, type 2, 10-second display.

Comments: If second-degree AV block is prolonged, escape beat may occur. Note the constant PR interval before dropped QRS in Figures 37-33 and 37-34. This may lead to a string of P waves without QRS complexes. This arrhythmia is worthy of a call to medical personnel according to protocol. Nonconducted P waves are indicated by the arrows in the preceding examples. This type of rhythm should be listed under second-degree AV Block (Mobitz II) in the report.

THIRD-DEGREE AV BLOCK, A-V DISSOCIATION

Features of Third-Degree Atrioventricular Block

P wave: Present, but has no relationship with QRS; often hidden in QRS and T waves
QRS complex: Present, appearance is the same
PR interval: Varies greatly
QRS interval: Less than 0.12 seconds if block is in a bundle of His; more than 0.12 seconds if block is in bundle branches.
P to QRS ratio: More than 1:1
Rhythm: Regular P-P and regular R-R but not at the same rate
Rate: 40 to 60 if bundle of His is blocked; 30 to 40 if bundle branches are involved.

Comments: Note the constant P-P interval and the constant R-R interval in Figures 37-35 and 37-36. That is, there is a regular atrial rhythm and a regular ventricular rhythm, just not at the same rate. P waves are noted at the arrows and are sometimes difficult to see when simultaneously occurring with other waveforms such as the T wave and QRS complex. This type of rhythm should be listed under third-degree AV Block in the report.

LEFT BUNDLE BRANCH BLOCK

Features of Left Bundle Branch Block

P wave: Normal
QRS complex: Present, widened, and notched (M-shaped pattern), best seen in V6, lead I, or AVL
PR interval: Normal, can be prolonged with first-degree block
QRS interval: More than 0.12 seconds

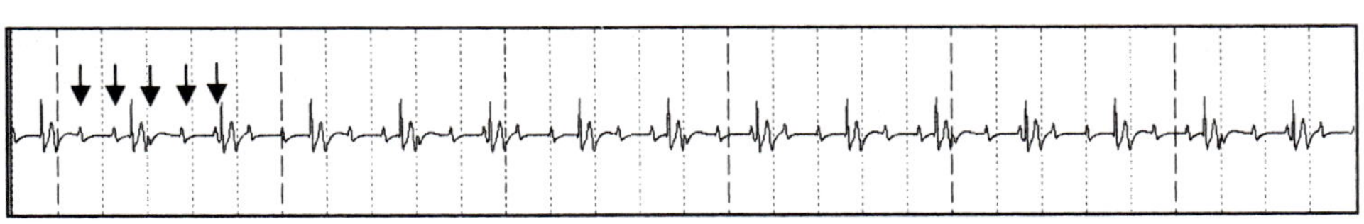

Figure 37-35 Third-degree atrioventricular block, 30-second display.

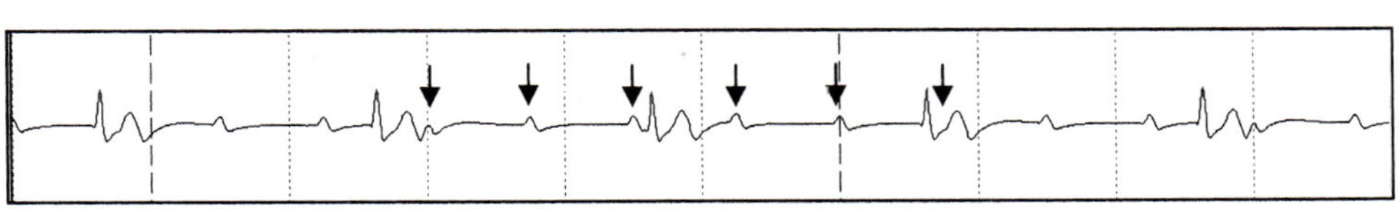

Figure 37-36 Third-degree atrioventricular block, 10-second display.

P to QRS ratio: 1:1
Rhythm: Regular
Rate: Usually 60 to 100 but can occur with slower or faster rates

Comments: The bundle branch blocks are difficult to visualize. The key is to use a 10-second display (or less) and look for the increased QRS interval and notching (may be quite subtle) (Figures 37-37 and 37-38).

RIGHT BUNDLE BRANCH BLOCK

Features of Right Bundle Branch Block

P wave: Normal
QRS complex: Present, widened, and notched (rabbit-eared appearance), best seen in V_1 or MCL_1; hence, not well seen in most sleep studies
PR interval: Normal, can be prolonged with first-degree block
QRS interval: More than 0.12 seconds
P to QRS ratio: 1:1
Rhythm: Regular
Rate: Usually, 60 to 100 but can occur with slower or faster rates

Comments: RBBB is often difficult to visualize during polysomnography. Use a 10-second screen and look for widened QRS. You might see W-shaped waves in lead I (Figures 37-39 and 37-40).

VENTRICULAR ARRHYTHMIAS

- PVCs
- Unifocal PVCs
- Multifocal PVCs
- Ventricular trigeminy
- Ventricular bigeminy
- Ventricular couplets
- Idioventricular rhythm
- Accelerated ventricular rhythm
- Ventricular tachycardia
- Runs of ventricular tachycardia
- Sustained ventricular tachycardia
- Ventricular fibrillation

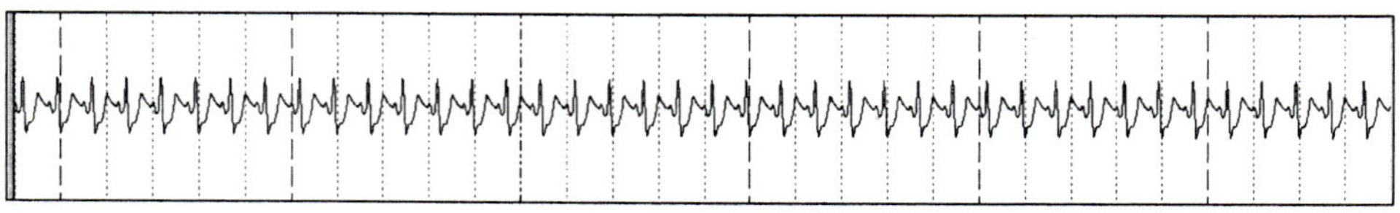

Figure 37-37 Left bundle branch block, 30-second display.

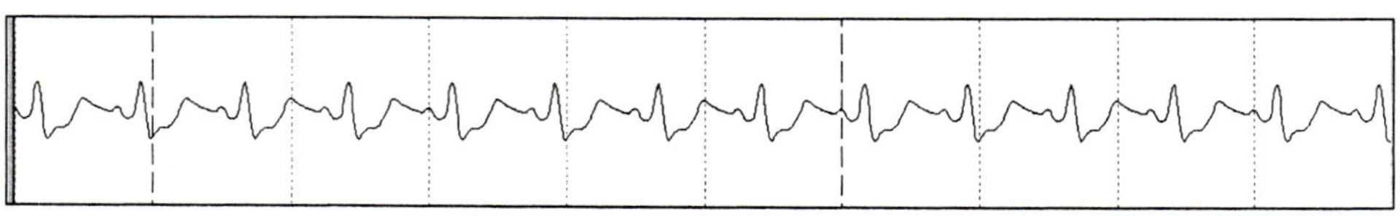

Figure 37-38 Left bundle branch block, 10-second display.

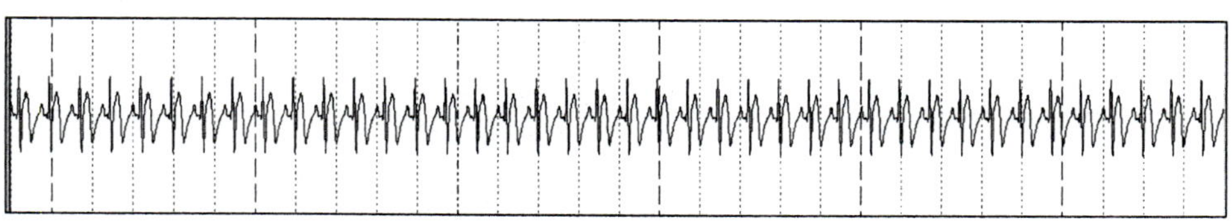

Figure 37-39 Right bundle branch block, 30-second display.

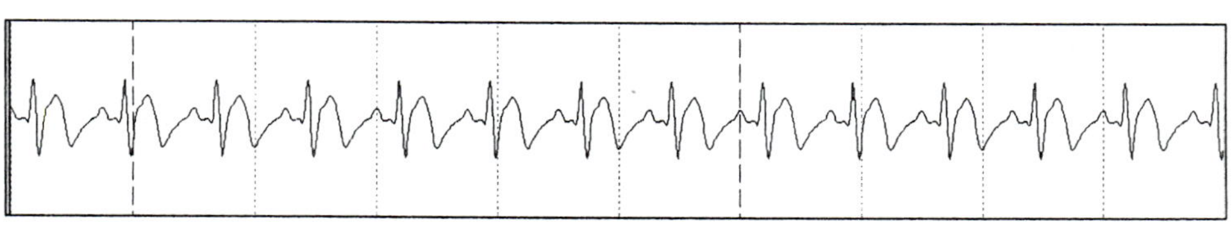

Figure 37-40 Right bundle branch block, 10-second display.

PREMATURE VENTRICULAR CONTRACTIONS, UNIFOCAL PVCS

Features of Premature Ventricular Contractions and Variants

P wave: Not present with abnormal beat
QRS complex: Occurs earlier than expected, widened and bizarre appearing in abnormal beat
PR interval: None
QRS interval: More than 0.12 seconds with abnormal beat
P to QRS ratio: Less than 1:1
Rhythm: Irregular
Rate: Usually, 60 to 100 but can occur with slower or faster rates

Comments: The arrows in Figures 37-41 to 37-50 indicate areas of ventricular ectopy (not all are annotated). Note that Figures 37-41 and 37-42 have different-appearing PVCs. This sample was taken from the same recording but using a different lead combination. Figure 37-41 is lead I and Figure 37-42 is lead II. Changing lead combinations may make the abnormality more apparent. In Figures 37-43 and 37-44, note the different appearance of the PVCs. Apply the *rule of differing morphology.* These beats originate from different areas of the ventricle (separate foci) and are therefore called "multifocal PVCs." Figures 37-45 and 37-46 display PVCs every third beat (ventricular trigeminy), and Figures 37-47 and 37-48 present PVCs every other beat (ventricular bigeminy). Note that the terms trigeminy and bigeminy can also refer to atrial and junctional extrasystoles bearing similar patterns. Figures 37-49 and 37-50 show paired PVCs (ventricular couplets). The aberrant waves have the same appearance; hence, they originate from the same location. Multifocal couplets are paired ventricular beats arising from different locations. These arrhythmias should be listed under Other Arrhythmias in the report if frequent or of clinical significance.

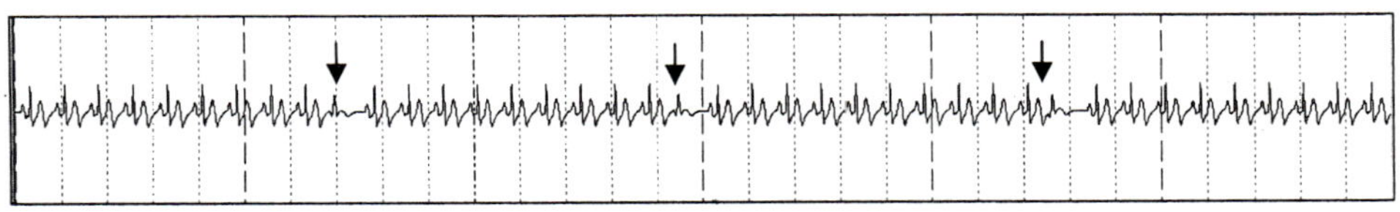

Figure 37-41 Unifocal premature ventricular contractions, 30-second display.

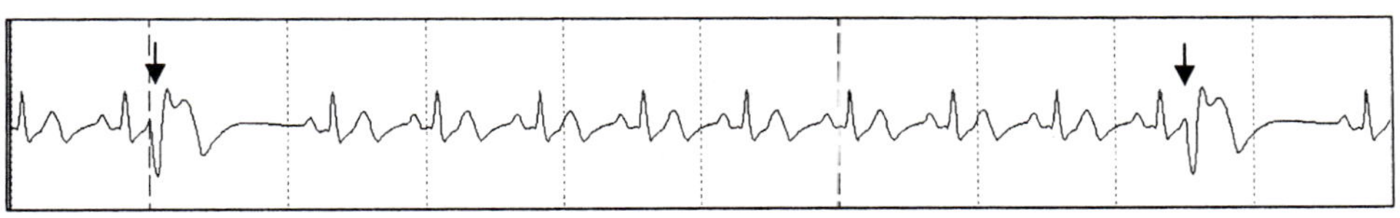

Figure 37-42 Unifocal premature ventricular contractions, 10-second display.

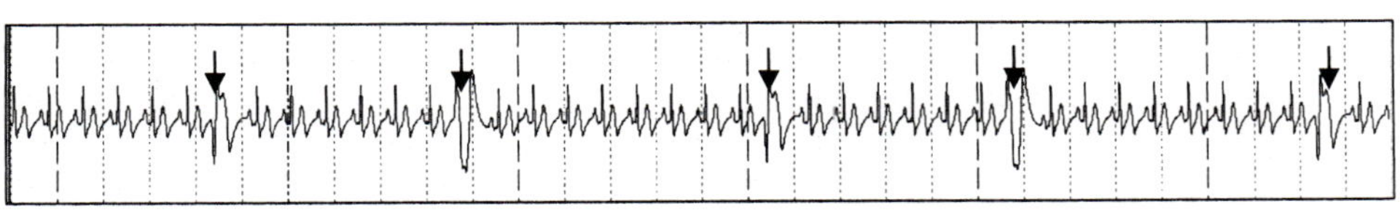

Figure 37-43 Multifocal premature ventricular contractions, 30-second display.

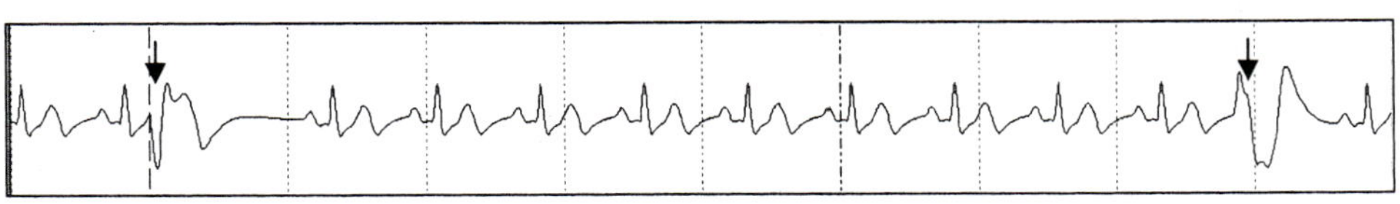

Figure 37-44 Multifocal premature ventricular contractions, 10-second display.

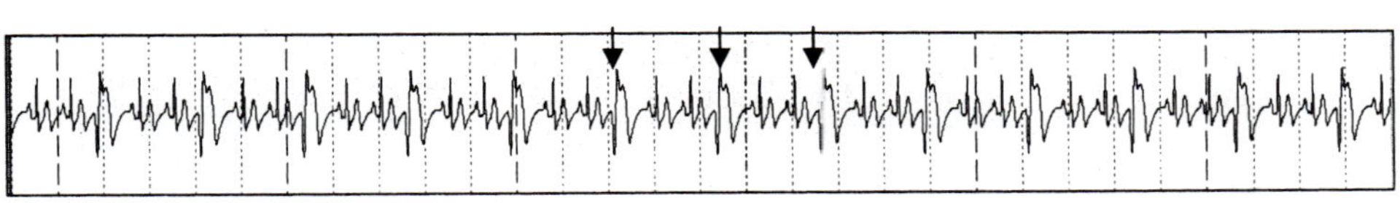

Figure 37-45 Trigeminal premature ventricular contractions, ventricular trigeminy, 30-second display.

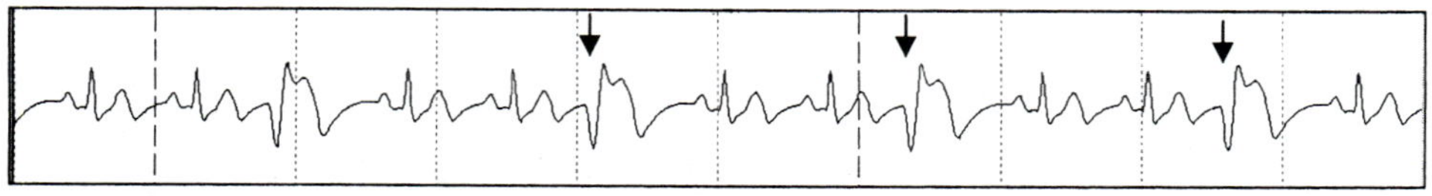

Figure 37-46 Trigeminal premature ventricular contractions, ventricular trigeminy, 10-second display.

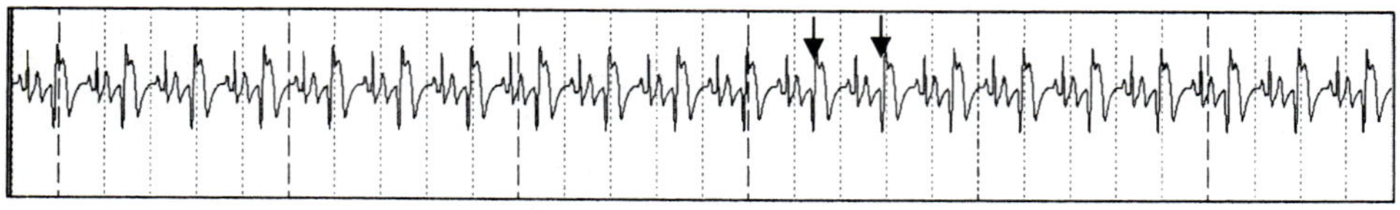

Figure 37-47 Bigeminal premature ventricular contractions, ventricular bigeminy, 30-second display.

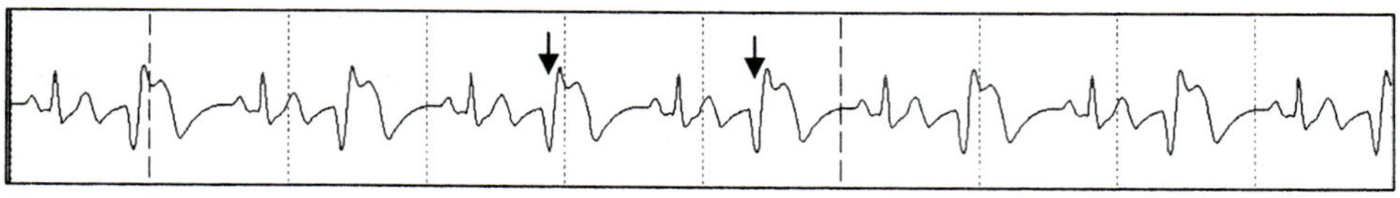

Figure 37-48 Bigeminal premature ventricular contractions, ventricular bigeminy, 10-second display.

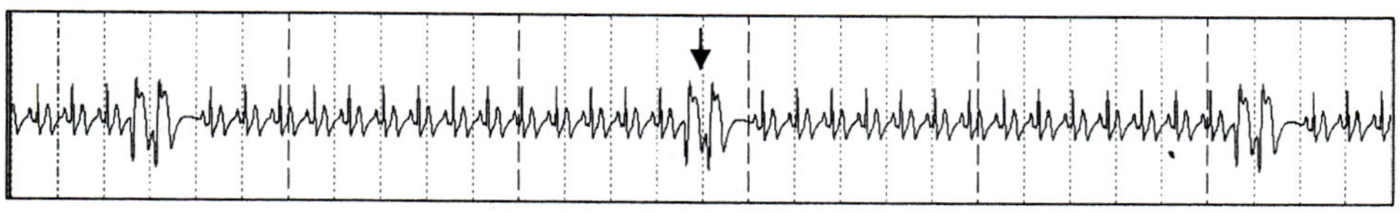

Figure 37-49 Ventricular couplets, 30-second display.

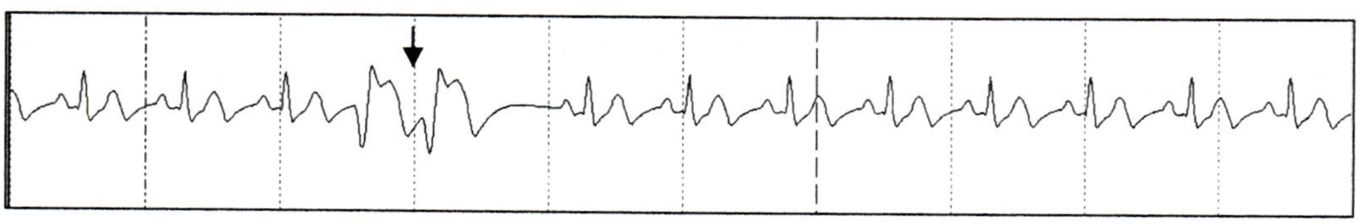

Figure 37-50 Ventricular couplets, 10-second display.

IDIOVENTRICULAR RHYTHM

Features of Idioventricular Rhythm

P wave: No P waves associated with abnormal
QRS complex: Wide and bizarre
PR interval: None
QRS interval: More than 0.12 seconds
P to QRS ratio: Less than 1:1
Rhythm: Regular
Rate: Less than 40 bpm

Comments: Idioventricular rhythm (Figures 37-51 and 37-52) is often seen as escape rhythm with sinus node and AV node dysfunction. If sustained, assess the patient and notify appropriate medical personnel according to

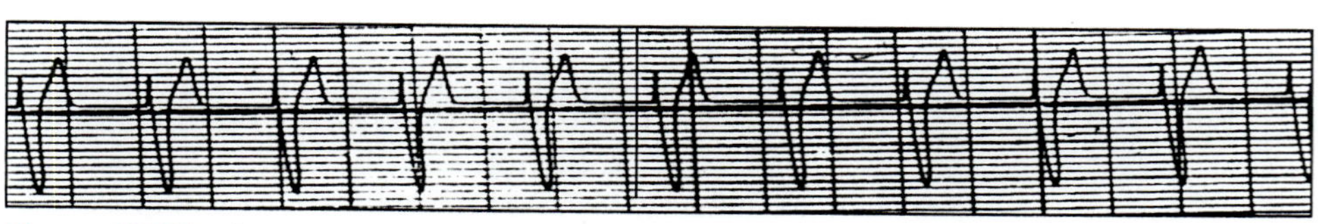

Figure 37-51 Idioventricular rhythm, 30-second timescale.

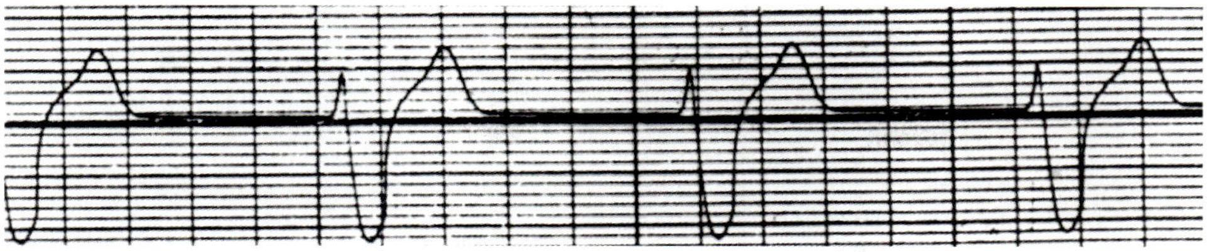

Figure 37-52 Idioventricular rhythm, 10-second timescale.

protocol. Indicate as Bradycardia on the polysomnographic report, although it may also be indicated under Other Arrhythmias.

ACCELERATED VENTRICULAR RHYTHM

Features of Accelerated Ventricular Rhythm

P wave: No P waves associated with abnormal
QRS complex: Wide and bizarre
PR interval: None
QRS interval: More than 0.12 seconds
P to QRS ratio: Less than 1:1
Rhythm: Regular
Rate: 37 to 100 bpm

Comments: Accelerated ventricular rhythm (Figures 37-53 and 37-54) is often seen as escape rhythm with sinus node and AV node dysfunction. Cardiac output is generally adequate. If sustained, assess the patient and notify medical personnel according to protocol. This type of rhythm should be listed under Other Arrhythmias in the report.

VENTRICULAR TACHYCARDIA

Features of Ventricular Tachycardia

P wave: No P waves associated with abnormal
QRS complex: Wide and bizarre
PR interval: None
QRS interval: More than 0.12 seconds
P to QRS ratio: Less than 1:1
Rhythm: Regular
Rate: 100 to 250

Comments: If ventricular tachycardia is not sustained, notify medical personnel according to protocol. If it is sustained, assess the patient and activate the emergency medical system (EMS) according to protocol (see Figures 37-55 to 37-58). This type of rhythm should be listed under Wide Complex Tachycardia in the report.

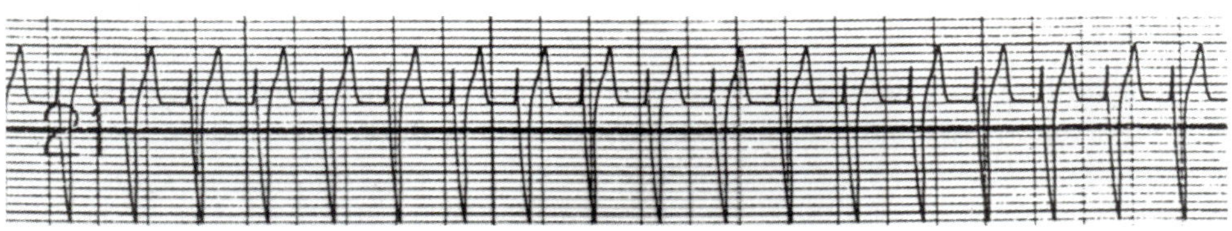

Figure 37-53 Accelerated ventricular rhythm, 30-second timescale.

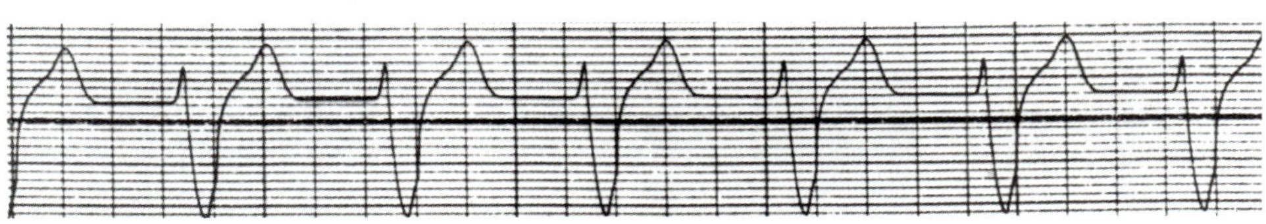

Figure 37-54 Accelerated ventricular rhythm, 10-second timescale.

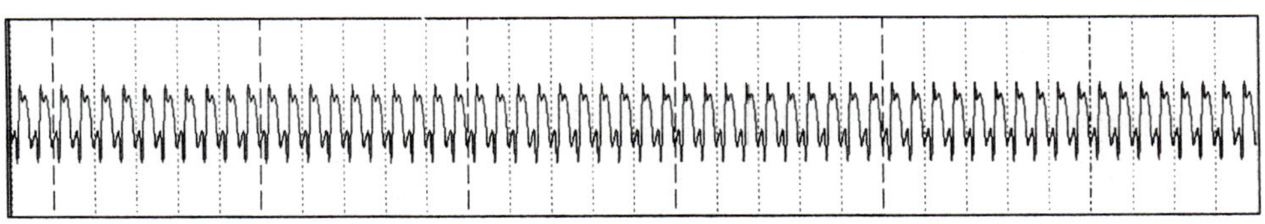

Figure 37-55 Sustained ventricular tachycardia, 30-second display.

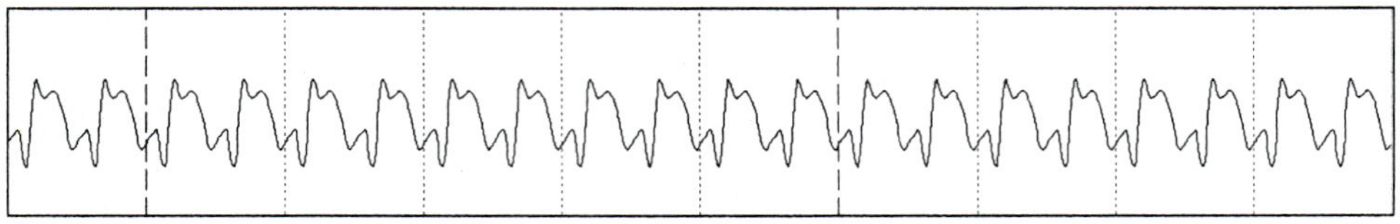

Figure 37-56 Sustained ventricular tachycardia, 10-second display.

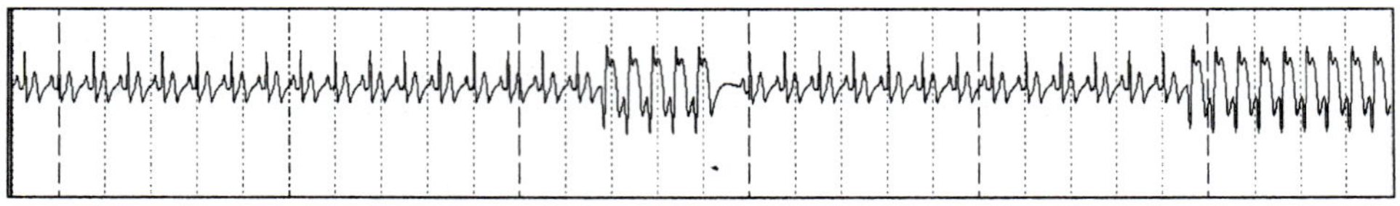

Figure 37-57 Runs of ventricular tachycardia, 30-second display.

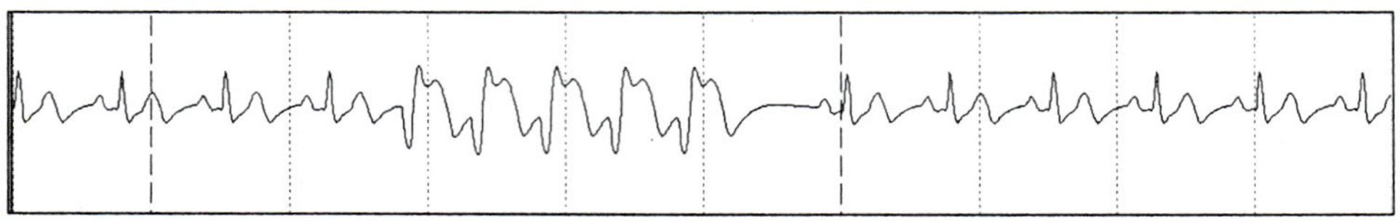

Figure 37-58 Runs of ventricular tachycardia, 10-second display.

VENTRICULAR FIBRILLATION

Features of Ventricular Fibrillation

P wave: No P waves seen
QRS complex: None; wave deflections are disorganized, chaotic, and varying in size and shape.
PR interval: None
QRS interval: Not measurable
P to QRS ratio: Not measurable
Rhythm: Chaotic
Rate: Not measurable

Comments: Ventricular fibrillation (Figures 37-59 and 37-60) is a medical emergency. Assess the patient and activate EMS. When the ECG looks like the EEG, take immediate action. This type of rhythm should be listed under Other Arrhythmias in the report.

INTERVENTIONS

Each facility should have a policy for dealing with significant arrhythmias. Sustained tachyarrhythmias (atrial or junctional tachycardias and ventricular tachycardias), atrial fibrillation and flutter with rapid ventricular response, and sustained ventricular arrhythmias (idioventricular or accelerated ventricular rhythm) require immediate assessment of the patient. Assessment should include the level of consciousness; dizziness or light-headedness; the presence of chest, arm, or neck pain; oxygen saturation; and blood pressure. Of course, emergency protocol for Code Blue or activating the EMS should be initiated in the case of unresponsiveness. Other arrhythmias such as nonsustained runs of ventricular tachycardia, asystole, second- and third-degree blocks, and previously undocumented atrial fibrillation

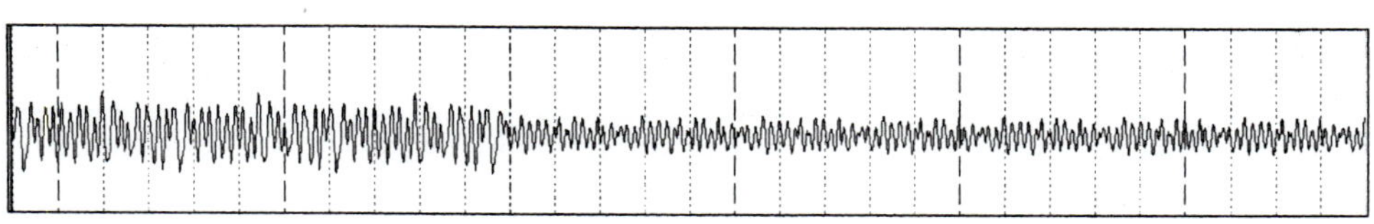

Figure 37-59 Ventricular fibrillation, 30-second display.

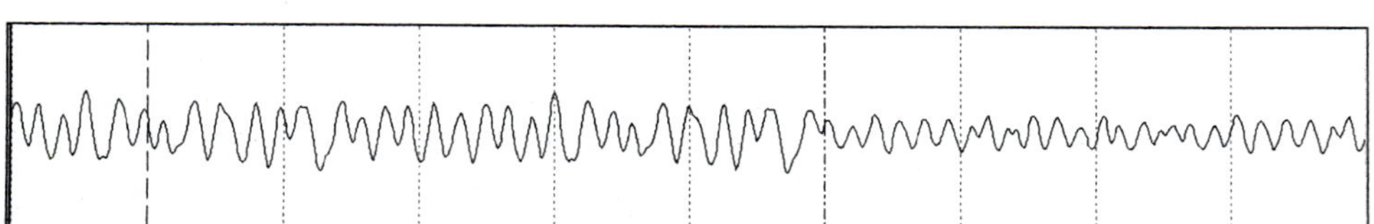

Figure 37-60 Ventricular fibrillation, 10-second display.

or flutter warrant a call to the medical director, referring physician, or house officer for direction, according to protocol.

RECORDING AND MONITORING TECHNIQUES

Many sleep centers have a prescribed electrode placement for recording the ECG. This usually involves recording from the right and left subclavicular areas (essentially lead I) or the right subclavicular area and the lower left thorax (essentially lead II, the AASM-recommended derivation). However, the chosen ECG derivation may not always demonstrate a good P wave and a QRS complex of adequate amplitude necessary for arrhythmia identification. The ECG quality should be observed before or during the physiologic calibration procedure. Different lead combinations should be sampled to provide the best ECG display before "lights out." Some recording systems have a dedicated paired input for the ECG. In this case, one must physically move the electrodes to another location. Other systems will allow the user to reference any recording electrode to any other using the system input selection panel. In this case, it is fairly simple to reference an ECG electrode to another recording electrode (such as a left leg electrode) and obtain a different view of the ECG.

A more advanced tactic is to routinely monitor two separate ECG leads (a lead I and a lead II, or a lead I and a lead III simultaneously). There are recording systems that have the capability to average recording signals. It is possible in these systems to provide a semblance of the precordial leads by averaging left arm, left leg, and right arm signals as a reference for any of the V leads. In addition, a reasonable facsimile of the augmented limb leads (aVR, aVL, and aVF) may be obtained by recording the right arm versus the average of the left arm and left leg (aVR), etc.

To ensure a quality recording, ECG electrodes should be applied with the same care and proper skin preparation as with any other electrodes used in the sleep study. The AASM guidelines recommend the use of standard ECG electrodes rather than EEG electrodes (1). High electrode impedances or sloppy application techniques will result in artifacts, which in some cases, may resemble ectopic beats. To avoid misinterpretation of the ECG, any questionable patterns should be confirmed by examining alternate derivations (as described earlier).

Viewing the ECG for arrhythmia recognition is facilitated by "spreading the recording out," utilizing a 10-second display or less (the author has used a 6-second display to try to find evidence of "hidden" P waves). Intervals are nearly impossible to assess using a standard 30-second screen width. Measurement of the PR and QRS intervals can be accomplished by printing the 10-second screen and then measuring the intervals with a millimeter ruler and dividing this measurement by the number of millimeters per second on the printout. Standard calipers can be used to determine regularity on these printouts. If the system is incapable of printing during recording, it is possible to measure the intervals and test regularity by using a stationary 10-second window and an index card. Make tick marks at the beginning and end of the interval of interest, measure this distance in millimeters, and divide by the number of millimeters per second provided by your display. Regularity can be checked by making tick marks at three successive R waves (or P waves) and then moving the card from R wave to R wave (or P wave to P wave). If the tick marks fall in line, the rhythm is regular.

At the end of the numbered references are a few web references that were recently accessed. The author has found them an interesting "challenge" and learning experience and would recommend them to the student or technologist as an additional learning resource after studying arrhythmias and developing a degree of confidence in arrhythmia identification.

REFERENCES

1. Iber C, Ancoli-Israel S, Chesson A, et al. *The AASM Manual for the Scoring of Sleep and Associated Events: Rules Terminology and Technical Specifications*. 1st ed. American Academy of Sleep Medicine; 2007.
2. Troester MM, Quan SF, Berry RB, et al; for the American Academy of Sleep Medicine. *The AASM Manual for the Scoring of Sleep and Associated Events: Rules, Terminology and Technical Specifications* [Version 3.0]. American Academy of Sleep Medicine; 2023.
3. Atkinson J. Cardiac arrhythmias. In: Lee-Chiong T, Brown W, eds. *Respiratory Clinics of North America*. Vol 11. W.B. Saunders; 2005:4.
4. Dubin D. *Rapid Interpretation of EKGs*. 6th ed. Cover Publishing; 2000.
5. Huff J. *ECG Workout: Exercises in Arrhythmia Interpretation*. 6th ed. Lippincott Williams & Wilkins; 2011.
6. Thaler MS. *The Only EKG Book You'll Ever Need*. 5th ed. Lippincott Williams & Wilkins; 2007.

WEB REFERENCES

EKG Academy. EKG practice drill. Accessed March 9, 2025. https://ekg.academy/ekg-interpretation-practice

Medical Intensive Care Nursing. Cardiology in critical care: EKG and arrhythmia recognition. Accessed March 9, 2025. http://www.micunursing.com/#Section_3_Cardiology_in_Critical_Care

Practical Clinical Skills. ECG practice. Accessed March 9, 2025. https://www.practicalclinicalskills.com/ekg-practice-drill

Chapter 38
Generating the Polysomnography Report

ELIZABETH Y. WIESEMANN

KEY CONCEPTS/LEARNING OBJECTIVES

The key concepts for this chapter include describing the purpose of the sleep study report, defining the parameters to be reported according to the American Academy of Sleep Medicine (AASM) guidelines set forth in *The AASM Manual for the Scoring of Sleep and Associated Events: Rules, Terminology and Technical Specifications Version 3.0*, citing the definitions and use formulae to calculate common sleep architectural parameters, definitions and use formulae to calculate common event parameters, deriving and utilizing histograms, developing derivations of unique/detailed event parameters and tables, validating the use of summary reports, describing archiving and data storage procedures, and describing the AASM reporting guidelines for home sleep apnea testing set forth in *The AASM Manual for the Scoring of Sleep and Associated Events: Rules, Terminology and Technical Specifications Version 3.0*.

KEY TERMS

Data analysis
Home sleep apnea testing (HSAT)
Polysomnography
Reporting

In the early days of sleep medicine, polysomnographic studies were recorded on paper. Utilizing a paper speed of 10 mm/s, these records usually contained 800 to 1,000 pages of data. The purpose of the polysomnographic report was to summarize these data, presenting an overview of the patient's sleep architecture and allowing for comparisons among sleep studies (1). In the late 1960s, a standard scoring system was developed to provide guidelines for staging human sleep, and this scoring system was the gold standard for decades (2). This document was based on data from normal, young adult subjects. As the practice of clinical sleep medicine evolved and a variety of sleep-related pathologies were recognized, it became clear that additional descriptive statistics were necessary to convey adequately the various aspects of normal and abnormal sleep. Guidelines for identifying and scoring arousals (3), periodic limb movements (PLMs) (4), and respiratory events (5) were then developed in an effort to standardize the tabulation of these data.

Manual scoring and data tabulation was a daunting task, even for a very experienced technologist, often consuming hours of time per recording. Before the advent of personal computers to assist with "number crunching," the tabulation of data and generation of the report summary sometimes involved more time than the identification of sleep stages and abnormal events. Today, a polished report representing the visual scoring of sleep and events, full of graphics and charts, can typically be produced within 1 to 2 hours (depending on the complexity of the recording and the severity of the patient's condition). This type of report would have been virtually impossible to produce in the formative years of polysomnographic technology.

The advent of digital polysomnography recording systems with intrinsic scoring and data tabulation has rendered the report generation task much less cumbersome. Although this represents a significant advance in technology, it has also given rise to several problems.

The digitization of polysomnographic data allows use of various automated functions, including computer-assisted or automated scoring. Many of the algorithms have not been validated and have inaccuracies. Automated scoring has become more accurate for sleep staging and abnormal event recognition. It still can make significant errors in the case of mechanical, physiologic, and medication-induced artifacts that can occur in unison or in combination. Computer-scored recordings must always be reviewed and edited by a competent technologist. This is not only for in-lab studies, but home sleep testing, as well. Current Medicare guidelines mandate that a Registered Polysomnographic Technologist (RPSGT) must score all in-lab and home sleep studies (6). In essence, the technologist must manually corroborate the sleep stage scoring and review/edit computer-scored abnormal events, such as apneas, hypopneas, oxygen desaturations, and limb movements.

Reliance on automated data tabulation and report generation built into these programs allows the technologist to be uninformed about the theory, concepts, and formulae involved in the generation of these reports. The knowledge base related to the theory, concepts, and formulae used to generate reports becomes very important when installing new systems and developing report templates or developing specialized reports or data points. The data points in a report must be checked for accuracy and appropriateness before the report is used to present patient data. It is not uncommon to find inaccurate numbers in the initial reports developed following a new installation.

Each software system has a different coding system to generate report statistics. Typically, the software company will assist in report template generation. Aside from the different languages between software, the terminology a specific software system uses to describe an event type or data range can vary.

Back in the days of analog paper-based recordings, the manual data tabulation theories, concepts, and formulae presented in this chapter were utilized many times daily. There was continuous reinforcement of this knowledge and a practical reason for learning and maintaining this information. Currently, many technologists have little exposure to this knowledge and do not spend time exploring its intricacies. It is important to be competent at manually calculating report statistics in order to detect inaccuracies in generated reports.

PURPOSE OF A SLEEP STUDY REPORT

The purpose of the polysomnographic report is dependent on the needs of the end user. This may be the interpreting physician, the referring physician, the homecare company, durable medical equipment (DME) supplier, or the third-party payer. With the advent of digital recordings, there is an ability to overanalyze and therefore produce reports with overwhelming, often superfluous amounts of data. Fortunately, it is also easy to develop multiple reports using the same data to meet the needs of multiple users.

For in-depth data analysis or research purposes, a report can contain multiple tables, statistics, graphs, and customized charts to meet the needs of the interpreter or research project. Visual summaries of data presented in the form of histograms can correlate events with sleep staging, body position, and treatment settings. Event tabulations, percentages, and indices can be provided for every conceivable condition encountered during the study. A report of this nature can be quite lengthy, but not necessarily practical. Figure 38-1 is an example of a Split-Night Study—Long Report for Sleep Center Use.

Split-Night Study (Long Report for Sleep Center Use)

Patient Name: Walker, Ima			
Gender	Female	**Study date**	September 13, 2011
D.O.B.	December 6, 1946	**Subject code**	98765
Age	64	**Referring physician**	Frequent referral, MD
Height	66.0 in	**Sleep specialist**	Sleep doctor, MD
Weight	190.0 lbs	**Recording tech**	IM Sleepy, RPSGT
BMI	30.7	**Scoring tech**	JW Atkinson, RPSGT

Study Indications:
Daytime complaints of EDS (ESS=9), loud snoring, nonrestorative sleep. Sleep complaints of breathing/snoring stops in sleep, wakes for unknown reasons, restless sleep, somniloquy, occasional heartburn, and bruxism.

Recording/Collection Notes:
Insert recording/collection technician notes here.

Scoring/Analysis Notes:
Insert scoring/analysis technician notes here.

Hypopnea Rule:	VIII.4.A
Stage Scored by:	TECH
Hypoventilation:	NO
Cheyne–Stokes Breathing:	NO
Arrythmias:	NO

Figure 38-1 Split-night study. CPAP, continuous positive airway pressure; PLM, periodic limb movement; REM, rapid eye movement; TIB, time in bed; TST, total sleep time; WASO, wake after sleep onset (long report for Sleep Center use and third-party payer).

Channel information Chart

Channel Input Label	Channel Name	Channel Type	Frequency
Snore (Amp 1)	Snore	Snore	256
Chest (Amp 1)	Chest	Chest	32
Abd (Amp 1)	Abdomen	Abdomen	32
C3 (Amp 1)	C3	EEG,C3,CZ	256
C4 (Amp 1)	C4	EEG,C4,CZ	256
O1 (Amp 1)	O1	EEG,O1,CZ	256
L Eye (Amp 1)	E1	Ocular, Left	256
R Eye (Amp 1)	E2	Ocular, Right	256
O2 (Amp 1)	O2	EEG,O2,CZ	256
A1 (Amp 1)	M1	EEG,A1,CZ	256
A2 (Amp 1)	M2	EEG,A2,CZ	256
L EMG (Amp 1)	EMG1	EMG, Left	256
R EMG (Amp 1)	EMG2	EMG, Right	256
L EKG (Amp 1)	ECG1	EKG,1	256
R EKG (Amp 1)	ECG2	EKG,2	256
L Leg+ (Amp 1)	L-Leg1	Legs, Left,1	256
L Leg– (Amp 1)	L-Leg2	Legs, Left,2	256
R Leg+ (Amp 1)	R-Leg1	Legs, Right,1	256
R Leg– (Amp 1)	R-Leg2	Legs, Right,2	256
Thermistor (Amp 1)	Airflow	AirFlow	32
Pressure (Amp 1)	Nasal pressure	Nasal canula	32
Body position (Amp 1)	Body position	Body position	1
OP. 1+ (Amp 1)	F3	EEG,F3,CZ	256
OP. 2+ (Amp 1)	F4	EEG,F4,CZ	256
OP. 3+ (Amp 1)	EMG3	EMG, Submental	256
SpO_2 (Amp 1)	SaO_2	SaO_2	16
Pulse (Amp 1)	Pulse	Pulse	16
Pleth (Amp 1)	Pleth	Pleth	16
DC X1 (Box 1)	CPAP flow	CPAP (flow)	16
DC X2 (Box 1)	CPAP	CPAP (pressure)	16
DC X3 (Box 1)	CPAP leak	CPAP (leak)	16

Figure 38-1 *(continued)*

Sleep Architecture	
Lights out clock time (h:min)	9:47:00 p.m.
Lights on clock time (h:min)	12:50:56 a.m.
Total recording time (TRT; in min)	183.9
Sleep period time (SPT)*	3:03:03
Total sleep time (TST; in min)	161.0
Sleep efficiency (SE)	87.5%
Sleep latency (SL)	0:00:54
Total stage changes (after sleep onset [SO])	84
Awakenings (after SO)	19
WASO	22.0
REM periods	2
REM latency*	1:35:00
REM latency (less wake time)*	1:32:30

*Time formats are in h:min:s

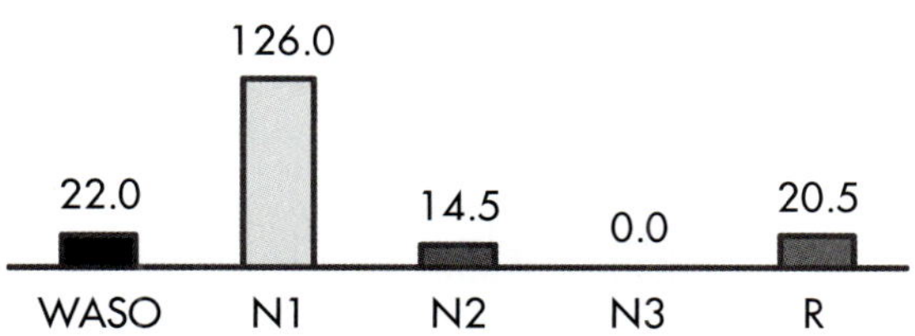

Stage Distribution (min)

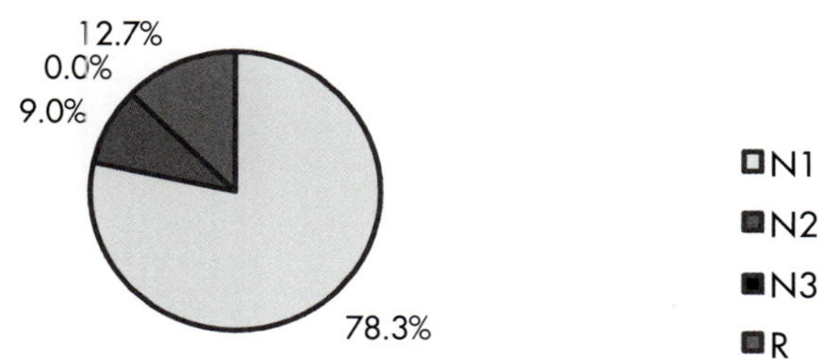

Sleep Stage (%TST)

Sleep Stage	Latency (min)
N1	0.0
N2	30.5
N3	N/A
R	95.0

Stage latency = 0.0 denotes start of sleep.

Figure 38-1 (*continued*)

Respiratory Events	Cen. Apneas	Obs. Apneas	Mxd. Apneas	Hypopneas	Total Apneas	Apnea+ Hypopnea	RERA	All Resp. Events*
Count:	0	52	0	155	52	207	0	207
Index (events/h)	0.0	19.4	0.0	57.8	19.4	**77.1**	0.0	77.1
Mean duration (s)	N/A	29.4	N/A	24.0	29.4	25.3	N/A	25.3
Longest event (s)	N/A	66.1	N/A	81.9	66.1	81.9	N/A	81.9
REM count	0	10	0	7	10	17	0	17
Non-REM count	0	42	0	148	42	190	0	190
REM index	0.0	29.3	0.0	20.5	29.3	49.8	0.0	49.8
Non-REM index	0.0	17.9	0.0	63.2	17.9	81.1	0.0	81.1

*Note: Does not contain Cheyne–Stokes breathing, hypoventilation, or periodic breathing.

Respiratory Events	Supine Sleep		Prone Sleep		Left-Side Sleep		Right-Side Sleep		Upright Sleep	
(by body position)	Count	Index	Count	Index	Count	Index	Count	Index	Count	Index
Duration (h:min:s)	2:40:50		0:00:00		0:00:00		0:00:00		0:00:00	
Obstructive apneas (OA)	52	19.4	N/A	N/A	N/A	N/A	N/A	N/A	N/A	N/A
Central apneas (CA)	0	0.0	N/A	N/A	N/A	N/A	N/A	N/A	N/A	N/A
Mixed apneas (MA)	0	0.0	N/A	N/A	N/A	N/A	N/A	N/A	N/A	N/A
Hypopneas	155	57.8	N/A	N/A	N/A	N/A	N/A	N/A	N/A	N/A
RERAs	0	0.0	N/A	N/A	N/A	N/A	N/A	N/A	N/A	N/A
Total	207	77.2	N/A	N/A	N/A	N/A	N/A	N/A	N/A	N/A

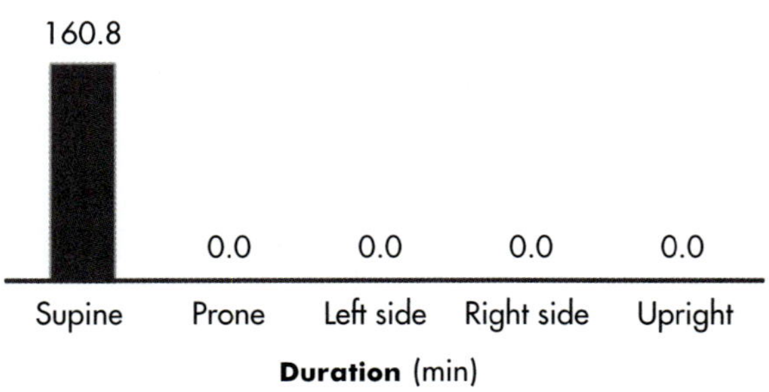

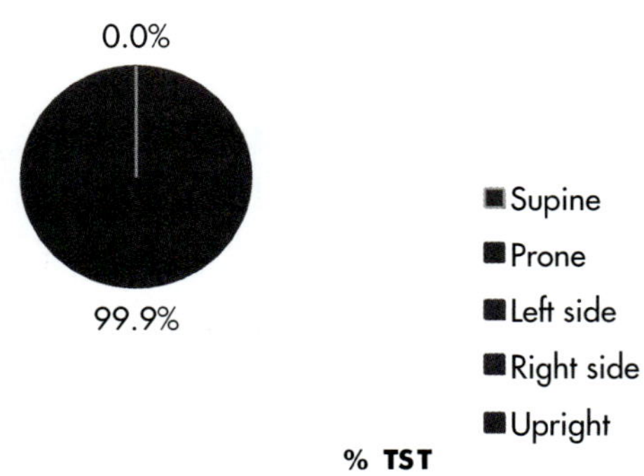

Body Position Results

Arousals	Resp. Count	Resp. Index	Spontaneous Count*	Spontaneous Index*	Total Count	Total Index
TST	153	57.0	25	9.3	178	66.3
Non-REM	141	60.2	25	10.7	166	70.9
REM	12	35.1	0	0.0	12	35.1

*EEG arousal activity *not* associated with *respiratory* or *PLM* events.

Figure 38-1 (*continued*)

Limb Movements (by sleep stage)	LM w Arousals Count	LM w Arousals Index	LM w/o Arousals Count	LM w/o Arousals Index	Total LMs Count	Total LMs Index	PLM Series Count	PLM Series Index
TST	0	0.0	0	0.0	0	0.0	0	0.0
N1	0	0.0	0	0.0	0	0.0	0	0.0
N2	0	0.0	0	0.0	0	0.0	0	0.0
N3	N/A	N/A	N/A	N/A	N/A	N/A	N/A	N/A
R	0	0.0	0	0.0	0	0.0	0	0.0

Oxygen Desaturation Events	Count	Index
TST	200	74.5
Wake (after SO)	5	13.6
Non-REM	181	77.3
REM	19	55.6

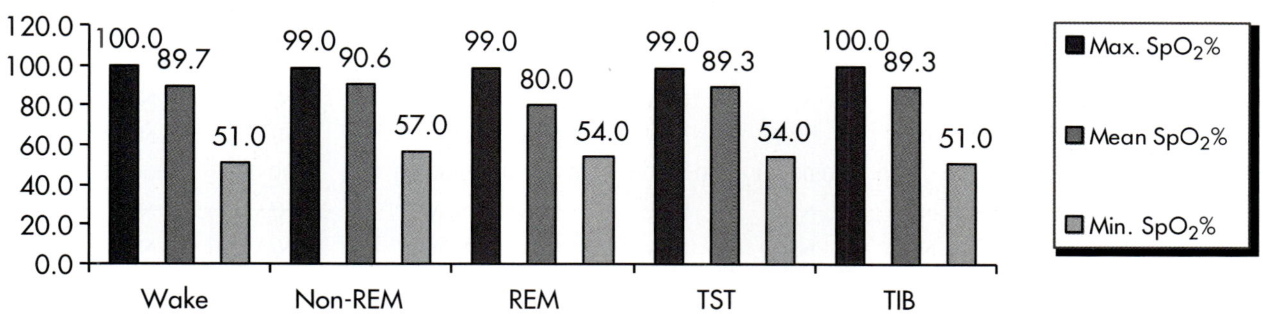

Oximetry Trend Graph

Oxygen Saturation	Wake	Non-REM	REM	TST	TIB
Max. SpO_2%	100.0	99.0	99.0	99.0	100.0
Mean SpO_2%	89.7	90.6	80.0	89.3	89.3
Min. SpO_2%	51.0	57.0	54.0	54.0	51.0
SpO_2% ≤ 89% (min)	0.1	49.3`	14.5	63.8	67.7
% Time in range					
90–100%	36.7%	59.6%	26.6%	55.4%	53.0%
80–89%	12.7%	35.3%	23.3%	33.7%	31.1%
70–79%	1.0%	3.9%	23.9%	6.4%	5.7%
60–69%	3.2%	0.8%	21.5%	3.4%	3.4%
50–59%	1.0%	0.1%	4.7%	0.7%	0.8%
<50%	0.0%	0.0%	0.0%	0.0%	0.0%
% Artifact/bad data	45.4%	0.4%	0.0%	0.3%	6.0%

Figure 38-1 (*continued*)

Heart Rate (HR) Results	Wake	Non-REM	REM	TST	TIB
Max. HR (bpm)	79.0	79.0	81.0	81.0	81.0
Mean HR (bpm)	64.6	61.7	60.7	61.4	61.6
Min. HR (bpm)	9.0	54.0	49.0	49.0	9.0
	% Time in range				
>100 (bpm)	0.0%	0.0%	0.0%	0.0%	0.0%
90–100 (bpm)	0.0%	0.0%	0.0%	0.0%	0.0%
80–89 (bpm)	0.0%	0.0%	0.1%	0.0%	0.0%
70–79 (bpm)	7.4%	1.7%	0.9%	1.5%	1.9%
60–69 (bpm)	48.1%	55.0%	51.4%	54.0%	53.6%
50–59 (bpm)	10.9%	43.2%	47.6%	44.3%	42.1%
<50 (bpm)	2.1%	0.0%	0.0%	0.0%	0.1%
% Artifact/bad data	31.4%	0.2%	0.0%	0.1%	2.2%

Cardiac Events	Brady.	Asystole	Tachy.	Narrow Complex Tachy.	Wide Complex Tachy.	Atrial Fibrillation	Accel.	Decel.
Count	0	0	0	0	0	0	0	0
Shortest event (min:s)	N/A	N/A	N/A	N/A	N/A	N/A	N/A	N/A
Longest event (min:s)	N/A	N/A	N/A	N/A	N/A	N/A	N/A	N/A
Sum duration (min:s)	0:00:00	0:00:00	0:00:00	0:00:00	0:00:00	0:00:00	0:00:00	0:00:00
Absolute max. rate (bpm)	N/A	N/A	N/A	N/A	N/A	N/A	N/A	N/A
Absolute min. rate (bpm)	N/A	N/A	N/A	N/A	N/A	N/A	N/A	N/A

Sleep Architecture	
Lights out clock time (h:min)	12:52:00 a.m.
Lights on clock time (h:min)	5:36:59 a.m.
TRT (in min)	285.0
SPT*	4:44:36
TST (in min)	278.0
SE	97.5%
SL	0:00:24
Total stage changes (after SO)	64
Awakenings (after SO)	10
WASO	6.6
REM periods	3
REM latency*	0:15:30
REM latency (less wake time)*	0:15:30

*Time formats are in h:min:sec

Figure 38-1 (*continued*)

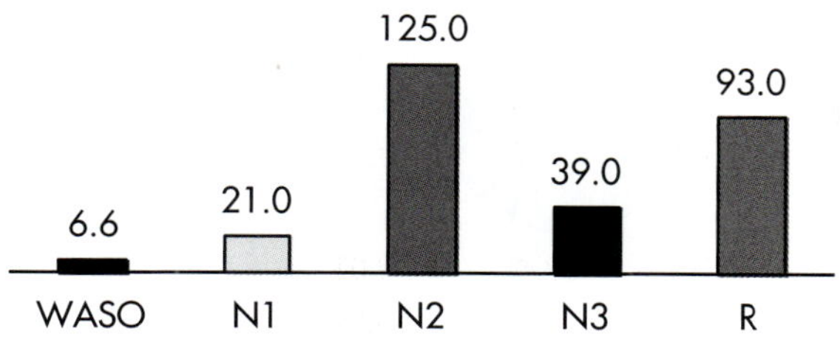

Stage Distribution (in min)

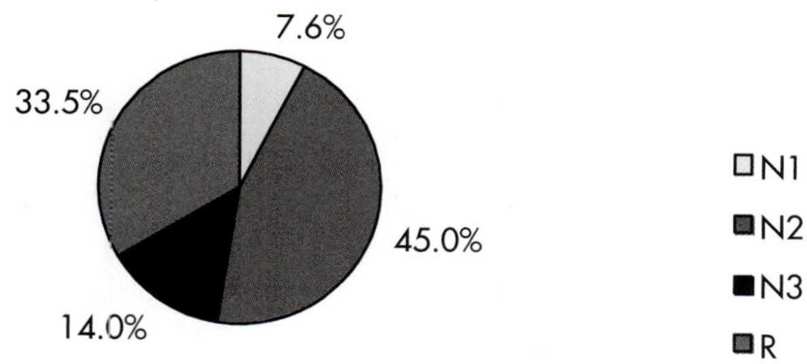

Sleep Stage (%TST)

Sleep Stage	Latency (min)
N1	0.0
N2	2.0
N3	13.0
R	15.5

Stage latency = 0.0 denotes start of sleep.

Respiratory Events	CA	OA	MA	Hypopneas	Total Apneas	Apnea+ Hypopnea	RERA	All Resp. Events *
Count	3	0	0	19	3	22	0	22
Index (events/h)	0.6	0.0	0.0	4.1	0.6	4.7	0.0	4.7
Mean duration (s)	13.5	N/A	N/A	28.5	13.5	26.4	N/A	26.4
Longest event (s)	18.4	N/A	N/A	56.3	18.4	56.3	N/A	56.3
REM count	0	0	0	14	0	14	0	14
Non-REM count	3	0	0	5	3	8	0	8
REM index	0.0	0.0	0.0	9.0	0.0	9.0	0.0	9.0
Non-REM index	1.0	0.0	0.0	1.6	1.0	2.6	0.0	2.6

*Note: Does not contain Cheyne–Stokes breathing, hypoventilation, or periodic breathing.

Respiratory Events	Supine Sleep		Prone Sleep		Left-Side Sleep		Right-Side Sleep		Upright Sleep	
(by body position)	Count	Index	Count	Index	Count	Index	Count	Index	Count	Index
Duration (h:min:s)	4:38:00		0:00:00		0:00:00		0:00:00		0:00:00	
OA	0	0.0	N/A	N/A	N/A	N/A	N/A	N/A	N/A	N/A
CA	3	0.6	N/A	N/A	N/A	N/A	N/A	N/A	N/A	N/A
MA	0	0.0	N/A	N/A	N/A	N/A	N/A	N/A	N/A	N/A
Hypopneas	19	4.1	N/A	N/A	N/A	N/A	N/A	N/A	N/A	N/A
RERAs	0	0.0	N/A	N/A	N/A	N/A	N/A	N/A	N/A	N/A
Total	22	4.7	N/A	N/A	N/A	N/A	N/A	N/A	N/A	N/A

Figure 38-1 (*continued*)

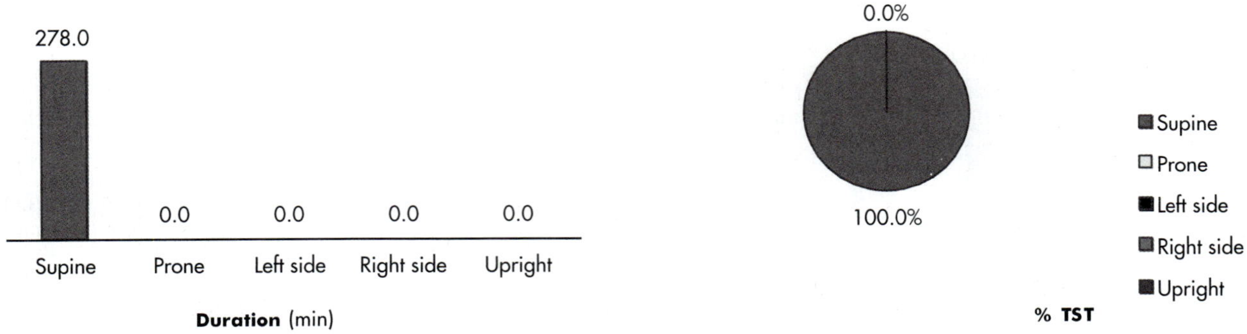

Body Position Results

Arousals	Resp. Count	Resp. Index	Spontaneous Count*	Spontaneous Index*	Total Count	Total Index
TST	1	0.2	27	5.8	28	6.0
Non-REM	1	0.3	21	6.8	22	7.1
REM	0	0.0	6	3.9	6	3.9

*EEG arousal activity *not* associated with *respiratory* or *PLM* events.

Limb Movements	LM w Arousals		LM w/o Arousals		Total LMs		PLM Series	
(by sleep stage)	Count	Index	Count	Index	Count	Index	Count	Index
TST	0	0.0	2	0.4	2	0.4	0	0.0
N1	0	0.0	1	2.9	1	2.9	0	0.0
N2	0	0.0	1	0.5	1	0.5	0	0.0
N3	0	0.0	0	0.0	0	0.0	0	0.0
R	0	0.0	0	0.0	0	0.0	0	0.0

Oxygen Desaturation Events	Count	Index
TST	28	6.0
Wake (after SO)	0	0.0
Non-REM	12	3.9
REM	16	10.3

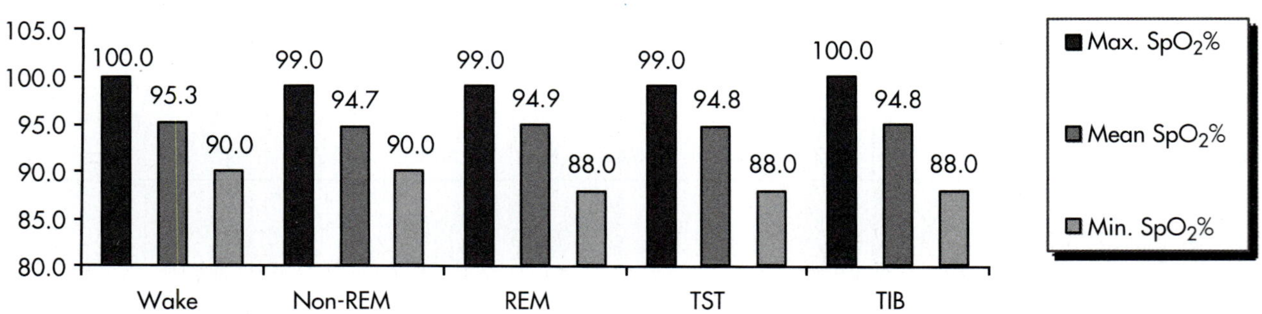

Oximetry Trend Graph

Figure 38-1 (*continued*)

OXYGEN SATURATION	Wake	Non-REM	REM	TST	TIB
Max. SpO_2%	100.0	99.0	99.0	99.0	100.0
Mean SpO_2%	95.3	94.7	94.9	94.8	94.8
Min. SpO_2%	90.0	90.0	88.0	88.0	88.0
$SpO_2\% \leq 89\%$ (min)	0.0	0.0	0.6	0.6	0.6
	% Time in range				
90–100%	99.0%	100.0%	99.0%	99.6%	99.6%
80–89%	1.0%	0.0%	1.0%	0.4%	0.4%
70–79%	0.0%	0.0%	0.0%	0.0%	0.0%
60–69%	0.0%	0.0%	0.0%	0.0%	0.0%
50–59%	0.0%	0.0%	0.0%	0.0%	0.0%
<50%	0.0%	0.0%	0.0%	0.0%	0.0%
% Artifact/bad data	0.0%	0.0%	0.0%	0.0%	0.0%

HR Results	Wake	Non-REM	REM	TST	TIB
Max. HR (bpm)	79.0	79.0	81.0	81.0	81.0
Mean HR (bpm)	64.6	61.7	60.7	61.4	61.6
Min. HR (bpm)	9.0	54.0	49.0	49.0	9.0
% Time in range					
>100 (bpm)	0.0%	0.0%	0.0%	0.0%	0.0%
90–100 (bpm)	0.0%	0.0%	0.0%	0.0%	0.0%
80–89 (bpm)	0.0%	0.0%	0.1%	0.0%	0.0%
70–79 (bpm)	7.4%	1.7%	0.9%	1.5%	1.9%
60–69 (bpm)	48.1%	55.0%	51.4%	54.0%	53.6%
50–59 (bpm)	10.9%	43.2%	47.6%	44.3%	42.1%
<50 (bpm)	2.1%	0.0%	0.0%	0.0%	0.1%
% Artifact/bad data	31.4%	0.2%	0.0%	0.1%	2.2%

Cardiac Events	Brady.	Asystole	Tachy.	Narrow Complex Tachy.	Wide Complex Tachy.	Atrial Fibrillation	Accel.	Decel.
Count	0	0	0	0	0	0	0	0
Shortest event (min:s)	N/A	N/A	N/A	N/A	N/A	N/A	N/A	N/A
Longest event (min:s)	N/A	N/A	N/A	N/A	N/A	N/A	N/A	N/A
Sum duration (min:s)	0:00:00	0:00:00	0:00:00	0:00:00	0:00:00	0:00:00	0:00:00	0:00:00
Absolute max. rate (bpm)	N/A	N/A	N/A	N/A	N/A	N/A	N/A	N/A
Absolute min. rate (bpm)	N/A	N/A	N/A	N/A	N/A	N/A	N/A	N/A

Figure 38-1 (*continued*)

CPAP/Bilevel Titration Chart

Treatment Level (cm H_2O)	TIB	Time: REM (h:min:s)	Time: Non-REM	Respiratory: OA	CA	MA	All Hypn's	A + H TOTAL	AHI	RERA	All Resp	RDI	Oximetry: Max. SpO_2%	Min. SpO_2%	Mean SpO_2%
CPAP 8	0:21:54	0:05:30	0:15:30	0	1	0	3	4	11.4	0	4	11.4	98.0	88.0	93.8
CPAP 9	0:11:52	0:11:52	0:00:00	0	0	0	3	3	15.2	0	3	15.2	98.0	90.0	94.3
CPAP 10	1:36:40	0:19:10	1:16:30	0	1	0	6	7	4.4	0	7	4.4	98.0	90.0	94.6
CPAP 11	1:07:10	0:45:58	0:18:12	0	1	0	4	5	4.7	0	5	4.7	98.0	91.0	95.2
CPAP 12	1:27:54	0:10:30	1:14:48	0	0	0	3	3	2.1	0	3	2.1	99.0	90.0	95.1

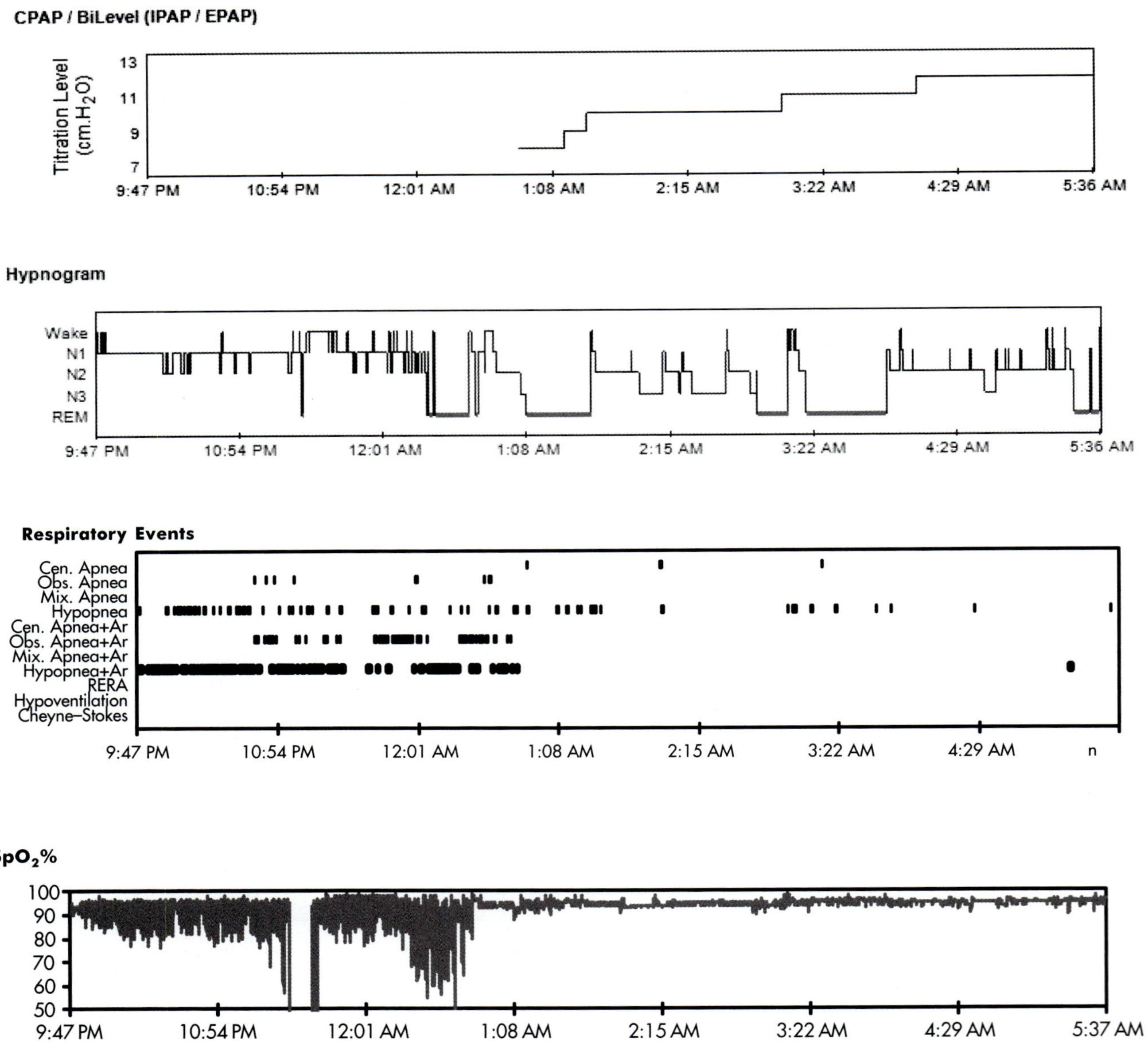

Figure 38-1 (*continued*)

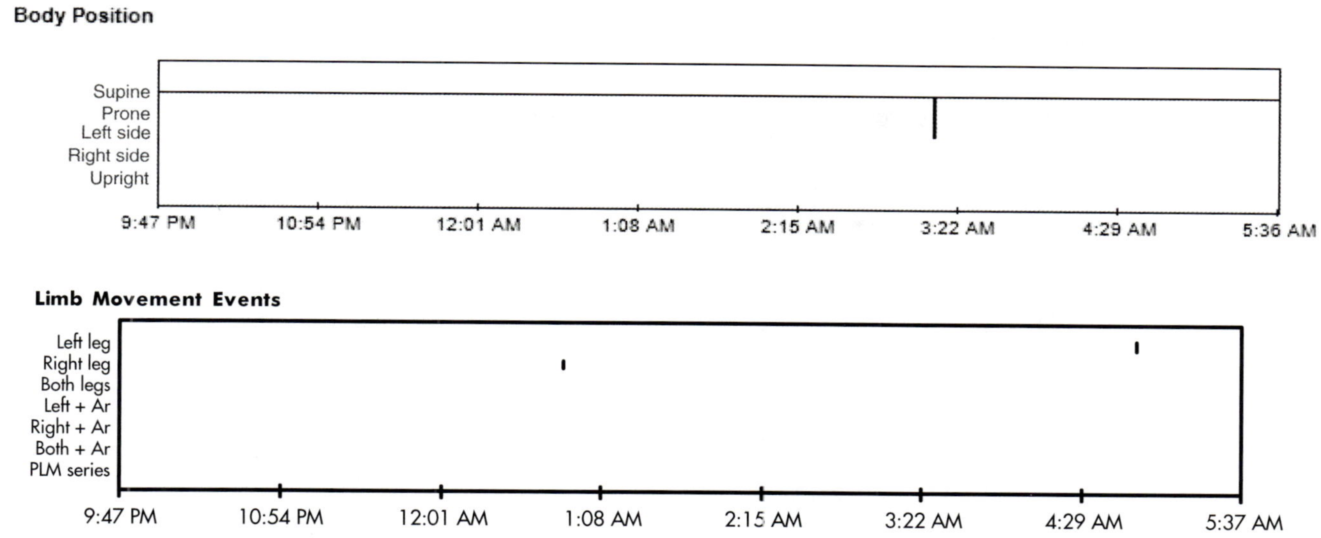

Figure 38-1 (*continued*)

A report generated for clinical use should be relevant, concise, and easily understood by the referring physician (7). This type of report generally serves the needs of the third-party payer as well. It typically includes a summary of sleep architecture, respiratory events, oxygen saturation levels, limb movements, arousals, and heart rate (HR) in a tabular form. A graphic summary is usually also presented. This report should not exceed two or three pages at the most. Figure 38-2 is an example of a Split-Night Study—Referring Physician Report.

Split-Night Report (Referring Physician Report)

Patient Name: Walker, Ima			
Gender	Female	**Study date**	September 13, 2011
D.O.B.	December 6, 1946	**Subject code**	98765
Age	64	**Referring physician**	Frequent referral, MD
Height	66.0 in	**Sleep specialist**	Sleep doctor, MD
Weight	190.0 lbs	**Recording tech**	IM Sleepy, RPSGT
BMI	30.7	**Scoring tech**	JW Atkinson, RPSGT

Study Indications:
Daytime complaints of EDS (ESS=9), loud snoring, nonrestorative sleep. Sleep complaints of breathing/snoring stops in sleep, wakes for unknown reasons, restless sleep, somniloquy, occasional heartburn, and bruxism.

Figure 38-2 Split-night report. CPAP, continuous positive airway pressure; PLM, periodic limb movement; REM, rapid eye movement; RERA, respiratory effort-related arousal; TIB, time in bed; TST, total sleep time; WASO, wake after sleep onset (referring physician report).

Diagnostic Analysis

Sleep Architecture	
Lights out clock time (h:min)	9:47:00 p.m.
Lights on clock time (h:min)	12:50:56 a.m.
TRT (in min)	183.9
SPT*	3:03:03
TST (in min)	161.0
SE	87.5%
SL	0:00:54
Total stage changes (after SO)	84
Awakenings (after SO)	19
WASO	22.0
REM periods	2
REM latency*	1:35:00
REM latency (less wake time)*	1:32:30

*Time formats are in h:min:s

Respiratory Events	CA	OA	MA	Hypopneas	Total Apneas	Apnea+ Hypopnea	RERA	All Resp. Events*
Count	0	52	0	155	52	207	0	207
Index (events/h)	0.0	19.4	0.0	57.8	19.4	**77.1**	0.0	77.1
Mean duration (s)	N/A	29.4	N/A	24.0	29.4	25.3	N/A	25.3
Longest event (s)	N/A	66.1	N/A	81.9	66.1	81.9	N/A	81.9
REM count	0	10	0	7	10	17	0	17
Non-REM count	0	42	0	148	42	190	0	190
REM index	0.0	29.3	0.0	20.5	29.3	49.8	0.0	49.8
Non-REM index	0.0	17.9	0.0	63.2	17.9	81.1	0.0	81.1

*Note: Does not contain Cheyne–Stokes breathing, hypoventilation, or periodic breathing.

Arousals	Resp. Count	Resp. Index	Spontaneous Count*	Spontaneous Index*	Total Count	Total Index
TST	153	57.0	25	9.3	178	66.3
Non-REM	141	60.2	25	10.7	166	70.9
REM	12	35.1	0	0.0	12	35.1

*EEG arousal activity not associated with respiratory or PLM events.

Figure 38-2 (*continued*)

Limb Movements	LM w Arousals		LM w/o Arousals		Total LMs		PLM Series	
(by sleep stage)	Count	Index	Count	Index	Count	Index	Count	Index
TST	0	0.0	0	0.0	0	0.0	0	0.0
N1	0	0.0	0	0.0	0	0.0	0	0.0
N2	0	0.0	0	0.0	0	0.0	0	0.0
N3	N/A	N/A	N/A	N/A	N/A	N/A	N/A	N/A
R	0	0.0	0	0.0	0	0.0	0	0.0

Oxygen Desaturation Events	Count	Index
TST	200	74.5
Wake (after SO)	5	13.6
Non-REM	181	77.3
REM	19	55.6

Oxygen Saturation	Wake	Non-REM	REM	TST	TIB
Max. SpO_2%	100.0	99.0	99.0	99.0	100.0
Mean SpO_2%	89.7	90.6	80.0	89.3	89.3
Min. SpO_2%	51.0	57.0	54.0	.0	51.0
$SpO_2\% \le 89\%$ (min)	0.1	49.3	14.5	63.8	67.7
	% Time in range				
90–100%	36.7%	59.6%	26.6%	55.4%	53.0%
80–89%	12.7%	35.3%	23.3%	33.7%	31.1%
70–79%	1.0%	3.9%	23.9%	6.4%	5.7%
60–69%	3.2%	0.8%	21.5%	3.4%	3.4%
50–59%	1.0%	0.1%	4.7%	0.7%	0.8%
<50%	0.0%	0.0%	0.0%	0.0%	0.0%
% Artifact/bad data	45.4%	0.4%	0.0%	0.3%	6.0%

HR Results	Wake	Non-REM	REM	TST	TIB
Max. HR (bpm)	79.0	79.0	81.0	81.0	81.0
Mean HR (bpm)	64.6	61.7	60.7	61.4	61.6
Min. HR (bpm)	9.0	54.0	49.0	49.0	9.0
	% Time in range				
>100 (bpm)	0.0%	0.0%	0.0%	0.0%	0.0%
90–100 (bpm)	0.0%	0.0%	0.0%	0.0%	0.0%
80–89 (bpm)	0.0%	0.0%	0.1%	0.0%	0.0%
70–79 (bpm)	7.4%	1.7%	0.9%	1.5%	1.9%
60–69 (bpm)	48.1%	55.0%	51.4%	54.0%	53.6%
50–59 (bpm)	10.9%	43.2%	47.6%	44.3%	42.1%
<50 (bpm)	2.1%	0.0%	0.0%	0.0%	0.1%
% Artifact/bad data	31.4%	0.2%	0.0%	0.1%	2.2%

Figure 38-2 (*continued*)

Cardiac Events	Brady.	Asystole	Tachy.	Narrow Complex Tachy.	Wide Complex Tachy.	Atrial Fibrillation	Accel.	Decel.
Count	0	0	0	0	0	0	0	0
Shortest event (min:s)	N/A	N/A	N/A	N/A	N/A	N/A	N/A	N/A
Longest event (min:s)	N/A	N/A	N/A	N/A	N/A	N/A	N/A	N/A
Sum duration (min:s)	0:00:00	0:00:00	0:00:00	0:00:00	0:00:00	0:00:00	0:00:00	0:00:00
Absolute max. rate (bpm)	N/A	N/A	N/A	N/A	N/A	N/A	N/A	N/A
Absolute min. rate (bpm)	N/A	N/A	N/A	N/A	N/A	N/A	N/A	N/A

Treatment Analysis

Sleep Architecture	
Lights out clock time (h:min)	12:52:00 a.m.
Lights on clock time (h:min)	5:36:59 a.m.
TRT (in min)	285.0
SPT*	4:44:36
TST (in min)	278.0
SE	97.5%
SL	0:00:24
Total stage changes (after SO)	64
Awakenings (after SO)	10
WASO	6.6
REM periods	3
REM latency*	0:15:30
REM latency (less wake time)*	0:15:30

*Time formats are in h:min:s

Respiratory Events	CA	OA	MA	Hypopneas	Total Apneas	Apnea+ Hypopnea	RERA	All Resp. Events*
Count	3	0	0	19	3	22	0	22
Index (events/h)	0.6	0.0	0.0	4.1	0.6	**4.7**	0.0	4.7
Mean duration (s)	13.5	N/A	N/A	28.5	13.5	26.4	N/A	26.4
Longest event (s)	18.4	N/A	N/A	56.3	18.4	56.3	N/A	56.3
REM count	0	0	0	14	0	14	0	14
Non-REM count	3	0	0	5	3	8	0	8
REM index	0.0	0.0	0.0	9.0	0.0	9.0	0.0	9.0
Non-REM index	1.0	0.0	0.0	1.6	1.0	2.6	0.0	2.6

*Note: Does not contain Cheyne–Stokes breathing, hypoventilation, or periodic breathing.

Figure 38-2 (*continued*)

Respiratory Events (by body-position)	Supine Sleep		Prone Sleep		Left-Side Sleep		Right-Side Sleep		Upright Sleep	
	Count	Index	Count	Index	Count	Index	Count	Index	Count	Index
Duration (h:min:s)	4:38:00		0:00:00		0:00:00		0:00:00		0:00:00	
OA	0	0.0	N/A	N/A	N/A	N/A	N/A	N/A	N/A	N/A
CA	3	0.6	N/A	N/A	N/A	N/A	N/A	N/A	N/A	N/A
MA	0	0.0	N/A	N/A	N/A	N/A	N/A	N/A	N/A	N/A
Hypopneas	19	4.1	N/A	N/A	N/A	N/A	N/A	N/A	N/A	N/A
RERAs	0	0.0	N/A	N/A	N/A	N/A	N/A	N/A	N/A	N/A
Total	22	4.7	N/A	N/A	N/A	N/A	N/A	N/A	N/A	N/A

Arousals	Resp. Count	Resp. Index	Spontaneous Count*	Spontaneous Index*	Total Count	Total Index
TST	1	0.2	27	5.8	28	6.0
Non-REM	1	0.3	21	6.8	22	7.1
REM	0	0.0	6	3.9	6	3.9

*EEG arousal activity not associated with respiratory or PLM events.

Limb Movements (by sleep stage)	LM w Arousals		LM w/o Arousals		Total LMs		PLM Series	
	Count	Index	Count	Index	Count	Index	Count	Index
TST	0	0.0	2	0.4	2	0.4	0	0.0
N1	0	0.0	1	2.9	1	2.9	0	0.0
N2	0	0.0	1	0.5	1	0.5	0	0.0
N3	0	0.0	0	0.0	0	0.0	0	0.0
R	0	0.0	0	0.0	0	0.0	0	0.0

Oxygen Desaturation Events	Count	Index
TST	28	6.0
Wake (after SO)	0	0.0
Non-REM	12	3.9
REM	16	10.3

Oxygen Saturation	Wake	Non-REM	REM	TST	TIB
Max. SpO_2%	100.0	99.0	99.0	99.0	100.0
Mean SpO_2%	95.3	94.7	94.9	94.8	94.8
Min. SpO_2%	90.0	90.0	88.0	88.0	88.0
$SpO_2\% \leq 89\%$ (min)	0.0	0.0	0.6	0.6	0.6
% Time in range					
90–100%	99.0%	100.0%	99.0%	99.6%	99.6%
80–89%	1.0%	0.0%	1.0%	0.4%	0.4%
70–79%	0.0%	0.0%	0.0%	0.0%	0.0%
60–69%	0.0%	0.0%	0.0%	0.0%	0.0%
50–59%	0.0%	0.0%	0.0%	0.0%	0.0%
<50%	0.0%	0.0%	0.0%	0.0%	0.0%
% Artifact/bad data	0.0%	0.0%	0.0%	0.0%	0.0%

Figure 38-2 (*continued*)

HR Results	Wake	Non-REM	REM	TST	TIB
Max. HR (bpm)	79.0	79.0	81.0	81.0	81.0
Mean HR (bpm)	64.6	61.7	60.7	61.4	61.6
Min. HR (bpm)	9.0	54.0	49.0	49.0	9.0
% Time in range					
>100 (bpm)	0.0%	0.0%	0.0%	0.0%	0.0%
90–100 (bpm)	0.0%	0.0%	0.0%	0.0%	0.0%
80–89 (bpm)	0.0%	0.0%	0.1%	0.0%	0.0%
70–79 (bpm)	7.4%	1.7%	0.9%	1.5%	1.9%
60–69 (bpm)	48.1%	55.0%	51.4%	54.0%	53.6%
50–59 (bpm)	10.9%	43.2%	47.6%	44.3%	42.1%
<50 (bpm)	2.1%	0.0%	0.0%	0.0%	0.1%
% Artifact/bad data	31.4%	0.2%	0.0%	0.1%	2.2%

Cardiac Events	Brady.	Asystole	Tachy.	Narrow Complex Tachy.	Wide Complex Tachy.	Atrial Fibrillation	Accel.	Decel.
Count	0	0	0	0	0	0	0	0
Shortest event (min:s)	N/A	N/A	N/A	N/A	N/A	N/A	N/A	N/A
Longest event (min:s)	N/A	N/A	N/A	N/A	N/A	N/A	N/A	N/A
Sum duration (min:s)	0:00:00	0:00:00	0:00:00	0:00:00	0:00:00	0:00:00	0:00:00	0:00:00
Absolute max. rate (bpm)	N/A	N/A	N/A	N/A	N/A	N/A	N/A	N/A
Absolute min. rate (bpm)	N/A	N/A	N/A	N/A	N/A	N/A	N/A	N/A

CPAP/Bilevel Titration Chart

Treatment Level	Time			Respiratory									Oximetry		
(cm H_2O)	TIB	REM (h:min:s)	Non-REM	OA	CA	MA	All Hypn's	A + H Total	AHI	RERA	All Resp	RDI	Max. SpO_2%	Min. SpO_2%	Mean SpO_2%
CPAP 8	0:21:54	0:05:30	0:15:30	0	1	0	3	4	11.4	0	4	11.4	98.0	88.0	93.8
CPAP 9	0:11:52	0:11:52	0:00:00	0	0	0	3	3	15.2	0	3	15.2	98.0	90.0	94.3
CPAP 10	1:36:40	0:19:10	1:16:30	0	1	0	6	7	4.4	0	7	4.4	98.0	90.0	94.6
CPAP 11	1:07:10	0:45:58	0:18:12	0	1	0	4	5	4.7	0	5	4.7	98.0	91.0	95.2
CPAP 12	1:27:54	0:10:30	1:14:48	0	0	0	3	3	2.1	0	3	2.1	99.0	90.0	95.1

Figure 38-2 (*continued*)

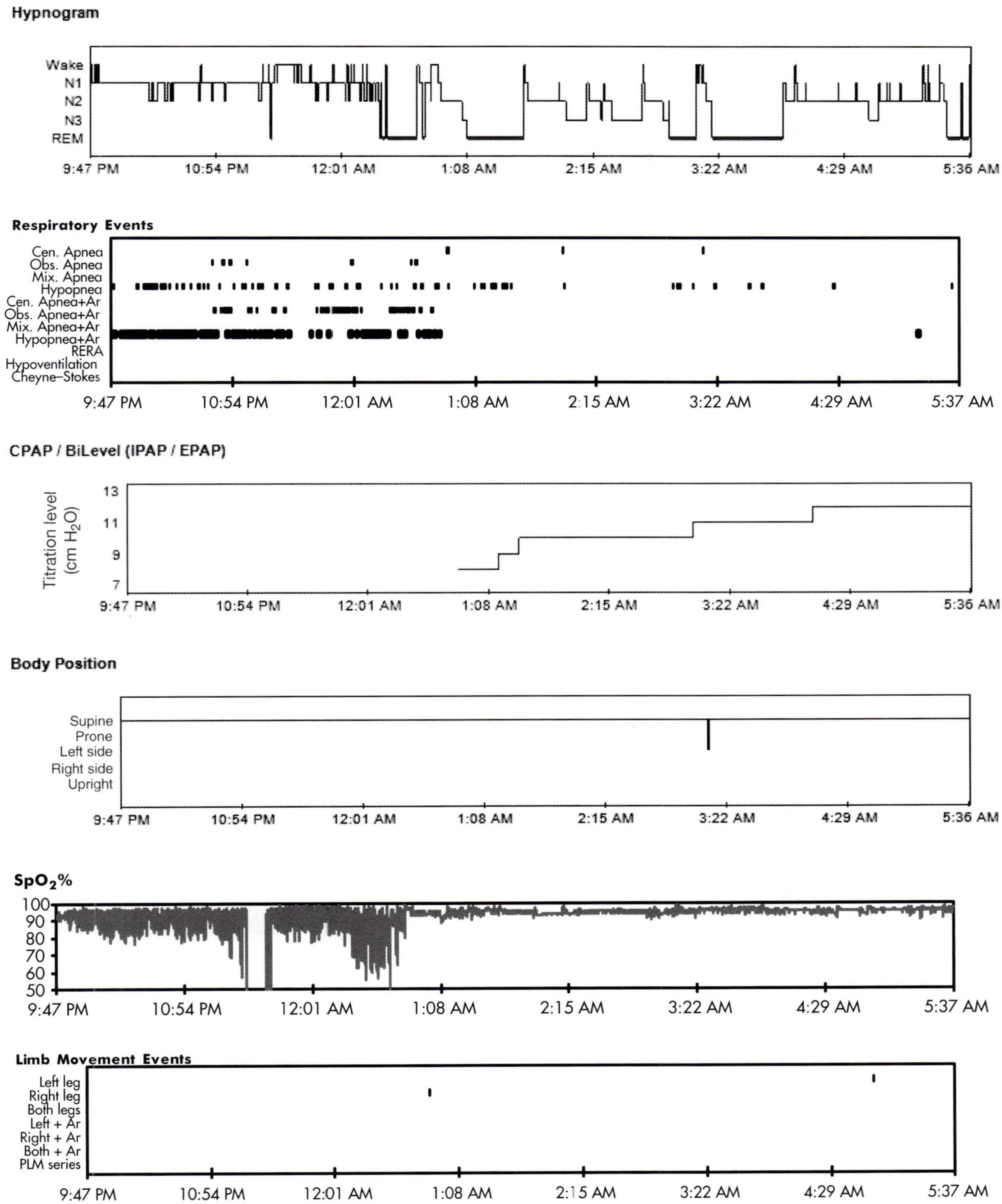

Figure 38-2 *(continued)*

A report to the homecare company or DME provider may be even more abbreviated information limited to basic sleep architecture, respiratory events, arousals, and oxygen saturation summaries. For basic positive airway pressure (PAP) treatment, the primary requirements for DME reimbursement are total recording time (TRT), total sleep time (TST), the apnea-hypopnea index (AHI), and the oxygen (O_2) saturation nadir. Figure 38-3 is an example of a Split-Night Report—DME/Insurance Co. Report.

The AASM Manual for the Scoring of Sleep and Associated Events: Rules, Terminology and Technical Specifications includes scoring rules for sleep stages, arousals, respiratory events, cardiac events, and movement events and provides the recommended minimum information to be included in a polysomnographic report. The following summarizes the AASM manual's recommended parameters for inclusion in the polysomnographic report (7).

Split-Night Report (DME/Insurance Co. Report)

Patient Name: Walker, Ima			
Gender	Female	**Study date**	September 13, 2011
D.O.B.	December 6, 1946	**Subject code**	98765
Age	64	**Referring physician**	Frequent referral, MD
Height	66.0 in	**Sleep specialist**	Sleep doctor, MD
Weight	190.0 lbs	**Recording tech**	IM Sleepy, RPSGT
BMI	30.7	**Scoring tech**	JW Atkinson, RPSGT

Study Indications:
Daytime complaints of EDS (ESS=9), loud snoring, nonrestorative sleep. Sleep complaints of breathing/snoring stops in sleep, wakes for unknown reasons, restless sleep, somniloquy, occasional heartburn, and bruxism.

Diagnostic Section

Sleep Architecture	
Lights out clock time (h:min)	9:47:00 p.m.
Lights on clock time (h:min)	12:50:56 a.m.
TRT (in min)	183.9
SPT*	3:03:03
TST (in min)	161.0
SE	87.5%
SL	0:00:54
Total stage changes (after SO)	84
Awakenings (after SO)	19
WASO	22.0
REM periods	2
REM latency*	1:35:00
REM latency (less wake time)*	1:32:30

*Time formats are in h:min:s

Figure 38-3 Split-night report (durable medical equipment/Insurance Co. report). CPAP, continuous positive airway pressure; PLM, periodic limb movement; REM, rapid eye movement; TIB, time in bed; TST, total sleep time; WASO, wake after sleep onset.

Respiratory Events	CA	OA	MA	Hypopneas	Total Apneas	Apnea+ Hypopnea	RERA	All Resp. Events *
Count	0	52	0	155	52	207	0	207
Index (events/h)	0.0	19.4	0.0	57.8	19.4	**77.1**	0.0	77.1
Mean duration (s)	N/A	29.4	N/A	24.0	29.4	25.3	N/A	25.3
Longest event (s)	N/A	66.1	N/A	81.9	66.1	81.9	N/A	81.9
REM count	0	10	0	7	10	17	0	17
Non-REM count	0	42	0	148	42	190	0	190
REM index	0.0	29.3	0.0	20.5	29.3	49.8	0.0	49.8
Non-REM index	0.0	17.9	0.0	63.2	17.9	81.1	0.0	81.1

*Note: Does not contain Cheyne–Stokes breathing, hypoventilation, or periodic breathing.

Oxygen Desaturation Events	Count	Index
TST	200	74.5
Wake (after SO)	5	13.6
Non-REM	181	77.3
REM	19	55.6

Oxygen Saturation	Wake	Non-REM	REM	TST	TIB
Max. SpO_2%	100.0	99.0	99.0	99.0	100.0
Mean SpO_2%	89.7	90.6	80.0	89.3	89.3
Min. SpO_2%	51.0	57.0	54.0	54.0	51.0
$SpO_2\% \leq 89\%$ (min)	0.1	49.3	14.5	63.8	67.7
	% Time in range				
90–100%	36.7%	59.6%	26.6%	55.4%	53.0%
80–89%	12.7%	35.3%	23.3%	33.7%	31.1%
70–79%	1.0%	3.9%	23.9%	6.4%	5.7%
60–69%	3.2%	0.8%	21.5%	3.4%	3.4%
50–59%	1.0%	0.1%	4.7%	0.7%	0.8%
<50%	0.0%	0.0%	0.0%	0.0%	0.0%
% Artifact/bad data	45.4%	0.4%	0.0%	0.3%	6.0%

Figure 38-3 (*continued*)

TREATMENT SECTION

Sleep Architecture	
Lights out clock time (h:min)	12:52:00 a.m.
Lights on clock time (h:min)	5:36:59 a.m.
TRT (in min)	285.0
SPT*	4:44:36
TST (in min)	278.0
SE	97.5%
SL	0:00:24
Total stage changes (after SO)	64
Awakenings (after SO)	10
WASO	6.6
REM periods	3
REM latency*	0:15:30
REM latency (less wake time)*	0:15:30

*Time formats are in h:min:s

Oxygen Desaturation Events	Count	Index
TST	28	6.0
Wake (after SO)	0	0.0
Non-REM	12	3.9
REM	16	10.3

Respiratory Events	CA	OA	MA	Hypopneas	Total Apneas	Apnea+ Hypopnea	RERA	All Resp. Events*
Count	3	0	0	19	3	22	0	22
Index (events/h)	0.6	0.0	0.0	4.1	0.6	**4.7**	0.0	4.7
Mean duration (s)	13.5	N/A	N/A	28.5	13.5	26.4	N/A	26.4
Longest event (s)	18.4	N/A	N/A	56.3	18.4	56.3	N/A	56.3
REM count	0	0	0	14	0	14	0	14
Non-REM count	3	0	0	5	3	8	0	8
REM index	0.0	0.0	0.0	9.0	0.0	9.0	0.0	9.0
Non-REM index	1.0	0.0	0.0	1.6	1.0	2.6	0.0	2.6

*Note: Does not contain Cheyne–Stokes breathing, hypoventilation, or periodic breathing.

Figure 38-3 (*continued*)

Oxygen Saturation	Wake	Non-REM	REM	TST	TIB
Max. SpO_2%	100.0	99.0	99.0	99.0	100.0
Mean SpO_2%	95.3	94.7	94.9	94.8	94.8
Min. SpO_2%	90.0	90.0	88.0	88.0	88.0
$SpO_2\% \leq 89\%$ (min)	0.0	0.0	0.6	0.6	0.6
		% Time in range			
90–100%	99.0%	100.0%	99.0%	99.6%	99.6%
80–89%	1.0%	0.0%	1.0%	0.4%	0.4%
70–79%	0.0%	0.0%	0.0%	0.0%	0.0%
60–69%	0.0%	0.0%	0.0%	0.0%	0.0%
50–59%	0.0%	0.0%	0.0%	0.0%	0.0%
<50%	0.0%	0.0%	0.0%	0.0%	0.0%
% Artifact/bad data	0.0%	0.0%	0.0%	0.0%	0.0%

Figure 38-3 (*continued*)

Recording Parameters

The AASM manual recommends listing the recording parameters employed during the sleep study in the report. These include the following:

a. Electroencephalogram (EEG) derivations
b. Electrooculogram (EOG) derivations
c. Chin electromyogram (EMG)
d. Leg EMG derivations
e. Airflow parameters
f. Effort parameters
g. Oxygen saturation
h. Body position
i. Electrocardiogram (ECG)

These are the typical parameters recorded. Although not specifically addressed, additional parameters such as carbon dioxide (CO_2) monitoring (end-tidal or transcutaneous) and esophageal pH monitoring should also be included in the list of recording parameters if they are utilized.

I. Sleep scoring data
 Lights out (off) time in hour: minute format
 Lights on time in hour: minute format
 TRT; lights off time to lights on time given in minutes
 TST; summation of all epochs of sleep given in minutes
 Sleep latency (SL); the time in minutes from lights out to the first epoch of sleep given in minutes (calculated by subtracting the lights out epoch number from the epoch number of the first epoch of sleep and dividing by 2)
 Stage R latency, RL; the time in minutes between the first epoch of sleep and the first epoch of stage R in minutes (calculated by subtracting the first epoch of sleep from the first epoch of stage R and dividing by 2)
 Wake after sleep onset (WASO); stage W in TRT minus the SL in minutes
 Percent sleep efficiency (SE); 100 × TST/TRT
 Time in each stage in minutes
 Percent of TST for each stage, %N1, %N2, and so on; 100 × time in each stage/TST
II. Arousal events
 The number of arousals
 Arousal index (ArI); 60 × # of arousals/TST
III. Respiratory events
 Number of obstructive apneas (OA)
 Number of mixed apneas (MA)
 Number of central apneas (CA)
 Number of hypopneas (H)
 Number of apneas and hypopneas
 Apnea index (AI); 60 × (OA + MA + CA)/TST
 Hypopnea index (HI); 60 × (H/TST)
 AHI; 60 × (OA + MA + CA + H)/TST
 Number of respiratory effort-related arousals[1] (RERA)
 Respiratory effort-related arousal index[2] (RERAI); 60 × (RERA/TST)
 Number of oxygen desaturations ≥3% or ≥4%[3]
 Oxygen desaturation index (ODI) ≥3% or ≥4%[4]; 60 × (O_2 desats/TST)
 Mean continuous oxygen saturation
 Minimum oxygen saturation in sleep (nadir)
 Occurrence of hypoventilation (a "yes/no" response)[5]

[1]These are optional statistics.
[2]These are optional statistics.
[3]These are also optional and depend on the hypopnea rule employed; 3% desaturation or arousal (AASM alternate rule), or 4% desaturation (AASM-recommended rule).
[4]These are also optional and depend on the hypopnea rule employed; 3% desaturation or arousal (AASM alternate rule), or 4% desaturation (AASM-recommended rule).
[5]These are optional statistics.

Occurrence of Cheyne-Stokes breathing (a "yes/no" response)

IV. Cardiac events
- Average HR during sleep
- Highest HR during sleep
- Highest HR during the recording
- The presence of the arrhythmias listed in the following paragraph should be acknowledged by responding "yes" if they occur and providing the HR or the duration of the pause.
- Bradycardia (yes/no); report lowest HR observed (defined as HR less than 40 bpm, asleep)
- Asystole (yes/no); report longest event observed (defined as pause greater than 3 seconds)
- Sinus tachycardia during sleep (yes/no); report highest HR observed (defined as sinus HR greater than 90 bpm, asleep)
- Narrow complex tachycardia (yes/no); report highest HR observed
- Wide complex tachycardia (yes/no); report highest HR observed
- Atrial fibrillation (yes/no)
- Other arrhythmias (yes/no); report the arrhythmia such as heart block or significant ectopy

V. Movement events
- Number of periodic limb movements of sleep (PLMS)
- Number of PLMS with arousals
- PLMS index (PLMSI); 60 × (PLMS/TST)
- PLMS arousal index (PLMSArI); 60 × (PLMS w arousal/TST)

VI. Summary statements
- Findings related to the diagnosis
- EEG abnormalities
- ECG abnormalities
- Behavioral observations
- Sleep hypnogram (this is optional)

The minimum recommended parameters will be expanded upon in the following sections.

COMMON SLEEP ARCHITECTURAL DEFINITIONS AND FORMULAE

Sleep architecture parameters generally include latencies, summation of time spent in each sleep stage and body position, and the percentage of TST spent in each sleep stage. Latencies are defined as the time periods from one hallmark event, such as "lights out" or sleep onset (SO), to another hallmark event, such as rapid eye movement (REM) onset or SO. The classic reporting parameters are TRT, TST, WASO, time spent in each sleep stage, and time spent in each body position. Computers can now subclassify these time frames to a much more stratified level. For example, a continuous positive airway pressure (CPAP) titration report may include a time value for each pressure setting, relative to every combination of sleep stage and body position (back/REM/CPAP × time). If you can define a parameter, it can be tabulated and reported!

Table 38-1 Common Sleep Architectural Terms With Definitions and Formulae

Term	Definition/Formula
%Stage N1	The percentage of TST spent in stage N1 sleep (Minutes of N1/TST) × 100 May also be presented as the percentage of TRT spent in N1, in which case the formula is: (Minutes of N1/TRT) × 100 Because TRT almost always includes some WASO, these presentations will always give a lower value than that of TST. Tables should clearly define the denominator for the statistic.
%Stage N2	The percentage of TST spent in N2 sleep (Minutes of N2/TST) × 100 May also be presented as the percentage of TRT spent in N2, in which case the formula is: (Minutes of N2/TRT) × 100
%Stage N3	The percentage of TST spent in N3 sleep (Minutes of N3/TST) × 100 May also be presented as the percentage of TRT spent in N3, in which case the formula is: (Minutes of N3/TRT) × 100

Table 38-1 Common Sleep Architectural Terms With Definitions and Formulae (*continued*)

Term	Definition/Formula
%Stage R	The percentage of TST spent in REM sleep $(\text{Minutes of R/TST}) \times 100$ May also be presented as the percentage of TRT spent in REM, in which case the formula is: $(\text{Minutes of R/TRT}) \times 100$
%Wake time, stage W	The percentage of time spent awake. This statistic can be based only on TRT. $(\text{Minutes of W/TRT}) \times 100$ Tables including this statistic should clearly define the denominator.
SO	The first epoch of sleep
Latency to stage R	The period of time from SO to the first epoch of stage R sleep This could be 0.0 min if the first epoch of sleep is REM. To calculate in minutes, count the number of epochs and divide by two $\frac{(\text{Criterion epoch} - \text{SO epoch})}{2}$
Latency to N2	The period of time from SO to the first epoch of N2 sleep. This could indeed be 0.0 min if the first epoch of sleep is N2. To calculate in minutes, count the number of epochs and divide by two $\frac{(\text{Criterion epoch} - \text{SO epoch})}{2}$
Latency to N3	The period of time from SO to the first epoch of N3 sleep $\frac{(\text{Criterion epoch} - \text{SO epoch})}{2}$
SE	The portion of the TRT spent asleep. Usually expressed as a percentage $(\text{TST/TRT}) \times 100$
SL	The time from lights out to SO (first of any epoch of sleep) $\frac{(\text{SO epoch} - \text{lights out epoch})}{2}$
TRT	The time from "lights out" to "lights on." To calculate in minutes, count the number of epochs and divide by two $\frac{(\text{"Lights on" epoch} - \text{"lights out" epoch})}{2}$
TST	The total amount of sleep recorded during the TRT. The basis for many of the additional statistics and indices. Derived by summing the total of all the minutes of N1, N2, N3, and R sleep $\text{Sleep time}_{\text{Total}} = \text{N1}_{\text{Total}} + \text{N2}_{\text{Total}} + \text{N3}_{\text{Total}} + \text{R}_{\text{Total}}$
TWT	Total time spent awake during the TRT. It is the sum of SL, WASO, and WASP $\text{TWT} = \text{SL} + \text{WASO} + \text{WASP}$
Unequivocal sleep	Primarily used to determine the end point of a maintenance of wakefulness test. Unequivocal sleep is defined as follows: 1. The first of three consecutive epochs of N1 sleep 2. The first epoch of N2, N3, or R (eg, unequivocal sleep occurs at the underscored stage R in the following sequence: W W W 1 W W R) 3. The first epoch of N1 that is contiguous with a non-N1 stage of sleep (eg, unequivocal sleep is at the underscored stage N1 in the following sequence: W W W 1 W W 1 2)
WASO	Wakefulness occurring between the SO and the last epoch of sleep
TIB or TRT	The time from "lights out" to "lights on." To calculate in minutes, count the number of epochs and divide by two $\frac{(\text{"Lights on" epoch} - \text{"lights out" epoch})}{2}$

REM, rapid eye movement; SE, sleep efficiency; SL, sleep latency; SO, sleep onset; TIB, time in bed; TRT, total recording time; TST, total sleep time; TWT, total wake time; WASO, wake after sleep onset; WASP, wake after the sleep period.

Another reported parameter is the percentage of time spent in each sleep stage, relative to TST. In addition, the percentage of TST relative to TRT establishes the SE. Variations from established normative data are often reported to help identify pathology and provide insight into the patient's clinical condition.

Table 38-1 presents common sleep architectural terms with definitions and formulae where indicated.

Abnormal Event Definitions and Formulae

In addition to the above-mentioned information, a reporting of abnormal events (apneas/hypopneas, limb movements, arousals, and indicated cardiac events) occurring during the polysomnogram provides the data to support the absence or presence and severity of sleep pathology. The number of event types and the data analysis statistics available to describe these events are practically limitless, depending only on one's needs and imagination. Traditionally, events commonly included in the sleep report are apneas and hypopneas, arousals, limb movements, and O_2 desaturations. The statistics reported can include any or all of the following:

- Number of events
- Maximum duration of events
- Average (mean) duration of events
- %TST occupied by a given event type
- Number of events of a given type per unit time, that is, TST (index)
- The lowest value of a given event type (nadir)

The number of events is self-explanatory; once the events have been described, simply count the number of events meeting the definition criteria.

The maximum duration is the longest event matching the definition criteria.

The mean duration of the event is determined by adding the durations of all the events and dividing by the total number of events.

The percentage of the TST occupied by a given event is the total of the durations of all the events divided by TST × 100.

The calculation of an *index* represents the average number of a specific event per hour of sleep time. Utilizing a standard epoch length of 30 seconds per epoch, the total number of epochs scored as sleep is counted and divided by two. This provides the total number of minutes of sleep. The events of interest are then counted, multiplied by 60, and divided by the total minutes of sleep.

The *nadir* is the lowest value recorded of an event type.

Table 38-2 presents common event parameters and formulae where indicated.

Table 38-2 Common Event Parameters and Formulae

Term	Definition/Formula
Total apneas	The total of all apneas recorded $Apneas_{Total}$ = obstructive $apneas_{Total}$ + mixed $apneas_{Total}$ + central $apneas_{Total}$
Total hypopneas	The total of all hypopneas recorded $Hypopneas_{Total}$ = obstructive $hypopneas_{total}$ + mixed $hypopneas_{total}$ + central $hypopneas_{total}$
AI	The number of apneas per hour of sleep AI = # apneas/hour of sleep or AI = (# apneas/minutes of sleep) × 60
Hypopnea index	The number of hypopneas per hour of sleep AI = # hypopneas/hour of sleep or AI = (# hypopneas/minutes of sleep) × 60
AHI	The number of apneas and hypopneas per hour of sleep. This statistic is useful to compare baseline with treatment conditions and one treatment condition to another because the time base is the same. or AHI = # apneas + # hypopneas/hour of sleep or AHI = (# apneas + # hypopneas) × (60)/minutes of sleep

Table 38-2 Common Event Parameters and Formulae (*continued*)

Term	Definition/Formula
Polysomnography RDI	Formerly synonymous with AHI; more recently, it has come to mean number of apneas and number of hypopneas and number of RERAs per hour of sleep RDI = (apneas) + (# hypopneas) + (RERAs)/hours of sleep or RDI = (# apneas + # hypopneas + RERAs) × (60)/minutes of sleep
Home sleep apnea testing RDI	Ever since the recognition of type III home sleep testing, RDI has been defined by the Centers for Medicare & Medicaid Services as the number of apneas and hypopneas per hour of recording time because sleep staging parameters are not recorded. RDI = # apneas + # hypopneas /hours of recording time or RDI = (# apneas + # hypopneas) × (60)/minutes of recording time
Mean duration apnea	The sum of all apnea durations (Σ apnea duration) per number of apnea events $\text{Mean duration apnea} = \frac{\Sigma \text{ apnea duration}}{\text{No. apnea}}$
Mean duration hypopnea	The sum of all hypopnea durations (Σ hypopnea duration) per number of hypopneic events $\text{Mean duration hypopnea} = \frac{\Sigma \text{ hypopnea duration}}{\text{No. hypopneas}}$
Maximum duration apnea	The longest apneic event recorded
Maximum duration hypopnea	The longest hypopneic event recorded
DI	The number of desaturation events per hour of sleep or DI = # desaturation events/hours of sleep or DI = (# desaturation events/minutes of sleep) × 60
Saturation nadir	The lowest saturation recording during the recording
PLMI	The number of PLMs per hour of sleep or PLMSI = #PLMS/hours of sleep or PLMSI = (#PLMS/minutes of sleep) × 60
Total PLM	The number of period limb movement events scored
Total PLM with arousal	The number of PLMs with corresponding arousals
PLMArI	The number of PLMs with arousal per hour of sleep or PLMArI = #PLMS with arousal/hours of sleep or PLMArI = (#PLMS with arousal/minutes of sleep) × 60
Desaturation events	The number of desaturation events meeting the criterion

AHI, apnea + hypopnea index; AI, apnea index; DI, desaturation index; PLMArI, PLM with arousal index; PLMI, periodic limb movement index; PLMS, periodic limb movements of sleep; PLMSI, PLMS index; RDI, respiratory disturbance index; RERA, respiratory effort-related arousal.

HISTOGRAMS

The old adage "A picture is worth a thousand words" holds true for polysomnographic reports. Graphic representation of the sleep histogram aligned with the representation of oxygen saturation levels, body position, abnormal respiratory events, PLMs, arousals, and CPAP treatment levels provides a wealth of valuable information even to the inexperienced viewer. Most polysomnographic recording systems provide this reporting capability.

The graph (or histogram) included with the reports shown in Figures 38-1 and 38-2 shows repetitive apneas and hypopnea with severe desaturations and limited sleep other than N1 in the baseline portion of the recording. The treatment condition shows scattered respiratory events, mostly in stage R and marked improvement in oxygen saturation. Significant amounts of N2 and N3 sleep are also present compared with the baseline condition.

DEVELOPING OTHER RELEVANT STATISTICS

Digital recording systems and their data manipulation abilities make it possible to develop statistics and reports that can provide significant amounts of data for the end user. As an example, it is common to report the AHI in both the baseline and the treatment segments of a split-night protocol recording. Understanding the concept of indices (the number of events per unit of time for a given condition) makes the derivation of the requisite formulae a relatively simple task. The key is to define the conditions, calculate the time spent in that condition, and then tabulate the events occurring in that condition. To obtain the relevant index, the number of events is multiplied by 60 and then divided by the minutes of time. For example, to calculate the AHI before and after CPAP initiation, the following formulae would be used:

$$AHI_{baseline} = (\#\ apneas_{baseline} + \#\ hypopneas_{baseline})/TST\ (hours)_{baseline}$$

or

$$AHI_{baseline} = (\#\ apneas_{baseline} + \#\ hypopneas_{baseline}) \times 60/TST\ (minutes)_{baseline}$$

and

$$AHI_{treatment} = (\#\ apneas_{treatment} + \#\ hypopneas_{treatment})/TST\ (hours)_{treatment}$$

or

$$AHI_{treatment} = (\#\ apneas_{treatment} + \#\ hypopneas_{treatment}) \times 60/TST\ (minutes)_{treatment}$$

To take this concept a bit further, suppose you are interested in finding the AHI for a given treatment condition such as a CPAP level of 10 cm H_2O in the supine position. Again, define the condition and tabulate the number of events and sleep time spent in that condition.

$$AHI_{CPAP\ of\ 10/SUPINE} = (\#apneas_{CPAP\ of\ 10/S} + \#hypopneas_{CPAP\ of\ 10/S})/TST\ (hours)_{CPAP\ of\ 10/S}$$

or

$$AHI_{CPAP\ of\ 10/SUPINE} = (\#apneas_{CPAP\ of\ 10/S} + \#hypopneas_{CPAP\ of\ 10/S}) \times 60/TST\ (minutes)_{CPAP\ of\ 10/S}$$

It may be that you would like to see the AHI for each CPAP or bilevel treatment level. As aforementioned, define the treatment condition, calculate the number of events for each level of treatment, and divide by the sleep time spent in that condition.

As another example, if you are interested in determining the percentage of apnea relative to the total AHI, the following formula is applied:

$$\%apnea = (\#apneas \times 100)/(\#\ apneas + \#\ hypopneas)$$

As can be seen from these few examples, the number of statistical data points is limited only by the imagination and the need of the user. Most equipment manufacturers provide the capability of tailoring reports to the specific requirements of the customer and have prescribed fields that may be used to generate customized statistics and reports. It is interesting to consider the number of hours that would be necessary to calculate something such as the AHI for each CPAP treatment level in the days before digital recordings.

Combining Fragmented Reports

Many errors can occur during the acquisition of data. A computer might lock up, and a computer restart may be necessary. The sleep study software can fail, causing portions of the study to be separated and not able to be merged. It is important to contact your software vendor for all options before undertaking manually combining reports from multiple study segments. This is a very time consuming and tedious process, so if the software vendor can repair the data sets to merge into one study, it is well worth the effort to get their assistance. Even if the segments are not able to be merged, some software vendors will combine the reports on your behalf either as a paid service or as a part of an existing service contract.

If study segments cannot be merged, each segment must be scored separately and the reports resulting from those scored segments must be manually combined to give a full representation of the study. Depending on the situation, data from 2, 3, 4, or more study segments may need to be merged to one report. Most data can be calculated manually with simple addition. For instance, if you have a study split into two separate reports, to find the TST for the entire study, add the TST from the first scored segment to the second scored segment.

$$TST_1 + TST_2 = TST_{total}$$

As you calculate time-dependent values, the equations you use become slightly more complex.

To calculate the percentage of REM sleep for the entire study, add the REM total from the first scored segment to the second scored segment and divide it by the TST you calculated.

$$REM_1 + REM_2 = REM_{total}$$

$$REM_{total}/TST_{total} = \%REM_{total}$$

It is important to keep in mind when combining data from two (or more) reports that indices are based on different time measurements. For instance, the AHI from first segment may have a TST of 3 hours and the AHI from the second segment may be based on 5 hours. One cannot just add the two indices together to get the overall AHI for the study. The AHI must be calculated using the combined number of apneas and hypopneas divided by the total study hours. It is best to derive any index on the combined report from the raw data from both segments. For instance, to get a new AHI from data of two report segments, add the total number of apneas and hypopneas from the first segment and add that to the total number of apneas and hypopneas from the second segment. Next, divide that total by the total number of hours from both segments.

$$TotalAH_1 + Total\ AH_2 = AH_{total}$$

$$TST_{total}/60 = TST_{total}\text{ in hours}$$

$$AH_{total}/TST_{total}\text{ in hours} = AHI_{total}$$

Typically, you will not be able to combine sleep histograms, such as the overall sleep architecture, into one full night graphic. You typically can copy and paste the histograms from each segment into one report so the interpreting physician has a representation of the entire night in a graphical format.

When combining multiple segments of reports into one combined report, it is important to double check your results. It is very easy to confuse different values. If possible, have a colleague double check your final report before submitting it for interpretation. Also, note that the values were manually calculated.

THE DICTATED SUMMARY

The dictated summary of the recording should be presented in an orderly manner. The following outline is generally accepted:

I. Findings related to sleep diagnosis include the following:
  Patient history and indications for the study
  A description of the monitoring parameters and recording montage
  A description of the sleep architecture
  Respiratory events and O_2 saturation levels
  PLMs
  Arousals
II. Cardiac events
III. Other events (EEG abnormalities and parasomnias/behavioral observations)
IV. Impression
V. Comments
VI. Recommendations

Note that much of the report can be obtained from the information derived directly from the demographics and the recording data from the sleep study. See Figure 38-4 as a good example of a Split-Night Report—Dictated Final Report.

Split-Night Report (Dictated Final Report)

Patient's Name: Ima Walker

Date of Study: September 13, 2011
Referring Clinician: Frequent Referral, MD
Date of Interpretation: September 15, 2011

Demographics:
The patient is a 64-year-old, 66.0 tall, 190.0 pound female with a BMI of 30.7, who completed a split-night study. The patient presents to the sleep lab with complaints of excessive daytime sleepiness (ESS=9), loud snoring, nonrestorative sleep. Sleep complaints of breathing/snoring stops in sleep, wakes for unknown reasons, restless sleep, somniloquy, occasional heartburn, and bruxism. Patient previously smoked for 15 years, she quit Dec. 1984. She drinks two alcoholic drinks per week and 2 to 4 diet sodas daily. She is being treated for HTN, Heart Cath in June '06, Neck circumference=16".

Figure 38-4 Split-night report (dictated final report) Sample report D.

Current Medications:
Lipitor, Tricor, Ramipril, Triamterene/HCTZ, Levocetirizine, Buspirone HCl, Metoprolol Tartrate, Nabumetone, Aspirin, Fish Oil, Niacin, Centrum Silver MVI.

Study Methods:
The polysomnography study included recording and monitoring of EEG, EMG, ECG, pulse oximetry, respiratory effort and flow, body position, and snoring. Video recordings were obtained as needed. A qualified sleep technologist continuously monitored the patient throughout the night. Sleep staging and respiratory events were scored manually using the AASM standards. The data were digitally collected using XXX software.

Diagnostic Period:
The diagnostic period took place from 9:47:00 p.m. to 12:50:56 a.m. The patient took 0.9 minutes to fall asleep, and slept for a total of 161.0 minutes out of 183.9 minutes of TRT, which resulted in a SE of 87.5%. REM latency is recorded at 92.5 minutes.

The patient's sleep architecture consisted of	Stage N1 (NREM 1): 78.3%	(126.0 minutes)
	Stage N2 (NREM 2): 9.0%	(14.5 minutes)
	Stage N3 (NREM 3): 0.0%	(0.0 minutes)
	Stage R (REM) : 12.7%	(20.5 minutes)

The patient had an average AHI of 77.1, with oxygen saturation falling to a low of 51.0%. The patient had a mean oxygen saturation of 89.3% throughout the diagnostic period of the study. The patient experienced 0 PLM events, resulting in a PLM index of 0.0 (events per hour).

Treatment Period:
The treatment period took place from 12:52:00 a.m. to 5:36:59 a.m. The patient took 0.4 minutes to fall asleep, and slept for a total of 278.0 minutes out of 285.0 minutes of TRT, which resulted in a SE of 97.5%. REM latency is recorded at 15.5 minutes.

The patient's sleep architecture consisted of	Stage N1 (NREM 1): 7.6%	(21.0 minutes)
	Stage N2 (NREM 2): 45.0%	(125.0 minutes)
	Stage N3 (NREM 3): 14.0%	(39.0 minutes)
	Stage R (REM) : 33.5%	(93.0 minutes)

With PAP therapy, the overall AHI was recorded as 4.7, with oxygen saturation falling to a low of 88.0%. The patient had a mean oxygen saturation of 94.8% throughout the treatment period of the study. With PAP therapy of 12 cm H_2O, the AHI was reduced to 2.1. The patient experienced two PLM events, resulting in a PLM index of 0.4 (events per hour).

Interpretation:
Severe sleep apnea was treated with PAP therapy of 12 cm H_2O. The Periodic Limb Movement Index of 0.3 is considered to be insignificant.

Recommendations:

1. Sleep hygiene information.
2. Avoid the use of depressant medication and alcohol in the evenings.
3. The patient may benefit from upper airway evaluation if clinically indicated.
4. Avoid sleeping in the supine position.
5. The patient may benefit from weight loss.
6. Begin CPAP therapy of 12 cm H_2O using heated humidification and optional use of pressure relief.

Sleepy Doctor, MD

Figure 38-4 *(continued)*

TECHNOLOGIST COMMENTS

A key component of the polysomnographic report is the attending and scoring of the technologist's comments. These key individuals, who have spent the most time with the patient and the data, respectively, can add further insight into the study. Examples may include an account of the patient's physical and emotional status, a description of audible breathing or snoring sounds, and any atypical findings that are not evident in the routine tabulation of sleep stages and events, such as alpha intrusion, medication effects on the EEG, atypical motor activity during REM sleep, or any other pertinent observations of parasomnia-like activity. When describing events like snoring, leg movements, etc, it is important to describe the magnitude, for example mild/moderate/severe, and the frequency occasional/frequent/very frequent. This documentation is important to provide appropriate context for the data acquired in the study and to provide information gaps when there are technical equipment failures such as video loss or bioelectric signal data losses during the study.

It is important to document in a way that is concise, descriptive, and objective. This type of information may only be intended for the interpreting physician but may also appear on the technical report to be a part of the patient's medical record.

DATA ARCHIVING AND STORAGE

Once record scoring and report generation are completed, the data must be archived and stored for a period of time. This period may vary, but typically this is regulated by state statute. A typical period required to keep records is 7 years or 7 years beyond the age of majority for unemancipated minors. The required length of time can vary based on your country, state, and accreditation standards.

The archiving process usually involves moving the data and video/audio recording to a remote server for long-term access. Many sleep labs store data on a virtual cloud server, whether self-managed or outsourced. Other alternatives involve archiving to external hard drives or CD/DVD media. Some facilities will remove video data to reduce storage size. Check on your facility's policies on retaining video data before making that decision.

When archiving the recording, one should always make a copy rather than move the record from the recording device to the storage device. Copying provides a safety net to prevent loss of data due to corruption during the transfer. The move process deletes the data from the original device as the transfer is being completed and hence risks data loss if the data become corrupt during the transfer process. Check the integrity of the data on the archival medium before deleting the recording from the original device. This can include cloud servers, and some sleep software systems have built-in archival processes. Be sure to be familiar with the storage settings and archive options in your software before moving studies.

Home Sleep Apnea Testing

The following rules for scoring and reporting home sleep apnea testing (HSAT) have been developed and are included in *The AASM Manual for the Scoring of Sleep and Associated Events: Rules, Terminology and Technical Specifications Version 3.0* for recording devices that utilize respiratory flow and effort parameters or peripheral arterial tonometry (PAT).

Reporting Home Sleep Apnea Testing Using Respiratory Flow and/or Effort Parameters

I. General reporting parameters
  - Type of device
  - Type of airflow sensor(s)
  - Type of respiratory effort sensor(s)—could be single or dual
  - Oxygen saturation
  - HR (from ECG or from pulse oximetry)
  - Body position—optional
  - Sleep/wake or monitoring time (MT) (if sleep/wake is reported, EEG, EOG, and chin EMG must be recorded; if MT is used, the method of determining the recording time should be specified)—optional
  - Snoring (from nasal pressure cannula, piezo, or acoustic sensor)—optional

II. Recording data required to be reported
  - Start time of the recording (hour: minute)
  - End time of the recording (hour: minute)
  - TRT in minutes including wake and artifact
  - MT in minutes (the divisor used to calculate the respiratory event index [REI])
  - TST in minutes if EEG, EOG, and chin EMG are recorded (the divisor for calculating AHI if sleep is recorded and scored)
  - HR (maximum, minimum, average)
  - Number of respiratory events (REs)
    - Number of apneas
      - Number of central mixed and obstructive events (Phenotyping of apneic events is optional.)
    - Number of hypopneas
  - REI 60 × (apneas + hypopneas/MT)
  - AHI 60 × (apneas + hypopneas/TST) if sleep is recorded
  - REI and AHI, supine and nonsupine—optional
  - Central apnea index (CAI = 60 × # CA/MT)—optional

A measure of oxygen desaturation using at least one of the following three parameters:

ODI ≥3% or ≥4%; ODI = 60 × # of desaturation events ≥3% or ≥4% per MT in minutes. The employed threshold level ≥3% or ≥4% must be specified.

Sp_{O_2} saturation (maximum, minimum, and mean values)

Sp_{O_2} saturation (% time at or below 88% or other designated thresholds

Presence of snoring (if recorded)—optional

III. Summary statements

Testing date/interpretation date

Study technical adequacy (as defined in sleep center policies and procedures)

Document repeat studies caused by technical failure

Limitations of the study

Interpretation of REI (based on MT) or AHI (if sleep recorded)

Occurrence of snoring, if recorded

Interpretation

Whether or not the study supports the diagnosis of obstructive sleep apnea

Statement of diagnostic severity, if applicable

If study is nondiagnostic, recommendation of in-laboratory polysomnogram, if indicated by clinical history

Printed name and signature of interpreting physician (verification of raw data review)

Recommendation for management of patient meeting AASM clinical practice guidelines and practice parameters

Chain of custody, if applicable—optional

Reporting Home Sleep Apnea Test Using Peripheral Arterial Tonometry

I. General reporting parameters

Type of device

Sleep, wake, REM times derived from actigraphy

Airflow/effort surrogate signals (based on peripheral arterial tone)

Oxygen saturation

HR

Body position—optional

Snoring, if recorded—optional

II. Recording data required to be reported

Start time of the recording (hour: minute)

End time of the recording (hour: minute)

TRT in hours: minutes

Estimated sleep time (in minutes)

Estimated % REM, light sleep, deep sleep—optional

HR (maximum, minimum, average)

Number of RE

REI (use PAT AHI [pAHI] as a surrogate for REI)

ODI ≥4%, ODI = 60 × # of desaturation events ≥4% per MT in minutes

III. Summary statements

Testing date/interpretation date

Study technical adequacy (as defined in sleep center policies and procedures)

Document repeat studies caused by technical failure

Limitations of the study

Interpretation of estimated sleep time

Occurrence of snoring, if recorded—optional

Interpretation

Whether or not the study supports the diagnosis of OSAS

Statement of diagnostic severity, if applicable

If study is nondiagnostic, recommendation of in-laboratory polysomnogram, if indicated by clinical history

Printed name and signature of interpreting physician (verification of raw data review)

Recommendation for management of patient meeting AASM clinical practice guidelines and practice parameters

Chain of custody, if applicable—optional

REFERENCES

1. Aldrich M. Approach to the patient. In: Aldrich M, ed. *Sleep Medicine*. Oxford University Press; 1999:95-110.
2. Rechtschaffen A, Kales A. *A Manual of Standardized Terminology, Techniques, and Scoring System for the Sleep Stages of Human Subjects*. UCLA BIS/BRI Publications; 1968.
3. Bonnet M, Carley D, Carskadon M, et al. ASDA report: Atlas and scoring rules: EEG arousals; scoring rules and examples. *Sleep*. 1992;15(2):174-184.
4. Bonnet M, Carley D, Carskadon M, et al. ASDA report: Atlas and scoring rules: Recording and scoring leg movements. *Sleep*. 1993;16(8):749-759.
5. American Academy of Sleep Medicine. Sleep related breathing disorders in adults: Recommendations for syndrome definition and measurement techniques in clinical research: The report of the American Academy of Sleep Medicine Task Force. *Sleep*. 1999;22:667-789.
6. CMS.gov. Polysomnography and sleep studies—medical policy article: A53019. Accessed November 8, 2025. https://www.cms.gov/medicare-coverage-database/view/article.aspx?articleId=53019
7. Troester MM, Quan SF, Berry RB, et al; for the American Academy of Sleep Medicine. *The AASM Manual for the Scoring of Sleep and Associated Events: Rules, Terminology and Technical Specifications* [Version 3]. American Academy of Sleep Medicine; 2023.

Chapter 39
Multiple Sleep Latency Test and Maintenance of Wakefulness Test

CARLOS TEIXEIRA

KEY CONCEPTS/LEARNING OBJECTIVES

The key concepts for this chapter include the consequences of excessive sleepiness, the difference between subjective and objective evaluation of sleepiness, when the multiple sleep latency test (MSLT) and the maintenance of wakefulness test (MWT) should be performed, and the specific protocols for performing and interpreting the MSLT and MWT.

KEY TERMS

Excessive daytime sleepiness (EDS)
Idiopathic hypersomnia
Narcolepsy
Sleep latency
Sleep-onset rapid eye movement period (SOREMP)

The American Academy of Sleep Medicine (AASM) has defined excessive daytime sleepiness (EDS) as sleepiness occurring in a situation when an individual would be expected to be awake and alert (1). Although related to the common notion of fatigue, sleepiness is a more precise term that reflects a universal physiologic homeostatic need state, comparable to hunger or thirst, associated with increased sleep pressure and that leads to a reduction in function (2). The amount of sleepiness one experiences can range from full alertness on one end to a debilitating state known as EDS on the other. Excessive sleepiness is then a complex issue that has a profound impact on society. Driving while sleepy regularly first increases the risk of motor-vehicle accidents (MVA), with a related estimated direct cost of \$139.4 billion to \$152 billion per year in the United States and 43 to 337 € billion in Europe, and also impairs the ability to work, resulting in an estimated indirect cost of sleepy driving on society for lost human lives of \$2,372 billion per year and an estimated cost of disability for insurance of \$2,580 to \$6,450 billion per year worldwide (3).

Sleepiness on the job may cause accidents in the workplace. Shift work is a prevalent practice in modern societies and is essential in various professions and industries to meet customer demands. In industrialized nations, 15% to 20% of the workforce is engaged in shift work (4). Shift work, particularly night shifts, disrupts circadian rhythms by causing circadian misalignment. This misalignment occurs when internal physiologic processes are out of sync with the external time of day (4). Considering that humans are not biologically wired to be nocturnal, attempting to work during one's biologically natural sleep time produces a tendency to be sleepy while at work. Additionally, shift workers often have to take extreme measures to sleep efficiently during the day. This leads to a generally sleepy working population at risk for accidents. Ironically, most sleep technologists have worked or currently work nights. It is not unusual to hear stories of fellow sleep technologists who have had trouble with sleepiness, including falling asleep while driving home.

Until recently, the issue of sleepiness in relation to accidents has not been routinely assessed, and in many cases, the individuals involved are unaware of falling asleep or will not admit to falling asleep at the wheel at the risk of assuming responsibility for an accident. Unlike in the case of alcohol-related accidents, there is no blood test to determine one's level of sleepiness when an accident occurs, and, therefore, sleepiness is often merely speculation. However, the association between sleepiness and MVA is undeniable. The National Highway Traffic Safety Administration reported 1,721 drowsy driving resulted in an average of 91,000 crashes, 50,000 injuries, and 800 deaths per year (5).

As sleepiness becomes a recognized problem in society, the role of the sleep center in documenting pathologic sleepiness has increased in importance. However, measuring sleepiness is a difficult and often an elusive task. Several scales, such as the Epworth Sleepiness Scale and the Stanford Sleepiness Scale, have been developed to subjectively measure sleepiness. Because of their subjective nature, these scales are used in conjunction with the sleep history and more objective measures to aid in the diagnosis of sleep disorders. Objective measures of sleepiness are the multiple sleep latency test (MSLT) and the maintenance of wakefulness test (MWT).

The MSLT's objective is to measure one's physiologic tendency to fall asleep under controlled conditions. It is used as part of the evaluation of patients with suspected narcolepsy and with suspected idiopathic hypersomnia (6). The MSLT consists of five-nap opportunities, each separated by 2 hours. A shorter four-nap test may be performed, but only when there is a clear diagnostic of narcolepsy, with mean latency less than 8 minutes, and two or more sleep-onset REM periods (SOREMPs) have occurred (either because of two or more SOREMPs during the nap trials or one in the nap trials and one during the night PSG) (6). The MWT's objective is to measures one's alertness and/or ability to stay awake. The MWT may be used to determine treatment success, whether it is with medication, continuous positive airway pressure (CPAP), or other treatment modality, and also to assess one's ability to remain awake as a measure of safety (6). The MWT consists of four 40-minute trials, each separated by 2 hours. Currently, the MSLT and MWT are the only objective measures available to the clinician to quantify sleepiness in a patient. They should be used in conjunction with other clinical information to determine the correct diagnosis and best course of treatment. The importance of quantifying sleepiness lies in the impact that sleepiness has on the patient and society as a whole. In this regard, technologists play an important role in the diagnosis of the disorders of excessive sleepiness.

INDICATIONS

The MSLT is indicated in the diagnosis of narcolepsy and idiopathic hypersomnia. The mean sleep latency (MSL), calculated as the arithmetic mean of the individual sleep latencies for the total number of naps or trials, is used as a component in the diagnosis of the disorders of excessive sleepiness. The difference in the MSL between controls and narcoleptics is statistically significant, with 84% of narcoleptics having an MSL less than 5 minutes (7). REM latency is defined as the time from sleep onset to the first epoch of REM sleep. A SOREMP is defined as an REM onset during an MSLT, with two or more SOREMPs being highly indicative of narcolepsy (7). However, other sleep disorders may produce similar results in an MSLT and, therefore, must be ruled out in the previous night's polysomnogram. Complications arise when attempting to use the MSLT to diagnose idiopathic hypersomnia. The MSL for idiopathic hypersomnia falls between that of narcoleptics and normal controls and is similar to that of sleepier normal controls (1).

The MWT may be indicated to investigate the effect of medications, substances, or other interventions compared to pretreatment or to determine the patient's nonpharmacologic state compared to controls (6). However, in both of these cases, normative data is sparse.

GENERAL CONSIDERATIONS AND PROCEDURES

Before the start of the MSLT or the MWT, several factors must be taken into account. A 2-week sleep diary is helpful in assessing the patient's sleep schedule before the study. Furthermore, actigraphy is a powerful tool in verifying the sleep diary. Used appropriately, actigraphy in coordination with a sleep diary will validate the patient's reported sleep, ensure adequate sleep is achieved, and rule out other disorders such as delayed sleep phase syndrome. The patient may use a smartwatch app to track their sleep, and this may assist the patient in completing their sleep diary. Once a history of adequate sleep has been obtained and circadian sleep disorders are ruled out as a possible differential diagnosis, an overnight polysomnogram must be performed before the MSLT to rule out other sleep disorders that would affect sleep architecture and produce excessive sleepiness. The prerequisites for the MWT are less stringent, and the need for a sleep diary or a prior polysomnogram is based on the clinician's judgment (6).

For both tests, a patient's normal sleep schedule should be considered. Shift workers may need a daytime polysomnogram before a nocturnal MSLT or MWT. Of course, one issue with such a schedule is that competition with the circadian rhythm may be affecting the MSLT or MWT. It may be quite normal, even after sleeping during the day, to experience sleepiness at 4 AM and have a lower than normal sleep latency on a nocturnal MSLT (8).

Medication use and discontinuation present significant challenges and should also be considered before the performance of the MSLT or MWT. Numerous medications may affect sleep and its architecture (in particular, REM sleep), including alcohol, caffeine, antihistamines, antidepressants, antipsychotic, benzodiazepines, steroids, stimulants, wake-promoting agents, and marijuana (9). The AASM task force, in the latest Recommended Protocol for MSLT and MWT, states that the agents listed in Table 39-1 should be gradually reduced before MSLT to minimize medication and effects of substances and that the patient is observed while outside the agents for a sufficient time before testing. Furthermore, a 2-week duration is normally sufficient in most patients, but it will depend on the half-life of the agent (6).

Selective serotonin reuptake inhibitors (SSRIs) suppress REM sleep, and, therefore, discontinuation of this medication should be considered before the

Table 39-1 Medications That May Interfere With Sleep Architecture

Drug Class	Example Agents
Acetylcholine modulators	Donepezil
Adenosine modulators	Theophylline, theobromine, caffeine
α-2-δ ligands	Gabapentin
Antidepressants	
SSRIs	Fluoxetine[a], escitalopram, sertraline, paroxetine
SNRIs	Venlafaxine, duloxetine
Bupropion	Bupropion
Tricyclic antidepressants	Nortriptyline, amitriptyline
MAOIs	Phenelzine
Antihistamine, sedating	Diphenhydramine, doxylamine
Antipsychotic agents	Quetiapine
Antihypertensives	Prazosin
Benzodiazepines/ NBRAs	Flurazepam[a], clonazepam, lorazepam, zolpidem, eszopiclone, zaleplon
Dopamine agonists	Pramipexole, rotigotine, ropinirole
Lithium	Lithium
Melatonin agonists	Ramelteon, tasimelteon
Opioid agonists	Morphine, hydrocodone, methadone, fentanyl
Orexin/hypocretin antagonists	Suvorexant
Sodium oxybate	Sodium oxybate
Steroids	Prednisone
Stimulants	Methylphenidates, amphetamines
Wake-promoting agents	Armodafinil, modafinil, pitolisant, solriamfetol
Marijuana	Tetrahydrocannabinol[a]

List of commonly encountered medications. A 2-week washout is generally recommended.
MAOIs, monoamine oxidase inhibitors; NBRAs, nonbenzodiazepine receptor agonists; SNRIs, serotonin noradrenergic reuptake inhibitors; SSRIs, selective serotonin reuptake agonists.
[a]Medication agents with long half-lives and longer washout (up to 6 weeks) may be needed.
Used with permission of American Academy of Sleep Medicine from Krahn LE, Arand DL, Avidan AY, et al. Recommended protocols for the Multiple Sleep Latency Test and Maintenance of Wakefulness Test in adults: guidance from the American Academy of Sleep Medicine. *J Clin Sleep Med.* 2021;17(12):2489-2498; permission conveyed through Copyright Clearance Center, Inc.

performance of an MSLT. From a technical standpoint, SSRIs may produce atypical eye movements throughout sleep. Every attempt should be made, in consultation with the patient's prescribing primary care physician or psychiatrist, to discontinue these drugs if feasible, practical, and safe in order to fully interpret the data obtained.

These considerations may not be necessary for the MWT, particularly if the purpose is to document the effectiveness of the stimulant. Although not required, a urine drug screen may be performed for any substance that might not have been reported. These general procedures should be followed before any MSLT or MWT. Omission of any of these preliminary considerations may lead to questions regarding the validity of the test and final diagnosis.

The recording montage for both the MSLT and the MWT is generally less complicated than a standard polysomnographic (PSG) montage, and in fact, it is more comfortable for the patient and also common practice to remove the unnecessary leads following the overnight polysomnogram. However, there are essential elements to each montage (Table 39-2). They include a frontal electroencephalogram (EEG [F3-M2 and/or F4-M1]), a central EEG (C3-M2 and/or C4-M1), an occipital EEG (O1-M2 and/or O2-M1), a left and right electrooculogram (EOG), a mental/submental electromyogram (chin EMG), and an electrocardiogram (6). For the MSLT, extra EOG leads may also be added to provide a clearer picture of lateral and vertical eye movements (a total of four EOG leads, including one above and one below the outer canthus of each eye). Although not routine, a snoring microphone and/or respiratory channels may be added if indicated (8).

Table 39-2 Multiple Sleep Latency Test and Maintenance of Wakefulness Test Montages

Minimally Required Channels
Frontal EEG (F3-M2 or F4-M1)
Central EEG (C3-M2 or C4-M1)
Occipital EEG (O1-M2 or O2-M1)
Left EOG (E1)
Right EOG (E2)
Chin EMG
ECG
Optional Channels
Vertical EOG
Additional frontal EEG
Additional central EEG
Additional occipital EEG
Snore microphone
Respiratory channels

ECG, electrocardiogram; EEG, electroencephalogram; EMG, electromyogram; EOG, electrooculogram.

MULTIPLE SLEEP LATENCY TEST

Beyond the general procedures that encompass both the MSLT and the MWT, specific criteria must be met to complete a valid MSLT. The previous night polysomnogram should mimic the patient's normal sleep schedule as much as possible with a minimum of 7 hours in bed and record at least a total sleep time (TST) of at least 6 hours (6). Performing an MSLT following a polysomnogram that is shorter than normal, longer than normal, or at a time that differs from the patient's routine sleep time may affect the overall results. Specifically, the MSLT should not be performed if the patient had insufficient sleep the night before the test.

The MSLT protocol consists of five-nap opportunities, each separated by 2 hours. A shorter four-nap test may be performed; however, it is not reliable for the diagnosis of narcolepsy unless at least two SOREMPs have been recorded, or a SOREMP period occurred in the overnight PSG and another one occurred during the MSLT. The first nap should be started 1.5 to 3 hours after the completion of the overnight polysomnogram. Each successive nap should be started 2 hours after the commencement of the previous nap (6). At the termination of each nap test, it is imperative—between naps—to keep the patient awake and out of the bed. The patient should be continuously monitored to ensure that sleep between naps does not occur. This can be a difficult task with a severely sleepy patient.

Original reports by Mitler et al (8) recommended having the patient wear street clothing during the MSLT. However, the current AASM practice parameters mention the patient's clothing should be comfortable, be appropriate to the environment, and not interfere with the performance of tests and also that a change in clothing is not required between the PSG and the MSLT (6). Allowing the patient to wear sleepwear all day may be psychologically associated with bedtime or sleep activity, potentially reducing sleep latency, and this issue should be considered when drafting policy and procedures. However, it is unclear whether this difference is clinically significant.

A breakfast and lunch are typically provided; however, it is important to note that caffeine should not be consumed at any point during the day of the study. Just before each nap, it is a good idea to make sure that the patient has used the bathroom recently, has turned off their cellular phone, and is generally ready for the nap. Any interruption in the nap has serious consequences for the entire study. Also, the time just before the first nap, or after breakfast, provides an ideal opportunity to obtain a urine specimen for drug screening if one has been ordered by the physician. Current guidelines allow the physician to determine whether a urine drug screen is needed and the conditions under which the sample is collected (6).

Additional considerations for the MSLT include the following: no vigorous physical activity during the day of the study, cessation of smoking, and cessation of any stimulating activity at least 30 minutes before each nap opportunity (6). It is important to note that different forms of nicotine delivery have different pharmacodynamics. Nicotine ingestion through inhalation is eliminated significantly faster than through other means of delivery (Figure 39-1) (10). Therefore, although it is acceptable for the patient to stop smoking 30 minutes before the nap, the use of items such as chewing tobacco, nicotine patches, and nicotine gum should not be allowed during the day of the study.

A recommended routine just before initiating each nap includes performing electrode impedance checks 10 minutes before lights out, performing biocalibrations 5 minutes before lights out, obtaining a subjective sleepiness assessment 45 seconds before lights out, requesting the patient to lie down in a comfortable position 30 seconds before lights out, and instructing the patient to "please lie quietly, keep your eyes closed, and try to fall asleep" at lights out (6,8).

Scoring and Ending Each Nap

Sleep onset for the MSLT is defined as the first 30-second epoch scored as any stage of sleep (6). Sleep latency is the elapsed time in minutes from lights out to sleep onset. If no sleep is achieved after 20 minutes, then the nap is ended, and the sleep latency for that nap is reported as 20 minutes. The MSL is calculated as the sum of the individual sleep latencies for each nap divided by the total number of naps. REM latency is defined as the elapsed time in minutes from the first 30-second epoch of sleep to the first 30-second epoch of REM sleep.

In order to assess for the occurrence of REM sleep, the clinical MSLT test is continued for 15 minutes after the first epoch of any stage of sleep (8). If any REM sleep occurs during this 15-minute window, it is considered a SOREMP (6). This differs from research-based MSLT protocols, where the nap is terminated after the onset of unequivocal sleep, which is defined as the first of three consecutive 30-second epochs of stage N1 sleep or the first 30-second epoch of any other stage of sleep. The research protocol ensures that sleep has been achieved but does not allow for accumulated sleep. The clinical protocol serves two purposes: it establishes a level of sleepiness by measuring sleep latency and allows time for SOREMPs to occur, which allows the diagnosis of narcolepsy.

Ending the Test and Interpretations

The MSLT can be ended after four or five naps have been completed. Only when the results are clearly diagnostic of narcolepsy after four naps with mean latency less than

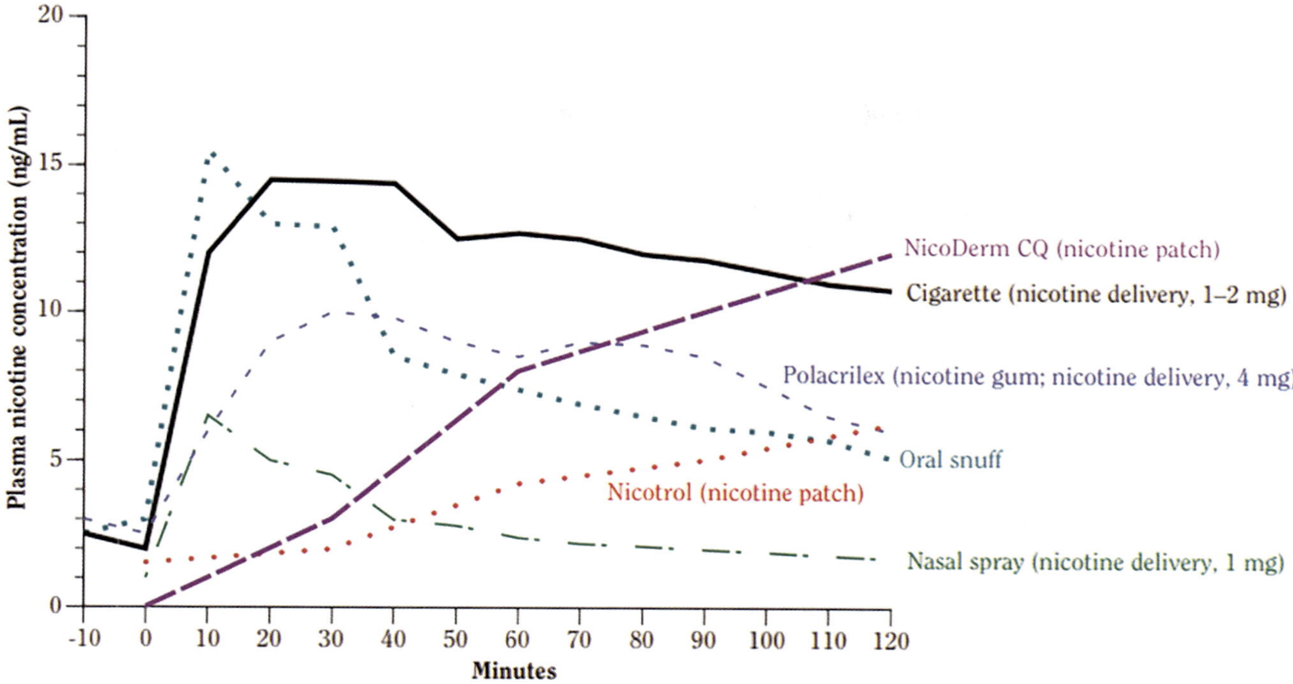

Source: Adapted from Fant et al. 1999 with permission from Elsevier, ©1999.
Note: **mg** = milligrams; **ng/mL** = nanograms per milliliter.

Figure 39-1 Venous blood nicotine levels using various forms of delivery. (From National Center for Chronic Disease Prevention and Health Promotion (US) Office on Smoking and Health. *The Health Consequences of Smoking—50 Years of Progress: A Report of the Surgeon General*. Centers for Disease Control and Prevention (US); 2014. Adapted from Fant RV, Owen LL, Henningfield JE. Nicotine replacement therapy. *Prim Care*. 1999;26(3):633-652. Copyright © 1999 Elsevier. With permission.)

8 minutes and two or more SOREMPs have occurred (either because of two or more SOREMPs during the nap trials or one in the nap trials and one during the PSG) should a shorter four-nap trial test be performed (6). However, there is a statistically significant difference in the MSL between a four-nap MSLT and a five-nap MSLT, with the latter generally producing a longer MSL. The number of naps was found to be one of four factors that significantly impact the MSL. The other factors were age, definition of sleep latency, and prior TST (7). MSL increases with age in adults. In fact, one analysis suggests that MSL will increase by 0.6 minute per decade (7). In general, an MSL less than 5 minutes is consistent with pathologic sleepiness. However, an isolated MSL value should not be used for diagnostic purposes outside of the clinical context (1,11). Normative MSL data may be found in Table 39-3.

MSL alone is generally not a good indicator of pathologic sleepiness in individuals suspected of idiopathic hypersomnia. This is due to the large overlap in MSL between individuals with idiopathic hypersomnia and controls in the normative data (1). Once the MSL is calculated, it is used in conjunction with other symptoms to determine the final diagnosis.

Special Considerations

Pediatric PSG presents unique issues and challenges that must be considered. The MSLT, validated for narcolepsy type 1, is widely used, but it has known limitations for

Table 39-3 Multiple Sleep Latency Test Mean Sleep Latency Based on Age

Age Range (y)	Mean Sleep Latency (SD)
10-19	10.0 (4.5)
20-29	10.4 (5.4)
30-39	10.8 (3.9)
40-49	11.7 (4.4)
50-59	12.1 (1.1)
60-69	11.2 (5.2)
70-79	No data
80-89	15.2 (6.0)

Data from Arand D, Bonnet M, Hurwitz T, Mitler M, Rosa R, Sangal RB. Review by the MSLT and MWT Task Force of the Standards of Practice Committee of the American Academy of Sleep Medicine. *Sleep*. 2005; 28(1):123-144.

narcolepsy type 2 and idiopathic hypersomnia diagnoses; this is especially true when conducting a pediatric MSLT.

Disorders of excessive sleepiness often go unnoticed or undiagnosed until early adulthood, but the onset of central disorders of hypersomnolence, including narcolepsy and idiopathic hypersomnia (IH), often occurs before 21 years of age (12). Children may simply be considered long sleepers or lazy.

MSLT is currently considered technically and clinically valid in developmentally normal children aged 5 years and older, but normative values differ depending on the pubertal Tanner stage (12). Normative MSL data may be found in Table 39-4.

The testing environment may be particularly unsettling for a child and could potentially produce a prolonged MSL, even in the most hypersomnolent child. For this reason, associated symptoms in a child may play a stronger role in diagnosis and treatment than in an adult. For example, an MSL of 12 to 14 minutes may be more pathologic in a child than in an adult. In general, prepubescent patients will have the longest MSL, whereas young adults will have the shortest MSL (7). Another consideration with pediatric patients is that narcolepsy tends to be an evolving disorder in childhood. Therefore, although SOREMPs may not be present, a child may still have narcolepsy with other classical symptoms such as cataplexy. For this reason, MSLTs may need to be repeated throughout childhood to account for developmental changes (13). Under these conditions, other symptoms are just as important as the MSLT in making a diagnosis in a pediatric patient.

Because of the possible comorbidity of obstructive sleep apnea (OSA) and narcolepsy, it may be necessary to perform an MSLT on a patient wearing CPAP. In fact, if a patient presents with a chief complaint of excessive sleepiness or any other narcolepsy symptoms and OSA is present on the polysomnogram, it is necessary to treat the OSA first, before attempting to perform the MSLT (6). However, if excessive sleepiness or any other narcolepsy symptoms persist after a history of compliant CPAP use, performing the MSLT with CPAP in place is advised. It is important that the patient wear CPAP during the preceding overnight polysomnogram at the optimal pressure setting and during the MSLT naps. If the MSLT is performed without CPAP, the patient's 15 minutes of sleep may be disrupted because of sleep-disordered breathing.

Table 39-4 Maintenance of Wakefulness Test Mean Sleep Latency Based on Age

Age Range (y)	Mean Sleep Latency (SD)
30-39	30.86 (2.04)
40-49	36.52 (1.88)
50-59	36.73 (1.59)
60-69	38.03 (1.06)

Data from Arand D, Bonnet M, Hurwitz T, Mitler M, Rosa R, Sangal RB. Review by the MSLT and MWT Task Force of the Standards of Practice Committee of the American Academy of Sleep Medicine. *Sleep*. 2005;28(1):123-144.

MAINTENANCE OF WAKEFULNESS TEST

In contrast to the MSLT, the MWT measures the ability to resist the urge to fall asleep. Instead of being used as a tool in diagnosing sleep disorders, MWTs are more commonly used to evaluate treatment response or assess one's ability to remain awake for safety purposes. Some authors state that it is reasonably appropriate to use the MWT in the evaluation of workplace, occupational, or driving safety (14). Increasingly, the transportation industry is recognizing the value of the MWT in assessing sleepiness, and in France, it is already part of the guidelines for driving license legislation for professional drivers(15). Unfortunately, there is less data available concerning standardized practices and normals for the MWT than for the MSLT. However, the practice parameters provided by the AASM make recommendations regarding the MWT collection and interpretation (6).

On the basis of clinical circumstances, the clinician should determine the necessity of a polysomnogram before the MWT. At present, no consensus has been reached regarding the use of a sleep diary; however, it is important to note that chronic sleep deprivation, or even a poor night's sleep before the test, may affect the outcome of the MWT. The AASM standards advise that if the patient reports having inadequate sleep before the MWT, if the patient does not feel normally alert, or if reliable information is unavailable, the MWT should not be performed (6).

Overall, the general procedures for the MSLT and the MWT are similar. The need to perform a preceding overnight polysomnogram is determined by the clinician (6). Similarly to the MSLT, the first trial should be started 1.5 to 3 hours after the individual wakes up, with no sleep occurring between the time the individual wakes up and the start of the first trial. The MWT is performed in a dimly lit room with the patient in bed in the seated position and the head and limbs fully supported. Subsequent trials are performed at 2-hour intervals (6). Breakfast is generally provided an hour before the first trial, and lunch should be provided immediately following the second trial. A urine drug screen may be collected, as in the MSLT protocol, just before the first trial.

There has been disagreement concerning the duration of each trial, with a 20-minute trial (similar to the

Table 39-5 Effect of Groups on Multiple Sleep Latency Tests (Time to Sleep Onset in Minutes)

Time of Test	Mean Values						
	Tanner 1	Tanner 2	Tanner 3	Tanner 4	Tanner 5	Older Adolescents[a]	*P* <
09:30	19,6	18,7	15,9	16,0	17,6	15,9	.002
11:30	19,0	18,8	13,3	15,2	18,3	15,4	.001
13:30	18,6	17,1	16,1	13,7	13,6	14,3	.001
15:30	18,5	17,9	16,1	14,0	12,5	11,8	.001
Daily mean	19,0	18,5	16,1	15,7	16,6	15,7	.001

[a]Older adolescents in the group with a bedtime of 22:00 to 08:00.
Data from Maski KP, Amos LB, Carter JC, Koch EE, Kazmi U, Rosen CL. Recommended protocols for the multiple sleep latency test and maintenance of wakefulness test in children: guidance from the American Academy of Sleep Medicine. *J Clin Sleep Med.* 2024;20(4):631-641.

MSLT) being used in some studies and a 40-minute trial in others. However, it has been shown that the use of a 40-minute trial avoids the "ceiling effect" produced by the 20-minute trial. For example, an individual who might fall asleep at minute 23 would show a sleep onset using the 40-minute protocol, whereas the same individual would show no sleep if the 20-minute protocol were used. For this reason, a four-trial, 40-minute protocol is recommended for maximizing sensitivity (16,17). One substantial difference between the MSLT and the MWT protocols is the test environment. Instead of a completely dark room, there should be a light of 0.10 to 0.13 lux positioned behind the patient's head, out of direct or peripheral vision at the level of the cornea. The patient should be sitting comfortably in bed with the back and head supported (6).

Before each trial, the general routine should be performed as in the MSLT. However, at the conclusion of the biocalibrations, the instructions differ significantly, whereby the individual should be instructed to "Please sit still and remain awake for as long as possible. Look directly ahead of you, and do not look directly at the light." Furthermore, it is usually necessary to ensure that the individual does not employ extreme measures to maintain wakefulness during the trials (6).

Scoring and Ending Each Trial

As in the MSLT, sleep onset for the MWT is defined as the first epoch of any stage of sleep as defined by the AASM practice parameters (6). However, other definitions for sleep onset have been used. Different protocols, including differing sleep-onset definitions, have been indicated for different clinical purposes as determined by the clinician (18). The trial is terminated if no sleep is achieved during the 40 minutes on the basis of the 40-minute MWT protocol recommended by the AASM or if the patient exhibits three consecutive epochs of stage N1 sleep or one epoch of any other stage of sleep (6).

Ending the Test and Interpretations

The MWT is terminated after four trials (6). Following the AASM-recommended 40-minute trial protocol, an MSL of less than 8 minutes is considered abnormal. As stated earlier, there are fewer normative data for the MWT than for the MSLT (Table 39-5) (18). The paucity of normative data, combined with the fact that the predictive value of the MSL in regard to safety issues has not been established, indicates the need to combine other clinical factors in making a determination of safety and occupational risk (1).

SUMMARY

The first guidelines for the MSLT and MWT were published by the AASM in 2005, while the current guidelines were published in 2021. Both the MSLT and the MWT are invaluable tools in diagnosing and evaluating disorders of excessive sleepiness when they are combined with a thorough sleep history and subjective measures of sleepiness. However, for all their merit, they are not without their weaknesses. Consequently, they should be part of the diagnostic process and not the process in its entirety. The impact of excessive sleepiness has become a societal issue, as evidenced by legislation addressing drowsy driving. The diagnosis of IH or narcolepsy has a far greater impact on the patient than ever before. To avoid false positives or negatives, strict guidelines must be followed not only by the clinician but also by the technologist performing these tests. For this reason, the MSLT and MWT guidelines outlined in the initial AASM practice parameters dictate: "sleep technologists who perform MSLTs (and MWTs) should be experienced in conducting the test" (1). Therefore, the role of the sleep technologist is crucial in the diagnosis of disorders of excessive sleepiness, and a thorough understanding of the test, its indications, procedures, and interpretation is essential in performing a valid test.

REFERENCES

1. Littner MR, Kushida C, Wise M, et al. Practice parameters for clinical use of the multiple sleep latency test and the maintenance of wakefulness test. *Sleep*. 2005;28(1):113-121. doi:10.1093/sleep/28.1.113
2. Roehrs T, Carskadon MA, Dement WC, Roth T. Daytime sleepiness and alertness. In: Kryger M, Roth T, Dement WC, eds. *Principles and Practice of Sleep Medicine*. 6th ed. Elsevier; 2017:39-48.e4.
3. Léger D, Pepin E, Caetano G. The economic burden of sleepy driving. *Sleep Med Clin*. 2019;14(4):423-429. doi:10.1016/j.jsmc.2019.07.004
4. Sweileh WM. Analysis and mapping of global research publications on shift work (2012-2021). *J Occup Med Toxicol*. 2022;17:22. doi:10.1186/s12995-022-00364-0
5. Tefft BC. Drowsy driving in fatal crashes, United States, 2017-2021. AAA Foundation for Traffic Safety. Published online March 6, 2024. Accessed January 25, 2025. https://aaafoundation.org/drowsy-driving-in-fatal-crashes-united-states-2017-2021
6. Krahn LE, Arand DL, Avidan AY, et al. Recommended protocols for the multiple sleep latency test and maintenance of wakefulness test in adults: guidance from the American Academy of Sleep Medicine. *J Clin Sleep Med*. 2021;17(12):2489-2498. doi:10.5664/jcsm.9620
7. Arand D, Bonnet M, Hurwitz T, Mitler M, Rosa R, Sangal RB. The clinical use of the MSLT and MWT. *Sleep*. 2005;28(1):123-144. doi:10.1093/sleep/28.1.123
8. Hirshkowitz M, Sharafkhaneh A. Evaluating sleepiness. In: Kryger M, Roth T, Dement WC, eds. *Principles and Practice of Sleep Medicine*. 6th ed. Elsevier; 2017:1651-1658.e3.
9. Schweitzer PK, Randazzo AC. Drugs that disturb sleep and wakefulness. In: Kryger M, Roth T, Dement WC, eds. *Principles and Practice of Sleep Medicine*. 6th ed. Elsevier; 2017:480-498.e8.
10. National Center for Chronic Disease Prevention and Health Promotion (US) Office on Smoking and Health. *The health consequences of smoking—50 years of progress: a report of the surgeon general*. Centers for Disease Control and Prevention; 2014. doi:10.1037/e510072014-001
11. Roth T, Roehrs TA. Multiple sleep latency test. In: Chokroverty S, ed. *Sleep Disorders Medicine: Basic Science, Technical Considerations and Clinical Aspects*. Springer; 2017:391-398.
12. Maski KP, Amos LB, Carter JC, Koch EE, Kazmi U, Rosen CL. Recommended protocols for the multiple sleep latency test and maintenance of wakefulness test in children: guidance from the American Academy of Sleep Medicine. *J Clin Sleep Med*. 20(4):631-641. doi:10.5664/jcsm.10974
13. Nisbet LC, Nixon GM, Anantharajah A, Davey MJ. Is there a role for repeating the multiple sleep latency test across childhood when initially non-diagnostic? *Sleep Med*. 2024;115:1-4. doi:10.1016/j.sleep.2024.01.022
14. Arand DL. The MSLT/MWT should be used for the assessment of workplace safety. *J Clin Sleep Med*. 2006;2(2):124-127. doi:10.5664/jcsm.26504
15. Sagaspe P, Micoulaud-Franchi JA, Coste O, et al. Maintenance of wakefulness test, real and simulated driving in patients with narcolepsy/hypersomnia. *Sleep Med*. 2019;55:1-5. doi:10.1016/j.sleep.2018.02.009
16. Mitler MM, Doghramji K, Shapiro C. The maintenance of wakefulness test: normative data by age. *J Psychosom Res*. 2000;49(5):363-365. doi:10.1016/S0022-3999(00)00182-3
17. Banks S, Barnes M, Tarquinio N, Pierce RJ, Lack LC, McEvoy RD. The maintenance of wakefulness test in normal healthy subjects. *Sleep*. 2004;27(4):799-802. doi:10.1093/sleep/27.4.799
18. Doghramji K, Mitler MM, Sangal RB, et al. A normative study of the maintenance of wakefulness test (MWT). *Electroencephalogr Clin Neurophysiol*. 1997;103(5):554-562. doi:10.1016/s0013-4694(97)00010-2

Chapter 40
Home Sleep Testing

CHAD EIKEN

KEY CONCEPTS/LEARNING OBJECTIVES

The key concepts for this chapter include a comparison of the use of polysomnography and home sleep testing, describing the various technologies used in home sleep testing, describing the clinical use of home sleep testing, and integrating the use of home sleep testing into overall patient care.

KEY TERMS

American Academy of Sleep Medicine (AASM)
Cardiopulmonary coupling (CPC)
Common procedural terminology (CPT)
G-codes
Local coverage determination (LCD)
Oxygen desaturation index (ODI)
Peripheral arterial tonometry (PAT)
Photoplethysmography (PPG)
Respiratory event index (REI)

The field of sleep medicine is undergoing many changes regarding technology and the clinical application of technology in the home to assist in the diagnosis of sleep disorders. As of 2026, home sleep testing (HST) is indicated only for the diagnosis of sleep-disordered breathing (SDB), but as technology evolves and new data/channels are incorporated into HST, there is ongoing discussion regarding the viability of expanding the use of HST to diagnose other sleep disorders beyond SDB. Readers are encouraged to refer to new guidelines related to the use of HST as they are released by professional health care associations.

Polysomnography (PSG) is the standard test for the diagnosis of suspected sleep disorders and for positive airway pressure (PAP) titration in patients diagnosed with SDB (1-4). Attended PSG requires highly trained personnel for adequate study performance and interpretation and can be costly. Timely access to PSG may be limited or delayed in many locales. Limited access and the high prevalence of SDB have prompted the use of limited channel monitoring outside the sleep center. Unattended limited channel testing can be performed in the sleep center or hospital, although it is nearly always performed in the patient's home.

At the advent of HST, the testing did not usually determine the amount of sleep time (no electroencephalogram [EEG] or peripheral arterial tonometry [PAT] recorded). Therefore, the names portable monitoring, out of center sleep testing, home sleep apnea testing, and HST were used interchangeably. This practice is not ideal as it creates ambiguity in the type of data recorded and analyzed when diagnosing. Technology has further evolved, creating increased variability in testing methods and channels used. This chapter will describe these technologies and the different ways data should be reported when using each (ie, respiratory event index or apnea/hypopnea index). The term home sleep testing (HST) will be used in this chapter to refer to the practice of testing for sleep disorders in the ambulatory or home environment and will include only technologies used clinically in the evaluation of sleep disorders during a verifiable sleep period. For instance, overnight oximetry would not be considered HST as it is measuring only oxygenation during a nocturnal period but not the patient's sleep state.

At the turn of the century, PSG was the most common test to diagnose SDB in the United States (1-4). However, in other locales, more limited studies have long been used in clinical practice. For example, Flemons et al (5) stated in 2004 that in the United Kingdom, PSG comprised approximately 10% of all sleep studies. Approximately two-thirds of the studies used oximetry alone, while the rest were limited channel studies. However, despite the widespread use of HST worldwide, such testing was only approved in the United States by the Centers for Medicare & Medicaid Services (CMS) to qualify patients for continuous positive airway pressure (CPAP) treatment in 2008 (6,7). Reimbursement for HST was subsequently approved in 2009 (8). Since then, the number of HST studies has continued to increase every year. In 2014, 845,569 sleep studies were completed by 1.4% of Medicare beneficiaries for a total cost of $189 million. Since 2010, annual expenditures for sleep studies have declined, whereas the number of studies performed has increased by 9.1%. In 2014, PSG, split-night PSG and unattended home sleep studies accounted for 40%, 48%, and 12%, respectively, of the total sleep studies. This represented a dramatic growth in the number of unattended sleep studies performed since 2000, when they represented only 0.9% of the total studies (9). Beginning in the early 2010s, many insurance providers mandated the use of HST for the diagnosis of obstructive sleep apnea (OSA) in all uncomplicated patients, and this has become more commonplace since. Presently, insurance providers will commonly require documentation of comorbidities that would indicate the need for in-lab PSG when evaluating a patient for SDB; otherwise, an HST is encouraged instead.

The prevalence of HST continued to grow and began to increase exponentially during the COVID-19 pandemic as PSG posed increased infection risk. As of 2024, roughly 51% of tests performed and billed to CMS bore CPT codes, reflecting HST, as opposed to PSG, which is a massive increase from 10 years prior at 12%. This demonstrates a significant degree of adoption and utility of HST in the overall diagnosis and management of sleep disorders.

ADOPTION OF HOME SLEEP TESTING IN THE UNITED STATES

The history of HST in the United States has been characterized by a slow acceptance of this type of testing as data supporting the use of the devices accumulated. CMS considered HST several times before finally approving the method for the diagnosis of sleep apnea. A detailed step-by-step description of the developments in evaluation and subsequent approval of HST for the diagnosis of OSA is provided in two of the references (10,11). An editorial discussing the rationale for the CMS decision to approve HST describes the final stages of the process (12). Early studies of the utility of HST for the diagnosis of OSA focused on a comparison of the ability of devices to rule in or rule out sleep apnea with that of PSG (13,14-19), and American Academy of Sleep Medicine (AASM) practice parameters recommended narrow indications for HST (20,21). However, in 2007, before the approval of HST by the CMS, the AASM did publish important clinical guidelines for the use of HST in a wider spectrum of indications (22) if certain evaluation and testing procedures were followed. The guidelines influenced the requirements for reimbursement of HSAT studies by insurance providers. The ultimate decision of CMS to allow HST for the diagnosis of OSA in patients to be treated with CPAP was heavily influenced by studies showing that clinical pathways using HST devices resulted in equivalent outcomes from CPAP treatment, including improvement in daytime sleepiness and the amount of adherence to treatment (23,24). In 2017, the AASM published updated evidence-based guidelines for the diagnosis of OSA, highlighting the well-studied ability to accurately diagnose OSA utilizing HSAT devices, using Type 3 or PAT.

The AASM clinical guidelines for the use of unattended portable monitors in the diagnosis of OSA in adults (22) provide important recommendations on how HST is to be performed and used. The guidelines provided a recommendation that HST be performed under the auspices of AASM-accredited sleep centers. Subsequent to the national carrier determination by CMS, a number of LCDs by regional durable medical equipment (DME) Medicare administrative contractors or private insurance providers were published, further defining requirements for the performance of HST. The requirements vary by region and funding entity but, in general, require HST following a clinical evaluation of the patient and should be performed under the auspices of an accredited sleep center (AASM, Joint Commission, or Accreditation Commission for Health Care). HST must be reviewed and interpreted by a physician who is either a board-certified/eligible sleep physician or a staff physician associated with an accredited sleep center. An AASM review of HST technology, AASM practice guidelines, and the AASM scoring manual also provide guidance on the technology to be used for HST (4,7,9).

TYPES OF HOME SLEEP TESTS

The commonly used classification of sleep testing was proposed by Ferber et al (25) in a 1994 American Sleep Disorders Association review (Table 40-1). This classification used the terminology Level I, II, III, and IV. This terminology was later modified to Type 1, 2, 3, and 4 (or Type I, II, III, and IV) (13). In 2008, CMS issued a decision to allow HST to qualify a patient for CPAP (6,7). CMS defined HST types slightly differently and created G-codes (G0398, G0399, and G0400) to describe HST services (Table 40-2) (7,8). The G-codes are found in the Healthcare Common Procedure Coding System Level II codebook and are maintained and valued by the CMS. G-codes are procedure codes developed by the CMS to identify products, supplies, and services that do not have an assigned Common Procedural Terminology (CPT) code for which there is a programmatic operating need to separately identify them on a national level. Reimbursement is determined regionally by the specific local coverage determination (LCD). Later HSTs were assigned CPT codes: 95800, 95801, and 95806. CPT codes are copyrighted and maintained by the American Medical Association. As of 2026, the AASM uses the HST CPT codes in their recommended standards for such testing (9,26).

Table 40-1 Classification of Sleep Testing

	Level I (Type 1)	Level II (Type 2)	Level III (Type 3)	Level IV (Type 4)
	Attended PSG	Unattended PSG	Cardiorespiratory monitoring	Continuous single or dual bioparameter recording
Parameters	Minimum of seven parameters: EEG, EOG, chin EMG, ECG, airflow, respiratory effort, and oxygen saturation	Minimum of seven parameters: EEG, EOG, chin EMG, ECG, airflow, respiratory effort, and oxygen saturation	Minimum of four: ventilation (at least two parameters of respiratory movement or respiratory movement and airflow), heart rate or ECG, and oxygen saturation	Minimum of one oxygen saturation: flow or chest movement
Body position	Documented or objectively measured	Possible	Possible	No
Leg movement	EMG or motion sensor desirable but optional	Optional	Optional	No
Personnel interventions	Possible	No	No	No

The terminology of Level I to IV was used, but recent terminology is Type I to IV or Type 1 to 4.
ECG, electrocardiogram; EEG, electroencephalogram; EMG, electromyogram; EOG, electrooculogram; PSG, polysomnography.
Adapted from Ferber R, Millman R, Coppola M, et al. Portable recording in the assessment of obstructive sleep apnea. ASDA standards of practice. *Sleep*. 1994;17(4):378-392. Reproduced by permission of American Sleep Disorders Association and Sleep Research Society.

Type 1 testing is a PSG performed in a facility or sleep center that is attended by a registered polysomnographic technologist (RPSGT). Type 2 testing (often referred to as unattended or ambulatory or in-home PSG) records similar parameters as Type 1, although the setting is typically in the patient's home or outside of a sleep center and is not attended by an RPSGT, although an RPSGT is required for the asynchronous analysis following the completion of the recording. Historically, Type 2 studies have not commonly been used in the United States because of the expertise required to apply the testing equipment. However, with the introduction of new, innovative, simplified designs from HST manufacturers that allow the patient to easily apply the equipment themselves, it is expected that Type 2 in-home PSG testing will become far more common. Additionally, in the past, there was a barrier to using Type 2 in-home PSG because of limited reimbursement when compared with Type 1 studies (many insurance companies provided no reimbursement at all). With the redesign of CPT codes (expected to be deployed in January 2027), Type 2 in-home PSG can be expected to gain popularity as it expands the potential parameters reported and channels recorded from the home setting. It also creates

Table 40-2 Centers for Medicaid and Medicare Classification of Sleep Testing

Code	Type	Setting	Monitoring
	I	Attended in facility	Minimum of seven channels, including EEG, EOG, EMG, ECG/heart rate, and oxygen saturation
G0398	II	Unattended in or out of a sleep lab facility or attended in a sleep lab facility	Minimum of seven channels, including EEG, EOG, EMG, ECG/heart rate, and oxygen saturation
G0399	III	Unattended in or out of a sleep lab facility or attended in a sleep lab facility	Minimum of four channels and must record ventilation, oximetry, and ECG or heart rate
G0400	IV	Unattended in or out of a sleep lab facility or attended in a sleep lab facility	Minimum of three channels, *one of which is airflow*
		Unattended in or out of a sleep lab facility or attended in a sleep lab facility	PAT, minimum of three channels: PAT, actigraphy, and oximetry

ECG, electrocardiogram; EEG, electroencephalogram; EMG, electromyogram; EOG, electrooculogram; PAT, peripheral arterial tonometry.
Based on Centers for Medicare and Medicaid Services. Decision memo for sleep testing for obstructive sleep apnea (CAG-00405N). 2009; Berry RB, Albertario CM, Harding SM, et al; for the American Academy of Sleep Medicine. The AASM manual for the scoring of sleep and associated events: rules, terminology and technical specifications [Version 3]. American Academy of Sleep Medicine. 2023.

the capacity for potential diagnosis/screening of sleep disorders other than SDB outside the sleep lab.

A Type 3 study consists of at least two channels of respiratory monitoring, oximetry, and electrocardiogram (ECG) or heart rate. Typically, airflow and respiratory effort (eg, chest and abdominal respiratory inductance plethysmography [RIP] or polyvinylidene fluoride [PVDF] belts) are used for respiratory monitoring. The CPT 95806 classification specifies monitoring of airflow and respiratory effort. Some of the simpler HST devices use only one respiratory effort belt. In most Type 3 devices, the heart rate is derived from the oximetry data. An example of a Type 3 study from a comprehensive HST device is shown in Figure 40-1.

In the 2017 AASM clinical practice guidelines for the diagnosis of OSA, the task force described the limitations of the Type I-IV classification system, the lack of context this system provides, and the inability to recognize all technologies being utilized in the diagnosis of OSA. At the time of publication, CMS has put forth new CPT codes to be utilized beginning January 2027. This new evaluation of HST procedures provides far more context regarding the physiologic data recorded and the parameters reported. There will be three levels of complexity (low, moderate, and high) as determined by the number of channels recorded, types of channels recorded, and the number of parameter categories reported. Six CPT codes will be used with three for the technical component and three for the professional components (each having three levels of complexity). These new codes will allow for new technologies to be utilized for HST with a focus on the data recorded rather than method of recording.

ACCURACY OF HOME SLEEP TESTING

Apnea-Hypopnea Index Versus Respiratory Event Index

In most HSTs, EEG is not recorded, which leads to the use of "recording time" or "monitoring time," as opposed to total sleep time (TST), as is used in PSG. Many technologies such as actigraphy and PAT can allow for the measurement of TST with high correlation to PSG; the accuracy of these devices should be considered by the clinician during interpretation. If a device can accurately assess sleep time, an apnea-hypopnea index (AHI) may be calculated in the same manner as PSG. However, if sleep time cannot be accurately assessed by the recording device (as is common in most Type 3 devices), the AASM suggests the use of a respiratory

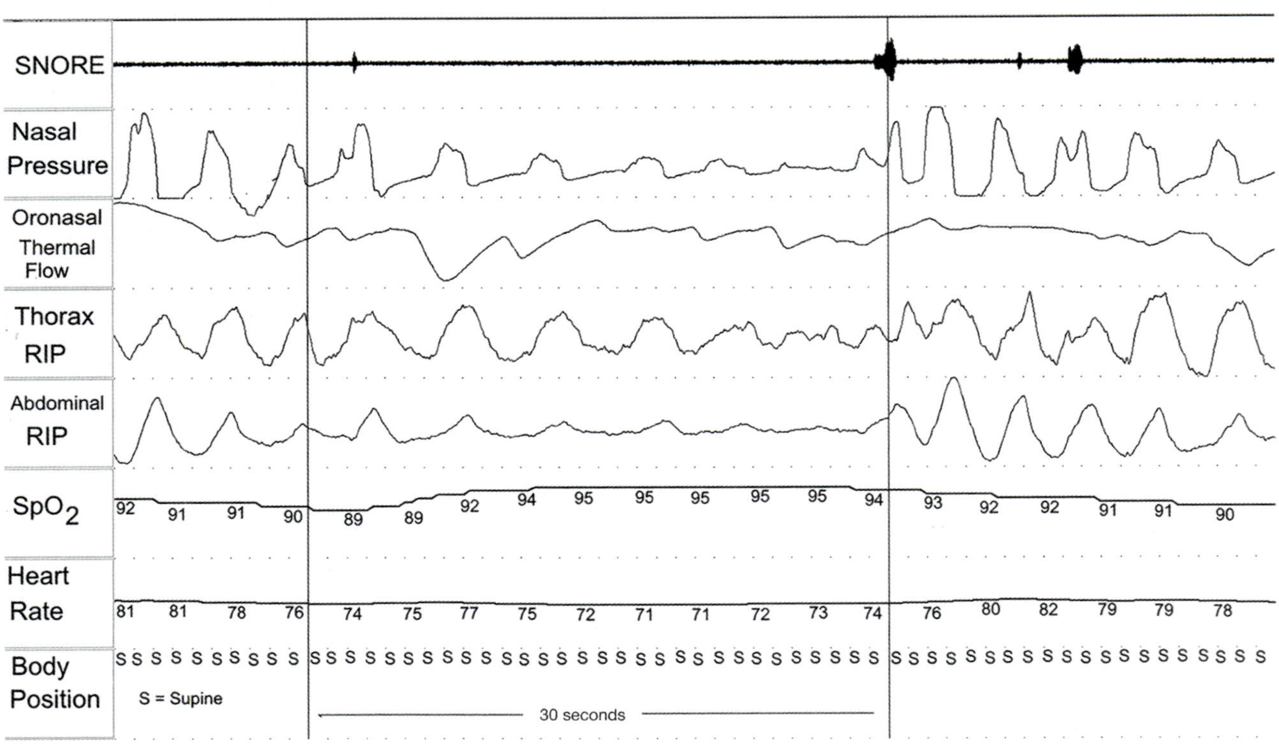

Figure 40-1 Tracings (120-second window) from a Type 3 home sleep apnea testing device (PDX, Philips Respironics) showing a hypopnea. In this study, the signal from the oronasal device was suboptimal. RIP, respiratory inductance plethysmography.

event index (REI) in lieu of an AHI. This is calculated by dividing the count of all respiratory events by the total hours of recording time. It is important to note that REI has the potential to underrepresent the severity or frequency of SDB as the recording time is always larger than the TST.

The TST is always less than or equal to the recording time and often shorter than the recording time by an hour or more. Thus, even if the same number of events is detected by PSG and HST devices, the AHI will be greater by PSG as the TST is less than the total recording time. For example, if 100 events are recorded and the TST is 5 hours and the recording time is 6 hours, the AHI for PSG is 20/h, but the AHI by HST will be 16.6/h.

Differences in Disease Severity Between Polysomnography and Home Sleep Testing

The AHI values may vary from HST and PSG studies if the respiratory sensors used in the studies are not the same. For example, a study by Dingli et al used a thermal sensor to detect apnea and hypopneas during PSG and nasal pressure during HST (14). If PSG and HST studies are done on different nights, night-to-night variability may also contribute to differences in AHI. Many patients have a much higher AHI in the supine position or during rapid eye movement (REM) sleep. In these patients, the relative amounts of supine and REM sleep contribute to night-to-night variability in the AHI. Of interest, a study by Levendowski et al (27) found greater night-to-night variability with PSG compared with HST. Another study, by Smith et al, comparing HST with PSG, found that patients had less supine sleep at home compared with the sleep center (28). Having less supine sleep at home would often result in a lower HST AHI compared with a PSG AHI. In addition, if some events are missed by HST because of sensor dislodgement for a portion of the night, this will also reduce the AHI. On the other hand, patients may sleep better at home and have a greater amount of REM sleep. Individuals may consume more alcohol at home, therefore changing the HST REI (AHI).

Exact agreement between AHI values by PSG and HST is less important than correct classification of a patient as either having SDB or not. Although AHI (REI) values of 30 and 50/h are quite different, both would clearly support a diagnosis of OSA. On the other hand, values of 3 and 8/h are very similar, but only one would support a diagnosis of OSA. It is not surprising that HSTs often have their greatest utility in patients likely to have a moderate-to-high AHI. Differences in AHI by HST and PSG usually have minimal impact on the diagnosis of OSA in patients with moderate-to-severe OSA who have a relatively high AHI by either technique.

OUTCOME STUDIES USING HOME SLEEP TESTING

The ultimate decision of the CMS (6) in 2008 to allow HST for the diagnosis of OSA in patients to be treated with CPAP was heavily influenced by studies showing that clinical pathways using HST devices resulted in equivalent outcomes from CPAP treatment, including improvement in daytime sleepiness and the amount of adherence to treatment (21,23). One of the Agency for Healthcare Research and Quality (AHRQ) evidence reviews published in 2007 focused on outcomes rather than agreement in AHI (29). Studies by Whitelaw et al (21) and Mulgrew et al (23) were two important evaluations that influenced the CMS decision. Ever since those outcome studies were published, others have also been published showing similar findings (27,30-34). Whitelaw et al (21) randomized 288 patients referred by a family physician to either standard PSG or a SnoreSat home monitor (only oximetry data were actually utilized). A randomly selected subset of eligible patients referred to the sleep center was studied. Inclusion criteria contained a history suggestive of OSA in association with somnolence or significant physiologic consequences of OSA. Only 44% of patients were considered eligible, and of those, only 11% actually completed the trial. All patients underwent treatment with an auto-titrating PAP (APAP). The patients were followed after a 4-week period to determine their improvement with treatment. There was no difference in the ability of the AHI by PSG and the RDI by HST (desaturations per hour) to predict the response to APAP treatment in terms of adherence to treatment or improvement in the quality of life. Mulgrew et al (23) compared a pathway using PSG (Dx PSG, CPAP PSG separate nights) with a pathway using autotitration followed by CPAP treatment (95% pressure determined during autotitration). CPAP was further adjusted on the basis of oximetry in this group. Patients were chosen on the basis of the Epworth Sleepiness Scale (ESS), Sleep Apnea Clinical Score, and desaturations per hour greater than 15. Thus, patients in both treatment pathways had a high probability of having moderate-to-severe OSA. Once patients met inclusion and exclusion criteria, they were randomized to the PSG pathway or to the APAP pathway (oximetry → autotitration → CPAP). At 3 months, the improvement in ESS and quality of life was similar between the two pathways. CPAP adherence was actually better with the pathway not using PSG (eg, oximetry → autotitration → CPAP). At the end of the study, PSG was performed on CPAP at the final pressure chosen for each patient. The two pathways had similar AHI values (similar treatment effectiveness).

Berry and coworkers (24) compared a pathway using HST, APAP titration, and CPAP treatment with a pathway utilizing PSG for diagnosis and titration (most PSGs were split studies) and CPAP treatment. Patients were required to have daytime sleepiness and a moderate-to-high probability of OSA on the basis of history. An AHI greater than 5/h was used to diagnose OSA (either by HST or by PSG), and all patients diagnosed with OSA were offered CPAP. After 6 weeks of CPAP treatment, the percentage of patients using CPAP, the mean CPAP adherence, and the improvements in ESS and quality of life did not differ between clinical pathways. The study used an HST device on the basis of PAT.

Antic and coworkers (30) identified a high-risk patient group for OSA with ESS greater than 8 and an oxygen desaturation index (ODI) (2% dips) greater than or equal to 27/h. Patients were randomized to a pathway using autotitration, CPAP at the 95th percentile pressure determined during autotitration, and treatment directed by a specialist nurse (visits at 1 and 3 months) OR a pathway consisting of diagnostic PSG, CPAP PSG, CPAP treatment, nurse visits, and MD visits if needed. At 3 months, the groups did not differ in ESS improvement or CPAP adherence.

Skomro and coworkers (31) randomized patients to a PSG arm or home monitoring (HM) arm. The patients in both arms had a PSG performed (usually, split night in PSG arm and diagnostic PSG in HM arm). The HST device was the Embletta (Embla, Denver CO). The HM arm underwent APAP for 1 week and then CPAP for 3 weeks on the basis of the APAP data. Patients in the PSG arm underwent CPAP treatment for 4 weeks. The pathways were equivalent in CPAP adherence, improvement in ESS, and quality of life. A large study in Veterans Association (VA) patients found a pathway using HST not to be inferior to one using PSG for diagnosis and PAP titration (33). Rosen and coworkers found a higher PAP adherence in patients diagnosed by HST (34) who underwent autotitration at home to determine an effective level of CPAP rather than PSG for diagnosis and PAP titration. Of note, in all the aforementioned studies, patients with significant comorbidities were excluded. The studies do suggest that diagnosis by HST in a group with moderate-to-high probability of having OSA (without comorbidity), followed by CPAP treatment based on APAP titration, results in equivalent outcomes compared with pathways using PSG.

CLINICAL USE OF HOME SLEEP TESTING

Advantages and Limitations of Type 3 Home Sleep Testing

HST has a number of potential advantages (Table 40-3), including sleep in the normal home environment with

Table 40-3 Potential Advantages and Limitations for Unattended Type 3 Home Sleep Testing

Advantages	Limitations
• Sleep in normal home environment (patients may sleep better) • Some patients may find HSAT more comfortable than PSG (fewer monitoring leads) • Good for patients who are immobile or who might find PSG challenging (claustrophobia) • Flexible setting: home, hospital room, hotel • HSAT monitoring less technically complex than PSG • Each device less costly than PSG equipment • Less expertise needed to set up HSAT device and sensors • Less expertise needed to score and interpret HSAT studies than PSG • Virtual sleep center—number of patients who can be studied is not limited by the size of a sleep center • Some locales may decrease wait time for diagnosis and treatment (depends on availability of PSG)	• Some patients very anxious about becoming disconnected without someone available for reconnection • Unattended—so potential for monitoring leads becoming unhooked or technically inadequate study • 10%-15% technically inadequate studies (up 30% in some studies if patient places the sensors) • TST and amounts of different sleep stages are not documented (Type III and IV HSAT). Were the TST and amount of REM sleep adequate? • Apnea + hypopnea index underestimated because of division by monitoring time, which is greater than total sleep time • May not determine amount of supine monitoring time (some HSAT devices) • HSAT device loss or damage can be a significant problem • Good-quality HSAT studies require trained personnel and have substantial costs (education, setup, download, cleaning units, analysis, report generation). • Less cost to perform HSAT but much less reimbursement • Need to perform PSG for negative studies in most sleepy patients • If diagnosis of significant obstructive sleep apnea is made—still need to perform PSG CPAP titration in most patients unless alternate approach used (APAP titration, APAP treatment, empiric CPAP level) • Cannot detect arrhythmias if pulse rate by oximetry rather than electrocardiogram recorded

APAP, autotitration positive airway pressure; CPAP, continuous positive airway pressure; HSAT, home sleep apnea testing; PSG, polysomnography; REM, rapid eye movement; TST, total sleep time.

fewer sensors (patients may sleep better), and ease of study for patients with immobility, those with special needs (claustrophobia), or unstable medical conditions requiring intensive care. HST may also be useful in verifying an adequate CPAP before discharge from the hospital, until a follow-up by PSG titration can be obtained. HST monitoring is less complex and requires less expertise than PSG devices. The number of diagnostic studies is not limited by the number of rooms in the sleep center. In locales with limited PSG capacity, the use of HST may reduce the wait time to study and treatment.

There are also a host of disadvantages to HST. Some patients are quite anxious about sensors becoming disconnected and would actually prefer an attended study. If sensors do become dislodged during an unattended study, it may be technically inadequate. In fact, a significant proportion of HST studies are technically inadequate (5%-30%) (35). HST is less cost-effective if a high proportion of studies must be repeated. HST devices are less expensive than PSG equipment but may not be returned or may be damaged in the patients' home. Type 3 (95806) HSAT studies typically do not determine the amount of sleep or the amount of REM sleep. It may be difficult to determine if a study underestimates the severity of OSA caused by limited amounts of sleep or REM sleep. Some HST devices determine body position. This is important if the patient has much more severe apnea in the supine position. Good-quality HST studies often require significant expertise in either education of patients to self-apply the sensors or hooking them up in the sleep center. Additionally, HST studies do require experienced RPSGTs to avoid a high percentage of technically inadequate studies. Golpe et al (35) found much higher rates of failed studies when the patients set up HSAT in the home (33%) versus having HSAT devices applied at the sleep center (7%). If the HSAT study is negative and the patient is sleepy, most patients will need a PSG. If the HST is positive, many patients will need a PSG CPAP titration, unless an alternate approach is available (APAP titration or APAP treatment). One could argue that a split study might be more cost-effective than diagnosis by HSAT, followed by a PSG titration. The relative cost of the two approaches will depend on the number of negative HSAT studies, the number of HST studies that need repeating, and the treatment algorithm once a diagnosis of OSA is made. In the private sector, in the United States, autotitration studies are not reimbursed, and DME suppliers receive the same reimbursement for CPAP and APAP devices, even though APAP devices are more expensive. These reimbursement issues limit the use of alternate approaches to CPAP treatment. However, as the cost differential between APAP and CPAP devices has decreased considerably, many DME providers are willing to supply APAP devices if specifically ordered by a physician.

Standards and Indications Unattended Home Sleep Testing

Clinical guidelines for portable monitoring (CGPM) were first published by the AASM in 2007 on the basis of an evidence review and consensus (22). The guidelines stated that HST "may" be used as an alternative to PSG for the diagnosis of OSA in patients with a high probability of OSA (provided certain conditions are met); in cases where PSG is not possible by virtue of immobility, safety, or critical illness; or to monitor the response to non-CPAP treatment of OSA (including oral appliance, upper airway surgery, and weight loss). However, as you will read further on, HST studies have been recommended in these cases of high probability of OSA *unless* the patient has comorbidities increasing the complexity of the diagnosis or treatment.

In 2017, an AASM task force published practice guidelines for diagnostic testing for adult OSA superseding/updating previous guidance (4). The task force recommended that PSG *or home sleep apnea testing* with a technically adequate device be used for the diagnosis of OSA in *uncomplicated adult patients* presenting with signs and symptoms that indicate an increased risk of moderate-to-severe obstructive apnea. The selection of "uncomplicated" patients is described in the following section.

Candidates for Home Sleep Testing

A comprehensive sleep evaluation should precede HST. Ideally, each patient should be seen by a board-certified/board-eligible sleep physician before sleep testing. If this is not possible, another physician or advanced practice provider may perform an evaluation consisting of questionnaires or an interview.

Review of the medical record to exclude patients with comorbidities that may complicate diagnosis or treatment is important. Comorbidities excluding patients from HST include severe pulmonary disease, neuromuscular disease, or congestive heart failure (CHF). The rationale is that such patients may exhibit hypoventilation without discrete respiratory events, or Cheyne-Stokes breathing. Guidelines for diagnostic testing for adult OSA published by a task force of the AASM (4) recommended PSG (rather than HSAT) for the diagnosis of OSA in complicated adult patients with *significant cardiorespiratory disease, potential respiratory muscle weakness due to neuromuscular condition, awake hypoventilation or suspicion of sleep-related hypoventilation, chronic opioid medication use, and a history of stroke or severe insomnia.*

One can argue that if HST devices use the same sensors used for PSG, then both types of testing should have a similar ability to detect central apnea, Cheyne-Stokes breathing (Figure 40-2), or hypoventilation (manifested

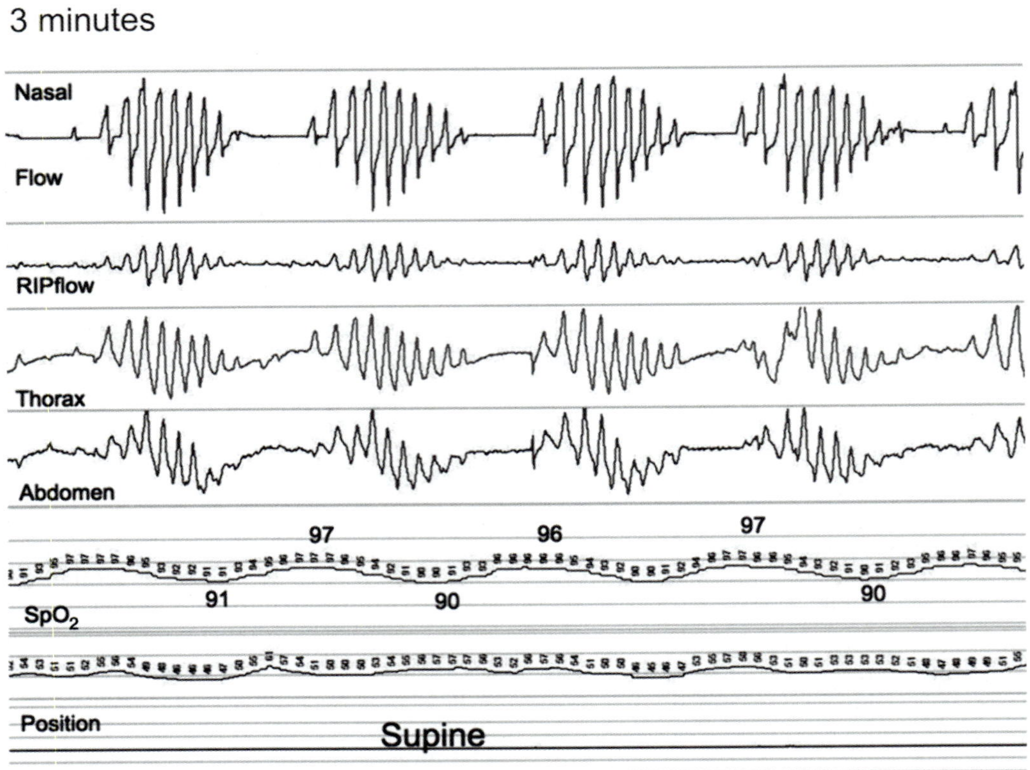

Figure 40-2 A 3-minute tracing from a home sleep apnea testing device that displays RIP flow, which is an estimate of airflow (here also measured by nasal pressure after a square root transformation). The thorax and abdomen channels are RIP effort belt signals at those locations. The figure shows an example of Cheyne-Stokes breathing central apnea. RIP, respiratory inductance plethysmography.

by a low Sa_{O_2} without discrete events). According to the AASM scoring manual (36), a diagnosis of hypoventilation should be based on measurement of arterial P_{CO_2} or an accurate surrogate. Hence, neither routine PSG nor HSAT can definitively document hypoventilation. Even if HST can detect Cheyne-Stokes breathing, central apneas not of the Cheyne-Stokes type, or arterial desaturations without discrete events, patients with these findings would not be good candidates for autotitration or treatment with an auto-titrating device. These patients would benefit from an attended PSG titration. Patients with a low baseline Sa_{O_2} will often need both supplemental oxygen and CPAP. In these situations, a split sleep study may be more cost-effective than HST followed by a PSG titration. Most HSAT devices would miss significant cardiac arrhythmias because typically, a heart rate signal is derived from the oximeter rather than ECG. However, many HST devices have incorporated ECG capability or arrhythmia detection through PAT. If patients with significant insomnia undergo HST, the morning time (MT) may tremendously overestimate TST, thus reducing the sensitivity of detecting sleep apnea when utilizing devices not validated to accurately determine TST. HSAT is also not indicated in patients in whom other sleep disorders are present and that would be better evaluated by PSG (coexistent OSA and parasomnias).

Recommended Home Sleep Testing Methodology

The AASM scoring manual (36) provides recommendations for the sensors and devices to be used in HST (Table 40-4).

- HST should be performed under the auspices of an AASM-accredited sleep center.
- Adequately trained staff should either place the monitoring equipment on the patient or instruct them on the application of the sensors. This is essential to avoid a high percentage of technically inadequate studies.
- The raw data tracings must be reviewed and edited for accuracy if an automated scoring system is used.
- For quality assurance, standard operating procedures for the HST process must exist.

Table 40-4 Recommended Methodology for Home Sleep Testing

Equipment (Scoring Manual and Accreditation Standards)
• FDA approved with unique identifier for each unit • Meets criteria for 9580, 95801, 95806 • Monitor at least three parameters: airflow, effort, and oximetry (or peripheral arterial tonometry, actigraphy, oximetry). • Ability to record oximetry and a measure of heart rate • Ability to display raw data for review, manual scoring, or editing of automated scoring • Ability to calculate an REI on the basis of monitoring time as a surrogate for the AHI determined by PSG • Airflow—at least one: nasal pressure, oronasal thermal airflow sensor, or alternate sensor (Recommended: RIPflow, RIPsum; Acceptable: PVDF sum) • Respiratory effort—Recommended: dual thoracoabdominal RIP belts, Acceptable: single RIP belt, single or dual PVDF belts, single or dual piezoelectric belts, single pneumatic effort belt • Device must provide an REI that approximates AHI by PSG.
Personnel and Setting

• HSAT should be performed by an AASM-accredited sleep center
  • Standard policies and procedures for HST
  • Quality assurance program
  • Interscorer reliability program
• Experienced sleep technician/technologist either places sensors or directly educates the patient on sensor application
• Review of all raw data and interpretation by BC/BE sleep physician

Scoring of Study
• Raw data are scored manually or edited if automated scoring • Scoring criteria according to AASM scoring manual
Follow-Up
• Sleep MD or referring MD/extenders discuss results with patient and plan treatment • Sleep center has a method to document adequate follow-up • If HST study is technically inadequate or fails to establish a diagnosis of obstructive sleep apnea in a patient with a high pretest probability, a diagnostic PSG should be performed.

The reader should review current accreditation standards for updates.
AASM, American Academy of Sleep Medicine; AHI, apnea-hypopnea index; FDA, U.S. Food and Drug Administration; HST, home sleep apnea testing; PSG, polysomnography; PVDF, polyvinylidene fluoride; REI, respiratory event index; RIP, respiratory inductance plethysmography.
Based on AASM accreditation standards, Kapur VK, Auckley DH, Chowdhuri S, et al. Clinical practice guideline for diagnostic testing for adult obstructive sleep apnea: an American Academy of Sleep Medicine clinical practice guideline. *J Clin Sleep Med*. 2017;13(3):479-504; Collop NA, Tracy SL, Kapur V, et al. Obstructive sleep apnea devices for out-of-center (OOC) testing: technology evaluation. *J Clin Sleep Med*. 2011;7(5): 531-548; Department of Health and Human Services. Decision memo for continuous positive airway pressure (CPAP) therapy for obstructive sleep apnea (OSA) (CAG#0093R2). Centers for Medicare & Medicaid Services. 2008. https://www.cms.gov/medicare-coverage-database/view/ncacal-decision-memo.aspx?proposed=N&NCAId=204

- To verify adequate scoring, interscorer reliability on scoring of HST studies should be performed on a routine basis and documented.
- If the HST recording is technically inadequate or if the study results are negative in a patient with a high pretest probability of having OSA, an attended PSG should be performed.
- In the AASM Scoring Manual, there is guidance for what parameters are required to be reported.

PRACTICAL CONSIDERATIONS FOR HOME SLEEP TESTING

There are a number of technical and economic factors to be considered in setting up a successful HST program. A system that works in one locale may not work in another. A systematic approach is indicated to avoid a high percentage of technically inadequate studies. The choice of the device and method of device application are major considerations. Devices with more sensors provide additional information (and backup sensors) but are more difficult to apply. Before selecting an HST device, one must carefully consider the method of device setup that is planned. The HST device software should provide the ability to review the raw data in detail. An accurate autoscoring algorithm that minimizes the amount of editing that is required is highly desirable, given the low reimbursement for the technical component of HST monitoring. If the software is similar to that used for PSG, this may be an advantage in reducing training costs. The durability of the device and the cost of expendables (nasal cannula, oximeter probes) should be considered.

HST devices can be placed on the patient in the sleep center, or patients can be trained on the HST device and asked to apply the sensors themselves at home. Adequate patient education is essential, and instructional videos along with simple instruction sheets can be very useful. One option is to have the patient come to the sleep center for education on device placement and practice sensor application. A rapid turnaround time reduces the number of HST devices that need to be purchased while also reducing time to diagnosis. If the HST device is simple to operate, mailing the device to the patient's home with instructions and having them apply it can work in some patient populations. Most HST devices require the patient to return the device before the data is uploaded and interpreted by a clinician. However, some HST devices have recently been introduced with smartphone capabilities allowing the patient to transfer the data from the device to the clinician via cloud storage. This results in rapid availability of data for interpretation and significantly reduces wait time for diagnosis/therapy.

There are a number of common sensor application problems that need to be addressed. Patients often have difficulty applying some types of oximeter probes as well as chest and abdominal belts. The physician, or sleep center, should be aware of the options before purchasing a device. During a home study, dislodgement of either the nasal cannula or oximeter probe as well as pulling sensor leads out of the HST device during movement are typical causes of technically inadequate studies. Patients can be trained to apply tape at strategic points to reduce these events. Many devices have the ability to inform the patient, or technologist, that sensors are working and that the device is recording data. It is also useful to have patients complete a brief sleep diary to record their estimate of how long they slept and if the night of sleep was fairly typical. An occasional patient will sleep very poorly with the sensors attached. If minimal sleep is recorded, a false-negative study is more likely. Devices that can record more than one night provide another monitoring night opportunity and may also reduce the influence of first-night variability.

HOME SLEEP TESTING TECHNOLOGIES

There are numerous devices available for HST monitoring, and many incorporate technologies found in PSG, especially Type 3 devices (Figure 40-3). These often include respiratory effort belts (RIP or PVDF), airflow via pressure transducer and cannula or thermistor, and a pulse oximeter. Some include AC channel inputs for the recording of ECG, EEG, or EMG if the clinician chooses. However, because the patient is often applying the recording equipment themselves, ease of use is of utmost importance. This has led to the innovation and utilization of new technologies that seek to record data typically gathered by PSG, but in a simple and patient accessible way. A few technologies often seen in HST more often than PSG are PAT and cardiopulmonary coupling (CPC). Additionally, software algorithms and artificial intelligence applied to oximetry (photoplethysmography [PPG]) data have been introduced as a low-cost way to utilize older recording technology common to all hospitals/clinics for the use of HST.

Peripheral Arterial Tonometry

PAT is an innovative approach to HST (Figure 40-4) that utilizes the vasomotor activity in the digit as a metric

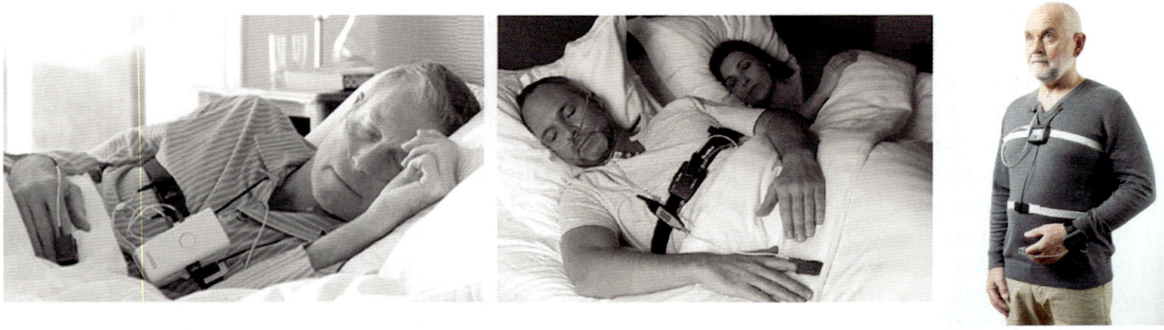

Figure 40-3 Three home sleep apnea testing monitors. In the left panel, an Alice Night-One device (Philips Respironics) is shown. In the center panel, ResMed's ApneaLink Plus (ResMed Ltd.) is shown. Both these devices use nasal cannula to monitor flow and a single effort belt. In the right panel, a Nox-T3 device (Nox Medical, Carefusion) is shown. The device uses chest and abdominal respiratory inductance plethysmography (RIP) belts and derived RIPsum (estimate of tidal volume) and RIPflow (estimate of airflow) tracings that provide additional information to the nasal pressure. An oximeter unit is worn like a watch and communicates with the main recording unit on the chest by Bluetooth wireless technology. (Used with permission from Koninklijke Philips N.V.; © Resmed. All rights reserved.; © Nox Medical. All rights reserved. This image is used with permission to reference Nox Medical. Any alteration or additional usage without prior written consent is prohibited.)

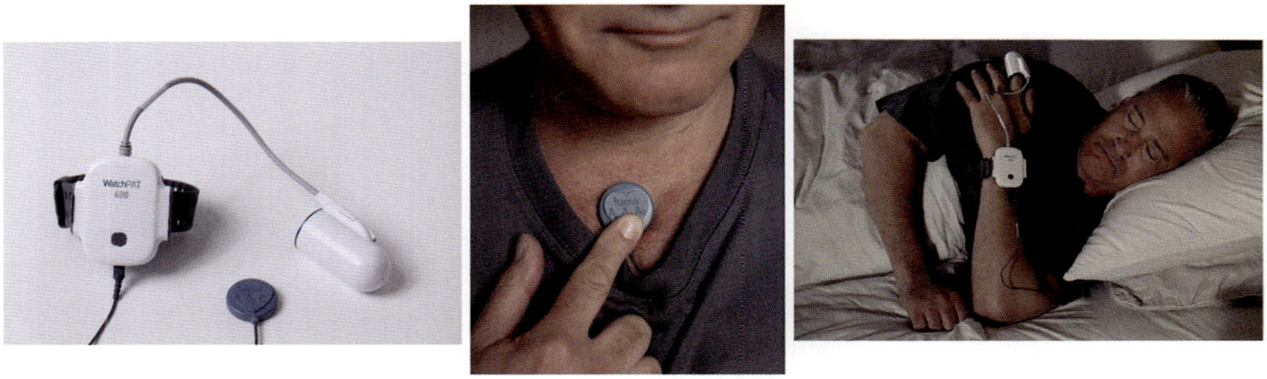

Figure 40-4 Images of the WatchPAT 400 device, which measures peripheral arterial tonometry, in addition to other signals discussed in this chapter. Used with permission from ZOLL, Itamar.

of sympathetic nervous system. This technology allows the clinician to determine a wealth of information including sleep stage and SDB. To measure peripheral arterial tone, a photoplethysmogram is used to measure changes in blood volume at the digit from one pulse to the next. This change in volume, called PAT amplitude, allows the clinician to observe vasoconstriction or vasodilation (narrowing or relaxation of the artery). The peripheral arteries of the fingertips are unique in comparison to the rest of the body as they are associated almost exclusively with α-1 receptors. When catecholamines (adrenaline and noradrenaline) bind to these receptors, it triggers the contraction of smooth muscle cells, resulting in an acute narrowing of the peripheral arteries, referred to as vasoconstriction. Conversely, when catecholamines bind to β-receptors, we see the opposite, a relaxation of the artery called vasodilation. Because of this, it is critical to measure PAT at the fingertip, as the closer we measure to the core or chest, the ratio of α-receptors to β-receptors reverses, reducing the ability to observe vasoconstriction associated with SDB events. Additionally, the ability to discern sympathetic activity (alerting) versus parasympathetic activity (rest promoting) is diminished when we have a higher concentration of β-receptors to α-receptors such as near the heart and lungs. A study in 2001 demonstrated via dose response curves in Figure 40-5 that α-adrenergic related vasoconstriction was more pronounced at the fingertip than even nearby at the forearm, but β-adrenergic related vasodilation was present at the forearm but not the fingertip (37). This shows that the fingertip is primarily, if not entirely, mediated by α-adrenergic receptors. Thus, the sympathetic activation (increase in catecholamines) associated with arousal, SDB response, and REM sleep is most pronounced or observed at the fingertip. To measure these changes in vasomotor activity accurately, it is important to measure PAT with a photoplethysmogram utilizing a wavelength monitoring an isosbestic point. An isosbestic point allows for the measurement of multiple substances equally. In the setting of PAT, changes in pulsatile blood volume are being measured as opposed to changes in oxygenation, as typically seen in oximetry PPG. As shown in the image in Figure 40-6, deoxygenated hemoglobin and oxygenated hemoglobin are best observed at separate wavelengths in the red/infrared spectrum. All oximeters utilize wavelengths similar to the ones shown to measure oxygen saturation. At 805 nm, between the two oximeter wavelengths, you will notice the isosbestic point where oxygenated and deoxygenated hemoglobin can be measured equally. While this spot would not be ideal for oxygen saturation, it is critical to measure PAT at this wavelength because it is not affected by changes in oxygen saturation. As you can see in Figure 40-7, the amplitude of the oximeter signals is affected by changes in oxygen saturation, while at the isosbestic point, the amplitude of the PAT signal is not.

For sleep staging via PAT, we focus on the relationship between sympathetic and parasympathetic nervous system activity. In the accompanying images in Figure 40-8, we can see a reduction or attenuation in PAT amplitude (decreased peripheral blood flow) during REM as well as an increase in the variability of the PAT signal, which easily differentiates wake and REM from nonrapid eye movement (NREM) sleep. This is also supported by an increase in baseline heart rate (HR) and variability of HR during REM. This is because REM sleep is associated with a profound increase in sympathetic nervous system activity. This contrasts with NREM sleep, where the parasympathetic nervous system is dominant with its most prominent activity during NREM stage 3 or slow-wave sleep. In the PAT signal, we see this as an increase in PAT amplitude (unaffected peripheral blood flow) and a decrease in variability. This is also supported by a reduction in baseline HR and less variability.

When measuring SDB with PAT technology, the body's response to each SDB plays a critical role in

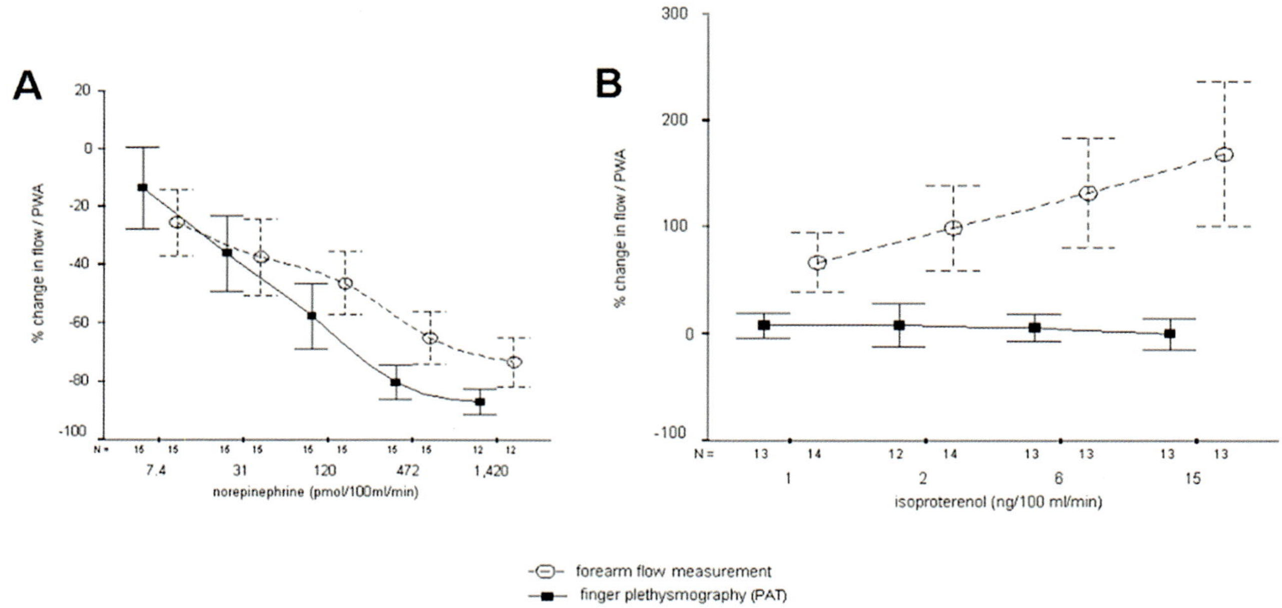

Figure 40-5 In this figure, we see the change in blood flow associated with increasing dosages of a vasoconstrictor, norepinephrine A: and a vasodilator, isoproterenol B: The graphs compare these changes at the fingertip, where there is a significantly higher prevalence of α-adrenergic receptors compared to β-receptors (shown as the solid black boxes) and at the forearm, where there are more β-adrenergic receptors comparatively (shown as the empty circles). A: demonstrates that arteries at the fingertip constrict more than the forearm norepinephrine dosage increases. Conversely, B: shows arterial vasodilation at the forearm in response to increasing isoproterenol dosage, but the arteries at the fingertip is not significantly affected. For this reason, it is critical to measure peripheral arterial tonometry at the fingertip, as opposed to the rest of the body, where β-adrenergic receptors are in higher prevalence.

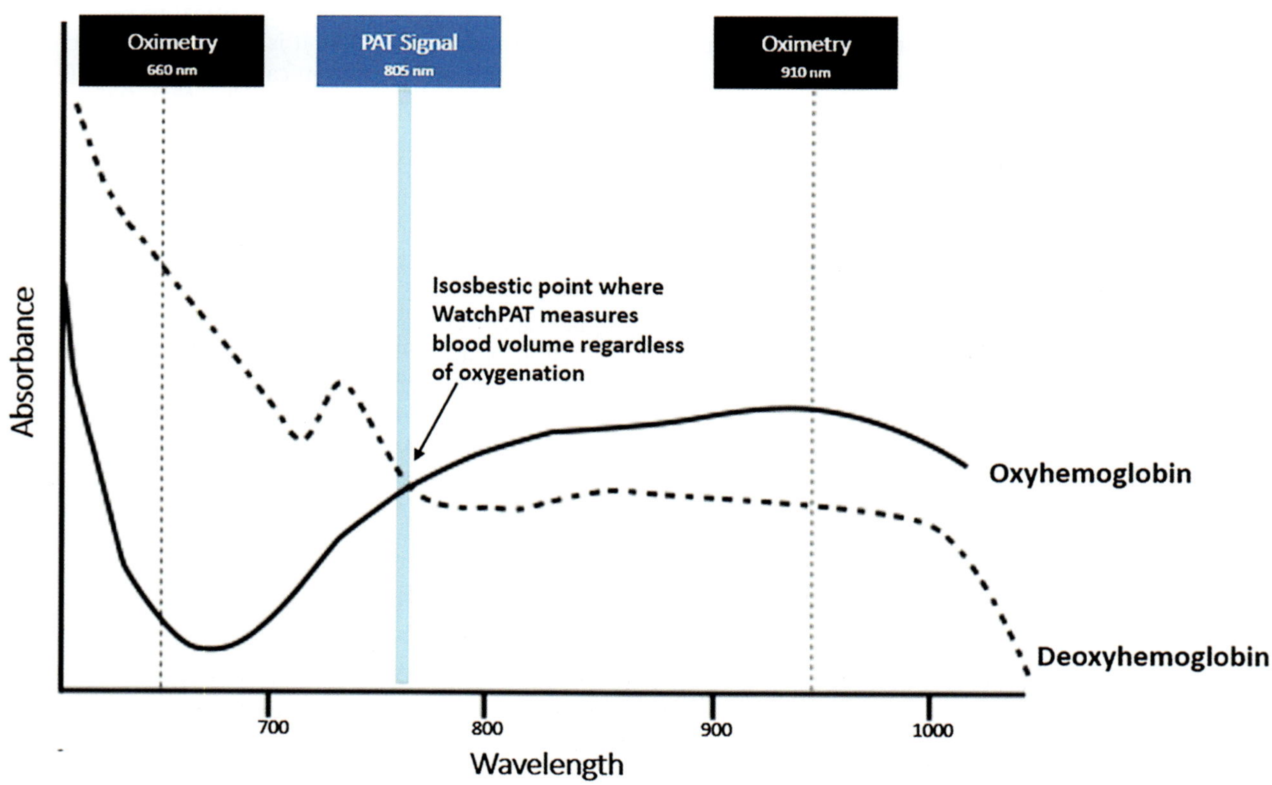

Figure 40-6 In this image, we compare the absorbance of light emitted from the PPG device across changing wavelengths in the x-axis. The isosbestic wavelength (PAT signal) will have the same absorbance of oxygenated and deoxygenated hemoglobin, as opposed to an oximeter, which will measure at two separate wavelengths to determine oxygen saturation. PAT, peripheral arterial tonometry; PPG, photoplethysmography.

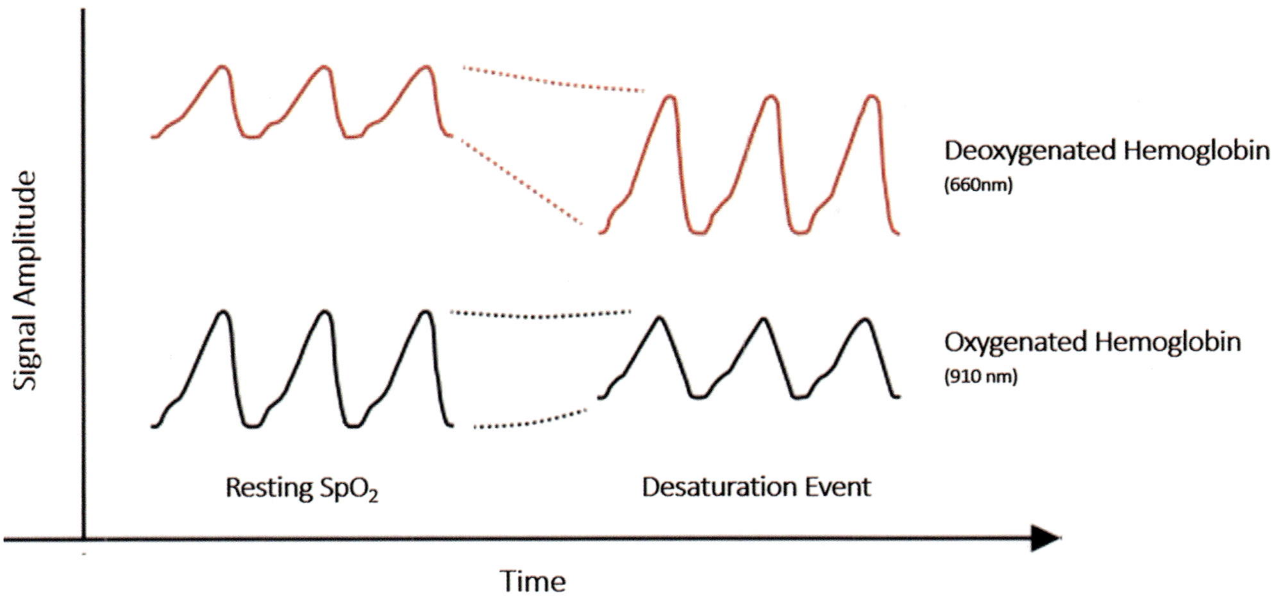

Figure 40-7 This image demonstrates the changes in amplitude of an oximeter-based signals during oxygen desaturation. Because of these changes, it is important to measure peripheral arterial tonometry with an isosbestic wavelength of 805 nm, which will capture both deoxygenated and oxygenated hemoglobin equally. Without an isosbestic wavelength from the recording device, the pulsatile volume changes will be affected by artifact from SDB events. SDB, sleep-disordered breathing.

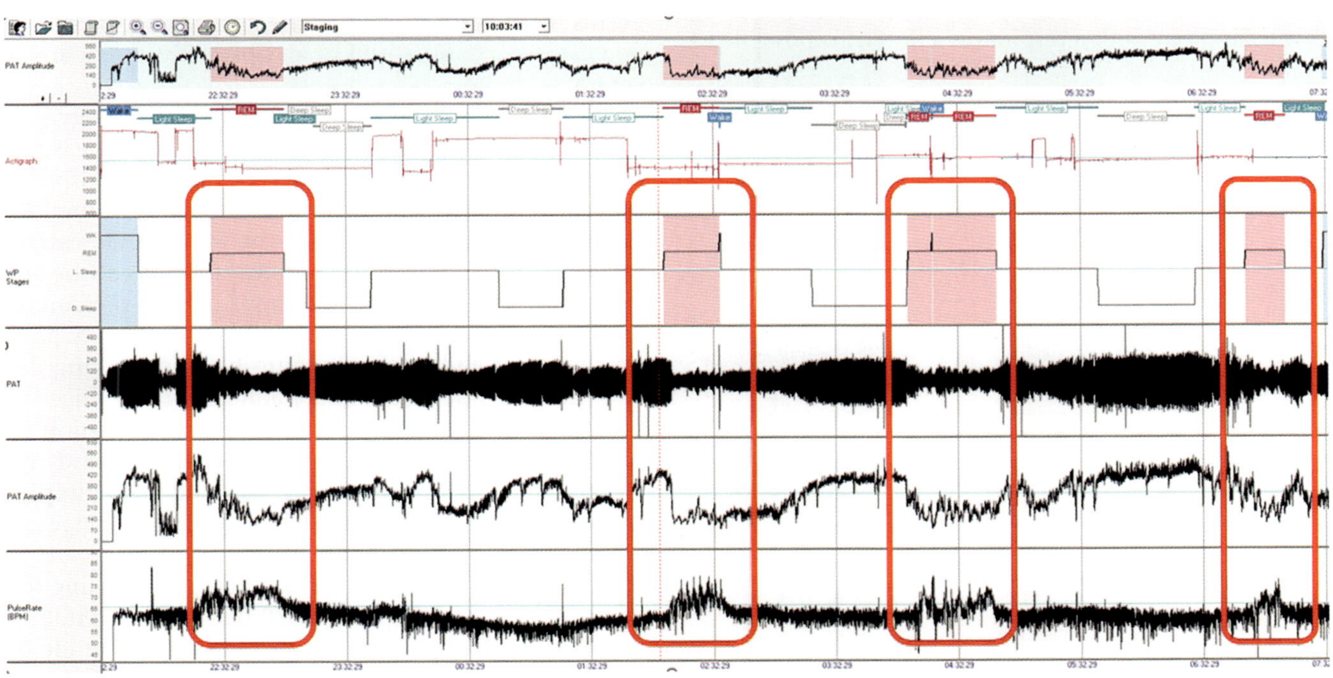

Figure 40-8 A limited WatchPAT montage demonstrates the following channels, Actigraphy, Sleep Stages, PAT, PAT Amplitude, and Pulse Rate. We can see during the REM periods, marked in red, the overall attenuation of the PAT signal, reduction in PAT amplitude, and increase in heart rate. Additionally, the variability of these signals increases. These values together demonstrate increased sympathetic nervous system activity indicative of REM sleep. Inversely, during NREM, we see an increase in PAT amplitude and a decrease in the variability of these signals, demonstrating parasympathetic nervous system activity indicative of NREM sleep. PAT, peripheral arterial tonometry; NREM, nonrapid eye movement; REM, rapid eye movement. Used with permission from ZOLL, Itamar.

detection of the event. In the termination of a SDB event, there is typically an increase in catecholamines (adrenaline), which is observed in the PAT signal as a decrease in amplitude. This phenomenon is advantageous as during a period of hypercapnia/hypoxia, the flow of newly ventilated blood is reduced to the peripheral arteries (fingertips and toes), allowing for increased prioritization of the core and brain; this is due to β-receptors in the core/chest promoting vasodilation, as discussed previously. In addition to this attenuation of the PAT amplitude, we also observe an acceleration in pulse. The combination of PAT amplitude reduction and acceleration in pulse is indicative of sympathetic activation. This sympathetic activation in conjunction with oxygen desaturation shows a high correlation with PSG reported apnea/hypopnea events Figure 40-9.

A PAT signal can also provide insight into whether an SDB event is obstructive or central by measuring the variability of the PAT upstroke during the systolic phase of the pulse. During inspiration, intrathoracic pressure increases, influencing the morphology of the PAT upstroke. Because our HR is much faster than our respiratory rate, we see variability in the curvature of the PAT upstroke from one pulse to the next as the intrathoracic pressure increases and decreases with respiration. When the variability of this morphology decreases, it is a great indicator that the diaphragm has become stagnant—such as in a central sleep apnea event. When coupling this technology with a respiratory effort, it is possible to

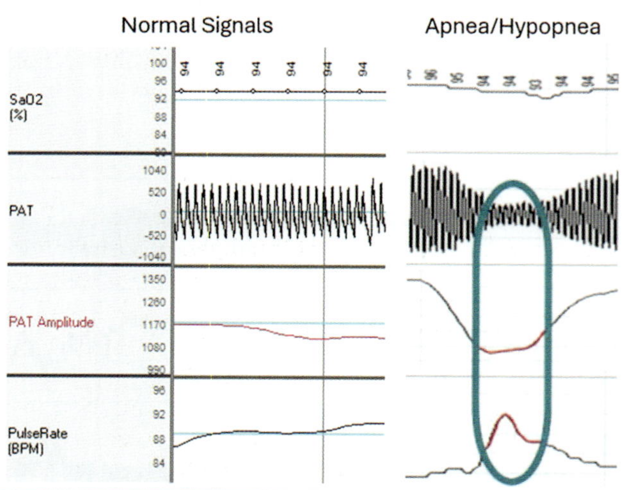

Figure 40-9 In this image, we look at only four channels of WatchPAT data, including Sao_2, PAT, PAT amplitude, and Pulse Rate. This image demonstrates the signals at rest and during an apneic/hypopneic event. During the apneic/hypopneic event, notice the concurrent acute attenuation of the PAT signal, the decrease in PAT amplitude, the acute acceleration of the pulse rate, and the associated oxygen desaturation. PAT, peripheral arterial tonometry.

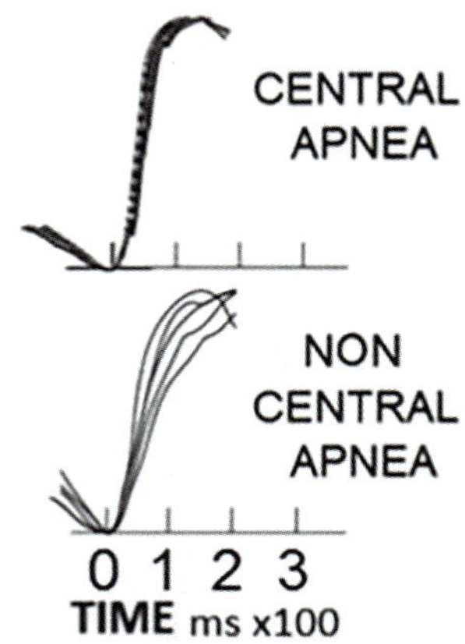

Figure 40-10 In this image, we compare the waveform morphology of the systolic phase of five consecutive heart beats. The waveforms have been transposed to the same point on the x-axis to easily visualize the variation in morphology. During the central apnea event, we see little to no variation in the morphology of the systolic phase from one beat to the next as the diaphragm is motionless and there is no change in intrathoracic pressure. In the noncentral apnea event, we see significant variability in morphology from one beat to the next. This is due to changes in intrathoracic pressure as the patient moves their diaphragm during respiration.

differentiate central SDB events from obstructive SDB events with great accuracy. In the image in Figure 40-10, you can see a comparison of an obstructive event and a central event.

Another important feature of PAT technology is a uniform counter pressure surrounding the measurement site at the digit. This serves multiple purposes but, most importantly, maximizes the range of the PAT signal amplitude, thereby allowing for accurate assessment. Measurement of vasomotor activity can be inhibited by venous blood pooling if uneven pressure is applied, such as in ring devices, where blood may pool on the distal end of the fingertip beyond the ring device. Inversely, devices that are adhered to the fingertip via adhesive tape may result in an overall reduction in blood flow if the adhesive tape is too tight. A study by Henriksen et al, published in 1976, found that by applying a uniform pressure to the fingertip, larger changes in volume were observed Figure 40-11 (38).

The AASM guidelines for the diagnostic testing for adult OSA support the use of PAT, but it is worth noting that this recommendation was based on a multitude of studies validating the WatchPAT devices manufactured by ZOLL Itamar (previously Itamar Medical). It is important to differentiate devices claiming to provide a PAT signal as not all devices provide a uniform counterpressure or isosbestic wavelength, as discussed, and the recommendations made by the AASM cited only studies with PAT technology, as described here. Some

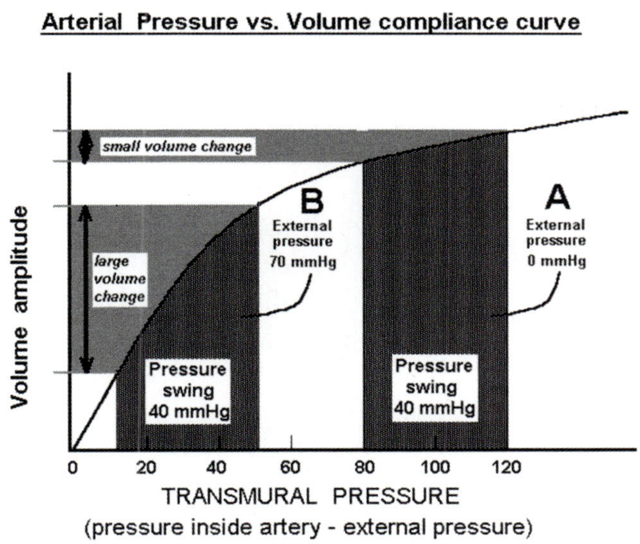

Figure 40-11 Demonstrates the relationship between transmural pressure (pressure inside the artery—external pressure applied to the fingertip) and the amplitude of the PAT wave. In A: no external pressure is applied to the fingertip, and we see that there is only a very small change in the amplitude of the PAT signal during each pulse. In B: after applying external pressure to the fingertip, we see a very large change in amplitude during each pulse. This demonstrates the importance of a counterpressure on the finger when measuring pulsatile volume changes via peripheral arterial tonometry.

device manufacturers claim to provide a PAT signal via an oximeter device which is not consistent with PAT as described here or in the AASM guidelines. These devices, often termed "PPG devices" will be described later in this chapter.

Cardiopulmonary Coupling

This technology also utilizes differences in sympathetic versus parasympathetic activity. CPC utilizes software algorithms to analyze data collected from ECG and/or oximeters to determine relationships between heart rate variability (HRV) and respiratory rate variability (RRV) via software-derived respirations. The coupling, or coherence, between these two metrics is analyzed by a software algorithm and designated as either high frequency coupling (HFC), which is suggestive of a parasympathetic dominant state (synchronized low variability), or low frequency coupling (LFC), which is suggestive of a sympathetic dominant state (asynchronous high variability). This insight allows for estimation of sleep/wake as well as REM/NREM stages (Figures 40-12 and 40-13).

When this technology is used in the diagnosis of SDB, this data is typically gathered via an oximeter as this allows for the monitoring of oxygen saturation as well. When significant oxygen desaturation is associated with LFC, this is suggestive of an SDB event and allows for estimation of AHI. Some CPC software analysis systems also monitor for periodicity of LFC, which may prompt the clinician to suspect that detected SDB events are central in nature.

While CPC technology often provides a channel for manual interpretation, the channels created are software derived as the only physical channel is the ECG or pulse wave from an oximeter. It is worth noting that many insurance companies do not allow the use of software-derived channels and require physical channels. The difference between these types of channels is described later in this discussion.

Photoplethysmography

This is a very commonly used technology for the assessment of oxygen saturation. Because of the widespread use of pulse oximeters, this technology is very accessible and inexpensive to acquire. While simple overnight oximetry alone has been deemed inadequate for the diagnosis of SDB in the past, new innovative technology has allowed for the data acquired by a pulse oximeter to be analyzed by software algorithms and provide data similar to that of PSG and other HST devices.

These software as a medical device (SaMD) applications analyze the PPG data through proprietary algorithms to report TST, sleep efficiency, sleep staging, SDB events, and HR. Some are able to utilize smartphone applications to also monitor snoring and acoustic flow. In most cases, these channels are available for manual interpretation but are also considered software-derived channels as opposed to physical channels, potentially making it problematic for certain insurance companies, as discussed next.

Physical and Software-Derived Channels

As new software and artificial intelligence is introduced to HST, a distinction has been made by some insurance companies (most notably, the Palmetto MAC) calling for a differentiation of physical and software-derived channels. For these insurance companies, they require that a channel be a physical channel, as opposed to a software-derived channel. To define the difference simply, a physical channel could be described as data that is measured directly from the patient via a sensor. For instance, respiratory effort can be physically measured in a variety of ways, such as RIP, PVDF, and thoracoabdominal accelerometry. These sensors all provide data measured at the chest or abdomen using technology that measures the movement or expansion of the thoracic cage and/or abdomen. A common example of respiratory effort or rate measured by a software-derived channel would be

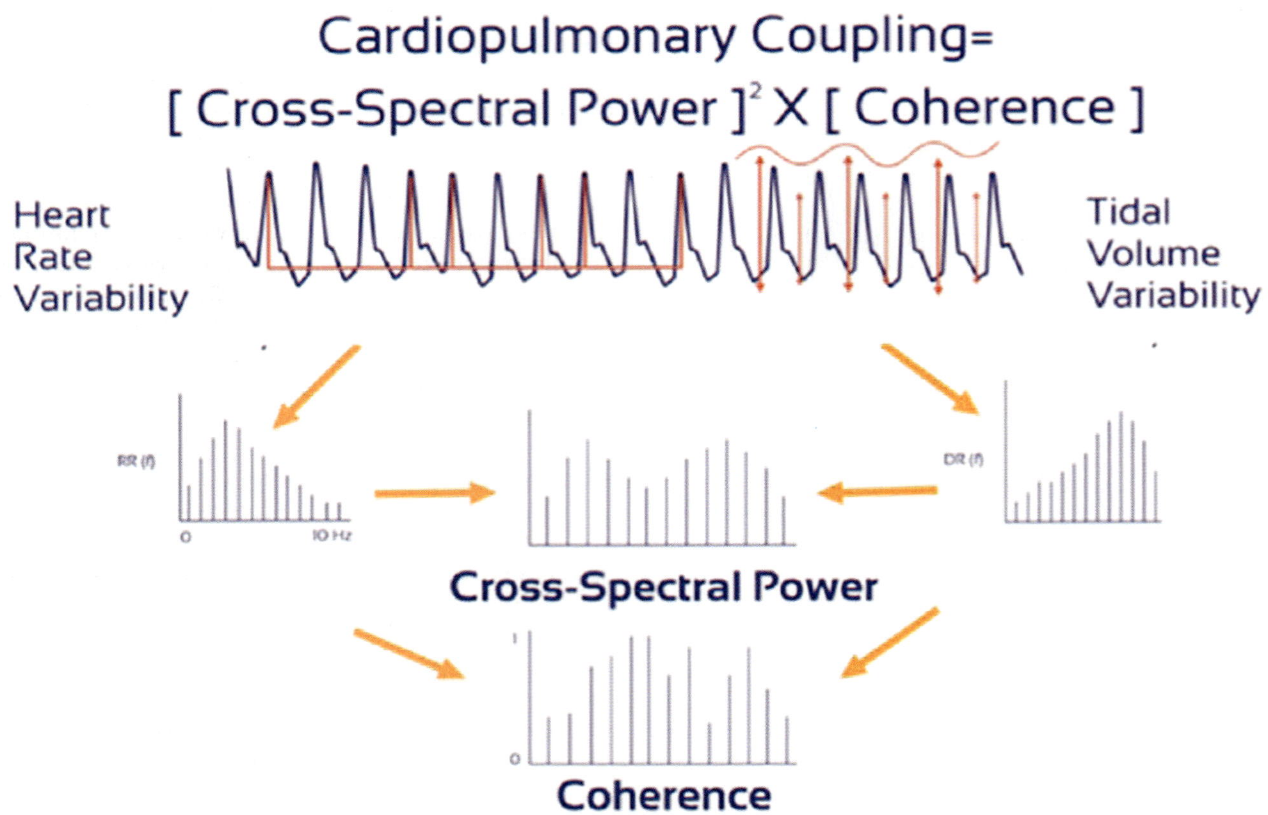

Figure 40-12 This figure shows how heart rate variability and tidal volume variability are calculated from an oximeter. The cardiopulmonary coupling equation then uses these values and their coherence to determine sleep stages as well as detect apneic events.

analysis, by software, of a PPG channel. In an unfiltered PPG channel, there is a slow undulating change in baseline that may be associated with inspiration/expiration. This method to gather respiratory rate is common in other fields such as emergency medicine. However, this is not a direct measurement of thoracoabdominal excursions, but rather an estimation provided by software analysis. It is important to be aware of this distinction when evaluating HST reimbursement by different insurance companies' criteria.

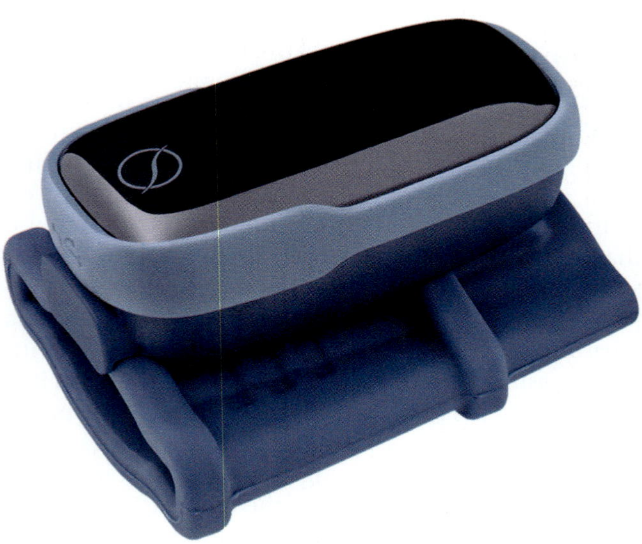

Figure 40-13 Sleep Image Ring CPC device. CPC, cardiopulmonary coupling.

SUMMARY

Similarly to all other diagnostic tools, HST requires expertise in selecting patients to be studied, proper interpretation of results, and decision-making concerning the need for treatment or other diagnostic studies. Many patients with sleep disorders and comorbidities will continue to benefit from PSG for the diagnosis, but, as has been demonstrated in recent years, HST allows for increased access and patient comfort in the diagnosis of SDB. HST may also help identify patients with sleep disorders who would otherwise have gone undiagnosed and untreated. As technology continues to evolve, it can be expected that HST will be indicated for the evaluation of sleep disorders other than SDB in some capacity.

REFERENCES

1. Polysomnography Task Force, American Sleep Disorders Association Standards of Practice Committee. Practice parameters for the indications for polysomnography and related procedures. *Sleep*. 1997;20:406-422.
2. Chesson AL Jr, Ferber RA, Fry JM, et al. The indications for polysomnography and related procedures. *Sleep*. 1997;20:423-487.
3. Kushida CA, Littner MR, Morgenthaler T, et al. Practice parameters for the indications for polysomnography and related procedures: an update for 2005. *Sleep*. 2005;28:499-521.
4. Kapur VK, Auckley DH, Chowdhuri S, et al. Clinical practice guideline for diagnostic testing for adult obstructive sleep apnea: an American Academy of Sleep Medicine clinical practice guideline. *J Clin Sleep Med*. 2017;13(3):479-504.
5. Flemons WW, Douglas NJ, Kuna ST, et al. Access to diagnosis and treatment of patients with suspected sleep apnea. *Am J Respir Crit Care Med*. 2004;169:668-672.
6. Department of Health and Human Services. Decision memo for continuous positive airway pressure (CPAP) therapy for obstructive sleep apnea (OSA) (CAG#0093R2). Centers for Medicare & Medicaid Services. 2008.
7. CMS Manual System. Pub 100-03 Medicare national coverage determinations. Transmittal 86. Centers for Medicare and Medicaid Services. 2008. Accessed November 8, 2025. https://www.cms.gov/transmittals/downloads/R86NCD.pdf
8. Centers for Medicare and Medicaid Services. Decision memo for sleep testing for obstructive sleep apnea (CAG-00405N). 2009. Accessed November 8, 2025.
9. Chiao W, Durr ML. Trends in sleep studies performed for Medicare beneficiaries. *Laryngoscope*. 2017;127:2891-2896.
10. Collop NA. Portable monitoring. *Sleep Med Clin*. 2009;4:435-442.
11. Chediak AD. Why CMS approved home sleep testing for CPAP coverage. *J Clin Sleep Med*. 2008;4:16-18.
12. Ross SD, Sheinhait IA, Harrison KJ, et al. Systematic review and meta-analysis of the literature regarding the diagnosis of sleep apnea. *Sleep*. 2000;23:519-532.
13. Collop NA. Portable monitoring for the diagnosis of obstructive sleep apnea. *Curr Opin Pulm Med*. 2008;14:525-529.
14. Dingli K, Coleman EL, Vennelle M, et al. Evaluation of a portable device for diagnosing the sleep apnoea/hypopnoea syndrome. *Eur Respir J*. 2003;21:253-259.
15. Calleja JM, Esnaola S, Rubio R, et al. Comparison of a cardiorespiratory device versus polysomnography for diagnosis of sleep apnoea. *Eur Respir J*. 2002;20:1505-1510.
16. ATS/ACCP/AASM Portable Monitoring Taskforce Steering Committee. Executive summary on the systematic review and practice parameters for portable monitoring in the investigation of suspected sleep apnea in adults. *Am J Respir Crit Care Med*. 2004;169:1160-1163.
17. Agency for Healthcare Research and Quality. Effectiveness of portable monitoring devices for diagnosing obstructive sleep apnea: update of a systematic review. 2004. Accessed November 8, 2025. https://www.cms.gov/Medicare/Coverage/DeterminationProcess/downloads/id24TA.pdf
18. Agency for Healthcare Research and Quality. Technology assessment: home diagnosis of obstructive sleep apnea-hypopnea syndrome. 2007. Accessed November 8, 2025. https://www.cms.gov/Medicare/Coverage/DeterminationProcess/downloads/id48TA.pdf
19. Agency for Healthcare Research and Quality. Obstructive sleep apnea-hypopnea syndrome: modeling different diagnostic strategies. 2007. Accessed November 8, 2025. http://www.cms.gov/determinationprocess/downloads/id50TA.pdf
20. Chesson AL Jr, Berry RB, Pack A. Practice parameters for the use of portable monitoring devices in the investigation of suspected obstructive sleep apnea in adults. *Sleep*. 2003;26:907-913.
21. Whitelaw WA, Brant RF, Flemons WW. Clinical usefulness of home oximetry compared with polysomnography for assessment of sleep apnea. *Am J Respir Crit Care Med*. 2005;171:188-193.
22. Collop NA, Anderson WM, Boehlecke B, et al; for the Portable Monitoring Task Force of the American Academy of Sleep Medicine. Clinical guidelines for the use of unattended portable monitors in the diagnosis of obstructive sleep apnea in adult patients. *J Clin Sleep Med*. 2007;3(7):737-747.
23. Mulgrew AT, Fox N, Ayas NT, et al. Diagnosis and initial management of obstructive sleep apnea without polysomnography: a randomized validation study. *Ann Intern Med*. 2007;146:157-166.
24. Berry RB, Hill G, Thompson L, et al. Portable monitoring and autotitration versus polysomnography for the diagnosis and treatment of sleep apnea. *Sleep*. 2008;31:1423-1431.
25. Ferber R, Millman R, Coppola M, et al. Portable recording in the assessment of obstructive sleep apnea. ASDA standards of practice. *Sleep*. 1994;17(4):378-392.
26. American Academy of Sleep Medicine. Standards for accreditation of out of center sleep testing (OCST) in adult patients. 2011. Accessed November 8, 2025. https://www.aasm.org/resources/pdf/ocststandards.pdf
27. Levendowski D, Steward D, Woodson BT, et al. The impact of obstructive sleep apnea variability

measured in-lab versus in-home on sample size calculations. *Int Arch Med*. 2009;2:2.

28. Smith LA, Chong DW, Vennelle M, et al. Diagnosis of sleep-disordered breathing in patients with chronic heart failure: evaluation of a portable limited sleep study system. *J Sleep Res*. 2007;16:428-435.
29. Standards of Practice Committee ASDA. Practice parameters for the use of portable recording in the assessment of obstructive sleep apnea. *Sleep*. 1994;17:372-377.
30. Antic NA, Buchan C, Esterman A, et al. A randomized controlled trial of nurse-led care for symptomatic moderate-severe obstructive sleep apnea. *Am J Respir Crit Care Med*. 2009;179:501-508.
31. Skomro RP, Gjevre J, Reid J, et al. Outcomes of home-based diagnosis and treatment of obstructive sleep apnea. *Chest*. 2010;138:257-263.
32. Kuna ST, Gurubhagavatula I, Maislin G, et al. Noninferiority of functional outcome in ambulatory management of obstructive sleep apnea. *Am J Respir Crit Care Med*. 2011;183(9):1238-1244.
33. Rosen CL, Auckley D, Benca R, et al. A multisite randomized trial of portable sleep studies and positive airway pressure autotitration versus laboratory-based polysomnography for the diagnosis and treatment of obstructive sleep apnea: the HomePAP study. *Sleep*. 2012;35(6):757-767.
34. Berry RB, Sriram P. Auto-adjusting positive airway pressure treatment for sleep apnea diagnosed by home sleep testing. *J Clin Sleep Med*. 2014;10(12): 1269-1275.
35. Golpe R, Jimenez A, Carpizo R. Home sleep studies in the assessment of sleep apnea/hypopnea syndrome. *Chest*. 2002;122:1156-1161.
36. Berry RB, Albertario CM, Harding SM, et al; for the American Academy of Sleep Medicine. The AASM manual for the scoring of sleep and associated events: rules, terminology and technical specifications [Version 3]. American Academy of Sleep Medicine. 2023.
37. Grote LB, Hedner J, Ding Z. Alteration of digital pulse amplitude reflects alpha-adrenoceptor mediated constriction of the digital vascular bed. *Sleep*. 2001;24(suppl):A79.
38. Henriksen O, Sejrsen P. Local reflex in microcirculation in human cutaneous tissue. *Acta Physiol Scand*. 1976;98:227-231.

Chapter 41
Actigraphy

SU JEONG LINSTROM

KEY CONCEPTS/LEARNING OBJECTIVES

The key concepts for this chapter include a review of the use, function, and purpose of actigraphy in sleep medicine, actigraphy's strengths and weaknesses, as well as threats to validity, and how actigraphy data are applied in a clinical setting.

KEY TERMS

Actigraphy
Accelerometer
Validity

An actigraph is a small device typically worn on the nondominant wrist. These devices are used to estimate sleep and wake patterns for multiple nights in a wide range of patients. For multiple reasons, the use of actigraphy has become very popular over the past 20 years (1). First, actigraphy can collect information for extended periods in the patient's natural environment. Second, it is relatively noninvasive as most devices are the size of a wristwatch. Third, the cost of performing an actigraphy study is significantly less than that of polysomnography (PSG). Although there are a host of devices available on the market, the decision about which one to use should be made based on the validity of the device, the cost of the equipment, and the populations to be studied. These issues vary by individual clinicians, researchers, and/or sleep centers, and thus, this chapter will not focus on which actigraph to use but rather provide an overview of actigraphy, when to use it, how it works, its validity compared with PSG, and its utility in clinical and research settings. There are also a host of consumer wearable devices that are marketed directly to consumers for detection of sleep and wake. However, for the purpose of this chapter, the focus will solely be on clinical grade actigraphy devices.

WHAT IS ACTIGRAPHY?

Most actigraphs are wristwatch-sized devices that use a piezoelectric accelerometer to measure activity levels of the person wearing the device. The use of motion as a measure is common in medical devices. For example, pacemakers have a mechanism that adjusts the rate in response to the patient's activity level, whereas pedometers use motion as a way to monitor the number of steps a person takes. The use of activity monitoring to estimate sleep-wake patterns has been around for many years (2). Early devices were self-contained activity counters with integrated circuits and memory that provided offline data retrieval (3). Over the years, actigraphs have become more compact and lightweight, with greater memory for data storage and a longer battery life (3). In addition to the newer models of actigraphs being noninvasive and compact, many include a watch capability on the device, so it is also functional to the user. These devices do not interfere with everyday activities, as most brands are water resistant or even waterproof.

WHEN TO USE ACTIGRAPHY

In 2018, the American Academy of Sleep Medicine (AASM) published updated guidelines for the use of actigraphy in the assessment of sleep and sleep disorders (4). Actigraphy should be used for a minimum of 72 hours to 14 consecutive days. It is recommended that actigraphy is conducted for 7 to 14 days before a multiple sleep latency test to ensure sufficient sleep duration. Actigraphy is recommended to be conducted for 2 to 3 weeks or more for insufficient sleep syndrome (4).

Actigraphy provides many benefits over PSG. During an overnight PSG, patients often have to travel to a center that may be a distance from their home. In addition, they sleep in an unfamiliar setting, removed from the comfort of their own bed, and required to wear numerous sensors placed on the head and body. The sensations from the sensors may be overstimulating and difficult to tolerate for some patients (eg, children with autism spectrum disorders or older adults). Furthermore, PSG most often only records one night of sleep, which may not be representative of the person's typical sleep due to the "first-night effect (5)." Actigraphy, on the other hand, can be worn in the patient's natural home/sleep environment and for an extended period.

However, actigraphy is not a substitute for PSG. PSG uses multiple channels to measure the different physiologic stages of sleep as well as the respiratory state of the patient during the night. Also, an in-lab PSG is performed with the sleep technologist monitoring the patient to ensure the signal quality is optimal, and any needed troubleshooting and interventions are performed during the PSG. These measurements are essential in accurately diagnosing sleep-related breathing disorders, movement-related sleep disorders, and narcolepsy. Actigraphy may be able to measure the disruptions in sleep caused by sleep-related breathing disorders or movement-related sleep disorders; however, it cannot accurately identify the causes of these awakenings. Information from actigraphy can be a useful tool in clinical and research settings, but it should not be used as a simple substitute for PSG.

There are Home Sleep Apnea Test (HSAT) devices with actigraphy integrated into them. In a comparison between HSAT that utilized actigraphy integration for sleep/wake detection, it was reported that actigraphy-integrated devices showed more accurate measurement of total sleep time (TST), thus generating a more accurate apnea-hypopnea index (AHI) for the detection of obstructive sleep apnea (4).

HOW DOES ACTIGRAPHY WORK?

Activity counts are measured per epoch in actigraphy. While some devices have a fixed epoch length of 1 minute, other devices allow the user to set the epoch length to 15 seconds, 30 seconds, 1 minute, or 2 minutes. Each device has a different way to digitize the signal. For some devices, the user can choose the data mode; for other devices, the data mode is automatically selected. When the user can select the data mode, three choices become available: time above threshold (TAT), zero crossing mode (ZCM), and proportional integration mode (PIM). TAT measures the amount of time per epoch the activity waveform is above the set threshold; ZCM measures the number of times per epoch the waveform crosses a threshold set close to zero; PIM, also known as digital integration, measures the area under the curve for each epoch (see ref 3 for more information). Newer devices allow for multiple modes to be used simultaneously. Different studies have provided support for different measurement modes (1). Owing to the variance in results, it is questionable whether there is one best method of measuring the digitalized signal from the actigraphy. Further study should be conducted on a wider range of user populations to see if one mode or a combination of modes yields the most accurate results.

When the actigraphs are returned by the patient, the devices are downloaded to a computer using a device-specific interface. Each brand of actigraph has proprietary software that uses device-specific scoring algorithms (eg, Sadeh and Cole-Kripke) or wake sensitivity (eg, medium, high, and low) thresholds to determine whether each epoch should be scored as sleep or wake. The selection of which algorithm to use should be based on the sample being studied (3,20). Once the data have been scored, the program will generate an actigram (a picture of the patient's sleep during the study; see Figures 41-1 and 41-2 for examples) as well as summary variables such as TST, actigraphic sleep onset

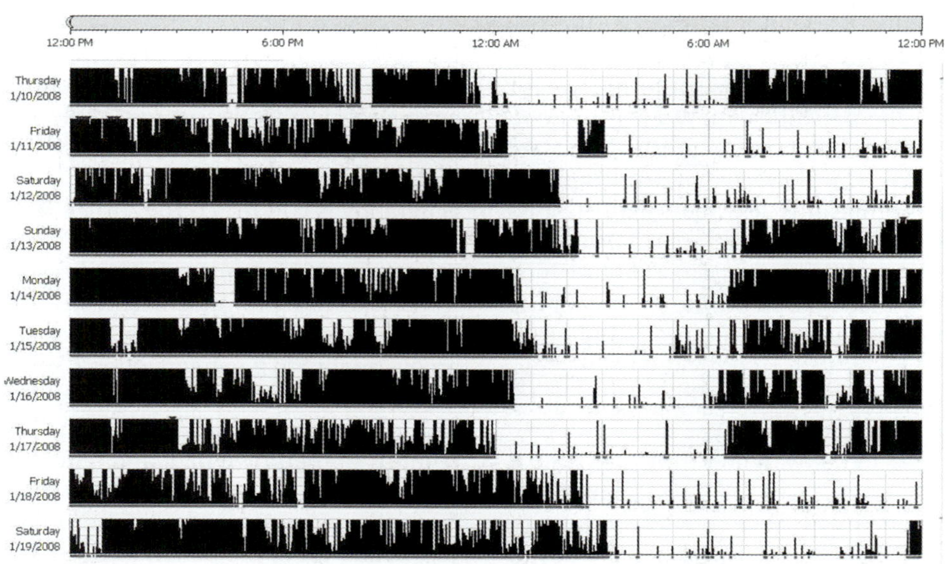

A

Figure 41-1 **A:** Actigram of a 17-year-old male who reported excessive daytime sleepiness. This patient typically fell asleep between 12 and 1 AM, waking between 6 and 7 AM, except on weekends, when he would sleep from 3 AM up to 12 PM.

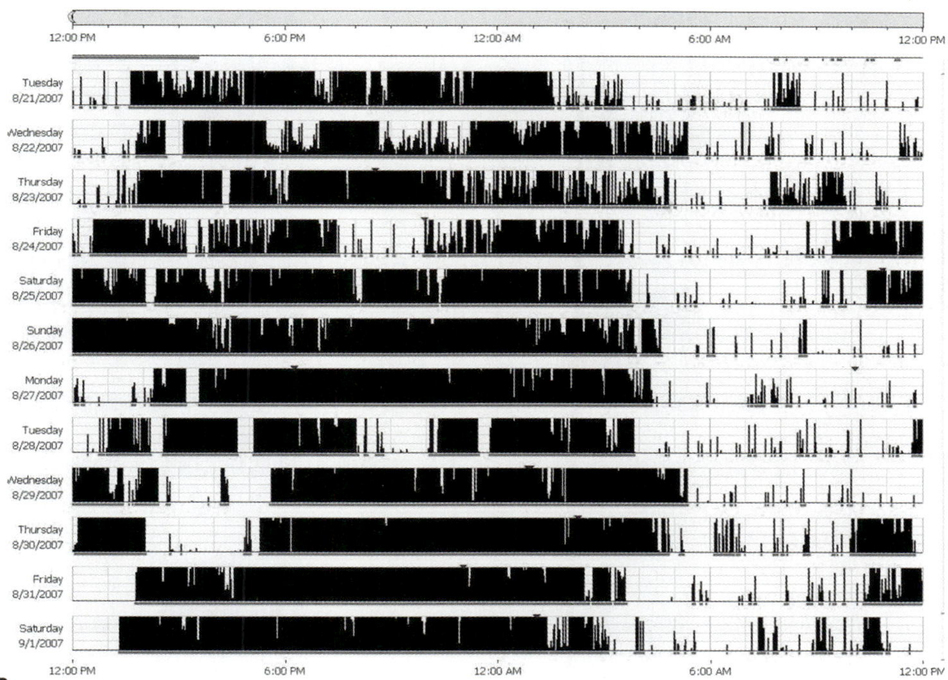

B

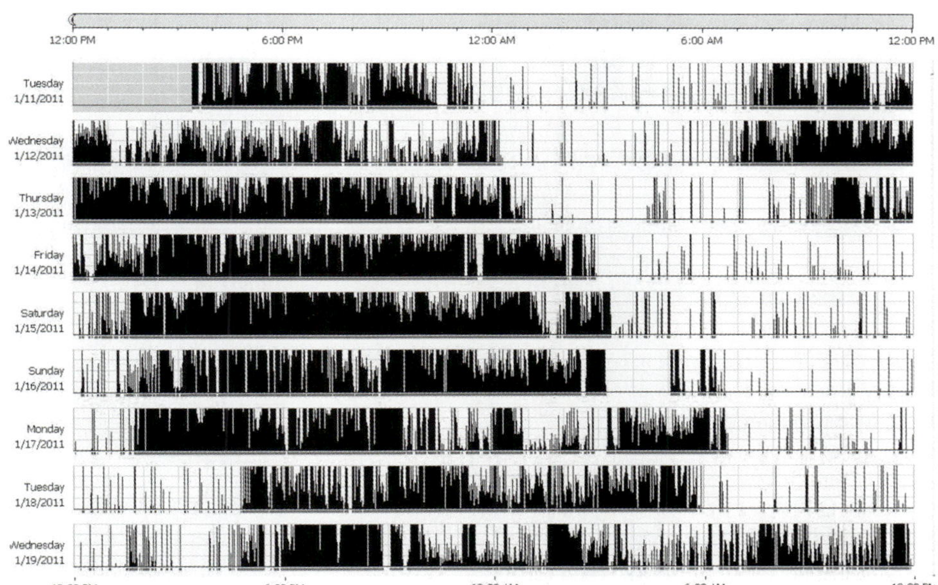

C

Figure 41-1 (*continued*) **B:** Actigram of a 14-year-old male who reported excessive daytime sleepiness and the inability to fall asleep before 3 AM. This patient typically fell asleep around 3 AM and woke up around 1 PM. C: Actigram of a 22-year-old female who reported excessive daytime sleepiness and an irregular sleep pattern. Actigraphy showed a circadian rhythm sleep disorder, free-running type with her sleep onset time starting at midnight, and then progressively getting later each night over the course of the study.

time, wake after sleep onset, and actigraphic sleep offset time. Variables such as bedtime, wake time, and sleep onset latency should be reported only if the patient also keeps a concurrent daily sleep diary (discussed further on) or uses the event marker feature included with some devices (1). Along these lines, sleep efficiency (SE) should be calculated only if a diary is included (providing bedtime and wake time; SE = minutes of sleep from actigraphic sleep onset to actigraphic sleep offset/minutes from bedtime to wake time × 100).

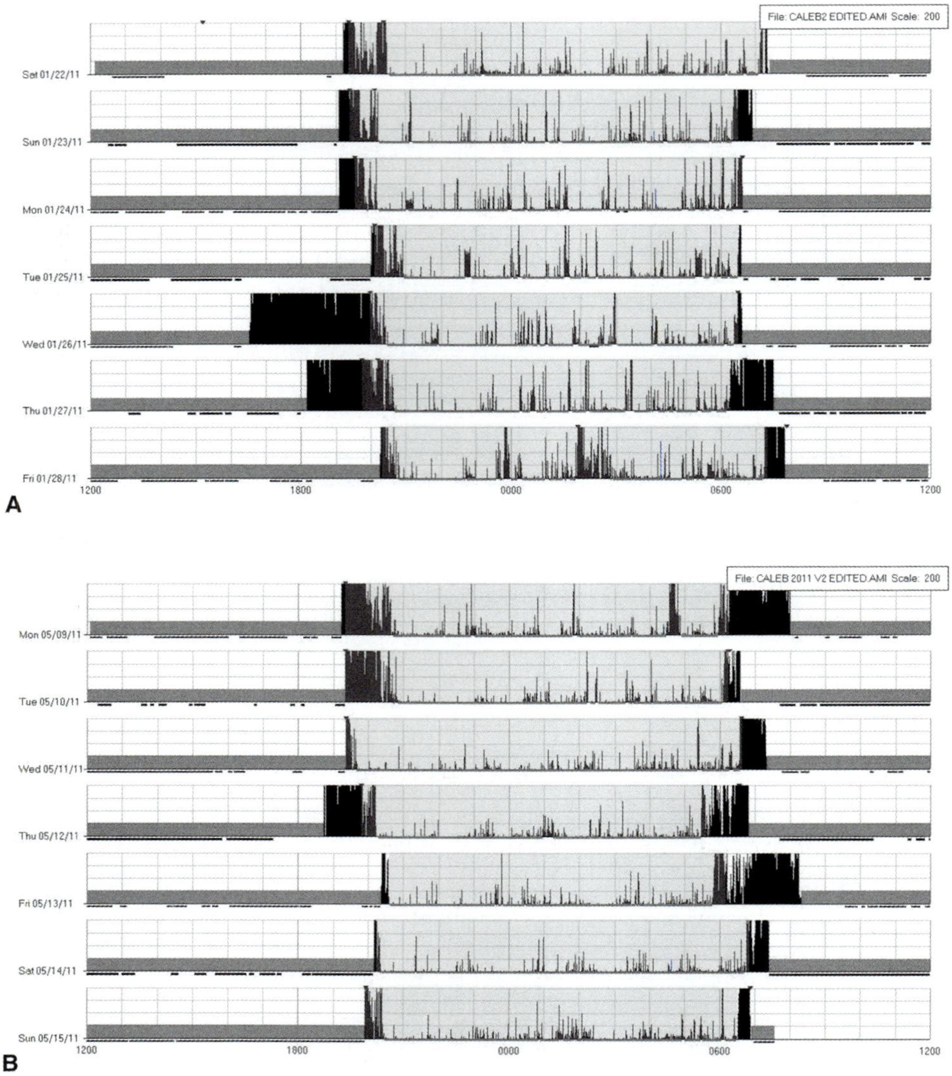

Figure 41-2 **A:** Actigram of a 7-year-old boy with high levels of activity during sleep. **B:** Actigram of the same 7-year-old boy following 3 months of iron supplementation showing reduced activity during sleep.

VALIDITY OF ACTIGRAPHY

Although actigraphy has several benefits over PSG (ie, relatively low cost, nonintrusive device that can be used for extended periods to estimate sleep-wake patterns), there are several concerns about validity that should be considered. The two primary areas of concern are (1) specificity to detect wake and (2) artifact.

Actigraphy in Comparison With Polysomnography

Several studies have compared the validity of sleep/wake data from actigraphy with a PSG or a videosomnography (6-9). When compared epoch by epoch, the sensitivity, or the ability of actigraphy to detect sleep when PSG scores sleep, is very good (typically >85%). However, the specificity, or the ability of actigraphy to detect wake when PSG scores wake, has been very low (typically below 70% but reported as low as 24%-44%). During a PSG, an accurate measurement of sleep and wake can be detected through multiple channels of electroencephalogram (EEG). Wrist actigraphy, on the other hand, relies on a single channel of information (movement), which results in this larger margin of error. Most commonly, this error results in an overestimation of TST and an underestimation of wake after sleep onset. Also, since the data retrieval does not occur until the actigraphy study has been completed, it is difficult to assess the quality of the recorded signals and data while the actigraphy study is being conducted.

Artifact

Artifact is the other primary threat to validity. Because actigraphy relies on the use of activity to estimate sleep-wake patterns, there are several instances when sleep and wake may be scored inappropriately. For example, actigraphy may identify a person lying in bed watching television as sleeping if there is a low level of activity. On the other hand, if the user were asleep as a passenger in a moving vehicle, the movement of the car would be detected as sufficient activity to estimate that the person is awake. Environmental causes of awakenings, such as a restless or snoring bed partner, or a pet jumping on the bed, can also alter the results. Finally, atypical days (due to illness, holidays, vacations, etc) can also result in artifacts since the study day would not be representative of that patient's typical sleep-wake patterns.

A daily sleep diary is needed in order to reduce artifact. Using such a diary (example in Figure 41-3) allows patients to record times when they removed the device, times with low activity when the person was awake, and times with high activity when the person was asleep. In addition, diaries can include questions about bed partners (or pets) that may have resulted in increased activity during sleep, medications used for sleep, subjective sleep quality, as well as whether it was a typical day/night of sleep. Daily sleep diaries are also necessary for clinicians/researchers to identify bedtime (time attempted to fall asleep) and wake time (time patient awakened for the day), allowing for the calculation of sleep onset latency. As mentioned, some devices have an event marker feature that allows patients to push a button at bedtime/wake time. However, one study found that 27% of actigraphy data were not valid due to participants' nonadherence to using the event marker (10). A combination of event markers and daily sleep diaries is recommended.

Special Populations

An important consideration for the validity of actigraphy is the population being studied. With the AASM guidelines for the use of actigraphy with special populations (4), studies have examined the validity of actigraphy on different clinical populations, including infants, toddlers, or preschoolers (11), children and adolescents with or without sleep-disordered breathing (1), and older adults (12). Although there have been mixed findings in the literature about the use of actigraphy in patients with insomnia, several articles suggest the benefit of actigraphy in this population (1,13).

Other devices are being developed with applications beyond sleep-wake estimates, including the detection of periodic limb movements in sleep (PLMs). Studies found that actigraphic devices specially designed for PLMs were useful in detecting PLMs in adults (14,15). However, updated recommendation from the AASM shows that there is a potential for the overestimation of PLM with actigraphy alone, and for proper measurement and detection of PLMs, an EMG during PSG is the gold standard (4).

Length of Actigraphy Study

The duration of an actigraphy study should be carefully considered. For most people, sleep patterns differ from weekday to weekends; thus, a minimum of 7 to 10 days of actigraphy would be needed to capture these differences. Another consideration is the amount of data lost to artifact. As previously mentioned, some days/nights from an actigraphy study may not be valid if the participant does not wear the device or complete the sleep diary, the device has a technical failure, or the night is atypical. One study reported that due to the loss of data from artifact, a minimum of seven nights of data collection are needed to gain information for five nights of sleep (16). The final consideration is billing, with a minimum of three nights required (see next section) in order to bill for an actigraphy study.

CLINICAL APPLICATION

In 2009, actigraphy became a category 1 current procedural terminology (CPT) code. The description for this service is "testing, recording, analysis, interpretation, and report (minimum of 72 hours to 14 consecutive days of recording, requires the patient to wear a home monitor for 24 hours a day for 3-14 days)." Although Medicare may reimburse for this service, most other insurances do not provide reimbursement, stating that actigraphy is investigational, experimental, or not medically necessary (3).

Despite the lack of insurance coverage, the information about sleep-wake patterns gathered from actigraphy can be an essential tool in clinical settings. As previously stated, wrist actigraphy is minimally invasive and does not interfere with normal routines and is recommended for use in the diagnosis of difference sleep disorders (4). Beyond diagnostic utility, the following provides a description of the most common clinical uses of actigraphy in the sleep center: (1) to identify potential causes of daytime sleepiness (eg, frequent night wakings and prolonged sleep onset latency), and (2) to monitor the patient's adherence to treatment recommendations (eg, maintaining a consistent sleep schedule).

Excessive daytime sleepiness (EDS) is a common complaint in sleep clinics. Once physiologic sleep disorders (eg, obstructive sleep apnea and PLMs in sleep) are ruled out by a clinical interview or overnight PSG, other potential causes for EDS need to be evaluated, including circadian rhythm sleep disorders, poor sleep hygiene,

Fill this form out JUST BEFORE going to bed

Today is __________ Today's Date ____/____/____

What time is it now? ____________ a.m./p.m. Did you go to work/school today? ____ Yes ____ No

Were you sick today? ____ Yes ____ No If yes, with what? ____________________

Write times the following occurred (and circle a.m. or p.m.)	START	END
Removed the actigraph	a.m. p.m.	a.m. p.m.
Nap (or accidentally fell asleep)	a.m. p.m.	a.m. p.m.
Very quiet activity (e.g., going to the movies)	a.m. p.m.	a.m. p.m.

Fill this form out FIRST THING in the morning

Today is __________ Today's Date ____/____/____

	Circle a.m. or p.m.
Last night—got into bed at:	a.m. p.m.
Last night—tried to fall asleep at:	a.m. p.m.
Last night it took________minutes to fall asleep	Min
After falling asleep—woke up____times during the night (circle one choice)	0 1 2 3 4 5 or more
Woke up this morning at:	a.m. p.m.
Finally got out of the bed this morning at:	a.m. p.m.

Figure 41-3 Example of a daily sleep diary to be used with actigraphy studies.

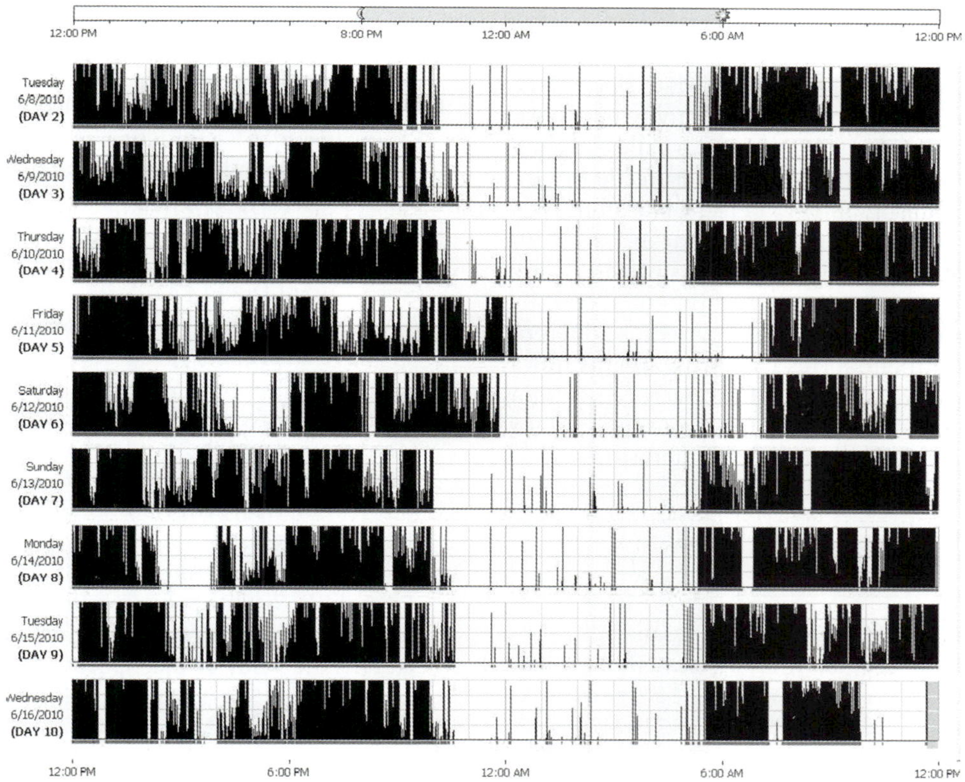

Figure 41-4 Actigram of 57-year-old female with circadian rhythm sleep disorder, delayed sleep phase type after chronotherapy treatment. Patient was able to maintain consistent sleep schedule from 10/11 PM to 6/7 AM.

or insufficient sleep. By monitoring sleep-wake patterns for 1 or 2 weeks, the clinician can examine whether a patient has a consistent sleep schedule and is getting enough sleep. For example, Figure 41-1 includes three actigrams of patients complaining of EDS. Figure 41-1A is a 17-year-old boy who reported EDS but denied symptoms of sleep-disordered breathing or movement during sleep. His actigraphy study revealed that he was obtaining six or less hours of sleep on school nights, with significant oversleep on the weekends. This was suggestive of insufficient sleep and poor sleep hygiene rather than an underlying physiologic sleep disorder. Figure 41-1B is a 14-year-old boy reporting EDS and the inability to fall asleep before 3 AM, regardless of bedtime. His actigraphy study revealed circadian rhythm sleep disorder, delayed sleep phase type, with a sleep schedule of approximately 3 AM to 1 PM Figure 41-1C is a 22-year-old female who reported EDS due to an erratic sleep schedule. Her actigraphy study revealed circadian rhythm sleep disorder, free-running type. Actigraphy can also help determine the need for an overnight PSG when sleep center availability is limited or the patient may not tolerate a PSG. For example, as seen in Figure 41-2A, a 7-year-old boy with autism complained of EDS but denied symptoms of sleep-disordered breathing. His mother reported that he was "twitchy" during sleep, but this child would not tolerate a PSG. The high level of activity during sleep resulted in the recommendation for a serum ferritin level to be drawn, which was found to be low (20 ng/mL).

Actigraphy can also help monitor treatments and clinical recommendations. For example, actigraphy can help determine whether a treatment (eg, iron therapy) is effective. As seen in Figure 41-2B, following 3 months of supplemental iron therapy, along with a clinical report of improvements in daytime functioning, there was a significant reduction in activity during sleep for the same 7-year-old boy with autism. For a patient with circadian rhythm sleep disorder, delayed sleep phase type, actigraphy can help monitor whether the patient is adherent to adjusting their sleep-wake schedule as recommended (eg, moving schedule forward by 3 hours each day). For example, Figure 41-4 is a 57-year-old female following chronotherapy to regulate her sleep-wake schedule. Her actigraphy study showed a consistent sleep schedule, with a bedtime of 10 PM on weekdays and 11 PM on weekends, and a wake time of 6 AM on weekdays and 7 AM on weekends. Figures 41-2B and 41-4 are excellent examples of "normal" actigraphy studies. In addition, if the actigraph has a light sensor, the clinician is able to monitor whether the patient is obtaining a sufficient amount of light in the morning and restricting light late in the day.

CONCLUSION

Actigraphy is a noninvasive way to estimate sleep-wake patterns through the measurement of activity levels. Although actigraphy has been reported as a valid estimate of sleep-wake patterns, additional work is needed to increase the ability of actigraphy to detect wake after sleep onset (17). In a clinical setting, actigraphy can assist with the diagnosis of sleep disorders, as well as provide a significant amount of information about potential reasons for daytime sleepiness and whether a patient is adherent to treatment recommendations (4). Actigraphy is not a substitute for PSG, but when used properly (eg, with a daily sleep diary and event marker), it is a useful tool for evaluating the sleep-wake patterns of patients.

REFERENCES

1. Meltzer LJ, Montgomery-Downs HE, Insana SP, Walsh CM. Use of actigraphy for assessment in pediatric sleep research. *Sleep Med Rev*. 2012;16(5):463-475. doi:10.1016/j.smrv.2011.10.002. PMID: 22424706; PMCID: PMC3445439.
2. Tryon WW. *Activity Measurement in Psychology and Medicine*. Plenum; 1991.
3. Ancoli-Israel S, Martin JL, Blackwell T, et al. The SBSM guide to actigraphy monitoring: clinical and research applications. *Behav Sleep Med*. 2015;13(suppl 1): S4-S38. doi:10.1080/15402002.2015.10463564
4. Smith MT, McCrae CS, Cheung J, et al. Use of actigraphy for the evaluation of sleep disorders and circadian rhythm sleep-wake disorders: an American Academy of Sleep Medicine clinical practice guideline. *J Clin Sleep Med*. 2018;14(7):1231-1237.
5. Toussaint M, Luthringer R, Schaltenbrand N, et al. First-night effect in normal subjects and psychiatric inpatients. *Sleep*. 1995;18(6):463-469.
6. Benson K, Friedman L, Noda A, Wicks D, Wakabayashi E, Yesavage J. The measurement of sleep by actigraphy: direct comparison of 2 commercially available actigraphs in a nonclinical population. *Sleep*. 2004;27(5):986-989.
7. Pollak CP, Stokes PE, Wagner DR. Direct comparison of two widely used activity recorders. *Sleep*. 1998; 21(2):207-212.
8. Tonetti L, Pasquini F, Fabbri M, Belluzzi M, Natale V. Comparison of two different actigraphs with polysomnography in healthy young subjects. *Chronobiol Int*. 2008;25(1):145-153.
9. Weiss AR, Johnson NL, Berger NA, Redline S. Validity of activity-based devices to estimate sleep. *J Clin Sleep Med*. 2010;6(4):336-342.
10. Ustinov Y, Lichstein KL. Actigraphy reliability. *Sleep*. 2011;34:A330.
11. Bélanger MÈ, Simard V, Bernier A, Carrier J. Investigating the convergence between actigraphy, maternal sleep diaries, and the child behavior checklist as measures of sleep in toddlers. *Front Psychiatry*. 2014;5:158. doi:10.3389/fpsyt.2014.00158. PMID: 25426082; PMCID: PMC4226151.
12. Mehra R, Stone KL, Ancoli-Israel S, Litwack-Harrison S, Ensrud KE, Redline S. Interpreting wrist actigraphic indices of sleep in epidemiologic studies of the elderly: the Study of Osteoporotic Fractures. *Sleep*. 2008;31(11):1569-1576.
13. Natale V, Léger D, Martoni M, Bayon V, Erbacci A. The role of actigraphy in the assessment of primary insomnia: a retrospective study. *Sleep Med*. 2014;15(1): 111-115. doi:10.1016/j.sleep.2013.08.792. PMID: 24325809.
14. Sforza E, Johannes M, Claudio B. The PAM-RL ambulatory device for detection of periodic leg movements: a validation study. *Sleep Med*. 2005;6(5):407-413.
15. King MA, Jaffre MO, Morrish E, Shneerson JM, Smith IE. The validation of a new actigraphy system for the measurement of periodic leg movements in sleep. *Sleep Med*. 2005;6(6):507-513.
16. Acebo C, Sadeh A, Seifer R, et al. Estimating sleep patterns with activity monitoring in children and adolescents: how many nights are necessary for reliable measures? *Sleep*. 1999;22(1):95-103.
17. Meltzer LJ, Montgomery-Downs HE, Insana SP, Walsh CM. Use of actigraphy for assessment in pediatric sleep research. *Sleep Med Rev*. 2012;16(5):463-475. doi:10.1016/j.smrv.2011.10.002. PMID: 22424706; PMCID: PMC3445439.

Chapter 42
Artificial Intelligence in Sleep

CARLOS TEIXEIRA

KEY CONCEPTS/LEARNING OBJECTIVES

The key concepts for this chapter include understanding artificial intelligence (AI) fundamentals in the context of sleep medicine, recognizing key benefits of AI (eg, improved scoring accuracy, efficiency, personalized care), identifying limitations and risks (eg, bias, privacy, clinician overreliance), and applying critical thinking when integrating AI tools into sleep labs.

KEY TERMS

Artificial intelligence (AI)
Confusion matrix
Deep learning
Machine learning (ML)

OVERVIEW

Artificial intelligence (AI) is rapidly transforming the field of sleep medicine, offering new opportunities to enhance diagnostic accuracy, improve efficiency, and personalize patient care. At its core, AI refers to computer systems capable of performing tasks that typically require human intelligence, such as recognizing patterns, classifying data, and making predictions. In the sleep lab, this translates into powerful tools that can potentially assist technologists and clinicians across various aspects of sleep diagnostics and therapy.

One of the most significant applications of AI in sleep medicine is the automated analysis of polysomnography (PSG) data. Machine learning (ML) algorithms, particularly deep learning (DL) models, have demonstrated performance levels comparable to those associated with expert human scorers in tasks such as sleep staging, respiratory event detection, and limb movement classification. This can significantly reduce the time required for manual scoring while improving interscorer reliability, a persistent challenge in traditional workflows. Additionally, AI systems can flag uncertain or borderline segments, guiding technologists toward more targeted review and correction, thus optimizing workflow efficiency.

The American Academy of Sleep Medicine (AASM) has taken a proactive stance on the role of AI in the field. In its official position statement published in 2020, the AASM emphasizes that AI should be viewed as a supportive tool rather than a replacement for human expertise (1). It recommends that AI outputs should always be reviewed and validated by trained professionals and highlights the importance of transparency, reproducibility, and fairness in AI system development. The AASM has also established a dedicated committee on AI in sleep medicine, which aims to guide ethical integration, promote education, and foster innovation in this space.

Despite its promise, integrating AI into clinical sleep medicine is not without limitations. One major concern is algorithmic bias: if AI systems are trained on datasets that lack diversity, their performance may not generalize well across different populations or clinical settings. This could lead to misclassification or underdiagnosis in certain groups. Furthermore, many AI models function as "black boxes," offering little insight into how decisions are made—a challenge for clinicians seeking explainable and trustworthy outputs. Privacy and data security are also critical, as the use of large datasets—including sensitive biometric and behavioral data—demands strict adherence to ethical and regulatory standards. Finally, there is a risk of overreliance on AI, where clinicians may place undue trust in algorithmic results without sufficient oversight.

INTRODUCTION

What Is Artificial Intelligence?

AI refers to the ability of machines to emulate human cognitive functions such as learning, reasoning, and decision-making (2). Since its conceptual origin in 1955, AI has moved beyond theoretical exploration and now plays a tangible role in various fields of health care. Its growth has been propelled by a combination of factors: the rapid accumulation of health care data, advances in computational power, and increasingly sophisticated algorithms capable of analyzing complex datasets (3).

In health care, AI is already transforming how diseases are diagnosed, monitored, and treated. AI applications range from cancer detection and diabetic retinopathy screening to personalized treatment recommendations and hospital workflow optimization, and AI-based tools are being applied successfully to tasks like disease screening, triage, risk stratification, and therapy selection across multiple medical conditions (4).

AI operates through various branches, the most relevant to medicine being ML and DL. ML refers to the creation of algorithms that learn from data patterns and make predictions with minimal human intervention. DL, a specialized form of ML, uses neural networks to extract insights from unstructured data, making it especially effective at analyzing the vast and complex datasets produced in clinical environments (2,5). Sleep medicine stands at a particularly promising intersection with AI. PSG, the gold-standard diagnostic tool for sleep disorders, generates large volumes of multichannel physiologic data overnight, which makes it an ideal candidate for AI-based analysis. In addition, the growing prevalence of consumer wearables has led to a surge in long-term sleep data from real-world settings (3,6).

As a result, AI is now being explored to automate labor-intensive tasks like sleep staging and event scoring. But the potential of AI in sleep medicine extends far beyond automation. AI algorithms are being developed to diagnose sleep apnea with portable devices (7), identify individual endotypes of sleep disorders (8), predict treatment adherence (9), and even forecast long-term health outcomes based on sleep patterns (10).

The relevance of AI in sleep medicine also aligns with broader challenges in clinical care. Traditional metrics like the apnea-hypopnea index (AHI) are increasingly recognized as insufficient to capture the heterogeneity of sleep-disordered breathing (11). AI can help identify subtle patterns and clusters within physiologic data, potentially leading to more individualized, data-driven approaches to diagnosis and therapy, a cornerstone of precision medicine.

Despite its promise, AI integration into clinical workflows is not without obstacles. These include ethical concerns, the need for transparency in algorithm decision-making, regulatory requirements, and clinician trust (12). Therefore, understanding how AI works and how to critically assess its performance is essential for sleep technologists and clinicians who wish to harness its benefits responsibly.

DIFFERENT MODELS

AI in sleep medicine mainly includes two key areas: ML and DL (12). In traditional ML approaches, domain experts, such as sleep clinicians, identify relevant physiologic characteristics (known as features) based on clinical knowledge. This manual process of selecting and quantifying informative inputs is referred to as feature engineering or feature extraction. These curated features are then used to train models for specific tasks, such as automated sleep staging.

In contrast, DL eliminates the need for hand-crafted features. DL models are capable of learning directly from raw data by autonomously identifying patterns through multilayered neural network architectures. With the advent of large-scale datasets, enhanced computational power, and improved learning algorithms, DL models now consist of thousands to millions of parameters, enabling them to handle highly complex tasks (13). This automated process of learning internal data representations is known as representation learning. A key advantage of such learned representations is their robustness to irrelevant variations—such as noise artifacts or filter distortions—that do not affect the underlying physiologic meaning (14).

Both ML and DL have their respective strengths and limitations. ML benefits from transparency; since features are manually selected, they often carry clear biomedical meaning. However, this reliance on human-defined features may limit the discovery of novel or hidden patterns. Furthermore, ML algorithms typically show limited performance gains when trained on larger datasets compared to DL approaches.

DL, on the other hand, thrives on large amounts of data and is capable of automatically constructing effective features that often lead to higher predictive accuracy. However, these features are frequently not interpretable in biologic terms, posing a challenge for clinical understanding. As illustrated in Figure 42-1, the general pipeline of AI in sleep medicine involves feeding input data into either ML or DL models to produce outputs. These AI-generated outputs are typically objective, reproducible, and significantly faster than human-generated results.

A key distinction in the use of AI lies in whether the learning is supervised or unsupervised. In supervised learning, the model is trained using labeled data, where the correct output is provided for each input during training. The objective is to minimize the discrepancy between the model's predictions and the known answers. Sleep staging is a prime example of supervised learning: data are segmented into 30-second epochs and labeled by experts following AASM sleep scoring rules (15). These labeled epochs are then used to train models to replicate human scorers. Similarly, in sleep apnea detection, the exact start and end times of apneas, as scored by experts, serve as the ground truth during model training.

In unsupervised learning, the data are unlabeled; no predefined answers are provided. The goal in this case is to

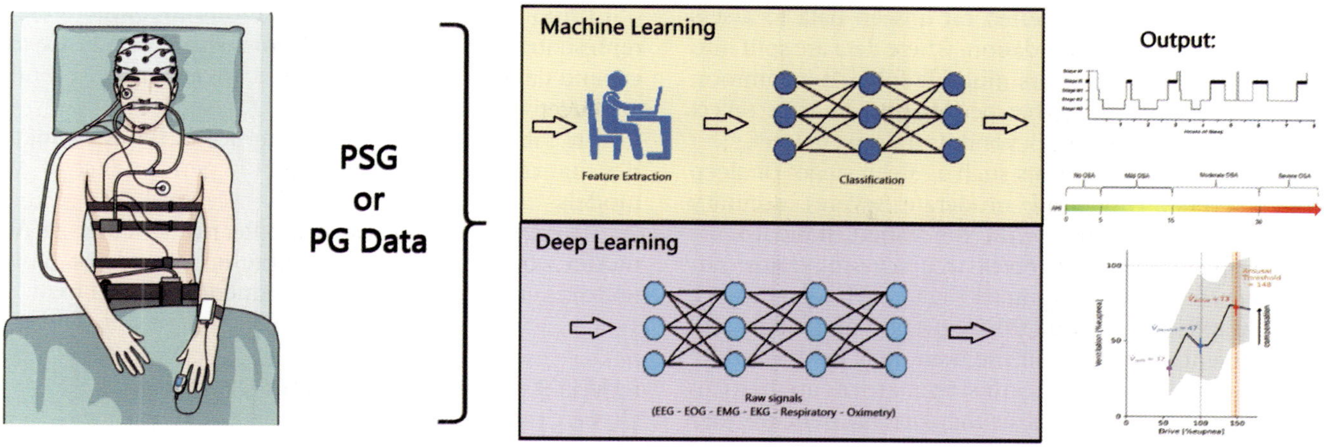

Figure 42-1 Illustration of the general pipeline of AI in sleep medicine. It involves feeding input data (polysomnography or polygraphy data) into either ML or DL models to produce outputs. And then the output can vary; it can be a hypnogram (showing sleep microstructure), apnea-hypopnea index (AHI), oxygen desaturation index (ODI), hypoxic burden (HB), sleep apnea endotypes (with an endogram), sleepiness; this all depends on the model—what it was trained or designed to do. (Illustration created by Carlos Teixeira.)

uncover hidden structures, detect patterns, or learn useful data representations. For example, the task of sleep apnea phenotyping, identifying subgroups of patients with shared clinical or physiologic traits, can be approached using clustering techniques in an unsupervised learning framework (8,16). These models can reveal important patient subtypes that may correlate with outcomes, comorbidities, or treatment response. When selecting models for clinical use, it is necessary to assess qualitatively each model's complexity and interpretability.

EVALUATION OF DIFFERENT MODELS

Assessing the performance of AI algorithms in sleep medicine typically involves comparing model predictions against expert-labeled ground truth values. To measure performance on sleep stage classification, we use the overall classification accuracy, and classification accuracy broken down by stage, shown as a confusion matrix (17). These are often 5×5 in size, corresponding to the five standard sleep stages: Wake, N1, N2, N3, and rapid eye movement (REM) (Figure 42-2). In respiratory event detection, a simpler 2×2 matrix is used, reflecting binary classification (event vs no event). These matrices display either the percentage or absolute number of epochs and summarize model performance across classes.

In these matrices, the actual (expert-labeled) classes are shown in rows, and the predicted classes by the AI are displayed in columns. Each row sums to 100%, showing the proportion of each true class predicted as various classes. This detailed layout enables clear identification of specific misclassification trends.

While confusion matrices provide a class-by-class overview, Cohen's kappa offers a single summary metric of agreement, adjusting for chance agreement. It ranges from −1 (complete disagreement) to +1 (perfect agreement), with 0 indicating random predictions. Although some literature segments kappa into qualitative levels (eg, moderate, substantial agreement), these thresholds remain debated.

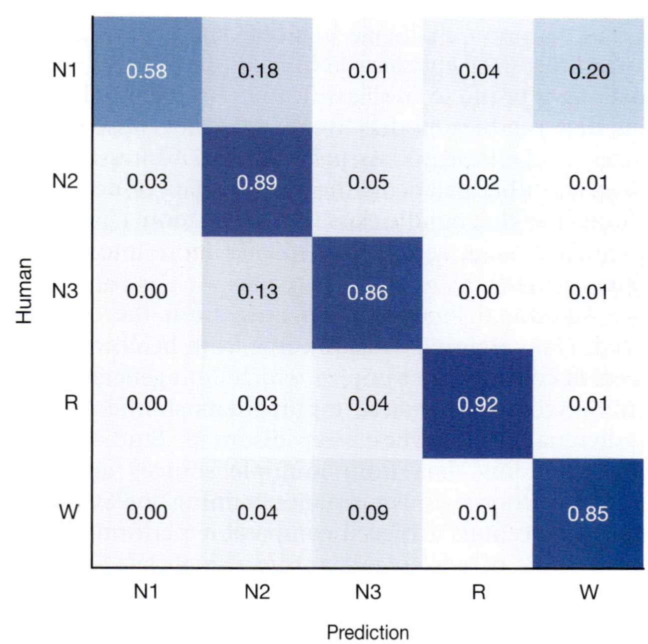

Figure 42-2 Example of a confusion matrix. (Adapted from Biswal S, Sun H, Goparaju B, Westover MB, Sun J, Bianchi MT. Expert-level sleep scoring with deep neural networks. *J Am Med Inform Assoc.* 2018;25(12):1643-1650. Reproduced by permission of Oxford University Press.)

AI models must be tested on unseen data to assess generalizability. Cross-validation, where data are split into training and test sets across multiple folds, is a common technique. This ensures that performance metrics reflect how the model performs beyond its training dataset.

For categorical outputs such as sleep stages or sleep apnea severity (no, mild, moderate, severe), accuracy and percent agreement with the expert standard are commonly reported. However, accuracy can be misleading when data are imbalanced (ie, unequal class sizes). For example, a model might frequently misclassify underrepresented classes, but the issue may be masked by a high overall accuracy. Confusion matrices are particularly helpful in such cases, as they display per-class performance and errors.

In binary classification tasks (eg, detecting obstructive sleep apnea), additional performance metrics are derived from 2×2 tables: true positives (TP), false positives (FP), true negatives (TN), and false negatives (FN). These enable calculation of:

- **Sensitivity (Recall)** = TP/(TP + FN), reflecting how well the model identifies positive cases
- **Specificity** = TN/(TN + FP), measuring how well the model avoids false alarms
- **Precision** = TP/(TP + FP), showing the accuracy of positive predictions
- **F1 Score** = harmonic mean of precision and recall
- **Accuracy** = (TP + TN)/(TP + TN + FP + FN), representing overall correct classification

A common challenge in sleep data is class imbalance. Most sleep epochs are N2 or REM, while N1 is rare, making it prone to misclassification. Imbalanced training data can bias models toward majority classes, compromising minority class performance. Addressing this involves either balancing the training data or designing algorithms that handle class imbalance more effectively. In such settings, sensitivity becomes more informative than accuracy.

Additional complications arise from the datasets used. Many training datasets come from healthy volunteers or convenience samples, which limit generalizability. For clinical relevance, training data should include individuals with diverse sleep disorders. Studies show that including data from multiple sources improves model performance. For instance, training on PSGs from five sleep centers achieved comparable performance to using 100% of available data from a single site (7).

Moreover, testing on datasets from the same center as the training data (same equipment, scorers, protocols) can inflate performance metrics. Using external, independent datasets offers a more realistic assessment (18,19). There's a growing need for standardized test datasets and performance metrics to allow meaningful comparisons across AI models.

Importantly, pediatric populations are often underrepresented in training data. Efforts should be made to expand datasets that include children, ensuring AI tools are effective across age groups.

In Table 42-1, we have compiled a series of metrics that can be used to evaluate the performance of AI models.

These metrics help evaluate not just whether an AI model works but how and where it succeeds or fails, which is critical for clinical implementation and trust.

LIMITATIONS OF ARTIFICIAL INTELLIGENCE IN SLEEP MEDICINE

AI is rapidly reshaping sleep medicine, offering exciting new possibilities—from automated diagnostics to personalized treatments. However, despite this promise, AI still faces significant hurdles that limit its integration into routine clinical care. Understanding these challenges is essential to ensuring that AI systems are not only accurate but also fair, ethical, and usable in real-world settings.

One of the biggest limitations lies in the quality and diversity of the data used to train AI models. Like any other tool, AI is only as good as the information it learns from. Unfortunately, many sleep datasets are relatively narrow in scope. They often include only certain types of patients, collected in specific environments, with annotations made by just one or a few technicians. This introduces the risk that the AI model may "learn" a particular scoring style or population profile, making it less effective when applied to different clinical settings. For instance, a model trained entirely on

Table 42-1 Key Performance Metrics for Artificial Intelligence Models in Sleep Medicine

Metric	Formula	Description
Accuracy	(TP + TN)/(Total)	Overall correct predictions
Precision	TP/(TP + FP)	Correct positive predictions
Sensitivity	TP/(TP + FN)	Ability to detect true positives (recall)
Specificity	TN/(TN + FP)	Ability to identify true negatives
F1 Score	2 × (Precision × Recall)/(Precision + Recall)	Balance between precision and recall
Cohen's Kappa	Adjusted agreement score	Accounts for chance agreement across classes

FP, false positives; TN, true negatives, TP, true positives.

healthy adults might underperform when used with patients with complex sleep disorders or underrepresented community backgrounds. This issue of bias and limited generalizability is not just a technical flaw but can have real consequences in terms of equity and patient outcomes (5).

Then, there's the question of interpretability. Many of the most powerful AI models today, especially those based on DL, operate as black boxes. They might produce accurate predictions but often fail to explain how they arrived at those conclusions. In medicine, this lack of transparency can be a serious barrier. Clinicians need to understand and trust the tools they use, especially when making decisions affecting patient care. From a practical perspective, integrating AI into existing sleep clinics presents its own set of logistical and technical barriers. DL, in particular, often require robust IT infrastructure and high processing power, resources that not every clinic can afford. AI systems also need to be compatible with current electronic health records, PSG systems, and clinical workflows. Without seamless integration, there's a risk that these tools become more of a burden than a benefit (20). On top of that, user interfaces need to be intuitive and actionable. Clinicians should not need to be data scientists to interpret the output of an AI system. Ideally, the technology should fit naturally into clinical decision-making, providing support rather than complexity.

Data imbalance is another technical issue that often gets overlooked. In many sleep studies, certain stages like N1 or particular patient subtypes are underrepresented. Standard ML models may perform poorly on these minority classes, skewing results and potentially missing critical diagnoses. Strategies like class rebalancing and more sophisticated training algorithms can help, but again, it underscores the need for careful dataset design and thoughtful model evaluation (20).

Finally, as we embrace AI's potential, we must also consider broader ethical and societal concerns. AI should never replace the human connection that defines good health care. Rather, it should support clinicians, helping them make better, more informed decisions. To do this responsibly, we need to ensure patient privacy, establish clear guidelines for clinical use, and continuously evaluate whether these technologies are truly improving care.

In summary, AI holds considerable potential to enhance the practice of sleep medicine, especially when applied thoughtfully and ethically. Sleep professionals are uniquely positioned to play a central role in this transformation, ensuring that AI tools are used to complement, not replace, human expertise. As the field evolves, ongoing education and engagement with AI technologies will be essential for sleep professionals to remain at the forefront of innovation and to uphold the highest standards of patient care.

REFERENCES

1. Goldstein CA, Berry RB, Kent DT, et al. Artificial intelligence in sleep medicine: an American Academy of Sleep Medicine position statement. *J Clin Sleep Med*. 2020;16(4):605-607.
2. BaHammam AS. Artificial intelligence in sleep medicine: the dawn of a new era. *Nat Sci Sleep*. 2024;16:445-450. doi:10.2147/NSS.S474510
3. Watson NF, Fernandez CR. Artificial intelligence and sleep: advancing sleep medicine. *Sleep Med Rev*. 2021;59:101512. doi:10.1016/j.smrv.2021.101512
4. Kelly JL, Ben Messaoud R, Joyeux-Faure M, et al. Diagnosis of sleep apnoea using a mandibular monitor and machine learning analysis: one-night agreement compared to in-home polysomnography. *Front Neurosci*. 2022;16:726880. doi:10.3389/fnins.2022.726880
5. Verma RK, Dhillon G, Grewal H, et al. Artificial intelligence in sleep medicine: present and future. *World J Clin Cases*. 2023;11(34):8106-8110. doi:10.12998/wjcc.v11.i34.8106
6. Jonasdottir SS, Minor K, Lehmann S. Gender differences in nighttime sleep patterns and variability across the adult lifespan: a global-scale wearables study. *Sleep*. 2021;44(2):zsaa169. doi:10.1093/sleep/zsaa169
7. Brennan HL, Kirby SD. Barriers of artificial intelligence implementation in the diagnosis of obstructive sleep apnea. *J Otolaryngol Head Neck Surg*. 2022;51(1):16. doi:10.1186/s40463-022-00566-w
8. Finnsson E, Arnardóttir E, Cheng WJ, et al. Sleep apnea endotypes: from the physiological laboratory to scalable polysomnographic measures. *Front Sleep*. 2023;2:1-13. doi:10.3389/frsle.2023.1188052
9. Wickwire EM, Bailey MD, Somers VK, et al. CPAP adherence is associated with reduced inpatient utilization among older adult Medicare beneficiaries with pre-existing cardiovascular disease. *J Clin Sleep Med*. 2022;18(1):39. doi:10.5664/jcsm.9478
10. Williamson AA, Zendarski N, Lange K, et al. Sleep problems, internalizing and externalizing symptoms, and domains of health-related quality of life: bidirectional associations from early childhood to early adolescence. *Sleep*. 2021;44(1):zsaa139. doi:10.1093/sleep/zsaa139
11. Malhotra A, Ayappa I, Ayas N, et al. Metrics of sleep apnea severity: beyond the apnea-hypopnea index. *Sleep*. 2021;44(7):zsab030. doi:10.1093/sleep/zsab030
12. Goldstein CA, Berry RB, Kent DT, et al. Artificial intelligence in sleep medicine: background and implications for clinicians. *J Clin Sleep Med*. 2020;16(4):609-618. doi:10.5664/jcsm.8388

13. LeCun Y, Bengio Y, Hinton G. Deep learning. *Nature*. 2015;521(7553):436-444. doi:10.1038/nature14539
14. Mohsenvand MN, Izadi MR, Maes P. Contrastive representation learning for electroencephalogram classification. Presented at: Proceedings of the Machine Learning for Health NeurIPS Workshop. PMLR; 2020:238-253. Accessed June 17, 2025. https://proceedings.mlr.press/v136/mohsenvand20a.html
15. Olesen AN, Jørgen Jennum P, Mignot E, Sorensen HBD. Automatic sleep stage classification with deep residual networks in a mixed-cohort setting. *Sleep*. 2021;44(1):zsaa161. doi:10.1093/sleep/zsaa161
16. Zinchuk AV, Jeon S, Koo BB, et al. Polysomnographic phenotypes and their cardiovascular implications in obstructive sleep apnoea. *Thorax*. 2018;73(5):472-480. doi:10.1136/thoraxjnl-2017-210431
17. Biswal S, Sun H, Goparaju B, Westover MB, Sun J, Bianchi MT. Expert-level sleep scoring with deep neural networks. *J Am Med Inform Assoc*. 2018;25(12):1643-1650. doi:10.1093/jamia/ocy131
18. Stephansen JB, Olesen AN, Olsen M, et al. Neural network analysis of sleep stages enables efficient diagnosis of narcolepsy. *Nat Commun*. 2018;9(1):5229. doi:10.1038/s41467-018-07229-3
19. Patanaik A, Ong JL, Gooley JJ, Ancoli-Israel S, Chee MWL. An end-to-end framework for real-time automatic sleep stage classification. *Sleep*. 2018;41(5):zsy041. doi:10.1093/sleep/zsy041
20. Bandyopadhyay A, Goldstein C. Clinical applications of artificial intelligence in sleep medicine: a sleep clinician's perspective. *Sleep Breath*. 2023;27(1):39-55. doi:10.1007/s11325-022-02592-4

SECTION V

Interventions and Therapeutics

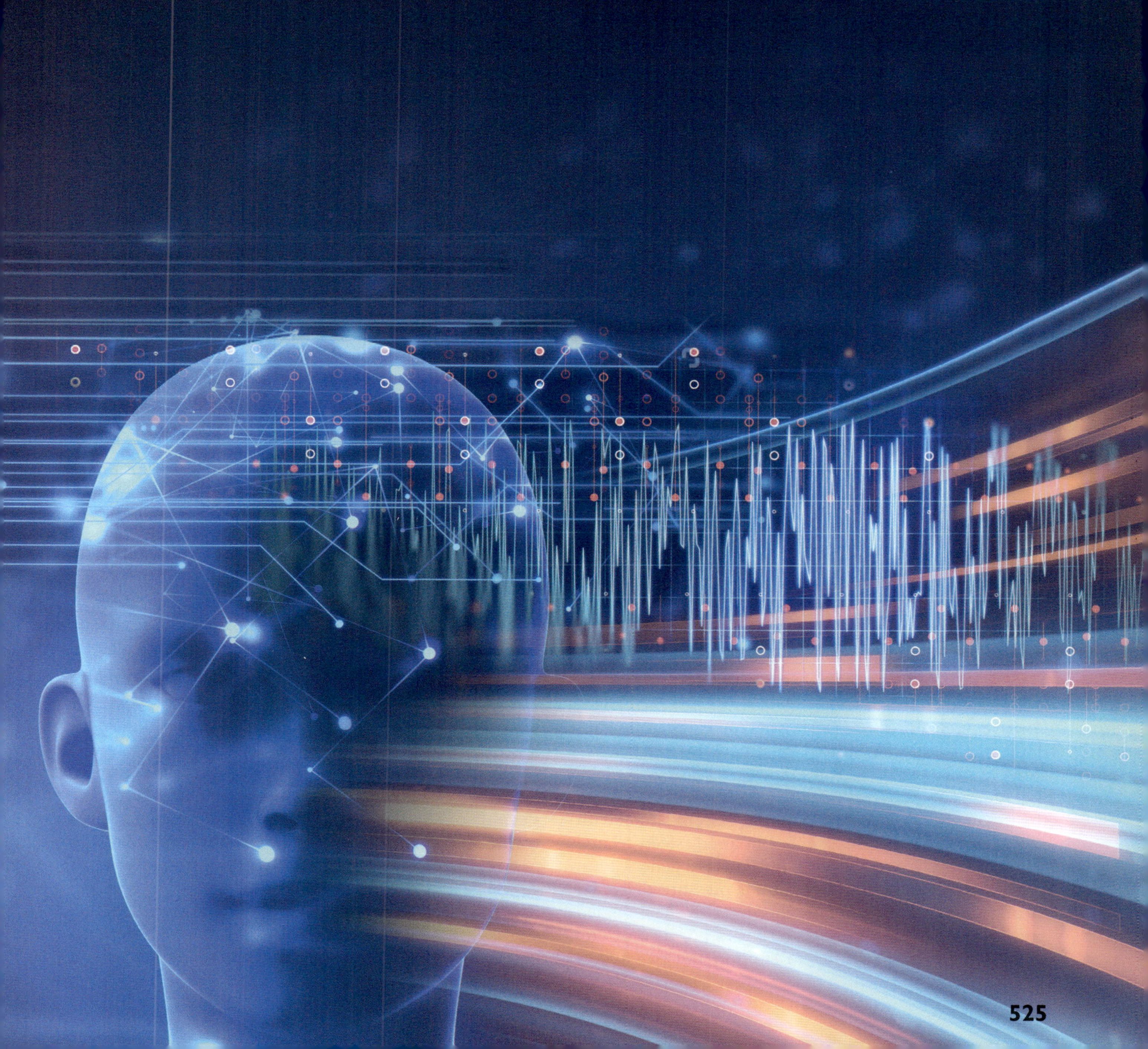

Chapter 43
Positive Airway Pressure Therapy: Basic Principles

JAMES A. REHILL

KEY CONCEPTS/LEARNING OBJECTIVES

The key concepts for this chapter include describing the anatomy and function of the upper airway, defining the principles of positive airway pressure (PAP) therapy, explaining how PAP therapy restores patency in the upper airway, and listing the various PAP treatment modalities.

KEY TERMS

Adaptive servo-ventilation (ASV)
Automatic bilevel positive airway pressure (ABPAP)
Automatic positive airway pressure (APAP)
Bilevel positive airway pressure (BPAP)
Cheyne-Stokes respiration
Continuous positive airway pressure (CPAP)
Crescendo-decrescendo pattern
Epiglottis
Expiratory pressure relief (EPR)
Pharynx
Volume-assured pressure support (VAPS)

OVERVIEW

Positive airway pressure (PAP) therapy is the gold standard and most widely used treatment for obstructive sleep apnea (OSA). PAP therapy is recommended by the American Academy of Sleep Medicine (AASM) in the treatment of properly diagnosed OSA in adults with excessive daytime sleepiness, impaired sleep-related quality of life, or hypertension (1). PAP is a generic term applied to all therapies that use air pressure delivered through the upper airway of patients with sleep-related breathing disorders (SRBDs) with the purpose of creating a "pneumatic splint" to support the patency of anatomic structures of the upper airway by opening and thus allowing an uninterrupted flow of air to the lungs during sleep.

In this chapter, we will establish a framework for how the anatomy of the upper airway contributes to SRBDs and introduce the different types of PAP therapy developed to restore normal breathing. We will also provide an understanding of how these devices interact with the upper airway to produce salutary health benefits on sleep apnea and diseases comorbid with the disorder.

BASIC PRINCIPLES OF POSITIVE AIRWAY PRESSURE THERAPY

The term apnea is derived from ancient Greek etymology, which means "absence of breathing." When obstructive, apnea results in *cessation* of breathing due to the closure of the upper airway. Hypopnea originates from the ancient Greek word for "underbreathing" and, in OSA, refers to a reduction in breathing due to a narrowing of the upper airway. Both apneas and hypopneas are breathing events that can be treated safely using PAP therapy. Snoring is also an obstructive breathing event that can have clinical implications. It is associated with OSA but can occur independently due to airway vibrations that typically range from 60 to 80 dB in intensity. As a point of reference, a vacuum cleaner typically emits a decibel level of 70 and a chainsaw 100. Hearing damage can result from prolonged exposures greater than 80 dB. A grandmother of four in the United Kingdom was recently recorded with a snoring level of 111.6 dB! In comparison, most modern CPAP machines produce less than 30 dB or the equivalent of a soft whisper.

Respiratory effort–related arousals (RERAs) are another important clinical manifestation of obstructive sleep-disordered breathing (SDB) that are often treated with PAP therapy. These events, like snoring events, do not rise to the level to meet the clinical definition of an apnea or hypopnea but are characterized by a reduction in airflow that leads to a pattern of arousals from sleep. Central apneas and central hypopneas are events that can be differentiated from obstructive apneas and obstructive hypopneas in their cause: Central events originate not because of a narrowing or obstruction in the upper airway but instead result from a lack of proper signal from the central nervous system to breathe adequately that can occur in coordination with conditions like heart failure and stroke and involves an area of the brain called the "brainstem" that triggers breathing. Sleeping at altitude can also cause central events in a breathing pattern called "periodic breathing." The use of opioid-based medications can also trigger central events and a "crescendo-decrescendo" pattern of central events called Cheyne-Stokes respiration.

Although the first modern use of the word "apnea" can be traced to 1719, and the symptoms of the disease first appeared in a fictional description of a Charles Dickens character in the Pickwick Papers in 1836 (2), it was not until 1965 that sleep apnea was first documented in the medical literature, and it was another 16 years (1980) until the first noninvasive ventilation device, a positive-pressure breathing circuit connected to the nose using plastic tubing and silicone sealant, was used on a patient by Dr Colin Sullivan. By the end of the 1980s, continuous positive airway pressure (CPAP) had been developed into a more sophisticated treatment for sleep apnea, and by the 1990s, bilevel positive airway pressure (BPAP) had been in use (3), followed by autotitrating devices that are continuing to evolve and use more sophisticated treatment algorithms to respond to breath-by-breath changes in patient respiration (Figure 43-1).

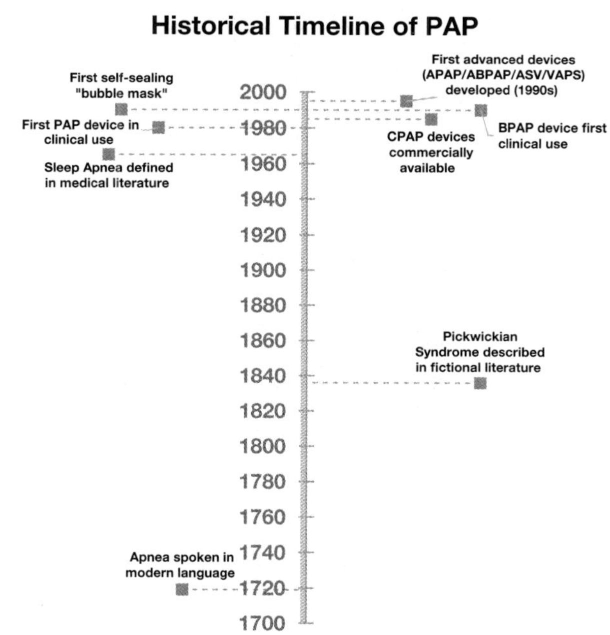

Figure 43-1 Historical timeline of positive airway pressure therapy (PAP). ABPAP, automatic bilevel positive airway pressure; APAP, automatic positive airway pressure; ASV, adaptive servo-ventilation; BPAP, bilevel positive airway pressure; CPAP, continuous positive airway pressure; VAPS, volume-assured pressure support.

The first CPAP machine was a simple device using a reversed vacuum motor to provide positive pressure to the patient. Early PAP machines and ancillary equipment were noisy, cumbersome, and not adaptable to each patient's individual needs. Modern PAP machines incorporate microprocessors, cellular modems, ambient temperature monitoring, and Bluetooth for smartphone integration. Other features intended to improve comfort, compliance, and efficacy include:

- **Pressure ramps** allow the user to start at a low initial PAP setting, which gradually increases over a set time to reach a preset therapeutic pressure.
- **Heated humidifiers** include a heated chamber for distilled water that the pressurized air passes through, thus moistening the air to prevent oronasal and upper respiratory dryness.
- **Heated hoses** prevent the warm, moist air exiting the heated humidifier from cooling in the hose, causing "rain out" or water to condense in the tubing.
- **Expiratory pressure relief (EPR)** is a comfort feature that provides a fraction of a second drop in expiratory pressure, decreasing the effort to exhale and making breathing against high pressure feel more comfortable.

A classification system for sleep apnea is used in the diagnosis and is useful in guiding treatment through the clinical pathway: Mild sleep apnea is defined as the occurrence of 5 to 14 respiratory events per hour, on average, throughout the sleep period; moderate sleep apnea is defined as 15 to 30 events per hour; severe sleep apnea is defined as greater than 30 events per hour (Figure 43-2).

It is not unusual for a sleep technologist to observe hundreds of respiratory events during a single night of sleep testing. Typically, the total number of obstructive and central apneas and hypopneas is combined to yield an apnea-hypopnea "index" (AHI), which is the average number of events per hour during a sleep period based on polysomnography (PSG) recording. For patients with a high pretest probability of sleep apnea as a result of associated subjective and objective sleep-related symptoms but who do not reach the clinically defined minimum for diagnosis by AHI, RERAs are often scored and added to the index to yield a respiratory disturbance index (RDI). RDI can be utilized to make a diagnosis of sleep apnea and qualify some

Mild: $\geq 5 \leq 15$ per hour
Moderate: $>15 \leq 30$ per hour
Severe: > 30 episodes per hour

Figure 43-2 Classification system for sleep apnea severity. AHI, apnea-hypopnea index.

patients for related follow-up care. Centers for Medicare and Medicaid Services (CMS) requires an AHI or RDI greater than or equal to 15 events per hour in the United States. However, CMS criteria for reimbursement coverage also extend to an AHI or RDI between 5 and 14 events per hour if a patient demonstrates documented objective or subjective sleepiness symptoms or suffers from comorbid conditions such as hypertension, stroke, or heart disease. PAP therapy has been shown to have positive clinical outcomes in patients with moderate-to-severe sleep apnea or patients with mild sleep apnea with associated comorbidities or disorders.

During therapeutic PSG, a sleep technologist fits a mask to seal over the openings of the nose and/or mouth of a patient with known sleep apnea and integrates with a medical PAP device that delivers room air at a pressure set by the technologist or determined through an internal device algorithm using the appropriate mode and settings to normalize a patient's breathing. Inside this box is also a chamber filled with heated water through which the air travels before being sent through plastic tubing to a mask interface and ultimately to the lungs, where oxygen enters the blood through sacs called "alveoli."

Depending on the physiologic, logistic, and psychological needs of the patient, there are a variety of PAP therapy modes to choose from. Most populations with SRBDs experience a reduced or blocked flow of air because of an obstruction by muscles and tissues of the upper airway behind the mouth and the throat. For these patients, a fixed flow of positive air, called CPAP, is typically applied. Alternatively, a PAP device with independently fixed inspiratory and expiratory positive airway pressures (IPAP and EPAP, respectively), known as BPAP, can also be effective. BPAP uses two pressures, and IPAP is applied during inhalation and is higher than the EPAP, which is applied during exhalation. In a version called auto-CPAP or auto-bilevel, an internal algorithm within the machine can be used to "auto-titrate" effective pressures.

More advanced titration approaches are needed to treat more complex forms of sleep apnea that involve a reduced airflow as a result of underlying neurologic conditions, lung disease, chronic obstructive pulmonary disease (COPD), or medication effect. Adaptive servo-ventilation (ASV) and volume-assured pressure support (VAPS) are two primary examples. The ASV device algorithm automatically adjusts IPAP, EPAP, and pressure support (PS), which is the difference in pressure between IPAP and EPAP (ie, IPAP minus EPAP equals PS) settings in response to patient breathing within a set range that is established by a technologist on the basis of a physician's order. The aim of VAPS is to maintain an optimal level of the patient's tidal volume (V_T), which is the volume of air displaced through normal inhalation and exhalation. With VAPS, the target tidal volume is determined based on a patient's body size, age, lung physiology, and underlying medical conditions. For adults, a common initial target tidal volume is 6 to 8 mL/kg of ideal body weight. The appropriate VAPS setting for V_T is equal to 7 mL/kg of ideal body weight. With VAPS, the inspiratory phase switches to exhalation settings only after a preset V_T is delivered to the patient (4).

SDB has a significant impact on society. The AASM contracted a global research and consulting firm to uncover the economic costs of untreated sleep apnea for payers, employers, and patients (5). Their 2016 report estimates that undiagnosed OSA cost the United States approximately $149.6 billion in 2015 alone. Between 2% and 4% of the adult US population is affected by sleep apnea, but of the estimated 22 million with the disorder, 80% are undiagnosed, and of those that are diagnosed and treated, compliance on PAP therapy is approximately 50%. This means that less than 10% of those suffering from sleep apnea are being effectively treated! This has significant implications for society because of the known, wide-reaching effects that sleep deprivation, or the lack of quality sleep, has on public health, workplace productivity, and safety. A case can be made that sleep apnea is a hidden health crisis of our time.

ANATOMY AND FUNCTION OF THE UPPER AIRWAY

The upper airway is quite complex (Figure 43-3). For the sleep technologist, the most important areas are the nasopharynx, the oropharynx, and the laryngeal pharynx. In terms of preventing snoring, hypopnea, and OSA, the goal of PAP therapy is to prevent collapse at any point in these three areas of the upper airway.

A useful model of the upper airway is the Starling resistor, invented by Ernest Starling while working on blood vessels in the heart. This model has been applied to analysis of airway collapse in OSA. It represents the complicated upper airway with just three sections—(1) "upstream," or the area of the nose and nasal cavity (2), the collapsible portions of the upper airway itself, and (6) "downstream" or the trachea and lungs. At its most basic, a formula can be used that allows prediction of airway collapse dependent on the pressure inside the upper airway and the pressure outside of the upper airway. This is the critical closing pressure. The likelihood of reaching this critical pressure and airway collapse is higher when the pressure outside of the upper airway is increased. This occurs when there is submucosal fat or edema present. Collapse is also more likely when the diameter of the airway is reduced, which can also be caused by the accumulation of submucosal fat. Finally,

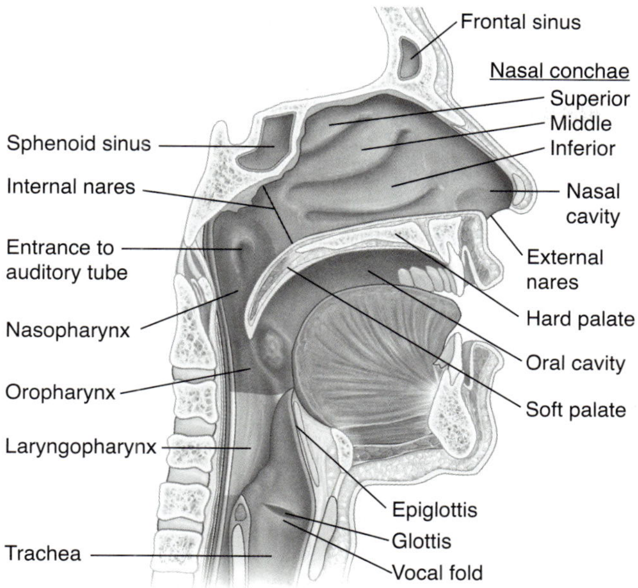

Figure 43-3 Upper respiratory system. (Modified with permission from Moore KL, Dalley AF II, Agur AMR. *Clinically Oriented Anatomy*. 7th ed. Wolters Kluwer Health/Lippincott Williams & Wilkins; 2014. Figure 7.83.)

collapse of the upper airway is more likely when flow through the airway is reduced. This can occur upstream when there is nasal congestion or blockage. Reduced flow may also occur downstream when lung function is impaired. When the pressure inside the airway is less than the pressure outside the airway, the critical closing pressure is achieved, and the airway collapses.

Unfortunately, the relationship between pressures inside and outside of the upper airway and the effect on airway collapse is not linear. Before closing, the upper airway may oscillate, leading to snoring and flow restriction. The more important nonlinearity is that once the upper airway is closed, increased pressure below the point of closure will not cause the airway to open. This means that once the airway has collapsed, it will stay closed until something in the relationship between pressures is changed. For patients with OSA, this usually means that the airway diameter must be increased, and this occurs when the patient wakes up and muscle tone in the upper airway is increased.

The Starling resistor predicts that several methods will reduce the likelihood of upper airway collapse. One method is to change the anatomy of the upper airway. Surgical options for increasing flow include removal of soft tissue such as tonsils and adenoids that may cause upstream blockage. The diameter of the upper airway may be increased by mandibular advancement, either surgically or with an oral appliance. More recently, methods for increasing muscle tone in the upper airway using surgically implanted stimulators have been shown to be effective in reducing the number of episodes of nonconcentric airway collapse.

The most common method for reducing the likelihood of airway collapse is to increase airway pressure. When the upstream pressure is increased and the external pressure remains the same, the ratio is changed, and collapse is prevented. PAP therapy provides extra upstream pressure and acts as a pneumatic "splint" to keep the airway open.

Although it is possible to calculate the additional pressure needed to prevent the airway from reaching the critical closing pressure, human airways are not Starling resistors. Pressure requirements change on the basis of elasticity of the upper airway, airway diameter, and flow rate. Tongue position and size are important elements in the equation. These factors change with age, obesity, and tissue swelling. During the night, the pressure requirement may change because of changes in body position. And because pressure is a key part of the discussion and pressure decreases with elevation above sea level, moving from Detroit to Denver will change pressure requirements as well. This makes titration of PAP an important part of the therapeutic process. The airway is complex, but the model of the Starling resistor explains how providing positive pressure at the nose and/or mouth can reduce or eliminate OSA.

MECHANISMS OF POSITIVE AIRWAY PRESSURE THERAPY DELIVERY

Given the complexity of the upper airway, the mechanism by which PAP therapy restores patency is remarkably straightforward. In its simplest form, PAP establishes a positive pressure outside of the airway to the negative pressure inside. This disequilibrium encourages the upper airway (if narrowed or blocked) to expand, thus allowing positive and negative sides to equalize. It is basically a physiologic example of homeostasis, one breath at a time.

PAP therapy introduces positive pressure to the airway by first delivering pressurized air to the nose and/or mouth through what is called an "interface," a mask that covers the nose and/or mouth that is held in place by straps that form the "headgear" (Figure 43-4). This air is first humidified and typically heated, and the amount of pressure needed to maintain an open airway, measured in centimeters of water (cm H_2O), is established by the technologist (during a manual titration) or machine (using an autotitrating device) before it is sent to the patient. The measurement cm H_2O refers to the number of centimeters in height that the pressure of the air will push a column of water to, using a detection device called a "manometer." Relatively speaking, each "one" cm H_2O equals much less than "one"

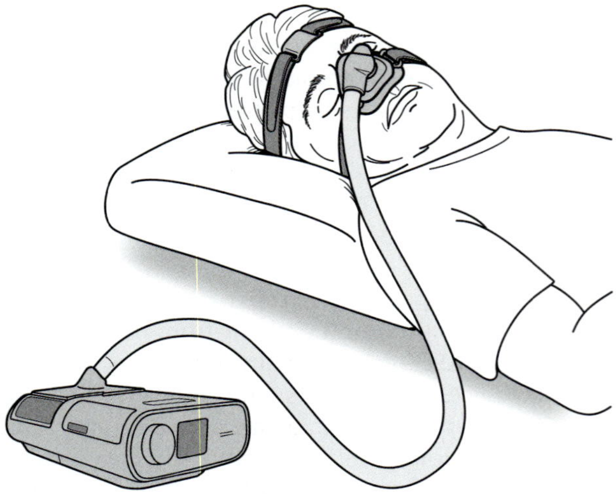

Figure 43-4 Positive airway pressure therapy introduces positive pressure to the airway by first delivering pressurized air to the nose and/or mouth through an *interface,* a mask that covers the nose and/or mouth held in place by straps, referred to as *headgear*. This air is first humidified and typically heated before it is sent to the patient.

atmosphere or pound per square inch (PSI): 1 cm H_2O = 0.142,233 PSI, to be exact! For example, the amount of pressure from a PAP machine at 25 cm H_2O would provide a similar pressure on the lungs during exhalation as standing in the deep end of a pool with the water line up to the chin. If we assume that 25 cm is roughly 10 in or the height above the center of the lungs that air must travel through during exhalation, then 25 cm H_2O is comparable to the pressure one must exert to expand the chest against the water in a pool to exhale.

The internal effect of this pressure on the airway follows a similar mechanical progression, as illustrated in Figure 43-5. As air enters through the nose, it travels through the nasal cavity and past the structures of the hard palate and soft palate to the areas that are most crowded in the upper airway, such as the epiglottis, and to the trachea, and eventually fills the alveoli of the lungs.

POSITIVE IMPACTS OF POSITIVE AIRWAY PRESSURE THERAPY

The goals of this section are to summarize the negative impact of untreated OSA and describe the beneficial effects of PAP therapy. In a recent clinical practice guideline (5), the AASM notes the factors that are documented during sleep studies in patients with OSA, including fragmented sleep, pressure swings in the thorax, increased sympathetic nervous system activity, and changes in blood gases.

The AASM cites "wide-ranging" consequences of untreated OSA. These include fatigue and sleepiness during the day, impairment of the ability to stay awake, poor concentration, and diminished quality of life. These "can translate into higher rates of job-related and motor vehicle accidents" (7).

Untreated OSA is associated with an increased risk of cardiovascular disease, including heart failure, arrhythmias, and stroke. There are also associations with

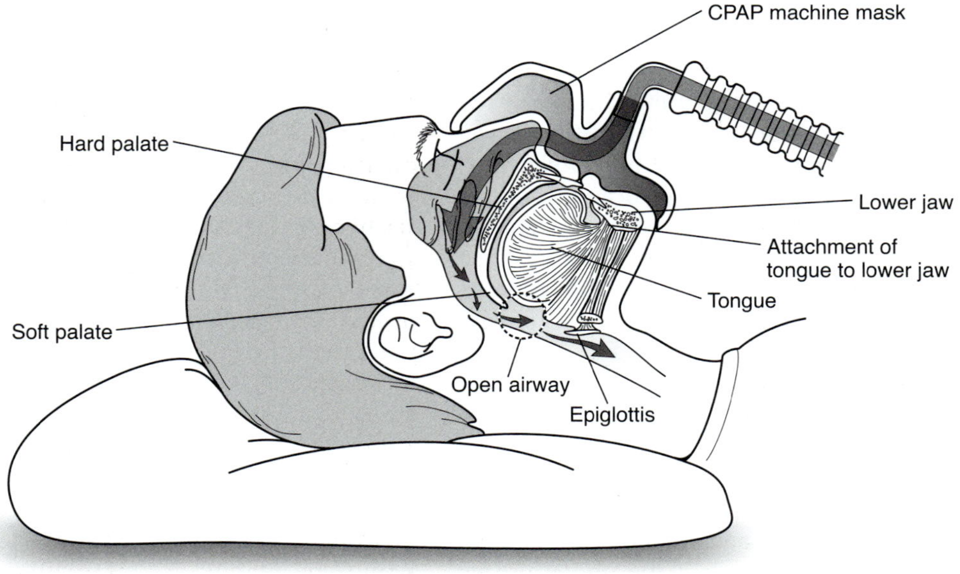

Figure 43-5 Continuous positive airway pressure (CPAP) therapy. Air enters through the nose, travels through the nasal cavity, past the hard palate and soft palate to the areas most crowded in the upper airway, the epiglottis, oropharynx, laryngopharynx, to the trachea, and eventually fills the alveoli of the lungs.

metabolic dysregulation and risk of diabetes. Studies have documented increased health care utilization in patients who have untreated OSA. A limited number of long-term follow-up studies have found increased mortality in patients with OSA who are not treated.

These associations are based on correlation, and as students of statistics frequently hear, correlation does not imply causality. This is an important factor in evaluating the effects of PAP therapy on medical disorders. Patients who choose to use PAP and are adherent to treatment are most likely to adhere to other treatment advice from their physician, such as weight loss, exercise, and avoiding high-cholesterol foods. If these patients have lower levels of cardiovascular disease, can we say that it is due to the use of PAP therapy and not to the other lifestyle changes that patients have made?

In order to establish a cause-and-effect relationship and provide strong evidence that untreated OSA causes these consequences, an experiment must be performed. Patients with OSA must be randomly assigned to treatment or no treatment groups. Successful treatment of OSA must result in reduction or elimination of the wide-ranging consequences.

Unfortunately, randomized controlled trials are few and far between. Short-term studies have documented changes in frequency of apnea and blood pressure, but these are not the important consequences that concern patients and physicians. Evidence that PAP therapy reduces cardiovascular events and mortality would be more important, but such studies require long-term follow-up and placing patients in the control, or untreated, group for the duration of the study. In one trial, CPAP provided no benefit for patients with OSA in the prevention of cardiovascular events with a mean follow-up of 3.7 years (8). Other trials are ongoing.

In one carefully controlled study (9), a group of patients with central sleep apnea (CSA) who were treated with a form of PAP therapy (ASV) actually had more cardiovascular events than the control group, forcing the investigators to discontinue the study before the intended date.

With regard to sleepiness and quality of life, the results have been more consistent. For example, the "BestAIR" study (10) found that CPAP improved several quality-of-life measures in patients with moderate-to-severe OSA when compared with "sham CPAP."

In an exhaustive review (11), the US Preventive Services Task Force concluded, "There is uncertainty about the accuracy or clinical utility of all potential screening tools. Multiple treatments for OSA reduce AHI, ESS scores, and blood pressure. Trials of CPAP and other treatments have not established whether treatment reduces mortality or improves most other health outcomes, except for modest improvement in sleep-related quality of life" (11).

Nevertheless, the position of the AASM has been and continues to be that "Positive airway pressure (PAP) is the treatment of choice for mild, moderate, and severe OSA and should be offered as an option to all patients" (12).

POSITIVE AIRWAY PRESSURE TREATMENT MODALITIES AND SUMMARY

The goals of PAP titration are airway management, breathing stabilization, and patient adherence to therapy. There are many PAP machine settings, generally called "modes," by which PAP therapy can individualize the treatment approach to a patient's breathing abnormality and address each of these treatment goals.

The AASM recommends a starting pressure of 4 cm H_2O to treat sleep apnea with CPAP (13). This starting pressure is then increased in a stepwise procedure in response to a continuation of SDB, until all events and symptoms are abolished. CPAP therapy is typically sufficient to normalize breathing and abolish respiratory events, but there are three main cases when it is advantageous to switch a patient to BPAP after a failed attempt to treat a patient using only CPAP (Figure 43-6).

After selecting an optimal interface, if a patient is simply unable to tolerate CPAP, especially in cases where exhaling against the pressure is uncomfortable, BPAP mode may be initiated and titrated beginning at 8/4 cm H_2O (IPAP set at 8 cm H_2O; EPAP set at 4 cm H_2O). A second case where a switch to BPAP is recommended occurs when high CPAP is necessary to control events: if higher pressures are not effective in eliminating events, the AASM practice parameters recommend switching to BPAP of 16/8 when a titration reaches 16 cm H_2O. The third scenario for switching to BPAP is in treatment-emergent CSA, which is a phenomenon whereby the CPAP treatment itself is thought to have a causal effect on the transition from obstructive to central apneas or hypopneas. This phenomenon occurs in approximately 10% of sleep apneics treated with CPAP (14).

BPAP is differentiated from CPAP, which provides a constant pressure, whether a patient is in the inhalation or exhalation phase of respiration or airflow. The advantage of BPAP is that it can provide a reduction in pressure, or PS, during exhalation. PS is typically 4 cm H_2O less than IPAP, and at most, a 10 cm H_2O difference is recommended between the two pressures for patients with OSA, although PS up to 20 cm H_2O is sometimes used for chronic stable hypoventilation patients. PS can address our goals for BPAP therapy by alleviating the pressure that a patient breathes against while keeping inhalation pressure high to address airway obstruction.

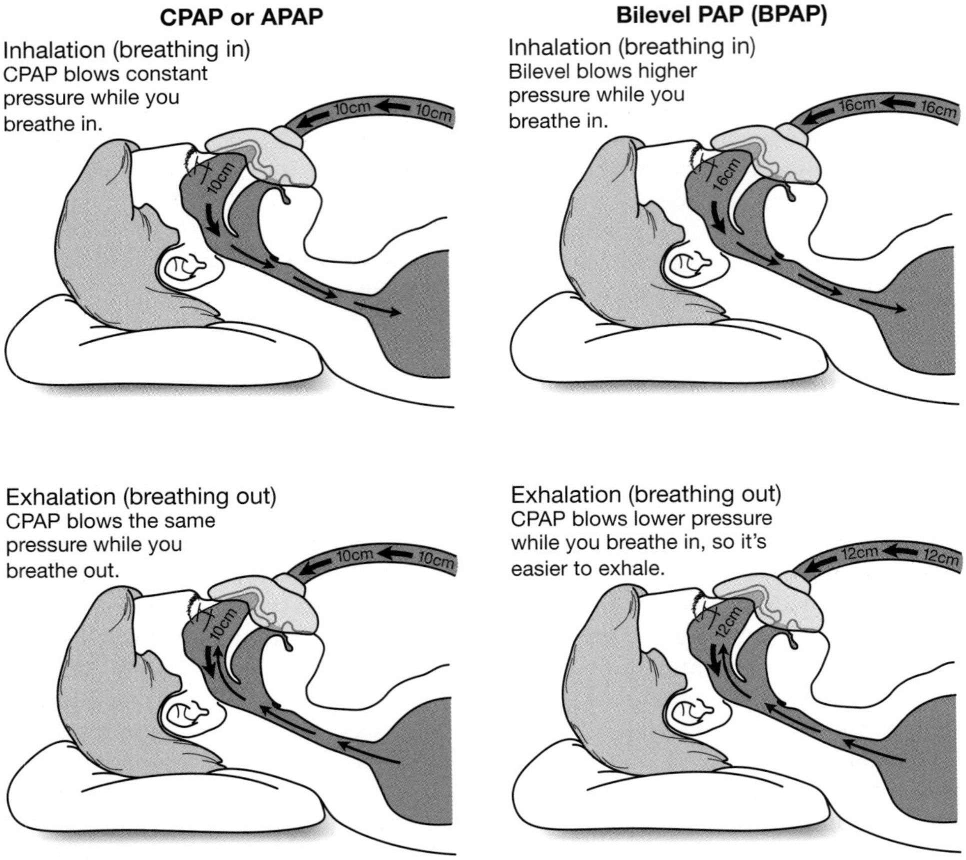

Figure 43-6 Continuous positive airway pressure (CPAP) delivers a continuous prescribed pressure, whereas bilevel positive airway pressure (BPAP) delivers two sets of prescribed pressures, one inspiratory positive airway pressure and the other a lower expiratory positive airway pressure. APAP, automatic positive airway pressure.

This makes BPAP a first-line mechanical intervention to address patient compliance. It also allows for improved airway management at high pressures and with treatment-emergent CSA.

BPAP can be set for spontaneous, timed, or spontaneous/timed (ST) modes depending on patient need. In the most common mode, spontaneous, the patient's change from exhalation to inhalation triggers a change in pressure from the device. Less commonly, a timed mode can be set to establish the timing of IPAP/EPAP delivery, which is independent of a patient's own breathing effort. This can lead to patient discomfort. ST mode uses the patient's spontaneous breathing effort to trigger pressure changes but will step in to trigger a breath at a previously set rate if a patient does not self-trigger (15).

ST mode is most often used for primary central apnea or central apneas caused by respiratory depression. ST mode may also be used for patients with neuromuscular disease, whose respiratory efforts reduce during rapid eye movement (REM) sleep, which may make them unable to trigger inspiration. Timed mode is most often used for patients with severe neuromuscular weakness or spinal cord injury and who are unable to trigger inspiration.

Auto-adjusting CPAP (AutoCPAP) machines measure flow and vibration-based snoring many times per second to tailor treatment pressure to the changing needs of a patient during a therapeutic PSG or home PAP trial. AutoCPAP can be used to determine the optimal fixed treatment pressure for a patient. Typically, AutoCPAP is set to a range of pressures, and the machine titrates between these pressures depending on the level of pressure needed at various points throughout the night. This pressure range is usually informed by the results of a previous PAP titration. The advantages of AutoCPAP include the ability to adjust to sleep apnea severity that is greater during Stage R sleep or in certain positions, typically supine. In patients with REM-related or positional events, higher levels of pressure are needed, and a patient can more comfortably use PAP at a lower effective pressure at other times.

AutoBPAP adds an adjusting PS feature between the IPAP and EPAP settings, which can also be set to a maximum range (usually 10 cm H_2O). With AutoBPAP, an internal algorithm calculates the PS needed in addition to IPAP and EPAP levels (16).

Because higher PAP and high PS can induce treatment-emergent CSA, periodic breathing, and Cheyne-Stokes respiration, devices have been developed to try to even out breathing over several breaths. ASV is an example of this type of device (17). ASV uses an algorithm that senses the patient's breathing patterns and provides subtle changes in pressure to restore normal breathing. The hope is that by stabilizing breathing, the periodic breathing pattern will subside.

VAPS machines adjust PS in order to maintain a target average ventilation. This mode of PAP is often helpful for patients with respiratory insufficiency caused by neuromuscular and restrictive conditions in which respiratory effort varies during sleep or who need PAP during the day. It may also be useful in patients with COPD with risk of hypoventilation and for patients with obesity hypoventilation who may need compensation on the basis of positional and sleep stage changes.

The upper airway is a critical space in the management of effective breathing and is important for the healthy function of an individual. Although the identification of conditions that affect proper breathing is relatively recent in the field of medicine, a variety of effective treatment options are available that can be used in the approach to treatment in an effort to provide precision therapy for OSA.

REFERENCES

1. Patil SP, Ayappa IA, Caples SM, Kimoff RJ, Patel SR, Harrod CG. Treatment of adult obstructive sleep apnea with positive airway pressure: an American Academy of Sleep Medicine Clinical Practice Guideline. *J Clin Sleep Med.* 2019;15(2):335-343.
2. Dickens C. *The Posthumous Papers of the Pickwick Club.*Chapman and Hall; 1836.
3. Gokcebay N, Salepci B, Parmaksiz ET, et al. Effects of heated humidification on CPAP compliance and symptoms in patients with obstructive sleep apnea. *Respir Med.* 2010;104(1):99-105.
4. Amato MB, Barbas CS, Bonassa J, et al. Volume-assured pressure support ventilation. *Chest.* 1992;102(4):1225-1234.
5. Watson NF. Health care savings: the economic value of diagnostic and therapeutic care for obstructive sleep apnea. *J Clin Sleep Med.* 2016;12(8):1075-1077.
6. Sanders MH, Kern N. Obstructive sleep apnea treated by independently adjusted inspiratory and expiratory positive airway pressures via nasal mask. *Chest.* 1990;98(2):317-324.
7. Kapur VK, Auckley DH, Chowdhuri S, et al. Clinical practice guideline for diagnostic testing for adult obstructive sleep apnea: an American Academy of Sleep Medicine clinical practice guideline. *J Clin Sleep Med.* 2017;13(3):479-504.
8. McEvoy RD, Antic NA, Heeley E, et al. CPAP for prevention of cardiovascular events in obstructive sleep apnea. *N Engl J Med.* 2016;375(10):919-931.
9. Cowie MR, Woehrle H, Wegscheider K, et al. Adaptive servo-ventilation for central sleep apnea in systolic heart failure. *N Engl J Med.* 2015;373(12):1095-1105.
10. Zhao YY, Wang R, Gleason KJ, et al. Effect of continuous positive airway pressure treatment on health-related quality of life and sleepiness in high cardiovascular risk individuals with sleep apnea: Best Apnea Interventions for Research (BestAIR) trial. *Sleep.* 2017;40(4):zsx040. doi:10.1093/sleep/zsx040
11. Jonas DE, Amick HR, Feltner C, et al. Screening for obstructive sleep apnea in adults: an evidence review for the U.S. Preventive Services Task Force (Report No. 14-05216-EF-1) [Internet]. Agency for Healthcare Research and Quality (US). 2017. https://pubmed.ncbi.nlm.nih.gov/28211654/
12. Epstein LJ, Kristo D, Strollo PJ, et al. Clinical guideline for the evaluation, management and long-term care of obstructive sleep apnea in adults. *J Clin Sleep Med.* 2009;5(3):263-276.
13. Kushida CA, Chediak A, Berry RB, et al; Positive Airway Pressure Titration Task Force of the American Academy of Sleep Medicine. Clinical guidelines for the manual titration of positive airway pressure in patients with obstructive sleep apnea. *J Clin Sleep Med.* 2008;4(2):157-171.
14. Edwards BA, Malhotra A, Sands SA. Adapting our approach to treatment-emergent central sleep apnea. *Sleep.* 2013;36(8):1121-1122.
15. Johnson KG, Johnson DC. Treatment of sleep-disordered breathing with positive airway pressure devices: technology update. *Med Devices (Auckl).* 2015;8:425-437.
16. Berry RB, Parish JM, Hartse KM. The use of auto-titrating continuous positive airway pressure for treatment of adult obstructive sleep apnea. In: *Database of Abstracts of Reviews of Effects (DARE): Quality-Assessed Reviews* [Internet]. Centre for Reviews and Dissemination (UK); 2002.
17. Donovan LM, Boeder S, Malhotra A, et al. New developments in the use of positive airway pressure for obstructive sleep apnea. *J Thorac Dis.* 2015;7(8):1323-1342.

Chapter 44
Personalizing the Selection of Interfaces

JILL WEST

KEY CONCEPTS/LEARNING OBJECTIVES

The key concepts for this chapter include recognizing the different types of interfaces available, selecting the proper interface option to optimize comfort and fit to enhance patient adherence, describing obstacles to effective positive airway pressure (PAP) therapy, PAP desensitization, and the role of the technologist in optimizing patient outcomes in PAP therapy.

KEY TERMS

Acclimation
Adherence
Desensitization

The American Association of Sleep Technologists (AAST) guidelines indicate that all potential positive airway pressure (PAP) titration candidates (including those candidates before a diagnostic study where the clinical suspicion of obstructive sleep apnea [OSA] is high and a split-night study is a possibility) should receive adequate PAP education, hands-on demonstration, careful mask fitting, and acclimatization before titration (1).

Studies have shown that educational, supportive, and behavioral interventions have shown positive effects on patient adherence (2).

INTERFACE FITTING

It is best to introduce a patient to PAP therapy before the titration night in the sleep center. An education session should include a discussion of the rationale for the use of PAP therapy, side effects, mask fitting, and a hands-on demonstration with acclimatization; this is of particular importance for pediatric patients. Acclimating a patient to PAP therapy with positive feedback, patience, understanding, and empathy will help maximize future outcomes.

A well-fitting comfortable interface is critical for patient adherence. A patient who is uncomfortable with a mask for any reason will not use it regularly. For this reason, it is important that patients be included in the selection of their PAP interface. Among the considerations in selecting an appropriate interface are nasal patency, nasal or facial abnormalities, facial hair, whether the patient wears dentures or is missing teeth, full or shallow cheeks, hand-eye coordination, finger strength, impaired vision, manual dexterity and cognitive abilities, or a history of claustrophobia. There are several varieties of mask styles and sizes from which patients may choose. No single mask is ideal for all patients. The patient may select one type of mask at the beginning of the study that seems to fit comfortably and then during the study awaken and request a different mask. It is important to let patients know that there are alternatives if they have any issues during or after the study.

BREATHING DURING WAKEFULNESS AND SLEEP

Humans are obligate nose breathers during wakefulness and mainly during sleep independently of sleep stage or position. However, many patients with untreated sleep apnea will state that they are "mouth breathers" during sleep. Mouth breathing during sleep typically occurs when the airway collapses. This is caused by an increase in negative intrathoracic pressure, creating thoracic traction (also known as "thoracic tug") that pulls the jawbone down, leading to mouth opening and an increased breathing effort. For this reason, a nasal mask should be the first mask of choice. A nasal mask is effective at decreasing mouth openings and prevents overuse of oronasal masks, increasing patient adherence (3).

TYPES OF POSITIVE AIRWAY PRESSURE INTERFACES

There are several types of PAP interfaces, including nasal masks, nasal pillow, nasal cushion, oronasal (full-face) masks, oral masks, and total-face masks.

When selecting the proper interface, there are several factors to consider: mask size and weight, strap types, the patient's ability to move, and their preferred sleep position.

Nasal masks traditionally cover only the nose while resting on the upper lip, sides of the nose, and the nasal bridge. With any type of nasal interface, there is a chance of air leaking from the patient's mouth. In such instances, a nasal mask may be used with a chinstrap. A chinstrap is an elastic fabric band that applies upward pressure on the jaw to keep the mouth closed.

Nasal pillow masks rest on the inside rim of the nostril. They are light and require minimal headgear. They are appropriate for patients who experience claustrophobia with a nasal mask and may work well for a patient with facial hair that prevents an adequate seal with other types of masks. However, the patient must be able to tolerate the inserts resting in the nostrils.

Nasal cushion masks have minimal contact under the nose cushions that prevent discomfort from or irritation in the nostril or on the bridge of the nose. However, modern nasal mask designs include minimalist cushions that cradle the base of the nostrils rather than cover the nose.

Oronasal masks (full-face) cover the nose and the mouth while resting on the chin, sides of the nose, and mouth and bridge of the nose. This interface is heavier than nasal masks or pillows but may be required in patients without a patent nasal airway.

Oral masks fit in the mouth between the lips and the teeth. They have a tongue stabilizer, which holds the tongue forward to prevent airway obstruction. Oral masks are not often used in the sleep center. Limitations with this interface include upper airway dryness, rainout associated with heated humidification, and air leakage from the nose.

Total-face masks cover the entire face. It is an alternative for patients unable to obtain a good seal with other masks. It is preferably indicated for patients with facial deformities and those suffering from skin breakdown around the facial area.

Also available are combination devices that include an oral appliance and PAP interface (3). Combination PAP and oral appliance therapy may be an alternative approach for patients unable to tolerate PAP therapy due to high pressures (4).

Most manufacturers provide a size guide for clinicians to use to obtain an accurate mask fit. Using the guide provides a good starting point for finding the right mask for the patient. However, faces and noses are all different, and sometimes it is necessary to try more than one size or type of mask to get an optimal fit. Also, mask sizes differ between manufacturers; a medium-wide mask from one manufacturer may be quite different than a medium-wide mask from another.

Mask selection may also include three-dimensional and two-dimensional facial scanning applications. These applications utilize artificial intelligence and machine learning to provide patients with recommended masks after accounting for patient preferences such as facial hair, preferred sleeping position, as well as nasal congestion and claustrophobia (5).

ORONASAL (FULL-FACE) MASK VERSUS NASAL MASKS AND UPPER AIRWAY OBSTRUCTION

Upper airway resistance and the likelihood of developing OSA is higher when breathing through the mouth than when breathing through the nose. The oronasal (full-face) mask applies positive pressure equally to the nasopharyngeal and oropharyngeal compartments, thus eliminating the pressure gradient that allows the soft palate and tongue to relax and cause an obstruction. Higher PAPs are required, and leaks are significantly higher in patients wearing oronasal (full-face) masks than nasal mask interfaces. Additionally, oronasal (full-face) masks reflect a lower PAP adherence rate. Sleep efficiency, slow-wave sleep, and rapid eye movement sleep are greater during titration with a nasal mask. Patients wearing the nasal pillows mask and those wearing the nasal masks have both reported improved Epworth Sleepiness Scale score and quality of life. The nasal mask and the nasal pillows are equally as effective when treating patients with OSA requiring high pressures (3). Oronasal masks are associated with higher PAPs, higher residual apnea-hypopnea index (AHI), and poorer adherence than nasal masks. Therefore, patients using oronasal (full-face) masks should be closely monitored. Nasal interfaces should *always* be the first choice. There is evidence that the prolonged use of nasal PAP reduces mouth opening and oral breathing. Therefore, even patients with OSA who claim to be mouth breathers could be initiated with nasal masks. Another clinical implication is that sleep studies for PAP titration must be performed with the same type of mask that the patient will use at home. It is highly recommended that nasal masks or nasal pillows be used instead of oronasal (full-face) masks in patients with OSA unless there is a clear indication otherwise (2,5).

CONTRAINDICATIONS FOR ALL MASK TYPES

1. History of allergy to any of the materials used in the mask
2. Acute trauma, infection, or inflammation of the face or head that is in contact with the mask or headgear, respectively
3. Recent surgery of the face, nose, or head until medically cleared for use

CAUTION FOR ALL MASK TYPES (DURING POSITIVE AIRWAY PRESSURE THERAPY)

1. History of trabeculectomy or tube shunt procedure for glaucoma
2. Recent eye surgery until medically cleared to use PAP therapy
3. Uncontrolled glaucoma, or dry eyes
4. Hiatal hernia, impaired lower esophageal sphincter function, or gastric surgery
5. Impaired cough reflex

ADDITIONAL CAUTION FOR FULL-FACE MASKS (DURING POSITIVE AIRWAY PRESSURE THERAPY)

1. Inability to remove the mask without assistance
2. Increased risk of aspiration, including vomiting, excessive gastroesophageal reflux tube feeding, or copious respiratory secretions

CHINSTRAP AND POSITIVE AIRWAY PRESSURE ADHERENCE

Delivery of PAP requires an adequate seal that prevents leakage. Unintentional air leak in the system results in the development of an open circuit that may reduce the pressure of air delivered to the site of obstruction, with associated recurrence of respiratory events. Air can leak from around a mask that does not fit properly. Leaks can also be caused by mouth opening. A chinstrap may be used to reduce mouth leaks by supporting and restricting lower jaw movement (6). Chinstraps are compatible with a wide range of PAP interfaces and typically made from comfortable, adjustable material. An alternate mask for these patients is an oronasal (full-face) mask. Some patients may prefer this kind of mask even without air leakage issues. However, because the full-face mask comes into contact with more of the facial area, it can be difficult to maintain a seal, leading to increased leakage, especially as the pressure is increased. A full-face mask should not be offered as a first choice if the patient has a patent nasal airway.

It is impossible to tell if a mask fits properly when it is not pressurized. Therefore, after ensuring proper measurement, mask selection, and patient comfort, it is critical to initiate a low PAP during the mask-fitting process. Most PAP machines provide a measure of unintentional air leakage. A small amount of leakage is expected, and the value varies by manufacturer and is specific to the mask at a defined pressure. Large leaks can cause irritation of the skin or eyes and prevent delivery of an adequate therapeutic pressure. Leaks can often be remedied by reseating the mask on the face and with minor adjustments of the head strap.

The mask should fit snug and the straps firm but not tight. Masks fitted too tightly can cause excessive air leaks, pressure sores, and discomfort. Tight straps may produce abrasions and, in some patients, cause headache, neck pain, and pressure points in the upper gums and teeth. The well-fitted mask should be loose enough to be pulled away from the face about one-half inch and reseated. If a mask has an acceptable leak level only when the straps are tight, then it may not be an appropriate-sized mask for the patient. When you and the patient are convinced that the mask is comfortable, and the leak level is acceptable, the titration can begin (6).

POSITIVE AIRWAY PRESSURE DESENSITIZATION

Mask comfort is a key factor that can significantly impact a patient's use of PAP therapy, especially in the early stages of therapy, potentially affecting long-term PAP adherence (2). Common complaints may be the interface or therapeutic pressure. Patients should return to the sleep center or PAP supplier for reevaluation. A skilled, knowledgeable, and patient technologist should be able to solicit constructive feedback from the patient to better facilitate a successful treatment plan.

DESENSITIZATION TECHNIQUES

1. Evaluate and measure the patient's face and head carefully and select an appropriate interface and headgear.
2. Allow the patient to handle the mask themself, holding it to the patient's face to assess fit and comfort before connecting the mask to the hose or PAP instrument.

3. Connect the hose to the mask and PAP instrument and allow the patient to hold the mask to the face, gradually introducing pressure at 4 cm H_2O. It is important to allow the patient to have control of the mask.
4. When the patient is comfortable holding the mask as described and breathing with PAP at a low pressure, turn the pressure off and fit the mask and headgear. Show the patient how to disconnect the hose from the mask and have them recline in a recliner or lie supine on a bed.
5. Reinitiate pressure at 4 cm H_2O using heated humidity while the patient is lying down. Offer encouragement, such as "It looks like you are breathing comfortably at this pressure" or "You are doing fine; remember that this is going to help your breathing while you sleep."
6. If the patient is having any difficulty at this low pressure, refrain from increasing the pressure. In some cases, distraction techniques such as watching TV or reading may help the patient tolerate the procedure.
7. If the patient is tolerating the low pressure well, inform them that you will gradually increase the pressure. Remind the patient that they can disconnect the hose if the pressure becomes intolerable. This allows the patient to remain in control of the process.
8. Verify there are no interface leaks or other issues before beginning to increase PAP.
9. Increase pressure gradually in 1-cm increments in a ramping fashion, carefully monitoring patient reaction and tolerance. In general, pressure should be increased to about 8 cm H_2O during the desensitization process.
10. Check for leaks and adjust interface fit, if necessary, and change interface styles as needed. Utilize a chinstrap or oronasal (full-face) mask if mouth breathing is occurring.
11. If the patient has difficulty tolerating higher pressures, particularly exhaling against the pressure, try using pressure relief or bilevel PAP.
12. Remember to continue to reassure the patient and reinforce their success, for example, "You are doing well, keep it up." It is vital to make this a positive experience for the patient.
13. When the patient is able to tolerate 8 cm H_2O for approximately 15 minutes, the desensitization is considered successful. If desensitization is successful, the patient should be able to tolerate a PAP titration study.
14. At the conclusion of the desensitization, ask the patient to summarize their experience. Document your assessment as well as the patient's responses as well as which masks and sizes were trialed.
15. If the patient has difficulty with the mask/interface or does not tolerate the desensitization procedure in the sleep clinic or sleep center, consider sending the patient home with the PAP equipment to continue the process at home for a period of 1 to 2 weeks. Give the patient specific written instructions for the process to follow at home. Some patients become more tolerant of the mask in their own home or surroundings. This can be accomplished by instructing the patient to wear the mask in the evening, with or without pressure as tolerated while watching TV until they can tolerate it for at least 30 minutes. Once the mask is tolerated, desensitization in the sleep clinic or sleep center can be attempted again.
16. If the patient tolerated the mask but had difficulty with the pressure, consider sending them home with a PAP device set to approximately 8 cm H_2O and a 30-minute ramp time. Instruct the patient on how to reset the ramp to lower the pressure at any time and encourage them to practice outside of the sleep period, perhaps while reclining and watching TV in the evening, until they are able to tolerate the pressure at 8 cm H_2O. Once this is accomplished, the patient can be scheduled for a PAP titration study (1).

The desensitization process may be challenging yet very rewarding for the technologist. Through continued support and encouragement, most patients can tolerate and benefit from PAP therapy. Desensitization techniques, interface options, pressure relief technology, and humidification along with support, empathy, and understanding from the technologist will have a considerable effect on successful patient outcomes.

TIPS TO HELP YOUR PATIENT ADJUST TO COMMON POSITIVE AIRWAY PRESSURE PROBLEMS

1. **Difficulty wearing a PAP interface**
   Have the patient wear the mask for short periods during the day when watching TV, reading a book, or surfing the Internet. When the patient is comfortable with the mask, have him or her wear the mask and hose with the device turned on during the day while they are awake. Once the patient feels comfortable with the mask on the face, ask the patient to start wearing the PAP mask every time they sleep, whether it is at night or during a nap (7,8).
2. **Uncomfortable interface**
   Refit the patient with a different interface, paying attention to the size and style of the mask to ensure a proper fit.

3. **Intolerance of air pressure**
The inability to tolerate the air pressure may be alleviated by using the ramping feature on the PAP machine. This feature allows therapy to begin with low air pressure, which is then followed by an automatic, gradual increase that eventually sets itself to the prescribed pressure. If this feature does not help, bilevel PAP may be a treatment of choice.
4. **Dry or stuffy nose**
Check for proper mask fit and for mask leaks. A mask leak can dry out the nose. Check to make sure the patient is using the heated humidifier and that it is functioning properly.
Additionally, the use of a nasal saline spray at bedtime may help prevent irritation from dry nasal passages.
5. **Mask leak, skin irritation, or pressure sores**
A leaky or an ill-fitting mask may be irritating to the patient's skin, causing pressure sores or directing air into the eyes, triggering dryness or tearing. You may need to refit the patient with a different size or style of mask, particularly if their weight has changed significantly. Changing to a different interface style, such as a nasal pillow mask, may be helpful. Provide patient education on intentional mask leak, that is, air originating from the exhalation port. It is important to note that PAP mask leaks can occur and set an appropriate expectation that masks may temporarily exhibit leaks with position changes.
6. **Difficulty falling asleep**
Assure the patient that this is not uncommon, but also confirm whether the patient is practicing good sleep hygiene and using the ramp feature on the PAP device. The clinical overlap of patients with insomnia and OSA is approximately 30% to 50%. It is important for clinicians to document the patient's reported difficulty initiating or maintaining sleep to improve acceptance and long-term continuous positive airway pressure (CPAP) adherence (9).
7. **Dry mouth**
Air leaks and oral breathing may dry the mouth of a patient wearing nasal PAP. The use of a chinstrap may alleviate this problem by helping keep the patient's mouth closed.
8. **Unintentional removal of PAP during the night**
It is not uncommon for a patient to unintentionally remove the PAP interface during sleep. This may be a result of nasal congestion. On such occasions, confirming a good mask fit and adding a heated humidity may help. A chinstrap may also help keep the mask on the patient's face. If this removal is a consistent problem, have the patient set an alarm for a few hours after bedtime to check whether the device is still on. The patient can then progressively set the alarm for later in the night as the device is tolerated longer. If the patient removes the mask following prolonged periods of wake succeeding sleep onset, the patient my benefit from cognitive behavioral therapy (9).
9. **Bothersome noise**
The newest generation of PAP devices is virtually silent. However, if the patient finds the device disturbing, confirm whether the device's air filters are clean and unblocked. If they are, have the PAP supplier check the device to ensure it is working properly. If it is and if the noise is still bothersome, earplugs can be helpful, or a fan or "white noise" machine can disguise the noise of the PAP machine.
10. **Bed partner acceptance**
Adherence to PAP is positively influenced by bed partner acceptance. When applicable, a patient's bed partner should be included in the educational process, including the importance of PAP therapy and follow-up care related to sleep disordered breathing (9). Listening to and addressing concerns a bed partner may have about PAP therapy are an important part of the process. Concerns such as machine noise or disruption to their sleep may be avoided through proper education and early intervention.

CONCLUSION

Biomedical engineers have been working to optimize the PAP interface to enhance comfort and adherence. Various masks are available that use different anchor points on the face and different strategies to hold the mask in place. Innovative methods allowing patients to sleep on their stomachs while using PAP have been developed. Hose holders, special pillows, and pressure relief devices have been developed to assist patients in achieving their goals.

The PAP acclimation and choice of interface are integral facilitators of the continued health and well-being of our patients and should therefore be afforded the time and consideration needed to promote successful outcomes.

REFERENCES

1. American Association of Sleep Technologists. Positive airway pressure acclimation and desensitization. 2022. https://aastweb.org/wp-content/uploads/2025/03/Positive-Airway-Pressure-Acclimation-and-Desensitization-Guideline-2022.pdf

2. Luyster FS. Impact of obstructive sleep apnea and its treatments on partners: a literature review. *J Clin Sleep Med*. 2017;13(3):467-477. doi:10.5664/jcsm.6504
3. BaHammam AS, Singh T, George S, et al. Choosing the right interface for positive airway pressure therapy in patients with obstructive sleep apnea. *Sleep Breath*. 2017;21(3):569-575.
4. Tong BK, Tran C, Ricciardiello A, et al. CPAP combined with oral appliance therapy reduces CPAP requirements and pharyngeal pressure swings in obstructive sleep apnea. *J Appl Physiol (1985)*. 2020;129(5):1085-1091. doi:10.1152/japplphysiol.00393.2020
5. Spear L. Remote CPAP mask fittings are easier now, due to the launch of new technologies. Sleep Review. Published August 5, 2020. Accessed February 11, 2025. https://sleepreviewmag.com/sleep-treatments/therapy-devices/cpap-pap-devices/remote-cpap-mask-fittings-easier-technologies/
6. Rowland S, Aiyappan V, Hennessy C, et al. Comparing the efficacy, mask leak, patient adherence, and patient preference of three different CPAP interfaces to treat moderate-severe obstructive sleep apnea. *J Clin Sleep Med*. 2018;14(1):101-108.
7. Andrade RGS, Viana FM, Nascimento JA, et al. Nasal vs oro-nasal CPAP for OSA treatment: a meta-analysis. *Chest*. 2018;153(3):665-674.
8. Brooks R. Top 10 most common CPAP mask problems and discomfort (& how to solve them). American Association of Sleep Technologists. 2015. https://aastweb.org/top-10-most-common-cpap-mask-problems-and-discomfort-how-to-solve-them/
9. Sweetman A, Lack L, Bastien C. Co-Morbid Insomnia and Sleep Apnea (COMISA): prevalence, consequences, methodological considerations, and recent randomized controlled trials. *Brain Sci*. 2019;9(12):371. doi:10.3390/brainsci9120371

Chapter 45
Titration of Continuous Positive Airway Pressure and Bilevel Positive Airway Pressure

CHRISTOPHER SPEIGNER AND BYRON JAMERSON

KEY CONCEPTS/LEARNING OBJECTIVES

The key concepts in this chapter include applying positive airway pressure devices when appropriate to adult and pediatric patients, optimizing pressure settings to eliminate respiratory events and improve sleep pattern, and troubleshooting patient complaints that might interfere with tolerance of treatment.

KEY TERMS

Obstructive sleep apnea
Positive airway pressure (PAP)
RERA (respiratory effort–related arousal)
Split-night
Titration
Treatment-emergent central sleep apnea

No procedure is more challenging for the sleep technologist than positive airway pressure (PAP) titration. Although challenging, PAP titration is also the most potentially rewarding procedure that the technologist will perform in the sleep center. An adequate PAP titration can dramatically improve the health and quality of life for the patient. The technologist must use social skills to prepare the patient for titration and reduce their fears. The technologist interacts with the patient to ensure that a proper mask is chosen and is appropriately fit for comfort and safety. Once the titration begins, the technologist must recognize sleep stages, arousals, and sleep-related breathing events "on the fly" to determine when to change the pressure to normalize respiration. As changes to the pressure level are made, the technologist must evaluate patient responses. All of this must occur within the patient's sleep period, which may be shortened by patient anxiety, resulting in prolonged sleep-onset latency or awakenings.

Most sleep centers have a "split-night" protocol in which the first half of the night is used to make or confirm a diagnosis of obstructive sleep apnea (OSA) and the second half of the night is available for PAP titration. This requires the sleep technologist to closely monitor the patient's sleep and respiratory patterns as well as body position and accomplish the goals of PAP titration in a limited time. Split-night studies are not recommended for pediatric patients less than 12 years of age.

The American Academy of Sleep Medicine (AASM) has provided guidelines for the titration process (1). These guidelines were developed through literature review and consensus. One important conclusion of this review was that appropriate pressure cannot be determined using mathematical models that use height, weight, neck size, airway size, or other measures. The only approved way to determine the pressure needed to normalize breathing is to monitor respiration during a titration study.

The primary goal of PAP titration is to eliminate obstructive respiratory events, including apneas, hypopneas, respiratory effort–related arousals (RERAs), and snoring. A secondary goal of PAP titration is to improve the patient's sleep architecture. There is a window of acceptable pressures for most patients, rather than one absolutely correct pressure. Pressure that is too low will not treat the patient's respiratory events, and pressure that is too high may cause arousals and central respiratory events. These challenges require the sleep technologist to find an optimal pressure level that normalizes breathing without disrupting sleep.

From the moment the patient enters the sleep center, the technologist begins building a rapport with the patient to ensure a positive experience during PAP titration. A positive initial experience with PAP therapy has been shown to predict future adherence to the treatment (2).

Even the best treatment is useless if the patient does not use it. The initial impression of the patient to PAP therapy is an essential factor in treatment adherence. The technologist should work to find the best PAP platform for each patient (within the bounds of the sleep center's policies and procedures) and the most comfortable mask and headgear, and, if necessary, provide heated humidification. Ideally, the titration study provides all the information needed to guide the physician in prescribing the most appropriate treatment for each patient.

Regular meetings between the technologist, the interpreting physician, and the sleep center team provide an opportunity to discuss cases and challenges in determining when to perform a split-night study and address issues that do occur during PAP titrations. The decision to perform a split-night procedure is usually outlined in the sleep center policy manual.

To determine a final pressure for the patient, detailed technologist notes are of utmost importance during PAP titration studies. The technologist is expected to explain why PAP was started, which is typically based on an estimate of the patient's apnea-hypopnea index (AHI). The technologist should always document changes in PAP and the reasons that changes were made. In addition, it is sometimes helpful to note why changes were not made. The technologist may be giving the patient a few minutes to adjust to a change in pressure or waiting to see if sleep-onset central apneas will resolve. A brief note will let the interpreting physician know that the technologist is aware of all aspects of the situations that occur during the titration study and provide insight into the decisions that were made.

PREPARING THE PATIENT FOR POSITIVE AIRWAY PRESSURE TITRATION

Let us look at a split-night study scenario. Put yourself in the patient's shoes (or slippers) for a moment. It is 1 AM and you have been sleeping soundly in the sleep center. The lights go on suddenly, and Bob, the sleep technologist, is at the bedside. He mumbles something about starting treatment. You have no idea what he means. He looks at your face, says "Medium Wide," and begins rummaging in a closet. He pulls out a plastic bag with a contraption inside, connects it to a vacuum cleaner hose, connects the hose to a machine on the bedside table, and tells you to sit up. Looming over you, he presses a plastic mask onto your nose and starts wrapping straps around your head. Can you expect a successful titration? I think not.

Most patients undergoing full-night titrations will have reviewed their diagnostic study with the sleep physician and had a discussion about PAP therapy. Receiving a diagnosis of OSA can cause anxiety, and patients may not remember what they were told in the office. There should be a copy of the diagnostic report in the patient's chart, which the technologist can review with the patient and answer questions the patient might have. The discussion should include an explanation of why PAP is important, device options, and a review of the masks that are available in your sleep center.

When a split-night study has been ordered, the technologist should review the patient's chart thoroughly before their hookup. The AASM recommends that all potential PAP titration candidates receive adequate PAP education, hands-on demonstration, careful mask fitting, and acclimation before titration (1). Surprises may be OK for birthday parties, but they should be avoided whenever possible in the sleep center. The technologist should inform the patient that if the protocol for a split-night study is met, the technologist will come in during the night to initiate PAP.

ANTICIPATING PATIENT CONCERNS

It is best to introduce a patient to PAP therapy before the night of titration in the sleep center. An education session should include a discussion of the rationale for the use of PAP therapy, side effects, mask fitting, and a hands-on demonstration with acclimatization; this is of particular importance for pediatric patients. However, because of time and reimbursement issues, this is not always possible. The technologist may be providing the first introduction the patient has about the PAP device. If this is the case, the technologist should be as comprehensive as possible and allow plenty of time for questions. It may not be clear what a patient is feeling, and for the titration to be successful, you must maintain a positive, "can do" attitude. Explain that the device uses room air and contains a fan that speeds up to produce increased air pressure when the airway is obstructed. Let the patient know that you will be controlling the pressure from another room. Describe the mask options that are available. Reassure the patient that the mask is clean or new and that procedures are in place to reduce infection. One approach to patient education is:

- If possible, allow the patient to watch a video that follows a patient through diagnosis and treatment.
- Show the patient the equipment and describe how it works.
- Let the patient handle the equipment and the mask. Have the patient hold the PAP mask in place (at the lowest pressure of 4 cm H_2O) without strapping the mask on. Allow the patient to practice breathing through the mask until they feel comfortable (a minimum of 2-3 minutes). Next, have the patient

try PAP with the straps holding the mask in place. Demonstrate how to release the headgear in the event the patient panics and needs to remove the mask quickly. Allow the patient to remove the mask.
- Explain that they will be exhaling against the PAP. Explain that a nasal mask works best with the mouth closed and that when the patient opens their mouth, the air will rush out, making it difficult to talk. Slowly raise the pressure to between 8 and 10 cm H_2O in order to demonstrate a higher level of pressure to the patient.

The most common question encountered before PAP titration is "how will I sleep with that on my face?" Telling the patient "almost everyone sleeps" is often not enough. It is more helpful to address the patient's concerns directly. Ask if the patient is concerned about the mask, the pressure, or the newness of the situation. Patients often ask about going to the bathroom during the night, waking with the mask off, feelings of suffocation, and noise. Some technologists provide answers to these questions even before they are asked. It is also helpful to explain that you will be adjusting the pressure throughout the night with the goal of eliminating the patient's respiratory events. Explain that on awakening, the pressure may feel different from the way it did when they fell asleep. Similarly, it is important to be open about the fact that the patient may still have breathing problems during the titration night, as the technologist needs to see respiratory events before increasing PAP. Reviewing this information with the patient before lights out can be beneficial and reduce the patient's apprehension. It is not uncommon for patients to have difficulty falling asleep with PAP in place for the first time.

If a patient is tense or anxious, it may be necessary to let the patient take a break from PAP for a brief time and sit up for a while, instead of having them continue to try to sleep. By having the patient sit quietly, they are likely to calm down and relax, thus increasing the chance that the patient will be able to continue with the PAP titration and be able to sleep. While the patient is sitting up, the technologist can work with the patient to practice using PAP again. The technologist should reduce the pressure before reapplying the mask.

For patients who awaken during the night and have difficulty tolerating PAP while awake, reduce the PAP pressure setting until the patient returns to sleep. Most PAP devices that the patient will have at home will have a ramp feature to allow them to lower the pressure and return to sleep after awakening during the night. Once the patient is asleep, gradually increase to the pressure titrated before the awakening and continue the titration.

With experience, technologists develop techniques and skills to respond to patient concerns and reassure patients in order to get an optimal titration.

Adjustment of Positive Airway Pressure

During a full-night titration, adjustment of pressure begins at lights out. For split-night titrations, the sleep center policy and procedures manual should define the criteria that must be met before beginning titration. The AASM practice parameters (3,4) recommend titration guidelines but do not set a standard for when to begin the titration portion of a split-night study. The basic recommendation is that PAP titration should be started if an AHI higher than 40 is documented during 2 hours of a diagnostic study. Titration may be considered for an AHI between 20 and 40 based on the clinical judgment of the ordering physician. Because this is a recommendation and not a standard, some centers use different thresholds for initiation of a split-night titration. Some sleep centers set thresholds for the AHI that will cover PAP device reimbursement by Medicare. At the time of this writing, the Medicare requirement is an AHI of at least 15 or 5 or more with associated clinical symptoms such as high blood pressure and daytime sleepiness. Sleep centers should have a policy that delineates the cutoff time for starting a split-night titration. In AASM-accredited centers, the medical director is required to provide clear and detailed instructions for all procedures, including PAP titration, in a policy and procedures manual.

Recognizing Inadequate Titration

The core concept of PAP titration is simple: change the pressure until the goals of titration are met (Figure 45-1). The primary goal of PAP titration is the elimination of obstructive respiratory events, including apneas, hypopneas, RERAs, and snoring. A secondary goal of PAP titration is to improve the patient's sleep architecture.

Inadequate pressure is defined by the AASM guidelines (1) as two or more obstructive apneas, three or more hypopneas, five or more RERAs, or three or more minutes of loud snoring in adults. Scoring of these respiratory events during titration is somewhat different

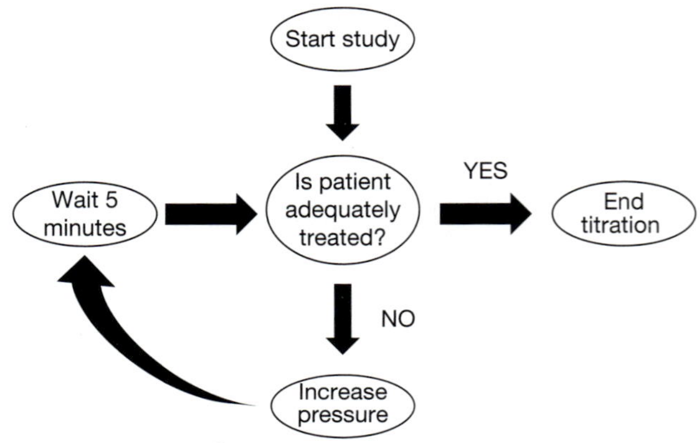

Figure 45-1 Basic titration flow chart.

than during the diagnostic portion of the study because the oronasal thermal sensor and the nasal pressure transducer are typically replaced by a flow measure output from the PAP machine. Scoring of both apneas and hypopneas is therefore based on the PAP device flow signal. According to the AASM scoring manual (5), score a respiratory event as an apnea when there is a drop in the peak signal excursion by 90% or more of the pre-event baseline and the duration of the *90% or more drop in flow* signal is 10 seconds or more. Two rules for scoring of hypopnea are provided:

- Rule 1A Score a respiratory event as a hypopnea when there is a drop in the peak signal excursion by ≥30% of the pre-event baseline, the duration of the ≥30% drop in flow signal is ≥10 seconds, there is a ≥3% oxygen desaturation from pre-event baseline, or the event is associated with an arousal.
- Rule 1B Score a respiratory event as a hypopnea when there is a drop in the peak signal excursion by ≥30% of the pre-event baseline, the duration of the ≥30% drop in flow signal is ≥10 seconds, and there is a ≥4% oxygen desaturation from pre-event baseline.

When scoring a hypopnea, either rule 1A or 1B should be specified in the polysomnography report.

Score the hypopnea as obstructive if there is snoring, an increased inspiratory flattening of the PAP device flow signal compared to baseline, *or* an associated thoracoabdominal paradox that occurs during the event but not during the pre-event.

Score the hypopnea as central if there is no snoring, no increased inspiratory flattening of the PAP device flow signal, *and* no associated thoracoabdominal paradox that occurs during the event but not during the pre-event (5).

The PAP device flow signal will show flattening of the waveform if there is flow restriction, much like the nasal pressure transducer output. If there is a 10-second or more period of signal flattening or an increasing respiratory effort leading to an arousal from sleep, a RERA can be scored. Increasing effort measured by respiratory inductance plethysmography may also be used to score RERAs. Indicators of inadequate titration are shown in Figure 45-2, which demonstrates a flattened flow signal, even without an arousal, and Figure 45-3, which demonstrates a RERA on the basis of the PAP flow channel. Snoring may be difficult to evaluate with a microphone during titration because the PAP device produces noise, which may mask the snoring. A well-placed sensor on the neck that measures vibration is very helpful for proper titration. At times, a "sawtooth" pattern in the PAP flow signal provides an indication of snoring.

The AASM guidelines (1) also outline criteria for an optimal, good, adequate, and unacceptable PAP titration. The overall goal of PAP is to control the patient's

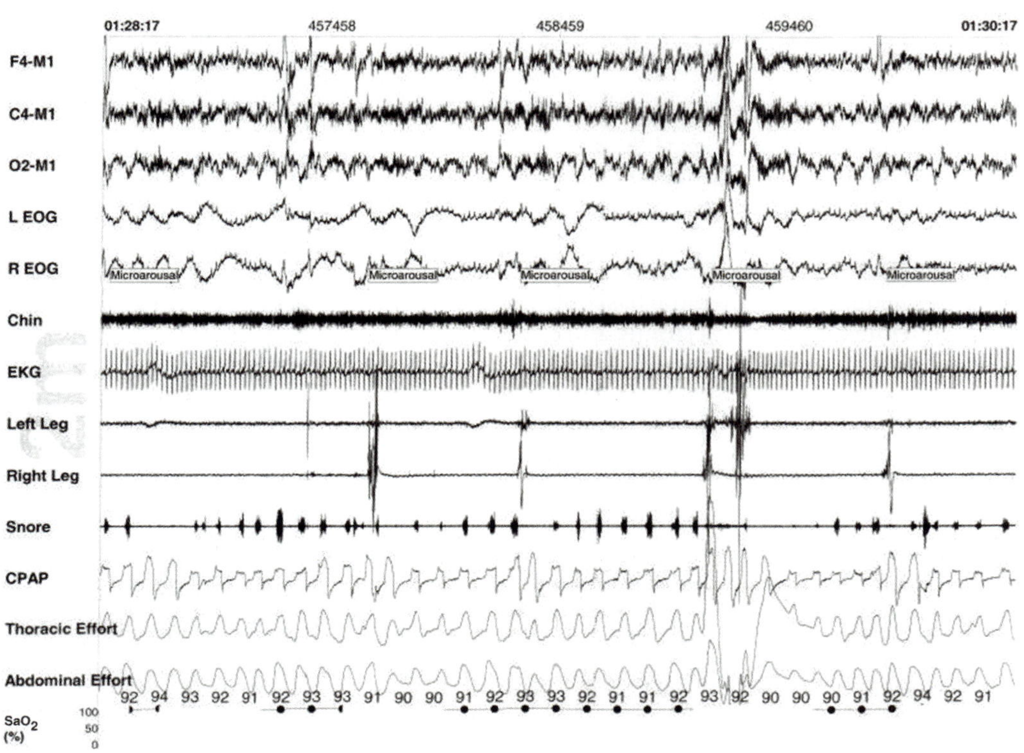

Figure 45-2 A sample of a 2-minute epoch of inadequate titration. CPAP, continuous positive airway pressure; EKG, electrocardiogram; EOG, electrooculography.

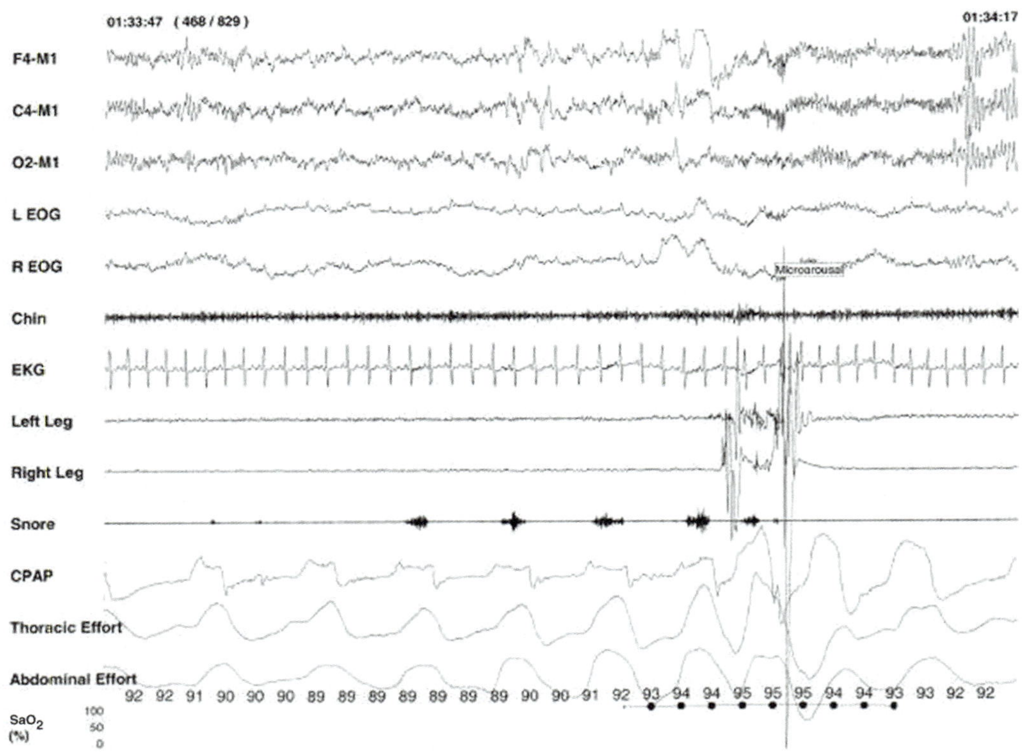

Figure 45-3 A sample of a 30-second epoch with respiratory effort–related arousal indicating inadequate titration. CPAP, continuous positive airway pressure; EKG, electrocardiogram; EOG, electrooculography.

obstructive respiratory events while maintaining Spo_2 above 90%, with acceptable leak parameters at the selected pressure.

- In an *optimal* PAP titration, the selected pressure keeps the Respiratory Disturbance Index (RDI) below 5 for at least 15 minutes while the patient is supine and in stage R sleep without spontaneous arousals or awakenings.
- In a *good* PAP titration, the selected pressure keeps the RDI below 10 or reduced by 50% if the baseline RDI was below 15, while the patient is supine and in stage R sleep without spontaneous arousals or awakenings.
- In an *adequate* PAP titration, the RDI may be above 10 but is reduced by 75% from the baseline study. A PAP titration is also considered *adequate* if it meets the criteria for *optimal* or *good* without evaluation of rapid eye movement (REM) sleep in the supine position.
- An *unacceptable* PAP titration is one that does not meet any of the aforementioned criteria (1).

Increasing Pressure

The AASM guidelines recommend 4 cm H_2O as the starting pressure for continuous PAP (CPAP) (1). This is a very low pressure that is usually ineffective in treating apnea but allows the patient to fall asleep comfortably. The recommended maximum CPAP is 20 cm H_2O for adults and children who are 12 years or older. The maximum recommended CPAP for children under 12 years is 15 cm H_2O.

The guidelines recommend increasing pressure in response to inadequate titration in at least 1 cm H_2O increments. Larger increases are appropriate during retitration of patients who have previously been determined to have high-pressure requirements or if there are other reasons to suspect high pressure will be needed. The guidelines recommend waiting a minimum of 5 minutes between changes in PAP, allowing time to confirm that the pressure is inadequate based on the criteria indicated earlier. It is best to increase the pressure during inspiration, because the patient is less likely to notice the change. At times, a change in pressure may cause an arousal or change in sleep stage. Allowing a few minutes for the patient to settle down also provides a better assessment of the patient's response to the increased pressure.

For pediatric patients, CPAP should be increased by at least 1 cm H_2O with an interval of no less than 5 minutes.

- CPAP should be increased if at least one obstructive apnea is observed in patients younger than 12 years or if at least two obstructive apneas are observed in patients 12 years of age or older.

- CPAP should be increased if at least one hypopnea is observed in patients younger than 12 years or if at least three hypopneas are observed in patients 12 years of age or older.
- CPAP should be increased if at least three RERAs are observed in patients younger than 12 years or if at least five RERAs are observed in patients 12 years of age or older.
- CPAP may be increased if 1 minute of loud or unambiguous snoring is observed in patients younger than 12 years or at least 3 minutes of loud or unambiguous snoring is observed in patients 12 years of age or older.

Reduction of airway resistance has been demonstrated by increasing PAP; however, do not increase the pressure higher than 5 cm H_2O over what is required to control obstructive events.

Ideally, patients should be recorded in supine REM sleep for at least 15 minutes at the designated optimal pressure during the PAP titration study. If the patient is in REM sleep but not in the supine position while at the designated optimal pressure, the patient may be awakened and instructed to lie in the supine position.

Note that the titration process is circular (Figure 45-1). After increasing the pressure, assess the patient to see if the pressure is still inadequate. If the pressure is still inadequate, increase the pressure by at least 1 cm H_2O, wait for 5 minutes, and reassess the patient. The recommended 5-minute rule is a minimum. If the patient has evidence of inadequate titration in the first 2 minutes, wait for at least 5 minutes before making another increase. If the patient does not have evidence of inadequate titration, just wait. The patient may have three RERAs in the first 5 minutes and not have the other two RERAs for 30 minutes. The patient would then meet criteria for inadequate titration at the 30-minute mark, and the pressure should be increased at that point. Remember to document all changes in PAP and the reason for the change on the recording.

The AASM guidelines also recommend exploration of higher pressure levels. In patients who no longer have apneas, hypopneas, RERAs, and snoring, an additional increase in pressure may provide benefits, including resolution of flow limitation (as evidenced by elimination of flow signal flattening) and improved sleep continuity. The guidelines recommend increasing pressure by 2 cm H_2O and no more than 5 cm H_2O over the pressure needed for resolution of respiratory events and snoring (1) in the exploratory phase of PAP titration. Part of this exploration should occur during REM sleep with the patient supine. In most patients, this is the condition during which OSA is at its worst and pressure requirements are greatest. To test patients during REM in a supine position, it may be necessary to enter the patient's room and ask that they try sleeping on their back.

Switching to Bilevel Positive Airway Pressure

Bilevel PAP (BPAP) provides PAP at one level during inspiration (IPAP) and at a lower level during expiration (EPAP). This modality is useful for patients who cannot tolerate CPAP or who complain of trouble exhaling during CPAP therapy (3). To change from CPAP to BPAP during a titration, set the EPAP at the pressure that resolved obstructive events, and set the IPAP 4 cm H_2O higher. BPAP may improve compliance, especially in patients requiring a high pressure. Some sleep centers limit the technologist to CPAP during the initial titration study. Other centers provide guidelines for switching to BPAP in their policy and procedures manual.

To perform a BPAP titration, the AASM guidelines recommend starting at an IPAP of 8 cm H_2O and an EPAP of 4 cm H_2O (1). The maximum recommended BPAP is IPAP of 30 cm H_2O, and the recommended maximum difference between IPAP and EPAP is 10 cm H_2O. Increasing BPAP in patients with inadequate titration is slightly more complicated than CPAP titration. The recommendation is that IPAP and EPAP should be increased in response to apneas, whereas only IPAP should be increased in response to hypopneas, RERAs, and snoring (1). As with CPAP, increases of at least 1 cm H_2O with an interval of at least 5 minutes are recommended.

For pediatric patients, BPAP should be increased by at least 1 cm H_2O with an interval of no less than 5 minutes.

- BPAP should be increased if at least one obstructive apnea is observed in patients younger than 12 years or if at least two obstructive apneas are observed in patients 12 years of age or older.
- BPAP should be increased if at least one hypopnea is observed in patients younger than 12 years or if at least three hypopneas are observed in patients 12 years of age or older.
- BPAP should be increased if at least three RERAs are observed in patients younger than 12 years or if at least five RERAs are observed in patients 12 years of age or older.
- BPAP may be increased if 1 minute of loud or unambiguous snoring is observed in patients younger than 12 years or at least 3 minutes of loud or unambiguous snoring is observed in patients 12 years of age or older.

Reduction of airway resistance has been demonstrated by increasing BPAP; however, do not increase the pressure higher than 5 cm H_2O over what is required to control obstructive events.

As is the case with CPAP titrations, during BPAP titrations, patients should be recorded in supine REM sleep for at least 15 minutes at the designated optimal pressure during the BPAP titration study. If the patient is in REM sleep but not in the supine position while at the designated optimal pressure, the patient may be awakened and instructed to lie in the supine position.

As an example, BPAP titration may proceed as follows: the patient begins the night at IPAP 8 cm H_2O and EPAP 4 cm H_2O. Within the first 30 minutes, two obstructive apneas are seen. The technologist raises the pressure to IPAP 9 and EPAP 5 and waits 5 minutes. During the next 5 minutes, two more obstructive apneas are recorded. The pressure is increased to IPAP 10 and EPAP 6. Additional apneas are observed, and the pressure is increased to IPAP 11 and EPAP 7. At this point, apneas resolve, but three hypopneas occur in the next 20 minutes. In response to the hypopneas, only the IPAP should be increased. IPAP should be increased to 12 and EPAP remains at 7. Over the next 20 minutes, three more hypopneas are seen. Pressure is increased to IPAP 13 and EPAP remains at 7. At this pressure, hypopneas resolve, but moderate snoring persists. After 3 minutes of continuous loud snoring, the IPAP is once again increased to 14 and EPAP remains at 7. At this pressure, the snoring resolves, and the patient sleeps soundly for the remainder of the night. For home use, BPAP is recommended at IPAP 14 and EPAP 7 for this patient.

Decreasing Pressure

Increasing pressure until the breathing becomes normal is one way to determine the appropriate pressure for a patient. Patients will have a "therapeutic window" of effective PAP. If the pressure is too low, the respiratory events will continue. If the pressure is too high, the patient may develop frequent arousals and/or treatment-emergent central sleep apneas (6).

The determination of the therapeutic window of PAP for a given patient may require a slightly different method than the one outlined earlier. The "staircase method" made famous by the psychophysicist Georg von Békésy, also referred to as an "up-down-up titration," involves starting the pressure low and increasing until it is clearly too high, then reducing the pressure until it is too low. The final step is to once again increase the pressure until it is too high. This process provides a more precise definition of the therapeutic window for each patient. Unfortunately, it takes more time than the standard methods and may not be possible to accomplish during a split-night study.

Indicators that PAP is too high include frequent arousals and the appearance of treatment-emergent central sleep apnea (Figures 45-4 and 45-5). The most certain indicator of excessive pressure is the patient waking up, complaining that the pressure is too high. When indicators of excessive pressure are seen, the pressure should be reduced in 1 cm H_2O increments until the indicators disappear. A larger decrease in pressure may be necessary when the patient is awake and complaining. In this case, the pressure should be decreased to a level that feels comfortable to the patient. After decreasing the pressure, it is critically important to monitor the

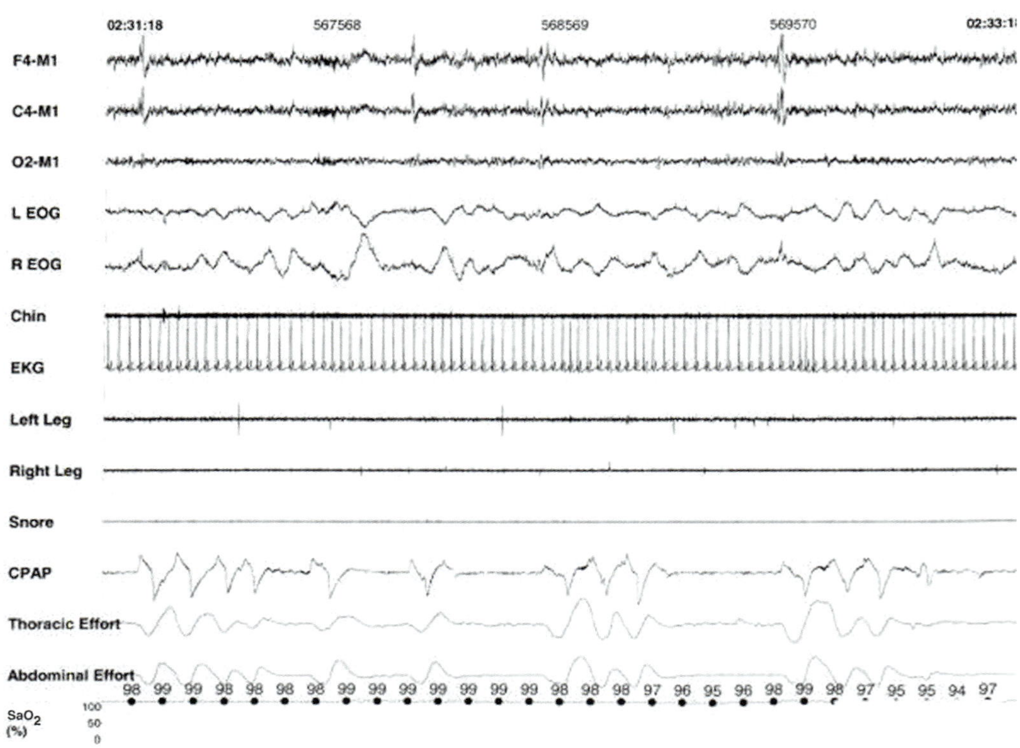

Figure 45-4 A sample of a 2-minute epoch of central apneas caused by overtitration. CPAP, continuous positive airway pressure; EKG, electrocardiogram; EOG, electrooculography.

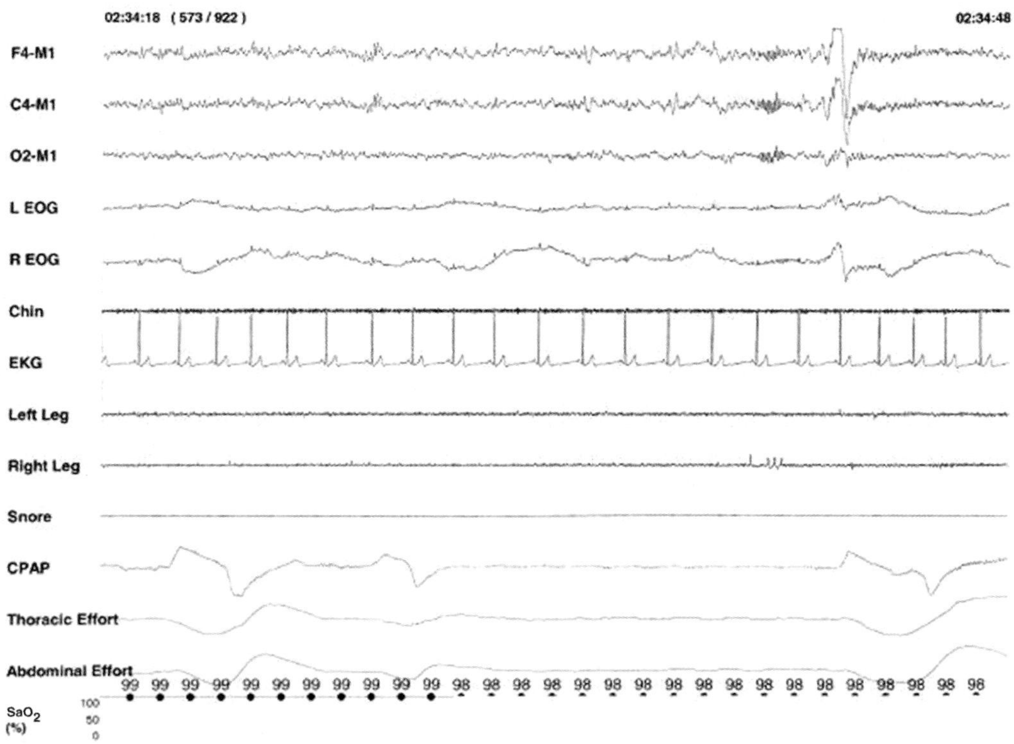

Figure 45-5 Sample 30-second epoch showing central apnea due to overtitration. CPAP, continuous positive airway pressure; EKG, electrocardiogram; EOG, electrooculography.

patient to be sure that the new pressure setting is adequate, particularly as the patient falls back to sleep. In a few patients, the pressure that adequately treats the OSA may be too high for patient comfort. In other words, the therapeutic window may be very narrow or may not even exist. In these cases, several trials of waiting for the patient to enter consolidated sleep using a low pressure and then gradually increasing the pressure until it is adequate provides the maximum information for the interpreting physician. Careful technologist documentation is an essential part of this process. These patients will usually tolerate PAP at home using a machine with a "ramp" feature that they can activate as needed. The ramp feature reduces the pressure and then gradually increases it over a preset time, allowing the patient to adjust over time to the higher pressure necessary to control their sleep-disordered breathing.

A flowchart that indicates appropriate increases and decreases in pressure, as well as a check for stage REM sleep with the patient supine, is shown in Figure 45-6.

Down titrating during a BPAP titration typically involves a 1 cm H_2O decrease in both the IPAP and EPAP at the same time. In cases where an increase in IPAP only was made in response to hypopnea, RERA, or snoring, which seems to lead directly to arousals, a decrease in IPAP alone may be considered. An attempt to monitor

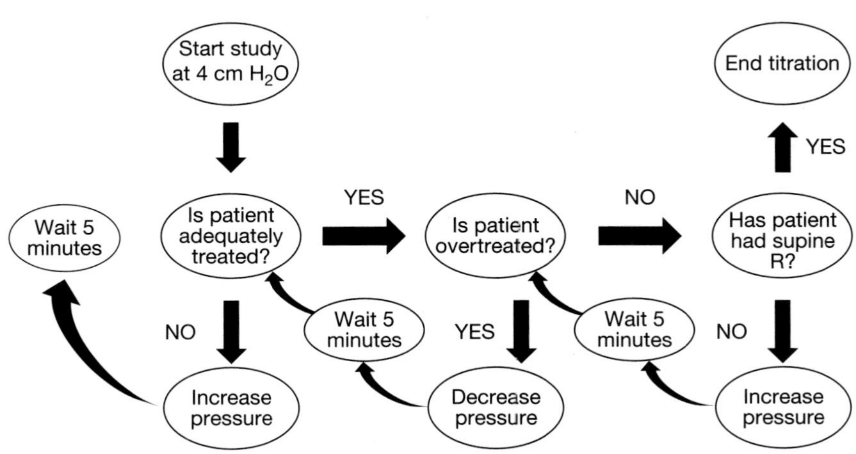

Figure 45-6 A sample of positive airway pressure titration flowchart.

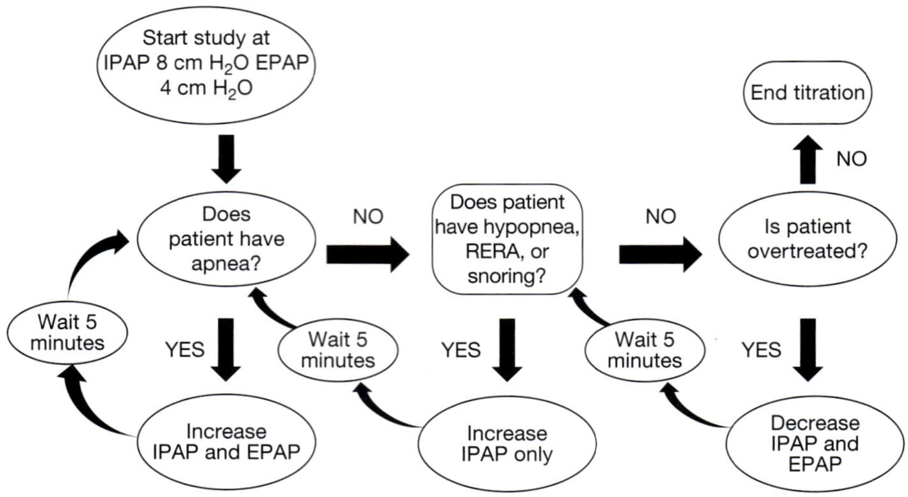

Figure 45-7 Sample bilevel positive airway pressure titration flowchart. EPAP, expiratory positive airway pressure; IPAP, inspiratory positive airway pressure; RERA, respiratory effort–related arousal.

the patient in stage REM sleep while supine is important during a BPAP titration as well. Figure 45-7 provides a sample flowchart for performing a BPAP titration.

Supplemental Oxygen

Supplemental oxygen should be added to the PAP titration in accordance with physician instructions and the Policy and Procedure manual for the center. For many centers, this occurs if the patient is awake, in the supine position, and the oxygen saturation (Spo_2) is less than 88%. During the titration, in the absence of obstructive respiratory events, oxygen (O_2) may be added when the Spo_2 is less than 88% for more than 5 minutes. In both situations, oxygen should be initiated at 1 L/min and titrated upward to achieve a Spo_2 range of 88% to 94%. O_2 should be increased by 1 L/min with at least a 15-minute time interval. The minimum starting O_2 rate should be 1 L/min for both pediatric and adult patients (1). Remember to always read the patient chart and note any comorbid conditions (chronic obstructive pulmonary disease, hypercapnia) that could be affected by the addition of supplemental oxygen. Refer to the center Policy and Procedure manual for specific instructions on titrating supplemental oxygen in those patients.

ALTERNATIVE POSITIVE AIRWAY PRESSURE PLATFORMS

Advances in technology have led to the development of several new PAP devices. Most of these build on the BPAP platform and provide changes in applied pressure that result from measured changes in flow. BPAP decreases applied pressure when patient expiration is detected. Flex-PAP or pressure relief provides a brief decrease in pressure when expiration is detected and, in some patients, may feel more comfortable than CPAP. Autotitrating positive airway pressure (APAP) therapy devices detect periods of apnea and hypopnea and increase pressure for a time in response.

APAP has been approved for several uses by the AASM:

1. In some centers, APAP is used to titrate pressure during an attended sleep study, with a final fixed CPAP determined for home use.
2. APAP can be used as a treatment device by patients requiring changes in pressure as determined by the device.
3. APAP may be used by the patient at home and a fixed pressure determined based on the information stored in the device. It is recommended that patients using APAP be evaluated on a regular basis to ensure that the treatment is adequate (7).

APAP devices have not been tested and therefore should not be used in patients with OSA who have significant comorbid conditions, such as chronic obstructive pulmonary disease, in patients with central sleep apnea, or in patients who do not snore. There are several devices that provide autotitration, and the parameters that can be changed vary from device to device. If APAP devices are used, centers are required to include autotitration protocols as part of their Policy and Procedure manual.

Adaptive servo-ventilation (ASV) monitors breathing on a breath-by-breath basis and continuously modifies pressure in response to changes. The advantage of ASV over other PAP platforms is that it can respond to hypoventilation (decreased airflow without apnea). There are some data that suggest that ASV may be useful in patients with central apnea or Cheyne-Stokes breathing pattern because it may counteract the waxing and waning of airflow. Most sleep specialists recommend a trial of standard CPAP before switching to ASV and close monitoring of patients once they are on treatment (7).

Troubleshooting

Studies have shown that APAP results in final pressure settings that are not statistically different from attended titrations (6). However, an experienced technologist can have an important impact on treatment by resolving mask and tolerance problems during the night of PAP titration.

MASK PROBLEMS

The most common problem requiring technologist intervention during titration is mask leak. Each mask will have an *acceptable leak* value that arises mainly from the CO_2 port of the mask and increases with increasing pressure. Most manufacturers have published guides that identify acceptable leaks for their masks at various pressures. Two factors that often lead to the development of unacceptable leakages during the course of a titration are movement-related problems and pressure-related problems. For further details, see Chapter 44.

HUMIDIFICATION

During normal breathing, room air is warmed, moistened, and cleaned in the nose before it is inhaled into the lungs. PAP devices push air quickly through the nose and sinuses, which can prevent the usual warming, moistening, and cleaning. This often results in a sensation of cold and dryness in the throat for patients using PAP, which is especially problematic in areas where the air is already cold and dry. Saliva production is decreased during sleep, and heated humidification is particularly necessary when using a full-face mask. It is important to have adequate humidification to reduce patient arousals and complaints caused by a dry mouth. A heated humidification unit, which is available as an add-on to PAP devices, is typically a "pass over" device in which the air going to the patient passes over a pool of warmed water. The temperature of the water must be regulated to avoid excessive warming and humidification, which causes water to pool in the tubing that connects the machine to the PAP interface.

After the heated humidification process occurs at the PAP device, the air must travel 6 to 8 ft (1.8-2.4 m) through a plastic tube before it reaches the mask. If tubing is exposed to room air, it will cool during its journey. Cooling can be reduced by directing the tubing under the bedcovers or by wrapping the tubing in a sheath. Tubing sheaths come in various materials and colors and may provide some benefit for patients. In addition, some manufacturers have developed heated tubing, which has served to improve adherence in some patients.

FOLLOW-UP

Technologists should be involved in the sleep center's efforts to improve PAP adherence. Studies have shown that early intervention may be the most effective method for improving adherence to therapy. Some insurance carriers require demonstration of adherence 3 months after treatment begins, and the technologist may be involved in this process as well. Key elements of follow-up include documentation of usage (usually by a download from the PAP device), response to questions and concerns, replacement of masks and tubing when indicated, and a discussion of alternatives when appropriate.

A useful quality improvement exercise is to provide feedback to the titration technologist on the successful and unsuccessful treatment of patients. Over time, it is possible to evaluate the effectiveness of policies and strategies. Procedures can be modified to improve adherence—keep doing what works and stop doing what does not work. Working together, the sleep center team can provide optimal treatment for patients. Proper titration, appropriate equipment adjustments, and timely follow-up are key elements of the evaluation and treatment of patients with OSA.

REFERENCES

1. Kushida CA, Chediak A, Berry RB, et al. Clinical guidelines for the manual titration of positive airway pressure in patients with obstructive sleep apnea. *J Clin Sleep Med*. 2008;4(2):157-171.
2. Budhiraja R, Parthasarathy S, Drake CL, et al. Early CPAP use identifies subsequent adherence to CPAP therapy. *Sleep*. 2007;30(3):320-324.
3. Epstein LJ, Kristo D, Strollo PJ Jr, et al. Clinical guideline for the evaluation, management and long-term care of obstructive sleep apnea in adults. *J Clin Sleep Med*. 2009;5(3):263-276.
4. Kushida CA, Littner MR, Morgenthaler T, et al. Practice parameters for the indications for polysomnography and related procedures: an update for 2005. *Sleep*. 2005;28(4):499-521.
5. Troester MM, Quan SF, Berry RB, et al; for the American Academy of Sleep Medicine. *The AASM Manual for the Scoring of Sleep and Associated Events: Rules, Terminology and Technical Specifications. Version 3*. American Academy of Sleep Medicine; 2023.
6. American Academy of Sleep Medicine. *International Classification of Sleep Disorders*. 3rd ed. American Academy of Sleep Medicine; 2014.
7. Morgenthaler TI, Aurora RN, Brown T, et al. Practice parameters for the use of autotitrating continuous positive airway pressure devices for titrating pressures and treating adult patients with obstructive sleep apnea syndrome: an update for 2007. *Sleep*. 2008;31(1):141-147.

Chapter 46
Advanced Positive Airway Pressure Therapies for Sleep-Disordered Breathing

CYNTHIA D. MATTICE

KEY CONCEPTS/LEARNING OBJECTIVES

The key concepts for this chapter include the use of advanced positive airway pressure devices in the sleep center setting, including adaptive servo-ventilation, spontaneous timed, and volume-assured pressure support, including the indications and limitations of these therapy modes and the operation and algorithms for the titration of both ResMed and Philips Respironics model devices.

KEY TERMS

Adaptive servo-ventilation (ASV)
Alveolar ventilation (Va)
Central sleep apnea syndrome (CSAS)
Congestive heart failure (CHF)
Minute ventilation (MV)
Sleep-related hypoventilation disorder
Spontaneous breathing
Spontaneous timed (ST)
Volume-assured pressure support (VAPS)

INDICATIONS FOR ADVANCED POSITIVE AIRWAY PRESSURE THERAPY MODES

Positive airway pressure (PAP) technology has advanced dramatically since continuous positive airway pressure (CPAP) was first offered as a treatment for sleep-disordered breathing (SDB) in 1983 (1,2). One of the many reasons for these advancements is the increase in the understanding of SDB. Conditions that were once frustrating and baffling to both sleep technologists and physicians are now treatable by specific PAP therapy modes utilizing advancements in technology and algorithms (2). This chapter focuses on advanced PAP therapy modes applicable to a typical sleep disorders center: adaptive servo-ventilation (ASV), volume-assured pressure support (VAPS), and spontaneous timed (ST). This chapter will cover the indications for their use and the specific devices used in the sleep disorders center at the time of this writing. The two primary manufacturers of these advanced PAP devices, ResMed and Philips Respironics, each offer training and documentation with every major release in technology; however, the mode types and principles of their instructions have been consistent since their development. The technologist must have a clear understanding of each modality and their indications to properly perform testing using these therapies.

Adaptive Servo-Ventilation for Central Sleep Apnea Syndrome

ASV is a PAP therapy mode specifically intended for central sleep apnea syndrome (CSAS) (3). The *International Classification of Sleep Disorders (ICSD) 3* identifies eight different forms of central sleep apnea (CSA): central sleep apnea with Cheyne-Stokes breathing, central apnea due to medical disorder without Cheyne-Stokes breathing, central sleep apnea due to high-altitude periodic breathing, central sleep apnea due to medication or substance, primary central sleep apnea, primary sleep apnea of infancy, primary sleep apnea of prematurity, and treatment-emergent central sleep apnea (4). CSAS is described thoroughly in Chapter 11. ASV was first introduced by ResMed and was first validated as a treatment for CSAS with Cheyne-Stokes breathing in 2001 (5). Philips Respironics soon produced their own version (2,6). By 2012, ASV was an American Academy of Sleep Medicine (AASM)–recommended treatment option (7). Before the availability of ASV, treatment of CSAS was especially difficult. CPAP, bilevel positive airway pressure (BPAP), BPAP ST, and oxygen therapy were long-standing treatment options for CSAS with varying levels of success (2,8). The primary function of ASV is to respond to irregular ventilation caused by CSA to maintain proper respiration. ASV is indicated only for CSA (2,3,5-7).

Variable-Assured Pressure Support for Hypoventilation Syndromes

VAPS is a type of PAP therapy that is applicable to patients diagnosed with hypoventilation disorders (9,10). Sleep-related hypoventilation disorders include obesity hypoventilation syndrome, congenital alveolar hypoventilation syndrome, late-onset central hypoventilation with hypothalamic dysfunction, idiopathic central alveolar hypoventilation, sleep-related hypoventilation due to a medication or substance, and sleep-related hypoventilation due to a medical disorder (4). Therefore, indication for VAPS in the sleep center setting may include patients with diagnosed chronic hypoventilation syndromes such as neuromuscular/restrictive disorders, chronic obstructive pulmonary disorder, or obesity hypoventilation. There is a full explanation of obesity hypoventilation syndromes in Chapter 12. Although there are many similar terms and setting descriptions between ASV and VAPS, the two modalities are not interchangeable (10,11). VAPS uses variable pressure support to achieve a target tidal volume (VT), in contrast to ASV, which performs a quick constant breath-by-breath response and does not augment the patient's VT consistently (10,11). VAPS is an AASM-recommended option for patients with chronic hypoventilation receiving PAP therapy adjustment in the sleep center (12).

Bilevel Positive Airway Pressure Spontaneous-Timed Mode for Hypoventilation Syndromes

BPAP ST mode refers to a BPAP with an added backup inspiratory rate. Like VAPS, it is indicated for SDB in patients with chronic alveolar hypoventilation syndrome (13,14). The ST mode can be applied to standard BPAP or VAPS modes, and AASM guidelines recommend its use in patients with alveolar hypoventilation syndromes with central hypoventilation, having a significant number of central apneas or an inappropriately low respiratory rate (RR), and who unreliably trigger inspiration PAP (IPAP)/expiration PAP (EPAP) cycles because of muscle weakness (15). It is also enabled in ASV mode and assists the ASV algorithm with resolving central apnea (3). Regular BPAP in ST mode is not indicated for the treatment of CSAS; however, there is a history of the mode being used for that purpose, and it is listed within AASM guidelines as an optional treatment modality when ASV, CPAP, and oxygen therapies are exhausted (15).

FUNDAMENTALS OF THERAPEUTIC MODES

Adaptive Servo-Ventilation

In contrast to standard BPAP that provides static IPAP and EPAP, ASV delivers variable inspiratory pressure support to maintain respiration (3). Although auto CPAP and auto BPAP have varying pressure outputs, those modes increase or decrease on the basis of the detection of upper airway obstruction. ASV uses an algorithm to detect unstable ventilation and compensate with a variable pressure support. Pressure support is the amount of inspiratory pressure above the exhalation pressure. For example, consider a standard BPAP set to IPAP 10/EPAP 6, that is, the expiratory pressure is 6 cm, and the inspiratory pressure is 10 cm. Therefore, the pressure support (Ps) is 4 cm (EPAP 6 cm + 4 cm Ps = 10 cm IPAP). This term is sometimes interchangeable with delta (Δ) pressure, or delta P (ΔP).

Both the Philips Respironics version of ASV, called BPAP autoSV Advanced, and the ResMed version, AirCurve 11 ASV, follow the same general principle explained in the preceding paragraph but have different proprietary algorithms.

The BPAP autoSV monitors the inspiratory peak flow rate (IPFR) of the patient on a breath-by-breath basis. IPFR is the highest amount of liters per minute (L/min) inhaled during a respiratory cycle. Every 4 minutes of monitoring, the device calculates an average peak flow for the patient. This is regarded as a moving 4-minute window, because the most current data continuously override previous data. Once this average peak flow is calculated, the device delivers pressure support to compensate for breathing that falls short of the average peak flow on a per-breath basis. By default, the devices provide an ST backup rate that synchronizes with the patient's spontaneous breathing; however, the setting can be overridden and set to a specific rate. Because a patient's SDB often includes an obstructive component even when predominantly central in nature, the ASV models must also be able to compensate for obstruction. The EPAP can be set to a static setting or an auto setting, in which the EPAP uses Philips Respironics–patented auto PAP algorithm to increase and decrease pressure according to the detection of upper airway obstruction (13).

The ResMed AirCurve 11 ASV algorithm differs in that rather than focusing on peak flow rate, its algorithm focuses on minute ventilation (MV). MV is the total amount of air that moves in and out of the ventilation system, and it is calculated by multiplying the RR by VT. The device monitors MV on a breath-by-breath basis and uses a moving 3-minute window of monitoring to calculate target MV. The device then delivers pressure support to compensate for breathing that falls short of the target MV. AirCurve 11 ASV incorporates an ST backup rate somewhat differently than its Philips Respironics counterpart. The backup rate is set to a minimum of 15 breaths per minute (BPM) and is not adjustable by the clinician. The rate may occur during the first 3 minutes of therapy. The EPAP can be set to a static setting or an auto setting, in which the EPAP uses a ResMed-patented auto PAP algorithm to increase and decrease pressure according to the detection of upper airway obstruction (16).

Volume-Assured Pressure Support

Like ASV, VAPS delivers variable inspiratory pressure support to maintain respiration. However, the algorithms and intended purposes are much different. VAPS uses its algorithm to detect insufficient volume or ventilation and compensate with a variable pressure support. Key to the ability of VAPS to adequately perform its function is the input of applicable patient parameters by the technologist performing the titration so that the algorithm of the device can properly calculate the target volume or ventilation (11,17). Because the respiratory needs of a patient with hypoventilation can vary through the night, this type of PAP is often helpful for these patients because it is able to constantly adapt throughout the night. These needs can vary significantly according to body position, sleep stage, or sleep versus wake for patients required to use PAP during the day because of the severity of disease (2).

The two versions of VAPS devices available to the sleep center are the ResMed intelligent volume-assured pressure support (iVAPS) mode and the Philips Respironics average volume-assured pressure support (AVAPS). ResMed iVAPS utilizes an algorithm on the basis of a target alveolar volume set by the clinician (2). Alveolar volume is inspired air that reaches the alveoli. The volume of inspired air that does not reach the alveoli is referred to as "dead space ventilation." The dead space gas in the conducting airways (the nose, mouth, pharynx, larynx, and lower airways down to, but not including, the respiratory bronchioles) is referred to as "anatomic dead space." The iVAPS algorithm calculates alveolar ventilation by measuring the volume of each breath and subtracting an approximated value of anatomic dead space. From this, a continuous estimate of alveolar ventilation is calculated, and pressure support is then appropriately applied to achieve this target. With Philips Respironics AVAPS, the algorithm depends on a set target VT (2). VT is the volume of air that normally moves into and out of the lungs in one quiet breath. The set VT can be input by the clinician according to ordering provider suggestion, patient comfort, or ideal body weight. Both devices may incorporate ideal body weight into their settings and calculations. The device manufacturer recommends that ideal body weight in kilograms be multiplied by 6 mL/kg (ResMed) or 8 mL/kg (Philips Respironics) to find a target VT setting (2).

Spontaneous-Timed Mode

ST mode is a combination of spontaneous mode and timed mode. Spontaneous mode is the term commonly referred to as BPAP. The term "spontaneous" refers to the fact that the patient's own natural breathing triggers the change from EPAP to IPAP. Timed mode refers to a set rate in BPM that triggers the change from EPAP to IPAP. Timed mode would be applicable to patients completely unable to initiate a breath without the assistance of the device. ST, then, is a combination of the two methods: the patient's natural breathing triggers the change from EPAP to IPAP, unless the patient's natural breathing rate falls below a rate set by the clinician. The rate set during ST mode is referred to as a backup rate because the timed function is essentially a backup used when the patient's natural breathing falls below a certain rate (18).

CONTRADICTIONS, LIMITATIONS, AND ALTERNATIVES

CSAS has several pathologies, including heart failure. Heart failure is characterized by the heart's inability to pump an adequate supply of blood to the body. Congestive heart failure (CHF) refers to the stage in which fluid builds up around the heart and causes it to pump inefficiently. Severity of CHF is commonly determined by left ventricular ejection fraction (LVEF). LVEF is the percentage of blood that is pumped out of a filled left ventricle with each heartbeat. In 2015, a clinical trial called the *Treatment of Predominant Central Sleep Apnoea by Adaptive Servo Ventilation in Patients with Heart Failure (SERVE-HF)* tested the hypothesis that ASV would reduce incidences of heart failure such as all-cause mortality, life-saving cardiovascular interventions, or unplanned hospitalizations for worsening heart failure. The trial was, however, cut short after a discovery that ASV treatment caused a 34% increase in cardiovascular mortality in patients who have heart failure with a reduced ejection fraction. These findings resulted in ResMed, which had funded the trial, issuing a Field Safety Notice that same year stating that ASV therapy is contraindicated in patients who have CHF with an LVEF equal to or less than 45%. Two possible explanations were suggested by the study. One is a theory that has been previously suggested, namely, that CSA may be a compensatory mechanism for patients with heart failure, while the other is that PAP can impair cardiac function in certain patients with heart failure (19).

This information led to an update of AASM CSAS treatment guidelines in 2016 regarding the implementation of ASV for patients with heart failure. The updated guidelines state that ASV for the treatment of CSAS related to CHF *should not be used in adults with an ejection fraction equal to or less than 45%* and *can be used for the*

ASV is an appropriate modality for patients with moderate to severe predominantly central sleep apnea who ***do not have heart failure***. The following are steps to assess patients for ASV therapy:

- Verify the patient is not at risk for heart failure (HF).
  - Does the patient have signs or symptoms of heart failure?
  - Is there a history of cardiovascular disease?
  - Does the patient take medications used to treat heart failure?
- Consider an echocardiogram to determine left ventricular ejection fraction (LVEF) if there is any suspicion of heart failure.

ASV can also be used appropriately *in some patients with possible or definite heart failure with a documented LVEF of > 45%*. Cardiology assessment is essential including an echocardiogram to assess LVEF.

*ASV is **not** appropriate for use in patients with heart failure with a documented left ventricular ejection fraction (LVEF) of ≤ 45%*. Cardiology assessment is essential including an echocardiogram to document the LVEF.

Figure 46-1 Assessment of patients with moderate to severe predominant central sleep apnea for consideration for adaptive servo-ventilation therapy.

treatment of CSAS related to CHF in adults with an ejection fraction over 45%. ASV is still recommended for CSAS not related to heart failure (Figure 46-1).

In the sleep lab setting, it is, of course, ideal that a comprehensive policy and procedure manual and thorough patient history exist, leaving the technologist with a clear course of action for patients with CSAS. ResMed's sleep lab titration guide contains a flowchart that may be useful to the technologist lacking a clear direction (13).

Guidelines for the treatment of CSAS related to heart failure indicate ASV for patients failing an initial trial of CPAP and BPAP ST, as an optional treatment if there is no response to adequate trials of CPAP and oxygen therapies. Oxygen therapy is an indicated treatment for CSAS related to CHF. Of note, these guidelines explain that in studies testing the effectiveness of CPAP and BPAP in CSAS, BPAP ST has been used more frequently; however, data that support BPAP ST being more than just an optional treatment (or not) are limited (15).

Treatment of CHF, including pharmaceutical treatment, is recommended for CSAS related to heart failure in any case. AASM guidelines state that acetazolamide and theophylline, if accompanied by close clinical follow-up and after optimization of standard medical therapy, are options for the treatment of CSAS related to CHF if PAP therapy is not tolerated (15).

VAPS is not recommended for patients with CSAS. Treatment of CSAS requires a variable, breath-by-breath response, so that respiration stabilizes quickly. Breath-by-breath response prevents overshooting or undershooting; VAPS does not have this quick variable response to changes in respiration. It is designed to adjust and maintain a constant VT with each breath over time (11).

ASV is not recommended to address chronic hypoventilation or for patients with neuromuscular disease having sleep-related hypoventilation. ASV's frequent variable adaptation to respiration is not designed for hypoventilation and could potentially worsen the occurrence as the night progresses (11).

CONCLUSION

The advancement of PAP technology, as well as clinical research and understanding of sleep-related breathing disorders over the past decade, has been vast. This allows sleep clinicians to treat patients and improve quality of life in ways not possible in the past. As technology continues to advance, manufacturers of the said technology strive to provide training for sleep medicine professionals to keep them up to date in advancements. It is the responsibility of the sleep technologist to ensure that they have a sound understanding of the fundamentals of these technologies. Thorough knowledge of key respiratory principles and terminology and the PAP settings that affect these is required. The greater the understanding, the more prepared the technologist will be to provide exceptional patient care.

REFERENCES

1. Sullivan CE, Issa FG, Berthon-Jones M, et al. Reversal of obstructive sleep apnoea by continuous positive airway pressure applied through the nares. *Lancet*. 1981;1(8225):862-865.
2. Johnson KG, Johnson DC. Treatment of sleep-disordered breathing with positive airway pressure devices: technology update. *Med Devices (Auckl)*. 2015;8:425.

3. Javaheri S, Brown LK, Randerath WJ. Positive airway pressure therapy with adaptive servoventilation: Part 1: operational algorithms. *Chest*. 2014;146(2): 514-523.
4. American Academy of Sleep Medicine. *International Classification of Sleep Disorders*. 3rd ed. American Academy of Sleep Medicine; 2014.
5. Teschler H, Döhring J, Wang YM, et al. Adaptive pressure support servo-ventilation: a novel treatment for Cheyne-Stokes respiration in heart failure. *Am J Respir Crit Care Med*. 2001;164(4):614-619.
6. Allam JS, Olson EJ, Gay PC, et al. Efficacy of adaptive servoventilation in treatment of complex and central sleep apnea syndromes. *Chest*. 2007;132(6): 1839-1846.
7. Aurora RN, Chowdhuri S, Ramar K, et al. The treatment of central sleep apnea syndromes in adults: practice parameters with an evidence-based literature review and meta-analyses. *Sleep*. 2012;35(1):17-40.
8. Verbraecken J. Complex sleep apnoea syndrome. *Breathe*. 2013;9(5):372-380.
9. Oscroft NS, Smith IE. A bench test to confirm the core features of volume-assured non-invasive ventilation. *Respirology*. 2010;15(2):361-364.
10. Selim BJ, Wolfe L, Coleman JM, et al. Initiation of noninvasive ventilation for sleep related hypoventilation disorders: advanced modes and devices. *Chest*. 2018;153(1):251-265.
11. Philips Respironics. DreamStation BiPAP S/T and AVAPS user manual. Published 2025. Accessed March 5, 2025. https://www.philips.com/c-dam/b2bhc/master/landing-pages/src/update/replacement-devices/dreamstation-advanced/en-us/philips-dreamstation-avaps-st-user-manual.pdf
12. Berry RB, Chediak A, Brown LK, et al; NPPV Titration Task Force of the American Academy of Sleep Medicine. Best clinical practices for the sleep center adjustment of noninvasive positive pressure ventilation (NPPV) in stable chronic alveolar hypoventilation syndromes. *J Clin Sleep Med*. 2010;6(5):491.
13. Philips Respironics. Titration protocol reference guide. 2025. Accessed March 5, 2025. https://www.documents.philips.com/doclib/enc/9792335/BiPAPAutoSVAdvanced_Protocol.pdf
14. Aurora RN, Bista SR, Casey KR, et al. Updated adaptive servo-ventilation recommendations for the 2012 AASM guideline: "the treatment of central sleep apnea syndromes in adults: practice parameters with an evidence-based literature review and meta-analyses". *J Clin Sleep Med*. 2016;12(5):757.
15. ResMed. Sleep lab titration guide. 2025. Accessed March 5, 2025. https://document.resmed.com/documents/products/titration/s9-vpap-tx/user-guide/1013904_Sleep_Lab_Titration_Guide_amer_eng.pdf
16. Thomson R, Richards GN, Woehrle H. *Pacewave Therapy: An Overview of Minute Ventilation Targeted Adaptive Servo-Ventilation (MV ASV)*. ResMed Science Center; 2012.
17. ResMed. S9 VPAPTM ST-A with iVAPS. ResMed. 2013. Accessed March 5, 2025. https://support.resmed.com/en-in/sleep-devices/vpap-sta-with-ivaps
18. Des Jardins TR. *Cardiopulmonary anatomy & physiology: essentials of respiratory care*. 7th ed. Cengage Learning; 2019.
19. Cowie MR, Woehrle H, Wegscheider K, et al. Adaptive servo-ventilation for central sleep apnea in systolic heart failure. *N Engl J Med*. 2015;373(12):1095-1105.

Chapter 47

Noninvasive Ventilation in Patients With Respiratory and Neuromuscular Disease

DANIEL L. HEROLD

KEY CONCEPTS/LEARNING OBJECTIVES

On completion of this chapter, the reader should be able to identify the main types of lung disease and how they impact breathing, outline the purpose of noninvasive ventilation (NIV) and how it works, identify the goals for delivering NIV to a patient with a respiratory or neuromuscular disease, and define modes, settings, and other terms used to implement NIV as well as state the relationship between carbon dioxide levels and ventilation, the relationship of tidal volume and respiratory rate to alveolar ventilation and be familiar with new technologies that can be utilized to track therapy and automatically adjust settings to maintain a desired level of ventilation.

KEY TERMS

Alveolar minute ventilation
Amyotrophic lateral sclerosis (ALS)
Chronic obstructive pulmonary disease (COPD)
Continuous positive airway pressure (CPAP)
Dead space
Expiration
Hypercapnia
Hyperventilation
Hypocapnia
Hypoventilation
Inspiration
Minute ventilation
Muscular dystrophy (MD)
Noninvasive ventilation (NIV)
Obesity hypoventilation syndrome (OHS)
Obstructive sleep apnea (OSA)
Respiratory rate
Restrictive thoracic disorder
Tidal volume

Sleep technologists see a wide range of patients coming into the sleep laboratory for diagnosis and treatment. These patients will range in complexity from simple obstructive sleep apnea (OSA) to patients exhibiting complex periodic breathing. Between these extremes of the sleep-disordered breathing spectrum are those patients with some form of underlying lung disease. Some of these patients will also have the complication of upper airway obstruction.

Healthcare professionals often categorize lung disease into two main types of disease processes. These are restrictive and obstructive disorders. Recognizing the differences in these disease processes will aid the sleep technologist in understanding how noninvasive ventilation (NIV) is used to improve the quality of sleep and life for patients with these diseases.

RESTRICTIVE THORACIC DISORDERS

The term "restrictive thoracic disorder" is used instead of restrictive lung disease because most of the diseases in this category are not really disorders of the lung. These disorders normally involve some problem with the thorax or chest. These patients may have relatively normal healthy lungs but still have a problem breathing. These disorders are characterized by processes that limit the patient's ability to take a normal-sized breath, something that "restricts" the ability to inspire fully. A few of the more common types of restrictive disorders are discussed in the following paragraphs.

Amyotrophic lateral sclerosis (ALS), also known as Lou Gehrig disease, is an example of a restrictive disorder.

This disease is characterized by a gradual destruction of motor neurons in the brain and spinal cord. As these motor neurons are gradually destroyed, the patient loses the ability to move voluntarily, speak, swallow, and breathe. Because this is a progressive disease, it is also an excellent example illustrating the need for monitoring therapy after initiation and then adjusting therapy as needed. These patients will get worse after they are seen in the sleep laboratory, and their therapy may need to be adjusted to manage their weakening condition.

Muscular dystrophy is the name for a group of genetically inherited muscle diseases that are characterized by a loss of muscle protein. This loss of muscle protein weakens the muscle to the extent that it can no longer do its assigned task. This is also a progressive disorder like ALS and may lead to inability to perform activities of daily living and could ultimately lead to breathing difficulty as the muscles of breathing become affected.

Obesity hypoventilation syndrome (OHS) is another type of disorder that exhibits restrictive characteristics. Patients with this disorder are obese and exhibit daytime alveolar hypoventilation. These patients do not have chronic obstructive pulmonary disease (COPD) as a cause of their alveolar hypoventilation. Consequences of this daytime alveolar hypoventilation include hypercapnia and hypoxemia. The mechanisms causing the hypoventilation are complex and involve reduced chest wall compliance, impaired respiratory drive, and severe OSA. Treatment of the OSA component with continuous positive airway pressure (CPAP) is beneficial to these patients, but if they continue to have persistent hypercapnia and oxygen desaturation, then bilevel therapy or noninvasive ventilation (NIV) may have to be utilized (1).

All of these patients with restrictive lung disease have the potential to have difficulty maintaining a normal level of ventilation while they are awake. These patients lose voluntary control of ventilation when sleeping, and their breathing can become compromised to the point where serious health consequences can occur.

OBSTRUCTIVE LUNG DISEASE

Unlike most of the restrictive thoracic disorders, obstructive lung disease does involve destructive changes to the lung tissue itself. Obstructive lung disease is more commonly referred to as chronic obstructive pulmonary disease, or COPD. COPD is not the only type of obstructive lung disease, but it is the most common one. It typically results from cigarette smoking or in some cases, industrial exposure to dust or fumes. Asthma is also a type of obstructive lung disease.

Like OSA, there is an obstruction or airflow limitation occurring in these patients, but COPD is very different from OSA in two primary ways. The airflow limitation occurs during the expiratory phase of breathing instead of the inspiratory phase, as is the case with OSA. The other way by which COPD differs from OSA is that the obstruction to flow occurs in the distal airways and alveoli of the lung instead of the upper airway. COPD is not diagnosed during a sleep study but with a pulmonary function test called "spirometry."

These patients have trouble exhaling the air out of their lungs. In extreme cases, this will cause the patient to inhale before all the air in the previous breath is exhaled. This causes the patient to gradually hyperinflate their lungs over time until, eventually, they can no longer inhale properly because there is no more room for air in the lungs.

The patient with COPD and OSA is referred to as an "overlap patient" and, like the patient with OHS, will usually benefit from a resolution of OSA symptoms but may still experience persistent hypercapnia and oxygen desaturations that may need to be treated using bilevel ventilation or NIV. The patient with COPD in need of NIV presents unique challenges to the sleep technologist. Although these patients need additional alveolar ventilation, the sleep technologist needs to be aware that these patients may present with significant airflow limitation, not on inspiration, but on expiration. It is not simply a matter of turning up the respiratory rate or increasing the amount of pressure delivered in order to increase alveolar ventilation. Although it is always important to deliver the properly sized breath to a patient, in patients with COPD who have hyperinflated lungs, it is just as important to allow the breath to be exhaled.

NONINVASIVE VENTILATION

NIV has been used successfully for decades in acute care environments to assist patients to avoid intubation in cases of acute respiratory failure. The evidence for using NIV for the successful treatment of chronic respiratory failure caused by neuromuscular disease in home care environments is also well documented. The use of NIV to treat chronic respiratory failure due to COPD has been the focus of several recent studies. The practice of placing these patients with COPD on minimal levels of NIV is changing. Recent studies into the use of NIV with patients with COPD have focused on the use of higher pressures, or high-intensity NIV, in order to increase ventilation to the point where carbon dioxide (CO_2) reductions in blood gases are produced (2).

One of the main differences in the use of NIV in the acute care environment, and for chronic care at home, is the different quality of monitoring and intervention by trained healthcare professionals. This makes the initial setup and effective titration of NIV in the sleep laboratory all the more critical to the successful treatment of the patient with chronic respiratory failure in the home environment. The patient who has an OSA component in addition to chronic respiratory failure has two strikes against them when they sleep. Although eliminating the upper airway component is always helpful, these patients will often require the assistance of NIV to mitigate the impact of their chronic respiratory condition on their sleep, health, and quality of life.

GOALS OF NONINVASIVE VENTILATION TREATMENT

The goal of NIV is to reduce the work of breathing and to normalize or improve the patient's blood gases. Regardless of whether the patient has a restrictive or obstructive disorder, the goal is the same, although there are some subtle differences in how NIV is applied for these disorders. Complete normalization of blood gases is not always attained, but reducing the work of breathing is essential, and if not attained, it is less likely that the patient will be compliant with the therapy. The consequences of a lack of compliance with NIV therapy can be worse than CPAP noncompliance. If the patients do not use the therapy, there is no benefit.

Anyone who routinely initiates and titrates NIV on patients should experience it for themselves, at least briefly, so they can better relate to what patients feel like. NIV uses pressure support to provide ventilation. Properly adjusted pressure support therapy should follow the patient's breathing pattern and provide assistance with inspiration and allow for comfortable exhalation. Most often, patients should be able to control both their respiratory rate and tidal volume if the therapy is titrated properly. Easing the work of breathing for someone is one of the most critical and rewarding things a clinician can do.

BASICS OF NORMAL VENTILATION

The basics of normal ventilation should be reviewed before delving into the details of treatment methods. Knowing what normal ventilation is important before attempting to bring the patient back toward normal ventilation. Some of the terms the clinician should be familiar with include the following: inspiration, expiration, respiratory rate, tidal volume, dead space, minute ventilation, and alveolar minute ventilation.

INSPIRATION

In normal healthy people, *inspiration* is achieved when the diaphragm contracts. This causes the diaphragm to flatten out and drop down in the chest cavity. The result is that the amount of space or available volume in the chest cavity increases. This increase in space causes the pressure in the chest to decrease. If the upper airway is not obstructed, then air will move from outside the chest to fill the lungs. The diaphragm is the primary muscle involved in breathing, but the diaphragm can be supplemented by the use of accessory muscles in the ribs, neck, and chest, to help elevate the rib cage upward and outward to further increase the dimensions of the chest cavity, thus creating more negative pressure to draw more air into the lungs.

EXPIRATION

Expiration is normally passive, with the elastic nature of the diaphragm and lungs providing the recoil to push air out of the lungs. Like inspiration, expiration can also be supplemented by the use of accessory muscles if necessary to facilitate expiration. This is most commonly seen in obstructive lung disease, where the distal airways collapse and trap air in the lungs. Patients with obstructive lung disease have to work to inhale and to exhale. They have to actively *push* air out of their lungs in addition to the normal work of breathing to inhale. These patients expend a great deal of energy on just breathing.

RESPIRATORY RATE

The number of times a person breathes each minute is their *respiratory rate*. Respiratory rate can vary from person to person, according to their metabolic needs at the time. Normal respiratory rates are about 10 to 12 breaths per minute.

TIDAL VOLUME

The amount of air that is drawn into the lungs on any single breath is called *tidal volume*. The size of the tidal volume can vary greatly from person to person on the basis of their size and metabolic activity. Normal tidal volumes are in the range of 6 to 8 mL/kg of body weight. Higher tidal volumes delivered by NIV may be uncomfortable, whereas lower tidal volumes are not efficient for achieving alveolar ventilation.

DEAD SPACE

A portion of each inhaled tidal volume does not participate in gas exchange. This portion of the breath is called *dead space*. There are two types of dead space. The first is *anatomic dead space*. Every person has a certain amount of anatomic dead space, which comprises the larger airways in the lungs and portions of the upper airway. On inspiration, this dead space is the last portion of air from outside of the body that cannot reach the gas exchange areas. On expiration, the anatomic dead space is flushed out and filled with air leaving the alveoli. This air has a high CO_2 content and is then pulled back into the alveoli on the next inspiration. The average person has about 150 mL of anatomic dead space (2). Of course, larger people will have larger amounts of dead space volumes and smaller people smaller dead space volumes.

The other type of dead space is known as *physiologic dead space*. This is air that is inhaled and that *does* reach the areas where gas exchange is supposed to occur but that for some reason does not fully participate in gas exchange. Proper respiration relies on ventilation matching up with good blood flow to the lungs. Mismatches of ventilation to perfusion can lead to increased amounts of dead space. Physiologic dead space is more of an issue in obstructive lung disorders than with restrictive lung disorders. Physiologic dead space is difficult to calculate, and, in any event, it is not always necessary to know what the volume of physiologic dead space is in order to provide adequate therapy.

MINUTE VENTILATION

A person's average tidal volume multiplied by their respiratory rate determines their *minute ventilation*. Another way to describe minute ventilation is that it is all the air the patient moves in and out of their body in a minute.

ALVEOLAR VENTILATION/ALVEOLAR MINUTE VENTILATION

Alveolar ventilation is the effective ventilation. Once dead space is known, then alveolar ventilation is the next calculation that can be made. Alveolar ventilation is calculated simply by taking the tidal volume of the patient and subtracting the dead space from it. This is the alveolar tidal volume. Multiply the alveolar tidal volume by the respiratory rate to determine the alveolar minute ventilation.

RELATIONSHIP OF TIDAL VOLUME TO ALVEOLAR MINUTE VENTILATION

The average amount of anatomic dead space and its relationship to alveolar minute ventilation becomes important when considering assisting a person's breathing with mechanical ventilation. There are numerous ways to get to an adequate level of alveolar ventilation. Start with the delivery of an adequate tidal volume that is comfortable to the patient, and then assure that this tidal volume is provided at the correct frequency. That frequency or breath rate should be sufficient to provide the minimum alveolar minute ventilation for that patient. See Figures 47-1 and 47-2 for an illustration of the importance of tidal volume and the impact to alveolar ventilation.

$$450\ \text{mL} \times 10\ \text{bpm} = 4.5\ \text{L}/\text{min}$$

$$\frac{-150\ \text{mL dead space}}{300\ \text{mL} \times 10} = 3.0\ \text{L}/\text{min alveolar ventilation}$$

Figure 47-1 The example assumes that the patient weighs 70 kg. A tidal volume of 450 mL would be equal to 6.4 mL/kg of body weight, which is in the normal range for tidal volumes (6-8 mL/kg). Delivery of 450 mL would yield a minute ventilation of 4.5 L/min, but if the anatomic dead space is considered, the effective tidal volume is only 300 milliliter per breath. The display on the device might indicate a minute ventilation of 4.5 L/min, but the effective level of ventilation is actually less because of the impact of anatomic dead space.

These changes to tidal volume and rate have not changed minute ventilation, but, in reality, the alveolar ventilation has been reduced by 10%, and a rise in CO_2 levels may occur as a result. It can get pretty confusing thinking in terms of alveolar ventilation, dead space, tidal volume, and minute ventilation. The simplest way to approach ventilation is to get the supported breath volume needed correct. Know the patient's weight and use the guideline of 6 to 8 mL/kg as a starting point for determining tidal volume. The tidal volume calculation is based on body size, and there is no need to add any extra volume to account for anatomic dead space (Table 47-1). Tidal volumes larger than 8 mL/kg should be avoided unless ordered by a physician. Larger tidal volumes may produce effective increases in alveolar ventilation and reductions in CO_2, but they do create a risk of discomfort and noncompliance with therapy (3).

$$375\ \text{mL} \times 12\ \text{bpm} = 4.5\ \text{L}/\text{min}$$

$$\frac{-150\ \text{mL dead space}}{225\ \text{mL} \times 12} = 2.7\ \text{L}/\text{min alveolar ventilation}$$

Figure 47-2 If the same 70 kg patient is ventilated with a smaller tidal volume, the impact to alveolar ventilation should be considered. Decreasing the delivered tidal volume to 375 mL and increasing the respiratory rate to 12 breaths per minute may still display a minute ventilation of 4.5 L/min, but alveolar ventilation has actually decreased.

Table 47-1 Conversion Table for Tidal Volume (VT)

Height (m)	Calculated Ideal Weight (if BMI = 23) (kg)	Target VT (mL) if 8 mL/kg	Target VT (mL) if 10 mL/kg
1.50	52.0	410	520
1.55	55.0	440	550
1.60	59.0	470	590
1.65	62.5	500	620
1.70	66.5	530	660
1.75	70.5	560	700
1.80	74.5	600	740
1.85	78.5	630	780
1.90	83.0	660	830

Calculated with an ideal body mass index of 23 kg/m^2 (BMI = weight/height^2).

Guidelines/values developed for use with Philips Respironics products only. Variations may occur with other manufacturers' products. Please consult specific manufacturers' guidelines for specific product information and operational guidelines.

CARBON DIOXIDE AND VENTILATION

The common thread between all types of lung disease is that these patients tend to have some degree of hypoventilation. Hypoventilation occurs when a patient breathes either too shallowly or too slowly to remove the CO_2 that they are producing. The end result is that CO_2 levels build up in their bodies, producing something called "hypercapnia," or elevated CO_2 levels.

Why is CO_2 so important? Think of CO_2 as the cellular metabolic by-product of life. All of our cells are continually busy metabolizing or "burning" sugars to produce energy. One of the waste products of this process is CO_2. It is released from the cells into the bloodstream and is carried to the lungs, where the lungs try to vent this CO_2 into the air that enters and leaves the lungs. Thinking of this CO_2 as "smoke" from the burning sugar will help in understanding why it is important for it to be removed from the body. When CO_2-rich blood reaches the lungs, it is passively transported from the lungs to the air sacs or alveoli. The lungs then need to exchange this CO_2-laden air with fresh air from outside the body in order to get rid of the CO_2. At a higher rate of ventilation, the CO_2 levels in the blood are usually lower. Conversely, if the amount of air being moved through the lungs is reduced, then the CO_2 level in the blood usually increases. Another way of stating this is that CO_2 levels in the blood are *inversely* proportional to ventilation. This is one of the most important concepts needed to fully understand ventilation.

The normal range for CO_2 is between 35 and 45 mm Hg. Simply put, if the patient's measured CO_2 is above the normal range, then they are not getting enough alveolar ventilation, or are hypoventilating (Figure 47-3). If the measured CO_2 is below the normal range, then the patient is getting too much alveolar ventilation, or hyperventilating. Hyperventilation is unusual to see during sleep, except during periods of periodic breathing such as with Cheyne-Stokes respirations. Most of the time, hypoventilation/hypercapnia will present clinically.

This brings the discussion full circle back to tidal volumes and the impact they have on alveolar ventilation and CO_2 levels. In critical care, it is common to have CO_2 levels readily available to the clinician with the use of arterial blood gas (ABG) analysis. Respiratory therapists rely heavily on CO_2 measurements to titrate and

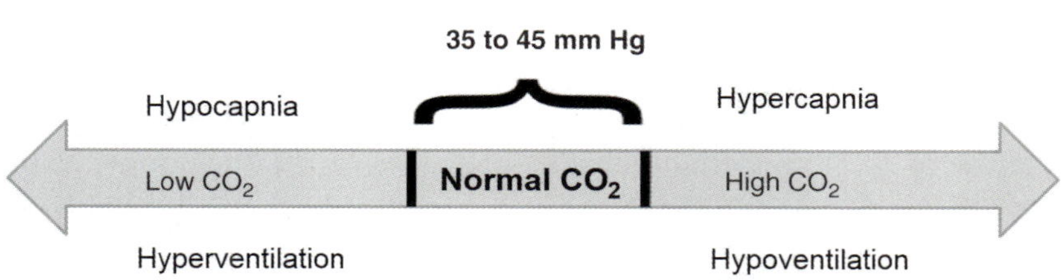

Figure 47-3 *Hypo*ventilation (low ventilation) is associated with *hyper*capnia (high CO_2), and *hyper*ventilation (high ventilation) is associated with *hypo*capnia (low CO_2).

adjust ventilation. The clinician in the sleep laboratory may not have access to ABG data. Special lab equipment and qualified clinicians are required to obtain the sample and perform ABG analysis. ABG blood draws are also very painful and would have a negative impact on sleep.

Capnography, or end-tidal CO_2 readings, can be used to estimate what the CO_2 levels are in the blood, but they are never the same as ABG data. The accuracy of end-tidal CO_2 readings obtained during NIV is also impacted by the leak that is a normal component of NIV. Most NIV devices use a leak circuit, just like CPAP, instead of a closed circuit. Capnography may be useful to track how end-tidal CO_2 readings are trending, but clinicians should always be cautious when using capnography as a guide for titration during NIV.

Transcutaneous CO_2 readings are not impacted by the use of NIV and may be a more reliable measure of what the true CO_2 level is in the blood. It can be useful as a trending tool to see if CO_2 levels are decreasing as increases in ventilation are made during an NIV titration.

NONINVASIVE VENTILATION

NIV is the practice of delivering ventilatory assistance without the use of an endotracheal or tracheostomy tube. It is most often delivered via a nasal or full-face mask but can also be delivered via a mouthpiece in some situations. The mouthpiece assembly allows the patient to place their lips firmly around the mouthpiece and initiate a breath, triggering the ventilator to deliver a breath of air, assisting with both inhalation and exhalation, therefore providing breathing support. This allows the patient increased mobility and independence as the patient can disconnect from the ventilator for activities like speaking, eating, and socializing, improving their quality of life.

NIV or noninvasive positive pressure ventilation can lead to some confusion with terminology. This is compounded by the distinction that insurance providers make between the NIV devices that have the capability to provide a backup rate and those that do not. Discussions about NIV and NIV devices in this chapter will refer to those devices with the ability to deliver a backup breath in the absence of patient effort.

Most NIV devices are not intended to be used as life support devices. The patients who use them should be able to safely discontinue therapy with the device for short periods of time without harm. Some life support devices have NIV modes, but the use of an NIV device in those modes does not make the mode a life support mode.

Most NIV ventilators are designed to be used by adult patient populations and will have age and/or weight restrictions in their intended use statements. Pediatric patients will frequently be placed on life support ventilators that are approved for pediatric patients in NIV modes in order to avoid any use contrary to the intended use statement.

PRESSURE VENTILATION VERSUS VOLUME VENTILATION

There are two common types of ventilation in use today: *volume ventilation* and *pressure ventilation*.

Volume ventilation delivers a specific tidal volume with each breath. Although the volume is consistent for each breath delivered, the pressure generated in the patient's lungs can, and often will, change with each breath. This consistent tidal volume allows clinicians using volume ventilation to control the level of ventilation easily using the tidal volume and rate. The use of volume ventilation can sometimes generate high pressures in the lungs that can cause damage in the form of barotrauma.

Pressure ventilation delivers specified pressures during the breathing phase, one pressure for inspiration and one pressure for expiration. These are the inspiratory positive airway pressure (IPAP) and the expiratory positive airway pressure (EPAP) settings. The difference between the EPAP and IPAP settings is the amount of pressure support delivered. Figure 47-4 provides an example of pressure support of 5 cm H_2O. Pressure ventilation is like a mirror image of sorts to volume ventilation. Pressure ventilation delivers a precise pressure during each inspiration, but the volume delivered by that pressure breath can and often will vary from breath to breath. This possibility of inconsistent tidal volume with pressure ventilation is both good and bad, depending on the situation.

PRESSURE SUPPORT VENTILATION: THE GOOD AND THE BAD

One of the best reasons to use pressure support ventilation is that it is a very comfortable way to support the patient's effort. Because the device is targeting a pressure, it allows the patient to inspire a larger breath if they desire. If the patient wants to take a smaller breath, they are able to reject the breath when using pressure ventilation. Once the pressure reaches the selected pressure level, the breath is terminated and the patient can exhale. These aspects of pressure ventilation give the patient a great deal of control over how much ventilation they receive, making it more comfortable for them.

The drawback of using pressure ventilation is once again a mirror image of the advantage. NIV using pressure ventilation does not assure a minimal level of ventilation. Patients change over time. Some get better, but most tend to get worse. Patients with neuromuscular disease will almost certainly get worse. Pressure settings

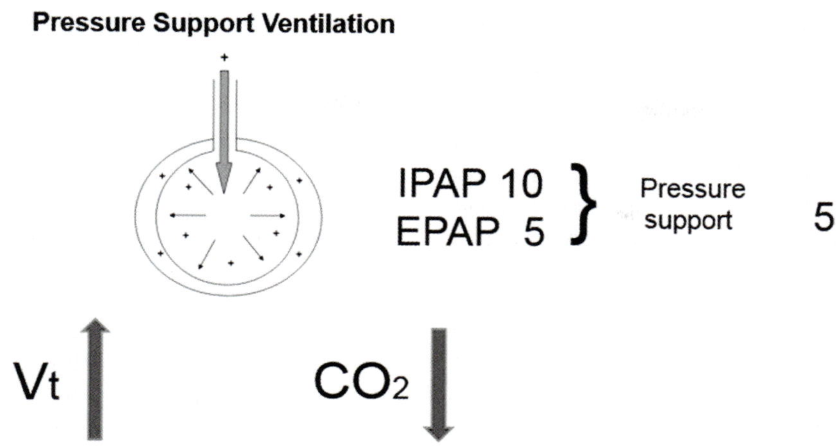

Figure 47-4 With settings of an inspiratory positive airway pressure (IPAP) of 10 cm H_2O and an expiratory positive airway pressure (EPAP) of 5 cm H_2O, the result is a pressure support of 5 cm H_2O.

that generate tidal volumes of 500 mL in January may generate only 400 mL in July. Therapy will need to be monitored and adjusted because even though the settings on the device do not change, the resulting ventilation can change on the basis of changes occurring in the patient. Never forget that the patient is a big variable that a clinician has little to no control over. NIV devices are almost exclusively pressure ventilators, but many are also capable of "targeting" a tidal volume or alveolar ventilation with their pressure. This "targeting" will be discussed in more detail later.

HOW DOES NONINVASIVE VENTILATION AND PRESSURE SUPPORT VENTILATION WORK?

The foundation of NIV is that air flows from areas of higher pressure to areas of lower pressure. As discussed earlier, normal ventilation occurs when we decrease the pressure in our chest by contracting the diaphragm, causing air to flow from outside the chest into the lungs. With NIV, we don't reduce the pressure in the chest but rather increase the pressure at the opening of the airway in order to affect ventilation. We do this with a flow generator in the NIV device. NIV devices generate a pressure differential between inspiratory and expiratory phases of the breath. This pressure differential is commonly referred to as "the level of pressure support," or simply as "*pressure support.*" The goal of pressure support is to increase the tidal volume above what one would normally inspire on one's own without assistance. The level of pressure support is controlled by the level of IPAP and EPAP. Some advanced NIV devices allow for setting a pressure support instead of individually setting the EPAP and IPAP.

A pressure support of 5 cm H_2O should generate a larger tidal volume than an unsupported breath, which, in turn, should generate more alveolar ventilation, resulting in lower CO_2 levels. If this level of pressure support does not generate enough of an increase in tidal volume or a decrease in CO_2 (remember that ventilation and CO_2 are *inversely* related), then the IPAP can be increased to increase the pressure support and tidal volume. Increases in pressure support may not always result in increases in tidal volume and ventilation. Remember, the patient is on the other end of the NIV device, and if they are uncomfortable with the pressure being supplied, then they may resist the ventilation, and the end result could be decreased ventilation.

If upper airway obstruction is still present with an EPAP of 5, the EPAP can be increased as needed, but the IPAP will have to be increased by the same amount to maintain the same level of pressure support. The level of *pressure support* is what drives ventilation, and EPAP is used for airway control. These two concepts are the most important ones to understand in order to apply NIV successfully.

NONINVASIVE VENTILATION TERMINOLOGY

A review of common NIV terminology is warranted before a discussion of therapy concerns about specific patient types. Some of the terms to be familiar with include the following:

(Note to the reader: There are no nomenclature standards for NIV devices. The terms discussed in the following paragraphs are used by a majority of manufacturers, but beware of some potential differences in them.)

Mode is the precise manner by which a device produces breaths to a patient, controlling the pressure or volume, and/or the timing during each breath. There are several modes available on NIV devices. The mode can determine if there is a backup rate setting and could also define how spontaneous breaths are delivered. Spontaneous-timed (ST) mode is one of the most frequently used modes. Once ST mode is understood, it is easier to grasp the details of spontaneous (S) mode, pressure control (PC) mode, and timed (T) mode. Most manufacturers provide these modes but may use different terminology. Figure 47-5 identifies the various settings in the NIV device.

Bilevel therapy is another way to describe pressure support therapy. This is the application of two different pressure levels during the breath cycle. Ideally, if the pressures are applied at the proper times, they will follow the patient's own breathing pattern and increase pressure to increase the size of the inhaled breath and then decrease to allow for exhalation while maintaining a patent upper airway. Pressures are measured in cm H_2O unless indicated otherwise. Many devices are sold internationally and may therefore support the ability to change pressure settings to hectopascals (hPa).

EPAP is the pressure level set for the expiratory phase of the breath. It is lower than the inspiratory pressure to allow the inhaled breath to be easily exhaled. This pressure is typically titrated to maintain an open upper airway at the transition point between end exhalation and beginning of inspiration. EPAP can also be increased to improve oxygenation in some cases.

IPAP is the higher of the two pressure settings and is used to support the inspiratory phase of the breath. Increasing only IPAP will also increase pressure support at the same time. Increasing the IPAP will normally increase the tidal volume of the breath. At some point, increasing the IPAP or pressure support may not yield higher tidal volumes because of discomfort or asynchrony.

Pressure support is what drives ventilation in NIV. Pressure support may not be a setting on the device, so it is important to know that it is the difference between the IPAP and EPAP settings. Increase the IPAP if an increase in pressure support is needed. Increases in EPAP will necessitate an increase in IPAP if the pressure support is to be maintained. Increasing the level of pressure support will usually increase the tidal volume for each breath, which, in turn, increases the level of ventilation that normally reduces the CO_2 level in the blood.

Trigger is the transition point between the expiratory phase of the breath and the inspiratory phase. It is the beginning of the breath. During NIV, the patient is at the EPAP during exhalation, and the device is waiting for a "trigger" to tell it to transition to IPAP. Devices with trigger settings may refer to them as a "sensitivity setting." When triggering occurs, the device targets the higher pressure level (IPAP) and increases flow to do this. This provides the additional flow necessary for the patient's tidal volume. Most of the devices on the market use some type of flow trigger. During use, the device is continually monitoring flow and will determine if the patient is trying to inspire, which will then initiate a transition to IPAP. Flow triggering on NIV devices normally uses settings from 1 L/min to as high as 9 L/min. A trigger setting of 1 L/min means that if the device detects an increase of 1 L/min of flow over what it is delivering, it will initiate the transition to the inspiratory phase. Low trigger settings, such as 1 L/min, are the most sensitive and may need to be used in pediatric patients or, possibly, adult patients with neuromuscular disease in order to detect faint inspiratory efforts. In patients with normal inspiratory capability, a setting of 1 L/min may be too sensitive and may induce false or premature triggering. This will induce asynchrony and should be avoided. At the other end of the spectrum, a less sensitive trigger setting, such as 9 L/min, may be too difficult for the patient to trigger. Missed trigger events can also induce asynchrony between the patient and the

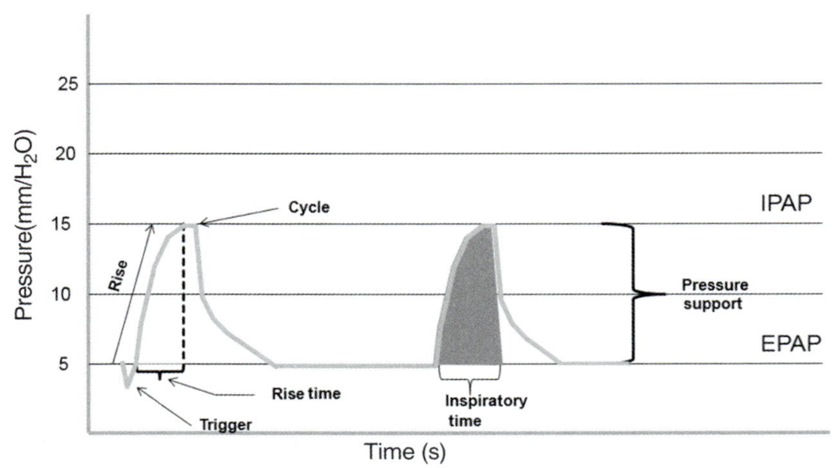

Figure 47-5 The various settings on the noninvasive ventilation device. EPAP, expiratory positive airway pressure; IPAP, inspiratory positive airway pressure.

device. Triggering needs to be adjusted to meet each individual patient's needs.

Rise time is the amount of time the device takes to transition from EPAP to IPAP. After the breath is triggered, the pressure starts to rise from EPAP to IPAP. Some devices have time settings for rise time, whereas other devices just use a setting that is correlated with a specific time. In either case, the setting determines how fast the device transitions from low to high pressure. A short time or a low setting initiates a very quick rise to pressure, and a longer time produces a more gradual rise to pressure. Manipulating this setting can affect patient comfort with the therapy. A very short rise time can create a very ballistic feel to the change in pressure, and the patient may not be comfortable with that sensation. A longer rise time may feel more comfortable to some patients, but longer rise times can affect overall ventilation. Longer rise times mean less time at higher pressures. This could translate into smaller tidal volumes. It may be more important to get the patient comfortable on the therapy than to maximize tidal volume. Longer rise times could be uncomfortable for some patients as well. They may feel a need for a faster breath and prefer shorter rise times.

Clinicians should try to determine a comfortable rise time setting for the patient that can be relayed to the home care team. Rise time settings typically range from 0.1 to 0.9 seconds. As an example, think of settings of EPAP 5 and IPAP 15. When inspiration is triggered, the pressure will increase from 5 to 15 cm H_2O. If the rise time is set to 0.1 seconds, the pressure will rise from 5 to 15 in 0.1 seconds. Changes to the rise time will affect how the breath delivery feels to the patient and may also impact the amount of ventilation achieved by the breath (Figure 47-6).

Cycling is the opposite of triggering. The device transitions from IPAP back to EPAP at the cycle point. Knowing when to terminate the inspiratory phase of the breath is as important as knowing when to initiate the breath.

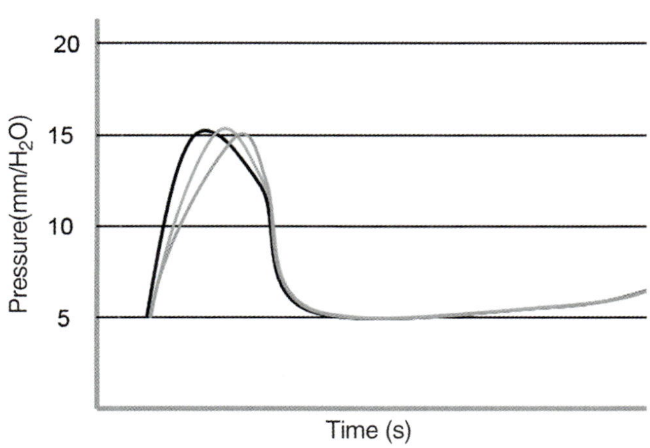

Figure 47-6 The impact of changing rise time on the pressure-time curve. The black line shows a fast rise time of 0.1 seconds. The gray (light) line shows a rise time of 0.2 seconds, and the gray (dark) line is a rise time of 0.3 seconds.

Reaching the cycle point or "cycling" is done using flow-based algorithms just like triggering does. Cycling settings are percentages. The percentage refers to the peak flow of the current breath. When the patient inspires, the device is targeting a higher pressure by generating more flow. When the patient inhales, the device has to deliver much more flow than it does during exhalation. When the patient begins to end the breath, the flow needed to deliver the higher IPAP starts to decrease. When the patient starts to decrease their inspiratory effort, or the lungs have started to fill, the peak flow point has already been reached, and the device will have recorded it for cycling purposes. For example, if the peak flow on the breath reaches 100 L/min and cycling is set to 40%, then the device will provide flow to maintain the IPAP until the delivered flow reaches 40 L/min. At that point, the device will "cycle" and stop delivering the IPAP and start delivering a lower flow to maintain the EPAP. If the device does not properly detect when the patient wants to exhale, it will not cycle at the right time. If it cycles too soon, the breath will be too small and the patient may become short of breath and may need to breathe faster. If the device cycles too late, the patient will be trying to exhale against the higher pressure, and this will cause asynchrony issues as well. NIV devices have limits on how long the device will stay in IPAP. This limit is usually 50% of the cycle time, so even if the device misses the patient's request to cycle the breath, it will not stay in IPAP excessively long.

Triggering and cycling are extremely important, and device manufacturers spend a lot of time and effort working on algorithms to make sure the devices they make do these things properly. Proper triggering and cycling are key to patient synchrony. *Synchrony* is essential to patient comfort and adherence to therapy. If the patient attempts to inspire and the device does not detect the effort, known as a "missed trigger," it will not provide the extra flow needed for a comfortable inspiration. Determining the right settings for triggering and cycling requires some skill and experience. Some devices offer automated algorithms that do this for the clinician. Is something like this better than manually titrating a trigger and cycle setting? That probably depends largely on the skill level of the clinician. Flow triggering and cycling settings (Table 47-2) offer the possibility of customization to the patient needs, but they can also be set incorrectly and lead to asynchrony issues for the patient.

BREATH TYPES: PRESSURE SUPPORT VERSUS PRESSURE CONTROL

One of the subtle things to know about NIV delivery is that there are two different types of breath that can be supplied by NIV devices. There are important differences between a pressure controlled breath (PC) and a

Table 47-2 Breath Rates and Corresponding Cycle Times

Breath Rate	Cycle Time (s)
8	7.5
10	6
12	5
15	4
20	3

pressure support breath, and these differences can become critical when choosing a mode of ventilation for some patients.

The discussion of the different modes of therapy builds on how these two different breath types are used. Pressure support breaths are the most common type of breath delivered during NIV. A pressure-supported breath is a completely spontaneous breath. The downward spike on the pressure channel may not always be seen because the device may be using flow triggering, and the response time of devices in use today is too fast for a drop in pressure to occur. The length of the breath is determined essentially by the patient, with some limits imposed by the cycling algorithm of the device. This type of breath offers a great deal of flexibility for the patient. The patient is able to initiate the breath and also terminate it. The device will essentially monitor the inhaled flow and look for indications as to whether the patient is trying to cycle or terminate the inspiration. This allows the patient to control the length of the breath and the amount of air they inspire, making this a very comfortable breath for the patient. This type of breath may not be the best for all patients, however. Patients with a neuromuscular disease may be unable to sustain an inspiratory effort long enough to attain an adequate tidal volume. In this case, the patient may benefit more from receiving PC breaths. Figure 47-7 demonstrates these various breaths.

Pressure-controlled or timed breaths use device-controlled pressures, just like a pressure support, but the device also controls the amount of time that the inspiratory pressure is delivered. Controlling the amount of time the pressure is delivered requires the use of another control parameter, called inspiratory time (I time). This setting determines the amount of time that the device will remain in the inspiratory phase of the breath. Once the breath is initiated, the device will transition from the lower pressure (EPAP) to the higher pressure (IPAP) and stay at the higher pressure for the set I time. PC breaths are also usually delivered by a timed trigger instead of a patient trigger, so PC breaths are found in modes of therapy that employ a backup rate. These are the breaths that are delivered when the patient's own breathing rate falls below the backup rate that is set on the device.

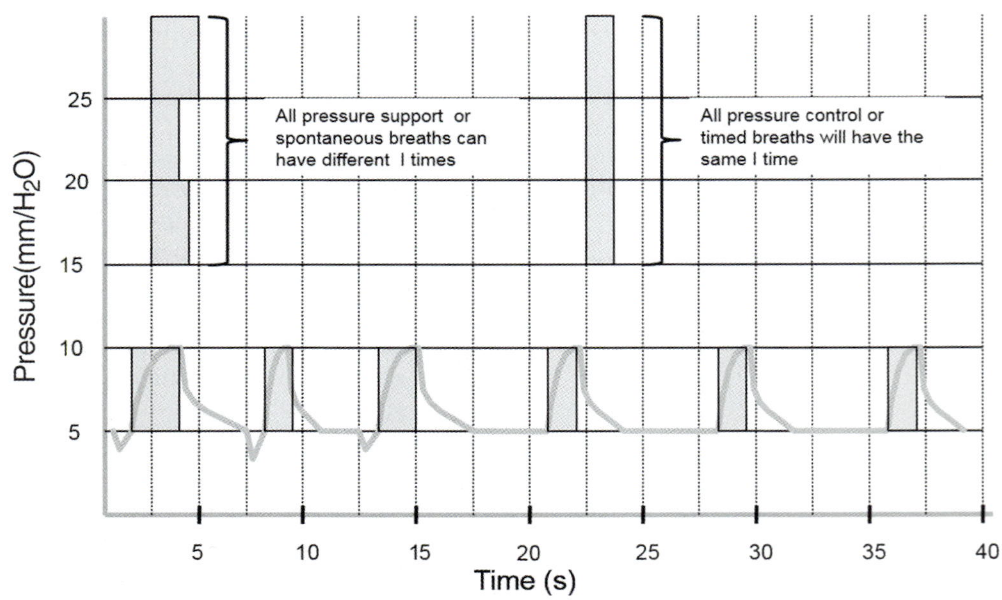

Figure 47-7 The difference between pressure support or spontaneous breaths and pressure control or timed breaths. The first three breaths are pressure support breaths. The breath was initiated by the patient, and the device supports that breath with the pressure support set by the clinician. Note the trigger event as the downward spike in pressure just before the pressure rises. The trigger event is shown to highlight the fact that the breath is a spontaneously triggered pressure support breath. Pressure control breaths, shown as the last three breaths, are also sometimes called "timed breaths." I time, Inspiratory time.

CYCLE TIME AND RESPIRATORY RATE

One additional concept needs to be addressed before therapy modes are introduced. This is the concept of cycle time. Depending on the mode selected, there are certain control parameters that will need to be set. EPAP, IPAP, and rise time are pretty straightforward. Even respiratory rate and I time appear to be pretty straightforward, but there are some subtle concepts that need to be understood. One of the subtleties is cycle time.

When using a mode of therapy with a backup rate feature, an I time and respiratory rate have to be set. When setting a respiratory rate, a cycle time is automatically being set in the background. Calculate the cycle time by dividing 60 seconds by the respiratory rate. Cycle time is the amount of time devoted to a full inspiratory and expiratory phase of the breath. In modes that support a backup rate function, the cycle time is the maximum amount of time allowed between breaths. See Table 47-3 for an inspiratory time conversion table.

ST mode allows the patient to start a spontaneous breath before the end of the cycle time, but if they fail to do so, a timed breath will be delivered (Figure 47-8). Another way of thinking about cycle time is that it is a timer that is counting down. If the patient does not trigger a breath spontaneously before the timer reaches zero, then the device will deliver a timed breath. The timer then restarts with each breath, either timed or spontaneous.

The respiratory rate selected multiplied by the average tidal volume will determine the minimum minute ventilation. It should be understood that the set rate is a minimum rate. Most modes of therapy allow for additional breaths if the patient triggers or "asks" for a breath by starting a spontaneous breath. This is why setting an appropriate trigger is important. Most of the time, the respiratory rate is set as a safety net backup to the patient's own rate. The patient should be able to trigger and essentially set their own pace for breathing. Higher respiratory rates may be uncomfortable for the patient because the rate setting is a minimum, and breaths will be delivered when the cycle time expires. If the patient's own respiratory rate is adequate for their needs, then the backup respiratory rate is usually set just below the patient's own rate. High backup rates can be a source of *asynchrony*. The patient can always trigger and get additional breaths but will not be able to get fewer breaths than the set backup rate.

Table 47-3 Conversion Table for Inspiratory Time (I Time)

Set Backup Breath Rate (bpm)	I/E 1/3, Ti/Ttot 25% (s)	I/E 1/2, Ti/Ttot 33% (s)	I/E 1/1, Ti/Ttot 50% (s)
10	1.5	2.0	3.0
11	1.4	1.8	2.7
12	1.3	1.7	2.5
13	1.2	1.5	2.3
14	1.1	1.4	2.1
15	1.0	1.3	2.0
16	0.9	1.3	1.8
17	0.9	1.2	1.7
18	0.8	1.1	1.6
19	0.8	1.1	1.5
20	0.8	1.0	1.5
21	0.7	1.0	1.4
22	0.7	0.9	1.3
23	0.7	0.9	1.3
24	0.6	0.8	1.2
25	0.6	0.8	1.2

Set the I time in seconds: Ti (seconds) = 60/respiratory rate × %Ti. I/E, inspiratory/expiratory; Ti/Ttot, inspiratory time to total cycle time.

Guidelines/values developed for use with Philips Respironics products only. Variations may occur with other manufacturers' products. Please consult specific manufacturers' guidelines for specific product information and operational guidelines.

SETTING INSPIRATORY TIME

Setting the respiratory rate automatically sets the cycle time. The inspiratory time now needs to be set. With a respiratory rate of 12 breaths per minute, the cycle time is 5 seconds. This means that the breath has to be delivered and exhaled within 5 seconds because the device will deliver the next breath 5 seconds after the last trigger. A normal breathing pattern uses 25% to 33% of the cycle time to inspire the breath. That leaves 67% to 75% of the cycle time for expiration.

I time is only a factor for timed or PC breaths. It has no bearing on spontaneous breaths. The setting for I time has a big impact on tidal volumes if the patient receives a high percentage of pressure-controlled breaths. Many devices that provide NIV will limit the amount of inspiratory time to 50% of the cycle time or less. This is a safeguard to ensure that the patient has sufficient time to exhale the breath before the next one is given. Normal respiratory rates are usually in the low-to-mid-teens, or 10 to 15 breaths per minute. Determine the cycle time and set the I time in the range of 25% to 33% of that cycle time. Patients with COPD have longer expiratory times because of obstruction in the distal airways. These patients may benefit from shorter I times in order to devote a larger portion of the cycle time for exhalation.

Another way to set I time is to review the patient's spontaneous breaths with good tidal volumes.

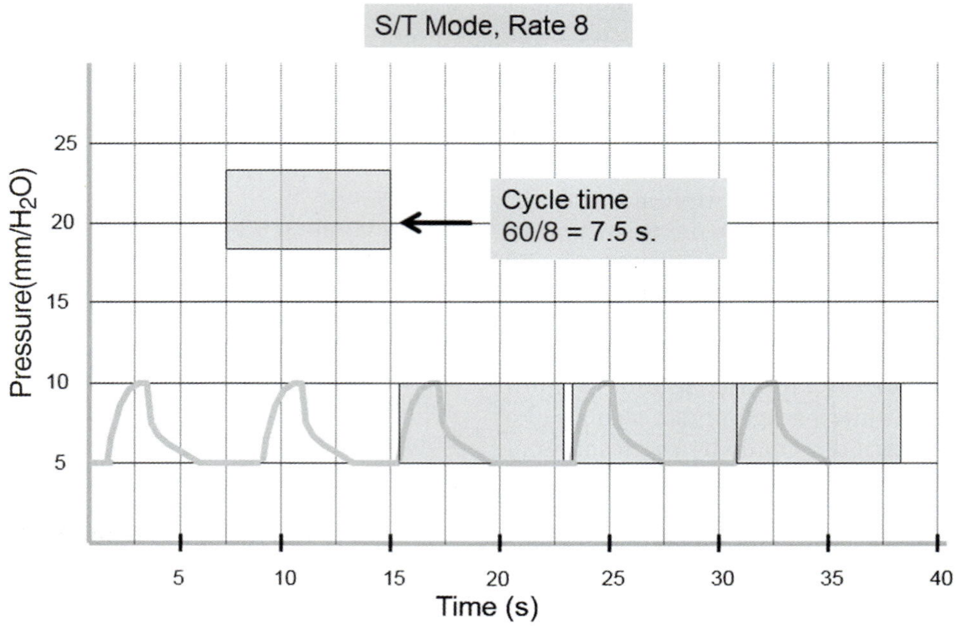

Figure 47-8 A respiratory rate setting of eight breaths per minute in spontaneous/timed mode shows a cycle time of 7.5 seconds. The gray-shaded area depicts the cycle time of 7.5 seconds.

Remember that spontaneous breaths do not use the set I time. The patient may inspire as long or short as they need. See how long the patient inspires with spontaneous breaths (Figure 47-9). If the spontaneous breath volumes are good, then the I time can be set similar to the patient's own spontaneous I times.

The tidal volumes should be reviewed during spontaneous breaths and, if they are acceptable, then the inspiratory time setting could be lowered to match the spontaneous breathing (Figure 47-9). The adjustment in this case would be very minor, and if the longer I time setting is not uncomfortable to the patient, it does not always need to be changed. If the situation were reversed and the set I time were shorter than the spontaneous I times, then the adjustment to match spontaneous I times should always be done.

BUILDING THE BREATH

Knowing how all the settings in NIV come together allows for tailoring those settings to the goals of reducing the work of breathing and normalizing blood gases. It allows the clinician to build the breath to meet the patient's needs. See Table 47-4 for setting guidelines.

NIV is a series of supported breaths given to the patient. Start by getting the breath adjusted to the patient's needs, and then decide how frequently to repeat it. NIV uses pressure support (IPAP−EPAP) applied over time (I time) to generate flow to the patient. This flow is the *tidal volume*. The applied pressure support is the most important control parameter because many of the delivered breaths will be spontaneous, and the patient will have complete control over the I time. When I time

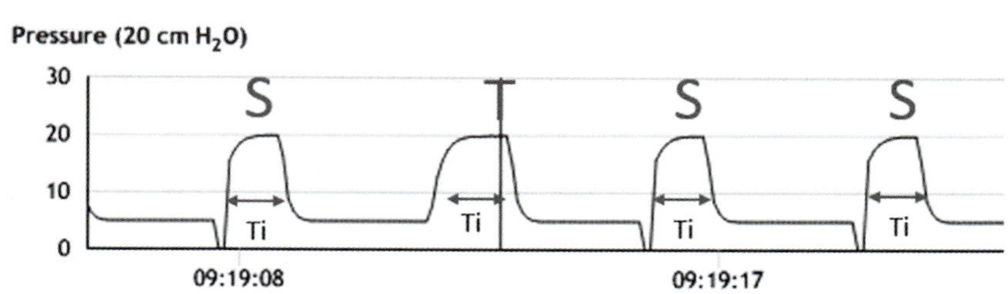

Figure 47-9 The first, third, and fourth breaths are spontaneous (S) breaths, whereas the second is a timed (T) breath. The T breath does not have a downward deflection on the pressure graph, denoting a trigger. The three S breaths stay in the inspiratory phase for a similar length of time. The patient has control over the I time for these S breaths, which appears to be shorter than the I time for the T breath. This may indicate that the I time setting is too long.

Table 47-4 Guidelines for Ventilation Settings[a]

Initial settings	• IPAP = 8-10 cm H_2O • EPAP = 4 cm H_2O • RR = 10-12 bpm		
IPAP	Increase IPAP if the patient wants more air, targeting patient tidal volume at 8 mL/kg of ideal weight		
EPAP	• Without obstructive sleep apnea (OSA) 4-5 cm H_2O • With OSA: intrinsic PEEP to remove obstructive apnea events • With intrinsic PEP (stable chronic COPD): 5-6 cm H_2O		
BPM	Set to 2-3 bpm under the patient's spontaneous frequency		
Rise time	• Obstructive patients prefer short rise time: from 1-4 (100-400 ms) • Restrictive patients prefer long rise time: from 3-6 (300-600 ms)		
Ti	• Obstructive patients: set Ti between 25% and 33% • Restrictive patients: set Ti between 33% and 50% • (Refer to table to set I time)		
AVAPS Only			
	OHS	**COPD**	**Other Restrictive Diseases (NMD, etc)**
VT target	The target tidal volume (VT) is 7-8 mL/kg of ideal body weight (IBW). Adjustments outside this range may be made at the discretion of the prescribing provider, depending on clinical indications		
IPAP window (IPAP min and IPAP max)	Allow a wide range of pressure variation to ensure the right pressure at the right time. IPAP min = EPAP IPAP max = 25-30 cm H_2O	Allow a more restrictive pressure window to combine comfort and efficacy. IPAP min = comfortable IPAP IPAP max = IPAP min + 5 cm H_2O	Allow a more restrictive pressure window to combine comfort and safety. IPAP min = efficient IPAP IPAP max = IPAP min + 5 cm H_2O
AVAPS rate	AVAPS rate setting depends on patient needs and clinical condition: • 0.5-3 cm H_2O/min so target tidal volume is reached smoothly • 3-5 cm H_2O/min so target tidal volume is reached more rapidly		

Check patient arterial blood gases ($PaCO_2$ and PaO_2) and oxygen saturation (SpO_2).

Important: Guidelines are intended to serve only as a reference. They shall be used only in conjunction with the instructions and/or protocol set forth by the physician and institution in which the assist device is being used. The guidelines are not intended to supersede established medical protocols.

AVAPS, average volume-assured pressure support; BPM, breaths per minute; COPD, chronic obstructive pulmonary disease; EPAP, expiratory positive airway pressure; IPAP, inspiratory positive airway pressure; NMD, neuromuscular disease; OHS, obesity hypoventilation syndrome; OSAS, obstructive sleep apnea syndrome; PEEP, positive-end expiratory pressure; PEP, positive expiratory pressure; RR, respiratory rate.

[a]Guidelines/values developed for use with Philips Respironics products only. Variations may occur with other manufacturers' products. Please consult specific manufacturers' guidelines for specific product information and operational guidelines.

must be set, refer to the patient's spontaneous breath I times, or keep the I time in the range of 25% to 33% of the cycle time.

The flow channel on a polysomnogram shows flow over time, which is more representative of tidal volume than a pressure-time graph. If the device in use reports tidal volumes, that may be used as well. In most cases, the majority of breaths will be spontaneous, so the only parameter that matters is the amount of pressure support applied (Figure 47-10). This does not mean that the I time is not important, because the patient may need timed breaths during the night, and the correct I time will matter then.

Always keep in mind that the patient must enough time to exhale all of the previous breaths before another breath is given. If settings do not allow full expiration, breath stacking can occur. Breath stacking causes gradually hyperinflated lungs because of an inability to completely exhale breaths. If this occurs, then the ventilation has to be decreased by reducing pressure, reducing I time, or decreasing the rate. Reducing pressure will reduce the inhaled volume. Reducing I time and respiratory rate will allow more time to exhale before the next breath.

MODES OF THERAPY

The mode of therapy used in NIV is usually the first point that is decided. There are several different modes that can be used, but in reality, the choice comes down to one of two modes.

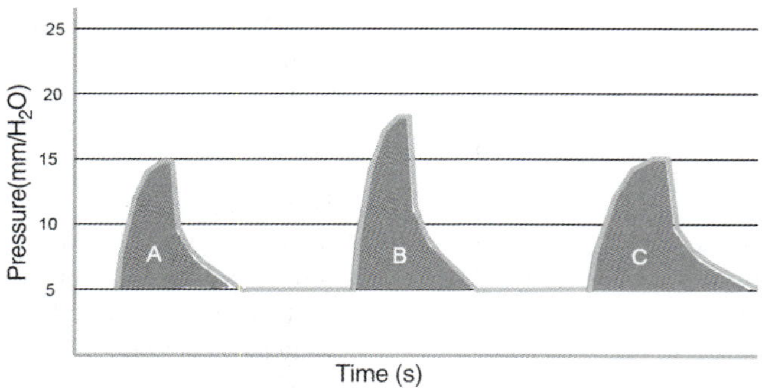

Figure 47-10 The shaded area under the curves represents the pressure support applied over time to the patient airway. This pressure/time representation is a way to demonstrate how to make changes to the settings. In breath A, the tidal volume was insufficient to meet patient needs. An increase in pressure support is shown in breath B. This increase in pressure should create additional flow during the I time and increase the delivered tidal volume. The other choice, shown in breath C, is to increase the I time. This too may increase the tidal volume by applying the pressure for a longer period of time.

S Mode

S mode is the simplest of the available modes because it has fewer settings. The only breath that is allowed is one that is triggered by the patient. The only parameters that the clinician can adjust are EPAP, IPAP, and rise time. S mode does not support a backup rate feature, so if the patient stops breathing for any reason, the device will not be able to deliver a timed breath. For this reason, it *should not* be used on patients who cannot or will not trigger a breath on their own consistently.

ST Mode

ST mode is the most frequently used mode. This mode of therapy supports a backup rate feature and can deliver all spontaneous, all timed, or a mixture of both spontaneous and timed breaths depending on the rate selected and the spontaneous rate of the patient. If the patient does not trigger breaths on their own, the device will deliver timed breaths at the exact rate set on the device. If the patient triggers breaths faster than the set rate on the device, they will receive all spontaneous breaths. The patient can also receive a mixture of spontaneous breaths and timed breaths.

The device in ST mode will use the cycle time window derived from the set respiratory rate to determine which type of breath to deliver. For example, with a rate of 12 breaths per minute, the cycle time is 5 seconds. The device will monitor the patient for 5 seconds after the last breath. If the patient triggers a breath before 5 seconds has elapsed, they will get a spontaneous breath. The device will then reset the cycle time window and start the 5-second timer again. If there is no patient trigger after 5 seconds, a timed breath will be given. Remember, these two breaths are different in that the timed breath has a duration based on the I time setting, and the spontaneous breath is terminated by the patient ending the breath. The rate setting in ST mode assures that the patient will receive at least that number of breaths, but what type of breath occurs depends on the number of breaths triggered by the patient.

T Mode

T mode is very seldom used. This mode looks just like ST mode in the settings except that there are no triggering and cycling settings. T mode delivers all timed breaths. Patient triggering and cycling are not allowed. If the rate is set to 12 breaths per minute, then the patient will get a breath from the device every 5 seconds. This mode is seldom, if ever, used.

PC Mode

The final mode is called PC mode. The settings of this mode are the same as those of ST, but all the breaths, even spontaneously triggered ones, are delivered for the specified I time. When using this mode, it is critical to get the I time set properly because all breaths delivered will use that I time. This mode is used on patients who are able to trigger breaths but who for some reason are unable to sustain the breath long enough to get an adequate tidal volume. A patient with a neuromuscular disease might be one such person. If the patient triggers a breath but is not strong enough to sustain it, the device may cycle the breath sooner than is acceptable. This is not an error of the device but rather a reflection of the patient's weakened state. For example, assume that a patient with a neuromuscular disease is being titrated to get to a desired tidal volume in ST mode. The patient is breathing faster than the set rate on the device, so they are getting all spontaneous breaths. If the patient is too weak to sustain an inspiratory effort, the device could terminate breaths too early. If the clinician does not note that the breaths are very short in duration, the clinician may be tempted to increase pressures in order to gain more ventilation. In this case, the patient may be better served by changing the mode to PC mode and setting an I time longer than what the patient is achieving during their own spontaneous breaths. This could result in longer breaths at lower pressures at slower rates that have adequate tidal volumes.

ADVANCED THERAPIES

Unfortunately, even the best titration is just a snapshot in time. There are just too many variables involved that can affect the desired therapy. Medication changes, alcohol use, and weight changes can impact the effectiveness of any titration. Patients with progressive diseases will almost certainly have changes that affect their therapy. At a minimum, NIV patients should have their therapy monitored and appropriate changes made as needed. Most devices in use today provide for monitoring therapy via proprietary software or cloud access provided by the manufacturer.

Medical device manufacturers have also developed automated technologies that allow the clinician to set a volume target for the device and allow it to operate within pressure boundaries in order to continually titrate therapy so as to maintain the desired level of ventilation. These technologies allow the clinician to set a target for ventilation, and the device will continually monitor the delivered therapy and adjust the delivered pressure support in order to stay at or above that level of ventilation.

Average volume-assured pressure support (AVAPS) technology provides settings similar to those of the ST mode, but instead of a single IPAP setting, there is a minimum IPAP and a maximum IPAP setting. There is also a target tidal volume setting. AVAPS will operate in all the modes outlined earlier: S, ST, T, and PC. AVAPS will monitor delivered tidal volumes and will raise IPAP if the tidal volume is below the target and decrease IPAP if the tidal volume is above the target. AVAPS keeps a running average of tidal volumes and makes small changes to IPAP in order to avoid arousing the patient with large pressure changes. This mode of therapy essentially continues the titration all the time while the patient is using the device. The IPAP is always at least the IPAP minimum and never more than the IPAP max. Care should be taken to set these pressures to assure a minimum level of pressure support at all times. The IPAP max is then set at a level that limits the maximum pressure the patient will receive but still ensures it is high enough to allow the device to achieve the desired tidal volume.

AVAPS with auto EPAP (AVAPS AE) is another mode of therapy that will also titrate EPAP in order to keep the upper airway patent and automatically adjust pressure support on the basis of the tidal volume target. This mode of therapy has settings for minimum and maximum levels of pressure support instead of IPAP. AVAPS AE also has minimum and maximum EPAP settings. This mode of therapy can compensate for changes in the upper airway in addition to changes in the level of ventilation.

Intelligent volume-assured pressure support (iVAPS) technology targets a set alveolar minute ventilation. The device will monitor delivered alveolar minute ventilation and compare it with the target alveolar minute ventilation. iVAPS adjusts pressure support and respiratory rate in order to maintain target alveolar minute ventilation. The alveolar minute ventilation that the iVAPS algorithm targets is minute ventilation with anatomic dead space subtracted from it. It does not account for any additional physiologic dead space.

These technologies were designed to keep the patient closer to their intended therapy while at home. The patient still needs to be monitored, and therapy may still need to be adjusted. These technologies may present some challenges to the sleep technologist in the laboratory. The sleep technologist may be used to increasing pressure when more ventilation is needed. If AVAPS or iVAPS is being used, it may be necessary to wait and let the algorithm do the work. Changes may need to be made if pressures are consistently being delivered at either the maximum or the minimum pressure settings. If delivered pressures are rising to the maximum setting, it may be necessary to increase the setting in order to allow the algorithm to reach the volume target. If delivered pressures have dropped to the minimum setting, it may mean that the minimum is set too high and the patient could be exposed to unnecessary pressures.

CURRENT TRENDS TREATING CHRONIC OBSTRUCTIVE PULMONARY DISEASE

Patients with COPD have historically been "rescued" from ventilatory failure in the intensive care unit by the use of NIV. These patients are then returned to the community, sometimes on NIV and sometimes not, only to return repeatedly to the hospital in respiratory failure.

Why does NIV work so well in an acute situation and then seem to fail when used chronically in a home care situation? Anecdotally, some physicians feel that one of the reasons is that the NIV is not targeting a high enough reduction in CO_2. However, it could be a whole host of issues normally observed with normal PAP and NIV issues occurring when the patient goes home.

High-intensity noninvasive positive pressure ventilation (HI-NPPV) has recently been utilized in patients with chronic hypercapnic COPD. This form of treatment uses NIV to maximize pressure support and respiratory rate to the highest level that the patient will tolerate. The goal is to gain the greatest reduction in CO_2 levels via arterial blood gas (ABG) analysis. IPAP levels of 30 cm H_2O are common, and respiratory rates approaching 20 breaths per minute are as well. The device is essentially taking over for the patient and doing most or all of the work of breathing while the patient is on the device.

This form of NIV has shown good results in CO_2 reduction and improvements in quality-of-life measures. These patients are usually titrated in a hospital or clinic setting in order to ensure that they are comfortable with the therapy and that CO_2 reductions are being achieved. These are not routine NIV titrations. Specific physician directions should be followed when attempting HI-NPPV (4,5).

SUMMARY

Neuromuscular disease and COPD are two of the most common disorders that are treated with NIV. Each of these disorders can present with or without coincident upper airway obstruction. Although these two disorders are very different in many ways, the goals of NIV therapy are very much the same. The primary goals are to reduce the work of breathing and to normalize blood gases.

Synchrony is another goal to add to these primary goals. Synchrony occurs when the patient is comfortable and accepting of the therapy that has been applied. Asynchrony is, of course, the opposite of synchrony. Asynchronous events happen all the time during NIV therapy. The job of the clinician setting up and titrating NIV is to minimize the number of these asynchronous events. These events include missed triggers, late triggers, missed cycles, early triggers, and late cycling. Asynchrony can occur because of incorrect I time settings and respiratory rates. Too slow or too fast rise times can also lead to asynchrony events. Too much or too little pressure support can cause asynchrony. If the breath is built properly and delivered with the proper timing, asynchronous events should be minimized.

To provide successful NIV therapy, break it down to the fundamentals. The EPAP is used to control the upper airway and keep it patent. It is the foundation for building a breath that is going to reduce the work of breathing for the patient. Pressure support is used to augment the patient's tidal volume to increase overall ventilation. CO_2 levels can be used as guidance to assure the proper amount of ventilation. ABG measurements of the CO_2 level are the gold standard. Transcutaneous CO_2 monitoring is useful as well. Capnography or end-tidal CO_2 measurements should be used cautiously with NIV. If CO_2 measurements are not available, or even if they are, ventilation can be improved by building a breath for the patient on the basis of the size of the patient. Use 7 to 8 mL/kg of body weight as a guide for the tidal volume and titrate the pressure support to get there (6). HI-NPPV for patients with COPD will override the standard 7 to 8 mL/kg guidance. Follow specific physician instructions if asked to deliver HI-NPPV.

Make sure that the triggering and cycling criteria are set appropriately. Most devices have automated algorithms that perform this function well. Some patients may need manually set flow triggering and cycling. Use caution because these criteria can also be set incorrectly, making it difficult for the patient to synchronize with the device.

Set the I time to provide a 1:2 to 1:3 inspiratory to expiratory ratio for the cycle time. As the backup rate is increased, the I time usually needs to be decreased in order to maintain the ratio. Remember that the air that goes into the lungs has to be fully exhaled before the next breath is given, or else breath stacking and asynchrony may result.

Respiratory rate is normally set just below the patient's own spontaneous rate. There are exceptions, of course. Patients with COPD on HI-NPPV will probably need higher rates to further reduce CO_2. Weaker neuromuscular patients may have trouble triggering spontaneously and need higher rates in order to maintain their current level of ventilation.

A patient tolerating NIV with adequate tidal volumes is a great start for NIV therapy. Some patients may need more aggressive forms of NIV therapy, but these patients may need frequent follow-up and adjustments, and only then will they get to the desired level of ventilation.

REFERENCES

1. Piper A, Grunstein R. Obesity hypoventilation syndrome, mechanisms and management. *Am J Respir Crit Care Med*. 2011;183(3):292-298.
2. Pruitt WC. Ventilation and oxygenation. In: Hess DR, MacIntyre NR, Galvin WF, et al, eds. *Respiratory Care Principles and Practices*. 3rd ed. Jones and Bartlett Learning; 2016:1131.
3. Gay PC. Complications of noninvasive ventilation in acute care. *Respir Care*. 2009;54(2):246-258.
4. Struik FM, Lacasse Y, Goldstein R, et al. Nocturnal non-invasive positive pressure ventilation for stable chronic obstructive pulmonary disease. *Cochrane Database Syst Rev*. 2013;2013(6):CD002878. doi:10.1002/14651858.CD002878.pub2
5. Weir M, Marchetti N, Czysz A, et al. High intensity non-invasive positive pressure ventilation for stable hypercapnic chronic obstructive pulmonary disease patients. *Chron Obstr Pulm Dis*. 2015;2(4):313-320. doi:10.15326/jcopdf.2.4.2015.0145
6. Selim B, Mokhlesi W, Randerath W, Javaheri S. Advanced modes of positive pressure therapy for sleep-disordered breathing. In: Kryger M, Roth T, Goldstein CA, Dement WC. *Principles and Practices of Sleep Medicine*. 7th ed. Elsevier; 2021:1363-1388.e5.

Chapter 48
Oxygen Administration in the Sleep Center

LAURA MCFARLAND

KEY CONCEPTS/LEARNING OBJECTIVES

The key concepts for this chapter include describing the various storage methods for oxygen, understanding how to regulate and control the flow of oxygen and choose an appropriate oxygen administration device, describing the limitations and inaccuracies of oxygen delivery, listing variables affecting oxygen therapy used with positive airway pressure therapy, recognizing the potential for creating increased nasal resistance, and understanding the importance of documenting oxygen administration.

KEY TERMS

Actual FIO_2
Delivered FIO_2
Entrainment
FIO_2
Hypoxemia
Hypoxia
lpm
$PaCO_2$
psi
$SpO_2\%$

Ambient or atmospheric air is comprised of nearly 21% oxygen gas. Oxygen is tasteless, colorless, odorless, and transparent. By itself, oxygen is not flammable but vigorously accelerates combustion. Oxygen is an elemental gas required for life, and while we can survive for days without food or water, we will only survive minutes without oxygen. Various respiratory and/or cardiac conditions result in the need for supplemental oxygen. With the surge in home sleep testing, the complexity of patients presenting to the sleep lab has increased 28% to 36% over the past decade (1). These patients are more likely to require advanced modalities, including the initiation and titration of oxygen therapy.

This chapter discusses the techniques and concerns of oxygen therapy, specifically, how supplemental oxygen is delivered in the sleep center environment. Common delivery devices and their inherent limitations are discussed.

Effective oxygen administration demands a technologist familiar with the physiology of respiration, ventilation, and gas exchange. Oxygen is considered a drug and is therefore administered in accordance with institution policy and procedure. Typically, oxygen therapy is prescribed by a physician through lab protocols or individual patient orders and administered by appropriately credentialed personnel. The reader is encouraged to review their particular workplace procedures, pertinent policies, and licensure.

Oxygen is one of the most commonly used drugs in hospitals. Interestingly, given the incidence and severity of hypoxemia encountered in the sleep center, the use of oxygen is relatively uncommon. Because hypoxemia occurring during sleep is most often caused by transient upper airway obstruction and/or hypoventilation, treatment is directed toward maintaining upper airway patency through a variety of methods, including continuous positive airway pressure (CPAP) and/or augmenting ventilation using bilevel positive airway pressure (BPAP). Supplemental oxygen is not considered an alternative to positive airway pressure (PAP) therapy for obstructive sleep apnea (OSA), however, in patients with congestive heart failure and central sleep apnea, it has been shown to reduce apnea-hypopnea index (AHI) due to central events (2).

OXYGEN STORAGE AND DISTRIBUTION

The use of medical grade oxygen requires a method of storage and means of delivery. Oxygen is commercially packaged as a compressed gas or in its liquid form. Alternatively, it can be separated and concentrated from room air using an "oxygen concentrator."

Manufactured oxygen is most often void of any humidity and is termed *anhydrous*, meaning without water. The gas is completely dry, which can irritate the upper airway mucous membranes. This is more of an issue with higher oxygen flows not often encountered in the sleep center.

Compressed Oxygen Gas

Medical gas cylinders (tanks) have been in use since 1888. Several medical/anesthetic gases, including pure (99%) oxygen, are packaged in cylinders, which are manufactured from seamless, high-quality, finely tempered steel or aluminum. For safety, cylinders are color coded. Oxygen tanks are colored white (or green). Although white is the international color code for oxygen, most cylinders in the United States are green. Despite color coding, the contents of a cylinder should be verified by its tag/label. If there is no tag, *do not use the cylinder*.

Numerous federal and industrial regulatory bodies govern cylinder manufacturing specifications, labeling, transportation, storage, and handling of medical gases. It is often an accreditation requirement that empty cylinders be labeled as "Empty" and stored separately from full cylinders to avoid confusion during emergency situations.

Oxygen cylinders are available in different sizes that contain various amounts of gas. Cylinder size is designated by single letters. For example, popular oxygen tanks are termed H (large) size and E (small) size (with several other sizes available). E-sized tanks are usually used for patient transport or in emergencies. H-sized tanks measure over 4½ ft (1.37 m) tall and are used more for stationary/long-term (bedside) applications. Oxygen cylinders are an expensive and bulky form of packaging for a relatively inexpensive substance; however, they are indispensable for patient transport.

Cylinders contain much more gas than their unpressurized internal volume. Regardless of the size of the oxygen cylinder, it is filled to a tremendous pressure (2,200 psi). As a comparison, most automobile tires contain less than 50 psi. By pressurizing the gas into cylinders, H and E cylinders, when full, contain 244 ft^3 (6.91 m^3) and 23 ft^3 (0.65 m^3) of oxygen, respectively. The reader is reminded that 1 ft^3 (0.0283 m^3) equates to 28.3 L and that, therefore, an E cylinder will provide 650 L of oxygen for patient use. At a common flow rate of 2 lpm, a full E cylinder would ideally provide 325 minutes of supplemental oxygen. To quickly calculate the remaining contents of an oxygen cylinder, we use a simple formula with the specific conversion factor (CF) for each cylinder size. The CF for E- and H-sized tanks is 0.28 and 3.14 L/psi, respectively. The sleep technologist should be able to calculate the remaining duration of an oxygen cylinder to ensure patient safety. An E cylinder with 1,000 psi × 0.28 should provide 280 L of oxygen. This quantity of oxygen should last 280 minutes (4.7 hours) at 1 lpm, or 140 min (2.3 hours) at 2 lpm.

$$\text{Duration of flow (minutes)} = \frac{\text{Cylinder pressure} \times \text{CF}}{\text{Oxygen flow (lpm)}}$$

A means of controlling the release of oxygen from the cylinder is necessary to permit safe and adjustable delivery to the patient. Typically, this includes three components:

- Cylinder valve
- Pressure-reducing valve
- Flowmeter

In most applications, the pressure-reducing valve and flowmeter are combined into a single assembly called a *regulator*.

Cylinder Valve

Cylinders come with an onboard needle valve, which allows the tank to be opened and closed but does not allow pressure reduction or flow measurement. This valve opens when turned counterclockwise and closes when turned clockwise, much like household water taps. The outlet of the cylinder valve is safety indexed for each type of gas; only a specific oxygen regulator will attach to an oxygen cylinder's valve. H cylinders use a threaded outlet to which a regulator is attached using a hex nut. E cylinders utilize a flat surface that receives a nipple from the oxygen regulator. This special type of regulator is not threaded but is pressed into position using a yoke-styled connection. Remember, only oxygen regulators will fit oxygen tanks. Generally, an appropriate hand tool (wrench) is required to connect and disconnect regulators from the cylinder valve. A special wrench is required to operate E cylinder valves, and a washer placed between the regulator and cylinder is necessary to prevent leaks.

Pressure-Reducing Valve

The cylinder valve is only a gross controller of flow, basically on or off. A pressure-reducing valve is used to reduce the extreme pressure within the cylinder to a working pressure, usually 50 psi. Fifty psi is still dangerously high for direct patient use but is a traditional working pressure for most ancillary oxygen therapy equipment (flowmeters, ventilators, nebulizers, etc).

There are differing types of pressure regulators (preset, adjustable, and multistage), and most incorporate a round (Bourdon) gauge that measures the gas pressure within the tank. A full tank registers 2,200 psi but gradually drops as the cylinder empties. The registered pressure is accurate only when the cylinder valve is open.

Flowmeter

Flowmeters control and indicate the flow rate of oxygen. Given a fixed working pressure of 50 psi, the outlet flow increases in proportion to the opening of a needle valve control. The most common flowmeter uses a Thorpe tube. A small indicator (often a black ball) floats on the flow of gas as it passes through the tapered Thorpe tube. The tube is graduated in increments of liters per minute (lpm). The greater the flow, the higher the float rises within the tube.

Flowmeters are specific to a particular gas. It is wise to ensure oxygen flowmeters are used to measure oxygen flow. Pediatric oxygen flowmeters are available for finer control of gas flow. These flowmeters display flow in increments of 0.5 or even 0.25 lpm. The flow rate is read with the flowmeter in an upright position with the graduation that bisects the ball float indicating the liter flow.

Flowmeters utilized on E tanks designed for patient transport are often of the dial/click meter variety. This type allows the user to use a dial to select a specific flow in increments without the requirement of having the cylinder in the upright position to verify the flow rate.

Flowmeters can be used to turn off gas flow; however, if the cylinder is not being used for a prolonged time, it should be turned off using the cylinder valve and the flowmeter left open.

Having two controls (cylinder valve and flowmeter) can cause confusion. For example, the regulator may register near full pressure but then quickly drop to zero when the flowmeter is turned on. This occurs when the regulator is pressurized yet the cylinder valve is turned off. The pressure drops quickly as the relatively small volume of oxygen contained within the regulator bleeds down. This happens when the flowmeter is turned off before the cylinder valve is turned off. For this reason, it is important to watch the flowmeter for a few moments after the flow of oxygen begins in order to ensure that cylinder pressure is maintained.

Liquid Oxygen

Oxygen can be stored as a liquid. This requires very low temperatures (−183 °C) maintained within a thermos-like cryogenic vessel. These systems operate under a pressure of approximately 20 psi. As pressure is reduced, the liquid oxygen is converted into a gas. The quantity of liquid gas contained within the vessel is measured in terms of weight, rather than pressure, and patient reservoirs have integrated scales to assist in calculating the remaining duration of oxygen. The storage advantage is obvious when considering that a single cubic foot of *liquid oxygen* is equivalent to about 860 ft^3 (24.35 m^3) of *oxygen gas*. Liquid oxygen vessels can be transfilled, that is, one liquid system can be used to fill another. Patients requiring long-term oxygen treatment may arrive at the sleep center with a portable liquid oxygen tank. Although the patient can easily be switched to the sleep center's oxygen source, the technologist should be aware that the liquid oxygen will slowly vaporize, and the vessel will empty even while not being used. This is similar to having a thermos of hot coffee that will slowly cool despite never being opened, the difference being that as liquid oxygen warms, it vaporizes to gas and escapes from the storage vessel, potentially creating an oxygen-rich environment.

Liquid oxygen is more expensive than compressed oxygen, and its primary advantage is storage and duration of portability. Most hospitals and other high-volume users store oxygen on-site in its liquid form in large industrial size tanks.

Oxygen Concentrators

These self-contained devices use electricity to power a compressor and filtration system. Filtering of room air through a molecular sieve bed or permeable plastic membrane produces concentrated oxygen. Oxygen concentrators supply 90% to 95% pure oxygen but are generally not capable of delivering high flows and are therefore not suited to emergency situations.

Modern oxygen concentrators are available in stationary and portable (battery operated) systems as well as models that can transfill oxygen cylinders. They are convenient, quiet, safe, and provide a reliable source of relatively inexpensive low-flow oxygen. Because of these benefits, concentrators are a good oxygen source for sleep centers located outside of hospitals. The reader is encouraged to become familiar with their respective oxygen concentrator in terms of flow rate capability and oxygen concentration specifications. Oxygen concentration should be checked as a part of the laboratory equipment quality assurance process.

OXYGEN DELIVERY IN THE SLEEP CENTER

Precautions

Pure oxygen itself presents potential *physical* dangers. First, oxygen cylinders contain very high pressures. It must be ensured that tanks are secured from falling or tipping to avoid tank or regulator breakage. Oxygen cylinders must be stored away from heat sources. Liquid oxygen is of extremely low temperature, and the vaporizing liquid can cause low-temperature burns to the skin. Oxygen itself is not explosive but vigorously supports combustion. Oxygen and materials that are flammable make for a very dangerous mix. For example, collodion, which is both volatile and flammable, should not be used in the vicinity of oxygen.

Oxygen also poses physiologic consequences. Prolonged high alveolar oxygen levels (>60%) are associated with the production of free radicals and lung damage (oxygen toxicity). Alveolar oxygen concentrations of more than 80% (with special circumstances) can be associated with regional microlung collapse (absorption atelectasis).

Oxygen and Ventilation

The theory of "hypoxic drive" has dominated the administration of supplemental oxygen for patients with pulmonary disease since the 1960s. This theory states that the stimulus to breathe in patients with lung disease (and associated high carbon dioxide levels) is hypoxia (low oxygen) rather than hypercapnia (high carbon dioxide), which is the main stimulus in normal patients. It was widely accepted that providing high levels of oxygen in these patients could actually suppress the stimulus to breathe or even cause them to become apneic. This theory was quickly adopted by a diverse cohort of medical professionals and has resulted in a general hesitancy to initiate or increase supplemental oxygen for patients with chronic obstructive pulmonary disease (COPD).

This theory has been re-evaluated in recent years, and it is now accepted that there are multiple mechanisms at work when oxygen is provided to chronic lung disease patients. It is now accepted that the Haldane effect and ventilation-perfusion mismatch are more likely to be the main drivers of physiologic response. These processes result in some brief, self-limited decreases in breathing (hypoventilation) and increased carbon dioxide levels ($Paco_2$). However apneic response is generally not seen until patients are approaching hypercapnic coma (3).

Ventilation-perfusion mismatch: The body strives to match the quality of ventilation (gas exchange) with perfusion (blood flow) at the alveolar level. When ventilation is impaired by lung disease, the blood vessels surrounding the affected alveoli become constricted so that blood flow will be directed to healthy areas where gases can exchange more efficiently. When a high Fio_2 (fraction of inspired oxygen) is introduced to these impaired regions, the blood vessels relax, but the alveoli are unable to effectively ventilate (exhale the carbon dioxide), and this results in a release of the elevated CO_2 into the bloodstream, increasing $Paco_2$.

Haldane effect: This mechanism is related to the affinity of hemoglobin (Hb) to CO_2 and O_2. Hemoglobin that is not bound to O_2 has a higher ability to bind to CO_2, and it is not unusual for our patients with chronic lung disease to maintain higher levels of CO_2 and lower levels of O_2 in their bloodstream on a daily basis. Once high levels of O_2 are introduced, the Hb molecules (which prefer to carry O_2 molecules) release their CO_2 molecules into the plasma, resulting in an increase in $Paco_2$ and potentially altering the acid-base balance.

The presence of lung disease impairs the body's ability to increase ventilation to remove increased levels of carbon dioxide in the bloodstream; therefore, it is essential that we find a balance between providing adequate levels of oxygen (required by every cell in the body), while limiting the unwanted increases in $Paco_2$. The solution is to target lower Spo_2 levels (88%-92%) in our patients with chronic lung disease.

Patients should be closely monitored, and the technologist should be mindful of potential physiologic changes when supplemental oxygen is initiated or increased. Since many patients with chronic lung disease remain undiagnosed, and/or may not have recent arterial blood gas (ABG) results to determine if they have chronically high CO_2 levels, it is best to closely observe every patient's response to supplemental oxygen. Oxygen should not be withheld from patients with pulmonary disease due to concerns over their ventilatory response; on the contrary, this patient population can greatly benefit from the data acquired and the skills employed by the sleep technologist.

Aims and Rationale of Intervention

The objective of treatment is to use the least amount of oxygen to bring about the desired therapeutic effect, which is often defined as a predetermined level of oxygen saturation. Various devices are available to deliver oxygen to patients, each with inherent advantages and limitations. Choosing the optimum delivery method is dependent on therapeutic goals, clinical status, and delivery device constraints.

It is advisable to establish both criteria and method for oxygen usage *before* performing polysomnography. Such guidelines are set by the physician via lab protocols or individual patient orders and are usually based on patient clinical circumstance. The sleeping patient is particularly challenging, because changes in blood oxygen saturation are common (during rapid eye movement [REM] sleep or supine position) and often transient. Setting limits of desaturation and appropriate intervention during polysomnography is a medical determination and must be clear to the technologist. Often, medical protocols related to the initiation of supplemental oxygen are related to insurance guidelines. If oxygen is initiated before we meet the associated reimbursement requirements, it will not be covered by insurance, and the patient will likely go untreated.

As the technologist prepares for testing, the patient's medical record should be reviewed for the presence of lung disease and/or medications that indicate the potential need for supplemental oxygen. The following predictors are independently associated with the requirement for supplemental oxygen with PAP therapy: a history of COPD, a body mass index (BMI) greater than 35 kg/m^2, age over 50 years, and those displaying more than 5% drop in SpO_2 between upright and supine positions (4). However, the presence of fewer than two of these factors has excellent negative predictive value for the need for supplemental oxygen.

Procedures describing "how" to add oxygen to CPAP/BPAP treatment should be set forth *in advance of testing*. For example, "when supplemental oxygen is required, the oxygen flow will be added as close as possible to the CPAP interface" or "oxygen requirements will be assessed 10 minutes after each 1 (one) lpm increment change."

In the sleep center, oxygen is most commonly administered in terms of flow rate measured in lpm. The flow of oxygen is controlled at the source, which is commonly located at the head of the bed or within the sleep room. Unfortunately, this requires the technologist to enter the patient's room to make oxygen flow adjustments. Ideally, the oxygen source and flowmeter would be located outside the sleep room, and the oxygen tubing would run to the patient. This can make for long runs of tubing, which should be avoided. It is best to administer oxygen in the sleep center as it is provided at home; however, the sleep technologist may well discover that patient needs have changed since oxygen was prescribed, and optimizing oxygen saturations is one of the goals of polysomnography. This may involve initiating, increasing, decreasing, or discontinuing supplemental oxygen during testing.

Oxygen can also be delivered in terms of concentration. Concentration is expressed as a percentage, such as 40% oxygen, or a fraction of inspired oxygen, termed FIO_2. For example, FIO_2 of 0.4 means 40% of the inspired air is oxygen (note that FIO_2 has no units of measure).

Both delivery device and liter flow determine FIO_2. In the sleep center, it is rare for the physician to request a specific FIO_2 or liter flow. Oxygen therapy is often ordered in advance by the physician without mention of actual dosage but based on therapeutic results. For example, "administer oxygen as required to maintain $SpO_2\% > 92\%$."

OXYGEN DELIVERY DEVICES

Oxygen delivery devices fall into two general categories: *high flow* and *low flow*.

High flow: The goal of these devices is to provide gas flows of specific oxygen concentrations at rates greater than the patient's inspiratory flow rate. These systems are designed to provide a specific FIO_2. However, *in practice*, if the patient's inspiratory flow exceeds the delivered flow, the *actual* FIO_2 diminishes as the patient draws in room air to compensate.

Venturi Masks (Air-Entrainment Masks)

This mask system incorporates larger mask ports (Figure 48-1) and assorted jet nozzle attachments to deliver specific FIO_2 levels. The nozzles are usually color coded and labeled with their specific oxygen flow requirement and resultant FIO_2. As the oxygen passes through the nozzle, it also pulls in room air, increasing inspiratory flow. The FIO_2 is dependent on the flow of gas (nozzle size) and the size of the nozzle entrainment port with higher FIO_2, requiring higher oxygen flows. This approach to delivering oxygen is useful for transportation of patients and in situations where precise FIO_2 levels are desired. Limitations include lack of humidity and inaccuracies should the jet nozzle entrainment ports become occluded or covered, for example, with bedsheets.

High-Flow Oxygen Nasal Cannula

The use of high-flow oxygen via specialized nasal cannula has overcome several challenges and gained increased acceptance in acute care. These systems (Figure 48-2) provide up to 60 lpm of flow, blenders to specify FIO_2, and heated humidity. This therapy may be utilized to stabilize patients pre and post intubation, to treat respiratory failure, and to address OSA in acute care patients when CPAP is not well tolerated (5).

For the most part, high-flow oxygen systems are impractical for long-term home use and are not often encountered in the sleep center.

Low-Flow Oxygen

Low flow: These systems deliver a specific, relatively low flow of 100% oxygen at less than the patient's inspiratory flow rate. During inspiration, the patient draws in room air mixing with the oxygen, which results in variable inspired oxygen concentrations. Actual FIO_2 depends on the amount of room air the patient draws in, making up the breath. Mouth breathing and high inspiratory flows result in greater dilution (lower FIO_2).

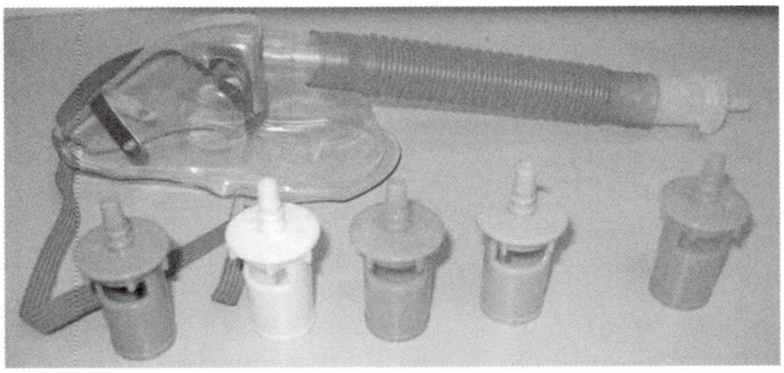

Figure 48-1 Venturi masks (air-entrainment masks).

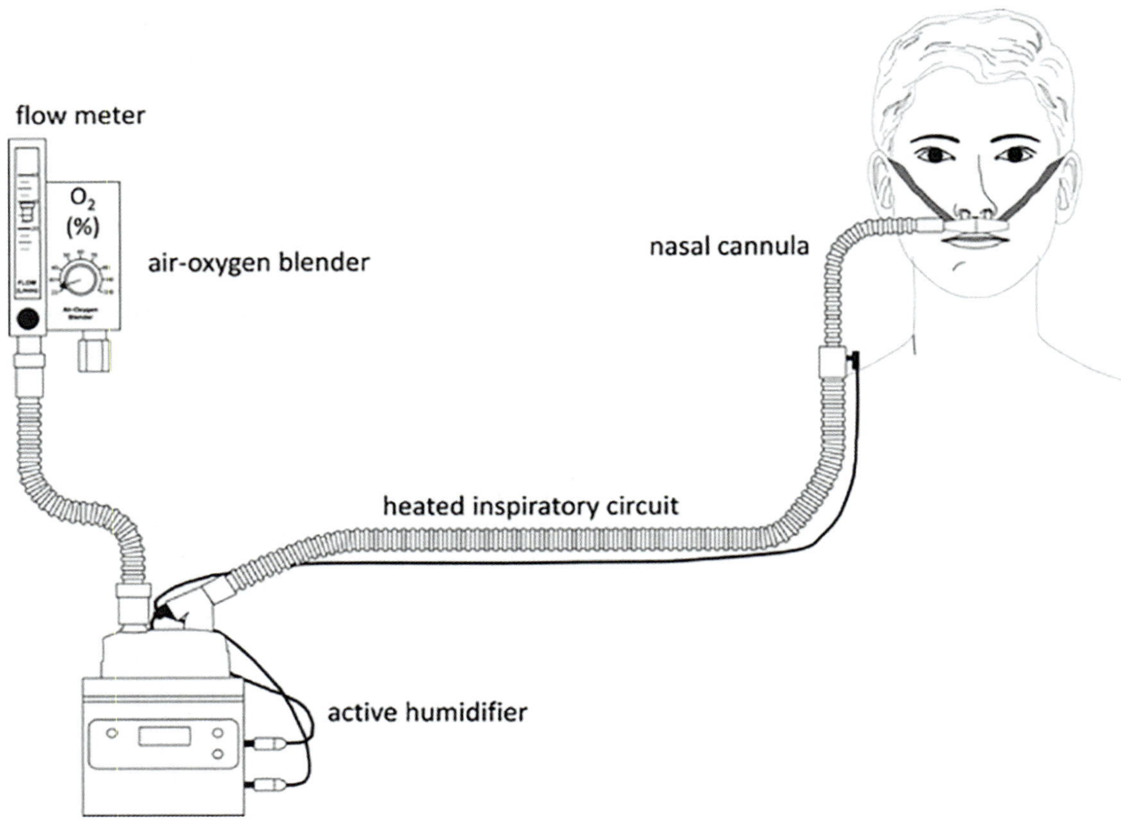

Figure 48-2 Principle setup of high-flow nasal cannula oxygen therapy. An air/oxygen blender, allowing from 0.21 to 1.0 FIO_2, generates up to 60 L/min flow. The gas is heated and humidified through an active heated humidifier and delivered via a single-limb heated inspiratory circuit. The patient breathes the adequately heated and humidified medical gas through nasal cannulas with a large diameter. (Reprinted from Nishimura M. High-flow nasal cannula oxygen therapy in adults. *J Intensive Care*. 2015;3(1):15. http://creativecommons.org/licenses/by/4.0)

Oxygen flow during inspiration is inhaled and therefore useful, but the oxygen flow is essentially wasted during exhalation. Considerable waste occurs because the typical patient exhales 2 to 4 times longer than they inhale. A number of oxygen conserving devices that limit delivery to a pulse of oxygen during the inspiratory phase only have been shown to deliver similar oxygen concentrations while using less oxygen. Other long-term, low-flow oxygen devices developed with the goal of conserving oxygen include transtracheal oxygen catheters as well as cannulae variants incorporating reservoirs and demand flow capabilities (6).

Low-flow devices may require supplemental humidity because the oxygen supply is anhydrous; however, typically, humidity is not required with low flows (<4 lpm). Alternatively, water based nasal lubricants can be utilized for patients with nasal dryness on low-flow oxygen and/or PAP therapy. When higher flow rates are required, common humidifiers used are bubble or jet type. These types of humidifiers are very inefficient and their value debatable. This is part of the reason that oxygen delivery devices such as a simple nasal cannula are generally not used when higher flow rates of oxygen are necessary to support blood oxygen levels.

Nasal Cannula

The nasal cannula is the most commonly used oxygen delivery device (Figure 48-3). The nasal cannula is relatively comfortable, inexpensive, and easily positioned with each prong of the cannula within the entrance of each nostril. A small tube runs over each ear, coming together below the chin, and running to the oxygen

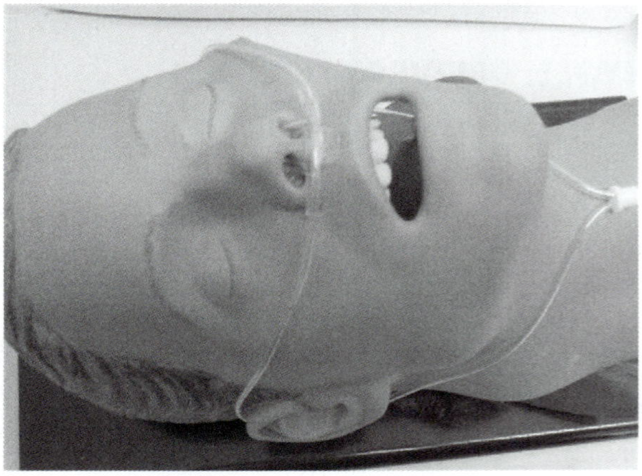

Figure 48-3 Nasal cannula.

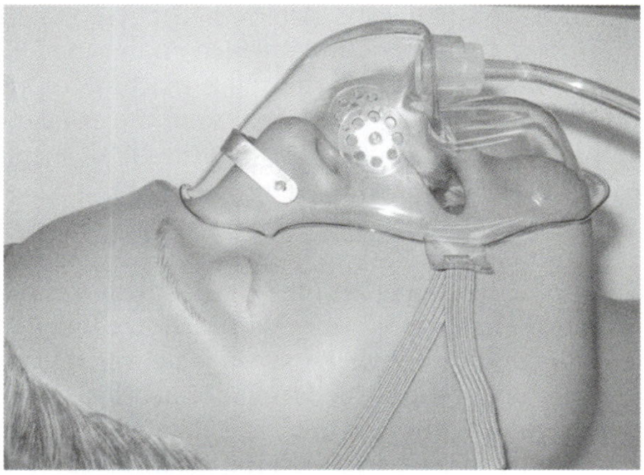

Figure 48-4 Simple oxygen mask.

source. Most problems are caused by kinked tubing, disconnection, or poor positioning within the nares.

The nasal cannula can provide 24% to 40% oxygen (depending on patient inspiratory flow rate) with oxygen flow rates up to 6 lpm for adults, and infants up to 2 lpm.

Simple Oxygen Mask

The simple oxygen mask is both inexpensive and easily applied (Figure 48-4). The mask is less well tolerated than the nasal cannula because it is more obtrusive, covering both nose and mouth. Oxygen flows should be greater than 5 lpm to prevent rebreathing of carbon dioxide (7). A maximum of 10 lpm oxygen can be used, and bubble-type humidifiers are often utilized. FIO_2 is variable but thought to be approximately 35% to 50%. Simple oxygen masks are usually used for short-term applications and emergencies requiring higher oxygen concentrations.

Miscellaneous Oxygen Masks

Other modified simple oxygen masks incorporate reservoirs and/or one-way valves to control the amount of rebreathing and thereby increase FIO_2 (Figure 48-5). These devices can be dangerous if not properly applied or monitored. It would be most unusual to encounter such devices in the sleep center aside from an emergency situation, and obtaining assistance from trained personnel is strongly recommended.

OXYGEN DELIVERY DEVICES AND POLYSOMNOGRAPHY

When patients arrive at the sleep center receiving supplemental oxygen, an effort should be made to maintain the type and style of device, as well as the set flow rate of oxygen before and after testing. Often, one of the purposes of the polysomnogram is to evaluate nocturnal oxygen requirements; therefore, unless otherwise ordered, it is the technologist's responsibility to make adjustments during testing. This can pose a problem, as monitoring sensors and CPAP requires unfettered access to the patient's face, nose, and mouth.

Oxygen is usually administered in the sleep center using a nasal cannula during the diagnostic portion of testing. Airflow is generally monitored using an oronasal thermal airflow sensor, and a nasal pressure transducer, and adding an additional cannula for oxygen administration raises various concerns.

Spontaneously Breathing Patients

Many technologists will simply place the oxygen cannula *in addition to* the flow-sensing devices. This practice is ill-advised (especially with pediatric patients) for two reasons:

- The added oxygen flow may interfere with airflow-monitoring techniques and result in a dampened airflow signal. The flow-sensing device signal is dampened by the added oxygen flow, artificially changing the actual temperature, pressure, and composition of the patient's breath and breathing.

Instrumentation occupying the nostrils can significantly increase nasal resistance (8). Given the relatively

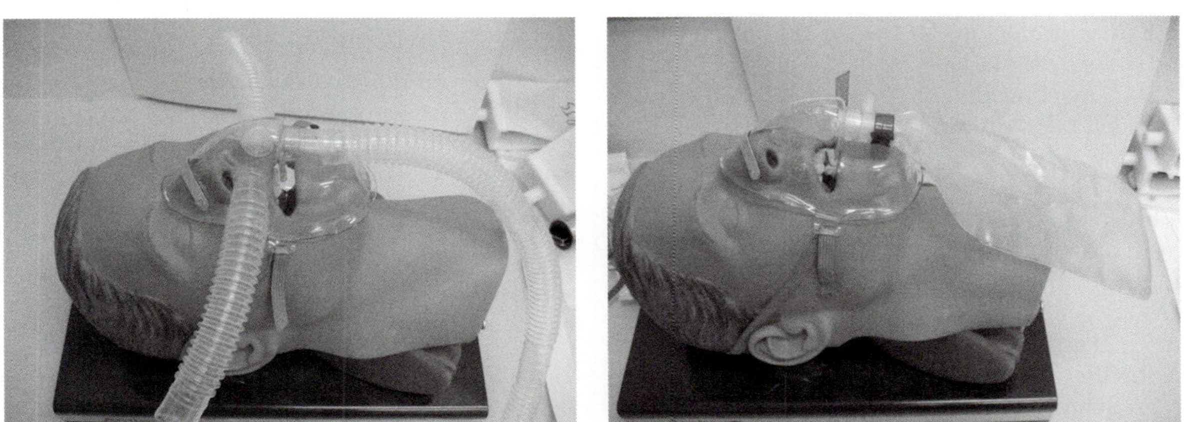

Figure 48-5 Other oxygen masks.

small cross-sectional area and large variants of patient nare(s), both the size (lumen) and the number of cannulae placed within the nostrils should be minimized. The relationship between increased nasal resistance and sleep-disordered breathing (SDB) has been recently and extensively reviewed (9). To avoid these shortcomings, bifurcated (dual lumen) cannulae allowing individual access to each nostril would be ideal. Because air pressure would be sampled from only one naris, and oxygen delivered to the other, equally patent nostrils are ideal but rarely encountered. Commonly available dual lumen cannulas have two luer lock (used in syringes) connectors (designed to attach to the PSG system and an end-tidal CO_2 device) or two oxygen connectors (to attach to an oxygen flowmeter and conserving device). To accomplish our goal of monitoring airflow and delivering oxygen, we would need one of each type of connector. Although this approach would minimize the occupying space of the cannulae, the proximity of the oxygen flow to nasal pressure/gas sampling may very well result in dampened flow signals.

In general practice, the nasal pressure cannula is removed and replaced by the oxygen cannula, and scoring of respiratory events relies on the oronasal thermal sensor. Fortunately, the American Academy of Sleep Medicine (AASM) also allows for the use of alternative sensors—RIPsum and RIPflow. Using two belts placed around the thorax and the abdomen, the RIP method allows semiquantitative assessment of volume changes (RIPsum) and/or airflow changes (RIPflow). The use of these signals can be invaluable when standard airflow signals are not functioning or reliable. Technologists are encouraged to become comfortable with the use and appearance of these signals so they can serve as a resource in the analysis of respiratory events.

Patient Using Continuous Positive Airway Pressure/Bilevel Positive Airway Pressure

Flow-monitoring sensors near or within the patient's nose interfere with the proper placement of CPAP interfaces and are typically removed when instituting CPAP. Flow and pressure signals can be derived from the sleep center CPAP machine remote control DC outputs or from an added inline flow transducer.

Oxygen is usually added directly into the CPAP circuitry by adding a pressure adapter that fits between the CPAP tubing and the CPAP mask and has a port for the connection of oxygen tubing running from the flowmeter. Some types of heated CPAP tubing come with an integrated oxygen port.

Oxygen is generally measured in terms of liter flow (lpm) with the least amount added, or "bled in" to achieve adequate saturations. However, the *actual* FIO_2 delivered to the patient is determined by several factors: the flow rate of oxygen, at which end of the CPAP hose the oxygen is added (near the machine or near the mask), mask leakage, the position of the exhalation port, the type of exhalation port, and the CPAP, inspiratory PAP, and expiratory PAP settings (10,11).

While some CPAP masks have provisions for adding oxygen, most do not have oxygen inlets, and the oxygen flow must be connected into the CPAP circuit upstream from the exhalation port. Studies have shown that delivered FIO_2 is optimized when oxygen is delivered via nasal cannula under the mask during noninvasive positive pressure ventilation (12); therefore it can be assumed that proximity to the nares is an important factor in the site of oxygen delivery. Future advances in mask design may well take these results into consideration by incorporating oxygen delivery. The sleep technologist needs to use equipment that will be readily available and comfortable for use in the home, and placing a cannula under a CPAP mask is not a long-term solution.

One safety-related consideration is keeping the added oxygen flow as distal to the machine as possible. It is generally advisable to keep gases that support or accelerate combustion away from electrical equipment. The only downside is the requirement of having another tube running to the patient.

OXYGEN DELIVERY DEVICES AND INTEGRATION WITH THE POLYSOMNOGRAPH

The author is unaware of any oxygen flowmeter capable of producing an electronic output signal allowing integration with a polysomnographic system. For this reason, the technologist almost always documents the administration of oxygen via tech comments within the sleep study and/or the addition of oxygen to PAP entry tags, which will allow the reading physician to visualize the oxygen levels on the PAP table and hypnogram. The information presented and referenced in the previous section clarifies the need for documenting more than only the liter flow of oxygen. Other factors include the following:

- Oxygen administration device
- Style of oxygen cannulae used
- Other instrumentation occupying the nostrils
- Site of oxygen entry into the CPAP/BPAP circuit
- Type and position of exhalation ports
- Type of CPAP interface (nasal or full-face mask)
- Measures of interface or oral air leak
- CPAP or BPAP settings

This all seems rather laborious, although necessary, because all these factors determine the actual concentration of oxygen delivered to the patient. The underlying objective of this documentation is to achieve accurate duplication in the home environment after the patient leaves the sleep center. It is simple to state CPAP/BPAP and oxygen liter flow rates were required during the sleep study to maintain a certain Spo_2%. However, it is an assumption to extrapolate the sleep center observation to the home without consideration or knowledge of the many determinants of *actual* Fio_2.

To minimize redundant documentation, a sleep center protocol should be established so that supplemental oxygen is provided consistently using the same tubing, cannulae, ports, site of interface, and so on. This would require documentation only for deviations from procedure. Ideally, the sleep center standard should be communicated to hospital respiratory therapy services and community durable medical equipment providers.

MONITORING AND REPORTING OUTCOMES

The goal of oxygen administration is usually the resultant change in blood oxygen levels. Blood oxygen levels are related to Fio_2—not lpm of oxygen. Although there is a relationship between the two, as previously discussed, there are many determinants of actual Fio_2.

Several methods of monitoring and measuring blood oxygen exist. The most common monitoring tool in the sleep center is the arterial oxygen saturation monitor (oximeter), which expresses blood oxygen levels in terms of Spo_2%.

Most pulse oximeters interface nicely with polysomnographic systems, allowing oxygen saturation to be continually displayed and recorded. As stated earlier, the technologist must manually document (annotate) the specific level of supplemental oxygen administration throughout the study.

Another common monitoring technique (ABGs) generally used in the acute care setting requires an arterial blood sample to measure the partial pressure of oxygen dissolved within the plasma expressed in units of mm Hg (torr). The blood sample is obtained from an artery in the patient's wrist using a needle and cannot be procured while the patient sleeps. Indwelling arterial lines that allow for quick access to arterial blood sampling are uncommon in the sleep lab. Blood gases obtained immediately after waking may have some value in detecting the presence of OSA and monitoring the effectiveness of supplemental oxygen (13,14). This is unlikely to be done in the sleep center.

Measuring transcutaneous oxygen ($Ptco_2$), which is typically done in conjunction with transcutaneous carbon dioxide—$Ptcco_2$, is another monitoring method. This approach is noninvasive, and the output is usually used as a trending tool. These monitors also easily interface with the polysomnograph. Since the application of supplemental oxygen may increase $Paco_2$ levels in patients with chronic lung disease, the use of transcutaneous monitoring could be helpful in determining target Spo_2 levels. If the baseline $Ptcco_2$ levels are increased, this indicates a disease state in which the patient retains CO_2 on a daily basis, and a target Spo_2 of 88% to 92% would be reasonable.

Each oxygen measurement/monitoring technique has advantages and inherent limitations. The technologist should become intimately acquainted with the equipment available in each sleep center. Even within a health care system with multiple sleep centers, there may be variations in equipment available for polysomnographic testing.

Reporting outcomes entails documentation throughout the recording and summarization of data at the conclusion of the sleep study. The acquisition technologist enters tags and/or comments within the recording to document the use of supplemental oxygen, but this may not be noticed until the study is opened by the scoring technologist. Since the unexpected need for supplemental oxygen could indicate a need for additional care, it is the responsibility of the acquisition technologist to ensure that this information is passed along to the day technologist, or appropriate surrogate. Some sleep centers have daily crossover between night and day staff, while others may have no day technologist on site, so it is important to understand and utilize the appropriate reporting structure for concerning clinical outcomes.

Although oxygen administration is commonly monitored by Spo_2%, there are numerous caveats. In certain situations, a patient can be hypoxic despite "normal" Spo_2% values. The technologist is urged to explore terms such as oxygen extraction, oxygen delivery, oxygen-carrying capacity, and regional perfusion. (See Suggested Readings.)

TROUBLESHOOTING OF OXYGEN DELIVERY DEVICES

Should oxygen administration fail to increase oxygen saturation, the first thing to check is the patient. In addition, a check of the monitoring device is prudent; it is important to ensure proper sensor placement and function. The possibility of erroneous or artifactual monitoring cannot be ignored.

Once the patient's oxygen level has been deemed accurate, the next thing to check is your plumbing. Simple checks for flowmeter function, tubing disconnection, cannula misplacement, and kinked tubing should be performed.

Other considerations include mouth breathing or nasal obstruction. If the patient is unable to inhale the oxygen from the delivery device, there may be little or no benefit. Similarly unappreciated, ongoing upper airway obstruction or hypoventilation may confound successful administration of oxygen.

If the patient's oxygen level cannot be maintained when asleep, the technologist may consider waking the patient for assessment. How these decisions are made and when testing ought to be interrupted should be determined in advance through the use of sleep center protocols. However, a patient not responding to increased FIO_2 may be presenting with a profound physiologic problem that should not be ignored.

WHEN TO GET HELP!

The sleep technologist should not hesitate to summon help and should have a good understanding of emergency policies. The ways and means of accessing assistance are varied, depending on the resources available to your sleep center. Once again, the reader is encouraged to explore their resources *before* the need becomes a crisis.

Assuming there are no technical problems, the sleep technologist would be generally advised to call for help in the following circumstances:

- The patient's oxygen saturation level cannot be maintained despite reaching the flow limits of the delivery system, sleep center protocol, or the physician's order.
- The patient is awake and hypoxic, experiencing respiratory distress and/or cardiac instability.
- The patient is hypoxic and unresponsive despite attempts to awaken.

FINAL CONSIDERATIONS

At first glance, a general review of oxygen delivery devices seems rather extraneous to the sleep center. However, with the increasing complexity of patients presenting to the sleep center, the need for supplemental oxygen is likely to rise. There are few studies examining oxygen delivery devices in the sleep center. Most studies have been done in postoperative recovery rooms, intensive care units, or in ambulatory patients with chronic lung disease. Nonetheless, one cannot ignore the wealth of information available, because many of the principles and relationships apply to the sleep center.

Challenges

Patients undergoing polysomnography begin the night with adjustments to their environment, routine, and comfort. Their upper airway quickly displays reduced nasal patency as soon as we ask them to lie down (15), and we add sensors that may trigger an afferent response, resulting in nasal congestion (16). If oxygen delivery becomes necessary, we may introduce a cannula reducing the cross-sectional area available for inspiratory flow (17) and dry the nasal passages—all factors that may further challenge our patients.

Newer CPAP modalities and other adjunct therapies pose other questions. It is reasonable to expect FIO_2 fluctuation depending on the amount and extent of interaction during "auto" or "smart" PAP treatment. The introduction of gas flows to systems equipped with adjuncts such as C-Flex, the impact on I → E and E → I phase triggering with bilevel machines, and the alterations in tidal volume with servo or volume-assured ventilation are all variables to consider in the interaction between supplemental oxygen and PAP therapy.

Opportunities

Despite the complex changes we introduce during testing, the sleep technologist has a unique role in diagnosis and treatment. Over the course of one night, we can positively impact our patient's lives by optimizing the "one-third" dedicated to sleep. When supplemental oxygen is needed, we can provide a calm, supportive atmosphere where the needs of the patient are assessed, addressed, and documented for the rest of the care team This can have immediate impact as our patients wake feeling better, the hypoxic burden on their organs is decreased, and they are potentially referred for further specialty care due to our findings.

REFERENCES

1. Colaco B, Herald D, Johnson M, Roellinger D, Naessens JM, Morganthaler TI. Analysis of the complexity of patients undergoing polysomnography in the era of HSTs. *J Clin Sleep Med.* 2018;14(4):631-639.
2. Zeineddine S, Rowley JA, Chowdhuri S. Oxygen therapy in sleep-disordered breathing. *Chest.* 2021;160(2):701-717.
3. Abdo WF, Heunks LM. Oxygen-induced hypercapnia in COPD: myths and facts. *Crit Care.* 2012;16(5):323.
4. Shetty S, Fernandes A, Patel S, Combs D, Grandner MA, Parthasarathy S. Unanticipated nocturnal oxygen requirement during positive pressure therapy for sleep apnea and medical comorbidities. *J Clin Sleep Med.* 2017;13(1):73-79.
5. Nishimura M. High-flow nasal cannula oxygen therapy in adults. *J Intensive Care.* 2015;3:15.
6. AARC Clinical Practice Guidelines. Oxygen therapy in the home or alternative site health care

facility—2007 revision and update. *Respir Care*. 2007;52(1):1063-1068.

7. AARC Clinical Practice Guidelines. Oxygen therapy for adults in the acute care facility—2002 revision and update. *Respir Care*. 2002;47(6):717-720.
8. Lorino AM, Lorino H, Dahan E, et al. Effects of nasal prongs on nasal airflow resistance. *Chest*. 2000;118:366-371.
9. Rappai M, Collop N, Kemp S, et al. The nose and sleep disordered breathing: what we know and what we do not know. *Chest*. 2003;124:2309-2323.
10. Schwartz AR, Kacmarek RM, Hess DR. Factors affecting oxygen delivery with bi-level positive airway pressure. *Respir Care*. 2004;49(3):270-275.
11. Yoder EA, Klann K, Strohl KP. Inspired oxygen concentrations during positive pressure therapy. *Sleep Breath*. 2004;8(1):1-5.
12. Mi S, Jiang C, Feng X, Zhang L. Effect of different oxygen delivery methods on transcutaneous oxygen pressure and fraction of inspired oxygen during non-invasive positive pressure ventilation. *Altern ther health med*. 2022;28(3):24-29.
13. Tarrega J, Guell R, Antón A, et al. Are daytime arterial blood gases a good reflection of nighttime gas exchange in patients on long-term oxygen therapy? *Respir Care*. 2002;47(8):882-886.
14. Guardiola J, Yu J, Hasan N, Fletcher EC. Evening and morning blood gases in patients with obstructive sleep apnea. *Sleep Med*. 2004;5(5):489-493.
15. Chang GH, Hsu CM, Huang EI, et al. Effects of supine and prone positions on nasal patency in healthy individuals. *Ear Nose Throat J*. 2023;102(7):460-466.
16. Baraniuk JN, Kim D. Nasonasal reflexes, the nasal cycle, and sneeze. *Curr Allergy Asthma Rep*. 2007;7:105-111.
17. Kjærgaard T, Cvancarova M, Steinsvåg SK. Relation of nasal air flow to nasal cavity dimensions. *Arch Otolaryngol Head Neck Surg*. 2009;135(6):565-570.

SUGGESTED READINGS

Berry RB, Chediak A, Brown LK, et al; NPPV Titration Task Force of the American Academy of Sleep Medicine. Best clinical practices for the sleep center adjustment of noninvasive positive pressure ventilation (NPPV) in stable chronic alveolar hypoventilation syndromes. *J Clin Sleep Med*. 2010;6(5):491-509. PMID: 20957853; PMCID: PMC2952756.

Lumb AB, Thomas CR. *Applied respiratory physiology*. 9th ed. Elsevier; 2020.

Stoller JK, Heuer AJ, Vines DL, Chatburn RL, Mireles-Cabodevila E. *Egan's Fundamentals of Respiratory Care*. 13th ed. Elsevier; 2024.

Troester MM, Quan SF, Berry RB, et al. *The AASM Manual for the Scoring of Sleep and Associated Events: Rules, Terminology and Technical Specifications. Version 3*. American Academy of Sleep Medicine; 2023.

Volsko TA, Chatburn RL, El-Khatib MF. *Equipment for Respiratory Care*. 2nd ed. Jones & Bartlett Learning; 2020.

Chapter 49
Dental Sleep Medicine: Oral Appliance Therapy (OAT) and Titration Management

JOSHUA ERIC SHORE

KEY CONCEPTS/LEARNING OBJECTIVES

The key concepts for this chapter include an introduction to the use of mandibular advancement devices for the treatment of obstructive sleep apnea, including a review of types of devices, essential features, compliance monitoring, clinical value, and effectiveness.

KEY TERMS

Mandibular advancement devices (MAD)
Obstructive sleep apnea (OSA)
Oral appliance therapy (OAT)
Temporomandibular joint (TMJ)

INTRODUCTION TO OBSTRUCTIVE SLEEP APNEA AND MANDIBULAR ADVANCEMENT DEVICES

Obstructive sleep apnea (OSA) is a chronic and prevalent disorder characterized by repeated episodes of partial or complete upper airway obstruction during sleep. These events result in intermittent hypoxemia, sleep fragmentation, and activation of sympathetic pathways, which collectively contribute to excessive daytime sleepiness, cognitive impairment, and increased risk for cardiovascular and metabolic disease (1). The estimated prevalence of OSA among US adults is approximately 15% to 30% in men and 10% to 15% in women, while a large proportion of cases remain undiagnosed (2).

Although continuous positive airway pressure (CPAP) remains the gold standard treatment for moderate-to-severe OSA, adherence to CPAP therapy is suboptimal, with long-term use rates frequently below 50% (3). This has prompted growing clinical interest in alternative and adjunctive treatments that are better tolerated and easier to integrate into patients' lifestyles.

Mandibular advancement devices (MADs) have emerged as a first-line treatment for primary snoring and mild OSA and a second-line therapy for moderate to severe cases when CPAP is not tolerated (4). MADs are intraoral appliances worn during sleep that mechanically advance the mandible to increase upper airway caliber and reduce collapsibility. Their therapeutic value lies in their ability to provide noninvasive, quiet, and portable therapy with relatively high patient adherence compared to CPAP.

The American Academy of Sleep Medicine (AASM) and the American Academy of Dental Sleep Medicine (AADSM) have collaboratively issued practice parameters and clinical guidelines detailing the indications, design specifications, and management protocols for oral appliance therapy (OAT) using MADs. The most recent standards highlight the use of custom, titratable MADs delivered by qualified dentists in collaboration with sleep physicians (4,5).

As of 2023, emerging evidence continues to reinforce the utility of MADs, not only in effecting symptom improvement but also in contributing to better cardiovascular metrics such as blood pressure reduction in certain patient populations (6). Moreover, technologic innovations like embedded compliance sensors and remotely titratable devices have further enhanced their clinical applicability.

This chapter will provide a comprehensive and clinically actionable overview of MAD therapy as applied in dental sleep medicine. Topics covered include device types, mechanisms of action, clinical efficacy, side effects, fitting and titration protocols, and long-term management strategies. Special emphasis will be placed on the latest AASM and ABDSM clinical guidelines (2020-2025), while acknowledging the historical foundation of sleep science laid by earlier seminal works, including Rechtschaffen and Kales (7).

In sum, MADs represent a key pillar of contemporary OSA management—especially when prescribed within a structured, interdisciplinary framework. Their appropriate use can lead to substantial improvements in patient outcomes, quality of life, and public health burden associated with untreated sleep apnea.

TYPES OF MANDIBULAR ADVANCEMENT DEVICES AND CHARACTERISTICS OF EFFECTIVE DESIGNS

MADs form the cornerstone of OAT for OSA and primary snoring. Their design, customization, and adjustability significantly affect both therapeutic success and patient adherence. In addition to traditional mechanical features, recent innovations—particularly smart MADs with embedded compliance monitors—are reshaping best practices and aligning OAT more closely with the objective tracking capabilities long associated with CPAP therapy.

Mandibular Advancement Devices Classification Framework

1. Custom versus Prefabricated
   - Custom-fabricated MADs are made using digital intraoral scans or dental impressions. These offer a highly retentive and comfortable fit, essential for long-term adherence. They also accommodate dental arch variations and reduce unwanted pressure points.
   - Prefabricated or "boil-and-bite" MADs, although cost-effective, lack long-term durability and are discouraged in clinical guidelines for OSA treatment (4).
2. Titratable versus Fixed (Monobloc)
   - Titratable MADs allow stepwise mandibular advancement (typically in 0.5-1 mm increments). These devices are ideal for individualized titration to balance efficacy with comfort, as per AADSM consensus recommendations (8).
   - Fixed-position MADs, which hold the jaw in a static position, are less adaptable and have a narrower therapeutic window. They are rarely used in modern clinical settings.

Essential Features of Clinically Effective Mandibular Advancement Devices

According to the AADSM Expert Consensus Statement (2019) and reinforced in the 2022 AADSM Clinical Practice Standards (5), a clinically effective MAD should:

- Be custom-fabricated for upper and lower dental arches.
- Include a reliable titration mechanism (≥1 mm adjustability).
- Allow retrusion and advancement for patient comfort and efficacy.
- Be durable and biocompatible, with a 3- to 5-year service life.
- Permit lip closure and adequate oral airflow during sleep.
- Include documentation for titration and position tracking.
- Be amenable to objective compliance tracking when indicated.

Smart Compliance-Recording Mandibular Devices

One of the most transformative advances in MAD technology is the integration of objective compliance tracking, enabled through embedded microsensors such as thermal sensing technology. This development responds to the growing demand for treatment verification—especially in medically monitored cases (eg, Department of Transportation [DOT], regulated commercial drivers, or patients with cardiovascular comorbidities).

CLINICAL VALUE

- Objective compliance data is especially valuable in populations where proof of adherence is medically or legally required.
- Research shows high accuracy: one study (9) demonstrated a mean nightly use of 6.4 hours, with 80% to 90% of patients meeting therapeutic adherence thresholds (≥4 hours on ≥70% of nights).
- Compliance monitors enable quantification of "mean disease alleviation" (a product of efficacy × adherence), a concept central to evaluating long-term OSA treatment success (10).

PRACTICE INTEGRATION

In 2022, the AADSM acknowledged smart MADs in its Clinical Practice Protocol, recommending their consideration in cases where monitoring use is essential or where insurance or regulatory entities demand objective evidence. These devices are particularly beneficial in commercial driver certification: Federal Motor Carrier Safety Administration (FMCSA), Federal Aviation Administration (FAA).

- Cardiovascular risk management (hypertension, atrial fibrillation)
- Sleep studies with unclear symptom correlation

Limitations and Considerations

- These devices tend to be more costly.
- Sensor data requires patient consent and secure handling.
- Not all labs offer sensor integration at the point of fabrication.

Despite these limitations, smart MADs represent a crucial step toward parity with CPAP therapy, aligning OAT with AASM guidelines for objective adherence monitoring.

Summary

In conclusion, the landscape of MADs has evolved beyond simple mechanical platforms. Today's best practices focus on custom, titratable, biocompatible designs with an increasing role for smart, compliance-recording technology. The integration of embedded sensors offers a significant advance in aligning OAT with precision medicine goals, data-driven treatment, and interdisciplinary accountability between dental and sleep medicine providers.

MECHANISM OF ACTION

MADs exert their therapeutic effect in OSA by biomechanically altering the upper airway anatomy to maintain patency during sleep. The core mechanism involves anterior repositioning of the mandible, which, in turn, displaces the tongue and associated soft tissues forward, increasing the caliber of the oropharyngeal and hypopharyngeal airway spaces and decreasing their propensity to collapse (11).

When the mandible is held in a protruded position by the MAD, it tethers the genioglossus muscle—the primary protrusor of the tongue—forward. This anterior displacement reduces posterior tongue base encroachment into the pharyngeal airway, a common site of obstruction in OSA. At the same time, the forward jaw posture exerts lateral tension on the palatoglossal and palatopharyngeal arches, which can reduce the collapsibility of the soft palate and lateral pharyngeal walls (3). This multilevel stabilization effect helps maintain airflow throughout the sleep cycle, particularly during rapid eye movement (REM) sleep, when muscle tone is reduced and airway collapse is more likely.

Advanced imaging studies, such as magnetic resonance imaging (MRI) and computed tomography (CT), have documented significant enlargement of both the retropalatal and retroglossal airway dimensions in patients using MADs (12). Furthermore, flow dynamics simulations suggest a reduction in pharyngeal airflow resistance due to changes in airway shape and cross-sectional area (13). These improvements are achieved without introducing external pressure, in contrast to the pneumatic splinting action of CPAP.

Electromyographic data also indicate that MADs may stimulate basal upper airway dilator muscle activity, possibly contributing to increased neuromuscular tone during sleep (14). However, the extent of neuromuscular involvement remains an area of ongoing research.

Critically, the therapeutic benefit of MADs is dose dependent: increasing mandibular protrusion generally correlates with greater reductions in apnea-hypopnea index (AHI), up to a point of diminishing returns or intolerance. The optimal protrusive position varies across individuals and must be determined through careful titration (4,5).

In sum, MADs function as intraoral splints that reconfigure upper airway structure and dynamics through anterior mandibular repositioning. By directly targeting the mechanical pathophysiology of OSA, these devices offer a potent alternative for patients who cannot tolerate CPAP, particularly when custom-fitted and titrated properly.

Clinical Efficacy of Mandibular Advancement Devices in Obstructive Sleep Apnea and Snoring

- MADs have demonstrated consistent clinical efficacy in reducing OSA severity, mitigating snoring, and improving quality-of-life outcomes. Although CPAP remains the gold standard treatment for moderate-to-severe OSA, OAT with MADs offers a viable, evidence-based alternative, especially in patients with mild-to-moderate disease or those intolerant of CPAP (4,5).

Obstructive Sleep Apnea Severity Reduction and Symptom Improvement

- Numerous randomized controlled trials (RCTs) and meta-analyses have validated the capacity of MADs to reduce AHI, arousal index, and oxygen desaturation events. In a pivotal comparative RCT by Gagnadoux et al (14), titrated MADs significantly reduced AHI from baseline (mean AHI reduced by >50% in many cases), and improved daytime sleepiness, as measured by the Epworth Sleepiness Scale (ESS). Similarly, a multicenter study by Sutherland et al (11) showed MADs to be noninferior to CPAP in terms of sleepiness and quality-of-life outcomes, despite CPAP achieving lower residual AHI values.
- This apparent paradox—greater physiologic efficacy with CPAP but similar patient-centered outcomes with MADs—is often explained by higher adherence rates to MAD therapy. According to Kuna et al (3), when considering both efficacy and adherence (termed "mean disease alleviation"), MADs deliver comparable overall therapeutic impact to CPAP in real-world usage.

Snoring Reduction

- MADs are particularly effective in addressing primary snoring and snoring associated with OSA. The mandibular protrusion mechanically stabilizes the upper airway, reducing tissue vibration and soft palate flutter. In a prospective study using both subjective reports and objective acoustic analysis, MAD use led to significant reductions in snoring frequency and intensity (12).
- This effect has important social and psychosocial implications, as bed partner–reported snoring often drives initial evaluation and therapy adherence. In clinical practice, improvement in snoring is often the first and most noticeable benefit experienced by patients and their partners, promoting therapy continuation.

Cardiovascular and Metabolic Outcomes

- Beyond symptom control, recent studies have investigated MADs' potential to favorably impact cardiovascular metrics. In a 12-month RCT, de Vries et al (6) found that MAD therapy led to modest reductions in 24-hour systolic and diastolic blood pressure in patients with OSA, comparable to the effect size observed with CPAP in similar populations. These findings suggest that MADs may confer cardiovascular benefits through improved nocturnal oxygenation and reduced sympathetic activation.
- Emerging data also explore potential benefits in glycemic control and metabolic syndrome management, although results are more variable and require further investigation.

Response Predictors and Outcome Variability

- Clinical efficacy varies across individuals. Predictors of favorable response include lower baseline AHI, supine-dependent OSA, younger age, lower body mass index (BMI), and absence of significant upper airway anatomic abnormalities (8). While MADs can significantly reduce AHI in patients with severe OSA, complete normalization is less likely than in mild-to-moderate cases.
- Polysomnographic or home sleep apnea test (HSAT) confirmation is recommended post titration to assess therapeutic success and guide ongoing management (4,5).
- In summary, MADs are effective in reducing AHI, alleviating sleepiness, and controlling snoring in a substantial proportion of patients. Their tolerability and adherence advantages further support their role as a cornerstone therapy in modern OSA management.

SIDE EFFECTS AND ADVERSE EVENTS OF MANDIBULAR ADVANCEMENT DEVICES THERAPY

MADs are generally well tolerated, especially when compared to CPAP therapy. However, their long-term use is not without risk. Understanding the potential side effects and adverse outcomes is essential for clinicians to optimize patient care, monitor appropriately, and address complications promptly.

Short-Term Side Effects

The initial adjustment period with MAD use can involve several mild, transient side effects. Common early complaints include:

- Excess salivation or dry mouth: Salivary response varies among users; some experience drooling, while others report xerostomia. These typically normalize within a few weeks (4,5).
- Oral and mucosal discomfort: Contact between the device and soft tissues may cause irritation of the gums, cheeks, or tongue. Modifications to the device or use of protective wax often alleviates this (5).
- Tooth soreness or pressure: This is often related to the force exerted on dentition by the appliance and usually resolves as adaptation occurs.
- Morning occlusal changes: Patients often wake up with a "misaligned bite" or temporary malocclusion. Morning exercises or repositioners are routinely recommended to re-establish normal occlusion (4).

Long-Term Dental and Skeletal Changes

Prolonged use of MADs may result in permanent occlusal changes due to the continuous anterior positioning of the mandible. Common findings include:

- Reduction in overjet and overbite
- Development of posterior open bite
- Tipping of incisors or slight tooth migration

These changes may not be symptomatic but are detectable during routine dental evaluations. A 5-year longitudinal study indicated that more than 60% of patients had detectable occlusal changes, although only a minority discontinued therapy because of them (8).

Temporomandibular Joint and Muscle Effects

MAD therapy can influence TMJ dynamics and masticatory muscles. Some patients may develop:

- TMJ soreness, particularly if the device is set too far forward too quickly

- Clicking or popping in the joint
- Masseter or temporalis muscle tenderness

However, studies show that most TMJ symptoms are transient and do not develop into clinically significant dysfunction if titration is gradual and well monitored (15). Patients with pre-existing temporomandibular disorders (TMD) should be managed cautiously and monitored more frequently.

Prosthodontic and Periodontal Considerations

Loose dental restorations, irritation of gingival tissues, and plaque accumulation around the appliance are possible, especially in patients with suboptimal oral hygiene. Regular professional dental cleanings and careful oral hygiene instruction are key.

Management and Monitoring

Routine dental follow-up is recommended every 6 to 12 months, per AADSM guidelines (5). Strategies to mitigate long-term effects include:

- Using morning occlusal guide appliances
- Documenting baseline occlusion and tracking changes
- Adjusting or remaking devices as needed based on dental changes or patient comfort

In summary, while MADs are safe and effective for most users, clinicians should remain vigilant for short-term discomfort and long-term occlusal or TMJ effects. A proactive management strategy ensures continued comfort and success with therapy.

Fitting Protocols and Clinical Workflow

Effective use of MADs in treating OSA requires a structured, interdisciplinary clinical workflow. The AASM and AADSM emphasize that OAT should be initiated only after a physician's diagnosis and delivered by qualified dentists (4,5).

Referral and Diagnosis

The workflow begins with a comprehensive medical evaluation and diagnosis of OSA by a sleep physician. Diagnostic confirmation is made through a Type I polysomnography or HSAT in accordance with AASM scoring standards. The physician determines the patient's suitability for OAT—generally indicated for:

- Primary snoring
- Mild-to-moderate OSA
- CPAP-intolerant or nonadherent patients with moderate-to-severe OSA

Following diagnosis, a formal prescription or referral is issued to a dentist trained in dental sleep medicine (preferably, an AADSM Qualified Dentist or ABDSM Diplomate).

Dental Evaluation and Records

At the initial dental visit, the clinician conducts an in-depth oral examination, evaluating:

- Number and stability of teeth
- Occlusion and overjet/overbite
- Periodontal status
- TMJ function and range of motion
- Gag reflex and oral anatomy

Baseline records, including intraoral scans or impressions and occlusal bite registrations, are collected. The patient is educated on the MAD mechanism, risks (eg, dental changes, TMJ effects), and expected course of therapy. Informed consent is obtained at this stage (5).

Device Selection and Fabrication

The dentist selects an appropriate custom, titratable MAD, based on oral anatomy and patient needs. Most US Food & Drug Administration (FDA) cleared devices meet AADSM criteria: bilateral coverage, titratability in increments of 1 mm or less, and documentation of the mandibular position (8). The impressions and bite registration are submitted to a dental lab for fabrication, with delivery in 2 to 3 weeks.

Device Delivery and Initial Titration Setup

At the delivery appointment, the appliance is checked for fit, retention, comfort, and ease of insertion/removal. The initial mandibular advancement is typically set at 50% to 70% of the patient's maximal comfortable protrusion. Instructions include:

- Daily wear routine
- Cleaning methods
- Start of titration (if patient controlled)
- Morning repositioning exercises

The patient is encouraged to report discomfort, pain, or looseness for timely adjustments.

Titration and Early Follow-Up

Follow-up occurs 2 to 4 weeks postdelivery to assess comfort and response. Titration (manual or remote) is tailored to symptom relief and tolerability. Regular check-ins ensure the patient is adjusting appropriately and tolerating the appliance. Communication with the referring physician is maintained throughout.

Verification of Efficacy

Per AASM/AADSM guidelines, efficacy should be confirmed with a post titration sleep study (typically HSAT). If residual OSA remains, further advancement, combination therapy, or alternative treatments may be discussed (4).

In summary, the fitting workflow for MADs is a collaborative process involving physicians, trained dentists, and the patient. When followed diligently, it ensures that therapy is personalized, effective, and well tolerated.

TITRATION METHODS—MANUAL, REMOTE, AND PREDICTIVE TOOLS

Titration is the process of adjusting a MAD to determine the optimal mandibular position that reduces obstructive events while maintaining patient comfort. The efficacy of MAD therapy is highly dependent on achieving this balance, and titration remains a critical clinical step following device delivery.

Manual Titration

Manual or subjective titration is the most common approach used in clinical practice. Patients begin therapy with the MAD set to an initial mandibular advancement position, typically 50% to 70% of their maximum comfortable protrusion (4,5). The patient is instructed to incrementally advance the device (usually by 0.5-1 mm) every few nights or weekly, depending on symptom persistence and comfort.

The endpoint of manual titration is reached when:

- Snoring and apneic symptoms resolve
- Further advancement causes discomfort
- Maximal advancement is reached

Regular follow-up with the dental provider (often, every 2-4 weeks) is critical during this period to ensure proper technique, troubleshoot discomfort, and monitor response. While manual titration is straightforward and cost-effective, its reliance on subjective symptom reporting may limit precision.

Remote-Controlled Titration and In-Lab Prediction

Remote-controlled mandibular positioning (RCMP) is an emerging method that provides objective titration during a single overnight polysomnogram (PSG). Devices such as the MATRx Plus (Zephyr Sleep Technologies) allow for precise control of mandibular position during sleep. A sleep technologist adjusts jaw advancement in real time while monitoring the reduction of apneas, hypopneas, and snoring (11).

Advantages of RCMP include:

- Real-time determination of optimal mandibular advancement
- Identification of likely responders to MAD therapy
- Shortened treatment time to therapeutic effect

Despite its accuracy, RCMP remains limited by high cost, device availability, and access to in-lab testing.

Drug-Induced Sleep Endoscopy-Guided Titration

Drug-induced sleep endoscopy (DISE) involves administering sedation to simulate natural sleep while a flexible scope visualizes the airway. Mandibular advancement is manually applied (eg, with a protrusion jig), and airway changes are assessed. This method provides valuable insight into airway collapsibility and the mechanical impact of jaw advancement (16). DISE is especially useful in complex or refractory cases.

PREDICTIVE AND EMERGING TECHNOLOGIES

Predictive modeling using cephalometric, anthropometric, or sleep data is under development to estimate MAD effectiveness and titration needs. Technologies such as machine learning algorithms and artificial intelligence aim to guide titration strategy and identify responders before treatment initiation (17).

Smart Titration Tools and Auto-Adjusting Devices

A recent innovation includes smart MADs capable of autonomous titration based on physiologic feedback. Prototypes are being tested with embedded sensors that adjust mandibular protrusion in response to detected snoring or airway resistance during sleep. While not yet commercially mainstream, these technologies may revolutionize OAT by reducing reliance on subjective patient feedback.

In conclusion, titration methods have evolved from manual, trial-and-error strategies to more objective and technology-driven approaches. When tailored to the patient's clinical profile and preferences, they enhance therapeutic precision and improve outcomes.

LONG-TERM FOLLOW-UP, MONITORING, AND COMPLIANCE

The long-term success of MAD therapy depends not only on device design and titration but also on structured follow-up and adherence monitoring. Sustained efficacy, minimal side effects, and patient satisfaction are achievable only when MAD use is supported by ongoing care, interprofessional collaboration, and patient education.

Follow-Up Protocols

According to AADSM Clinical Practice Guidelines (2022) and AASM/AADSM Joint Guidelines (2015), (4,5) follow-up begins within 3 to 6 weeks of device delivery and should continue at regular intervals—typically at 6-month and annual visits. These evaluations assess:

- Comfort and tolerance
- Dental and occlusal changes
- Presence of TMJ symptoms
- Device integrity and wear
- Continued symptom control (eg, snoring, daytime sleepiness)

Dentists trained in sleep medicine are advised to use standardized documentation, such as the AADSM's template forms, to track progress, titration settings, and any side effects.

Efficacy Verification and Re-Evaluation

Objective verification of MAD therapy efficacy is recommended through post titration sleep testing. This can be performed via PSG or HSAT after titration has stabilized. The AASM endorses this approach for all patients, especially those with moderate-to-severe OSA or comorbid conditions (4,5).

In cases of suboptimal response, treatment alternatives may include:

- Additional mandibular advancement
- Combination therapy, for example, MAD + positional therapy or positive airway pressure (PAP)
- Transition back to CPAP for severe or refractory cases

Re-evaluation is also needed when patients undergo major dental work or TMJ treatment or report symptom recurrence.

Compliance Monitoring and Smart Devices

Historically, one limitation of OAT was the lack of objective adherence data—unlike CPAP, which includes built-in compliance tracking. However, the introduction of thermistor-based sensors now allows for precise recording of nightly MAD wear time (9).

These systems:

- Detect intraoral temperature to confirm wear
- Log usage data for up to 100 days
- Generate compliance reports in accordance with AASM standards

Objective compliance data is particularly important for:

- Commercial drivers; DOT, FAA, etc.
- Patients in research trials
- Medico-legal documentation (eg, surgical clearance)

Recent studies report high adherence rates to MAD therapy—often exceeding CPAP in real-world settings (3). When both efficacy and adherence are considered, MADs may offer equivalent long-term benefits through a metric known as "mean disease alleviation."

PATIENT ENGAGEMENT AND RETENTION

Key to long-term success is ongoing patient education. Patients should be reminded about the risk of dental changes, device wear, and symptom recurrence. Encouraging regular dental hygiene, informing about when to seek re-evaluation, and involving bed partners in feedback all help to sustain engagement.

In conclusion, long-term follow-up transforms MAD therapy from a static intervention to a dynamic, monitored process. With structured reviews, smart device integration, and interprofessional collaboration, OAT can deliver sustainable, evidence-based outcomes for patients with OSA.

CONCLUSION AND FUTURE DIRECTIONS

MADs have evolved from a niche treatment option into a foundational modality in the management of OSA and primary snoring. Their growing acceptance and integration into clinical care are supported by evidence-based guidelines, sustained research, and rising patient preference. MADs offer a highly valuable alternative for patients who are unable or unwilling to tolerate CPAP, while also serving as a viable first-line treatment for mild-to-moderate OSA.

Recent updates from the AASM and AADSM reaffirm the clinical legitimacy of OAT, especially when delivered by trained dentists in collaboration with board-certified sleep physicians. The emphasis on custom-fitted, titratable devices, objective follow-up sleep testing, and long-term occlusal and TMJ surveillance reflects a maturing field that values precision and multidisciplinary oversight (4,5).

Technology has further propelled MAD therapy forward. Compliance-tracking microsensors now allow dentists and physicians to verify adherence—once a major limitation in evaluating OAT success. Additionally, RCMPs and DISE are helping predict treatment responders, optimize titration, and reduce time to efficacy. Meanwhile, smart oral appliances—featuring real-time snoring feedback, automated adjustments, and cloud-connected dashboards—are in early-stage development, offering a glimpse into a future of digital, responsive sleep therapy.

However, despite these advances, several areas require continued attention:

- Standardized definitions of treatment success that go beyond AHI to include sleep quality, cardiovascular risk reduction, and patient-reported outcomes.
- Longitudinal data on the impact of dental and skeletal changes associated with years of MAD use.
- Personalized prediction algorithms that integrate anatomic, polysomnographic, and biometric data to guide device selection and jaw advancement targets.

Moreover, access and education remain critical. Expanding the number of trained dental sleep medicine providers through programs like the AADSM Mastery Series and ABDSM Diplomate certification is essential to meeting demand. Encouraging collaboration between sleep physicians, dentists, and registered polysomnographic technologists (RPSGTs) ensures that patients benefit from a cohesive, evidence-based approach.

In conclusion, MADs are no longer a secondary or experimental therapy—they are an established, effective, and increasingly sophisticated solution for managing OSA and snoring. As the field advances through better technology, interdisciplinary training, and research-guided protocols, MADs will continue to play a vital role in the evolving landscape of sleep medicine. For general dentists, dental sleep medicine fellows, sleep physicians, and technologists, mastering MAD therapy is a critical competency in the pursuit of better patient sleep and long-term health outcomes.

REFERENCES

1. Patil SP, Ayappa IA, Caples SM, Kimoff RJ, Patel SR, Harrod CG. Treatment of adult obstructive sleep apnea with positive airway pressure: an American Academy of Sleep Medicine clinical practice guideline. *J Clin Sleep Med.* 2019;15(2):335-343. doi:10.5664/jcsm.7640
2. Peppard PE, Young T, Barnet JH, Palta M, Hagen EW, Hla KM. Increased prevalence of sleep-disordered breathing in adults. *Am J Epidemiol.* 2013;177(9):1006-1014. doi:10.1093/aje/kws342
3. Kuna ST, Gurubhagavatula I, Maislin G, et al. Noninferiority of functional outcome in ambulatory management of obstructive sleep apnea. *Am J Respir Crit Care Med.* 2011;183(9):1238-1244. doi:10.1164/rccm.201011-1770OC
4. Ramar K, Dort LC, Katz SG, et al. Clinical practice guideline for the treatment of obstructive sleep apnea and snoring with oral appliance therapy: an update for 2015. *J Clin Sleep Med.* 2015;11(7):773-827. doi:10.5664/jcsm.4858
5. American Academy of Dental Sleep Medicine. Guideline for the assessment and follow-up of dental side effects of oral appliance therapy for sleep-disordered breathing. 2022. Accessed November 8, 2025. https://www.aadsm.org
6. de Vries GE, Wijkstra PJ, Houwerzijl EJ, Kerstjens HA, Hoekema A. Cardiovascular effects of oral appliance therapy in obstructive sleep apnea: a systematic review and meta-analysis. *Sleep Med Rev.* 2018;40:55-68. doi:10.1016/j.smrv.2017.10.004
7. Rechtschaffen A, Kales A. *A Manual of Standardized Terminology, Techniques and Scoring System for Sleep Stages of Human Subjects.* U.S. Government Printing Office, National Institutes of Health; 1968.
8. Marklund M, Verbraecken J, Randerath W. Non-CPAP therapies in obstructive sleep apnea: mandibular advancement device therapy. *Eur Respir Rev.* 2012;39(5):1241-1247. doi:10.1183/09031936.00144711
9. Almeida EO, Freitas Júnior AC, Bonfante EA, Rocha EP, Silva NRFA, Coelho PG. Effect of microthread presence and restoration design (screw versus cemented) in dental implant reliability and failure modes. *Clin Oral Impl Res.* 2013;24(2):191-196 doi:10.1111/j.1600-0501.2012.02437.x
10. Phillips CL, Grunstein RR, Darendeliler MA, et al. Health outcomes of continuous positive airway pressure versus oral appliance treatment for obstructive sleep apnea: a randomized controlled trial. *Am J Respir Crit Care Med.* 2013;187(8):879-887. doi:10.1164/rccm.201212-2223OC
11. Sutherland K, Vanderveken OM, Tsuda H, et al. Oral appliance treatment for obstructive sleep apnea: an update. *J Clin Sleep Med.* 2014;10(2):215-227. doi:10.5664/jcsm.3460
12. Huang Z, Zhou N, Lobbezoo F, et al. Dental sleep-related conditions and the role of oral healthcare providers: a scoping review. *Sleep Med Rev.* 2023;67:101721. doi:10.1016/j.smrv.2022.101721
13. Chen H, Eckert DJ, van der Stelt PF, et al. Phenotypes of responders to mandibular advancement device therapy in obstructive sleep apnea patients: a systematic review and meta-analysis. *Sleep Med Rev.* 2020;49:101229. doi:10.1016/j.smrv.2019.101229
14. Gagnadoux F, Fleury B, Vielle B, et al. Titrated mandibular advancement versus positive airway pressure for sleep apnea. *Eur Respir J.* 2009;34(3):914-920. doi:10.1183/09031936.00148208
15. de Britto Teixeira AO, Abi-Ramia LB, de Oliveira Almeida MA. Treatment of obstructive sleep apnea with oral appliances. *Prog Orthod.* 2013;14:10. doi:10.1186/2196-1042-14-10
16. Rodriguez-Bruno K, Goldberg AN, McCulloch CE, Kezirian EJ. Test-retest reliability of drug-induced sleep endoscopy. *Otolaryngol Head Neck Surg.* 2009;140(5):646-651. doi:10.1016/j.otohns.2009.01.012
17. El-Solh AA, Lawson Y, Wilding GE. Impact of low arousal threshold on treatment of obstructive sleep apnea in patients with post-traumatic stress disorder. *Sleep Breath.* 2021;25:597-604. doi:10.1007/s11325-020-02106-0

Chapter 50
Introduction to Orofacial Myofunctional Therapy for Sleep Apnea

KEVIN ADLEY

KEY CONCEPTS/LEARNING OBJECTIVES

The key concepts for this chapter include the use of orofacial myofunctional therapy for sleep apnea, a review of the anatomy and physiology of the orofacial and airway structures involved in airway function and their pathophysiology in sleep apnea, and the principles of orofacial myofunctional therapy as therapeutic modality for patients with mild-to-moderate obstructive sleep apnea.

KEY TERMS

Genioglossus
Mandibular
Maxillary
Oral appliance therapy (OAT)
Orofacial myofunctional therapy (OMT)
Pharyngeal walls
Soft palate

INTRODUCTION TO OROFACIAL MYOFUNCTIONAL THERAPY FOR SLEEP APNEA

Obstructive sleep apnea (OSA) is a prevalent sleep disorder characterized by recurrent episodes of upper airway obstruction during sleep, leading to intermittent hypoxia, fragmented sleep, and increased cardiovascular risk. Traditional treatment modalities, including continuous positive airway pressure (CPAP) and oral appliance therapy (OAT), aim to maintain airway patency but do not address a neuromuscular dysfunction that is sometimes present. Orofacial myofunctional therapy (OMT) has emerged as a complementary approach targeting the functional deficits contributing to airway collapse in OSA.

First described in 1918 by Alfred Rogers, DDS (1), for proper tongue positioning in the oral cavity to improve mandibular growth, nasal breathing, and facial appearance, OMT was proposed as a treatment of OSA by Guimaraes (2) to improve upper airway (UA) dilator function. Puhan et al (3) reported that UA muscle training, by means of didgeridoo playing, reduced OSA severity. Historically, OMT has been used to address speech and swallowing disorders, but its application in sleep medicine has gained traction in recent years. Research indicates that OMT can lead to reductions in the apnea-hypopnea index (AHI), which measures the severity of sleep apnea. A narrative review highlighted that OMT not only decreases AHI but also reduces snoring and daytime sleepiness, while improving oxygen saturation and overall sleep quality in both pediatric and adult patients during sleep (4).

OMT consists of a structured regimen of exercises designed to retrain the muscles of the tongue, soft palate, oropharynx, and face to optimize airway stability during sleep. The therapy is rooted in the understanding that oropharyngeal muscle tone plays a critical role in maintaining upper airway patency. Weakness or maladaptive positioning of these muscles has been implicated in the pathophysiology of OSA, particularly (but not limited to) in patients with anatomic predispositions such as retrognathia, macroglossia, and high arched palates. By improving muscle tone and coordination, OMT aims to reduce airway collapsibility and enhance neuromuscular control of breathing during sleep (5).

Clinical interest in OMT has grown due to its noninvasive nature and potential to serve as an adjunct or alternative to conventional OSA treatments. A growing body of evidence supports its efficacy in reducing AHI, improving oxygen saturation, and enhancing patient-reported sleep quality (6). Additionally, OMT may benefit patients who are unable to tolerate CPAP or oral appliances, providing a viable therapeutic option to improve compliance and outcomes.

The implementation of OMT for treating OSA in clinical practice requires a multidisciplinary approach involving sleep medicine specialists, dentists, speech-language pathologists, and orofacial myologists. Comprehensive assessment and individualized therapy plans are essential to optimize effectiveness and long-term adherence (7). However, disparities in health care access pose a significant challenge to the widespread implementation of specialty care services. Many patients, particularly those in underserved or rural areas, may have limited access to trained specialists, creating barriers to care (8). As research continues to explain the mechanisms and efficacy of OMT, efforts should be made to improve accessibility and affordability, ensuring that all patients can benefit from this emerging therapy. Its integration into sleep medicine holds promise for broadening the therapeutic landscape for OSA management.

ANATOMY AND PHYSIOLOGY OF OROFACIAL STRUCTURES AS THEY RELATE TO THE PATHOPHYSIOLOGY OF SLEEP APNEA

Understanding the role of orofacial anatomy in the pathophysiology of OSA is essential for recognizing how structural and functional abnormalities can contribute to airway compromise. The upper airway is a collapsible, muscular tube that relies heavily on proper tone and coordination of surrounding structures to remain open during sleep. When these systems are impaired, partial or complete obstruction may occur, leading to sleep-disordered breathing.

The Tongue and Genioglossus Muscle

The tongue occupies a substantial portion of the oral cavity and has a direct influence on the airway space. The genioglossus muscle plays a crucial role in maintaining airway patency by stabilizing and advancing the tongue during inspiration. In OSA, diminished tone or inappropriate resting posture (low or posterior placement) of the tongue can allow it to collapse against the posterior pharyngeal wall during sleep (Figure 50-1) (9).

The Soft Palate and Pharyngeal Walls

The soft palate is a muscular structure that must elevate and seal properly during swallowing and speech but also maintain appropriate tone during sleep to prevent airway obstruction. In many patients with OSA, especially those with redundant soft tissue or neuromuscular hypotonia, the soft palate becomes a site of collapse. The lateral pharyngeal walls, likewise, can contribute to narrowing or complete occlusion when muscular tone decreases in sleep.

Mandibular and Maxillary Position

Craniofacial structure has a profound effect on airway dimensions. Retrognathia (posteriorly positioned mandible) or maxillary underdevelopment reduces the available space for the tongue and soft tissue structures, leading to a narrowed oropharyngeal airway. This structural crowding is especially common

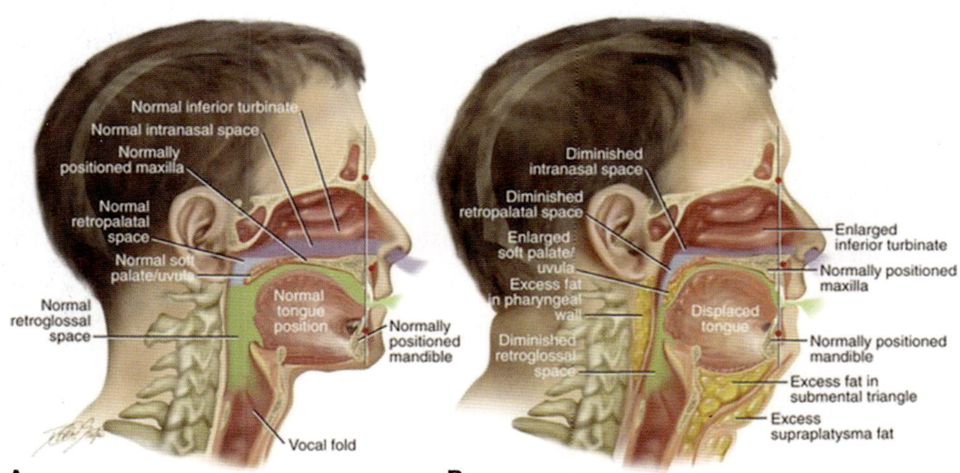

Figure 50-1 Sagittal view of the upper airway showing the tongue in A: proper versus B: obstructive posture. (Reprinted with permission from Posnick JC. *Pocket Dentistry. Obstructive Sleep Apnea. Evaluation and Treatment.*)

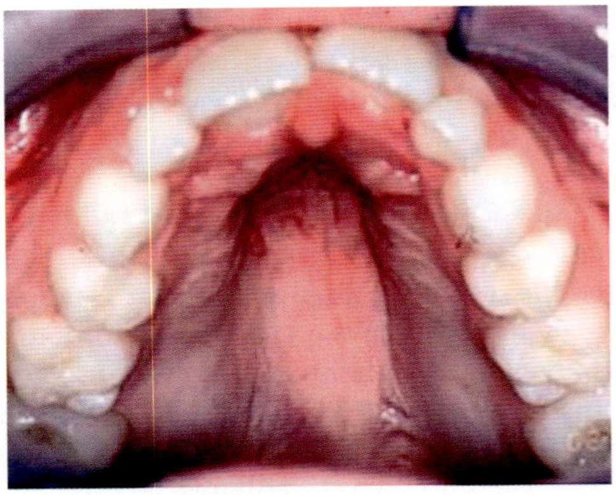

Palate, High

Figure 50-2 Patients with narrow palates and high vaulted palates often demonstrate compromised nasal breathing and are at higher risk for developing OSA. (Courtesy of National Human Genome Research Institute. https://elementsofmorphology.nih.gov/index.cgi?tid=c606b0119d4a894ebd5ee0242c136e29)

in patients with persistent mouth breathing habits or orofacial myofunctional disorders during childhood (Figure 50-2).

Lips, Cheeks, and Buccinator Function

The lips and cheeks contribute to oral competence and the maintenance of a closed-mouth posture. Lip incompetence, hypotonia of the buccinator muscle, and poor neuromuscular control often result in open-mouth posture and chronic mouth breathing. These habits alter tongue resting position, disrupt nasal breathing, and lead to adaptive changes in craniofacial growth that further reduce airway volume (7).

Nasal Airway and Breathing Patterns

Normal nasal breathing promotes optimal tongue posture and supports healthy craniofacial development. Obstruction of the nasal airway, due to hypertrophied turbinates, deviated septum, or allergies, often leads to compensatory mouth breathing. Over time, this can potentially result in downward and backward growth of the face, a narrow maxilla, and posterior tongue positioning, all of which reduce airway size and contribute to OSA risk(10).

Disruption of normal orofacial function, whether due to poor tone, incorrect posture, or structural anomalies, can impact the airway and contribute to the development or worsening of OSA. Understanding these relationships underscores the value of assessing orofacial function in patients with sleep-disordered breathing and highlights the potential of OMT to restore balance, improve muscle tone, and support upper airway stability during sleep.

PRINCIPLES OF OROFACIAL MYOFUNCTIONAL THERAPY

OMT is a neuromuscular re-education approach aimed at correcting dysfunctional habits of the oral and facial muscles that contribute to upper airway collapse, especially during sleep. In the context of OSA, the primary goals of OMT are to improve airway patency, enhance upper airway muscle tone, and retrain proper orofacial function to support more stable breathing during sleep.

Improving Airway Patency

By targeting muscles involved in maintaining airway openness, particularly the tongue, soft palate, lips, and pharyngeal wall, OMT can reduce the collapsibility of the upper airway. Through consistent, targeted exercises, patients can achieve improved resting posture and dynamic muscle engagement that facilitates better airflow during sleep. Some studies suggest that OMT is associated with a reduction in AHI, particularly in mild-to-moderate OSA, and can be used adjunctively with CPAP or OAT to enhance outcomes (6,10).

Enhancing Muscle Tone and Function

The pharyngeal dilator muscles, including the genioglossus and palatoglossus, are essential in preserving upper airway patency. OMT has been shown to improve baseline tone and responsiveness of these muscles, which may otherwise become hypotonic during sleep, especially in rapid eye movement (REM) stages. Enhanced muscle coordination reduces upper airway resistance and can lead to sustained improvements in daytime function and sleep quality (9).

Overview of Therapeutic Exercises

OMT programs typically consist of daily, guided exercises that strengthen and coordinate the tongue, lips, and facial muscles. Therapy is often supervised by trained myofunctional therapists, with home exercises reinforcing skills over several weeks to months. Adherence and consistency are key determinants of success.

- **Tongue posture and strength training**
  Exercises to train the tongue to rest against the palate, rather than on the floor of the mouth, help promote forward positioning and reduce posterior collapse. Strengthening the intrinsic and extrinsic tongue muscles, such as through resistance training or suction holds, has been shown to contribute to better airway dynamics during sleep (6,11).
- **Lip seal exercises**
  Restoring lip competency encourages nasal breathing and supports proper tongue posture. Lip seal

exercises, such as isometric contractions, aim to retrain orbicularis oris function, which may be underdeveloped in chronic mouth breathers (12).

- **Breathing retraining**
  Nasal breathing is foundational to proper orofacial and airway function. OMT often incorporates elements of breathing retraining, such as diaphragmatic breathing, paced respiration, and nasal breathing awareness. These techniques not only improve oxygenation but also promote physiologic airflow and craniofacial development in pediatric populations (10).

CHALLENGES IN CLINICAL PRACTICE AND RESEARCH

Despite promising outcomes, the clinical adoption of OMT varies widely, and this inconsistency presents challenges for both implementation and research. There is no universally accepted standard of care, and therapeutic approaches often differ significantly depending on practitioner background, training, and regional practices. This heterogeneity complicates the ability to generalize findings across studies and makes it difficult to compare intervention outcomes. As the field matures, the development of standardized protocols and credentialing frameworks will be essential to increase the credibility and accessibility of OMT as part of interdisciplinary care for sleep-disordered breathing (6,11).

Evidence-Based Applications of Orofacial Myofunctional Therapy

OMT has gained increasing attention as a complementary or, in select cases, stand-alone intervention in the management of OSA. Over the past decade, a growing body of evidence has supported its efficacy in improving upper airway stability, reducing AHI, and enhancing patient adherence to primary treatments such as CPAP and OAT.

REVIEW OF CLINICAL STUDIES SUPPORTING OROFACIAL MYOFUNCTIONAL THERAPY FOR OBSTRUCTIVE SLEEP APNEA

Numerous studies and meta-analyses have demonstrated the positive impact of OMT on sleep-disordered breathing outcomes. Camacho et al conducted a systematic review and meta-analysis encompassing over 250 patients, concluding that OMT significantly reduced AHI, improved oxygen saturation, and lessened subjective symptoms such as snoring and daytime sleepiness (6). These findings were consistent across both pediatric and adult populations, suggesting that neuromuscular retraining of the orofacial complex can yield structural and functional improvements in airway patency.

Guimarães et al conducted one of the earliest randomized controlled trials (RCTs) showing that a structured program of oropharyngeal exercises reduced AHI by approximately 39% in adults with moderate OSA, in addition to reducing snoring frequency and improving sleep quality (11). Other studies have corroborated these findings, emphasizing the importance of targeted muscle activation, particularly of the tongue and soft palate, as a key factor in treatment efficacy (13).

EFFECTIVENESS AS A STAND-ALONE TREATMENT VERSUS ADJUNCTIVE THERAPY

While OMT has demonstrated stand-alone benefit in some individuals with mild-to-moderate OSA, its most consistent and meaningful application appears to be as an adjunctive therapy. As a stand-alone, OMT is generally insufficient for patients with severe OSA or those with significant anatomic obstruction (14). However, when used in conjunction with other therapies, such as CPAP or OAT, OMT has been shown to enhance treatment effectiveness, reduce required pressure settings, and improve long-term adherence (15).

Impact on Mild, Moderate, and Severe Obstructive Sleep Apnea

The greatest benefits of OMT have been observed in patients with mild-to-moderate OSA. Studies have shown clinically significant reductions in AHI, with corresponding improvements in quality-of-life metrics, such as daytime fatigue and sleep-related performance (11). In severe cases, OMT alone is rarely curative, but it may contribute to improved outcomes when integrated into a multidisciplinary treatment plan. Moreover, OMT may offer a pre- or postsurgical rehabilitation option in cases involving upper airway surgery.

Synergy With Other Treatments

OMT demonstrates a notable synergistic effect when combined with other treatment modalities. In patients using CPAP, OMT has been shown to reduce mask leak, promote better tolerance, and improve adherence by reinforcing nasal breathing and oral muscle coordination (15). In those treated with mandibular advancement devices, OMT can help maintain proper tongue posture and minimize relapse or regression of benefits over time (4). Furthermore, with OAT, it can assist in providing more protrusive movement to maximize therapy outcomes as well as prevent side effects such as jaw joint discomfort and bite migration. These findings support the integration of OMT into comprehensive treatment planning, particularly for patients with residual symptoms or low adherence to standard therapies.

FUTURE DIRECTIONS AND RESEARCH OPPORTUNITIES

As the field of sleep medicine continues to evolve, OMT is gaining traction as a promising adjunct in the management of OSA. Several emerging trends are shaping its future integration into multidisciplinary care models.

Emerging Trends in Orofacial Myofunctional Therapy

Innovations in digital health platforms have enabled remote delivery of OMT via telehealth and mobile applications, increasing access and adherence. Additionally, the development of standardized training programs and credentialing bodies, such as the Academy of Orofacial Myofunctional Therapy and the International Association of Orofacial Myology, aim to improve clinical consistency and evidence quality (14). Technologic advances in objective assessments, such as tongue strength dynamometry and 3D imaging, may further enhance individualized treatment planning (16).

Integration in Standard Sleep Apnea Care Pathways

A growing number of sleep centers are exploring the inclusion of OMT into standard OSA care pathways, particularly in pediatric populations and in patients with residual symptoms despite CPAP or OAT (17). Formal referral relationships between sleep physicians, dentists, and myofunctional therapists are being piloted to facilitate a more cohesive, interdisciplinary approach. Integration with orthodontics and ENT care is also gaining attention, especially in cases involving craniofacial or airway structural abnormalities (18).

Areas Needing Further Research

Despite encouraging outcomes, significant research gaps remain. There is a need for larger, high-quality RCTs to better understand the long-term efficacy of OMT in both adult and pediatric populations. Questions remain about ideal patient selection, the most effective exercise protocols, and maintenance strategies for sustained benefit (6). Standardization of diagnostic and outcome measures is critical to enabling meta-analyses and comparison across studies. Additionally, the cost-effectiveness of OMT in reducing long-term health burden from untreated OSA is an important area for future exploration.

CONCLUSION

OMT offers a compelling, noninvasive strategy for improving upper airway function and supporting the management of OSA. While not a universal solution, OMT has demonstrated benefit, particularly as an adjunctive therapy, for patients with mild-to-moderate OSA and those with suboptimal adherence to CPAP or oral appliances.

The successful implementation of OMT requires interdisciplinary collaboration among sleep physicians, dentists, speech-language pathologists, myofunctional therapists, and sleep professionals. As the evidence base grows and clinical practice evolves, integrating OMT knowledge into routine care can offer patients a more comprehensive and tailored treatment approach.

Sleep technologists and clinicians are encouraged to become familiar with the principles of OMT, advocate for its inclusion in patient care when appropriate, and collaborate with trained providers to optimize long-term outcomes for patients with sleep-disordered breathing.

REFERENCES

1. Rogers AP. Exercises for the development of muscles of face with view to increasing their functional activity. *Dental Cosmos*. 1918;59:857-876.
2. Guimaraes KC. Soft tissue changes of the oropharynx in patients with obstructive sleep apnea. *J Bras Fonoaudiol*. 1999;1:69-75.
3. Puhan MA, Suarez A, Lo Cascio C, Zahn A, Heitz M, Braendli O. Didgeridoo playing as alternative treatment for obstructive sleep apnoea syndrome: randomized controlled trial. *BMJ*. 2006;332:266-270. doi:10.1136/bmj.38705.470590.55
4. Ieto V, Kayamori F, Montes MI, et al. Effects of oropharyngeal exercises on snoring: a randomized trial. *Chest*. 2015;148:683-691. doi:10.1378/chest.14-2953
5. Koka V, De Vito A, Roisman G, et al. Orofacial myofunctional therapy in obstructive sleep apnea syndrome: a pathophysiological perspective. *Medicina (Kaunas)*. 2021;57(4):323. doi:10.3390/medicina57040323 PMID: 33915707; PMCID: PMC8066493.
6. Camacho M, Guilleminault C, Wei JM, et al. Myofunctional therapy to treat obstructive sleep apnea: a systematic review and meta-analysis. *Sleep*. 2015;38(5):669-675. doi:10.5665/sleep.4652

7. Rueda JR, Mugueta-Aguinaga I, Vilaró J, Rueda-Etxebarria M. Myofunctional therapy (oropharyngeal exercises) for obstructive sleep apnoea. *Cochrane Database Syst Rev*. 2020;11(11):CD013449. doi: 10.1002/14651858.CD013449.pub2 PMID: 33141943; PMCID: PMC8094400.
8. Schuldt R, Jinnett K. Barriers accessing specialty care in the United States: a patient perspective. *BMC Health Serv Res*. 2024;24:1549. doi:10.1186/s12913-024-11921-0
9. Isono S, Tanaka A, Tagaito Y, Sho Y, Nishino T. Contribution of the genioglossus muscle to pharyngeal airway maintenance during sleep in normal subjects. *Am J Respir Crit Care Med*. 2002;166(10):1448-1453. doi:10.1164/rccm.2102062
10. Harari D, Redlich M, Miri S, Hamud T, Gross M. The effect of mouth breathing versus nasal breathing on dentofacial and craniofacial development in orthodontic patients. *Laryngoscope*. 2010;120(10):2089-2093. doi:10.1002/lary.20991
11. Guimarães KC, Drager LF, Genta PR, Marcondes BF, Lorenzi-Filho G. Effects of oropharyngeal exercises on patients with moderate obstructive sleep apnea syndrome. *Am J Respir Crit Care Med*. 2009;179(10):962-966. doi:10.1164/rccm.200806-981OC
12. Guilleminault C, Huang YS, Monteyrol PJ, Sato R, Quo S, Lin CH. Critical role of myofascial reeducation in pediatric sleep-disordered breathing. *Sleep Med*. 2013;14(6):518-525. doi:10.1016/j.sleep.2013.01.013
13. Diaferia G, Badke L, Santos-Silva R, et al. Effect of oropharyngeal exercises on snoring: a randomized trial. *Chest*. 2017;152(3):533-540. doi:10.1016/j.chest.2017.06.025
14. de Felício CM, da Silva Dias FV, Trawitzki LVV. Obstructive sleep apnea: focus on myofunctional therapy. *Nat Sci Sleep*. 2018;10:271-286. doi:10.2147/NSS.S160894
15. Villa MP, Evangelisti M, Martella S, et al. Can myofunctional therapy increase adherence to CPAP? A randomized controlled trial. *Sleep Breath*. 2022;26(3):1149-1156. doi:10.1007/s11325-021-02535-w
16. Kim JA, Koo DL, Lee J, Kim D. Quantitative assessments of tongue muscle strength in patients with obstructive sleep apnea. *J Clin Sleep Med*. 2022;18(1):149-157. doi:10.5664/jcsm.9560
17. Villa MP, Rizzoli A, Miano S, Malagola C. Efficacy of myofunctional therapy in children with sleep-disordered breathing. *Sleep Breath*. 2014;18(4):891-895. doi:10.1007/s11325-014-0963-3
18. Guilleminault C, Huseni S, Lo L. A frequent phenotype for paediatric sleep apnoea: short lingual frenulum. *ERJ Open Res*. 2016;2(3):00043-2016. doi:10.1183/23120541.00043-2016

Chapter 51 Technical-Surgical Interventions for Sleep Apnea

EDWIN M. VALLADARES

KEY CONCEPTS/LEARNING OBJECTIVES

The key concepts for this chapter include a review of technical-surgical therapies for obstructive sleep apnea using hypoglossal nerve stimulation and phrenic nerve stimulation, the anatomy of the airway associated with obstructive sleep apnea, upper airway collapse as shown by drug-induced sleep endoscopy, and the role of the sleep technologist in technical-surgical interventions.

KEY TERMS

Central sleep apnea
Hypoglossal nerve stimulation
Implant
Inspire upper airway stimulation therapy
Obstructive sleep apnea
Phrenic nerve stimulation
Sleep apnea

Continuous positive airway pressure (CPAP) has been the first-line intervention for treating patients with moderate-to-severe sleep apnea since 1981 (1). However, with approximately 29% to 83% of adult patients unable to meet minimum CPAP therapy adherence criteria (4 hours or more per night for 70% of nights), technical-surgical alternatives have emerged for select patients (2-5). Thus, sleep medicine continues to move toward personalized interventions for optimal therapy. Technical-surgical interventions are one such example. These therapies can be called technical-surgical interventions because they involve a surgical implantation of a device and technical therapy management.

With the advent of new U.S. Food and Drug Administration (FDA)–approved implantable stimulators for treating sleep-disordered breathing in a fraction of noncompliant positive airway pressure (PAP) therapy patients, the landscape of sleep medicine and sleep technology is changing to narrow the gap between compliant and noncompliant patients (6,7). The Inspire therapy for treating obstructive sleep apnea (OSA) and the **rem**edē System for treating central sleep apnea (CSA) are providing new tools for sleep physicians, thus elevating the expertise of sleep technologists and paving the way for personalized medicine.

TECHNICAL-SURGICAL INTERVENTION FOR OBSTRUCTIVE SLEEP APNEA

In 2014, the FDA approved the Inspire therapy for the treatment of OSA. This therapy provides a feasible option for treating a subset of patients with OSA (7). Although these devices will not be appropriate for all of the PAP-intolerant patients, careful selection criteria make the Inspire therapy a viable option for a small but growing percentage of patients (8).

The Inspire therapy is for patients with moderate-to-severe OSA (apnea-hypopnea index [AHI] 15-100 events per hour) who have not been able to tolerate CPAP therapy and do not have concentric collapse of the upper airway. In addition, Inspire therapy is also indicated for pediatric patients with Down syndrome who are 13 to 18 years of age, have severe OSA (AHI of 10-100 events per hour), and adenotonsillectomy has not been successful in treating the OSA and cannot use CPAP consistently (9). The Inspire therapy stimulates the hypoglossal nerve during inspiration and moves the tongue base forward to open the upper airway. The therapy stimulates on the basis of signaling from the sensing lead's breathing information. The patient uses an external wireless remote to turn the therapy "on," "off," "pause," and to control stimulation intensity across a limited programmed range.

Inspire Therapy: Components, Function, and Indication

The Inspire therapy is composed of a neurostimulator with 1-stimulating lead to provide coordinated tongue protrusion and 1-monitoring sensing lead. The stimulator lead is connected to the hypoglossal nerve (XII), specifically on the medial-XII branch, and the sensing lead is connected to the upper border of the underlying rib in the fourth intercostal region to gate the hypoglossal nerve stimulation to inspiration. The device is accessed through an electronic tablet or computer where the SleepSync Programmer Application (2740S) has been downloaded on a customer-owned Windows-based laptop with interrogation component, and it is interfaced by the patient with the Inspire Sleep Remote (10). The estimated battery life of the neurostimulator is 10.9 years (11). Moreover, technical training for physicians and sleep technologists is easily accessible through Inspire's Healthcare Professionals website (9).

The criteria for being implanted are as follows: (1) have tried CPAP and failed, (2) have drug-induced sleep endoscopy (DISE) to rule out concentric collapse at the palate, (3) have an AHI 15 to 100/h, and (4) have a body mass index of less than 32 kg/m^2. This has been further extended to pediatric patients with Down syndrome who are 13 to 18 years of age with severe OSA (10-100/h) (9). These criteria narrow the therapy to a subset of patients with noncompliant PAP therapy. Contraindications for implanting the Inspire therapy are as follows: central + mixed apneas greater than 25% of total AHI, any anatomic finding that would compromise the performance of the therapy (eg, concentric collapse), any condition or procedure that has compromised the neurologic control of the upper airway, patients who are unable or do not have the necessary assistance to operate the sleep remote, pregnancy or plan to become pregnant, implantable device that may unintentionally interact with the Inspire System, and patients requiring magnetic resonance imaging (MRI) other than the specified MR conditional labeling (Inspire System implant manual) (11).

Airway evaluation through DISE has become a good predictor of success for Inspire therapy (12). DISE is conducted in an operating room where sleep is induced using a sedative, such as Propofol, to mimic airway collapse during sleep and characterize the airway collapse using a fiber-optic laryngoscope. The sedative is used at the lowest dose, which elicits loss of consciousness as measured by loss of response to normal conversational voice stimulation, while monitoring vital signs. Because this is a procedure conducted in an operating room, a team of nurses assist with monitoring the patient's vitals (13). It has been shown that patients with concentric collapse of the palate do not do well with Inspire therapy, as opposed to other types of collapse,

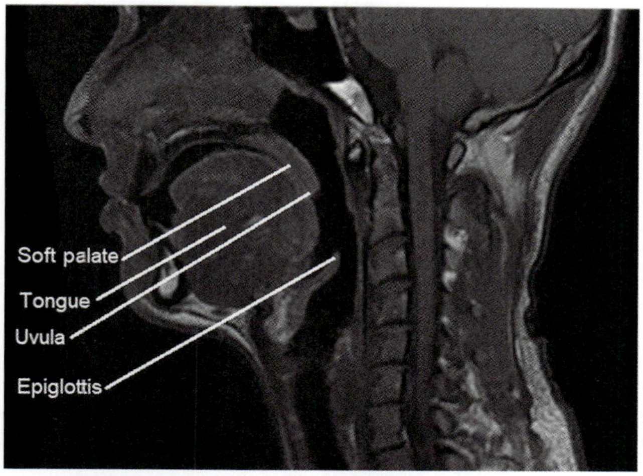

Figure 51-1 Anatomy of the upper airway. (Image courtesy of Krishna Nayak, PhD, Professor, Ming Hsieh Department of Electrical Engineering, Viterbi School of Engineering, University of Southern California.)

thereby suggesting that tongue protrusion from stimulation is insufficient to overcome airway obstruction in concentric collapse (Figures 51-1 and 51-2) (12). Figure 51-2 demonstrates examples of (a) an open airway, (b) lateral wall collapse, and (c) concentric collapse.

Inspire Therapy: Patient Process

A trained otolaryngologist implants the Inspire therapy and is subsequently followed at the sleep clinic by a sleep physician. The patient meets with a trained sleep physician and a trained sleep technologist to activate the device 1-month postimplant. This is the visit when the patient feels the stimulation for the first time, and two major parameters are established. The first parameter is the sensing threshold. The sensing threshold is the lowest voltage at which the patient "senses" an impulse from the device. The second parameter is the functional threshold, which is the voltage where the patient's hypoglossal nerve is stimulated enough to protrude the tongue past the lower teeth. The patient is then sent home with a range of "functional threshold + 10 tenths of a voltage" (eg, 2.1-3.0 V). The patient is asked to try to increase the voltage by 0.1 V every three to four nights to become acclimated to the therapy. A month after this activation visit, the patient comes into the sleep lab to be formally titrated by a trained sleep technologist (9,11). The Inspire therapy has a stimulation range from 0.1 to 5.0 V. Settings for each patient can vary, given differences in upper airway physiology (11,14).

Inspire therapy titration has an immediate effect on the upper airway when compared with CPAP titration. This immediate effect is due to the change in the physical upper airway evoked by hypoglossal nerve stimulation,

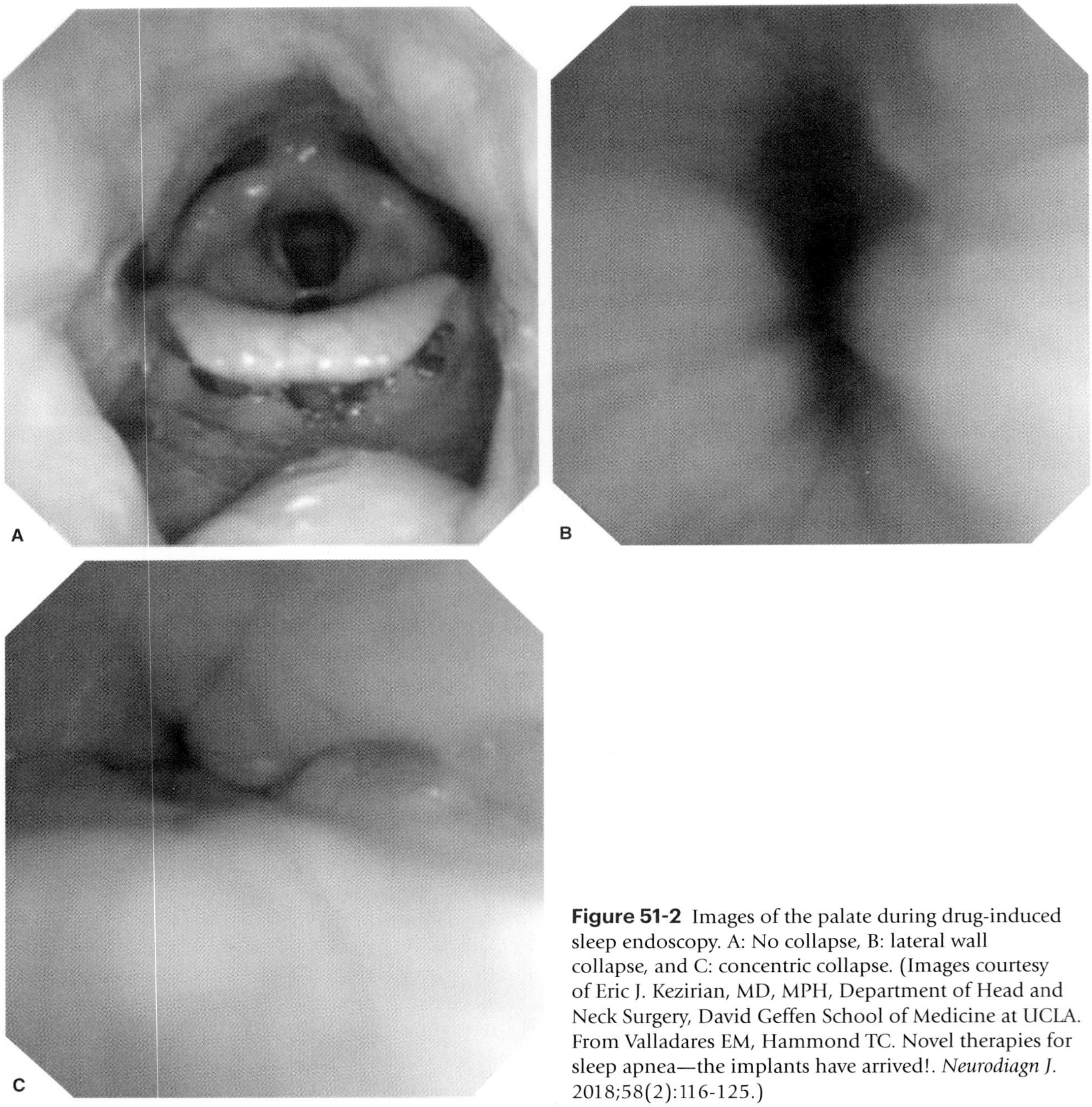

Figure 51-2 Images of the palate during drug-induced sleep endoscopy. A: No collapse, B: lateral wall collapse, and C: concentric collapse. (Images courtesy of Eric J. Kezirian, MD, MPH, Department of Head and Neck Surgery, David Geffen School of Medicine at UCLA. From Valladares EM, Hammond TC. Novel therapies for sleep apnea—the implants have arrived!. *Neurodiagn J.* 2018;58(2):116-125.)

as opposed to a more gradual effect from a CPAP setting increase (15). Although supine sleep during a titration is always ideal to eliminate respiratory events as a worst-case scenario, most of the emphasis during an Inspire titration is in identifying the optimal voltage when the patient is sleeping in a comfortable position because the patient has not been able to use CPAP (9). This may result in the patient being sent home with lateral sleep settings. However, stimulation can be raised at a later time once the patient acclimates to the therapy and shows the need for supine titration. Once the patient is sent home with a range of voltages, the patient meets with the sleep physician to further discuss settings, expectations, and follow-up (11).

On June 5, 2017, Inspire Medical, Inc. announced FDA approval for the next generation of Inspire therapy device, the Inspire 3028 neurostimulator (16). It has received conditional MRI labeling, allowing patients to undergo MRI testing safely (16). The Inspire Sleep Remote has also been simplified to include features where patients can easily visualize therapy settings, including "on" and "off" buttons via green and white lights.

Inspire Therapy: Clinical Effectiveness and Safety Findings

Inspire Medical, Inc. conducted a multicenter, prospective, single-group cohort design study to evaluate the clinical effectiveness and safety of the Inspire therapy (21). Their primary measures were the AHI and oxygen desaturation index (ODI). The study implanted 126 participants with a mean age of 54.5 years (83% male). At 12 months, the study showed a 68% decrease in the median AHI, from 29.3 to 9.0/h. A similar response was seen in the median ODI with a 70% decrease from 25.4 to 7.4/h. Secondary outcomes included the Epworth Sleepiness Scale score (range 0-24) to measure subjective sleepiness and the Functional Outcomes of Sleep Questionnaire (FOSQ; range 5.0-20.0) to evaluate quality of life and percentage of sleep time with oxygen saturation below 90%. Median Epworth decreased from 11 to 6, median FOSQ scores increased from 14.6 to 18.2, and median percentage of sleep time with oxygen saturation below 90% decreased from 5.4% to 0.9%. Less than 2% procedure-related serious adverse events were reported (10). Given the relatively recent FDA approval, long-term studies are yet to be available. However, in the latest 5-year outcomes report published in 2018, patients were reported to have continuous improvement in sleepiness and AHI, with serious adverse events being uncommon (17,18). Moreover, emerging data continue to show the Inspire therapy's effectiveness (19).

A common question regarding nerve damage caused by neurostimulation is yet to be established. However, decades of information from other neurostimulators (eg, used in pain management) show that nerve damage is not usually due to long-term stimulation but most commonly, lead movement (20).

Inspire Therapy: How Does It Affect Polysomnography Recordings?

These systems, unlike neural stimulators for seizures and depression, do not significantly affect polysomnography (PSG) signals, given their implant location. Artifact can be seen in the submental electromyogram (EMG) more than the electroencephalogram (EEG; Figure 51-3). PSG scoring is not significantly hindered, and the American Academy of Sleep Medicine (AASM) scoring rules can still be implemented (22). Moreover, scoring of rapid eye movement (REM) sleep is not hindered, because EMG artifact is periodic. Other PSG signals are not impacted by these implants; however, it is recommended that piezoelectric belts be used during PSG to eliminate any source of artifact (19,23).

Clinically, EEG measured sleep has been shown to be improved post Inspire therapy implant. Hofauer et al. showed a decrease in non-REM 1 sleep and an increase in REM sleep (24).

TECHNICAL-SURGICAL INTERVENTION FOR CENTRAL SLEEP APNEA

The **remedē** System is a feasible option for treating a subset of patients with CSA because it received FDA's approval in late 2017, and Zoll Medical Corporation acquired Respicardia Inc., the manufacturer of the **remedē**

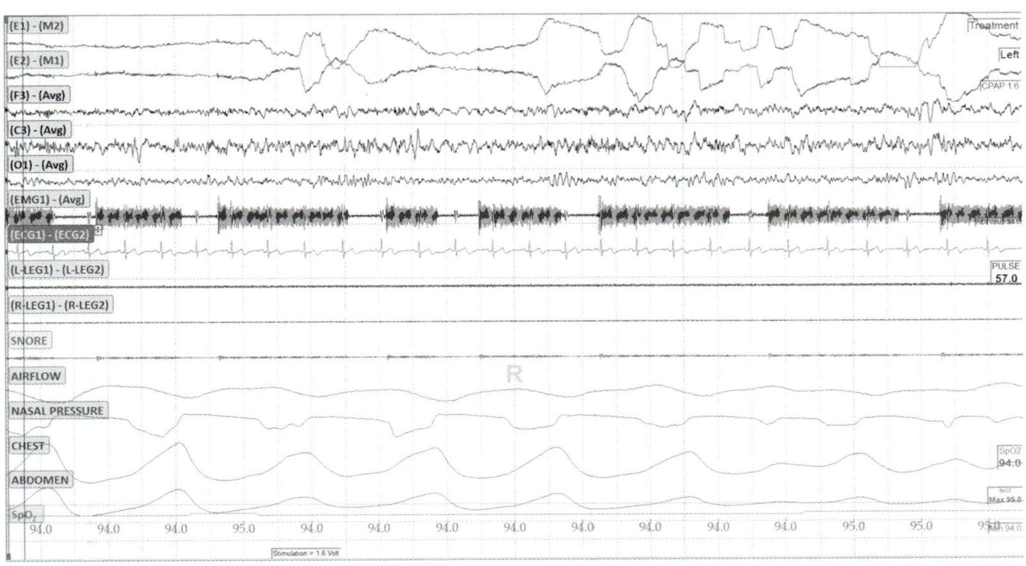

Figure 51-3 Hypoglossal nerve stimulation effect on polysomnography—Epoch (30 seconds) during hypoglossal nerve stimulation acquired using Sandman 10.1 software and Sandman 32+ amplifier. (Image courtesy of Edwin M. Valladares, MS, RPSGT, USC Sleep Disorders Center, Keck Medical Center of USC, University of Southern California.)

System in 2021(6). Although not everyone with CSA will require a **rem**edē System, careful selection criteria can make it a viable and novel alternative, for the most difficult-to-treat patients do not qualify for or tolerate PAP therapy (25,33). The system utilizes a transvenously placed pacemaker like lead to stimulate the phrenic nerve unilaterally, usually on the left side, to activate breathing on the basis of signaling information. Stimulation intensity is titrated to a setting where breathing is entrained to a target minute ventilation. The system is minimally invasive and is implanted by specially trained electrophysiologists (EPs). The device is activated at the programmed bedtime when the patient is recumbent and works continuously throughout the entire night without volitional patient effort until the programmed end time or continuous upright posture (26).

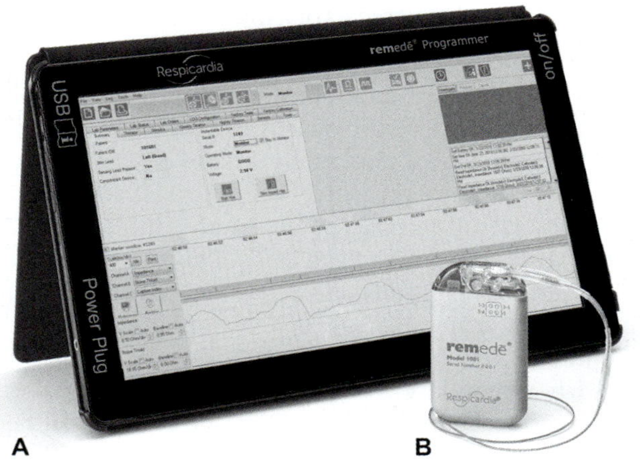

A B

Figure 51-4A and 4B Zoll remedē System components for treatment of central sleep apnea. Figure 4A demonstrates the interface tablet, and Figure 4B demonstrates the latest generation of implants, the remede EL-X System. (Courtesy of Zoll Medical Corporation.)

The remedē System: Components, Function, and Indications

This new system uses one lead, which acts as both for stimulation and sensing (26). The stimulator lead is placed in the left pericardiophrenic vein or the right brachiocephalic vein to stimulate the phrenic nerve and produce "diaphragmatic contractions thereby creating negative intrathoracic pressure that mimics normal breathing" (26). A preprogrammed computer tablet that is paired with an electronic wand serves as the interface unit, which is used to interrogate and make setting changes to the implanted device (27). All components have specific serial numbers. The implantable pulse generator (IPG) has a radiopaque identification marker inside it, allowing for the model number and manufacturing date to be visible through x-ray techniques. The device is accessed through an electronic tablet and interrogation component (Figure 51-4) (28). The original **rem**edē System has an estimated battery life of 41 to 55 months, depending on pulse generation, but the new **rem**eded EL-X system has a 40% more life expectancy (26,28).

The **rem**edē System received FDA approval to treat adult patients with moderate-to-severe CSA, which is broad and nonspecific to the type of CSA (28). Respicardia, Inc. recommends the use of selection criteria during their pivotal trial. During the pivotal trial, patients were 18 years of age or older, with a PSG test conducted within the last 40 days evidencing an AHI of at least 20/h, central apneas being at least 50% or higher of all apneas, 30 or more central apnea events throughout the night, and an obstructive apnea index of 20%. Contraindications for device implantation are active infection and the need for MRI (28). The pivotal study's exclusion criteria also included the following: phrenic nerve palsy, stage D heart failure, cerebrovascular event within the past 12 months, CSA secondary to opioids, and advanced renal disease (26). It has been shown to be just as effective in women as in men, with no adverse events reported in women compared to only 10% in men (25,33).

The remedē System: Patient Process

The **rem**edē System is implanted by a cardiologist who is an experienced electrophysiologist (EP) in cardiac resynchronization therapy. The system is activated 1 month post implant to allow time for healing. The device is activated by a trained sleep physician and sleep technologist. In the pivotal study, the device was titrated in the sleep lab 1 month post activation. A clinical protocol for implantation and activation based on the pivotal trial is currently being finalized.

The system functions independent of the patient's volition. The system is programmed to turn on and off according to the patient's usual sleep schedule. However, for times when the patient goes to bed later or awakens earlier than usual, the IPG does not actively stimulate if the patient is upright, regardless of clock time. The IPG has a programmable setting for pause time that is activated when the patient changes position (27).

The remedē System: Clinical Effectiveness and Safety Findings

The **rem**edē System Pivotal Trial evaluated the effectiveness and safety of the therapy. These data were used to apply for FDA approval. The study was a prospective, multicenter, randomized controlled trial, where clinical investigators across the United States and Europe randomized 151 patients to treatment (n = 73) or control (n = 78) groups. Five participants were excluded from each group, given unrelated deaths (n = 4), lost to follow-up ($n = 1$), missed appointments/medical issues ($n = 2$), and patients exiting the study ($n = 3$), with final groups of treatment ($n = 68$) and control ($n = 73$) (26).

The study showed that 35 (51%) of 68 treatment patients achieved a 50% or more reduction in their AHI at the 6-month mark. Moreover, 91% of the 151 patients did not have any serious adverse events at 12 months, and 27 of the 73 treatment group patients reported "nonserious therapy-related discomfort." Twenty-six of the 27 patients reporting discomfort had resolution with "simple system reprogramming" (26). At 12 months, patients continue to show sustained efficacy, and these effects have been shown to continue well into 5 years (26,28).

Like the Inspire therapy, questions regarding nerve damage caused by neurostimulations have not been established.

The remedē System: How Does It Affect Polysomnography Recordings?

Like the Inspire therapy, the **rem**edē System does not significantly affect PSG signals. Because the **rem**edē System is implanted closer to the heart when compared with the Inspire therapy, it affects the electrocardiogram (ECG) more than any other signal when stimulation is activated (Figure 51-5). As a result, PSG scoring is not hindered and AASM scoring rules can still be implemented, but ECG signals are limited (22). Effects on objective EEG sleep are not available, given this is an emergent technology.

INSURANCE COVERAGE AND COST

Both the Inspire therapy and the **rem**edē System are covered by insurance companies (29,30). The Current Procedural Terminology (CPT) codes are provided by the respective company to be used when implanting, activating, titrating, and managing the therapy.

The CPT codes for activating and titrating the Inspire therapy in a sleep lab setting are as follows: 95970 for interrogation of the device with no setting changes, 95974 for interrogation for the device with setting changes, and 95810-TC + 95974 for a PSG titration of the Inspire therapy. The CPT codes for activating and titrating the **rem**edē System in a sleep lab setting are as follows: 0434T for interrogation of the device with no setting changes, 0435T for interrogation of the device with setting changes, and 0436T for PSG and interrogation (CPT code 95810 is not to be used). Because CPT code updates occur from time to time, suitable CPT codes should be periodically verified with the corresponding manufacturer.

A model-based projection for the long-term cost-effectiveness of the Inspire therapy has been found to be beneficial when comparing it with nontreatment from a third-party US perspective (31). Inspire Medical has reported the approximate cost of its device to be $20,000 plus the cost of surgery (30). A cost-effectiveness analysis of the **rem**edē System is not available to the knowledge of the authors.

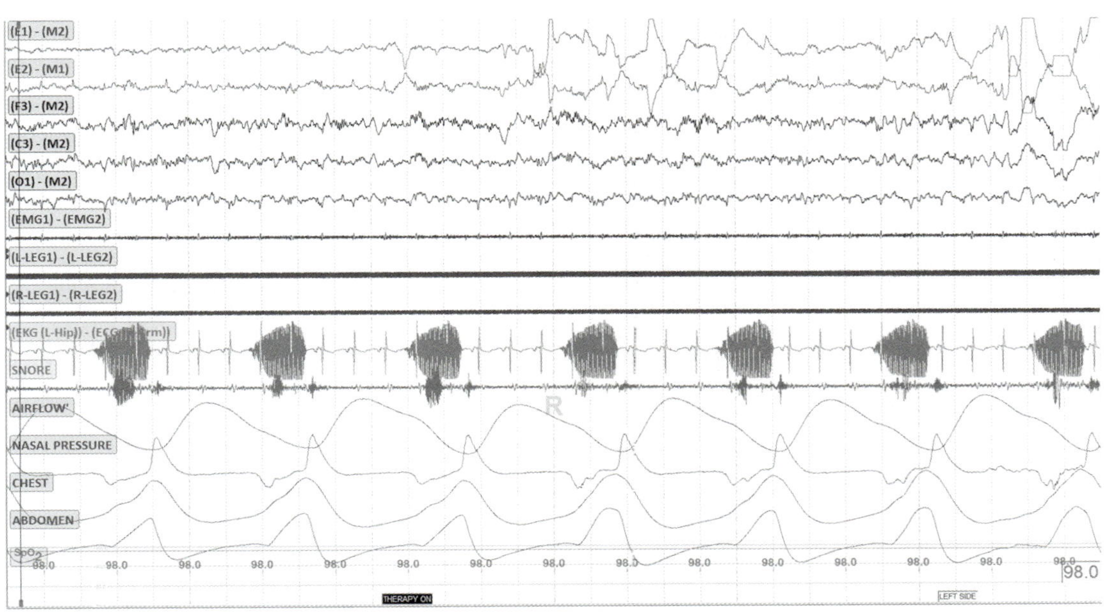

Figure 51-5 Phrenic nerve stimulation effect on polysomnography—Epoch (30 seconds) during phrenic nerve stimulation acquired using Sandman 10.1 software and Sandman 32+ amplifier. (Image courtesy of Edwin M. Valladares, MS, RPSGT, USC Sleep Disorders Center, Keck Medical Center of USC, University of Southern California.)

SUMMARY: EFFECT OF TECHNICAL-SURGICAL INTERVENTIONS TO THE FIELD OF SLEEP MEDICINE AND ROLE OF THE SLEEP TECHNOLOGIST

Technical-surgical interventions, such as the Inspire therapy and **rem**edē System, provide alternative therapies for a subset of patients with OSA and CSA who cannot benefit from traditional PAP therapies, respectively. These therapies are also expanding the role of the sleep technologist because they are needed to activate, interrogate, and make technical setting changes to these therapies during clinic visits and at night during PSG device titrations. The role of the sleep technologist is evolving as technology intersects with the changing landscape of health care. In an era where less complicated patients are being diagnosed using home sleep apnea testing units and more complicated patients are being tested in the sleep lab, the role of the sleep technologist is increasingly requiring highly skilled technologists (32). Sleep technologists are required to be ambitious and flexible to learn new facets of our field. Specific training for these devices is provided by the particular device company once a site is identified as having all the required team members (eg, sleep physician(s), otolaryngologists for Inspire therapy, and cardiac EP for the **rem**edē System). These implantable devices also provide sleep physicians more weapons in their arsenal against sleep-disordered breathing, resulting in an even more specialized sleep physician role. Lastly, the increase in available therapies is also paving the way for more personalized sleep medicine care as researchers connect endotypes with specific therapies to maximize efficacy and efficiency for individualized care (14).

REFERENCES

1. Sullivan CE, Issa FG, Berthon-Jones M, et al. Reversal of obstructive sleep apnoea by continuous positive airway pressure applied through the nares. *Lancet.* 1981;1(8225):862-865.
2. Weaver TE, Grunstein RR. Adherence to continuous positive airway pressure therapy: the challenge to effective treatment. *Proc Am Thorac Soc.* 2008;5(2): 173-178.
3. Wolkove N, Baltzan M, Kamel H, et al. Long-term compliance with continuous positive airway pressure in patients with obstructive sleep apnea. *Can Respir J.* 2008;15(7):365-369.
4. Campos-Rodriguez F, Martinez-Alonso M, Sanchez-de-la-Torre M, et al. Long-term adherence to continuous positive airway pressure therapy in non-sleepy sleep apnea patients. *Sleep Med.* 2016;17:1-6.
5. Senior BA, Rosenthal L, Lumley A, et al. Efficacy of uvulopalatopharyngoplasty in unselected patients with mild obstructive sleep apnea. *Otolaryngol Head Neck Surg.* 2000;123(3):9-82.
6. Respicardia, Inc. Respicardia's remedē system receives FDA approval. Press release, CISION PR Newswire. Published October 10, 2017. Accessed November 22, 2025. https://remede.zoll.com/press-releases/respicardias-remede-system-receives-fda-approval/
7. Inspire Medical Systems, Inc. FDA approves inspire upper airway stimulation (UAS) therapy for obstructive sleep apnea. Press release, American Academy of Sleep Medicine. Published May 1, 2014. Accessed November 22, 2025. https://aasm.org/fda-panel-recommends-approval-for-inspire-upper-airway-stimulation-system/
8. Inspire Medical Systems, Inc. Inspire Medical Systems, Inc. announces third quarter 2024 financial results and updates 2024. Published November 4, 2024. Accessed November 22, 2025. https://investors.inspiresleep.com/news/news-details/2024/Inspire-Medical-Systems-Inc.-Announces-Third-Quarter-2024Financial-Results-and-Updates-2024-Outlook/default.aspx
9. Inspire® Therapy. Indications for Inspire ® Therapy. Published 2025. Accessed April 27, 2025. https://professionals.inspiresleep.com/en-us/indications-and-contraindications/
10. Strollo PJ, Soose RJ, Maurer JT, et al. Upper-airway stimulation for obstructive sleep apnea. *N Engl J Med.* 2014;370(2):139-149.
11. Inspire Medical Systems, Inc. *System Implant Manual (200-236-101 RevB)*. Inspire Medical Systems, Inc; 2017.
12. Vanderveken OM, Maurer JT, Hohenhorst W, et al. Evaluation of drug-induced sleep endoscopy as a patient selection tool for implanted upper airway stimulation for obstructive sleep apnea. *J Clin Sleep Med.* 2013;9(5):433-438.
13. Charakorn N, Kezirian EJ. Drug-induced sleep endoscopy. *Otolaryngol Clin North Am.* 2016;49: 1359-1372.
14. Subramani Y, Singh M, Wong J, et al. Understanding phenotypes of obstructive sleep apnea: applications in anesthesia, surgery, and perioperative medicine. *Anesth Analg.* 2018;124(1):179-191.
15. Chen W, Gillett E, Khoo MCK, et al. Real-time multislice MRI during continuous positive airway response to pressure change. *J Magn Reson Imaging.* 2017;46:1400-1408.
16. Inspire Medical Systems, Inc. Inspire Medical Systems announces FDA approval of inspire 3028 neurostimulator for the treatment of obstructive sleep apnea. Published June 5, 2017 Inspire Medical Systems,

Inc. Accessed November 22, 2025. https://www.globenewswire.com/news-release/2017/06/05/1008171/0/en/Inspire-Medical-Systems-Announces-FDA-Approval-of-Inspire-3028-Neurostimulator-for-the-Treatment-of-Obstructive-Sleep-Apnea.html

17. Woodson BT, Soose RJ, Gillespie MB, et al. Three-year outcomes of cranial nerve stimulation for obstructive sleep apnea: the Star trial. *Otolaryngol Head Neck Surg.* 2016;154(1):181-188.
18. Woodson BT, Strohl KP, Soose RJ, et al. Upper airway stimulation for obstructive sleep apnea: 5-year outcomes. *Otolaryngol Head Neck Surg.* 2018;159(1):194-202.
19. Gillespie MB, Soose RJ, Woodson BT, et al. Upper airway stimulation for obstructive sleep apnea: patient-reported outcomes after 48 months of follow-up. *Otolaryngol Head Neck Surg.* 2017;156(4):765-771.
20. Eldabe S, Buchser E, Duarte RV. Complications of spinal cord stimulation and peripheral nerve stimulation techniques: a review of the literature. *Pain Med.* 2016;17(2):325-336.
21. Inspire Medical Systems, Inc. Inspire Medical Systems' inspire therapy for reducing obstructive sleep apnea demonstrates long-term safety and sustained benefit following 5-years of treatment. Published September 20, 2017. Inspire Medical Systems, Inc. Accessed November 22, 2025. https://www.globenewswire.com/news-release/2017/09/20/1125163/0/en/Inspire-Medical-Systems-Inspire-Therapy-for-Reducing-Obstructive-Sleep-Apnea-Demonstrates-Long-term-Safety-and-Sustained-Benefit-Following-5-Years-of-Treatment.html
22. Berry RB, Albertario CL, Harding SM, et al. *The AASM Manual for the Scoring of Sleep and Associated Events: Rules, Terminology and Technical Specifications. Version 2.5.* American Academy of Sleep Medicine; 2018.
23. Inspire Medical Systems, Inc. *Programmer Manual. (200-081-101 RevD).* Inspire Medical Systems, Inc; 2017.
24. Hofauer B, Philip P, Markus W, et al. Effects of upper-airway stimulation on sleep architecture in patients with obstructive sleep apnea. *Sleep Breath.* 2017;21:901-908.
25. Cowie MR, Woehrle H, Wegscheider K, et al. Adaptive servo-ventilation for central sleep apnea in systolic heart failure. *N Engl J Med.* 2015;373(12):1095-1105.
26. Zoll Remede® System. The latest advancement in remedē® system technology. Published 2025. Accessed April 27, 2025. https://remede.zoll.com/clinicians/about-remede/
27. Costanzo MR, Augostini R, Goldberg LR, et al. Design of the remedē® system pivotal trial: a prospective, randomized study in the use of respiratory rhythm management to treat central sleep apnea. *J Card Fail.* 2015;21:892-902.
28. Respicardia. *Remedē® System Implant and Clinician Use Manual.* Respicardia; 2010.
29. Costanzo MR, Ponikowski P, Javaheri S, et al. Sustained 12 month benefit of phrenic nerve stimulation for central sleep apnea. *Am J Cardiol.* 2018;121(11):1400-1408.
30. Inspire Medical Systems, Inc. (November 2015). *About obstructive sleep apnea & Inspire upper airway stimulation (UAS) therapy.* Inspire Medical Systems, Inc.
31. Pietzsch JB, Liu S, Garner AM, et al. Long-term cost-effectiveness of upper airway stimulation for the treatment of obstructive sleep apnea: a model-based projection based on the STAR trial. *Sleep.* 2015;38(5):735-743.
32. Brooks R, Trimble M. The future of sleep technology: report from an American Association of Sleep Technologists summit meeting. *J Clin Sleep Med.* 2014;10(5):589-593.
33. Samii S, Meyer TE, Shah N. Analysis by sex of safety and effectiveness of transvenous phrenic nerve stimulation. *Sleep Breath.* 2024;28(1):165-171. doi:10.1007/s11325-023-02882-5

Chapter 52
Other Treatments for Obstructive Sleep Apnea

PAMELA DEYOUNG

KEY CONCEPTS/LEARNING OBJECTIVES

The key concepts for this chapter include a review of therapies for anatomic compromise other than continuous positive airway pressure (CPAP), oral appliances, and upper airway surgeries based on the endotypes underlying obstructive sleep apnea.

KEY TERMS

Anatomic compromise
Endotypes
Low arousal threshold
Pharyngeal dilator muscle dysfunction
Unstable ventilatory control

Positive airway pressure (PAP) is the gold standard for obstructive sleep apnea (OSA). However, research suggests that after the first night of continuous positive airway pressure (CPAP), 8% to 15% of patients with OSA refuse further usage; furthermore, 50% of patients terminate CPAP usage within 1 year of treatment initiation (1-3). Other therapies have been clinically validated and may be offered to remedy the need for alternative therapy due to intolerance.

In order to understand the treatment alternatives, we need to understand the causes of sleep apnea. We now know that OSA is a heterogeneous disease—there are multiple mechanisms that cause OSA that are different from person to person. We will refer to these different mechanisms as endotypes, which is the language used in the sleep medicine field to help categorize patients with sleep apnea based on the causes of their condition. To date, we have identified four main endotypes: anatomic compromise, unstable ventilatory control (ie, increased loop gain), pharyngeal dilator muscle dysfunction, and low arousal threshold (4). While these are the most widely accepted endotypes, there are other factors, such as fluid redistribution, arousal intensity, negative effort dependence, hormonal imbalances, and lung volume, that can also contribute to OSA (4).

OSA endotypes are important because they guide providers to determine which treatments may work best for each individual patient. An individual's OSA is usually caused by a combination of endotypes; providers will attempt to find treatment options that address each endotypic, or mechanistic, concern. We will next discuss each main endotype and the treatment options that address their concerns.

ANATOMIC COMPROMISE

Anatomic compromise refers to the increased collapsibility of the upper airway, which restricts air from reaching the lungs during sleep (5). This airway collapse is due to two anatomic features of patients with OSA that make them more susceptible to airway collapse than patients without OSA: increased soft tissue (ie, tonsils and soft palate) and increased fatty tissue in the genioglossus and pharyngeal walls (5) (Figure 52-1). CPAP therapy, oral appliances, and surgical interventions are effective methods of treating anatomic compromise; they do this in a variety of ways that will be covered in chapters to follow. In this section, we will focus on therapies for anatomic compromise other than CPAP, oral appliances, and upper airway surgeries.

Weight Loss

As mentioned previous, increased fatty tissue in the areas surrounding the upper airways is a key contributor to anatomic compromise. Upper airway collapsibility is increased as fat deposits narrow the upper airway and abdominal fat masses reduce tracheal tension. A 2024 meta-analysis (a review of literature that combines multiple independent studies) looked at 27 studies from

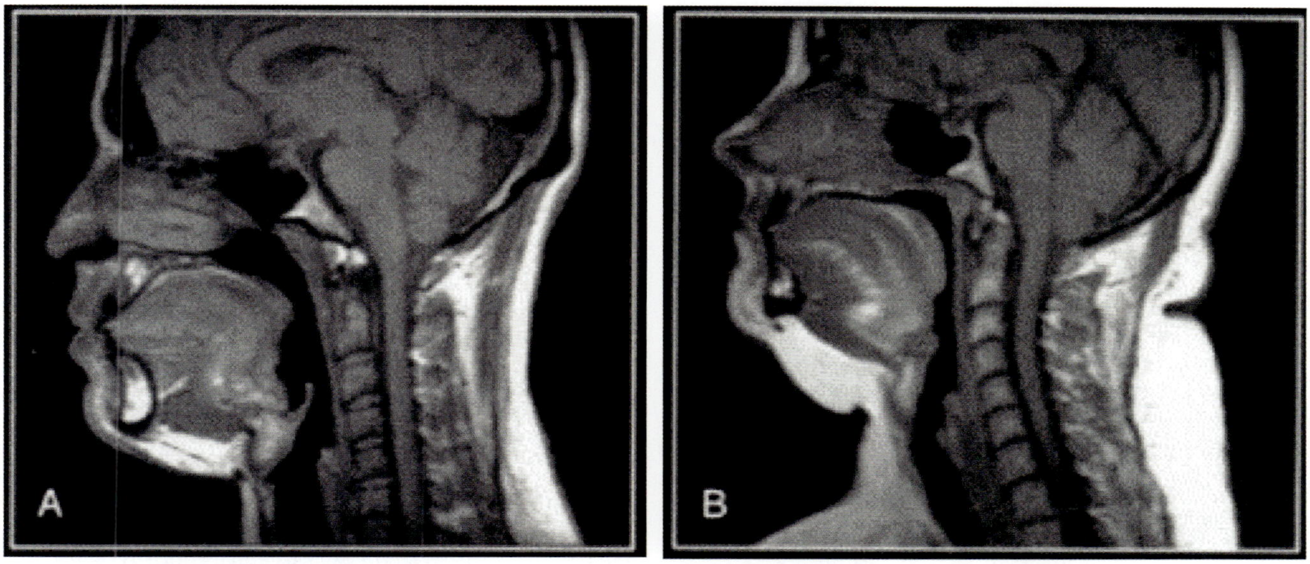

Figure 52-1 Comparison of a midsagittal MR image of a normal subject (A) and a patient with sleep apnea (B). Soft palate and tongue area are larger in the patient with apnea. (Reprinted from Schwab RJ. Upper airway imaging. *Clin Chest Med.* 1998;19(1):33-54. Copyright © 1998 Elsevier. With permission.)

2000 to 2023 to quantify the relationship between weight loss and OSA severity. They found that that a body mass index (BMI) reduction of 20% was associated with an apnea-hypopnea index (AHI) reduction of 57% (7). As someone loses weight, they lose fat everywhere, including in the upper airway.

When approaching weight loss, the patient should review their options and decide with their health care provider which is best for them. Evidence-based obesity treatments include dietary and lifestyle modifications, pharmacotherapy, and bariatric procedures (8). Research shows that obesity is best managed by a multidisciplinary clinical team that integrates diet, exercise, and pharmacotherapy, while bariatric surgery should be considered only for select patients (9).

Diet and Lifestyle Changes

The addition of behavioral interventions, different nutritional approaches, and physical activity fall under the umbrella of diet and lifestyle changes. Some behavioral interventions include technologic applications that monitor lifestyle changes, coaching, cognitive behavioral therapy, and peer support. There is a wide array of nutritional approaches to weight loss, including increasing fruit and vegetable intake, reducing caloric intake, and eliminating ultra-processed foods (8). Research shows that in choosing the best dietary approach, providers should choose based on the likelihood of adherence long-term, patient preference, and metabolic risk (8). Physical activity in conjunction with dietary changes helps with weight maintenance, although it is not a stand-alone treatment for obesity. These interventions are appropriate for both patients who are overweight and patients with obesity. While diet and lifestyle are important for weight loss, research shows that other treatment options, listed in what follows, may be more effective (8).

Metabolic and Bariatric Surgery

Bariatric surgery is a term that includes a variety of surgical procedures that reduce the amount of food the stomach can hold and cause malabsorption of nutrients. Recent guidelines recommend that they should be considered for patients with a BMI of 30 to 34.9 who have coexisting metabolic diseases or for patients with a BMI of 35 or greater (10). The most common metabolic and bariatric surgeries are laparoscopic sleeve gastrectomy (LSG), in which about 85% of the stomach is removed, and Roux-en-Y gastric bypass (RYGB) surgery, where nutrient absorption is decreased from bypassing a large segment of the intestine and connecting it to a small gastric pouch instead of the stomach (8).

While metabolic and bariatric surgery has been shown to effectively reduce AHI in patients with OSA, recent research has shown that the complete resolution of OSA is achieved in less than half of the patients who receive them (11). Furthermore, although these surgeries have long been considered effective interventions for weight loss, recent advancements suggest that pharmacotherapy may have caused reevaluation of treatments for obesity (12).

Pharmacotherapy

While there are a variety of antiobesity medications (AOM) available for weight loss, we will focus on AOMs that have been shown to improve sleep apnea specifically. Until recently, there was limited evidence of two AOMs potentially decreasing sleep apnea metrics: Liraglutide (a GLP-1 receptor antagonist) and a combination of phentermine (an appetite suppressant) with topiramate (13). However, a recent landmark study (SURMOUNT-OSA) followed nondiabetic patients diagnosed with OSA who had weekly injections of the weight loss medication tirzepatide, a dual antagonist of GIP and GLP-1 receptors. The study found that those patients with OSA had a 58.7% decrease in their AHI (14). This study resulted in tirzepatide, marketed under the brand Zepbound, being the first pharmacologic treatment that is Food and Drug Administration (FDA) approved to treat moderate to severe sleep apnea in adults with obesity. While tirzepatide is the only approved drug to treat OSA currently, there are ongoing trials testing similar weight loss medications.

Positional Therapy

While weight loss is an important method of treating sleep apnea, not all patients with sleep apnea are overweight or obese. Another treatment for sleep apnea that can resolve anatomic compromise is positional therapy, where patients are instructed to sleep on their sides rather than lying in the supine position. This position helps to prevent the upper airway from collapsing, by reducing pressure due to gravity on the airway (15).

Whether a patient with OSA has positional sleep apnea is a significant consideration when reviewing treatment options. Positional sleep apnea is defined as supine AHI 2 times the nonsupine AHI. Reports on the prevalence of positional sleep apnea vary, but it is estimated that approximately 56% to 75% of patients with OSA exhibit an increase in severity in the supine position (16).

Methods for Positional Therapy

Perhaps the most well-documented method of positional therapy is known as the "tennis ball technique." As the name implies, this method originated from the use of a tennis ball. A tennis ball would be sewn into the front pocket of a t-shirt, and then the patient would wear the t-shirt backward to bed. When the patient would attempt to move to the supine position, the discomfort from the tennis ball would prompt the patient to roll off the back. The term has since been associated with any device that includes a mass strapped to the patient's back, causing them not to lie supine. Although this method has efficacy, compliance is unsatisfactory. Compliance is estimated to be 40% to 70% in the short term but as low as 10% in the long term (16).

Newer devices exist with promising results to date, but there are limited data on long-term compliance. These devices strap to a person's chest or neck and give off vibrations or auditory alarms when the patient moves to the supine position (16). When considering a device, one should consider whether it has FDA approval and whether clinical studies have shown effectiveness.

POOR PHARYNGEAL MUSCLE RESPONSIVENESS

As mentioned previously, patients with genioglossi (tongues) that are anatomically large or that have extra fatty tissue can affect upper airway collapsibility. In patients with OSA, the genioglossi along with the surrounding pharyngeal walls are activated during the day to compensate for their collapsible upper airway anatomy. However, during sleep, some patients with OSA lack the ability to continue to recruit the muscles that keep the airway open when they are awake. This is called poor pharyngeal muscle responsiveness (5). Treatment options that may target this endotype include hypoglossal nerve stimulation (HGNS), oral muscle exercises and stimulation, and, potentially, pharmacotherapy. The only approved HGNS treatment in the United States is a surgical intervention that uses an electrical lead to stimulate the tongue and move it forward; surgical interventions for OSA will be covered in chapters to follow.

Oral Muscle Exercises

Some research suggests that orofacial myofunctional therapy, or oral muscle exercises, may have positive treatment outcomes for OSA (17). They are hypothesized to do so by improving pharyngeal muscle endurance and pharyngeal muscle coordination. Other research has shown that singing, playing the didgeridoo, or other wind instruments may also aid oral muscle recruitment, and therefore OSA, via a similar mechanism (5,17). Strengthening the muscles in the oral cavity during the day has some evidence to show that it will aid in improving the pharyngeal muscle responsiveness during sleep.

Transoral Neuromuscular Electrical Stimulation

The only currently FDA-approved device for daytime treatment of OSA is the eXciteOSA transoral neuromuscular electrical stimulation (NMES) device (Figure 52-2). Patients are instructed to insert the device into their oral cavity for 20 minutes every day, at any time of day. The device delivers electrical stimulation to the genioglossus, which has been shown to increase muscle strength and decrease upper airway collapsibility during the night. The device is approved to treat only mild OSA (AHI 5-14.9) and has been shown in some studies to decrease AHI substantially (18).

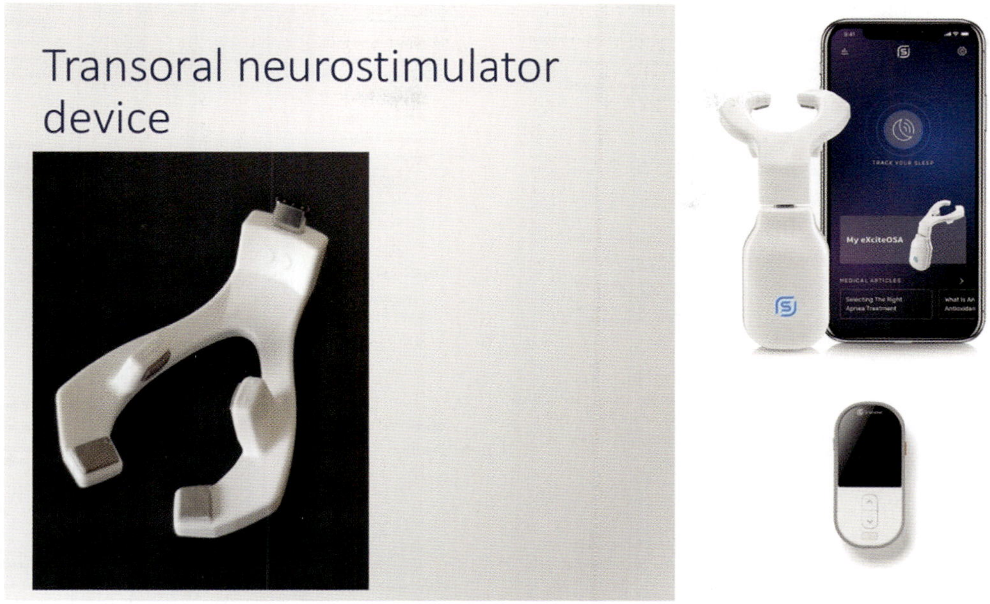

Figure 52-2 The eXciteOSA NMES device is the first approved by the Food and Drug Administration for daytime sleep apnea treatment. The device is shown along with the application interface (18). Patients usually pay out of pocket for the treatment, and it is only available by prescription. (Reprinted from Nokes B, Baptista PM, de Apodaca PMR, et al. Transoral awake state neuromuscular electrical stimulation therapy for mild obstructive sleep apnea. *Sleep Breath.* 2023;27(2):527-534. http://creativecommons.org/licenses/by/4.0)

FUTURE ALTERNATIVE TREATMENTS OPTIONS FOR OBSTRUCTIVE SLEEP APNEA

The remaining two endotypes, high loop gain and low arousal threshold, do not currently have any treatment options specifically FDA approved to target those endotypes. However, there are a variety of pharmacologic options that are being researched and that will likely be used to treat OSA in the near future. We will cover these options in the following section.

Unstable Ventilatory Control (High Loop Gain)

The amount of control that one has over their respiratory system can be quantified by a term called loop gain (5). Loop gain is an engineering term that describes a concept similar to a feedback loop. A common example is a thermostat: Say you set your home thermostat to 70° but that it is currently 69° in your house. If your temperature control system ends up blasting the heater, your house may end up at a temperature of 75° instead of the desired 70°, meaning that the control system has overcompensated. This is an example of a system with high loop gain. To relate it back to sleep apnea, when the receptors in your body detect higher than normal levels of carbon dioxide (CO_2), then the instinct is to ventilate more to compensate. Some patients with OSA are shown to overcompensate, resulting in hyperventilation and arousal during sleep (5). Research is looking into pharmacologic therapies such as acetazolamide and sulthiame in order to treat high loop gain (19).

Low Arousal Threshold

Respiratory arousal threshold is a term that describes how easily someone wakes up due to respiratory disturbance. A low respiratory arousal threshold describes a patient who arises from sleep easily, while a high threshold describes a patient who does not wake up easily from a respiratory event. A conceptual example of this is a mother and a father of a newborn baby.

Once the parents have gone to bed, say the newborn child starts babbling in its crib. If the mother wakes up to the first sound of the baby's whimpers while the father completely sleeps through the child's cries, this is an example of a low and high arousal threshold, respectively. Patients with low respiratory arousal threshold are extra sensitive to changes in the pressure of their upper airway, which causes them to wake up before the upper airway muscles can self-correct.

As discussed throughout this chapter, treatment of OSA is going in the direction of precision medicine—catering treatment options to each individual's needs—and endotypes will help us do just that. In the past,

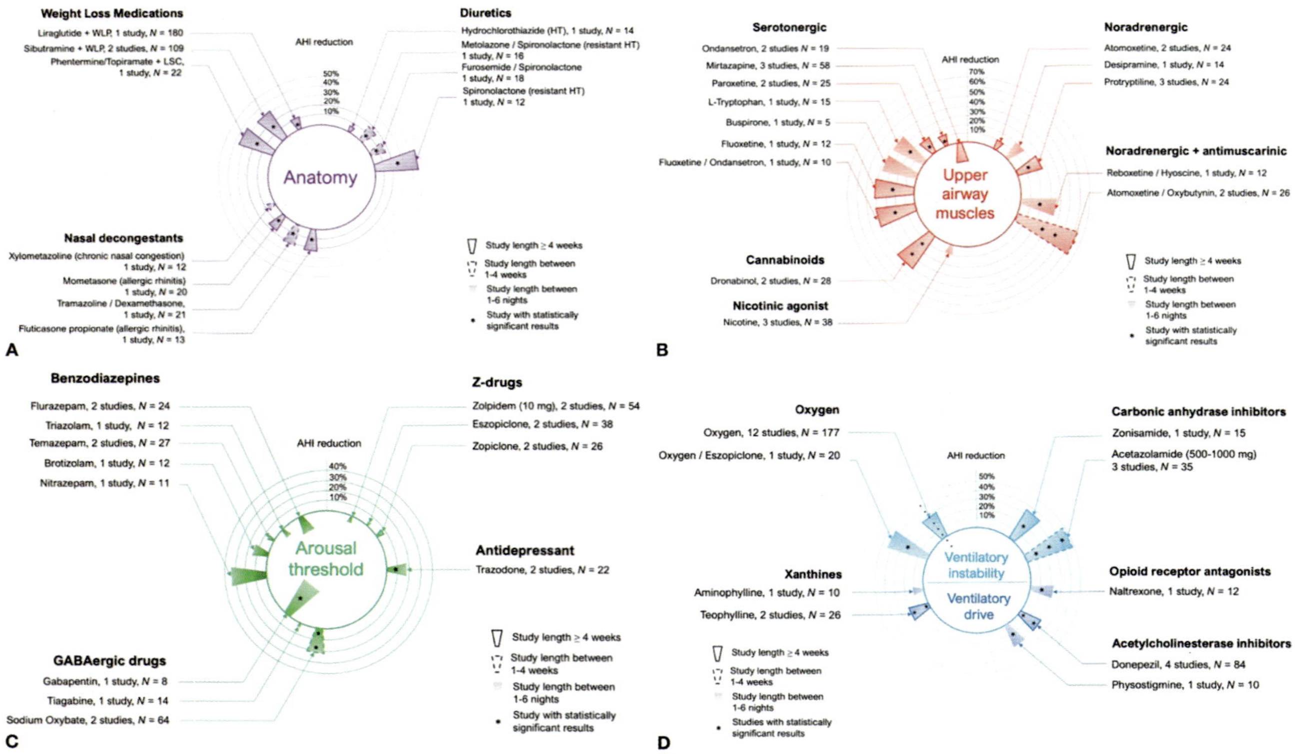

Figure 52-3 Circular bar plots from a review of studies targeting endotypic traits with medications for the pharmacologic treatment of obstructive sleep apnea by Taranto-Montemurro et al (20). A: A circular bar plot describing the studies performed using medications that modify anatomic traits in patients with OSA. B: Circular bar plot describing the studies performed using medications that modify upper airway muscle activity. C: Circular bar plot describing the studies performed using medications that modify the arousal threshold. When multiple doses of a medication were used in different studies, the dose considered is specified in the parenthesis. D: Circular bar plot describing the studies performed using medications that modify ventilatory instability (loop gain) or ventilatory drive. Drugs targeting more specifically ventilatory control instability (loop gain) are represented in the upper part of the circle; those that act more generically as ventilatory stimulants are represented in the lower part of the circle. (Reprinted from Taranto-Montemurro L, Messineo L, Wellman A. Targeting endotypic traits with medications for the pharmacological treatment of obstructive sleep apnea: a review of the current literature. *J Clin Med*. 2019;8(11):1846. http://creativecommons.org/licenses/by/4.0)

categorizing patients based on their endotypes was a very labor-intensive procedure requiring both a researcher and a sleep technician to manually manipulate the upper airway throughout the night. Currently, researchers can endotype overnight sleep studies using an algorithm, which further indicates the likelihood of artificial intelligence (AI) being used in clinical sleep studies in the near future (19).

Other treatment options for endotypes are also being heavily researched (Figure 52-3). Some examples include atomoxetine and other GLP-1 medications for anatomic upper way collapsibility, acetazolamide along with others for high loop gain, and noninvasive HGNS therapies for poor pharyngeal muscle recruitment.

Conclusion

Many of the therapies described in this chapter have the potential to treat OSA effectively or to be an effective adjunctive treatment option. It is extremely important that reports from patients about their symptoms be considered with these treatments and that patients be reevaluated to assess the efficacy of their treatment. No single treatment option is best for all patients. In fact, some treatments available to the patient population are not suited for a single individual or are not effective at all. Despite the constant advancements in PAP technology and adherence methods, other therapies are available and may be well suited for some individuals. As a vital participant in the patient's sleep medicine journey, the sleep technologist must be familiar with these other therapies and able to convey some general knowledge of validated treatment options.

REFERENCES

1. Borker PV, Carmona E, Essien UR, et al. Neighborhoods with greater prevalence of minority residents have lower continuous positive airway pressure adherence.

Am J Respir Crit Care Med. 2021;204(3):339-346. doi:10.1164/rccm.202009-3685OC

2. Contal O, Poncin W, Vaudan S, et al. One-year adherence to continuous positive airway pressure with telemonitoring in sleep apnea hypopnea syndrome: a randomized controlled trial. *Front Med (Lausanne)*. 2021;8:626361. doi:10.3389/fmed.2021.626361
3. Rotenberg BW, Murariu D, Pang KP. Trends in CPAP adherence over twenty years of data collection: a flattened curve. *J Otolaryngol Head Neck Surg*. 2016;45(1):43. doi:10.1186/s40463-016-0156-0
4. Malhotra A, Mesarwi O, Pepin JL, Owens RL. Endotypes and phenotypes in obstructive sleep apnea. *Curr Opin Pulm Med*. 2020;26(6):609-614. doi:10.1097/MCP.0000000000000724
5. Schmickl CN, Owens RL, Edwards BA, Malhotra A. OSA endotypes: what are they and what are their potential clinical implications? *Curr Sleep Medicine Rep*. 2018;4(3):231-242. doi:10.1007/s40675-018-0121-8
6. Schwab RJ. Upper airway imaging. *Clin Chest Med*. 1998;19(1):33-54. doi:10.1016/s0272-5231(05)70430-5
7. Malhotra A, Heilmann CR, Banerjee KK, Dunn JP, Bunck MC, Bednarik J. Weight reduction and the impact on apnea-hypopnea index: a systematic meta-analysis. *Sleep Med*. 2024;121:26-31. doi:10.1016/j.sleep.2024.06.014
8. Elmaleh-Sachs A, Schwartz JL, Bramante CT, Nicklas JM, Gudzune KA, Jay M. Obesity management in adults: a review. *JAMA*. 2023;330(20):2000. doi:10.1001/jama.2023.19897
9. Kheniser K, Saxon DR, Kashyap SR. Long-term weight loss strategies for obesity. *J Clin Endocrinol Metab*. 2021;106(7):1854-1866. doi:10.1210/clinem/dgab091
10. Eisenberg D, Shikora SA, Aarts E, et al. 2022 American Society for Metabolic and Bariatric Surgery (ASMBS) and International Federation for the Surgery of Obesity and Metabolic Disorders (IFSO): indications for metabolic and bariatric surgery. *Surg Obes Relat Dis*. 2022;18(12):1345-1356. doi:10.1016/j.soard.2022.08.013
11. Wyszomirski K, Walędziak M, Różańska-Walędziak A. Obesity, bariatric surgery and obstructive sleep apnea—a narrative literature review. *Medicina*. 2023;59(7):1266. doi:10.3390/medicina59071266
12. Gołacki J, Matyjaszek-Matuszek B. Obesity—standards, trends and advances. *Adv Med Sci*. 2024;69(1):208-215. doi:10.1016/j.advms.2024.04.001
13. Harding CD, Fuentes AL, Malhotra A. Tackling obstructive sleep apnea with pharmacotherapeutics: expert guidance. *Expert Opin Pharmacother*. 2024;25(8):1019-1026. doi:10.1080/14656566.2024.2365329
14. Malhotra A, Grunstein RR, Fietze I, et al. Tirzepatide for the treatment of obstructive sleep apnea and obesity. *N Engl J Med*. 2024;391(13):1193-1205. doi:10.1056/NEJMoa2404881
15. Srijithesh PR, Aghoram R, Goel A, Dhanya J. Positional therapy for obstructive sleep apnoea. *Cochrane Database Syst Rev*. 2019;5(5):CD010990. doi:10.1002/14651858.CD010990.pub2
16. Ravesloot MJL, White D, Heinzer R, Oksenberg A, Pépin JL. Efficacy of the new generation of devices for positional therapy for patients with positional obstructive sleep apnea: a systematic review of the literature and meta-analysis. *J Clin Sleep Med*. 2017;13(6):813-824. doi:10.5664/jcsm.6622
17. Koka V, De Vito A, Roisman G, et al. Orofacial myofunctional therapy in obstructive sleep apnea syndrome: a pathophysiological perspective. *Medicina*. 2021;57(4):323. doi:10.3390/medicina57040323
18. Nokes B, Baptista PM, De Apodaca PMR, et al. Transoral awake state neuromuscular electrical stimulation therapy for mild obstructive sleep apnea. *Sleep Breath*. 2023;27(2):527-534. doi:10.1007/s11325-022-02644-9
19. Kryger MH, Thomas RJ. The past and future of sleep medicine. *Sleep Med Clin*. 2025;20(1):1-17. doi:10.1016/j.jsmc.2024.10.012
20. Taranto-Montemurro L, Messineo L, Wellman A. Targeting endotypic traits with medications for the pharmacological treatment of obstructive sleep apnea. a review of the current literature. *J Clin Med*. 2019;8(11):1846. doi:10.3390/jcm8111846

SECTION VI

Patient Management

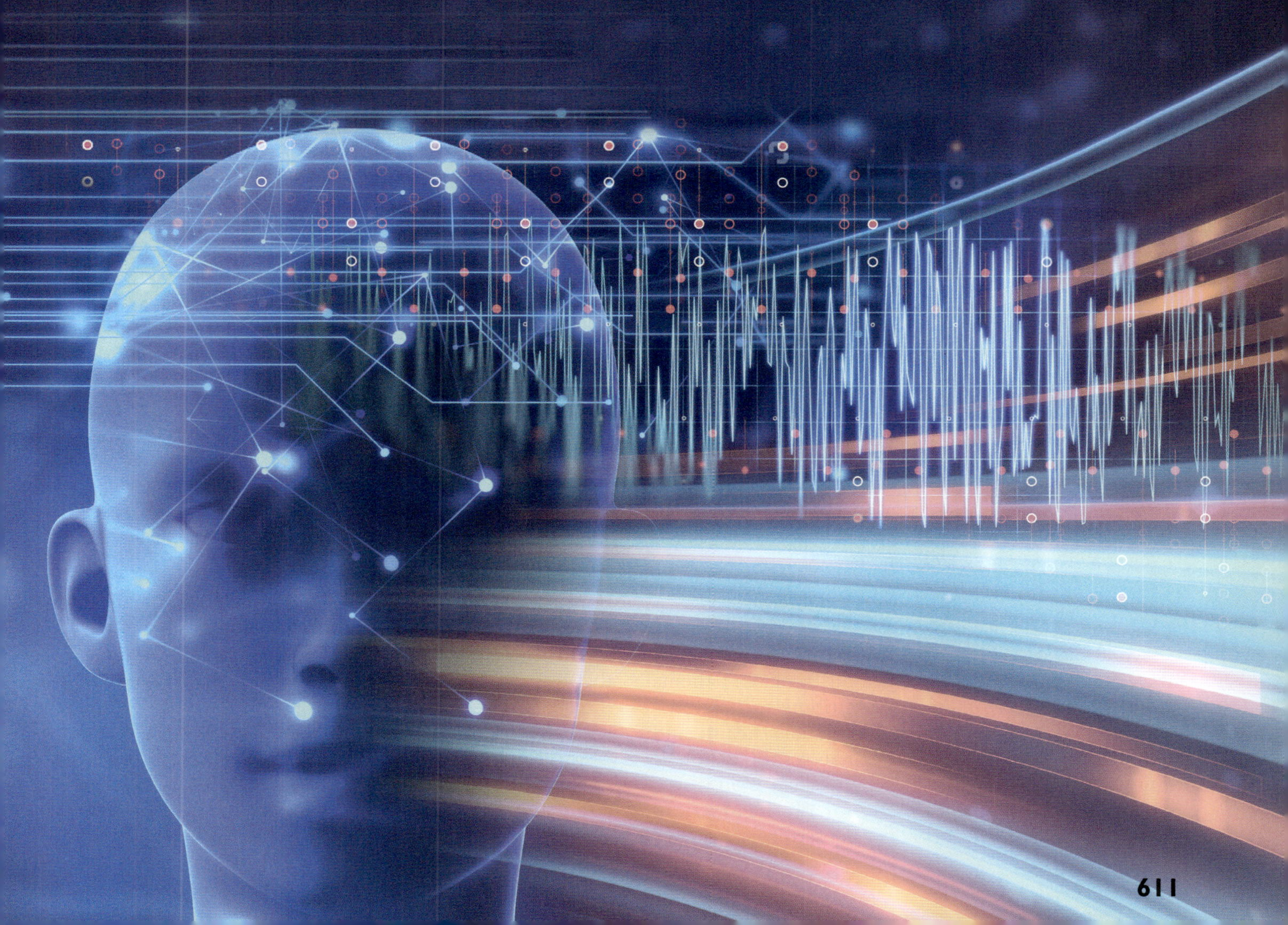

Chapter 53
Sleep Health Educator: Roles, Responsibilities, and Patient Management

ROBYN V. WOIDTKE

KEY CONCEPTS/LEARNING OBJECTIVES

The key concepts for this chapter include describing the roles and functions of a clinical sleep educator, employing concepts of patient self-management support in the continuum of care and as it relates to patient adherence, and implementing health literacy strategies in practice to improve patient outcomes.

KEY TERMS

Activation
Adherence
Behavioral intervention
Care coordination
Health literacy
Motivational enhancement (ME)
Patient engagement
Psychosocial
Shared decision making (SDM)

They may forget your name, but they will never forget how you made them feel.

Maya Angelou

Everyone needs a good night's sleep. Sleep health educators can make a meaningful difference in patients and the community. They can contribute their knowledge and skills to improving individuals' health and well-being community wide. Their role should not be limited to sleep disorders, as healthy sleep is an essential determinant of health benefits for all. The American Association of Sleep Technologists describes the role of the Clinical Sleep Educator. It provides an overview of competencies, including domains of practice, and a position summary, including promoting community sleep health.

THE ROLE OF THE CLINICAL SLEEP EDUCATOR

The role of the clinical sleep educator within sleep medicine continues to evolve, and there are many designated sleep educators in clinics, hospitals, and the community. This chapter may not encapsulate all the roles but will provide guidance anyone can embrace, including the concept of sleep stewardship. What is sleep stewardship? According to Gallegos in the AMA Journal of Ethics, sleep stewardship is "the responsible and ethical management of sleep resources and practices. It includes ethical, clinical, and cultural viewpoints." Throughout the United States, sleep education takes place in a variety of ways from full time sleep educator positions to the hybridization of the education within night and day technologist positions. Sleep education can also be integrated into medical assistant and nursing roles in sleep lab, practice, and hospital settings.

COMMUNITY SLEEP HEALTH EDUCATION

How can sleep education be disseminated throughout local communities? The American Academy of Sleep Medicine (AASM) offers numerous resources to help the sleep educator provide information. These materials include videos and various infographics on sleep topics, including sleep in the hospital, teen sleep, and access to sleep services. The sleep health educator can use these materials to promote healthy sleep and increase awareness of sleep disorders in their communities. Libraries, community organizations, and schools can be great conduits to conduct sleep education. When going into the community to educate about sleep, it is essential to also consider the social determinants of health on sleep and associated disorders. Social determinants of health include such concepts as homelessness, older adults, shift work, multiple jobs, family structure, and economic factors.

FOCUS ON THE PATIENT

Although the title for someone in this role may differ, the patient-centered goals should be the same: to provide the right care, to the right patient, at the right time. In addition, a goal is also to improve adherence to sleep treatment, regardless of the condition, by providing patients with the necessary tools for self-management at home. Although there is no single distinct definition for the role, core competencies exist for the sleep health educator, which include assessing the patient's educational needs and providing education appropriately, the ability to counsel patients concerning treatment options, providing access to community-based resources, and developing patient education materials.

For individuals in this role, it is not only about providing education about a specific topic or condition or training on a device but about completely understanding the patient's preferences, concerns, and limitations. When patients return home, it is often difficult for them to perform self-management, which is frequently expected of them, often without adequate tools and care. The sleep health educator can mitigate this issue by providing much-needed assistance.

Person- or patient-centered care refers to care incorporating many strategies: shared decision-making (SDM), care coordination and accessibility, top-down commitment to ensuring alignment with patient-centered goals, family inclusion, consideration of social determinants of health, and information sharing. By providing a more patient-focused approach rather than a one-size-fits-all approach, the patient may adhere more to therapy (1,2). Value in delivering patient-centered care has been demonstrated in improved patient satisfaction, clinician satisfaction, financial margins, and enhanced reputation of providers (2). The Agency for Healthcare Quality Improvement (AHRQ) (3) provides a good overview of several techniques surrounding SDM. These include the Three Talk Model, SHARE, and the Purposeful Approach.

The SHARE approach is Seek, Help, Assess, Reach, Evaluate. Each is different, but the goal is the same, namely, to find the best fit for the patient in terms of care and expectations. The AHRQ also offers free training on these communication techniques. Although physicians primarily use SDM, sleep health educators can provide foundational education to patients regarding their condition and options to elicit what is important to them. Such information gathering and education could be performed in conjunction with or following the physician providing the patient with a diagnosis and treatment options.

PATIENT EDUCATION

The role of patient education cannot be adequately summarized in a chapter—it is a complex intertwining of characteristics of the health care system, patient, and clinician, including gender, learning abilities, health literacy, age, patient-facing materials, and the social determinants of health. According to Barnason et al (4), therapeutic patient education can be defined as "an approach to facilitate patient and family learning about the treatment of disease and the adoption of self-management behaviors and lifestyles to improve physical and psychosocial health outcomes." Sleep health educators can be instrumental in educating sleep disorder patients to promote long-term adherence to sleep therapy.

HEALTH LITERACY

Health literacy is an issue for many patients. According to the Centers for Disease Control, in 2020, the definition of health literacy was updated to include organizations as well.

"*Personal health literacy is the degree to which individuals have the ability to find, understand, and use information and services to inform health-related decisions and actions for themselves and others.*

Organizational health literacy is the degree to which organizations equitably enable individuals to find, understand, and use information and services to inform health-related decisions and actions for themselves and others" (5).

Without adequate health literacy, self-care and management of their conditions become a burden not only to the patient but to the health care system at large.

Health literacy depends on the patient's ability to have such capacity, as well as the communication skills of the clinician, the patient's culture and belief systems, and the demands of the condition and health care system. Health literacy also includes skills such as numeracy. According to The National Center for Education Statistics, numeracy is "*the ability to access, use, interpret, and communicate mathematical information and ideas, to engage in and manage mathematical demands of a range of situations in adult life*" (6). This concept is fundamental as, in our field, numbers are used to communicate diagnosis, categories, and pressures for continuous positive airway devices. Patients may need additional time to understand these concepts fully.

According to a 2022 report by the Milken Institute (7), *"At least 88 percent of adults living in the US have health literacy inadequate to navigate the healthcare system and promote their well-being."* Older individuals, as well as those whose English is not their first language, pose additional barriers to understanding, and, hence, the ability to perform self-management in the home environment may be limited. The data regarding patients' ability to incorporate numeracy into daily care are similar to those of health literacy, but there are difficulties in determining how best to measure these data.

As noted, in sleep health care, many numbers are used to communicate with patients, such as the apnea-hypopnea index and percentages of sleep times and stages. Long-term health consequences should be explained to the patient, with particular emphasis on the impact on the individual. Both numbers and health information link back to the patient's health literacy ability. These types of information can confuse patients unless explained in a manner they understand. Thus, part of the sleep health educator's role is the individual's ability to translate these types of data into "plain language." In both written and spoken language, key elements of plain language include the following:

- Organizing information so that the most important behavioral or action points come first,
- Breaking complex information into understandable chunks,
- Using simple language or defining technical terms, and
- Providing ample white space so that pages look easy to read.

In spoken communication, in addition to using such techniques as the "teach-back method," limiting the use of medical jargon can also be helpful. The teach-back method is a health literacy tool that has been found useful to enhance communication. It is a mechanism that allows patients to put into their own words what was told to them. It provides an opportunity for the provider to correct information and ensure that the patient understands what is needed from them. The burden is on the clinician to ensure that they have communicated effectively.

PATIENT CARE COORDINATION

There are various definitions for care coordination. The Agency for Healthcare Research and Quality (8) describes care coordination as "the deliberate organization of patient care activities between two or more participants (including the patient) involved in a patient's care to facilitate the appropriate delivery of health care services. Organizing care involves the marshaling of personnel and other resources needed to carry out all required patient care activities. It is often managed by the exchange of information among participants responsible for different aspects of care." The role of the sleep health educator should be to act as an intermediary as needed and to help navigate patients through the fragmented health care quagmire.

PROVIDING PATIENT SELF-MANAGEMENT SUPPORT

Ultimately, the goal of sleep educator clinicians is to help patients along their therapeutic journey to achieve successful outcomes such as improving quality of life, reducing the burden of illness, and gaining control of their condition. This is typically accomplished by way of improved adherence to lifestyle modifications, treatment regimens, and routine follow-up care (9). Across all types of chronic conditions, behavioral intervention, education, and care coordination have been demonstrated to be effective ways to improve long-term adherence to therapy. Apps and other mobile health platforms enhance the opportunity for successful long-term management of chronic conditions such as insomnia, however, not all apps meet criteria for self-management. Alone, patient education has not been shown to be sufficient to make a difference (9-12).

Patient engagement, activation, and education are relevant to our goals. What is patient engagement and activation? These are actions that individuals must take to obtain the greatest benefit from the health care services available. Activation is a component of engagement and is defined as "understanding one's role in the care process and having the knowledge, skill, and confidence to manage one's health and health care" (13). These concepts are crucial in the patient's ability to perform successful self-management at home. For example, patients diagnosed with obstructive sleep apnea (OSA) are expected to acquire knowledge of their condition; learn how to obtain, use, and maintain a medical device in the home; and know when to seek help to overcome barriers. They should also understand when therapy is not working and when to contact their provider. This is not always easy, particularly if health literacy or social determinants of health impact one's ability to meet the objectives.

Another approach to self-management is to include a bed partner. A recent study found that motivation for continuous positive airway pressure (CPAP) use is enhanced when education and self-management support include the bed partner. The bed partner is often forgotten in terms of "needing to know" and also of their own sleep disruption, which can have a negative effect on a relationship (14).

One of the tools available for the sleep health educator, with additional training, is motivational enhancement (ME) or motivational interviewing (MI). One does not need an advanced degree to use these techniques, but they do require training. ME can be defined as follows *"The premise of the therapy is to honor the natural ambivalence that accompanies any change to behavior and to approach the patient in a thoughtful and empathetic manner that elicits critical thought to maximize behavior change"* (15), whereas MI "is a collaborative, goal-oriented style of communication with particular attention to the language of change. It is designed to strengthen personal motivation for and commitment to a specific goal by eliciting and exploring the person's own reasons for change within an atmosphere of acceptance and compassion." Both techniques have been demonstrated to be beneficial to patients with sleep apnea in several studies, resulting in better long-term adherence (16).

SUMMARY

The role of the sleep health educator addresses many aspects of the population: As an ambassador to the community at large, it is to provide clear, scientific information regarding sleep health in order to improve awareness and promote good sleep, while in a clinical setting, it is to provide education, counseling, and support. The sleep health educator, by working together with medical sleep specialists, dental sleep providers, and behavioral sleep practitioners, strives to shepherd the patient and, as appropriate, their families through the therapeutic journey.

REFERENCES

1. New England Journal of Medicine Catalyst. What is patient-centered care? Accessed February 8, 2025. https://catalyst.nejm.org/what-is-patient-centered-care/
2. Hilbert J, Yaggi HK. Patient-centered care in obstructive sleep apnea: a vision for the future. *Sleep Med Rev.* 2018;37:138-147. doi:10.1016/j.smrv.2017.02.004
3. Agency for Healthcare Research and Quality. Research in shared decision making. Accessed February 8, 2025. https://www.ahrq.gov/sdm/research/index.html
4. Barnason S, White-Williams C, Rossi LP, et al. Evidence for therapeutic patient education interventions to promote cardiovascular patient self-management: a scientific statement for healthcare professionals from the American Heart Association. *Circ Cardiovasc Qual Outcomes.* 2017;10:e000025. doi:10.1161/HCQ.0000000000000025
5. Centers for Disease Control and Prevention. What is health literacy? Accessed February 8, 2025. https://www.cdc.gov/health-literacy/php/about/index.html
6. National Center for Education Statistics. Adult numeracy in the United States. Accessed February 8, 2025. https://nces.ed.gov/pubs2020/2020025/index.asp
7. Lopez C, Kim B, Sacks K. Health literacy in the United States: enhancing assessments and reducing disparities. Milken Institute. Accessed February 8, 2025. https://milkeninstitute.org/sites/default/files/2022-05/Health_Literacy_United_States_Final_Report.pdf
8. Agency for Healthcare Research and Quality. Care coordination measures Atlas update: Chapter 2: what is care coordination? Last reviewed June 2014. Accessed February 8, 2025. https://www.ahrq.gov/ncepcr/care/coordination/atlas/chapter2.html
9. Grady PA, Gough LL. Self-management: a comprehensive approach to management of chronic conditions. *Am J Public Health.* 2014;104(8):e25-e31. doi:10.2105/AJPH.2014.302041
10. Reilly ED, Robinson SA, Petrakis BA, et al. Mobile app use for insomnia self-management: pilot findings on sleep outcomes in veterans. *Interact J Med Res.* 2019;8(3):e12408. doi:10.2196/12408
11. Pfammatter AF, Hughes BO, Tucker B, Whitmore H, Spring B, Tasali E. The development of a novel mHealth tool for obstructive sleep apnea: tracking continuous positive airway pressure adherence as a percentage of time in bed. *J Med Internet Res.* 2022;24(12):e39489. doi:10.2196/39489
12. Choi YK, Demiris G, Lin SY, et al. Smartphone applications to support sleep self-management: review and evaluation. *J Clin Sleep Med.* 2018;14(10):1783-1790. doi:10.5664/jcsm.7396
13. Hibbard JH. Patient activation and the use of information to support informed health decisions. *Patient Educ Couns.* 2017;100(1):5-7. doi:10.1016/j.pec.2016.07.006
14. Luyster FS, Dunbar-Jacob J, Aloia MS, et al. Patient and partner experiences with obstructive sleep apnea and CPAP treatment: a qualitative analysis. *Behav Sleep Med.* 2016;14(1):67-84. doi:10.1080/15402002.2014.946597
15. Bakker JP, Wang R, Weng J, et al. Motivational enhancement for increasing adherence to CPAP: a randomized controlled trial. *Chest.* 2016;150(2):337-345. doi:10.1016/j.chest.2016.03.019
16. Rudilla D, Landete P, Zamora E, Román A, Vergara I, Ancochea J. MEntA program based on motivational interview to improve adherence to treatment of obstructive sleep apnea with continuous positive airway pressure (CPAP): a randomized controlled trial. *Open Respir Arch.* 2021;3(2):100088. doi:10.1016/j.opresp.2021.100088

ADDITIONAL READING/RESOURCES

American Association of Sleep Technologists. AAST core competencies: sleep health educator. 2017. https://www.aastweb.org/Portals/0/Docs/Career/Sleep%20Health%20Educator%20New%20Template.pdf

Gossard T. Sleep Stewardship. *AMA J Ethics*. 2024;26(10):E747-E748. doi:10.1001/amajethics.2024.747

Institute for Healthcare Advancement. Always use teach-back. Accessed November 11, 2025. https://teachbacktraining.org/

Motivational Interviewing Network of Trainers. Understanding motivational interviewing. Accessed November 22, 2025. https://motivationalinterviewing.org

The Patient Revolution. Our mission. Accessed November 22, 2025. https://www.patientrevolution.org/

Chapter 54
Developing and Maintaining Therapeutic Compliance

MELINDA O. TRIMBLE

KEY CONCEPTS/LEARNING OBJECTIVES

The key concepts for this chapter include the importance of education before and after a sleep study is performed, providing various educational opportunities, and the development of a process for providing patient education within the sleep center. The technologist's communication with the patient, and often the family, is a significant factor in improving positive airway pressure (PAP) compliance. Patient outcomes are improved by providing materials to reinforce compliance, setting up mechanisms for providing answers to patient questions, and communicating with the patient's family about the importance of PAP compliance along with providing education related to cleaning procedures and identifying potential problems.

KEY TERMS

Assessment
Compliance
Education
Intervention
Obstructive sleep apnea (OSA)
Outcomes
Positive airway pressure (PAP)

In an era in which there is increasing knowledge, sophistication, and technologic advances to prevent and/or control many diseases, it is alarming that large numbers of individuals continue to be incapacitated, debilitated by, or to succumb to conditions for which effective treatments or measures of prevention are available (1). Sleep disorders are no exception. Although few would disagree that education is an important component of patient care, the majority of health professionals have received no formal training to prepare them for conducting patient education. Often, it is assumed that anyone with a health care background is qualified to educate a patient.

Sleep health education is an essential component of overall patient care. The provision of education for all patients with sleep disorders is critically important. In 2014, the Board of Registered Polysomnographic Technologists created a new certification examination for sleep health professionals as a benchmark to assure that minimum competency levels for patient education are achieved. The Certification in Clinical Sleep Health (CCSH) is offered to health care professionals seeking a nontechnical sleep certification. Certification is not required but is an important component of the evolving field of sleep health.

In the sleep center setting, patient education can be one of the most rewarding and gratifying things a sleep technologist experiences. Unfortunately, this is not true for many sleep technologists. A lack of time to educate patients properly and/or a lack of tools to educate patients can be especially frustrating. In this chapter, we will provide you with tools and methodologies that are useful to teaching regardless of the setting (ie, hospital, home, or in daily lives).

Establishing a standard of care for positive airway pressure (PAP) therapy and education is essential to enhance therapeutic compliance. Managing patients with sleep apnea with consistent, standardized instruction and information about sleep-disordered breathing is an achievable goal. This involves educating patients during the initial contact with a sleep technologist at the time of the sleep study, as well as during subsequent treatment and follow-up.

Patient education is best defined as the process that evolves from an exchange between health professionals and patients. As a sleep technologist, one has many opportunities to provide patient education. Education may occur on the phone, during a chance encounter, after an office visit, or at the time of a procedure; it may even occur in a more public setting such as a support group or an outreach effort. Although recognizing opportunities for education is important, effective education requires establishing a rapport with the patient and acquiring trust.

Consider the individual who is unable to tolerate daytime sleepiness, who has a nagging worry over near-miss auto accidents, or who is worried about the distress that snoring causes to the family. The patient decides to see a physician and is referred to a sleep center for a consultation with a sleep specialist. The opportunity to build a rapport begins the moment the patient calls to make the appointment. The rapport that is established between the patient and the sleep center staff will establish a foundation of trust and contribute to the successful resolution of the patient's sleep issues. If patients have confidence in the staff and the physician, they are more likely to listen, ask questions, and follow instruction. Likewise, when the patient is referred to the sleep center, that initial contact with the scheduling staff will have an impact on how the patient perceives the entire sleep study process. In addition, if the patient is approached with a genuine concern for their well-being, they are more likely to become engaged in the efforts to successfully resolve sleep problems.

One of the most common diagnoses established in a sleep center is obstructive sleep apnea (OSA). Although there are no cures for this disorder, there are treatments, and one of the most effective forms of treatment available to date is PAP. There are many reasons why an individual may have trouble acclimating to the PAP device, and understanding the patient's concerns will be key to a successful titration. Consider the pretitration situation where the patient declares, "I will not be able to sleep with that mask on my face or use that machine." The sleep technologist should understand from the patient's perspective the fundamental reason(s) why the patient believes the device would not be tolerated and work to address the issues. As an example, if the patient is claustrophobic, consideration may be given to acclimation sessions. If PAP has been determined to be the primary therapeutic intervention for the patient, all efforts should be exhausted before alternative therapeutic options (if any) are considered. Knowing how well the patient tolerates the device during the titration is imperative, especially if the patient is resistant to using the device at home. Review the titration detail carefully. Look for positive as well as negative responses throughout the titration segment of the polysomnogram. The information gleaned from a titration is critical to establishing the starting point, as well as goals for the patient's adherence to therapy.

Structuring the educational program for the patient

1. How does the patient learn?
2. What is needed for the patient to learn?
3. Are there any priorities to the educational process (i.e., medical urgency)?
4. Include success measurements.

Patient assessment

1. What is the patient's attitude toward learning?
2. What is the patient's ability to learn?
3. What are the patient's priorities?

Putting the plan into action

1. Help the patient put together a plan to meet the goals.
2. Help the patient determine a reasonable time frame to achieve the goals.
3. Allow the patient to have ownership of the process.
4. The patient needs to share the responsibility for his or her success.
5. Use all the patient support resources (e.g., family).
6. Make the plan manageable for the patient according to medical priorities.

Outcome assessment

1. Did the patient reach the set goals?
2. If goals were not reached:
   a. Identify reasons.
   b. Develop appropriate solutions.
   c. Alter plan accordingly to get the patient back on track.

Figure 54-1 Worksheet for setting patient goals.

PATIENT EVALUATION

Setting Goals

Patient education is an effective approach to improving PAP adherence. The plan for education should include specific goals and outcomes (Figure 54-1), as these will determine the focus for the patient's adherence. Work with the patient to establish these goals; ensure that they are realistic and appropriate for the patient's unique situation. The sleep technologist's role is to enable the patient to act on their own behalf by providing information, assisting with the practical problems of carrying out recommendations, increasing awareness of alternatives, and supporting the patient in the general acceptance and integration of new knowledge (1).

To begin, the sleep professional must get to know the patient. It will be necessary to consider the patient's emotions, their personal and professional environments, and beliefs and values. A thorough review of the patient's chart should provide fundamental information about the patient; however, information beyond this source will need to be obtained. Talking with the patient will be necessary to identify any concerns the patient has about their own health condition as well as determine the value the patient places on personal health. With this basic understanding, the sleep technologist can begin to develop an appropriate patient-centered therapy adherence plan.

An assessment of resources and a determination of professional and personal support available to the patient will be necessary for plan development. Coordination of educational efforts will minimize the risk of redundancy and contradictions and prevent components of the plan from being overlooked. It is necessary to determine who from the sleep center will be involved in the adherence plan and identify specific responsibilities for each person. Every staff member has the opportunity to be involved in the patient's compliance. If not involved directly, the staff member should at least be familiar with the structure of the adherence plan.

Family and friends can influence the success or failure of a patient's medical outcome. As the sleep technologist becomes involved with the patient's therapy, the role of the family becomes increasingly apparent. The sleep technologist will need to understand the family's general lifestyle. A series of questions such as "Who talks to whom?" and "How does the family interact with each other?" will be important to assess the dynamics and the appropriateness of the family's involvement. If there are family or friends available for support and if it is appropriate that they be involved in the patient's therapy, permission to involve them will need to be obtained from the patient. The impact of OSA extends beyond the individual and may have significant effects on the family. As such, the family should be included in the education process whenever possible to ensure the best outcome for the patient.

More than 70 sleep disorders have been classified in the *International Classification of Sleep Disorders*—Third Edition (*ICSD*-3), with varying options for treatment. Whether the therapy is behavioral, psychological, pharmacologic, or surgical, education is a key component of the patient's success in improving the quality of life. For some, it may be a fairly expeditious process with relatively few steps; for others, it will be a lengthy process, and the steps will be minute and numerous. Understanding the patient, coordinating resources, and assessing their response to the prescribed therapy will be vital to structuring realistic achievable goals toward adherence to therapy.

Health Literacy

The patient's health literacy level is not always reflective of their educational level. Most of the health care information that is provided to patients is written at a high school level, as the average Medicare age patient reads at a sixth-grade level (2). A 1997 study stated that even college-educated individuals had difficulty using medical information (3). Many patients state that they feel inept and incapable of asking their health care provider questions or requesting clarification of information that has been provided (4).

Learning Styles

There are three types of learning styles: visual, tactile, and auditory (5). It is vital that the patient educator understand the patient's style in order to have successful outcomes. Approximately 55% of the general population are visual learners. Seeing information helps to aid the visual learner in processing and retaining information. The second most common learning style is tactile, also referred to as kinesthetic, and 30% of the population prefer that style of learning. They are doers or hands-on learners. Verbal and auditory learning is the third style, and 15% of the population prefer this method of learning. This type of learner needs to hear or have the information read aloud to best process the information (6). Understanding the patients' learning style and providing information based on their delivery needs will be helpful to the patients' educational experience. Using a mixed approach with multiple learning styles will ensure that the patient's personal preferences are included in the educational process.

Learning Needs

No matter how dire the situation, patient compliance is always a choice. It is a very important concept for the sleep technologist to understand in the process of patient education, and it is critical to recognize what is necessary for patients to learn and understand about their sleep disorder and the prescribed therapy to achieve long-term adherence.

Learning begins when the patient starts to ask questions and, conversely, when the patient does not have answers to the questions being asked by the health care professional. Initially, the patient will need to be made aware of the sleep disorder, its prognosis, possible treatment options, and consequences of noncompliance. Also, it will be helpful for the patient to understand who participates in the education plan and the roles and responsibilities of each individual. It should be clearly communicated that the health care professionals involved in this treatment compliance plan work on behalf of the patient and want to establish a partnership to ensure adherence and improve the patient's quality of life.

Participants in such a plan may include, but are not limited to, the

- patient
- durable medical equipment (DME) company staff
- sleep technologist
- clinical sleep specialist
- family
- primary care physician (PCP)
- payer (insurance company)
- sleep disorders center staff
- support group

Establishing a coordinated partnership with the patient is a group effort. Effective communication needs to be developed collectively among the participants as well as individually with the patient. The patient should realize that even with complete adherence, circumstances might develop that necessitate assistance or direction. A change in health status, a trip out of the country, or equipment problems will be issues that can be readily addressed by the sleep professional(s) concerned.

Learning Priorities

With most medical conditions, the prognosis generally dictates the path and the priorities for learning. The spectrum of sleep disorders is extremely broad, and consequences range from the merely troublesome day or two of mild jet lag to the tragic loss of life when someone falls asleep at the wheel of an automobile (7).

Health and safety risks associated with the patient's condition will be a priority in the learning process. For the sleep patient, this may involve the PCP in the assessment of health and the sleep specialist to evaluate the patient's complaints and symptoms. If an individual does not understand or comprehend the significance of the health condition, it will be difficult to convince that individual to proceed with diagnostic testing or to comply with treatment recommendations. Therefore, it is important that the patient understands why a PAP machine has been prescribed and what the therapy will involve.

Sleep professionals need to determine what type of information is appropriate for the patient, as well as what type of changes the patient will need to make in everyday life. The goal of the adherence plan should be to assist the patient in learning the skills and knowledge necessary to develop behaviors that will maximize the prospects of a positive health outcome.

Learning Assessment

Although an adherence plan involves many sleep professionals, one of the most influential roles is that of the sleep technologist responsible for the PAP titration. The sleep technologist has a very narrow window of opportunity to introduce the patient to PAP, titrate to an optimum therapeutic pressure, and influence the patient's willingness to consider PAP as a treatment option. This time constraint makes the interaction between the sleep technologist and the patient all the more essential to achieving long-term compliance.

Acquiring specific information as part of an assessment will maximize the opportunity for a successful titration and increase the probability of compliance. An appropriate assessment will provide the sleep technologist with insight into the patient's motivation, which is necessary before they can communicate effectively with the patient (Table 54-1). There are certain factors that influence a patient's motivation and how the patient responds to sleep testing and treatment; these factors may be classified as individual, social, and environmental.

Table 54-1 Assessment Questions for Positive Airway Pressure as a Therapeutic Intervention: Potentially Helpful Questions When Assessing the Patient With Sleep Apnea

Sample Questions	Helpful Information for Technologist
What can you tell me about your condition?	Helps indicate the patient's basic knowledge and level of understanding about the purpose of the overnight study and the potential treatment of the condition
Do you have help or support at home?	A lack of family support may reduce the patient's ability to achieve their goals or their potential for PAP adherence.
Do you think you can use the PAP device?	Helps assess the patient's knowledge level, attitude, and willingness to improve their condition
How did you do with the mask?	Helps identify potential problems with the interface device. It is important to work through these types of problems as early as possible to improve the chances of success.
Do you need help choosing a home care company?	Most patients will not have worked with a home care company. Helps the patient to understand home care service process in advance to avoid frustration later
Do you have questions about your treatment plan?	Allows the patient the opportunity to ask questions and gives the technologist information about the patient's attitude and comprehension of the information and treatment plan that has been recommended
What are your expectations?	Helps the patient set realistic goals

PAP, positive airway pressure.

Individual Factors: Determine the Patient's Learning Potential

Determining the knowledge level of the patient is part of the patient's assessment and critical to education and the learning process. Generally, a sleep technologist can identify an individual's level of knowledge through observation and conversation. If the patient's level of knowledge is unknown, it will be difficult for the sleep technologist to know if the patient understands the health condition, has sufficient knowledge to assume responsibility for treatment, or understands the consequences of not following the treatment recommendations. In addition to knowledge, skill level and attitude contribute to an individual's ability to learn. The sleep technologist needs to ascertain whether or not the patient has the appropriate skill level to adhere to the treatment regimen. If not, the sleep technologist may need to adjust or modify the teaching techniques used to enable the patient to understand the concepts needed to use the treatment device.

Social and Environmental Factors: Determine if These Factors Facilitate or Hinder Medical Care

Social factors such as family, religious beliefs, cultural values, and employers have the potential to facilitate or hinder patients from reaching their desired goals. As an example, a patient returned for a follow-up to the sleep center and during the appointment was asked if he had been using his continuous positive airway pressure (CPAP) machine. He stated that he had not, and upon further questioning, it was discovered that the reason he was not using it was that the noise bothered his wife. With this knowledge, the sleep technologist can start helping the patient by determining if the noise issue involves the mask or the device and suggest changing to a different mask or moving the device further away from the bed.

It is vital for the sleep technologist to understand the reaction of family members to the patient's condition and treatment. If family members appear hesitant or apprehensive about learning the skills needed to assist with the patient's care at home, then the success of the treatment may be compromised. Some family members may not be responsive or may not wish to play an active role.

Issues such as these can be identified only after the sleep technologist has had the opportunity to observe and communicate with the family. If issues are identified, support and guidance should be provided to assist the family in creating solutions. The sleep technologist must understand the significant impact that social factors (eg, family) may have on the desired goals and create an educational plan according to the patient's priorities.

The impact of environmental factors such as geographic location, employer and job requirements, work and social schedule, and living arrangements should also be considered. The sleep technologist will need to understand the availability of resources to the patient. Does the patient's work schedule hinder his ability to arrange follow-up appointments? Is transportation available to allow for participation with a support group? Issues such as these will need to be considered because the sleep technologist will need to work with the patient to look at solutions that will help establish and meet treatment goals.

Understanding the patient's priorities will allow the sleep technologist to determine which factors may facilitate the patient's progress and which factors may hinder it.

EDUCATIONAL OPPORTUNITIES

Education should start at the initial visit. The sleep technologist and the board-certified sleep specialist should codevelop the educational process used within the sleep center. This will ensure a consistent educational process. Patient education should be a multitiered process, consisting of pretest, test, posttest, and PAP setup instruction and information.

Pretest

When possible, the patient should have the opportunity to visit the sleep center before the sleep study. This offers the patient the opportunity to become familiar with the facility and the test process and minimizes any apprehension about sleeping in an unfamiliar environment. Written instructions should be provided before the study to ensure that the patient is appropriately prepared and that the information being recorded will be valid. Basic instructions are listed in Table 54-2.

Table 54-2 Pretest Instructions
• Arrival and departure time
• Facility policies regarding guests
• Comfortable and appropriate bed clothing
• Personal toiletry items
• Items to enhance the patient's comfort (eg, pillow)
• Bring scheduled medications
• List of medications taken in the past week
• Instruct not to nap on the day of the study
• Abstain from caffeine after 12 noon

The admission process as well as the testing process should be fully explained to the patient. While the patient is at the sleep center, there is an opportunity for them to experience the PAP device. This helps acclimate the patient to the device in case it is necessary to apply PAP during the study. The patient can also be introduced to a PAP interface to assure proper fit before titration, and notes can be made in the patient's chart to notify the night sleep technologist of any potential problems the patient may have acclimating to the device. If problems arise, the sleep technologist should make every effort to work through the issues before the test. Potential issues may include hard-to-fit faces, claustrophobia, nasal obstruction, and edentulous mouths.

This is the patient's opportunity to ask any questions before testing and the sleep technologist's opportunity to address any concerns. The sleep technologist should make the most of this time to ensure that the patient is comfortable with the facility and the procedure.

Test Night

When the patient arrives on the night of the study, the sleep technologist should orient and/or reorient the patient to the facility, the procedure, the hookup, and the PAP titration if applicable. In many instances, the patient will not have had a pretest visit to the sleep center, and the sleep technologist will be the sole educator for the patient before testing. The sleep technologist should always ensure that the patient understands the procedure(s) being performed. The patient should have ample opportunity to ask questions or express concerns. It is particularly important to fit the patient with a mask and acclimate them to the PAP therapy pretest if there is a possibility for a split-night study.

Posttest

Educating patients after a sleep study can sometimes present a challenge. The patient may become overwhelmed by information about a new diagnosis, treatment options, DME provider selection, insurance questions, and overall lifestyle changes. To alleviate information overload, it is helpful for patients to leave the sleep center with written materials. It is important to recognize and respect a patient's hesitancy toward therapy. The more positive, informative, and helpful the educator is with the instruction, the more receptive the patient will be to accept therapy, initially and in the future. If the patient is unable to remain in the sleep center for poststudy education, it is imperative that the sleep technologist contact the patient for follow-up and/or mail educational materials to the patient's home. Patients who do not receive poststudy information are at a disadvantage in regard to achieving success with PAP therapy. The sleep technologist should follow the sleep center's policy on what information is to be provided to the patient following the use of PAP therapy during the sleep study.

Durable Medical Equipment Setup

The peak of most patients' acceptance and enthusiasm for PAP therapy occurs immediately after a successful titration or physician visit. Capitalizing on this enthusiasm promotes improved adherence to therapy and ongoing success. Patient participation in selecting the DME provider and equipment may enhance adherence through shared ownership of the choices, although in some cases, sleep center protocols, location, and insurance guidelines may dictate the DME selection process. Patients should receive written information with the name of the DME provider and a contact number where they may call for questions, concerns, or delivery schedules. A smooth flow of information among the sleep center, DME provider, and patient will reduce delays in the initiation of therapy.

Acclimating to PAP and the mask interface may be enhanced by desensitization techniques to minimize pressure discomfort, claustrophobia, and aversion to the mask. For these reasons, it is especially important to be understanding and reassuring. If the patient is hastily fitted and as a result gets panicky, they may be reluctant to try PAP at a later date. For many patients, there is a negative connotation or stigma of "failing a PAP trial" during a sleep study. This negativity should be countered with positive feedback from the sleep technologist when the comments are made. Offer the patient reassurance and praise for PAP attempts and remind them that many patients require additional time for adjustment to PAP.

Minimizing discomfort and hastening adaptation to the mask pressure can be approached in various ways. Desensitization or acclimation techniques are beneficial during initial mask fitting before a split-night or titration study (Table 54-3). The goal of these techniques is to reduce the failure of adaptation to PAP.

TREATMENT REGIMEN

It is the sleep technologist's responsibility to advise the patient that a follow-up appointment with the referring physician is necessary to receive study results. The patient should always have the opportunity to review the sleep study with the sleep physician. This may or may not be done in the sleep center setting. If the patient was placed on a PAP device, the physician may also request the patient to have a follow-up visit with the sleep technologist at the sleep center to work through any problems the patient may be having with PAP therapy. This is an opportunity for the technologist to review the patient's adherence to therapy and explore any issues

Table 54-3 Desensitization and Acclimation Strategies

Complaint	Solution
I cannot breathe.	Increase the pressure.
I cannot exhale.	Start with a very low pressure or ramp with the patient in an upright position. Instruct the patient to exhale into the mask as soon as they feel the pressure and then slowly inhale through their nose.
It is smothering me. . .	Start with a very low pressure or ramp with the patient in an upright position. Instruct the patient to exhale into the mask as soon as they feel the pressure and then slowly inhale through their nose.
The pressure is too high. . .	Reduce to a lower pressure or ramp.
I cannot stand anything against my face. . .	Work with alternate interface styles to obtain a mask that will aid in patient comfort. Do not apply headgear or air pressure until the patient is comfortable. With the patient in an upright position, instruct them to hold the mask against the face and practice breathing. While performing this exercise, provide a distraction (eg, television) to minimize the patient's focus on the mask. Have the patient perform this exercise at home. Schedule additional acclimation sessions as necessary.
The mask is uncomfortable. . .	Verify mask fit. Readjust headgear. Replace mask as necessary.

the patient may be having with the interface and PAP device. Some sleep centers establish PAP clinics. PAP clinics provide the patient with an opportunity to work one-on-one with the sleep technologist to assure adherence as well as an avenue to express concerns and work through problems with the device. A follow-up visit after the sleep study is extremely beneficial to adherence and patient success with therapy.

Adherence

The most frequently used definition of adequate adherence to therapy (previously designated as compliance) was first proposed in 1993 in one of the earliest studies with objective measurement of CPAP use (8). In this study, the authors defined a minimal use criterion (>4 hours per night) and an optimal use criterion (>7 hours per night) and found that CPAP use met minimal criteria on about 50% of nights and optimal criteria on about 20% of nights. By consensus of the authors, regular users were those who used CPAP at least 4 hours per day on at least 70% of nights; 46% of patients met this criterion. Thus, the most frequently used definition of adherence is use for a minimum of 4 hours per night, 5 to 7 nights per week. This definition has been adopted by the Centers for Medicare and Medicaid Services as the minimum objective adherence/compliance a patient must demonstrate for continued reimbursement for PAP therapy (9). PAP adherence is a long-term, comprehensive process. It is important for the patient to learn as much as possible about their condition to successfully and proactively manage it.

Follow-Up Telephone Calls

Follow-up telephone calls to a patient beginning PAP therapy can enhance adherence. The 24- to 72-hour period after initiation of PAP therapy is the most critical time to be in contact with the patient. Some patients may be tired, frustrated, hesitant, or even angry about their struggles with PAP therapy. Others may feel fully rested and even be ecstatic about their therapy. In either situation, a follow-up call should be instructional, helpful, and full of encouragement. Follow-up calls should be made at intervals of approximately 1 to 2 days, 1 week, 2 weeks, 6 weeks, 6 months, and yearly. During the call, the patient should be asked about hours of usage, problems with the mask or pressure, equipment cleaning, nasal problems, and any continued presence of snoring or excessive daytime sleepiness. Sometimes, patients are hesitant to discuss certain issues, such as bed partner complaints or embarrassment about using the equipment. Expressing empathy, respect, and support builds positive relationships with patients that facilitate education. It is helpful to be understanding and empathetic and to listen to all the patient's concerns and problems at the beginning of the phone call and then give suggestions and solutions to them. Some patients need and want lots of help, whereas others want only the bare necessities. It takes an intuitive listener and educator to be able to fulfill the needs of all types of patients. Ultimately, better patient communication can increase both patient and clinician satisfaction, improve efficiency, enhance adherence to therapy, and improve patient health outcomes.

Personal Empowerment

Quality of life is contingent on a patient's willingness to take responsibility for positive choices for better health and living. Patients need to believe in their ability to achieve and maintain effective therapy. Goal setting gives patients an incentive to aim for, increasing adherence on a nightly basis and over the long term. Personal empowerment aids in mastering the challenges of PAP therapy acceptance. Turning struggles and conflicts into learning opportunities is a way of providing positive feedback to the patient. It is important to encourage patients to become their own advocates for promoting good health, achieving their goals, and maximizing adherence to therapy.

Technology

Modern technology has provided various tools and options that may enhance adherence and increase breathing comfort for patients on PAP therapy. These may be used as augmentation measures for an adherent patient or to identify and assist a nonadherent patient to become adherent. PAP manufacturers have developed technology that provides relief on exhalation, making PAP therapy more comfortable.

Occasionally, there are patients who cannot tolerate PAP therapy, even when enhanced by this technology. When all avenues with standard PAP therapy have been exhausted, a physician-ordered bilevel positive airway pressure (BPAP) trial could be attempted. Patients who qualify for BPAP treatment are those who are at high surgical risk, have multiple medical problems in addition to sleep apnea, or require unusually high PAP levels to overcome their apnea. Rescue/trial BPAP is a final attempt to achieve successful therapy. The BPAP settings may be determined from the patient's current CPAP or a separate BPAP titration study.

In clinical practice, it is important to measure, assist, track, and enhance adherence. Various manufacturers have created tools that assist patients, sleep technologists, physicians, and home health care providers with feedback or efficacy data to determine effective therapy and to measure outcomes. Compliance data tracking can be very useful in measuring PAP adherence. Judging one's sleep time is always subjective and generally inaccurate. Patients tend to either underestimate or overestimate the amount of time they spend using PAP therapy. A data tracking system provides accurate information when addressing an adherence issue. When tracking adherence, it is important to first inform patients about the capabilities of the device and then instruct them on how to use it for their situation.

Patients can react negatively to data tracking if they perceive it as negative feedback from the clinician. An example is the patient who feels that they are using the PAP device all night, every night. Then, on reviewing the data download, the usage is recorded as poor. Perhaps the patient is unknowingly removing the PAP mask early in the night, believing it is near morning. If adherence feedback is perceived as a reprimand or therapy failure, usage may actually reduce. Consequently, care should be taken not to discourage the patient but to help solve the problem and offer a solution. In contrast, some patients believe that they have not been using their machine as much as expected, although the data download confirms adequate use. In these cases, the patients can be reassured about their accomplishments and praised for their efforts.

Most PAP machines now have "true" adherence monitors that measure the actual time during which patients are breathing with the device in place. Data storage and retrieval technology that tracks usage hours, pressure, mask leak, and apnea-hypopnea index is available from most PAP system manufacturers. Detailed reports can be generated to share information with the patient's health care team.

Some devices provide the ability for the patient to track usage when the feature is enabled. Information for monitoring adherence is now available via wireless modules used within PAP devices. The wireless module transmits therapy data from the device to a centralized server for access by the sleep professional through the Internet and provides the sleep professional with timely, objective data for assessing the patient's adherence to therapy.

Questionnaires

Questionnaires and rating scales can be useful for measuring a patient's transition from diagnosis to treatment and for tracking long-term results. Baseline information should be collected before the initial sleep study. Subsequent questionnaires and rating scales can then be used during follow-up visits to determine how much symptomatic improvement the patient is experiencing.

The Functional Outcomes of Sleep Questionnaire (FOSQ) is a clinically validated, self-reporting measurement developed by Terri Weaver designed to assess the improvement of excessive sleepiness on the basis of multiple activities of daily living. This 30-item questionnaire, intended specifically for people with sleep disorders, allows sleep professionals to follow improvements in the patient's quality of life after treatment.

The Epworth Sleepiness Scale (ESS) is a very simple, self-administered questionnaire, used to assess a patient's own perception of sleepiness. The ESS was developed by Murray Johns, MD, from the Epworth Hospital in Melbourne, Australia. This questionnaire helps sleep professionals to recognize and measure excessive daytime sleepiness. Again, it is preferred that the ESS be completed before a sleep study and then repeated at subsequent clinical visits to measure improvement.

Education/Support Meetings

People with sleep disorders often report being labeled as lazy, depressed, or even as hypochondriacs. They are offered little sympathy about their tiredness. Many have been to doctors and complained of being tired "for years" to no avail. Having a diagnosis and a way to treat their disorder can be very empowering for them. Support groups can alleviate the feeling of isolation and provide emotional support and understanding between patients and their families. This also opens the door for discussion and validation of their treatment with bed partners and other family members. Promoting communication and positive support, a sleep technologist can bridge the gap between patients and their families.

Assisting patients to integrate into the network of PAP education and support groups is suggested. Keeping in contact with sleep professionals and networking with other PAP users can help patients maintain their long-term commitment to treatment. One such group is the A.W.A.K.E. (alert, well, and keeping energetic) network developed by Lucy Seger, RPSGT.

Positive Airway Pressure Information Line

A dedicated toll-free telephone information line for patients with PAP questions can be a very helpful tool. First and foremost, the facility gives patients a lifeline to PAP educators and reassurance that help is available to them with their therapy. Knowing that there are professionals staffing the phone line is therapeutic in itself. Sometimes, a patient will have questions; at other times simple reassurance or a pat on the back may be all that is needed. The phone line may also minimize calls to the sleep center, physician's office, and the medical equipment provider.

Messages should be checked frequently and calls returned in a timely manner, because patients who need help will get discouraged after a short time and adherence will reduce. Providing a toll-free number gives the traveling patient, or the patient who lives elsewhere during a part of the year, a familiar resource to access.

Behavioral Change and Sleep Hygiene

Behavioral change is an important part of beginning any new therapy. Beginning PAP therapy can force a patient to change a treasured or habitual lifestyle and may be perceived as an intrusion on bedtime and morning routines. Some of the required changes include washing the mask and humidifier in the morning, filling the humidifier chamber with distilled water, and washing their face before bed to remove makeup and oils from the skin to promote a good mask seal. Patients may also have to adjust to the emotional aspect of using a medical device such as a PAP machine in their home. These changes, although minor, may seem insurmountable to some patients. The patient should be reminded that these additional changes to their daily/nightly routine will help reduce skin irritation and prevent premature breakdown of the mask and equipment.

Patients should also be informed of the risks of using alcohol, tobacco, and sleeping pills before bedtime. These may increase upper airway instability during sleep and should be avoided. Finally, encouraging weight loss is important to promote better health and to possibly reduce the necessary PAP level. In some cases, considerable weight loss may even eliminate the need for PAP therapy. A repeat sleep study should be recommended after considerable weight loss, such as from bariatric surgery or use of a prescription weight-loss drug. Change is difficult for most people. However, implementing good sleep hygiene techniques along with PAP therapy can improve a patient's and bed partner's sleep. Most compliant patients will agree that the benefits of PAP therapy outweigh its inconveniences.

Techniques for promoting good sleep:

- Maintain a regular sleep schedule.
- Implement a bedtime routine.
- Use your bedroom for sleep and intimacy only.
- Go to bed only when drowsy.
- If you are unable to fall asleep, leave the bedroom and do something quiet in another room.
- Avoid clock watching.
- Perform a repetitious activity or something to distract your mind.
- Avoid caffeine 2 to 4 hours before bedtime.
- Avoid nicotine close to bedtime.
- Avoid alcohol 2 to 4 hours before bedtime.
- Avoid large meals before bedtime.
- Avoid strenuous exercise 4 or more hours before bedtime.
- Limit napping during the day, and do not nap after 3 PM.
- Minimize light, noise, television, and radio use in the bedroom.

Potential Problems, Setbacks, and Solutions

Initial Mask Fit

The initial mask fit for a patient is one of the most important tasks a technologist will undertake. Remaining cheerful and enthusiastic helps the initial mask fit begin on a positive note. It is imperative that a poor fit not dampen the patient's enthusiasm to using PAP at a later date.

Problem

The patient's mask does not fit well. It may leak, cause sore spots, or hurt the face.

Solution
- Adjust mask/interface straps, forehead pads, or nasal cushions.
- Do not overtighten the mask.
- Refit with a different mask or nasal pillow.
- Refit mask to a different size.
- If all else fails, a full-face mask trial may be attempted. Because of safety issues (possible aspiration) and potential leak problems, a full-face mask should be used only as a last resort, with physician approval.

Adapting to Pressure Complaints

Problem
The patient complains of too much air, too high a pressure, difficulty exhaling, or of the air coming too fast.

Solution
- Verify correct PAP setting using a manometer (significant discrepancies may be present among various PAP equipment pressure readouts).
- Instruct the patient to exhale while initially applying mask to face.
- Initiate relaxation skills and desensitization techniques.
- Use ramp or delay features.
- Increase ramp or delay time.
- Add cool or heated humidifier (this requires a written prescription from the patient's physician).
- Use pressure relief technology to enhance patient comfort.
- Consider an ENT (ear, nose, and throat) consultation to check for possible nasal obstruction. (This option would be determined by the patient's physician.)

Claustrophobia

Problem
The patient complains of being unable to breathe, unable to exhale, or of having a sense of suffocation.

Solution
- Ask the patient to hold the mask to face without air pressure while they sit on the edge of the bed and provide distractions such as television, music, or conversation.
- Start with a very low pressure or ramp.
- Instruct the patient to exhale into the mask as soon as they feel the pressure and then slowly inhale through the nose.
- Try alternate mask styles to aid in patient comfort.
- Apply the headgear once the patient is comfortable.
- Instruct the patient to lie down with the mask on.
- Instruct the patient to gradually increase usage time with each attempt.

Noise Complaints

Problem
The machine is too loud!

Solution
- Recommend that the patient and/or bed partner wear earplugs.
- Use a white noise machine (a device that produces continuous background sounds, such as ocean waves).

Air Hunger Complaints

Problem
The patient states that they cannot get enough air or feel as if they are suffocating.

Solution
- Check for mask/interface leak.
- If using a ramp feature, increase the starting pressure.
- Mouth opening with PAP while awake does not necessarily indicate a need for a chin strap—this is necessary only when mouth opening occurs during sleep.
- If using an autoPAP machine, increase the starting pressure (this requires verbal or written approval from the patient's physician).
- Consider an ENT consultation for surgical options (as determined by the patient's physician).

Removing Positive Airway Pressure Mask Unknowingly During Sleep

Problem
The patient wakes up to find the mask off and does not remember removing it.

Solution
- Check the efficacy data (if available) to determine actual PAP usage.
- Review desensitization techniques to make sure the patient is comfortable with wearing the mask.
- Check for proper mask fit (for the same reason noted previously).
- Ask the patient if they suffer from nasal congestion. This could be a possible cause of mask removal and should be addressed with the patient's physician.
- Avoid using a chin strap, because it is unlikely to prevent the patient from removing the mask.
- Activate the disconnect alarm (if available).
- Encourage the patient to keep trying. Sometimes, the mask is removed inadvertently during deep sleep. As the patient's sleep patterns normalize and the patient becomes accustomed to the treatment, the problem may resolve on its own.
- Avoid using a full-face mask, because using a full-face mask does not preclude the patient from

removing it during sleep. Full-face masks are more susceptible to leaks and may pose a potential aspiration hazard.

Mask Leak

Problem

Air leakage around the mask interface

Solution

- Make sure the patient is not overtightening the mask.
- Adjust mask/interface straps, forehead pads, or nasal cushions for proper fit.
- Refit to a different mask or nasal pillows.
- Refit mask to a different size.
- Apply mask to the face while air is blowing through the circuit to help seal the mask on contact.

Mouth Breathing

Mouth opening during sleep may cause significant pressure drops, leading to a resumption of obstructive breathing, as well as mouth dryness and discomfort. Instruct the patient to try to keep the mouth closed when applying the PAP mask. If the PAP level is properly set for the patient, in most cases, the mouth will remain closed during sleep. A common cause of mouth breathing may be unresolved nasal congestion or obstruction. Problems with mouth breathing may also be seen in older patients, in patients who wear dentures, and in those with a history of stroke. Mouth breathing may also be an indication of inadequate titration, with pressures set either too high or too low.

Strategies to combat mouth breathing during sleep include the following:

- Verifying correct PAP level using a manometer.
- Using a heated humidifier (to reduce nasal congestion).
- Increasing the temperature of the humidifier.
- Using a chin strap.
- Using a pressure relief technology to reduce pressure upon exhalation.
- Using a full-face mask (this should be used only as a last resort, with physician approval).
- Addressing any unresolved problems (such as nasal obstruction) with the patient's physician.

Eye Discomfort

Problem

The patient reports that their eyes feel dry, air is blowing into the eyes, or the eyes are bloodshot.

Solution

- Make sure the patient is not overtightening the mask.
- Adjust mask/interface, forehead pads, or nasal cushions.
- Refit to a different mask or nasal pillow.
- Refit mask and change to a different size.
- Advise the patient to consult the physician if the problem remains unresolved.

Skin Irritation

Problem

The patient develops an unremitting rash, pressure sore, or skin irritation at the mask contact points.

Solution

- Make sure the patient is not overtightening the mask.
- Check for proper mask fit.
- Refit to a different mask or nasal pillow.
- Review proper mask cleaning techniques with the patient.
- Remind the patient to clean the mask daily.
- Advise the patient to consult the physician about any unresolved skin problems.

Complaints of Feeling Tired/Fatigued

Problem

The patient reports using the PAP on a regular basis but continues to complain of sleepiness or fatigue.

Solution

- Reassess the patient's sleep-wake habits to make sure they have adequate sleep time.
- Ask if the patient has been snoring on PAP.
- Check for proper mask fit and the condition of the mask to make sure it is not leaking.
- Reassess the patient's sleep hygiene.
- Reassess PAP usage during the entire night.
- Evaluate possible environmental factors such as noise.
- Ask about bed partner or pet disturbances in the bedroom.
- Ask if the patient is taking naps during the day.
- Ask about leg movements or bruxism.
- Inquire if the patient is using alcohol before bed.
- Ask about mouth opening during the night and/or a very dry mouth.
- Advise the patient to consult the physician if the problem is unresolved.

Communication With Family Members

Although PAP therapy mostly affects the patient, it can also have a great impact on other family members. Patients and their families may lack open communication. Having the patient and family members learn together about sleep-disordered breathing and PAP therapy can help bridge that communication gap. If a patient or family member makes negative comments about sleep-disordered breathing or PAP therapy, it is important to acknowledge the comment and then to counter the negativity by noting a positive benefit that PAP therapy has brought to that patient and family. Bringing the focus back to a positive note should be a recurring theme. Never underestimate the power of encouragement from family members. Remember, often it is a family member or bed partner who encouraged the patient to seek medical attention in the first place. Family and bed partner support is just as important after diagnosis as before. Patients with families who are supportive and aware of the benefits of PAP therapy often use their PAP more consistently.

Bed Partners

Adjustment periods are not exclusive to the PAP patient. The patient's entire household will need time to adjust to PAP therapy, bed partners more so than other family members. Bed partners, as well as patients, may feel therapy is an intrusion on a cherished bedtime routine. Also, bed partners may need time to adjust to a medical device in the bedroom. A common complaint from bed partners is noise from the device. This noise is produced either by the blower or by the air exchange through the mask ventilation port. The noise is actually very minimal, but to a sensitive sleeper, or a bed partner who is just returning to the bedroom, it may seem loud. A good solution for noise intrusion is the use of earplugs or of a white noise machine. In other cases, the bed partner may actually complain that the patient is now too quiet without the familiar sound of snoring (although this is unusual, most bed partners welcome the change from loud, obnoxious snoring). Another common complaint is of air blowing toward the bed partner from the exhalation port. Using a blanket or a pillow as a barrier between the patient and the bed partner can help deflect the flow of air. Occasionally, there is a complaint that the machine indicator light is too luminous in the bedroom. This light can disturb the patient and the bed partner. On some PAP machines, the light can be turned off; on others, the light remains on for a short time and then turns off automatically. If the light does not turn off automatically, then covering the light with electrical tape will eliminate the brightness. Always caution patients not to cover the entire PAP unit because that would interfere with its function and present a potential hazard.

When patients are better rested and the routine of PAP therapy has been established, sometimes there is a reversal of complaints. Now it is the patient who complains about the bed partner's snoring or movements. The dynamics between a patient and a bed partner can fluctuate throughout this transition period.

Equipment Cleaning

Daily

- Emphasize daily mask cleaning.
- Caution the patient about the risks of skin irritation or infection due to poor mask fit or from using a dirty mask.
- Clean the mask and tubing as per the manufacturer's directions.
- Clean the mask in the morning with warm, mild soapy water; rinse well; and allow to air-dry.
- Do not use chemicals, soaps with perfume-like smells, or antibacterial soaps that can cause a breakdown of the mask cushions.
- Disinfect the mask and tubing with water and white vinegar mixture as per the manufacturer's directions.

Monthly

- Clean filters more frequently if soiled or if pets sleep in the bedroom.
- Clean nondisposable filters with warm mild soapy water, rinse well, and allow to air-dry.
- Discard and replace paper filters monthly.

Humidifiers

- Replace the distilled water daily.
- Clean in the morning with warm, mild, soapy water, rinse well, and allow to air-dry all day.
- Do not use chemicals or soaps with perfume-like smells.
- Clean and disinfect the humidifier with water and white vinegar mixture as per the manufacturer's directions.
- Use only distilled water in the humidifier. (Do not use tap water in the humidifier because it will result in mineral buildup in the water chamber.)

General Considerations

Travel

Travel requires advanced planning and leaving home well rested for the PAP patient. Optimal driving time is during the hours when alertness is at its peak. PAP patients are advised to avoid alcohol and sedating medications while traveling. Driving with a companion can help both the patient and the companion keep each other awake. It is recommended that patients carry their PAP equipment along with them on their trip. Even after one night without wearing PAP, patients may feel tired and experience a return of symptoms and the risks associated with untreated sleep-disordered breathing. These risks, combined with sleepiness, may make a vacation or business trip unpleasant and potentially hazardous. PAP equipment should be packed in the passenger compartment to minimize temperature extremes. The PAP travel bag should include a heavy-duty extension cord for hard-to-reach outlets and an extra fuse if specific PAP equipment requires it. Voltage converters and wall receptacle adapters are available for traveling internationally. Additionally, an external power source and supplies will need to be packed if traveling where electricity is not available.

A PAP machine is a medical device and usually comes with its own travel or carrying bag. To make sure the PAP equipment does not become lost or damaged, it is advisable to carry it on a plane; never check it as baggage. The limit of one carry-on bag for airline travel does not usually apply to medical supplies or equipment. It is recommended to separately pack the equipment manual and a copy of the prescription and/or letter of medical necessity from the physician. This information will help travelers if the PAP device is lost or broken and will assist them at airport checkpoints and customs.

Because of limited packing space, many patients may not be able to bring a humidifier while traveling. When using a humidifier while traveling, it is important to either carry distilled water to the destination or obtain distilled water on arrival. A temporary alternative when the humidifier is not available is an over-the-counter normal saline nasal spray or gel. Also, a water-soluble gel to help with nasal dryness can be used; both of these products are available without a prescription.

When patients travel internationally, it is important that they learn about the voltage output and types of wall receptacles used in the countries they plan to visit. Most PAP machines adjust to international voltages, either manually through voltage converters or automatically. It is also important to bring the appropriate wall receptacle adapter(s) in order to be able to plug the unit in.

When traveling and changing altitudes, such as living at sea level and traveling to 5,000 ft (1,524 m), it may be necessary to adjust the PAP levels to adapt the equipment to atmospheric pressure changes. Increasing the pressure setting is required at elevations above 2,500 ft (762 m) to maintain treatment efficacy. If these modifications are not made, the patient may begin to snore and experience partial airway obstruction. Usually, the patient can make these adjustments with simple instructions from the PAP manual. Typically, adjustments for three levels are available. A low-level elevation is considered below 2,500 ft (762 m), a medium level is 2,500 to 5,000 ft (762-1,524 m), and a high-level elevation is greater than 5,000 ft (1,524 m) above sea level. Always remember to instruct the patient to reset the altitude when returning from high elevations. Many PAP machines now adjust automatically for altitude changes.

Many patients enjoy camping and boating, but traveling without a power source can be a challenge. Patients should be encouraged to investigate an appropriate alternate source of power for their device. Some patients may also want an alternate source of power in the event of a power outage. A battery backup system with an inverter or a 12-V cigarette lighter adapter can be used with most PAP machines. If using a humidifier, a pure sine wave inverter is recommended. Patients should refer to their manuals for specific instructions. It is important to note that using an unapproved electrical source could void any warranty and possibly damage PAP equipment.

Hospital Admissions and Surgery

If patients using PAP are scheduled to have surgery, they should be instructed to check with the hospital about being able to bring their PAP equipment with them to the hospital. Most medical facilities have a biomedical department that will inspect the PAP equipment for electrical safety and cleanliness before allowing its use in the hospital. Nearly all PAP machines are double-insulated for electrical safety. Patients should be encouraged to share information about their sleep-disordered breathing and pressure requirements with the attending physician. Using PAP before and after surgery, or during a hospital stay, will ensure continuity of treatment and enhance the recovery process.

Logistical Challenges at Home

The placement of the PAP machine and tubing in a patient's bedroom is different in every home. The machine should be placed on a stable and safe surface that is at least 6 ft (1.8 m) away from a heat source, air conditioner, or room humidifier. Some patients place the machine on the bedside table and others near the floor. Tubing lengths of 6 to 12 ft (1.8-3.7 m) can be used with the circuit to facilitate movement in bed. Tubing lengths greater than 12 ft (3.7 m) are not recommended because of pressure drops within the circuit.

If the machine is near the floor, it is recommended that it be elevated at least 4 to 6 in (10.2-15.2 cm). If not, the machine could draw fibers and dust from the carpet and flooring, which could impede the air intake. It is also not recommended to place the PAP machine higher than the patient's head. There is a potential for condensation to accumulate in the tubing and flow back to the patient's face. Also, if the machine is above the patient's head, there is the risk of it falling and striking them. It is important to keep the machine air intake unobstructed and free from blockage that would impair its function. An example of this would be an item of clothing or a towel draped over the device.

Placement of the tubing should enhance the patient's movement in bed. This is a very individual choice. One option is to bring the tubing up between the mattress and the headboard, or up over the headboard, so it is centered behind the patient's head. Usually, two sections of tubing (12 ft [3.7 m]) are required for this placement. There are also a variety of holders and hooks available that support the tubing above the patient, connected to an extension arm that fits between the mattress and the box spring. These alternate placements reduce tension on the tubing and provide greater flexibility for unrestricted movement and body position changes during the night. Patients who try various placements are more likely to arrive at a satisfactory solution for their PAP situation than those who do not experiment.

PAP therapy can bring about unexpected challenges with pets that share a bedroom with the PAP user. Dogs and cats that sleep in the same bed as the PAP user may become mischievous or fearful of their owner because of the apparatus or the sound of the device. The exhalation port is a particularly intriguing or frightening aspect of the machine for some pets. Also, cats and dogs are curious about the equipment when it is not in use. The mask can be especially tempting because it smells like its owner. It is not uncommon to have a dog chew a face mask or a cat chew through the PAP tubing.

OUTCOME ASSESSMENT

Assessing outcomes for effective patient education and PAP compliance will involve a comparative analysis to previously collected data. The sleep technologist will need to compare, deduce, examine, differentiate, and question all data collected over the course of the patient's care and training. A quality assurance program may be set up to track different aspects of the educational process. The program itself should also be evaluated. The program evaluation should be conducted with an awareness of the program's setting as well as the cost of maintaining the program. Persons directly and indirectly related to the program should be reviewed as well. Because a program will need to operate within the department's budget, management will play a big role both in the development and in the operation of the program.

One to 3 Days

Long-term adherence to CPAP therapy can be predicted as early as 3 days after the initiation of CPAP therapy. The pattern of adherence to CPAP at 3 and 7 days strongly predicted longer-term (1 month) adherence. Eighty-four percent of those who used CPAP for more than 4 hours a day at day 3 used CPAP for an average of more than 4 hours a day at day 30 compared with only 26% of those who used CPAP for less than 4 hours a day at day 3 (3).

The most critical time during PAP initiation is the first 1 to 3 days. Patients may be tired, frustrated, hesitant, or even angry about the struggles with PAP therapy. Others may acclimate quickly and be fully rested and even ecstatic about their results. When patients are struggling with their treatment, it is important to be understanding and empathetic and to offer possible solutions to their problems. Remind them that sleeping even for a short time on PAP is a step in the right direction. Likewise, when patients are doing well, it is important to congratulate them on their success and encourage continued use of PAP. Remind all patients that they can call for help and reassurance and always reiterate the importance of any available educational opportunities and A.W.A.K.E. meetings.

Four Days to 8 Weeks

This period in PAP therapy is transitional. Patients who were initially successful with wearing PAP may express disappointment that they do not feel the exuberance that they did in the first few days of therapy. These patients need to be told that this is a normal transition of PAP therapy called "the rebound effect," which occurs when a patient who has been sleep-deprived because of sleep-disordered breathing uses PAP and catches up on lost slow-wave and rapid eye movement sleep. This rebound effect may cause the patient to feel much rested during the first 1 to 3 days; they may even feel euphoric. After the first few days, this effect tapers off, and the patient returns to a normal sleep architecture.

Patients may also complain about waking up at night during this transition period. They are often not aware of the frequent arousals that occur during untreated sleep-disordered breathing. But after the elimination of the problem, nighttime awakenings may become bothersome. Patients need to be reassured that it is normal to awaken during the night while rolling over, adjusting blankets, or repositioning during the night. If awakenings happen frequently and the patient feels tired, then intervention is needed. If the patient is intolerant of PAP, has been working with the PAP educators, and has exhausted all suggestions, they should be instructed to return to the physician to discuss progress and other treatment options. For the patient who has adjusted to PAP therapy, once again, remind them that they can call for help and reassurance. Also reiterate the importance of any available educational opportunities and A.W.A.K.E. meetings.

Six Months

At 6 months, most PAP patients are quite confident with their therapy. Patients should be reminded that most insurance companies allow for a new mask every 6 months (the mask cushion should be replaced every 3 months; this is generally covered by insurance). Continue to remind the patients that they can call for help and reassurance, and always reiterate the importance of any available educational opportunities and A.W.A.K.E. meetings.

One-Year and Long-Term Follow-Up

After 1 year, expect the PAP patient to be very confident with therapy. Many patients become very educated about sleep-disordered breathing and PAP during this time. Increases in available educational materials, Internet access, and the media have helped patients become more knowledgeable and compliant. Patients should be encouraged to continue their pursuit of knowledge about their disorder and remain updated in PAP technology. Again, remind the patient that most insurance companies will cover a new mask. The equipment company generally holds a long-term prescription for this purpose. Many physicians suggest that their patients schedule a follow-up with their sleep physician or their primary care physician (PCP) at 1 to 2 years or as needed. Communications with patients at the 1-year mark offer the opportunity to reiterate support and provide informational resources such as educational opportunities and A.W.A.K.E. meetings.

Success with PAP therapy often requires a team effort from the patient, the physician, and the sleep technologist and/or sleep educator. The sleep professional's role cannot be overestimated in reassuring their patients that any effort to lengthen their use of PAP therapy will improve their chances of success. Comprehensive education, patient communication, feedback, application of desensitization strategies, and long-term follow-up will improve outcomes and result in improved quality of life for the patient with sleep-disordered breathing.

CONCLUSION

Effective patient education and PAP adherence require more than giving the patient information and having them recite it back to you. To be effective, patient education must be based on a well-developed educational program that takes into account all of the patient's needs. The educational program must be conducted in a way that facilitates the patient's ability to carry out recommendations. Remember, communication in patient education is a two-way process. It is essential that the sleep technologist and the patient be able to communicate effectively. The sleep technologist must have the ability to recognize patient cues and respond accurately as well as to provide support and feedback. Such skills promote a sense of trust that helps maintain an open relationship with the patient. This is crucial if the sleep technologist hopes to elicit accurate information from the patient and identify any misconceptions or misunderstanding they may have (1).

REFERENCES

1. Falvo DR. *Effective Patient Education: A Guide to Increased Compliance.* Aspen; 1994.
2. US Government Accountability Office. MEDICARE: communications to beneficiaries on the prescription drug benefits could be improved. 2006. https://www.gao.gov/products/gao-06-654
3. Schwartz LM, Woloshin S, Black WC, Welch HG. The role of numeracy in understanding the benefit of screening mammography. *Ann Intern Med.* 1997; 127(11):966-972.
4. Lydon GM, Boulton M, Moynihan C, et al. Cancer patients' information needs and information seeking behavior: in depth study. *BMJ.* 2000;320(7239):909-913.
5. Avillion AE. *Learning Styles in Nursing Education: Integrating Teaching Strategies into Staff Development.* HCPro; 2009.
6. Minninger J. *Total Recall: How to Maximize Your Memory Power.* MJF Books; 1997.
7. Chokroverty S. *Sleep Disorders Medicine: Basic Science, Technical Considerations, and Clinical Aspects.* Butterworth-Heinemann; 1994.
8. Kribs NB, Pack AI, Kline LR, et al. Objective measurement of patterns of nasal CPAP use by patients with obstructive sleep apnea. *Am Rev Respir Dis.* 1993;147:887-895.
9. Arfoosh R, Rowley JA. Adherence to positive airway pressure therapy. *Sleep Med Clin.* 2010;5(3):321-334.

Chapter 55

At-Home Positive Airway Pressure Follow-Up: Therapy Assessment Tools, Interventions, and Equipment Maintenance

ANGLEICA BENITEZ

KEY CONCEPTS/LEARNING OBJECTIVES

Key concepts for this chapter include the mask-fit process for home usage of interface, the side effects of positive airway pressure (PAP) and how to intervene once the patient is on PAP therapy, and maintenance and replacement of equipment.

KEY TERMS

Assessment
Compliance
Equipment
Positive airway pressure (PAP)
Side effects

Obstructive sleep apnea (OSA) is a chronic disorder commonly treated with positive airway pressure (PAP) therapy. Proper follow-up for at-home PAP therapy is critical to ensuring treatment efficacy and patient adherence. Without structured monitoring and support, adherence rates remain suboptimal (1,2).

Early follow-up (within the first 1-2 weeks of therapy) is helpful for troubleshooting issues and optimizing comfort, as adherence in the initial weeks strongly predicts long-term usage (3). Key challenges in at-home continued positive airway pressure (CPAP) therapy include:

- Mask fit and air leaks: Poorly fitted masks can cause air leaks, reducing therapeutic pressure and causing discomfort (4).
- Nasal congestion and dry mouth: PAP airflow can dry the airway, exacerbating discomfort and leading to reduced adherence (5).
- Discomfort and skin pressure: Tight masks can cause pressure sores and skin irritation, particularly in older patients (6).
- Psychological barriers: Anxiety and claustrophobia may prevent patients from consistently using PAP therapy (7).
- Lack of education or support: Patients often require coaching to develop a nightly CPAP routine and properly maintain equipment (8).

Addressing these challenges through structured follow-up is essential for successful OSA management. At follow-up visits (whether in-person or via telemedicine), clinicians can review objective device data, assess the patient's comfort, and intervene early to improve compliance.

This chapter presents a case example of a home PAP follow-up in a 78-year-old OSA patient struggling with PAP adherence. We highlight assessment strategies, targeted interventions—including mask refitting, humidification adjustments, and behavioral support—and their impact on therapy adherence.

CASE PRESENTATION

Patient Profile

A 78-year-old female with a history of diverticulosis, hypercholesterolemia, and overweight (BMI ~28) was diagnosed with moderate OSA (apnea-hypopnea index [AHI]: 20 events/h, significant oxygen desaturation). She was prescribed CPAP at 11 cm H_2O with an oronasal mask and a humidifier.

Initial Therapy and Complaints

At a 1-month follow-up, the patient reported several difficulties:

- Dry mouth upon awakening, despite a full-face mask, indicating potential mouth leaks or inadequate humidification
- Mask discomfort and leak: Air leaked around the mask edges, especially when changing position, leading to poor sleep quality
- Daytime fatigue: Inconsistent CPAP use due to discomfort led to fragmented sleep
- Claustrophobia: The patient experienced anxiety when wearing the mask, occasionally avoiding therapy.

Her daughter, who accompanied her, confirmed inconsistent CPAP use. These issues signaled a need for a thorough therapy assessment and intervention plan to improve her comfort and compliance with PAP therapy.

Therapy Assessment

A comprehensive assessment was conducted, reviewing the patient's 30-day CPAP device report and subjective feedback. The data confirmed suboptimal adherence, with the patient using CPAP an average of 3.5 hours/night. The humidifier setting was moderate (2 out of 5), but persistent dryness indicated possible inadequate humidification.

High leak rates (~35 L/min) suggested air leakage was compromising therapeutic pressure delivery. Such leak magnitude can explain the patient's dry mouth and might also trigger the device's high leak alarm or disturb sleep. The leak was most likely coming from mouth breathing or an inadequate mask seal around the nose and mouth.

The pressure was fixed at 11 cm H_2O, which was the prescribed therapeutic level. Ramp was enabled, starting at 4 cm H_2O for 20 minutes, to help her fall asleep more comfortably at a lower pressure. The humidifier was set at a midrange level; however, given her significant dryness complaints, this setting might have been insufficient, or the leak was so high that humidification benefit was lost.

SUBJECTIVE ASSESSMENT AND MASK-FIT CHECK

In addition to the data, we revisited the patient's experience in detail. She reiterated that the mask would often "leak air," especially when she turned to her side. She had to tighten it to try to control the leak, which caused pressure on her nose and occasional skin irritation. The dry mouth each morning suggested that despite using a full-face mask, a substantial portion of air was escaping, or she was sleeping with her mouth open and drying out. She also described feeling anxious once the CPAP was on: "I feel I can't breathe naturally with it at first," indicating some level of panic or claustrophobia when starting PAP each night. This anxiety likely contributed to her prematurely removing the mask.

During the follow-up visit, we performed a mask-fit check at her therapeutic pressure. We had the patient put on her current oro-nasal mask and run the CPAP at 10 to 11 cm H_2O while awake. This reproduced a significant air leak around the top of the mask (near the nasal bridge and cheeks) when she moved her jaw or head. The mask's cushion did not seem to seal optimally to her face contours, even when adjusted. The patient also coughed a bit as the airflow felt drying within minutes, strongly indicating that the humidifier might be too low or ineffective with the current leak.

In summary, the assessment identified the following issues: (1) excessive mask leak due to suboptimal mask fit (leading to dry mouth and higher apnea-hypopnea index [AHI]), (2) limited usage stemming from discomfort and possibly anxiety, and (3) likely inadequate humidification for her needs. The therapeutic pressure of 11 cm H_2O itself appeared appropriate (given her moderate OSA and partial response), so efforts would focus on mask/interface adjustments, side-effect management, and desensitization to improve tolerance.

Interventions and Equipment Adjustments

Based on the previous findings, a multifaceted intervention plan was implemented to address both equipment-related problems and behavioral factors. The goal was to improve comfort, reduce leaks, and build the patient's confidence with CPAP. Key interventions included a PAP Nap desensitization session, mask refitting with alternative equipment, humidification optimization, patient education, and emotional support. Each component is detailed in what follows.

Positive Airway Pressure Nap Desensitization Session

A supervised PAP Nap (daytime CPAP exposure session) was conducted to reduce anxiety (9).

During this time, a technologist and therapist worked with her on mask desensitization and breathing exercises. We started the CPAP at a low pressure (4 cm H_2O) and gradually increased it to 11 cm H_2O in increments, allowing her to acclimate to the sensations. She was coached with calming techniques—deep breathing, eyes closed with relaxing music, and guided imagery—to reduce focus on the mask. She tolerated therapy for 3 hours without panic (Figure 55-1).

Throughout the PAP Nap, we monitored leak and comfort. Initially, with her original mask, leak was

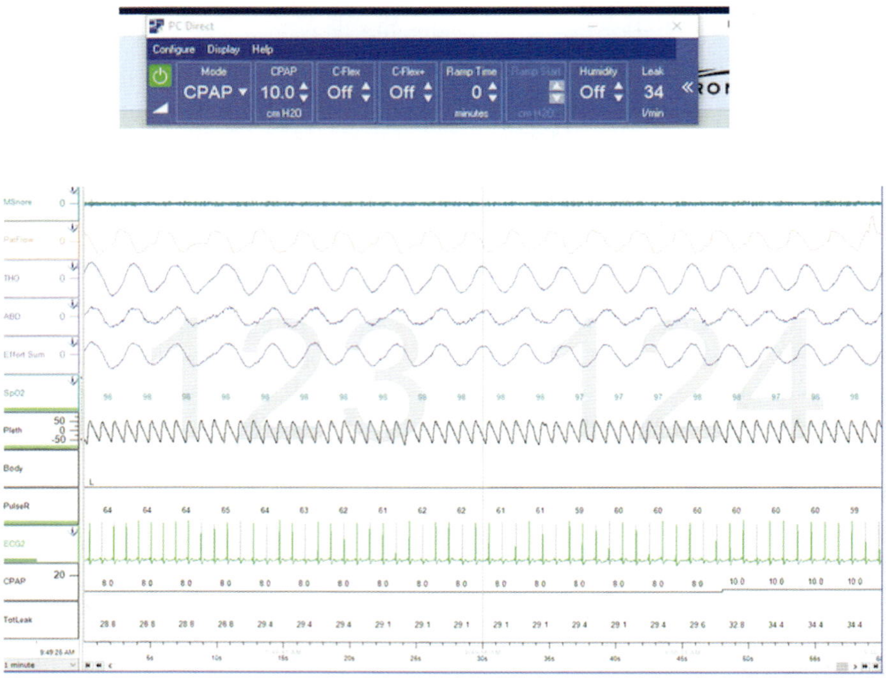

Figure 55-1 Supervised PAP Nap session. During a PAP Nap, the patient wears the CPAP while awake in a relaxed setting. The technologist incrementally raises the pressure and helps the patient practice breathing calmly with the mask on. This desensitization approach has been shown to improve comfort and subsequent nighttime adherence.

evident as pressure went up. Midway, we paused to try a different mask (see further on). By the end of the session, the patient was resting quietly at her full 11 cm H_2O pressure with minimal leak and reported feeling "much more comfortable" than when she started. Importantly, she experienced no panic during this trial; the gradual exposure and supportive coaching alleviated her anxiety. PAP Nap sessions have been reported in the literature to significantly improve subsequent CPAP use in patients with prior intolerance, so this session was a crucial step in building her confidence.

Mask Fitting Assessment With Artificial Intelligence-Powered Mask Fitting Tool and Interface Trials

Considering the observed issues with the current mask, a thorough mask refitting was performed. Using an AI-powered mask fitting tool, we scanned the patient's facial dimensions to objectively guide mask selection. This technology suggested that while a medium full-face mask was initially chosen, the patient's facial width and nasal structure might be better accommodated by a different mask model or size. The tool generated a list of masks ranked for her face (Figure 55-2).

We first fitted the new mask on the patient. On 4 and 6 cm H_2O, the leak was minimal, and she noted the mask felt lighter with no pressure on the nose bridge. As we raised it to 8 to 10 cm H_2O, a moderate leak appeared at the corners of her mouth. We then switched to a wider mask. This immediately improved the seal around her mouth.

We counseled her that every mask has a "break-in" period but that this one already felt better, which was promising. We also educated her on proper mask adjustment (not over-tightening the headgear; instead, allowing the cushion to inflate and form a seal) and advised replacing the mask cushion every few months as wear and tear can increase leaks.

Humidification and Dry Mouth Management

To address her dry mouth complaint, we adjusted the humidification settings on her CPAP. We increased the heated humidifier from 2 up to 4 (on a 0-5 scale) to provide more moisture. Adequate humidification helps alleviate nasal dryness and oral dryness, which, in turn, can improve comfort and possibly adherence.

We also verified that her CPAP had a heated tubing option and supplied a heated tube to maintain warm humidity all the way to the mask (this prevents condensation "rainout" while maximizing humidity). The patient was instructed to ensure the water chamber is filled nightly and to use only distilled water. We discussed that if dryness persists, we could consider using a chin strap even with the full-face mask, or a mouth moisturizer at bedtime, but we anticipated the new mask's better seal plus higher humidity would resolve the issue. Proper humidification has anecdotally helped many patients

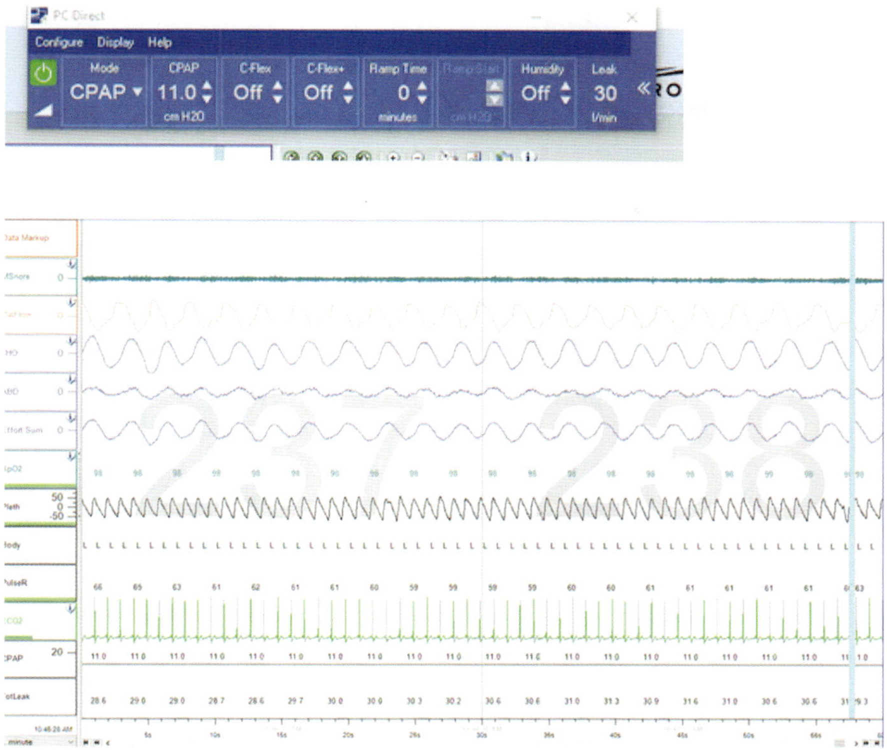

Figure 55-2 Mask-fitting trial.

use CPAP more comfortably, although evidence on its impact on adherence is mixed. In this patient's case, it was clearly indicated to combat a specific side effect.

Patient Education and Equipment Maintenance

An important part of the intervention was reeducating the patient on CPAP use and care (essentially, a refresher "CPAP clinic" session). We reviewed cleaning and maintenance of her equipment, as this can affect both comfort and health. The patient was taught to:

- Clean the mask cushion daily with mild soap and water or CPAP mask wipes. Oils from the skin can cause the mask to slip and leak; daily cleaning removes this film and can improve the seal. (We provided CPAP mask wipes for convenience.)
- Clean the humidifier chamber and tubing weekly and allow them to air dry. Also replace the disposable fine filter in the device every 2 weeks and rinse the foam filter if applicable. Regular cleaning not only protects from infections but also ensures optimal airflow and machine longevity.
- Inspect and replace mask components regularly: We explained that mask cushions wear out every 3 to 6 months and headgear straps can lose elasticity. Timely replacement (as covered by insurance schedules) will help prevent leak issues from recurring.

We emphasized the importance of these maintenance steps, noting that a well-maintained device and clean mask provide more effective therapy and a better experience. The patient was also reminded how to assemble/disassemble her mask and CPAP parts, and we observed her doing it to ensure confidence.

Emotional and Behavioral Support

Equally crucial was addressing the patient's emotional hurdles with PAP. During the PAP Nap and subsequent counseling, we employed techniques from behavioral sleep medicine to improve her PAP tolerance. We practiced relaxation breathing exercises that she could use at night when she first puts on the mask (slow deep breaths, progressive muscle relaxation).

We also employed a bit of motivational enhancement—discussing her personal health goals and how using CPAP could help (eg, improving her daytime energy and potentially protecting her heart and brain from OSA-related risks). By framing CPAP as a positive step she is taking for her health, we aimed to improve her mindset and commitment to therapy. We encouraged her to involve her family for support: for instance, having her daughter check in on her CPAP use or even sit with her for a few minutes in the evening when she puts the mask on, to reinforce the routine.

Additionally, cognitive reframing was used to counter her feelings of claustrophobia. We taught her to practice wearing just the mask (with no hose) during the daytime for 10 to 15 minutes while doing a calm activity (like reading or watching TV) as a desensitization exercise on her own. This kind of repeated exposure

Table 55-1 Summary of Interventions Addressing Each Problem and the Outcomes

Identified Issue	Intervention Implemented	Outcome/Result
Mask leak and poor fit	PAP Nap session with reevaluation; trial of alternative masks	Leak reduced (from ~35 to 40 L/min to ~30 L/min at 11 cm H_2O). New mask more comfortable; patient reports improved fit with no nose pressure.
Dry mouth (oral dryness)	Increased humidifier setting (2 → 4); provided heated tube. Educated on mask seal (to minimize mouth leak)	Moisture level improved; patient felt less dryness during trial. Better mask seal and humidity are expected to resolve morning dry mouth.
Claustrophobia/anxiety	PAP Nap desensitization with gradual pressure exposure and relaxation techniques. Taught breathing exercises and daytime mask practice	Patient became calmer with mask on; anxiety markedly decreased during session. Gained confidence to use CPAP at night
Limited usage (poor habit)	Motivational counseling (emphasized health benefits); involved family support; set up short-term goals. Education on CPAP benefits and adherence	Patient verbalized understanding of CPAP importance. Expressed commitment to use CPAP nightly. Family will help encourage use
Equipment maintenance gaps	Reviewed and demonstrated CPAP cleaning and part replacement schedule. Gave written instructions	Patient able to properly clean and assemble mask. Improved maintenance expected to enhance comfort (clean mask seals better, fewer leaks)

CPAP, continuous positive airway pressure; PAP, positive airway pressure.

can reduce anxiety over time. She was given a diary to log her CPAP use and any difficulties each night, with the understanding that these would be reviewed and addressed—this itself can boost adherence by adding accountability.

To summarize the interventions and their expected impact, see Table 55-1, which outlines each issue identified and the corresponding solution implemented.

FINDINGS AND RECOMMENDATIONS

After implementing the foregoing interventions, the patient's CPAP tolerance and performance showed notable improvement. During the in-clinic PAP Nap and mask fitting trials, she was able to tolerate her full pressure of 11 cm H_2O for an extended period without significant leak or panic. A new mask was supplied to her and the old mask retired.

The optimal CPAP pressure remains 11 cm H_2O, as her residual AHI and oxygen levels were acceptable at this setting once leaks were controlled. We did not see a need to increase pressure at this time—in fact, by eliminating leaks we effectively increased the delivered pressure to the airway, which should further reduce any residual events. We advised her to continue using the ramp feature if needed (starting at 4 cm H_2O for comfort), or even to extend the ramp duration a bit when first transitioning to the new mask at home, since the sensation might differ. The humidifier was set at level 4, and we recommended she keep it at this higher setting and ensure the room is not overly cold (to avoid rainout).

Patient Response

By the end of the session, the patient expressed relief and optimism. She remarked, "I never thought I could wear that machine for so long—now I see I can do it." She felt the new mask and tips gave her "a second chance" at making CPAP work. We reinforced her success during the trial to boost her confidence. She was encouraged to use the CPAP for the entire night, every night, and to apply the techniques learned (relaxation breathing, etc) at home.

Follow-Up Plan

We scheduled a follow-up contact 2 weeks after the interventions. Given the availability of modern PAP telemonitoring, we enrolled her CPAP device in a remote monitoring program. Her device was equipped with a cellular modem, so we set up access via the manufacturer's cloud platform. This allows us to track her nightly usage, leak, and AHI data in real time and intervene quickly if problems recur. We explained that someone from the clinic would check her data within the first week and call her if there were any red flags (eg, if her usage drops or large leaks are seen again). She also downloaded the patient app on her smartphone so she can see her own scores and get feedback each morning, which is intended to engage and motivate her. Studies have shown that such patient engagement tools and telemonitoring can improve adherence (eg, giving patients access to their PAP data and coaching can reduce therapy attrition rates).

At the 2-week follow-up call, we will review her subjective progress and the remote data. Key things to assess will be the following: Is she using the CPAP all night now? Is the dry mouth resolved? What is her leak report with the new mask? And how is her daytime alertness and comfort? We plan to reinforce any good trends and troubleshoot any remaining barriers. Additionally, we set a 1-month in-person follow-up (or via video visit if she prefers) to formally evaluate her adherence and clinical improvements (snoring eliminated, better sleep, etc). Long-term, she will be followed at least every 6 to 12 months once stable, with interim phone calls or telehealth check-ins as needed—consistent with guideline recommendations to provide ongoing support for PAP users.

Finally, our recommendations to the patient included continuing the current management with no new medications (she was using no sedatives or nasal meds—we noted that if nasal congestion became an issue, we might add a nasal steroid spray, but at this time her nasal patency was good). Weight management was encouraged as an adjunct to possibly reduce pressure needs in the future (although at 78, weight loss can be challenging). We also educated her on signs that would prompt reevaluation, such as if she could not tolerate PAP despite these changes (then we would consider alternatives like bilevel PAP or ENT referral). However, given her progress in this session, we were optimistic that these adjustments would significantly improve her adherence and OSA control.

REMOTE MONITORING AND ACCESS

It is worth highlighting how remote PAP therapy access was leveraged in this case and is recommended broadly. These platforms enable health care providers to view usage hours, leak, AHI, and even alter some settings remotely. The American Academy of Sleep Medicine suggests using telemonitoring-guided interventions, especially during the initial period of PAP therapy, to improve adherence (conditional recommendation). By using such systems, clinicians can intervene early—for instance, a simple phone coaching if a patient has not used the device for a few days or adjusting the humidity remotely if dryness is noted. In this patient's plan, remote monitoring is a key component to ensure she stays on track.

In summary, our final recommendations for this patient were as follows: (1) Switch to a new interface. (2) Continue CPAP at 11 cm H_2O with ramp and humidifier at level 4; use nightly for the entire sleep period. (3) Employ the learned strategies (relaxation, daytime practice) to overcome any discomfort. (4) Maintain the equipment with regular cleaning and part replacements. (5) Engage with follow-up, including remote monitoring check-ins and clinic visits, to sustain improvements. With these measures, the patient is expected to have improved symptom relief from OSA and better compliance, which will, in turn, contribute to the long-term effectiveness of her therapy.

DISCUSSION AND LITERATURE REVIEW

This case illustrates several important aspects of at-home PAP therapy follow-up and aligns with current literature and guidelines on optimizing CPAP adherence. Next, we discuss the broader evidence regarding mask fitting technologies, compliance-improvement strategies, and remote patient monitoring, as well as the role of PAP Naps, patient education, and behavioral interventions in PAP therapy.

MASK SELECTION AND ARTIFICIAL INTELLIGENCE-GUIDED FITTING

Choosing the right mask interface for a patient is often as crucial as selecting the right pressure. The American Thoracic Society (ATS) workshop on CPAP mask selection concluded that time and effort spent on initial mask fitting are invaluable (10). A well-fitted mask improves comfort and minimizes leaks, thereby enhancing adherence. Nasal masks are the preferred first option for most patients, as full-face (oronasal) masks can increase leak, residual AHI, and required pressure.

However, some patients (like the one in our case) need an oronasal mask due to habitual mouth breathing or jaw anatomy. In such cases, careful fitting and addressing contributing factors (eg, nasal congestion) are essential. AI-powered mask fitting tools represent an emerging solution to the challenge of mask fitting. These tools use artificial intelligence to match patient facial measurements with a database of mask models and sizes (11). By leveraging big data and machine learning, they can efficiently narrow down the best options, potentially reducing the trial-and-error period for finding the "right" mask. While formal studies on AI-driven mask selection are still limited, early adoption in sleep clinics and durable medical equipment (DME) companies has been promising. Such technology can be especially useful for remote setups where in-person mask fitting is not feasible—patients can scan their face via an app and receive personalized mask recommendations. This aligns with a trend in sleep medicine of using telehealth tools to enhance care.

Our case also underlines the importance of managing mask leaks. Large leaks not only disturb patients (noise, air blowing) but can also compromise therapy by reducing delivered pressure and causing arousals (12). Interventions for leak include refitting the mask, switching mask type, using chin straps, and managing mouth opening (12).

We pursued refitting and achieved significant improvement. Another factor is equipment maintenance—a mask cushion covered in facial oils will lose its tackiness and seal, so patient education on cleaning can directly translate into leak reduction. This is supported by expert recommendations that stress mask/interface problems (like skin irritation or leak) should be addressed by trying different masks or adjusting straps and that a *multidisciplinary approach to side-effect management* improves CPAP compliance.

TELEMONITORING AND POSITIVE AIRWAY PRESSURE ADHERENCE

Remote monitoring has revolutionized at-home PAP follow-up. Many CPAP devices can automatically upload usage data to secure cloud servers, allowing health care providers to monitor patients without waiting for them to bring in an SD card. The AASM 2019 guideline suggests that telemonitoring-guided interventions in the initial PAP period can be beneficial (conditional recommendation) (13). The rationale is that early identification of nonadherence or issues (via remote data) lets the care team intervene before the patient gives up. Several studies have explored telemonitoring's impact. For instance, a trial by Murase et al found that automated telemonitoring with feedback messages improved 90-day PAP adherence compared to standard care (12). Another study showed that providing patients with a web-based engagement tool in addition to clinician monitoring led to lower therapy termination rates than monitoring alone (13). However, not all studies show large differences, and a few have reported mixed results for long-term adherence (13). A meta-analysis indicated telemonitoring yields a modest increase in usage (~0.5-1 hours/night in the short term) (14,15). While this average gain may seem small, on a population level it is significant, and for an individual, it could mean the difference between meeting adherence criteria or not. Importantly, telehealth follow-up became even more crucial during the COVID-19 pandemic, where in-person visits were limited. Beyond monitoring data, telehealth platforms can enable video visits, remote mask fitting sessions, and digital education, which altogether form a "biopsychosocial telemedicine model" for OSA care (15).

In our practice, we use a combination of remote data and phone coaching as a standard for new PAP patients. This case was no exception, and we anticipate that the remote oversight will help sustain the patient's adherence by promptly catching any slip-ups.

POSITIVE AIRWAY PRESSURE NAP EFFICACY

The concept of the PAP Nap, as employed in our case, is supported by clinical experience and some studies. In a pilot study of patients with insomnia and OSA who were nonadherent to PAP, a daytime PAP desensitization protocol (the PAP Nap) significantly improved subsequent adherence: patients who underwent a PAP Nap had higher rates of completing titration and using CPAP for more than 4 hours/night compared to controls.

While sample sizes were modest, the results are compelling—67% of the PAP Nap group became regular PAP users versus ~23% in the control group in one report. PAP Naps are particularly useful for those with claustrophobia or high anxiety, as they allow exposure therapy in a safe environment. Guidelines have not formally mandated PAP Naps, but they are considered a reasonable clinical tool. Our patient clearly benefited from this approach, overcoming a major psychological barrier. The PAP Nap essentially combines multiple adherence strategies: dedicated coaching (one-on-one attention), mask fitting adjustments, relaxation techniques, and immediate positive reinforcement when the patient succeeds in using PAP calmly. This multidisciplinary method exemplifies the "integrated approach" recommended for managing PAP users who struggle.

CONCLUSION

At-home PAP therapy follow-up is a vital component of effective OSA management. This case demonstrated how a targeted follow-up visit, 1 month into therapy, uncovered the barriers to compliance and allowed for tailored interventions. By systematically assessing the patient's device data and listening to her difficulties, we identified correctable issues—chiefly, an ill-fitting mask and resulting discomfort. Interventions including a PAP Nap desensitization, mask refitting humidification adjustments, and thorough patient reeducation led to immediate improvements in her tolerance and a plan for sustained adherence.

Optimizing PAP therapy is often likened to "fine-tuning" a treatment over time. It requires collaboration between patient and provider and often multiple rounds of adjustments. Key lessons from this case and the broader evidence are as follows: ensure the mask is right for the patient, manage side effects proactively (dryness, leaks, etc), engage the patient with education and support from day 1, and utilize remote monitoring/telemedicine to keep a close eye on progress. With these strategies, even an older patient with initial CPAP intolerance can become a successful long-term user, reaping the health benefits of treated OSA.

In practical implementation, home care companies and sleep clinics should establish routine follow-up protocols—a call at weeks 1 to 2, an office visit by 1 month, and periodic reviews—to catch issues early. Tools like cloud-based PAP monitoring and AR-guided mask fitting can greatly enhance the efficiency of these follow-ups by providing actionable data and recommendations. Equally, investing time in patient-centric approaches (like desensitization sessions or motivational counseling) can pay dividends in adherence. As illustrated, our patient went from struggling with PAP to confidently using it, simply because we addressed her problems with a structured, compassionate approach. Going forward, continued follow-up and possibly refresher sessions will ensure she remains comfortable and compliant. This reflects the overarching principle: OSA is a chronic condition, and PAP therapy requires ongoing care and maintenance—both of the equipment and the patient's engagement—to achieve long-term success.

By sharing this case and linking it to current best practices, we hope to provide a template for clinicians in managing at-home PAP follow-up. With meticulous assessment, targeted interventions, and regular follow-up (in-person or remote), the common challenges in PAP therapy can be overcome, leading to improved adherence and better patient outcomes in OSA.

CLINICAL CASE

Key Finding

This case demonstrates how proper mask selection and a structured desensitization protocol can significantly improve patient comfort, reduce leak, and maintain optimal respiratory stability during CPAP therapy.

DreamWear Full Face—Left-Lateral Continuous Positive Airway Pressure Desensitization; Size Medium → Size Medium Wide

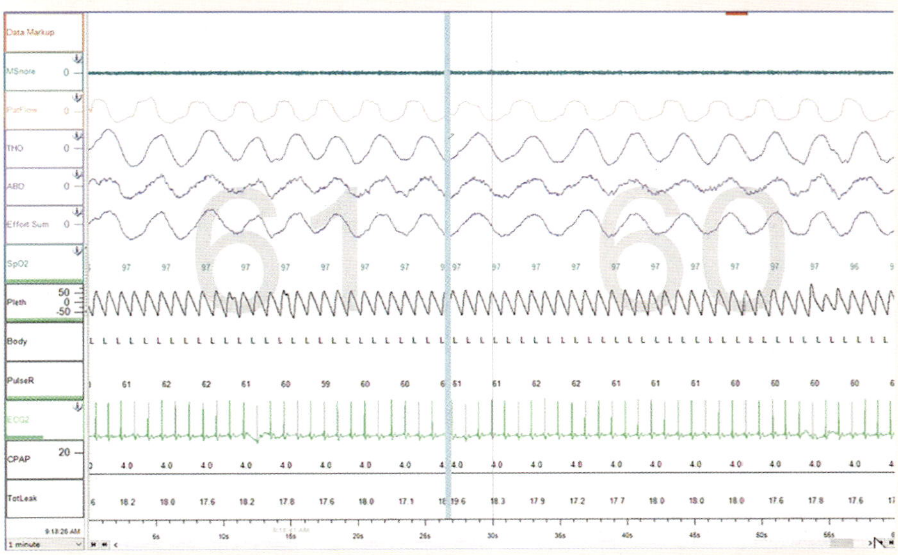

Epoch 61-60. Baseline—4 cm H_2O (Size M)

- Left-lateral; calm PatFlow; thoracic/abdomen (THO/ABD) synchronous
- Spo_2 96%-98%; leak minimal (~17 L/min)
- Interpretation: adequate baseline seal

Follow-up:

- Confirm comfort.
- Record baseline comfort (10).
- Plan rise to 6 cm H_2O.

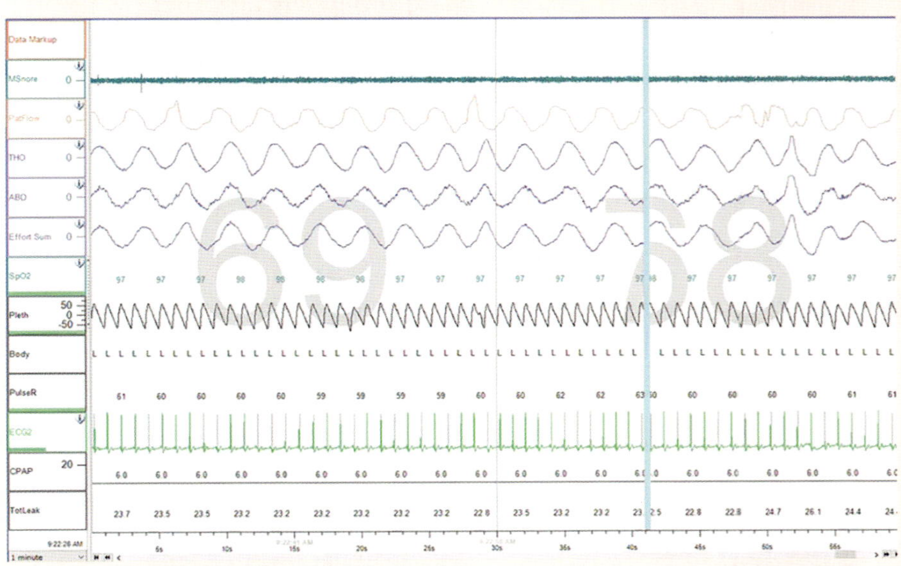

Epoch 68-69. Pressure rise—6 cm H_2O (Size M)

- Seal maintained; leak ~23-31 L/min
- No events; patient comfortable
- Continue desensitization.

Follow-up:

- Reassess cushion/straps.
- Note dryness/noise.
- Prepare 8 cm H_2O challenge.

(*continued*)

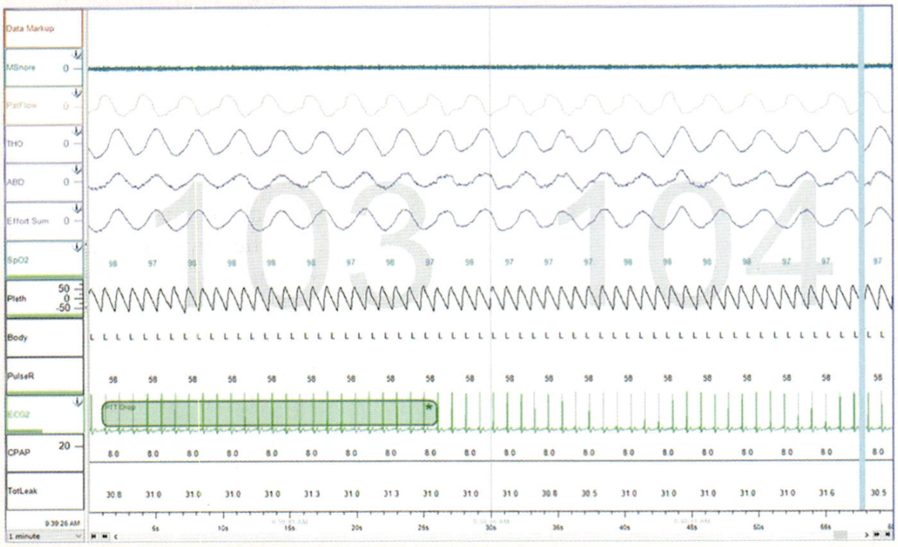

Epoch 103-104. Pressure rise—8 cm H_2O (Size M)

- Leak variable; peaks ~31 L/min
- Breathing smooth; comfort excellent

Follow-up:

- Recheck leak in favorite position.
- Document comfort and control leak.

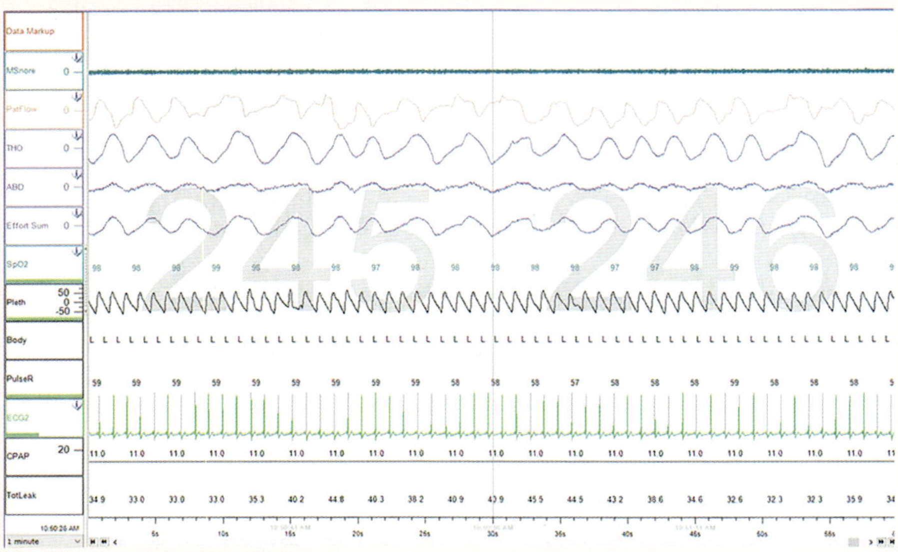

Epoch 245-246. Resizing seal—11.0 cm H_2O (Size MW)

- PatFlow: rounded, regular; no snore or flow-limitation
- THO/ABD: synchronous; no paradox
- Spo_2: ~98%; HR: sinus ~58-59 bpm
- TotLeak: low-to-mid 30s L/min (≈32-36; occasional 40s) after upsizing to MW

Interpretation: Since epoch 209 (switch to MW), leak control and comfort are improved at higher pressures, including 11 cm H_2O; Size M previously showed spikes up to ~50 L/min.

Follow-up:

- Maintain MW sizing; seal checks nightly.
- Reinforce cleaning routine.
- 1-2 week follow-up for leak/ compliance

Figure note: Left-lateral pressure challenge: leak controlled at 6-8 cm H_2O; at 11 cm H_2O, MW achieved better seal (~30-31 L/min) vs M (up to ~34-50 L/min). Breathing calm; Spo2 96%-98% throughout

Summary

MW sizing provided a more stable seal at approximately 11 cm H_2O. Emphasize strap symmetry, nightly cleaning, and left-lateral acclimatization to sustain comfort and control leak.

REFERENCES

1. Weaver TE, Grunstein RR. Adherence to continuous positive airway pressure therapy: the challenge to effective treatment. *Proc Am Thorac Soc.* 2008;5(2): 173-178. doi:10.1513/pats.200708-119MG
2. Patil SP, Ayappa IA, Caples SM, Kimoff RJ, Patel SR, Harrod CG. Treatment of adult obstructive sleep apnea with positive airway pressure: an American Academy of Sleep Medicine clinical practice guideline. *J Clin Sleep Med.* 2019;15(2):335-343. doi:10.5664/jcsm.7640
3. Richards D, Bartlett DJ, Wong K, et al. Increased adherence to CPAP with a group cognitive behavioral treatment intervention: a randomized trial. *Sleep.* 2007;30(5):635-640.
4. Bakker JP, Pack AI. CPAP treatment for obstructive sleep apnea: tackling the challenge of adherence. *Ann Am Thorac Soc.* 2020;17(10):1177-1185.
5. Bahammam AS, Alrajeh MS, Alamri Y, Al-Jahdali HH. Adherence to CPAP therapy. *Ann Thorac Med.* 2022; 17(suppl 1):S59-S66.
6. Krakow B, Melendrez D, Ferreira E, et al. Prevalence of insomnia symptoms in patients with sleep-disordered breathing. *J Clin Sleep Med.* 2008;4(3):212-222.
7. Thareja S, Mandapalli R, Shaik F, et al. Impact of obstructive sleep apnea on cardiovascular health: a systematic review. *Cureus.* 2024;16(10):e71940. doi:10.7759/cureus.71940
8. Balachandran JS, Yu X, Wroblewski K, et al. A brief behavioral measure of sleepiness. *Chest.* 2013;144(3): 565-573.
9. Li HP, Zhang XB, Wang YJ, et al. Telemedicine-based management of CPAP therapy improves adherence and outcomes. *Front Med (Lausanne).* 2022;9:876514.
10. Smith CE, Dauz E, Curbow B, et al. A telemedicine intervention to improve CPAP adherence in older adults. *Telemed J E Health.* 2006;12(3):289-296.
11. Kushida CA, Littner MR, Hirshkowitz M, et al. Practice parameters for the use of CPAP to treat obstructive sleep apnea in adults. *Sleep.* 2006;29(3):375-380.
12. Murase K, Yamamoto Y, Saito H, et al. Effectiveness of telemedicine for CPAP compliance in patients with obstructive sleep apnea: a randomized controlled trial. *Sleep Breath.* 2019;23(4):1223-1230.
13. Aloia MS, Arnedt JT, Stanchina M, et al. How early is early intervention? Predicting CPAP adherence patterns in newly diagnosed sleep apnea patients. *Sleep Breath.* 2001;5(1):13-21.
14. Schwab RJ, Badr SM, Epstein LJ, et al. An official ATS/AASM/ACCP clinical practice guideline: CPAP adherence. *J Clin Sleep Med.* 2009;5(3):263-276.
15. Likar LL, Panciera TM, Erickson AD. Predictors of CPAP adherence in sleep apnea patients. *Chest.* 1997; 111(5):1273-1276. doi:10.1378/chest.111.5.1273

Chapter 56
Treatment for Insomnia

ROBERT N. TURNER

KEY CONCEPTS/LEARNING OBJECTIVES

The key concepts for this chapter include insomnia treatment techniques and interventions, individual differences in insomnia therapy, and medications used to treat insomnia.

KEY TERMS

Bright light therapy
Cognitive therapy
Insomnia
Pharmacotherapy
Relaxation therapy
Sleep hygiene
Sleep restriction therapy
Stimulus control therapy

Treating insomnia can be challenging. Some patients presenting to the sleep disorders clinic have had trouble initiating and maintaining sleep for months or years; consequently, poor sleep-wake habits are often firmly established. Many "self-medicate," using alcohol or over-the-counter sleep aids for relief of insomnia. Dependency on sedative hypnotics also occurs. Others present with personality styles generally associated with enduring, maladaptive patterns of thinking and relating to others and their world. A multitude of characteristics, social and environmental factors as well as medical conditions can contribute to a persistent sleep-wake disturbance. Thus, it is essential to identify the disorder correctly as an initial step in specifying rational interventions for insomnia.

On a broader, conceptual scale, one may question whether nondrug treatments for insomnia are worthwhile or necessary. Although pharmacotherapy has been the mainstay of treatment for decades, patients accept cognitive-behavioral or other nondrug interventions when adequately prepared. Some patients express fears of "becoming addicted" to sleeping pills and prefer to rely on themselves rather than depend on a medication to sleep. Furthermore, it has become well known that sedative hypnotics may not be effective in the long-term treatment of insomnia and, if compounds have a short half-life, some can induce "rebound insomnia" when discontinued.

Sedatives can be helpful to those with specific types of insomnia, and many of these compounds are immediately effective in promoting sleep onset and sleep maintenance. If a patient presents with a disorder of hyperarousal, pharmacotherapy and/or relaxation training may be a rational first-line treatment, providing some quick relief to an overactive sympathetic nervous system (SNS). Both patients and physicians are accustomed to treating insomnia in this manner, although this is not necessarily helpful in the long run or to the patient's best benefit.

Details of evaluation prior to treatment are elaborated in Chapter 13. When necessary, referring patients to specialists is appropriate. However, presenting this to patients requires careful consideration. Some with insomnia firmly believe that they cannot be helped. This notion needs to be addressed rather than providing reinforcement when presenting the need for referral.

COGNITIVE AND BEHAVIORAL TREATMENTS FOR INSOMNIA

Once a detailed evaluation of underlying factors that could be contributing to difficulty initiating and/or maintaining sleep has been completed, a variety of techniques are available that have been shown to offer improvements (1).

The American Academy of Sleep Medicine's (AASM) practice parameters for psychological and behavioral treatment of insomnia recommend its use in patients with chronic insomnia (1).

Sleep restriction therapy is based on the homeostatic regulation of sleep, facilitating sleep initiation and maintenance through partial sleep deprivation. It is important to note that sleep restriction should not fall below 5 hours per night. Extreme caution should be used with patients for whom sleepiness presents a risk in their profession (eg, drivers, heavy equipment operators).

This process involves limiting the time a patient spends in bed until an improvement in sleep efficiency (SE) is seen. The amount of time allowed in bed can be viewed as the "time prescription." Calculation of how much to reduce the time in bed is based on findings from baseline sleep diaries. The goal is to achieve 85% SE. Sleep diaries are reviewed on a weekly basis, and if the SE goal is met, time in bed is increased by 20 minutes for a week. If the SE goal is not met and SE is less than 80%, time in bed is reduced by 20 minutes. Time in bed is kept stable if SE falls between 80% and 85%. Weekly adjustments in the sleep schedule are made until optimal sleep time and SE are reached (2).

Stimulus control therapy includes several instructions that target sleep-incompatible behaviors. Instructions to patients are as follows: Go to bed only when sleepy; get out of bed when unable to sleep, go to another room, and return to bed only when sleep is imminent; stop all nonsleep-promoting activities (ie, watching TV or problem-solving), only engage in nonstimulating activities. These steps may need to be repeated multiple times per night at first. The patient should get up at a regular time every morning despite any problems with sleep during the previous night.

Relaxation therapies center on reducing cognitive and/or somatic arousal. Progressive muscle relaxation techniques, diaphragmatic breathing, and biofeedback training have all been used among patients with insomnia. Cognitive interventions such as meditation or imagery may also be employed. These procedures may be most beneficial to patients who experience excessive muscular tension and/or ruminative thought patterns. Relaxation procedures are often described initially, and the patient chooses a preferred relaxation strategy. This strategy is encouraged and monitored for both compliance and effectiveness. The patient needs to be counseled that they are embarking on relaxation practice. This can, and should, include practice of an intervention or technique implemented during daytime waking hours. This can improve their ability to implement the intervention (practice) at nighttime while in bed. It is important for these methods to be employed over time (2-4 weeks at minimum) and practiced daily.

Progressive muscle relaxation training can be useful if the patient does not become more tense in response. This may be employed as a "body scan" or "tense and release" pattern. Teach the patient to focus first on their feet. One method is to focus on the area and determine if there is any tension. If tension is noted, focus on relaxation of that specific area. Alternatively, this same process may be taught by the patient tensing the area (feet), then releasing. Have the patient move up along the body with a similar focus on the next area as they go (eg, calves, thighs, hips). Some patients respond better to one approach than the other. The clinician should be flexible in allowing the patient to choose which technique they prefer to employ as part of their relaxation practice.

Diaphragmatic breathing is a process by which the patient is taught to focus on using their diaphragm to inhale. There are many patterns that can be used. Here is one example of how to teach diaphragmatic breathing. The patient is instructed to find a comfortable position, place one of the patient's hands on the diaphragm and the other on the chest to help the patient feel when the diaphragm moves, inhale slowly through their nose to a given count, pause at the end of inhalation, exhale through their mouth for a longer count than on the inhale, and repeat.

Cognitive therapy focuses on changing dysfunctional, arousing thoughts and beliefs regarding sleep and insomnia. Catastrophic thinking is challenged; maladaptive thoughts, which may perpetuate insomnia, are addressed; and faulty, unrealistic beliefs are discussed. Worry and rumination over the loss of sleep, unrealistic thoughts regarding the effects of partial sleep deprivation, and irrational expectations about sleep requirements are all relevant issues requiring careful examination and modification. Common examples of irrational beliefs might include "I cannot sleep at all," as well as "My day will be ruined if I do not sleep for at least 8 hours tonight." Because dysfunctional attitudes and thoughts about sleep can promote arousal, both anticipatory and performance anxiety can also occur, adding to difficulties with sleep onset. Offer suggestions to modify and replace these unrealistic or dysfunctional thoughts with rational ideation. This can be accomplished by educating the patient about thinking and the flaws contained in that thinking. This education needs to be based on scientifically proven sleep facts. Cognitive-behavioral therapy has been found to benefit various patients with insomnia (3).

Sleep hygiene education focuses on practices and patterns that can promote or disrupt sleep. The goal is to optimize sleep-wake patterns and habits. Encouraging patients to adopt a regular time of going to bed (with 1-2-hour variations) and, more importantly, instructing the patient to get up at about the same time every day are helpful. Patients need to avoid stimulants such as caffeine or tobacco several hours before bedtime, limit alcohol near bedtime, exercise regularly, provide for a time to wind down at least 1 hour before bedtime, and manage stress. Environmental variables, such as noise, light, sleep surface, and ambient temperature, can also be addressed. Specific instructions include moving the bedroom clock out of sight, not exercising too close to bedtime, and stopping intense efforts to try to sleep. The latter remains particularly important because the more one tries to sleep, the more aroused one becomes. It is, therefore, less likely that sleep will ensue easily (4).

It is important to remember that many patients have learned these recommendations with little support or other input. These patients may feel they have tried everything and have some resistance to further interventions since the sleep hygiene practices did not seem to help. Therefore, these and other sleep hygiene techniques should be viewed as adjuncts to cognitive-behavioral therapy for insomnia (CBTi).

Bright light therapy can be useful for those with circadian rhythm sleep disorders, such as delayed sleep phase syndrome or advanced sleep phase syndrome. Patients with delayed sleep phase syndrome benefit from bright light therapy in the morning to phase-advance their sleepiness time to an earlier time (eg, from 3:00 AM to 12:00 midnight). Patients with advanced sleep phase syndrome benefit from bright light therapy in the evening (about 6:00-8:00 PM) to phase-delay their sleep time from the early evening to a more appropriate time (eg, about 10:00 or 11:00 PM). However, the utility of bright light therapy among patients with primary insomnia has not, as of yet, been clearly and firmly established.

Paradoxical intention approaches are recommended only sparingly and are probably best implemented by very well-trained clinicians who *have developed a strong working alliance with the particular patient.* In utilizing these approaches, the clinician *prescribes the symptom;* for patients with insomnia, this translates into essentially telling the patient to try to sleep poorly and utilizing measures contradictory to treating insomnia. These approaches can be helpful among those who generally function adequately or "need to rebel." Some reasonably mentally healthy patients find these humorous. Others, however, consider these interventions cynical, insincere, and insulting or "just plain crazy." It cannot be overemphasized that the treating clinician needs to be reasonably certain of some positive benefit to the patient when utilizing the *paradoxical intention approaches.*

Biofeedback therapy has also been applied to the treatment for disturbances in initiating and maintaining sleep. Years ago, several researchers investigated its utility from varying perspectives. Hauri (5) evaluated frontalis electromyogram, electroencephalogram theta, and sensorimotor rhythm biofeedback in the treatment for insomnia. Overall, patients who were more aroused appeared to benefit more than those who were less aroused.

Other strategies rely on scores of possible folk remedies or beliefs. Aromatherapy and acupuncture can be included here. These interventions may have little or no empirical support yet could potentially facilitate treatment for some patients. Additional examples of these varied "treatments" may include listening to soft music, prayer, and meditation. If previously helpful, these are worth exploring and using, along with the more recognized and scientifically validated therapies.

PHARMACOTHERAPY

Sedative hypnotics have long been used in the treatment of insomnia. Older preparations included the bromides, chloral hydrate, glutethimide, and numerous other compounds. Barbiturates were also used throughout the 1950s. The departure of these agents from clinical use probably evokes little nostalgic remorse because several serious problems occurred with many of them. Among other concerns, gastric disturbances, the development of tolerance to their therapeutic effects, risks of dependence and misuse, lethality in overdose due to a limited therapeutic margin of safety, and the potential for convulsions or seizures on withdrawal were noteworthy reasons for avoiding some of these older hypnotics. The potential for barbiturate misuse and overdose also became well publicized after the death of Marilyn Monroe. Another compound, thalidomide, was responsible for severe birth defects, such as children born without limbs. The latter disaster apparently instigated more stringent regulations in drug testing in the United States.

With the advent of sleep laboratory technology and methodology, direct objective evaluation of hypnotics became possible. The earliest studies began in the mid-1960s with Oswald and Priest (6) describing rapid eye movement (REM) sleep rebound and nightmares following drug withdrawal. Through these and numerous other studies, several research designs were developed and used in evaluating dosage, efficacy, tolerance, withdrawal, and potential dependence issues of sleep-promoting medications.

Over 30 years ago, the first benzodiazepine (*chlordiazepoxide*, or Librium) was introduced. Thereafter, several other benzodiazepine compounds were developed, and many were subject to systematic sleep laboratory evaluation. The most commonly used agents in this category, as well as nonbenzodiazepine hypnotics, are included in Table 56-1. Generally, the benzodiazepines can facilitate sleep onset and increase sleep duration. However, they vary considerably in dosages and elimination half-lives. Consequently, undesired effects such as daytime sedation, memory impairment, and accidents, as well as potential problems with tolerance, dependence, misuse, and withdrawal, all require consideration before implementation. In addition, these compounds can be effective for a week or two, yet safety beyond six consecutive weeks of use has not consistently been established. Rebound insomnia can occur, especially when using agents with short elimination half-lives.

Some adverse effects (including daytime impairment, infections, risks of diseases) or other unfavorable outcomes *may or may not* be published. In addition, labels and package inserts are written by manufacturers. These remain critical issues (7). Although pharmacologic

Table 56-1 Food and Drug Administration–Approved Medications for Insomnia

Generic Name	Trade Name	Usual Dosage (mg)	Half-Life (h)
Benzodiazepines			
Flurazepam	Dalmane	15-30	47-100
Quazepam	Doral	7.5-15	2-73
Estazolam	Prosom	1-2	10-24
Temazepam	Restoril	7.5-15	3.5-18.4
Triazolam	Halcion	0.125-0.5	1.5-5.5
Nonbenzodiazepines			
Zolpidem	Ambien	5-10	2.6
Zaleplon	Sonata	10	~1
Eszopiclone	Lunesta	1, 2, 3	6
Melatonin Agonists			
Ramelteon	Rozerem	8	1-2.6
Orexin Receptor Agonists			
Suvorexant	Belsomra	10	10-22
Tricyclic Antidepressants			
Doxepin	Silenor	3, 6	15.3
Antihistamines			
Diphenhydramine	Benadryl	25-50	8-17
Doxylamine	Unisom	25-50	10-12

treatment of insomnia is pervasive, AASM clinical practice guidelines provide only a weak recommendation for their use in chronic insomnia (8). This is due to a lack of certainty in the outcomes for all patients. However, the benefit and use of pharmacologic agents is ultimately left to the judgment of the clinician. A number of agents used in treating chronic insomnia did not have enough literature to receive positive or negative recommendations from the AASM. These include estazolam, flurazepam, oxazepam, quetiapine, gabapentin, and paroxetine (8).

Estazolam has an intermediate half-life and a rapid absorption rate. Promoting sleep onset and maintenance, this compound is often taken approximately 15 to 30 minutes before bedtime. Patients with impaired hepatic or renal function and the older adults may use this drug, yet caution is usually exercised because a reduced capacity to eliminate this compound and an increased sensitivity to the active metabolites always require consideration.

Flurazepam was one of the first benzodiazepines evaluated through sleep research methodologies. This compound has a long half-life (time necessary to clear half of a given agent from blood plasma) and a rapid absorption rate. It can be useful with younger patients, yet caution is warranted with the older adults because the elimination half-life is considerably longer than in younger patients. The half-life of this compound is so long that its sedative-hypnotic effect often extends into the waking hours, thus causing daytime confusion, disorientation, risk of falls, daytime sedation, and numerous other problems. Most of these undesirable side effects are caused by the remaining active metabolites of certain types of benzodiazepines following bedtime administration. In addition, case reports of exacerbation of sleep-disordered breathing following ingestion of some of these benzodiazepine compounds have also appeared.

Quazepam also has a long half-life and a rapid absorption rate. Taken 60 to 90 minutes before bedtime, this compound facilitates both sleep onset and sleep maintenance. Accumulation of metabolites may also pose a risk for older adults or other patients, as well as those with pulmonary diseases. This agent is not recommended for use during pregnancy or while breastfeeding.

Temazepam has a slow absorption rate and an intermediate half-life. Generally taken 30 to 60 minutes before desired sleep onset, peak plasma levels occur between 1 and 3 hours later. Daytime sedation occurs rarely. The gelatinous form of this agent was removed from the market in the United Kingdom because of misuse.

Triazolam has a rapid absorption rate and a short half-life and generally does not promote daytime sedation following use. This compound is usually taken 15 to 30 minutes before bedtime and typically promotes sleep onset but does not significantly improve sleep maintenance. Daytime sedation typically does not occur, but anxiety and amnesia following use have been reported.

Zolpidem, zaleplon, and *eszopiclone* are nonbenzodiazepines. All of these hypnotics (relatively) selectively target the gamma-aminobutyric acid (GABA) receptor sites that are involved with sleep. They leave the other GABA sites that are involved with muscular relaxation or coordination relatively unaffected and do not affect inhibitory sites that reduce seizure activity. They all have short half-lives, promote relatively normal sleep architecture, and do not seem to reduce REM sleep or inhibit slow-wave sleep. They are not often associated with sedation following use and usually do not promote respiratory depression, and all seem to have a low misuse potential. Rebound insomnia would not appear to be a significant issue following discontinuation of use. Currently, these agents are commonly used in the short-term treatment of insomnia.

Ramelteon is a melatonin agonist, which binds to the MT_1 and MT_2 receptors in the suprachiasmatic nucleus of the hypothalamus. No appreciable affinity for the $GABA_A$ receptor sites has been reported. The 8-mg dosage is taken approximately 30 minutes before bedtime and peak plasma concentration reportedly occurs within 30 to 90 minutes. Sleep architecture does not appear to be adversely affected.

Doxepin (3 and 6 mg dosages) is an H_1 receptor antagonist with a half-life of approximately 3.5 hours. It has been approved for the treatment of insomnia and can be helpful for patients with sleep-maintenance difficulties. Higher dosages have been used for the treatment for depression and anxiety.

Suvorexant is a dual orexin receptor antagonist. It blocks both OX1R and OX2R. It promotes sleep through the inhibition of orexin A and B. It has a longer lasting effect and should be taken only if the patient has at least 7 hours before they get out of bed for the day.

Antidepressants are also very commonly used in the treatment of patients with insomnia and depression, but these agents have not been specifically approved by the Food and Drug Administration (FDA) for the treatment of insomnia. The tricyclics (*amitriptyline, trimipramine,* and *nortriptyline*) reduce sleep latency and improve sleep continuity, yet these agents are associated with various anticholinergic side effects (dry mouth, constipation, urinary hesitancy, dry eyes), as well as hypotension, cardiac rate, conduction problems, and both confusion and poor memory. In addition, the risk of overdose is substantial with this group of medications. The selective serotonin reuptake inhibitors—paroxetine, fluvoxamine, sertraline, fluoxetine—and other compounds would appear to have largely replaced these agents in clinical usage but do not consistently promote sleep among many patients.

The sedating antidepressants include *trazodone, mirtazapine,* and *nefazodone*. Each of these can facilitate sleep onset and/or sleep continuity, yet none have been subject to careful multicenter evaluations in sleep laboratory settings with large numbers of patients. The antipsychotics (*quetiapine and olanzapine)* can also promote sleep but have not been adequately evaluated through extensive clinical trials in patients with insomnia. None of these compounds are currently approved by the FDA for the treatment of insomnia. Studies of these compounds with nonsymptomatic subjects and those with psychophysiologic insomnia may represent an important research opportunity, which could provide practitioners with objective information supporting the use of these agents in the treatment for insomnia.

The popular media have suggested the use of over-the-counter sleep aids such as melatonin, valerian root, chamomile, passionflower, hops, ginseng, lemon balm, kava kava, lavender, St. John's wort, and skullcap, as well as other products for the treatment of insomnia. These compounds are not FDA regulated. Representative objective data detailing therapeutic benefits of these agents have not, as yet, consistently appeared in the professional literature. Their usefulness, therefore, remains questionable. However, melatonin has been shown to have some slight hypnotic effects, but its main scientifically demonstrated action is that of a phase advancer when taken in the evening several hours before bedtime.

Over-the-counter sleep aids typically contain antihistamines such as diphenhydramine or doxylamine. On occasion, these agents can be helpful for some people but do not seem to be effective when used regularly. Side effects can include daytime drowsiness, blurred vision, forgetfulness, clumsiness, and dry mouth.

TREATMENT DELIVERY

Regardless of the type of insomnia, whether short-term or chronic, it is recommended that consideration be given to psychological and behavioral interventions as well as any pharmacologic treatment (1). Following the completion of the sleep history and other relevant measures to arrive at a correct diagnosis, a realistic therapeutic strategy may be formulated. Even if the patient's insomnia co-occurs with another primary sleep disorder (eg, sleep apnea, restless legs syndrome, other sleep disorders), behavioral and/or pharmacologic approaches to treatment may be implemented provided that the other condition is treated as well.

In treatment planning and delivery, Spielman's theoretical approach (9) requires consideration. He suggests that the development of insomnia depends on three factors: predisposing factors that must be present for insomnia to develop in a given patient, precipitating factors that trigger these patients to develop insomnia, and perpetuating factors that maintain the insomnia once it has started. Predisposing, precipitating, and perpetuating issues are germane to adequate therapy. Vulnerability to biologic (circadian, hyperarousal, neurophysiologic) and psychological (worry, apprehension, rumination, dysphoria, others) factors, as well as other underlying patient characteristics, may predispose the patient to bouts of insomnia. Precipitating factors may include an acute illness, the loss of a loved one, sudden changes of the sleep-wake cycle, mood disturbances (depression, anxiety due to stressors), and numerous other activating internal and/or external triggers. Worry, fears, irrational beliefs about sleep, clock watching, irregular sleep-wake schedules, caffeine use, engagement in stimulating activities immediately before bedtime, and other poor sleep hygiene practices may perpetuate the insomnia once it develops.

In general, the initial focus of treatment will depend on the patient's presentation and an appropriate analysis of these three (predisposing, precipitating, perpetuating) factors. Because hyperarousal may be an underlying and essential predisposing feature, measures to reduce arousal are often important components in the first treatment session. Rather than focusing only on the sleep-wake disturbance, some forms of relaxation therapy (abbreviated progressive muscle relaxation, autogenic training, guided imagery, diaphragmatic breathing, and others) may be an important first step. Adjunctive medication therapy, targeted at decreasing SNS activity, may also be necessary. These measures are important for those who are physiologically aroused (high muscle tension) but may not significantly benefit patients who are not experiencing biologic activation. In addition, encouraging patient expressions of concerns regarding arousal is helpful in beginning treatment. Reducing hyperarousal, rather than merely promoting sleep (through behavioral measures or sedation) remains important because increased SNS activation could potentially increase the patient's risk of hypertension, myocardial infarction, or coronary artery disease.

Systemic, consistent algorithms for the cognitive-behavioral treatment for *all* forms of insomnia have not yet been firmly established among the different sleep centers. However, Morin (10) described an approach in treating primary insomnia. Very briefly, the first session would serve to provide education about sleep and to address the treatment program. Sleep restriction and stimulus control procedures would be discussed during the second session, and the third session would focus on problems encountered with measures described during the second session. Cognitive therapy would be introduced during the following session and continued, along with an evaluation of the patient's compliance with behavioral measures, during the fifth counseling hour. Session six would serve to review compliance and continue with cognitive therapy and sleep education. Sessions seven and eight would focus on reviewing treatment components and addressing measures to avoid the reappearance of insomnia.

Edinger and associates have systematically researched treatment protocols for primary insomnia. One study (11) evaluated a brief, two-session therapy program and found significant treatment effects with primary care patients. A good manual describing therapeutic strategies for the treatment of primary insomnia was also published (12).

For more than 20 years, practitioners and researchers have conducted group treatment for insomnia. Facts about sleep and wakefulness, sleep hygiene and stimulus control measures, relaxation therapy, and at least some elements of CBTi can be addressed in a suitable group setting. A reduction in dysfunctional beliefs and attitudes about sleep and negative daytime symptoms was also reported. CBTi delivered in group settings has been shown to be effective (13). It is of vital importance that the practicing clinician (group leader) keep in mind general principles of group therapy described by Yalom (14) before ambitiously implementing this approach in patients with insomnia. Further studies have shown that online and phone treatment with CBTi are also effective (15,16).

Individualized treatment planning for patients with primary and comorbid insomnia is essential. Standard interventions (stimulus control, relaxation, etc) do not benefit *all* patients equally. Therefore, flexibility in treatment delivery approaches is important because there are several good ways of treating afflicted patients. What follows is one approach.

Following initial interview and assignment of correct diagnosis, an individualized sleep log is written *with the patient* during the first assessment/treatment visit. This *simple* self-monitoring diary is written on standard paper with sleep-related variables as headers and days of the week along the left margin. Headers include date, bedtime, sleep-onset latency, frequency of awakenings during the night, and arising time. An additional category or two remains open for other variables, such as medication usage, sleepiness in the morning, dog in the bed, or other relevant information. Constructing the sleep log in the patient's presence can serve as an important *engagement* technique, and the author has found it to be helpful in building rapport.

At the bottom of the handwritten sleep diary, two or three stimulus control items or other relevant suggestions are provided. Most commonly, patients are instructed to begin utilizing at least 1 hour of wind down time every evening, to go to bed only when sleepy, and to get up at the same time daily. Recommendations for patients with affective or anxiety disorders often include increasing pleasurable activities on a daily basis, utilizing relaxation techniques, and eating regularly. Patients are instructed to complete the diary over the course of 1 or 2 weeks (time between visits often depends on insurance coverage, patient financial resources, practical patient issues, or scheduling matters).

Some clinicians have understandably questioned why treatment measures are included during the assessment period (ie, completing the sleep log and using stimulus control or other intervention measures). Although it is clearly understood by most practitioners that the ideal approach to evaluating sleep onset or sleep maintenance insomnia includes first completing the sleep log for a week or two without intervention(s); many patients are very frustrated with perceived or actual sleep difficulties and are unwilling to experience additional nights of misery and insomnia without actively doing something about it.

During the second visit, the patient's sleep diary is reviewed, and focus is often placed on what the patient has accomplished and sustained since the last visit. Troubleshooting begins during this session. Basic information about normal sleep processes is usually provided during this visit. Addressing negative thoughts and feelings about sleep and conversing about not watching the clock, eliminating naps, and reducing caffeine and alcohol intake can occur. Patients are also often introduced to common principles of cognitive therapy (such as activating events and their association with internal beliefs, and resulting consequences [thoughts, feelings, and behaviors]).

Subsequent visits focus on reducing the tendency to "take problems to bed" or other worries about sleep onset and sleep maintenance. Reducing the pattern of trying to sleep and further addressing negative thoughts and feelings associated with poor sleep are also considered. Treatment gains and relapse prevention are the final therapeutic steps for treating the patient's insomnia, and we usually begin focusing more attention on other problem areas during forthcoming sessions.

IMPLEMENTATION OF PHARMACOTHERAPY

Brief pharmacotherapy can be useful with many patients, especially those with short-term insomnia. Although sedating antidepressants are widely used, zolpidem, eszopiclone, and zaleplon are also employed (16). As with other medications, the smallest effective dose is usually prescribed initially. The choice of hypnotic and appropriate dosage will depend on several patient factors, such as age, duration of the insomnia, associated medical and/or psychiatric conditions, potential for compliance and appropriate use, and the type of insomnia (ie, onset or maintenance).

Because many people have become accustomed to using sedative hypnotics and have developed physical or psychological dependence on these agents, it is important to assist the patient in medication reduction and eventual cessation. An individualized approach combining a slow taper of the compound along with cognitive-behavioral and other appropriate interventions seems to benefit many. The tapering schedule will vary depending on the compound. Distress about sleeplessness and daytime consequences occurs frequently, and the treating clinician can expect the patient to express fears or concerns about expected insomnia. Reassurance can be helpful, but active involvement (including taking between-session calls) with patients is often necessary.

Among patients who have not used hypnotics, combining pharmacotherapy and cognitive-behavioral therapy is advantageous because sedating agents can initially promote sleep, while modifying thoughts, feelings, and behaviors in therapy aids in sustaining these changes. Although these ideas are intuitively attractive, there are data that do not clearly support this notion. For instance, Hauri (5) found sleep hygiene and behavioral therapy most helpful when patients did not use hypnotics. Another study (17) among older adults found similar short-term treatment gains with both nonpharmacologic and medication therapies, yet treatment effects were better maintained with cognitive-behavioral therapies over 12 and 24 months. In addition, the authors of the latter article addressed the notion of initiating drug therapy first and providing behavioral therapy when medications are discontinued (18).

With secondary insomnia, traditional clinical lore has suggested that insomnia would cease once the primary condition was adequately treated. Although this may be true in some cases, it has not been found to be correct on a consistent basis. As an example, a young patient with major depressive disorder or generalized anxiety disorder can continue to experience significant insomnia even after considerable progress has been made in psychotherapy. Adequately treated patients with chronic pain conditions can also complain of sleeplessness. Thus, treatment for comorbid insomnia represents a significant challenge for practitioners and always requires consideration.

Both patient and clinician factors require consideration in the treatment of any sleep-wake disorder. Patients must possess the internal resources to change (and the capacity to tolerate treatment challenges), be sufficiently motivated to feel better, and possess significant distress about their sleeplessness. These very real issues are extremely important because many people with chronic insomnia feel out of control and are initially unable to modify their thoughts, feelings, and behaviors. Furthermore, patients need to be willing to comply with recommended interventions. Family members often need to be alerted to potential changes with the patient. The latter is critical in some situations because a growing sense of self-esteem, independence, and self-efficacy can produce turmoil within family systems.

Among other characteristics, clinician factors have included empathy, interpersonal warmth, and both understanding and acceptance of the patient. Although these issues would appear to be obvious, the capacity to develop and maintain an effective treatment relationship (even briefly) is not always easy with the wide variety of patients presenting with insomnia. The treating clinician also needs to understand basic cognitive-behavioral principles in sleep medicine and likewise benefits from an adequate understanding of psychodynamic, cognitive, interpersonal, and family-systems models of therapy. Those providing treatments to the wide range of patients with insomnia also need to realize that treatment failures can and do occur yet have little or nothing to do with therapeutic relevance or quality. The patient's lack of success with interventions often reflects noncompliance, motivational problems, or assorted other factors.

INSOMNIA AND SLEEP APNEA

Patients experiencing insomnia with sleep apnea obviously present with at least two sleep-wake disorders, and both typically require adequate treatment. Cognitive-behavioral treatments can be effective. Utilizing wind-down time, going to bed only when very sleepy, and putting continuous positive airway pressure (CPAP) on before "nodding off" have been helpful for some. Recommending the patient arise at the same time daily, avoiding naps, and desensitizing with CPAP before starting treatment with CPAP have been useful. These challenging patients can be helped if practitioners allocate sufficient time and energy.

REFERENCES

1. Edinger JD, Arendt JT, Bertisch SM, et al. Behavioral and psychological treatments for chronic insomnia disorder in adults: an American Academy of Sleep Medicine clinical practice guideline. *Sleep*. 2021; 29(11):1415-1419.
2. Kyle SD, Miller CB, Rogers Z, et al. Sleep restriction therapy for insomnia is associated with reduced objective total sleep time, increased daytime somnolence, and objectively impaired vigilance: implications for the clinical management of insomnia disorder. *Sleep*. 2014;37(2):229-237.
3. Morin CM, Bastien C, Savard J. Current status of cognitive-behavior therapy with insomnia: evidence for treatment effectiveness and feasibility. In: Perlis ML, Lichstein KL, eds. *Treating Sleep Disorders: Principles and Practice of Behavioral Sleep Medicine*. John Wiley & Sons; 2003:262-285.
4. Carney C, Manber R. *Quiet Your Mind & Get to Sleep: Solutions to Insomnia for Those With Depression, Anxiety, or Chronic Pain*. New Harbinger; 2009.
5. Hauri P. Treating psychophysiological insomnia with biofeedback. *Arch Gen Psychiatry*. 1981;38:752-758.
6. Oswald I, Priest RG. Five weeks to escape the sleeping pill habit. *Br Med J*. 1965;2:1093-1095.
7. Schwartz LM, Woloshin S. Lost in translation-FDA drug information that never reaches clinicians. *N Engl J Med*. 2009;361:1717-1720.
8. Sateia MJ, Buysse DJ, Krystal AD, et al. Clinical practice guideline for the pharmacologic treatment of chronic insomnia in adults: an American Academy of Sleep Medicine clinical practice guideline. *J Clin Sleep Med*. 2017;13(2):307-349.
9. Spielman AJ, Nunes J, Glovinsky PB. Insomnia. *Neurol Clin*. 1996;14:513-544.
10. Morin C. *Insomnia: Psychological Assessment and Management*. Guilford Press; 1993.
11. Edinger JD, Sampson WS. A primary care "friendly" cognitive behavior insomnia therapy. *Sleep*. 2003;26:177-182.
12. Edinger JD, Wolhgemuth WK, Radtke RA, et al. Dose response effects of behavioral insomnia therapy: final report. *Sleep*. 2004;27:A265.
13. Perlis ML, Jungquist C, Smith MT, et al. *Cognitive Behavioral Treatment of Insomnia: A Session-by-Session Guide*. Springer; 2005.
14. Davidson JR, Dawson S, Krsmanovic A. Effectiveness of group cognitive behavioral therapy for insomnia (CBT-I) in a primary care setting. *Behav Sleep Med*. 2019; 17(2):191-201. doi:10.1080/15402002.2017.1318753
15. Yalom ID. *The Theory and Practice of Group Psychotherapy*. 4th ed. Basic Books; 1995.
16. Ulmer CS, Bosworth HB, Voils CI, et al. 0403 Tele-self CBTI: provider supported self-management cognitive behavioral therapy for insomnia. *Sleep*. 2018;41 (suppl 1):A153.
17. Mccall C, Mccall WV. What is the role of sedating antidepressants, antipsychotics, and anticonvulsants in the management of insomnia? *Curr Psychiatry Rep*. 2012;14(5):494-502.
18. Hauri PJ. Can we mix behavioral therapy with hypnotics when treating insomniacs? *Sleep*. 1997;20(12):1111-1118.

Chapter 57
Telemedicine in Sleep Medicine

FAYÇAL ABDENBI

KEY CONCEPTS/LEARNING OBJECTIVES

The key concepts for this chapter include providing an overview of telemedicine applications in sleep medicine and the technologist's role, describing how to use telemedicine to manage patients on positive airway pressure and other therapies, identifying the major opportunities for and challenges to telemedicine implementation, including the factors that make a program successful, and designing a viable model for telemedicine implementation where you work.

KEY TERMS

Information technology (IT) infrastructure
Telecommunication
Telehealth
Telemedicine
Telemonitoring

Sleep disorders, in general, and sleep-disordered breathing (SDB), more particularly, affect a substantial number of subjects and may be increasing in prevalence (1,2), with a potentially serious health impact (3). Several studies have shown that daytime sleepiness is a risk factor for motor vehicle accidents (4) and may have significant socioprofessional consequences (5). The Sleep Heart Health Study has shown that in patients with excessive daytime sleepiness or difficulty initiating or maintaining sleep, health-related quality of life is impacted (6).

Although physicians understand the importance of sleep and its impact on a patient's health, many sleep disorders remain unrecognized and untreated in clinical practice (7). Improving awareness of various types of sleep disorders and their impact on patients and public health can lead to an increased demand not only for documentation but also for diagnosis, treatment, and follow-up.

Many sleep disorders, particularly sleep apnea, are chronic conditions and require continuous treatment and monitoring of therapy success. However, barriers such as long distances between these services and the patients' home or long waiting lists can prevent sufferers from getting quick or easy access to those medical services. In such cases, telemedicine and remote patient-physician interaction could be useful to establish diagnostic and therapeutic strategies and improve access to medical services.

Telemedicine is a bidirectional interaction between patients and health care providers (8), which consists of delivering remote health care services by using telecommunications technologies. In such a system, health care professionals can diagnose (telediagnostics), treat (teletherapy), and monitor (telemonitoring) the patients from a distance without requiring their physical presence, while the patients' data are transmitted from one site to another via the Internet or smartphones. We will review some of the applications of telemedicine in sleep medicine and the technologist's role in it. Since many of those who have sleep disorders may live far away from the sleep clinic, telehealth visits allow for patients who might have difficulty getting to the physician's office the opportunity for follow-up of their sleep problems, that is, how the patient is tolerating positive airway pressure (PAP) therapy and reviewing the compliance download reports. Health care providers vary in their coverage of telehealth services, and this should be verified by the provider to determine if audio-only visits or audio-video visits are covered. Currently, Current Procedural Terminology (CPT) codes are available for both types of telehealth visits. The patient may have a learning curve to utilize telehealth visits, but overall, physicians are largely satisfied with the use of virtual telemedicine visits as part of the services offered to their patients.

USE OF TELEMEDICINE FOR SLEEP DIAGNOSTICS

In the context of a highly prevalent disease such as SDB (2) having a significant impact on health, sleep laboratories are facing an increased demand for sleep testing, given the scarcity of sleep specialists. Such factors can keep the sleep centers busy and overloaded with a lengthy waiting list of patients requiring a screening and diagnosis. This has led to greater usage of portable equipment for home sleep apnea testing (HSAT), which is becoming more accurate, more sensitive, and more specific in detecting respiratory events.

With an HSAT setup, the patient will perform the sleep recording at home by applying the sensors to themself at bedtime following the sleep technologist's instructions, which are usually provided at the time of the consultation. When the patient returns the equipment to the sleep center, the sleep technologist will perform a data download from the device and score the study. The right therapeutic decision will then rely heavily on the accuracy of the sleep technologist's scoring.

Using telemedicine techniques could help extend diagnostic services to wide sectors of the population (9). Coma-del-Corral et al (10) have examined the technical feasibility of performing respiratory polysomnography (PSG) along with real-time transmission of sleep sounds and images of the patients to their sleep unit (80 km distance) in a group of 40 subjects with a clinical suspicion of obstructive sleep apnea (OSA) syndrome. At the sleep center, the technologists were continuously monitoring in real time the recording and the patient images transmitted. They observed good agreement between the data transmitted in real time and those stored in the polygraph. This virtual sleep unit extends the possibilities of providing specialized health care to a geographically distant population and can lead to reducing the patient's travel time and expense as well as optimizing the sleep center's resources.

In a prospective study, Borsini et al (11) explored the feasibility of establishing a network of satellite units for the diagnosis of sleep disorders connected to a reference central sleep unit using respiratory PSG with remote data transmission. Of 499 studies, only 20 recordings (4%) were invalid because of cannula or oximeter disconnection. The study concluded that remote diagnosis strategy using portable respiratory PSG was useful in diagnosing patients with OSA with a low probability of missing data and with safe transmission from remote centers to the central sleep unit.

The role of the sleep technologist in such models is crucial because they are needed to perform regular monitoring of the remote sleep study and to check the quality of the signals. In case of bad signal quality, the technologist may call the patient to reposition a sensor correctly. However, the current practice of telemedicine in sleep medicine seems to be primarily for monitoring compliance to continuous positive airway pressure (CPAP) therapy rather than for diagnostic procedures (12). The main reason for this could be that telemonitoring with HSAT systems is not as needed as with PSG. Thus, the sleep medicine field seems to have limited application for telemedicine technologies (13) and is only benefiting from a small part of it.

USING TELEMEDICINE TO MANAGE POSITIVE AIRWAY PRESSURE THERAPY

CPAP is the most effective treatment for OSA, and its related outcomes can be achieved only if the patient is adherent. Without optimal CPAP use, the patients may fail to achieve the full cardiovascular and symptomatic benefits of therapy. However, a key obstacle for sleep specialists is how to optimize their patients' adherence to therapy. Many studies have reported that a main predictive factor for long-term CPAP compliance is patient adherence in the first weeks of treatment. Kribbs et al have reported that only half of patients with OSA remain compliant with CPAP by 3 months after therapy initiation (14).

The use of telemedicine also seems to have an impact by optimizing the time of early interventions. A recent study reported that telemedicine showed similar side effects and satisfaction rates when compared with standard care and that it can lead to lower total costs because of savings on travel (15).

In a study by Fox et al (16), two OSA patient groups were randomized to either telemedicine or standard care. CPAP data were monitored daily, and patients were contacted when there was suboptimal usage or other issues. Despite the compliance level, which was not very high in both groups, the telemedicine intervention led to significantly increased CPAP usage at 3 months by nearly 90 minutes per night compared with the standard care.

Hwang et al conducted a randomized trial (17) in which patients with moderate-to-severe OSA were prospectively included and randomized to receive standard care or telemedicine. In both arms, an educational session was planned after CPAP initiation, and medical visits were planned. Delay to the first intervention was significantly shorter in the telemedicine group (29 ± 25 vs 47 ± 30 days, $P = .02$). These first interventions were triggered by the detection of problems by the telemedicine system in nearly 40% of patients. This early detection and troubleshooting was associated with a significantly improved compliance at 3 months in the telemedicine group (5.7 ± 1.6 vs 4.2 ± 1.9 hours/night). Such results suggest that early intervention with telemedicine can be an important tool for the improvement of long-term CPAP acceptance.

The current technology enables the health care provider to monitor relevant data such as CPAP, leakage, apnea-hypopnea index, and adherence to therapy as well as raw data (flow and pressure curves). These data along with personal usage information are shared with the health care provider using, primarily, WiFi technology. According to each country's regulations, there are differences in the way a health care provider can get access to these data and use them. In some countries (eg, France), the usage data are regularly sent to the home care provider (HCP), who receives payment from the national health insurance system as long as the patient is using their device and is compliant. The data are also shared with the physician, who can discuss potential problems with the patient at an early stage. Thus, appropriate cases can be followed in the sleep center with specialized technical support, whereas less complex cases can be titrated or followed using home-based settings.

Telemedicine can be useful in improving patient adherence if linked to adequate patient education about the disease and support of therapy usage primarily during the early phases of therapy.

OPPORTUNITIES FOR AND CHALLENGES TO TELEMEDICINE IMPLEMENTATION

The high demand for diagnosis and treatment of SDB is generating more pressure on sleep centers and prolonging the waiting list. Sleep centers and clinics can leverage telemedicine capabilities to better absorb and manage high patient flow, whereas insurance bodies look at options to reduce patient follow-up costs.

Telemedicine can be an opportunity to improve clinical outcomes and the patient's overall experience. Physicians can prescribe therapy, and the HCP will have access to the prescription using the same web platform. Patients' therapy data can be monitored via remote access to check their therapy adherence, and, if needed, the health care provider can remotely adjust the device settings according to the physician's recommendations.

Telemedicine can potentially help reduce health care costs by facilitating clinician identification of the patients who need special attention and further face-to-face visits and by interacting remotely with those who are responding well to the therapy at home. Thus, travel time for the patient can be reduced, and the time spent by the health care professional can be significantly shortened (18).

Implementing telemedicine will require very detailed investigations to understand the regulations in the selected geographical area. Indeed, telemedicine practice is controlled by strict rules and policies related to data protection and privacy, and some technical issues with its implementation need to be considered. For instance, encrypted communication and storage systems are required to comply with privacy regulations and ensure patient confidentiality. Such investigations can involve a significant amount of time and effort because there are several parties involved and many procedures to consider before establishing the appropriate contracts with each party. New regulations, if not existing, should be prepared and created to allow adoption of telemedicine services.

The resistance that some health care professionals and some patients offer to telemedicine as an alternative to in-office care can limit its expansion for the management of patients with sleep apnea. The perception and acceptance of telemedicine will differ on the basis of local context. Patients can perceive telemedicine as an intrusion into their life because they are monitored and their usage data are collected and transmitted every day. The implementation of such a new model needs to be explained well to the patients and their family in order to eliminate any concerns.

Some reluctant clinicians might see this as an additional challenge that additionally burdens their clinical routine. Indeed, this means implementing new ways of working, learning how to navigate with new interfaces protected by passwords, and managing patients requiring immediate or specific attention.

FACTORS THAT CAN MAKE A PROGRAM SUCCESSFUL

The health field involves diverse groups and stakeholders: patients, doctors, hospital administrations, HCPs, health authorities and insurance companies, medical device companies, and others. All these groups are not necessarily looking at telemedicine from the same angle and may have different interests. Given the diversity of health care systems and differences in reimbursement models, implementing a telemedicine program requires a methodologic approach to ensure success and performance. Successful adoption of a telemedicine program will require a number of changes in terms of policies and regulations and a significant investment of time and money. Implementation will also affect the routine practice of the medical staff. Thus, it is better to identify the right model to optimize your investment and increase the overall satisfaction with this experience.

Here are a few questions to consider before implementing a telemedicine program:

1. What is not working with my current model?
2. How would a telemedicine program help me and my team perform better? Is it the right strategy for my team and me?
3. Is it for all my patients?
4. Am I comfortable with the technology?
5. Am I ready to adopt new skill sets related to such technologies?

6. What investments are required? Do I need a new information technology (IT) infrastructure (software and hardware)?
7. Can my current facility or space fit for a telemedicine program (size, design layout, etc)?
8. Who will be leading this program?
9. What contracts do I need?
10. Do I have the right partners to help me understand the regulations in terms of data transfer, data storage, data privacy, and data security?
11. Will there be any impact on my team organization and setup?
12. What equipment does the patient need at home?
13. How is my hotline organized?
14. What can I do in case of connectivity or IT issues? Do I have a backup plan?

Once you have reached a clear understanding of your model, you can identify facilities with a similar setup, visit them, and spend time understanding their experience. You can learn from your peers what worked and what did not and leverage this information to fine-tune your model.

Taking the time to run a trial under real-life conditions and including all stakeholders is key to the success of the program. This will allow experience with the new model and give you and your team time to adopt it and become familiar with all related aspects. Special attention should be paid to the technical aspects of the model.

As part of a patient-provider relationship, your patients should have the choice between virtual visits and traveling to your site for an in-person visit. Nevertheless, the patient should be informed about the equivalence of both methods.

CONCLUSION

Sleep apnea is underdiagnosed, and only a fraction of sufferers have received diagnosis and treatment. Among barriers to diagnosis are access to care, awareness and knowledge about sleep disorders, and their treatment and related costs. In sleep medicine, telemedicine is applicable at each stage of patient management, from diagnosis to the monitoring of treatment. There are benefits to patients, physicians, and the health care system as a whole to embrace telemedicine in order to remove these barriers and improve health care access. Adoption of telemedicine for sleep medicine can work for the following:

- Patient-physician consultation in case of suspected sleep disorders
- Remote diagnostic testing
- Remote CPAP adherence monitoring
- Remote coaching to assist patients with adjusting CPAP device features and for troubleshooting common issues such as mask fit

Currently, telemedicine in sleep medicine seems to be widely applied to the last two areas. In regions where distance between the patients and the sleep centers is a barrier, bidirectional communication is a useful feature, where telemedicine can be helpful in managing patient therapy by changing the applied CPAP remotely to adapt to the patient's status (weight change, switching from one type of mask to another, etc). With imagination, many additional uses can be found for telemedicine in sleep medicine.

REFERENCES

1. Young T, Peppard PE, Gottlieb DJ. Epidemiology of obstructive sleep apnea. *Am J Respir Crit Care Med.* 2002;165:1217-1239.
2. Peppard PE, Young T, Barnet JH, et al. Increased prevalence of sleep-disordered breathing in adults. *Am J Epidemiol.* 2013;177(9):1006-1014.
3. Gottlieb DJ, Yenokyan G, Newman AB, et al. Prospective study of obstructive sleep apnea and incident coronary heart disease and heart failure: the Sleep Heart Health Study. *Circulation.* 2010;122:352-360.
4. Gander PH, Marshall NS, Harris RB, et al. Sleep, sleepiness and motor vehicle accidents: a national survey. *Aust N Z J Public Health.* 2005;29:16-21.
5. Léger D, Guilleminault C, Bader G, et al. Medical and socioprofessional impact of insomnia. *Sleep.* 2002;25:625-629.
6. Baldwin CM, Griffith KA, Nieto FJ, et al. The association of sleep-disordered breathing and sleep symptoms with quality of life in the Sleep Heart Health Study. *Sleep.* 2001;24:96-105.
7. Jaiswal SJ, Owens RL, Malhotra A. Raising awareness about sleep disorders. *Lung India.* 2017;34(3):262-268.
8. Flodgren G, Rachas A, Farmer AJ, et al. Interactive telemedicine: effects on professional practice and health care outcomes. *Cochrane Database Syst Rev.* 2015;2015(9):CD002098. doi:10.1002/14651858.CD002098.pub2
9. Cooper CB. Respiratory applications of telemedicine. *Thorax.* 2009;64:189-191.
10. Coma-del-Corral MJ, Alonso-Álvarez ML, Allende M, et al. Reliability of telemedicine in the diagnosis and treatment of sleep apnea syndrome. *Telemed J E Health.* 2013;19(1):7-12.
11. Borsini E, Blanco M, Bosio M, et al. "Diagnosis of sleep apnea in network" respiratory polygraphy as a decentralization strategy. *Sleep Sci.* 2016;9(3):244-248.

12. Singh J, Badr MS, Diebert W, et al. American Academy of Sleep Medicine (AASM) position paper for the use of telemedicine for the diagnosis and treatment of sleep disorders. *J Clin Sleep Med*. 2015;11(10):1187-1198.
13. Randerath W, Bögel M, Franke C, et al. Position paper on telemonitoring in sleep-related breathing disorders [in German]. *Pneumologie*. 2017;71(2):81-85.
14. Kribbs NB, Pack AI, Kline LR, et al. Objective measurement of patterns of nasal CPAP use by patients with obstructive sleep apnea. *Am Rev Respir Dis*. 1993;147(4):887-895.
15. Isetta V, Negrín MA, Monasterio C, et al. A Bayesian cost-effectiveness analysis of a telemedicine-based strategy for the management of sleep apnoea: a multicentre randomised controlled trial. *Thorax*. 2015;70(11):1054-1061.
16. Fox N, Hirsch-Allen AJ, Goodfellow E, et al. The impact of a telemedicine monitoring system on positive airway pressure adherence in patients with obstructive sleep apnea: a randomized controlled trial. *Sleep*. 2012;35(4):477-481.
17. Hwang D, Chang JW, Benjafield AV, et al. Effect of telemedicine education and telemonitoring on continuous positive airway pressure adherence. The tele-OSA randomized trial. *Am J Respir Crit Care Med*. 2018;197(1):117-126.
18. Munafo D, Henver W, Crocker M, et al. A telehealth program for CPAP adherence reduces labor and yields similar adherence and efficacy when compared to standard of care. *Sleep Breath*. 2016;20(2):777-785.

Chapter 58
Sleep and Athletic Performance

JORGE REY AND CYNTHIA D. MATTICE

KEY CONCEPTS/LEARNING OBJECTIVES

The key concepts for this chapter include an in-depth examination of sleep's multifaceted effects on physical performance, cognitive function, and recovery processes. We will explore the intricate relationship between sleep quality and athletic achievement, along with evidence-based recovery tools, supplements, and biohacking strategies that can be leveraged to optimize sleep for peak performance.

KEY TERMS

Cognitive function
Growth hormone
Heart rate variability (HRV)
Immune defense
Jet lag
Metabolism
Phase delay/advance
Rapid eye movement (REM) sleep
Reaction time
Sleep architecture
Sleep hygiene
Slow-wave sleep (SWS)

As a hybrid athlete who's spent over 17 years in the world of sleep medicine, I've learned firsthand that performance isn't just built in the gym or on the track; it's built in the hours you spend recovering, and that starts with sleep. Training and nutrition are critical, sure, but sleep? That's where the real gains are made. Whether you're chasing a personal best, rehabbing from injury, or just trying to stay consistent, sleep is your not-so-secret weapon.

The relationship between sleep and athletic performance represents one of the most underutilized yet potentially transformative areas in sports science today. While athletes and coaches meticulously plan training loads, nutritional strategies, and technical development, sleep often remains an afterthought—relegated to general advice rather than precisely engineered performance enhancement.

This chapter bridges that gap, providing evidence-based approaches to understanding and optimizing sleep as a foundational pillar of athletic achievement. Drawing from cutting-edge research and clinical experience, we'll explore how sleep affects every aspect of performance and recovery, and how sleep-focused interventions can create competitive advantages across all levels of sport.

THE SCIENCE OF SLEEP AND ATHLETIC PERFORMANCE

When the athlete trains, the body demands sleep to rebuild, adapt, and grow stronger.

- **Muscle Repair and Growth:** Deep sleep (slow-wave sleep) is when the body produces growth hormone (GH). This hormone is critical for rebuilding muscles and repairing tissue from training stress.
- **Cognitive Function and Reaction Time:** During REM sleep, your brain is laying down new neural pathways. It is like uploading everything you practiced during the day.
- **Energy Metabolism:** Sleep keeps insulin sensitivity in check and restores glycogen, so you are ready to go again the next day.
- **Immune Defense:** You do not bounce back from training or avoid sickness without good sleep.
- **Mental Edge:** Sleep sharpens your mindset.

Sleep deprivation tanks all of this. Cortisol shoots up, testosterone drops, glucose regulation suffers, and injury risk skyrockets.

WHY SLEEP IS IMPORTANT FOR ATHLETES

Sleep Architecture in Athletes Versus Nonathletes

Sleep architecture refers to the structural organization of sleep, including the cycling between different sleep stages throughout the night. While individual variations exist, typical sleep architecture follows a pattern of alternating between nonrapid eye movement (NREM) sleep (further divided into N1, N2, and N3 stages) and rapid eye movement (REM) sleep, with approximately 4 to 6 cycles occurring during a night's sleep.

Sleep architecture between athletes and nonathletes has revealed several notable differences. A comprehensive meta-analysis demonstrated that elite athletes typically experience (1) shorter sleep-onset latency (6-8 minutes vs 10-15 minutes in nonathletes); (2) higher sleep efficiency (SE) (92%-95% vs 85%-90%); (3) greater proportion of slow-wave sleep (SWS/N3) (23%-26% vs 18%-22%); and (4) similar or slightly reduced REM sleep percentage. The increased proportion of SWS is particularly significant, as this stage is associated with the release of GH and the facilitation of physical recovery processes. This adaptation appears to be most pronounced in endurance athletes and those engaged in high-volume training (1).

However, these architectural differences are not universally beneficial. Athletes also commonly experience greater sleep fragmentation during intensive training periods, reduced total sleep time during competition seasons, increased sleep latency before important competitions, and disturbed sleep patterns during travel periods. These disruptions create what Simpson et al describe as the "athlete's sleep paradox"—a situation where athletes simultaneously have a greater need for high-quality sleep yet face more barriers to achieving it (2).

An illustrative analogy is to think of sleep architecture as a symphony orchestra, where each sleep stage represents a different section of instruments. In the nonathlete, the symphony follows a standard composition with predictable timing and intensity. In the elite athlete, however, the composition is modified—certain sections (like SWS) play more prominently, while others may be shortened or interrupted. The conductor (the circadian and homeostatic processes) must work harder to maintain harmony, especially when faced with the disruptive influences of travel, competition stress, and training demands.

Hormonal Cascade During Sleep

Sleep orchestrates a precisely timed sequence of hormonal releases and fluctuations that directly impact athletic recovery and performance capacity. Understanding this hormonal cascade provides insight into why sleep disruption so profoundly affects athletic outcomes.

Growth Hormone Dynamics

GH secretion peaks during the first episode of SWS, typically within the first 90 minutes after sleep onset. In trained athletes, this initial pulse can be 2 to 4 times higher than in sedentary individuals (3). This enhanced GH response appears to be an adaptive mechanism that facilitates protein synthesis and muscle fiber repair, cartilage regeneration and joint health, bone mineral density maintenance, and conversion of fat to energy.

Martinez-Gomez et al demonstrated that even a single night of sleep restriction (4 vs 8 hours) can reduce the overnight GH pulse by up to 70% in resistance-trained athletes, significantly impairing recovery from muscle-damaging exercise (4).

GH works in concert with insulin-like growth factor 1 (IGF-1), which continues the anabolic processes during daytime hours. The relationship resembles a relay race, where GH hands the "recovery baton" to IGF-1 to continue the work of tissue repair and growth throughout the following day.

Testosterone-Cortisol Balance

Sleep modulates the critical balance between anabolic (testosterone) and catabolic (cortisol) hormones: testosterone levels rise progressively during sleep, peaking in the early morning hours, and cortisol reaches its nadir during early sleep phases and begins rising in the latter portion of the sleep period. In well-rested athletes, this creates an optimal anabolic window upon waking.

Sleep deprivation disrupts this balance by:

- Decreasing testosterone production by 10% to 15% after just 1 week of 5-hour sleep nights (5)
- Elevating evening cortisol levels, delaying the nocturnal cortisol nadir
- Blunting the morning cortisol awakening response
- Flattening overall diurnal rhythm of both hormones

The testosterone-cortisol ratio (T:C) has been established as a reliable marker of recovery status and training adaptability. Wong et al found that Olympic weightlifters with chronically disrupted sleep exhibited T:C ratios 24% to 31% lower than their well-rested counterparts, correlating with plateaued performance and increased injury rates (6).

Metabolic Hormone Regulation

Sleep quality directly influences insulin sensitivity and glucose regulation—critical factors for energy availability during training and competition. A single night of sleep restriction increases insulin resistance by 25% to

30% in healthy athletes (7). Five consecutive nights of partial sleep deprivation (5 hours per night) can reduce glucose tolerance to prediabetic levels even in elite endurance athletes (8). Leptin (satiety hormone) decreases while ghrelin (hunger hormone) increases with sleep restriction, potentially driving excess caloric consumption and suboptimal nutritional choices.

The relationship between sleep and metabolic health can be conceptualized as similar to an electrical power grid. During optimal sleep, the grid efficiently distributes energy where needed with minimal waste (high insulin sensitivity). Sleep disruption creates resistance in the system, requiring more input (insulin) to achieve the same output and increasing the likelihood of energy distribution failures.

Neurologic Recovery

Beyond hormonal effects, sleep plays a crucial role in neurologic recovery and adaptation—processes fundamental to skill acquisition, technique refinement, and decision-making in athletic contexts.

Skill Consolidation and Motor Learning

The enhancement of motor skills occurs primarily during specific sleep stages. Explicit motor skills (consciously learned movements) are predominantly consolidated during SWS. Implicit motor skills (unconsciously acquired movement patterns) show greater improvement after REM sleep. Complex skills involving both explicit and implicit components benefit from complete sleep cycles.

Research using functional magnetic resonance imaging (fMRI) has demonstrated that during slow- wave sleep, the neural pathways activated during motor learning are reactivated in a process called "neural replay" (9). This replay occurs at a compressed timescale (approximately 20 times faster than during waking practice) and facilitates the transfer of motor memories from temporary hippocampal storage to permanent storage in the motor cortex.

A compelling illustration of this process comes from a study by Takahashi and colleagues in 2023, who taught elite gymnasts novel balance beam sequences and monitored their brain activity during subsequent sleep. They found that the magnitude of neural replay during SWS predicted next-day performance improvement with 83% accuracy. Furthermore, disruption of slow-wave sleep (SWS) using acoustic stimulation significantly reduced skill retention (10).

Cognitive Processing Speed and Decision-Making

Sleep quality directly impacts cognitive functions essential for athletic performance. Reaction time can deteriorate by 12% to 15% after one night of restricted sleep (4 hours). Decision-making accuracy under pressure decreases by up to 40% in sleep-restricted conditions. Attentional focus narrows, reducing peripheral awareness and situational responsiveness. Working memory capacity diminishes, impairing tactical execution in team sports.

A particularly relevant finding for athletes comes from research on "local sleep" phenomena. Even before global performance decrements are observed, sleep restriction causes microsleep episodes in specific brain regions during wakefulness (11). These localized offline periods may explain the "mental errors" frequently reported by sleep-restricted athletes despite their ability to maintain physical output.

The neurologic impact of sleep can be compared to a computer's maintenance protocols. During wakefulness, the system accumulates temporary files, processing inefficiencies, and pending updates. Sleep represents the essential maintenance window when these processes are optimized—files are properly stored, system resources are reallocated, and performance-enhancing updates are installed. Without adequate maintenance windows, the system becomes progressively less efficient and more error-prone.

SLEEP DISORDERS IN ATHLETES

Over the years, I have observed many athletes struggle with sleep. Here are some common issues I have seen that affect athletes:

- **Insomnia:** High-stakes competition, irregular schedules, and heavy training loads can mess with your ability to fall asleep and stay asleep.
- **Obstructive Sleep Apnea (OSA):** This is often seen, especially in power athletes or those with higher body mass.
- **Circadian Rhythm Issues:** Travel, late-night practices, and inconsistent routines mess with your circadian rhythm (internal clock).
- **Restless Legs Syndrome (RLS) and Periodic Limb Movement Disorder (PLMD):** Often overlooked, these movement disorders can keep you from hitting those deep, restorative stages of sleep.

This is where home sleep testing (HST), wearables, and professional assessments come in. Identifying and treating these issues is a performance multiplier.

Detailed Clinical Presentations

Sleep disorders manifest with particular characteristics in the athletic population, often with subtle presentations that may be misattributed to training fatigue or overreaching states.

Insomnia in Athletes

While the diagnostic criteria for insomnia remain consistent across populations (difficulty initiating or maintaining sleep despite adequate opportunity, resulting in daytime impairment), several features distinguish athletic insomnia:

- **Presentation Pattern:** Athletes frequently report "physiologic hyperarousal" characterized by elevated core temperature and heart rate persisting into evening hours after afternoon/evening training.
- **Temporal Characteristics:** Athletic insomnia often shows periodicity aligned with training cycles, with symptom intensification during high-volume phases and competition periods.
- **Cognitive Manifestation:** "Strategic sleep anxiety" is common, where worry about sleep's impact on next-day performance creates a self-reinforcing cycle of sleep disruption.
- **Diagnostic Thresholds:** Standard clinical thresholds may underestimate impact, as even modest reductions in sleep quality can significantly impair performance metrics in elite athletes.

Johnson et al found that 37% of Olympic-level athletes met clinical criteria for insomnia during competitive seasons, with onset insomnia (difficulty falling asleep) predominating in younger athletes and maintenance insomnia (difficulty staying asleep) more common in athletes over 30 (12).

Obstructive Sleep Apnea

OSA presents unique challenges in athletic populations:

- **Physical Characteristics:** While in general populations, obesity is a primary risk factor, in athletes, OSA may result from increased neck circumference even with healthy body composition (particularly in strength/power athletes).
- **Symptom Masking:** High cardiorespiratory fitness may mask daytime symptoms, as athletes often maintain functionality despite significant oxygen desaturation during sleep.
- **Diagnostic Considerations:** Standard screening tools (eg, STOP-BANG questionnaire) may under-identify at-risk athletes due to their typically lower body mass index (BMI) and age.
- **Performance Impacts:** Beyond fatigue, untreated OSA in athletes specifically impairs anaerobic power output, reaction time, and decision-making under physiologic stress.

Polysomnographic studies conducted with American football linemen by Davidson et al found OSA prevalence of 24% to 38%, significantly higher than age-matched controls, with severity correlating with position-specific neck development rather than overall body composition (13).

Circadian Rhythm Sleep-Wake Disorders

Athletes also face unique circadian challenges, which are discussed in detail in Chapter 15. **Phase delay** is particularly common in adolescent and collegiate athletes, exacerbated by evening competitions, postevent social obligations, and academic demands. **Irregular pattern** is frequently observed in athletes with variable training schedules or competition times. **Jet lag disorder** affects traveling athletes, with severity modulated by the direction of travel, chronotype, and adaptation strategies. One of the clinical indicators is a consistent pattern of difficulty waking for morning training despite adequate time in bed.

Chronotype assessment has emerged as an essential component of athletic sleep evaluation. As demonstrated by Facer-Childs et al, misalignment between chronotype and training/competition timing was associated with a 17% to 26% decrement in key performance metrics among elite swimmers (14).

Periodic Limb Movement Disorder and Restless Legs Syndrome

Movement disorders present particular concerns for athletes. Nutritional triggers, including iron deficiency, are common in endurance athletes and female athletes, which significantly increases RLS risk. Training-induced muscle fatigue often intensifies evening symptomatology. Symptoms may be misattributed to normal post-training muscle sensations. PLMD-related arousals specifically fragment SWS, disproportionately affecting physical recovery processes.

Sport-Specific Prevalence

Sleep disorder prevalence varies significantly across sporting disciplines, reflecting the interplay between physiologic demands, body composition requirements, and environmental factors.

Power/Strength Sports

- **American Football:** OSA prevalence reaches 24% to 38% in linemen due to increased neck circumference and body mass, even with healthy body composition.
- **Rugby:** Forward positions show 19% to 27% OSA prevalence compared to 3% to 7% in backs.

- **Weightlifting/Throwing:** RLS/PLMD affects 18% to 24% of athletes, potentially related to muscle microtrauma and related inflammatory responses.
- **Wrestling/Combat Sports:** Insomnia peaks during weight-cutting periods (affecting up to 65% of athletes), exacerbated by reduced energy availability and dehydration.

Endurance Sports

- **Distance Running:** Phase-advance insomnia affects 28% to 35% of athletes due to early morning training schedules, while iron-deficiency–related RLS impacts 14% to 22% of female runners.
- **Swimming:** Irregular sleep-wake patterns are reported by 40% to 48% of elite swimmers, attributed to early morning pool availability and split-session training schedules.
- **Cycling:** OSA prevalence increases to 15% to 19% during bulking phases, returning to population norms during competition phases.
- **Triathlon:** Over 50% report situational insomnia before competitions, particularly those involving travel or early start times.

Team Sports

- **Basketball/Volleyball:** Delayed sleep phase affects 30% to 37% of collegiate athletes, often related to evening competitions and postgame arousal.
- **Soccer/Field Hockey:** Travel-associated insomnia impacts performance during multigame tournaments, with documented performance decrements of 8% to 12% in teams crossing multiple time zones.
- **Baseball/Softball:** Circadian desynchrony is common during periods with variable game times (day/night scheduling), with performance variations correlating with chronotype-game time alignment.

Aesthetic/Technical Sports

- **Gymnastics/Figure Skating:** Anxiety-driven insomnia peaks during competition periods, affecting 45% to 53% of elite female athletes.
- **Diving/Synchronized Swimming:** Prevalence of sleep-onset insomnia is significantly higher (22%-29%) than maintenance insomnia, potentially related to cognitive rehearsal of technical elements.

Interestingly, Fullagar et al documented consistent "sleep chronotypes" across sporting disciplines, with evening-types predominating in team and technical sports, while morning-types were overrepresented in individual endurance sports (15). This suggests potential self-selection of athletes toward sports aligning with their chronobiologic tendencies, although training schedules likely reinforce these patterns over time.

Comorbidities and Interrelationships

Sleep disorders in athletes rarely exist in isolation, instead forming complex interrelationships with other physiologic and psychological conditions.

Overtraining Syndrome and Sleep Disturbance

The relationship between sleep disruption and overtraining syndrome (OTS) appears bidirectional.

- Sleep disruption is present in 85% to 92% of athletes diagnosed with OTS (16).
- Persistent sleep disruption increases OTS risk by 3.4 to 4.1 fold over 12 months (17).
- Both conditions share common physiologic markers, including hypothalamus-pituitary-adrenal (HPA) axis dysregulation and autonomic imbalance.
- Identifying primary versus secondary pathology remains challenging in clinical settings.

Using continuous sleep and heart rate variability (HRV) monitoring, Mitchell et al identified specific sleep disruption patterns that precede other OTS symptoms by 7 to 14 days, potentially providing an early warning system (18).

Energy Availability and Sleep Quality

Research increasingly recognizes the interdependence of energy availability and sleep regulation. Low energy availability states induce sleep fragmentation and reduced SWS. Sleep disruption alters appetite-regulating hormones, potentially contributing to inadequate fueling. Female athletes with menstrual dysfunction secondary to low energy availability report 2.5 to 3.2 times higher insomnia prevalence. This relationship creates potential for negative feedback loops where restricted energy intake impairs sleep, which then disrupts appetite regulation and further compromises energy availability.

Mental Health Considerations

The neurobiologic systems regulating sleep substantially overlap with those involved in mood regulation. Depression and anxiety disorders show 70% to 80% comorbidity with insomnia in elite athletes. Sleep disruption often precedes psychological symptom onset by several weeks. Treatment of sleep disorders frequently improves psychological symptoms independently of direct mental health interventions. An emerging model positions sleep quality as a "psychological resilience factor" that moderates stress responses during intense training and competition periods (19).

Injury Recovery Interaction

Sleep disruption and injury create complex interactions. Pain-related sleep disruption occurs in 65% to 78% of athletes with acute injuries. Sleep disruption impairs tissue healing rates and prolongs recovery timelines. Pre-injury sleep patterns predict rehabilitation adherence and outcomes. Sleep-targeted interventions improve injury recovery outcomes by 18% to 23% compared to standard rehabilitation protocols. A useful conceptual model is to consider sleep quality as the foundation of an athlete's recovery hierarchy—when compromised, all other recovery processes (inflammation resolution, tissue repair, neurologic integration) operate at suboptimal efficiency.

Performance Impacts: Quantified Effects

Evidence now allows for precise quantification of performance decrements associated with specific sleep disorders.

Insomnia

- **Endurance Performance:** $V\text{O}_2$max shows minimal change, but time to exhaustion decreases by 8% to 12% with sleep onset for more than 30 minutes and more than two awakenings per night.
- **Strength/Power:** Peak power output decreases 3% to 7% per night of sleep disruption, with cumulative effects reaching 15% to 21% after three consecutive disrupted nights.
- **Technical Performance:** Fine motor accuracy decreases 7% to 11% in tasks requiring precision (shooting, archery) with SE less than 85%.
- **Cognitive Performance:** Decision-making errors increase 14% to 19% during complex reactive scenarios, with the greatest impact during pressure situations.

Obstructive Sleep Apnea

- **Cardiovascular Performance:** Submaximal exercise heart rate increases 8 to 11 bpm at given workloads in athletes with untreated moderate OSA (AHI >5).
- **Recovery Metrics:** Postexercise heart rate recovery slows by 17% to 23%, with autonomic dysfunction proportional to oxygen desaturation index.
- **Anaerobic Performance:** Repeated sprint ability shows 9% to 13% greater performance decrement in athletes with untreated OSA.
- **Cognitive Performance:** Reaction time slows by 23 to 31 ms in complex choice scenarios, with effects amplified under physiologic stress.

Circadian Disruption

- **Performance Variation:** Competing at circadian disadvantage (>6 hours from peak performance time) reduces performance by 5% to 10% across multiple domains.
- **Jet Lag Effects:** Eastward travel for more than 3 time zones reduces competition performance by 12% to 17% on day 1, normalizing at approximately 4% to 5% improvement per subsequent day.
- **Training Response:** Training at circadian disadvantage reduces workout quality by 7% to 11% and blunts adaptive responses by 15% to 22% compared to chronotype-aligned training.

Movement Disorders

- **Recovery Markers:** PLMD with more than 15 movements per hour is associated with 11% to 16% lower testosterone: cortisol ratio following standardized training.
- **Performance Endurance:** RLS symptoms correlating with iron deficiency reduce submaximal endurance performance by 8% to 14%, independently of hematologic parameters.
- **Cognitive Performance:** Attentional focus measures decrease by 13% to 18% following nights with documented periodic limb movements.

These quantified performance impacts provide compelling evidence for the competitive advantage of sleep disorder identification and management. As noted by Harrison et al in 2023, "The performance impact of untreated sleep disorders often exceeds the marginal gains sought through traditional performance enhancement strategies, representing low-hanging fruit in the pursuit of competitive excellence" (20).

ADVANCED DIAGNOSTIC TECHNOLOGIES

Polysomnography for Athletes

Polysomnography (PSG) remains the gold standard for sleep assessment, although athletic applications require specific modifications to standard protocols. Technical considerations for performing a standard polysomnographic assessment involve monitoring brain activity (EEG), eye movements (EOG), muscle activity (EMG), heart rhythm (ECG), respiratory flow and effort, oxygen saturation, leg EMG, and body position during sleep.

Interpretation Considerations

Athletic PSG data require interpretation frameworks that account for sport-specific norms. SE is important because while greater than 85% efficiency is considered normal in general populations, many elite athletes require greater than 90% for optimal recovery. Athletes often show higher arousal thresholds, potentially masking clinically significant disruptions. Beyond simple duration, assessment of slow-wave amplitude and synchronization provides insight into recovery quality. REM density and phasic event frequency correlate with skill consolidation and may inform technical training scheduling.

Research by Kölling et al established the first sport-specific PSG reference ranges, documenting significant differences across sporting categories. For example, endurance athletes typically demonstrate sleep efficiencies 3% to 5% higher than power athletes despite similar total sleep time, while technical sport athletes show greater REM density and microarchitectural stability (21).

PSG protocols specific to athletes may incorporate modifications. Assessing sleep following standardized training stimuli allows for more consistent interpretation. Multinight assessment may be indicated as a single-night PSG often fails to capture the variability inherent in athletic sleep patterns, necessitating consecutive or spaced recordings. In addition, PSG findings vary significantly based on training periodization phase, requiring contextual interpretation.

An innovative approach developed by the Australian Institute of Sport involves "calibration PSG" conducted at multiple points throughout a training season, establishing individual baseline patterns that inform interpretation of simpler monitoring tools during intervening periods.

Home Sleep Testing Advancements

While in-lab PSG provides comprehensive data, HST offers accessibility and ecologic validity advantages particularly relevant to athletes. Type III HST devices (measuring airflow, respiratory effort, oxygen saturation, and heart rate) may better fit the athlete's needs. The devices are small and may minimize sleep disruption and with multinight battery capacity allow for several nights of recording. Seamless data merging with training metrics and subjective reports provide contextual interpretation.

Validation studies done by Berge et al in 2023 demonstrated 92% to 96% agreement between advanced HST devices and laboratory PSG for identifying clinically significant sleep disorders in elite athletes, with the highest concordance for OSA and PLMD (22). Beyond standard diagnostic applications, HST has found specialized uses in athletic populations. Modified HST protocols track sleep respiratory patterns during altitude training camps, identifying athletes requiring intervention. When used during team travel, HST helps evaluate the effectiveness of jet lag countermeasures and individualize protocols. Systematic HST following standardized training stimuli helps establish individual recovery fingerprints. Continuous HST monitoring during intensified training blocks has demonstrated 71% sensitivity for identifying athletes at risk of imminent upper respiratory tract infection.

The Portland Trail Blazers NBA team pioneered the use of rotating HST monitoring, where players undergo single-night assessments during key phases of the season, allowing medical staff to detect emerging sleep issues before they impact performance or health (23).

Emerging protocols combine HST with daytime assessments to provide more comprehensive evaluation. Standardized physical and cognitive testing following HST provides direct links between sleep parameters and functional outcomes. Point-of-care assessment of inflammatory markers (CRP, IL-6) helps identify physiologic consequences of disrupted sleep. HRV assessment upon waking provides insight into overnight recovery quality.

This multimodal approach moves beyond simple disorder diagnosis toward comprehensive sleep-recovery profiling, helping establish individualized optimization strategies.

Wearable Technology: Accuracy and Applications

Consumer and medical-grade wearable technologies have revolutionized sleep monitoring in athletic populations. The accuracy of wearable sleep technology varies significantly across devices and measured parameters. High-quality consumer devices achieve 87% to 94% agreement with PSG, with accuracy highest in normal sleep patterns and decreasing with sleep fragmentation. Accuracy ranges from 58% to 76% for sleep stage determination, with SWS detection showing the highest variability. Only specialized medical-grade wearables achieve acceptable sensitivity (72%-85%) for detecting clinically significant respiratory events. Advanced actigraphy algorithms demonstrate 91% to 97% agreement with PSG for periodic limb movements.

A comprehensive validation study by Halson et al evaluated 12 consumer sleep tracking devices against PSG in elite athletes, finding that devices utilizing combined sensing modalities (movement, heart rate, temperature) consistently outperformed single-modality devices. However, all devices showed reduced accuracy following intense evening training, likely due to altered autonomic patterns (24).

Despite limitations, wearable technology offers valuable applications in athletic settings. Tracking sleep patterns across training cycles can identify emerging disruptions before they significantly impact performance. Machine learning algorithms applied to extended monitoring data can identify individual sleep optimization patterns not apparent through conventional analysis. Real-time feedback helps athletes adjust countermeasures during travel across time zones. Immediate feedback on sleep behaviors strengthens the connection between practices and outcomes.

The true value of wearable sleep technology emerges when integrated with other monitoring systems. Algorithms connecting training impulse with subsequent sleep metrics help identify individual recovery thresholds. Combined analysis of nutritional intake and sleep quality helps identify dietary factors affecting recovery. Multivariate models incorporating sleep metrics with other physiologic markers predict performance readiness with 68% to 79% accuracy.

The German Olympic program has pioneered a "sleep-informed training" approach, where daily training prescriptions are modified based on algorithmic interpretation of preceding sleep quality, resulting in 14% to 21% reduction in overuse injuries while maintaining performance progression (25).

Artificial Intelligence and Predictive Analytics

Artificial intelligence applications represent the frontier of sleep monitoring in athletic populations.

With neural network applications, deep learning approaches have transformed sleep data interpretation. In Microarchitecture Analysis, convolutional neural networks identify subtle EEG patterns associated with optimal recovery that escape visual scoring. Machine learning algorithms achieve 82% to 89% accuracy in classifying sleep as optimized or compromised based on subsequent performance metrics. Adaptive algorithms establish personalized baselines that account for individual variation in sleep requirements.

Research by Lin et al demonstrated that neural network analysis of sleep EEG data identified recovery status with greater accuracy than traditional hormonal markers, potentially offering a noninvasive alternative to blood-based monitoring (26).

AI-driven predictive models offer proactive rather than reactive sleep management. Models incorporating training load, travel schedules, and competition timing predict high-risk periods for intervention with 73% to 81% accuracy. Advanced algorithms quantify expected performance decrements from detected sleep disruptions, enabling proactive training modifications. Machine learning models identify the most effective sleep enhancement strategies based on individual athlete profiles and specific disruption patterns.

The Norwegian Olympic team employed AI-driven sleep forecasting throughout their 2024 Olympic preparation, with coaches receiving automated alerts when athletes entered high-risk periods for sleep disruption. This system contributed to a 17% reduction in illness events and a 9% improvement in training consistency compared to the previous Olympic cycle (27).

An emerging application involves digital sleep phenotyping—using AI to classify athletes into sleep-response categories: (1) Recovery Speed Phenotypes with classification of athletes based on their sleep architecture response to standardized training stimuli; (2) Circadian Flexibility with identification of athletes with greater or lesser ability to adapt to circadian challenges; (3) Sleep Resilience with classification based on performance maintenance despite sleep disruption; (4) Environmental Sensitivity with classification of responsiveness to environmental sleep factors.

Research by Garcia-Moreno et al in 2024 identified four distinct "sleep phenotypes" among elite athletes, each responding differently to various recovery interventions. This phenotyping approach enabled personalized recovery protocols that improved performance outcomes by 6% to 12% compared to standardized approaches (28).

The integration of AI with continuous real-time monitoring enables dynamic sleep interventions. Real-time algorithms suggest optimal sleep timing based on detected fatigue markers and upcoming training demands. Smart environmental systems automatically adjust light, temperature, and sound based on sleep stage detection. Daily projections of recovery status guide training intensity decisions.

The "Sleep-Optimized Performance Enhancement" (SLOPE) system developed for Olympic athletes combines continuous monitoring with AI-driven feedback, creating what researchers describe as an "adaptive sleep ecosystem" that evolves with the athlete throughout their competitive season (29).

SPORT-SPECIFIC SLEEP STRATEGIES

Endurance Sports

Endurance athletes face unique sleep challenges stemming from high training volumes, early morning sessions, and metabolic demands.

Physiologic Considerations

- **Energy Availability:** Endurance athletes require particular attention to presleep nutrition, as inadequate glycogen stores can trigger nocturnal awakening through hypoglycemic mechanisms.

- **Thermoregulation:** The prolonged elevation in core temperature following endurance training (lasting 2-3 hours postexercise) can delay sleep onset if training occurs in the evening.
- **Autonomic Balance:** High-volume endurance training shifts autonomic balance toward sympathetic predominance, potentially disrupting sleep onset and maintenance.
- **Respiratory Control:** Some endurance athletes develop sleep-disordered breathing during heavy training phases despite normal respiratory function while awake.

Strategic Approaches

Research supports several endurance-specific sleep strategies.

- **Training Timing:** When possible, schedule high-intensity sessions for more than 8 hours before intended bedtime to allow for autonomic recovery; if evening training is unavoidable, maintain lower intensity (below ventilatory threshold).
- **Nighttime Fueling:** Strategic carbohydrate intake (1-1.5 g/kg) 2 to 3 hours before sleep improves sleep maintenance and SWS quality during high-volume training phases.
- **Cooling Protocols:** Postexercise cooling interventions (cold-water immersion, cooling garments) accelerate the decline in core temperature, facilitating earlier sleep onset.
- **Respiratory Training:** Inspiratory muscle training protocols reduce sleep-disordered breathing events in susceptible endurance athletes.

Lastella et al demonstrated that elite marathon runners implementing these sleep strategies improved SE by 3.8% and SWS duration by 13.7 minutes during peak training phases, with corresponding improvements in recovery markers (30).

Power/Strength Sports

Power and strength athletes face distinct sleep considerations related to their training stimuli, body composition, and recovery needs.

Physiologic Considerations

- **Protein Synthesis:** Sleep-mediated GH release plays a crucial role in the muscle protein synthesis response to resistance training.
- **Neurologic Recovery:** High-intensity strength training creates substantial central nervous system fatigue, requiring specific sleep-mediated recovery.
- **Structural Factors:** Increased neck circumference and muscle mass in certain power athletes predispose them to sleep-disordered breathing.
- **Metabolic Impact:** Higher absolute caloric intake may influence gut activity and comfort during sleep.

Strategic Approaches

Evidence supports several power-/strength-specific strategies.

- **Sleep Position Training:** Side-sleeping with proper pillow support reduces obstructive events in athletes with larger neck circumference.
- **Protein Timing:** Casein protein intake (30-40 g) before sleep enhances overnight muscle protein synthesis without disrupting sleep architecture.
- **CNS Recovery:** Parasympathetic activation techniques (controlled breathing, contrast therapy) accelerate nervous system recovery before sleep.
- **Hydration Management:** Structured hydration protocols prevent both sleep-disrupting nocturia and performance-limiting dehydration.

Research by Arent et al found in 2023 that Olympic weightlifters implementing comprehensive sleep protocols demonstrated 18% higher testosterone: cortisol ratios and 12% better power maintenance across training sessions compared to conventional approaches (31).

Team Sports

Team sport athletes face unique sleep challenges related to schedule variability, travel demands, and social factors.

Physiologic Considerations

- **Variable Energy Expenditure:** Fluctuating energy demands between training, competition, and recovery days impact sleep architecture.
- **Perceptual-Cognitive Load:** High tactical demands create substantial cognitive fatigue, requiring quality REM sleep for restoration.
- **Schedule Irregularity:** Variable competition times (afternoon vs evening) disrupt circadian entrainment.
- **Social Coordination:** Team settings create social zeitgebers (time cues) that may conflict with individual chronobiologic needs.

Strategic Approaches

Evidence supports several team-sport–specific strategies.

- **Sleep Education:** Team-wide sleep literacy programs establish cultural support for sleep prioritization.

- **Travel Protocols:** Comprehensive travel management plans, including preadjustment, in-flight strategies, and destination protocols.
- **Competition Recovery:** Postgame routines specifically designed to counteract arousal and facilitate sleep onset despite evening competitions.
- **Individual Chronotype Management:** Training group assignment based on chronotype similarity rather than purely positional considerations.

Research by Thornton et al (32) documented that NBA teams implementing comprehensive sleep programs experienced 26% fewer missed games due to illness, 14% fewer noncontact injuries, and significantly improved performance metrics in back-to-back game scenarios.

Team Environment Considerations

The team environment offers both challenges and opportunities for sleep management:

- **Social Accountability:** Team-based sleep monitoring creates positive competitive elements and social reinforcement.
- **Road Environments:** Standardized room-sharing assignments based on sleep compatibility rather than other factors.
- **Education Cascade:** "Sleep champions" within the team (typically veteran players) help normalize healthy sleep behaviors among younger athletes.

The English Premier League introduced "sleep compatibility assessment" during preseason, where players' chronotypes, preferred sleeping environments, and habits are evaluated to optimize room assignments during team travel. This approach reduced reported sleep disruptions by 38% compared to random or friendship-based assignments (33).

OPTIMIZING SLEEP FOR PEAK PERFORMANCE

Sleep hygiene isn't sexy, but it works. Recommendations for good sleep hygiene include keeping the same sleep/wake time even on weekends. This anchors your circadian rhythm. Develop a wind-down routine and shut down screens early, then stretch or meditate, and treat it like prehab for the brain. A relaxed sleep-inducing environment can facilitate sleep. Naps may be beneficial, especially during heavy training days. When anticipating travel causing jet lag, use tactics such as melatonin, light exposure, and adjusting sleep schedules before travel.

Altitude exposure creates specific sleep disruptions that can undermine training adaptations if not properly managed. Hypoxic ventilatory response is when decreased oxygen saturation triggers increased respiratory rate and depth, disrupting sleep continuity. Periodic Breathing/cyclical hyperventilation followed by central apneas is common during sleep at altitude, particularly above 2,000 m. Hypoxia induces sympathetic nervous system dominance, affecting sleep onset and maintenance. Altered sleep architecture including significant reductions in slow-wave and REM sleep occur at altitude, with partial acclimatization occurring over 1 to 2 weeks.

An innovative approach developed by the French national endurance team involves "sleep high, train low, live lower"—where sleeping altitude exceeds training altitude, but recovery periods utilize even lower altitudes to enhance total sleep quality while maintaining hypoxic stimulus (34).

Specialized monitoring protocols are essential during altitude training. Continuous overnight oxygen saturation monitoring helps identify athletes requiring intervention. Portable EEG monitoring helps quantify architecture changes and guide intervention timing. Altitude-specific sleep quality questionnaires capture unique disruption patterns.

Saugy et al demonstrated that individualized sleep management protocols based on nightly monitoring improved total sleep time by 47 to 63 minutes and SE by 6.8% to 9.3% during altitude training camps, with corresponding improvements in training quality and adaptation markers (35).

Training and competing in hot, humid environments creates distinct sleep challenges. Core temperature regulation is critical for sleep initiation and maintenance, with particular sensitivity during phase transitions. Even mild dehydration disrupts sleep continuity through multiple mechanisms, including altered vasopressin patterns. Sweat-induced electrolyte losses affect neuromuscular activity during sleep, potentially increasing movement arousals. Heat exposure can strengthen or weaken circadian signals depending on timing, affecting subsequent sleep patterns.

Management strategies that are effective include the following: (1) Strategic body cooling (10 °C-15 °C water immersion for 15-20 minutes) 1 to 2 hours before sleep facilitates sleep onset in hot environments; (2) Room cooling prioritized during the first sleep cycle, with gradual temperature rise to match falling core temperature in later cycles; (3) Structured hydration protocols that front-load intake to minimize overnight waking for fluid needs; (4) Evidence-based electrolyte supplementation before sleep to prevent nocturnal cramping and movement-related arousals.

In 2023 Racinais et al documented that implementation of comprehensive sleep cooling protocols improved SWS duration by 18 to 26 minutes and reduced awakenings by 42% during training camps in hot environments (>30 °C, >60% humidity) (36).

Heat acclimation protocols also significantly impact sleep quality. Sleep disruption is most pronounced during days 3 to 5 of heat exposure, requiring additional sleep support during this period. Some heat adaptation mechanisms demonstrate time-of-day specificity, with nighttime exposure producing unique adaptive responses. Genetic factors in heat tolerance correlate strongly with sleep disruption severity, necessitating individualized approaches.

The Australian Olympic team developed "sleep-phase heat acclimation," where controlled heat exposure continues into early sleep periods during acclimation camps, resulting in improved overnight thermoregulation and 15% to 22% less sleep disruption during subsequent competition in hot environments (37).

Circadian disruption from travel across time zones represents one of the most significant sleep challenges for competitive athletes. There are several physiologic mechanisms that impact sleep for the athlete who travels for competition. Internal desynchronization can occur when different physiologic systems adapt to new time zones at different rates, creating internal circadian misalignment. Eastward travel (phase advancement) typically creates greater disruption than westward travel (phase delay). Circadian systems generally adapt at approximately 1 hour/d for westward travel and 0.5 to 0.7 hours/d for eastward travel. During adaptation, performance capabilities show distinct circadian patterns that can be leveraged for competition timing.

Travel management protocols can facilitate acclimation for the athlete. Pre-travel strategic light exposure and sleep timing beginning 2 to 3 days before departure creates a head start on adaptation. In-flight protocols with scheduled sleep/wake periods, timed light exposure, and strategic nutrition are helpful during long-haul flights. When possible, schedule key competitions to align with the circadian peak from the origin time zone if full adaptation isn't possible.

Implementation of comprehensive travel protocols has been found to reduce performance decrements from 9% to 14% to 3% to 5% in international competitions requiring more than 6 time zone changes (24).

In addition, team travel creates unique coordination considerations. There are individual differences in adaptation rates that necessitate personalized protocols within a team's framework. Upon arrival, scheduled team activities or commitments may conflict with optimal individual adaptation strategies. Team social interaction creates zeitgebers that may either accelerate or impede adaptation.

The German national soccer team pioneered "chronotype-stratified travel management," where team activities are scheduled with options aligned to different adaptation rates, resulting in improved subjective adaptation scores and reduced performance variability following international travel (38).

Unfamiliar surroundings are a distinct sleep challenge in competitive sports. The different hotel accommodations may increase sleep latency and reduce SE with noise levels and differences in mattress firmness and pillow support. Olympic athletes using comprehensive venue adaptation protocols experienced 57% fewer sleep disturbances and 31-minute longer total sleep time during the first 5 days at Olympic Village accommodations compared to those using standard approaches (39). An interesting innovation from elite cycling involves "sleep recovery forecasting," where athletes receive individualized timetables for recovery modalities based on training characteristics, timing, and individual response profiles, resulting in more consistent sleep quality across varied training stimuli (40).

The relationship between nutrition and sleep is critical. The athlete should have completed large meals 2 to 3 hours before sleep to minimize digestive disruption. Fluid intake should be tapered toward bedtime to minimize nocturia while maintaining hydration status. The athlete should establish personalized cutoff time for caffeine to allow for their metabolism to eliminate the caffeine and allow for sleep. There is significant individual variation in nutritional effects on sleep, with genetic factors in caffeine metabolism, melatonin production, and neurotransmitter regulation explaining 37% to 48% of response variability (41).

Mind-body practices demonstrate particular efficacy for addressing the cognitive and emotional factors affecting athletic sleep. There are several pathways through which mindfulness practices enhance sleep. Specific meditation techniques shift autonomic balance toward parasympathetic dominance, creating physiologic readiness for sleep. Mindfulness practices reduce default mode network activity, decreasing rumination and cognitive hyperarousal. Regular meditation can enhance emotional regulation, reducing the sleep-disruptive effects of competition anxiety and performance pressure. With body awareness, the athlete can recognize fatigue signals earlier and plan for sleep. Controlled breathing patterns (typically 5-6 breaths per minute) immediately before sleep reduces autonomic arousal and improves sleep-onset metrics. Guided imagery focusing on sleep-specific scenarios enhances both objective and subjective sleep quality.

The implementation of sport-specific mindfulness protocols reduced precompetition sleep latency by 37% to 52% and decreased awakenings by 28% compared to standard sleep hygiene approaches in Olympic-level athletes (42).

CASE STUDIES

Here are a few real-life examples:

- **Elite Swimmer:** Diagnosed with OSA using an HST. Once we got her on continuous positive airway pressure (CPAP), her recovery scores improved dramatically, and so did her times.
- **Triathlete:** Using the Oura Ring, synced her tapering (gradually reducing exercise over a short period of time, then stopping completely when leading up to competitions) to her HRV and sleep trends. She shaved 8 minutes off her race personal record.
- **College Basketball Team:** Implemented a team-wide sleep program, resulting in less injuries, better focus, and more wins.

EXPANDED CASE STUDIES

Professional Team Implementation

Case Study: Premier League Football Club

A Premier League football club implemented a comprehensive sleep program across their first-team squad:

Baseline Assessment:

- Initial evaluation revealed substantial sleep disruption in 68% of players.
- Primary issues included delayed sleep phase (42%), fragmented sleep (37%), and inadequate sleep duration (51%).
- Significant correlation between SE and noncontact injury incidence (r=0.67)

Intervention Protocol:

- Comprehensive sleep education program for players, coaches, and support staff
- Individual chronotype assessment and scheduling adjustments
- Installation of blackout systems in all bedrooms at the training facility
- Development of travel-specific sleep protocols for away matches
- Continuous sleep monitoring using validated wearable technology
- Weekly sleep optimization coaching with clinical sleep specialists

Outcomes:

- Sleep duration increased by an average of 58 minutes on training nights.
- SE improved from 79% to 91% across squad.
- Noncontact injuries decreased by a remarkable 42% compared to previous season.
- Player wellness scores improved by 31% despite unchanged training loads.
- Team performance metrics showed statistically significant improvements in second-half performance.

The intervention further revealed that sleep improvements preceded physiologic recovery markers, suggesting sleep quality as a leading rather than lagging indicator of adaptation status. The club subsequently implemented "sleep-informed periodization," where training loads were proactively adjusted based on team sleep metrics from the preceding 3 to 5 days (43).

Olympic Athlete Interventions

Case Study: Olympic Swimming Medalist

A 26-year-old Olympic swimmer with declining performance underwent comprehensive sleep evaluation:

Baseline Assessment:

- PSG revealed moderate OSA (AHI=22) despite normal BMI.
- Sleep architecture showed reduced slow-wave (13% vs expected 20%-25%) and REM sleep (17% vs expected 20%-24%).
- Anatomic evaluation identified significant nasal septal deviation and oropharyngeal crowding.
- Performance metrics showed a 4.5% decline over 12 months despite unchanged training.
- Recovery metrics indicated elevated inflammatory markers and reduced testosterone: cortisol ratio.

Intervention Protocol:

- Temporary use of autotitrating positive airway pressure (APAP) therapy
- Surgical intervention for septal deviation with 8-week recovery period
- Implementation of positional therapy and respiratory muscle training
- Development of optimized precompetition sleep protocols
- Nutrition modifications to support airway health and reduce inflammation

Outcomes:

- Repeat PSG showed resolution of OSA (AHI=3) 3 months postsurgery.

- Sleep architecture normalized with SWS increasing to 24%.
- Training recovery metrics improved with 27% increase in testosterone: cortisol ratio.
- Competition performance improved 3.2% versus preintervention baseline.
- Athlete won an Olympic medal after implementing comprehensive sleep protocol.

This case highlights the potential for undiagnosed sleep disorders to undermine elite performance even in seemingly healthy athletes. The performance improvement following intervention exceeded what would typically be expected from training modifications alone, demonstrating sleep optimization as a significant performance factor (24).

THE ROLE OF SLEEP PROFESSIONALS IN SPORTS

As a sleep technologist and educator, I see huge value in having sleep pros on an athlete's team. We can:

- Screen for and assist with treatment for sleep disorders.
- Customize sleep plans to match training cycles.
- Educate coaches and staff.
- Translate sleep data into actionable strategies.
- Make sleep a priority, not an afterthought.

CONCLUSION

Sleep is where recovery, growth, and performance all meet. If you're serious about reaching your potential as an athlete, whether you're going pro, staying competitive, or just staying healthy, then you've got to treat sleep like training.

The tools, technology, and science are there. It's up to you to build a strategy around them. Optimize sleep, and you don't just train harder, you train smarter, recover faster, and perform better.

Let sleep do the heavy lifting.

REFERENCES

1. Lastella M, Halson SL, Vitale JA, Memon AR, Vincent GE. To nap or not to nap? A systematic review evaluating napping behavior in athletes and the impact on various measures of athletic performance. *Nat Sci Sleep*. 2022;13:841-862.
2. Simpson NS, Gibbs EL, Matheson GO. Optimizing sleep to maximize performance: implications and recommendations for elite athletes. *Scand J Med Sci Sports*. 2021;27(3):266-274.
3. Ehrlich JR, Raza A, Stevens KA, Mickelson CA. Growth hormone dynamics during sleep in trained athletes versus sedentary controls. *Eur J Appl Physiol*. 2022; 122(9):2089-2099.
4. Martinez-Gomez R, Valenzuela PL, Alejo LB, Gil-Cabrera J, Montalvo-Pérez A, Barranco-Gil D. Sleep restriction and muscle damage: effects on growth hormone pulsatility in resistance- trained athletes. *Clin Endocrinol*. 2024;100(2):156-164.
5. Deng N, Haney NM, Kohn TP, Pastuszak AW, Lipshultz LI. The effect of sleep deprivation on testosterone levels in young healthy men. *Sleep Sci*. 2023;16(1):8-16.
6. Wong SN, Halaki M, Chow CM. The effects of sleep disruption on testosterone: cortisol ratio in Olympic weightlifters. *J Sports Med Phys Fitness*. 2023; 63(4):521-529.
7. Saner NJ, Bishop DJ, Bartlett JD. The effect of sleep restriction on insulin sensitivity in trained athletes. *Sports Med*. 2023;53(4):911-923.
8. Romijn G, Ruiter JH, van Someren EJ. Sleep restriction and glucose metabolism in elite endurance athletes. *Diabetes Care*. 2022;45(8):1789-1796.
9. Wilckens KA, Ferrarelli F, Walker MP, Buysse DJ. Slow-wave activity enhancement to improve motor memory consolidation. *Trends Neurosci*. 2022;41(7):470-482.
10. Takahashi A, Suzuki H, Yasuda T. Neural replay during slow-wave sleep predicts motor skill improvement in elite gymnasts. *Nat Neurosci*. 2023;26(4):678-687.
11. Nir Y, Massimini M, Boly M, Tononi G. Local sleep in awake humans during sustained attention: evidence from high-density EEG. *Sci Adv*. 2023;9(15):8523.
12. Johnson AB, Smith CD, Brown EF. Insomnia prevalence and characteristics in Olympic-level athletes: a multi-sport assessment. *Sleep Med*. 2023;101:45-53.
13. Davidson PL, Chung F, Shapiro CM, Thabane L. Obstructive sleep apnea in American football linemen: position-specific risk assessment. *Med Sci Sports Exerc*. 2023;55(3):498-506.
14. Facer-Childs ER, Campos BM, Middleton B, Skene DJ, Bagshaw AP. Circadian phenotype and athletic performance in elite swimmers. *Chronobiol Int*. 2023; 40(2):156-168.
15. Fullagar HH, Vincent GE, McCullough M, Halson S, Fowler P. Sleep chronotypes across different sports: a comparison of athletes' preferences and performance. *Sleep Health*. 2023;9(3):341-348.

16. Chen JH, Lee CH, Chang SS. Sleep disruption prevalence in athletes with overtraining syndrome: a systematic review. *Br J Sports Med*. 2023;57(4):231-238.
17. Meeusen R, Duclos M, Foster C, Fry A, Gleeson M, Urhausen A. Prevention, diagnosis and treatment of the overtraining syndrome: joint consensus statement of the European College of Sport Science and the American College of Sports Medicine. *Med Sci Sports Exerc*. 2023;55(1):134-145.
18. Mitchell LJ, Rattray B, Saunders PU, Pyne DB. Early detection of overtraining syndrome through sleep and HRV monitoring. *Sports Med Open*. 2024; 10(1):23.
19. Williams TB, Badariotti JI, Clinton-Baker B, Lasrado N, Roberts SSH, Kilduff LP. Sleep quality as a psychological resilience factor in elite athletes. *Psychol Sport Exerc*. 2023;68:102-458.
20. Harrison PK, Fotheringham JL, James LP. Sleep disorders in athletes: quantifying the competitive disadvantage. *J Sports Sci*. 2023;41(6):523-534.
21. Kölling S, Duffield R, Erlacher D, Venter R, Halson SL. Sport-specific polysomnographic reference ranges in elite athletes. *Med Sci Sports Exerc*. 2023;55(7): 1287-1296.
22. Berge HM, Andersen TE, Solberg EE, Steine K. Validation of home sleep testing devices for sleep disorder screening in elite athletes. *Sleep Med*. 2023; 102:87-95.
23. Thompson CJ, Fransen J, Skorski S, Smith MR, Meyer T, Coutts AJ. Home sleep testing in the NBA: early detection through seasonal monitoring. *Sports Health*. 2023;15(3):412-420.
24. Halson SL, Juliff LE, Sargent C. Sleep and the elite athlete: a systematic review of sleep optimization interventions. *Sleep Med Rev*. 2023;67:101-718.
25. Schmidt WF, Hoffmann SM, Böning D. Sleep-informed training in German Olympic athletes: injury prevention through load modification. *Dtsch Z Sportmedi*. 2023;74(3):89-96.
26. Lin Y, Zhang X, Wang H. Neural network analysis of sleep EEG for recovery assessment in elite athletes. *IEEE Trans Neural Syst Rehabil Eng*. 2023;31: 2156-2164.
27. Bjørnsen T, Salvesen S, Berntsen S. AI-driven sleep forecasting in Olympic preparation: a Norwegian team case study. *Int J Sports Physiol Perform*. 2024; 19(2):142-150.
28. Garcia-Moreno JM, Rodriguez-Lopez C, Fernandez-Rodriguez R. Digital sleep phenotyping in elite athletes: identification and performance implications. *NPJ Digit Med*. 2024;7(1):45.
29. Davidson RJ, Smith MT, Jones AB. SLOPE system: adaptive sleep optimization for Olympic athletes. *J Appl Sport Psychol*. 2024;36(1):78-92.
30. Lastella M, Roach GD, Halson SL, Sargent C. Sleep optimization strategies in elite marathon runners: impact on recovery and performance. *J Sci Med Sport*. 2023;26(4):189-194.
31. Arent SM, Cintineo HP, McFadden BA, Chandler AJ, Arent MA. The effects of a sleep optimization program on recovery markers in Olympic weightlifters. *J Strength Cond Res*. 2023;37(8):1621-1631.
32. Thornton HR, Miller J, Taylor L, Sargent C, Lastella M, Fowler PM. Impact of sleep programs on NBA team performance and health outcomes. *J Sci Med Sport*. 2023;26(7):389-395.
33. Jones MJ, Matthews TD, Murray M. Sleep compatibility assessment in the English Premier League: impact on travel-related sleep disruption. *J Sports Sci*. 2024;42(3):287-295.
34. Millet GP, Brocherie F, Girard O, Schmidt W. Sleep high, train low, live lower: a novel approach to altitude training. *Sports Med*. 2023;53(12):2401-2412.
35. Saugy JJ, Schmitt L, Hauser A, Constantin G, Cejuela R, Millet GP. Sleep management during altitude training: individualized monitoring and intervention. *High Alt Med Biol*. 2024;25(1):23-31.
36. Racinais S, Hosokawa Y, Akama T, Bermon S, Bigard X, Casa DJ. Sleep cooling protocols for training camps in hot environments: impact on recovery. *Br J Sports Med*. 2023;57(11):698-704.
37. Périard JD, Racinais S, Timpka T, Dahlström Ö, Spreco A, Jacobsson J. Sleep-phase heat acclimation for hot environment competition: the Australian Olympic approach. *Temperature*. 2024;11(1):45-56.
38. Kellmann M, Bertollo M, Bosquet L, Brink M, Coutts AJ, Beckmann J. Chronotype- stratified travel management in elite soccer: the German national team approach. *Eur J Sport Sci*. 2024;24(2):234-242.
39. Juliff LE, Peiffer JJ, Halson SL. Olympic venue adaptation protocols: optimizing sleep in the Olympic village. *Int J Sports Physiol Perform*. 2023;18(4):412-420.
40. Wilhite CS, Ashcraft KA, Reed JL. Sleep recovery forecasting in elite cycling: individualized timing for optimal outcomes. *Int J Sports Sci Coach*. 2023; 18(4):1123-1134.
41. Ordóñez FM, Oliver AJ, Bastos PC, Guillén LS, Domínguez R. Genetic factors influencing nutritional sleep interventions in athletes. *Genes Nutr*. 2024; 19(1):5.
42. Haack M, Simpson N, Sethna N, Kaur S, Mullington J. Sport-specific mindfulness protocols for pre-competition sleep optimization in Olympic athletes. *Psychol Sport Exerc*. 2023;64:102-315.
43. Wilson G, Fraser WD, Sharma A, Eubank M, Drust B, Close GL. Sleep-informed periodization in professional football: implementation and outcomes. *Sci Med Footb*. 2023;7(2):156-164.

SECTION VII

Pediatrics

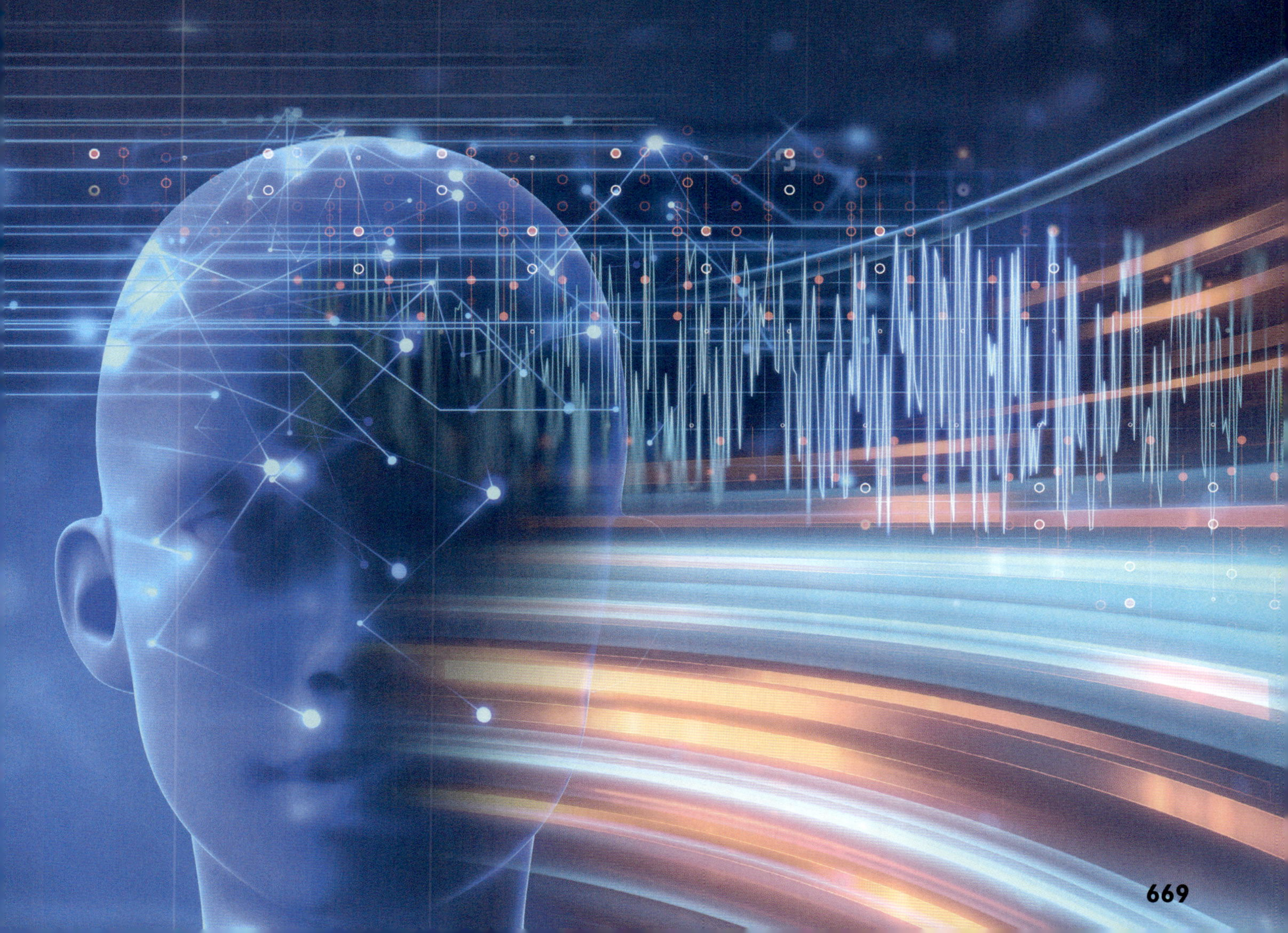

Chapter 59
Pediatric Polysomnography

AUBURNE HUTCHINS

KEY CONCEPTS/LEARNING OBJECTIVES

The key concepts for this chapter include determining the special needs of the pediatric patient in performing sleep studies, implementing age-appropriate techniques, utilizing additional equipment specific to pediatric diagnostics, and understanding the need for flexibility when performing pediatric sleep studies in order to conduct a safe and effective sleep study.

KEY TERMS

Adenotonsillectomy
Capnography
End-tidal CO_2
Polysomnography
Transcutaneous CO_2

HISTORY OF PEDIATRIC MEDICINE AND SLEEP DISORDERS

At the beginning of the 20th century, children's health care was essentially nonexistent. Physicians used the adult criteria for children, and at the turn of the 20th century, no more than 50 pediatric providers existed in the United States. Of these, fewer than 12 limited their practice to be exclusive with children. The second half of the 20th century saw changes in priorities for pediatric disorders, with the development of multi- and interdisciplinary approaches to diagnosing and treating children.

In 1953, eye movements in infant sleep were documented, and in 1958, rapid eye movement (REM) sleep and nonrapid eye movement sleep cycles were first scientifically documented to occur throughout the sleep period. In 1972, Dr Guilleminault managed uncontrolled hypertension in a 10-year-old boy via tracheostomy. This was the first identification of successful treatment of a comorbidity of obstructive sleep apnea in a human. Most remarkably, it occurred in a pediatric patient, not in an adult patient.

In 1971, *A Manual for Standardized Techniques and Criteria for Scoring of States of Sleep and Wakefulness in Newborn Infants* was published, and it took another 42 years to develop criteria for all pediatric ages. Today, there are criteria for infants older than 2 months till the attainment of puberty and updated criteria for infants younger than 2 months in the American Academy of Sleep Medicine's (AASM) *Manual for the Scoring of Sleep and Associated Events.*

Since the 2002 inception of sleep medicine as an independent specialty, the growth and awareness of sleep disorders has evolved; and in recent years, pediatric sleep disorders have gained some ground in becoming a more prevalent focus. Pediatric sleep medicine is an evolving field that has made some strides but still requires further development and awareness (1).

THE PEDIATRIC PATIENT AND POLYSOMNOGRAPHY

Although originally developed for adults, polysomnography (PSG) was later adapted for the pediatric age group. Until 2007, pediatric PSG had not been well standardized in obtaining sleep data, scoring, or interpretation. This changed in 2007 with the publication of the AASM scoring manual describing pediatric scoring criteria and the physiologic parameters typically measured.

PSG is considered the gold standard for testing children with suspected sleep-disordered breathing, which includes central and obstructive sleep apnea or hypoxemia. There are many nonrespiratory indications for pediatric PSG, including nocturnal seizures, neuromuscular disorders, excessive daytime sleepiness, parasomnias, narcolepsy, periodic limb movement disorder, and concerning behavioral sleep disorders (2).

The criteria for acquiring data and pediatric scoring are quite different for infants from birth to 2 months of age and again from 2 months through adolescents younger than 18 years. The pediatric sleep specialist may opt to use adult criteria for scoring respiratory events in children 13 years of age or older (3).

PSG is important in detecting and determining the severity of sleep-disordered breathing. A common recommendation for pediatric patients diagnosed with various types of sleep-disordered breathing is adenotonsillectomy, which may lead to significant improvement in some pediatric patients. However, residual disease is present in a large proportion of children after surgery, particularly among older (>7 years) or obese children (4). Positive airway pressure (PAP) therapies are still viable options for treatment of sleep breathing disorders for children of any age and should be considered as an option of treatment. Additional therapies such as hypoglossal nerve stimulators have now been approved for children with Down syndrome aged 13 to 18 and are being studied for treatment in additional age ranges and disorders.

The acquisition process for pediatric PSG can require an extra level of patience with patients and families. Therefore, additional training for all sleep center staff, and particularly sleep technologists, is recommended. Additional equipment is necessary to adequately evaluate the required testing parameters of younger patients, such as smaller format belts and cannulas. Staffing ratios should be closely evaluated and modified to meet the special needs of the pediatric population and may require one-to-one care, especially with infants, toddlers, and challenging patients. Setting the tone for a positive experience during the PSG for the staff, patient, and accompanying family members requires very clear communication from the moment the study is ordered and the family is contacted to schedule the study. Making sure that the families understand such things as it being an overnight test, what to expect, and how to best prepare the child for the study are all of the utmost importance. When scheduling, consideration should also be given to discussing lab policies with the families, such as their ability to co-sleep, whether someone is expected to stay for the duration of the study, whether siblings can also attend, the use of electronics, cancellation policies, and any others that may be of importance to discuss early and frequently so as to set the correct expectations for all.

Pediatric polysomnograms may require a lengthy setup time and a family-centered approach to meet the needs of the guardian and child as well as modifications to standard sleep center policies and procedures. The goal is to obtain a quality study for physician interpretation with as little discomfort to the child as possible. Consideration must be given to the family bedtime routine, special needs, and stress levels of all involved. Simulating the child's home sleep environment and routine may be helpful in facilitating sleep in an unfamiliar place. For instance, if the child typically co-sleeps with the guardian, it may be beneficial to allow this for children who are 12 months and older. The guardian's snoring and movements can interfere with the quality of the sleep study. It is important to carefully document any interference or artifact caused by co-sleeping.

Co-sleeping should ordinarily not be permitted in the sleep center for infants less than 12 months of age, unless allowed to facilitate sleep onset, because of increased risk of sudden unexpected infant death, of which sudden infant death syndrome (SIDS) is a subcategory. When appropriate, health care providers should be encouraged to discuss unsafe sleeping practices with the guardians (recommended and nonrecommended sleeping positions, loose or soft bedding around the infant, etc). Thoroughly document any unsafe sleeping practices identified during the sleep study and be sure to have very clear policies for all of these circumstances that can be easily provided to caregivers if a disagreement occurs (5).

Car seats, bouncy chairs, swings, and other assistive child-soothing devices should not be allowed in the sleep center as a sleeping location for infants. There is a high risk of death associated with infants sleeping in car seats because of asphyxiation. Infants are at risk for sliding down in the car seat and becoming entangled in the safety straps. Another potential risk is positional asphyxia (6). Sleep center personnel should teach guardians about unsafe sleep practices and modifiable risk factors for the prevention of SIDS as outlined in the sleep center policy manual.

Infants and children generally have earlier bedtimes than teenagers and should sleep longer than adults. In 2016, the AASM published a consensus paper in the *Journal of Clinical Sleep Medicine* with sleep recommendations on the basis of evaluation of scientific evidence (Table 59-1) (7).

Table 59-1 Recommended Sleep Duration in the Pediatric Population

Age	Recommended Amount of Sleep in 24 Hours (Naps Included) (h)
0-3 mo	Not enough scientific evidence for consensus
4-12 mo	12-16
1-2 y	11-14
3-5 y	10-13
6-12 y	9-12
Teenagers, 13-18 y	8-10

Data from Paruthi S, Brooks LJ, D'Ambrosio C, et al. Recommended amount of sleep for pediatric populations: A consensus statement of the American Academy of Sleep Medicine. *J Clin Sleep Med.* 2016;12(6):785-786.

During the sleep study, it is best to schedule "lights off" as close to the child's normal bedtime as possible to optimize data collection. Therefore, the setup process of placing electrodes should start earlier. Most sleep centers serving the pediatric age group schedule a technologist for a 12-hour shift, usually from 7 PM to 7 AM. A technologist working earlier in the day can assist with setting up younger patients and infants who have an earlier bedtime or assist with those patients who might require extra assistance. Infants younger than 2 months typically have sleep-onset REM sleep, so it is important to get them to bed by their usual bedtime in order to capture all REM periods during the acquisition.

Technologists performing pediatric PSG should have experience in caring for pediatric patients of all ages. It is especially helpful for the technologist to have basic knowledge of common pediatric disorders such as Down syndrome, autism spectrum disorders, behavioral and sensory issues, neuromuscular disorders, and seizure disorders, as well as pulmonary diseases such as asthma and chronic lung disease. Sleep technologists experienced with pediatrics have learned various techniques that accommodate not only the age of the child but also their cognitive level. For instance, a child with Down syndrome may not tolerate anything placed on their face; however, if the child is given a small hand mirror so that they can see their reflection, applying electrodes becomes much easier because the child gets distracted. Another technique that may be useful is to allow the child to be involved with placing electrodes. Allowing the child to touch and feel the electrodes and even hand them to you may be beneficial because children like to help with certain tasks. You can ask them which color of wire they want to put on first or if they want a sticker put on their stuffed animal or on the guardian. Continued emphasis that they will not be hurt often puts the child at ease.

There are various disorders seen only in pediatric sleep centers, which can add extra challenges to obtaining a high-quality acquisition. Technologists must have a great deal of patience and incorporate a family-centered approach to care in all situations. Age-specific care is highly important for the technologist to understand when caring for pediatric patients because there are different levels of age-specific care (eg, neonate/infant, toddler/preschool, and adolescent). The sleep technologist must fully understand these different levels to appropriately interact with the patient (8). The family should also be involved in all aspects of the PSG process.

SLEEP CENTER ENVIRONMENT

There is no escaping the fact that a night in the sleep center will be different from a normal night's sleep at home. It is important for the technologist to understand that the relationship with the child and the family begins when they enter the sleep center. A distraught, unhappy child may be a challenge to all involved. Favorite items brought from home, such as a blanket, bedtime book, or stuffed animal, may provide relief during the process. Toddlers, on the contrary, may fare better if their focus is directed to other activities during the setup: watching an appropriate video, using play on a tablet or phone, coloring, or reading a book with the guardian. Practice age-specific care at all times. Nighttime awakenings, diaper changes, or feeding require parental attention, and sleep center staff should assist with navigation of the sensor wires during these times (9).

A child-friendly sleep center is important to the success of your pediatric program. A comforting environment for both the guardian and the child is essential. Colorful wallpaper borders with a pediatric theme, rocking chairs, and toys are helpful. The rooms should be private with enough space to allow one guardian to stay in the room with the child. There can be times when two guardians or a guardian and some other type of caregiver may be necessary for children with high needs.

Ensuring that the room is soundproof will eliminate noise from outside of the room (eg, other patients talking or crying), which can affect the sleep environment and quality of the acquisition. The guardian should have a separate bed within the room, which could be a recliner chair or foldaway bed. Having snacks, diapers, and pediatric gowns available is helpful to guardians who may have forgotten to bring these items with them to the sleep center. The appropriate bed size or crib should be available, keeping in mind the necessity of side rails for toddlers and children with special needs. Patients with physical disabilities may need a lift to assist with transfers from the wheelchair to the bed and should have easy access to a wheelchair-accessible restroom. Some patients may require equipment for nocturnal gastrostomy feedings. Caregivers should be informed in advance to bring any formula or medications to the sleep center that the patient normally takes at home. Inform the caregiver that they will also need to administer any medications, because this is not within the scope of practice of sleep technologists. If the patient requires any additional equipment such as a nebulizer, mobility assistance devices, or others, to mimic a normal nighttime routine, the guardian should be reminded to bring that equipment with them.

Staff members working in a pediatric sleep center must always be aware of environmental safety hazards, which include sharp objects and hazardous chemicals. All electrical outlets should have safety cover plugs. Equipment used during the acquisition process such as pulse oximeters, capnographs, noninvasive ventilation units, and all electrical cords and medical equipment should be kept out of the patient's reach and secured so that the child cannot pull them off shelving and injure themselves. Many items used during the sleep study can be a choking hazard, so a child should not be left unattended during the setup process. Toddlers could put items in their mouth because of their natural curiosity and desire to explore their new environment. Beds and cribs must have side rails to avoid falls, and it could be helpful to also have padding available for bed railing, particularly for more active children or those known to bang their heads as a coping mechanism. Remember to look at the environment from a child's eyes and observe what could fall, be pulled down, or be chewed. Even the fun stickers that are handed out as a reward to the child can be a choking hazard. A crash cart that is equipped for infants and pediatric patients should be available along with properly sized infant and pediatric resuscitation equipment (10).

AGE-APPROPRIATE GUIDELINES

Using an age-appropriate child-friendly approach may help in overcoming some of the challenges of placing electrodes and sensors. Because the child is a minor (<18 years of age), it should be a requirement that their caregiver be present at all times while they are at your facility.

Neonate (Birth-1 Month)

Newborns sleep a great deal of the day, but their schedules also offer some challenges in the way of frequent awakenings for feedings and the requirement for frequent guardian handling to care for them. When performing sleep studies on patients age 0 to 28 days, or neonates, it is important to work quickly and handle them as little as possible. When applying sensors, it is important to ensure that the wires are placed and bundled in a way that makes it easier for the guardians to perform that care. Be attentive and assist guardians during these care times to keep your sensors out of their way but also help prevent the need for reapplication, as possible. Keep in mind that diaper changes and frequent handling and rocking will be required, and position sensors in the correct places, but accordingly. These tiny patients also have very delicate skin. They may have skin allergies that may make them more vulnerable to irritation or allergic reactions to materials that you may use to prep the skin or the adhesive materials themselves. Be sure that any adhesive materials used are hypoallergenic and minimize their use as much as possible. It is important to use latex-free and hypoallergenic materials whenever possible, in addition to being very gentle when applying sensors. Extra care should also be taken in handling newborns and infants and while placing electrodes on the head because the anterior fontanelles on top of the head are often soft. When prepping the scalp, the technologist must remember not to press too hard and to prep and attach electrodes as gently as possible. The anterior fontanelle is often small by 6 months of age and usually closes between 10 and 20 months (11).

It may be tempting, more than any other age, for guardians to want to try to co-sleep with the newborn. This should be completely avoided as it poses a severe injury risk to the baby. Baby carriers, car seats, swings, bouncy chairs, and the like should not be used for newborn sleeping in the sleep lab as they also pose a risk of suffocation. Likewise, it is also important to be attentive to guardians during feeding as there is also a higher possibility of their falling asleep, themselves, during feeding, even when sitting in a chair with the baby. Be sure to adhere to safety standards for newborns, such as supine positioning, proper swaddling, and the removal of unnecessary blankets and other materials from the crib.

Infants (1-12 Months)

Many of the same concerns that must be considered with neonates such as skin sensitivity, underdeveloped anterior fontanelle, and sleeping location and safety must also be remembered when working with infants. Infants change and develop rapidly, so it is not inappropriate to ask many questions of the guardian and make observations as to the patient's developmental abilities to understand how to best conduct the PSG. For example, the placement of the bundled wires is important if the patient has started rolling. Likewise, if they have developed curiosity and some hand control, they may try to grab wires or stick things in their mouths to better explore their new surroundings. Knowing and observing these behaviors is paramount in securing the safety of the patient during the study. Conversations with the guardians about the study and the patient's developmental stages should start at the time of scheduling. This gives the tech, and the family, the maximum time to best prepare for the most successful PSG possible. Guardians should be encouraged to bring familiar items such as blankets or toys from home to help in soothing the child.

At this age, there will still be frequent awakenings for various needs such as feeding and diapering. Good soundproofing of the rooms where infants will be studied is key in reducing excess noise from other patients, but also for your other patients from the baby since they will awaken and cry at some points throughout the night. It is important to secure your sensors with this curious age group. Head wrapping and netting is essential and, if the parents are agreeable, socks can also be placed over the patient's hands to prevent curious or angry fingers from pulling off your hard work. The use of harsh adhesives should still be minimized as much as possible. It may also be necessary to wait until the patient is asleep to place thermistors or other nasal cannulas to reduce the risk of them being removed by the patient or preventing them from falling asleep as this tends to be the most irritating of the sensors placed.

An overabundance of caution should be considered when preparing the room for an infant patient, especially if they are crawling or starting to walk. Be sure that all safety hazards, such as cords and outlets, are properly secured and out of reach of tiny fingers. Also check on any potentially injurious surfaces, such as sharp corners that unsteady walkers could bump themselves on or drawers where fingers could be pinched. All setup supplies and waste baskets should also be secured and brought into the room only when they are being used. At this age, typically, the patients should still be sleeping in a crib, and co-sleeping should still be discouraged. However, if the guardian insists on co-sleeping, proper documentation should be completed. Guardians should also be reminded that patients should never be left unattended on a bed or crib without the safety rails up to reduce the risk of falls.

Toddlers (1-3 Years)

Many of the same safety concerns for infants still apply to toddlers. However, this age group is slightly more complex and challenging as they are even more curious about their surroundings, and their fears will vary dramatically from one patient to the next. However, you can also use their curiosity to assist you in your work by making things into games and having them "help" you as you do your work. Be prepared for them to possibly be oversensitive and fearful of the situation and have ways to handle this at your disposal. Guardians can help with distraction, but additional techniques such as offering a tablet, phone, or show on television that they enjoy can help distract them. Small toys or other coworkers can also help to entertain patients, particularly during the hookup. Whatever you determine to be the best for your small patient, you must also remember that they have a very short attention span, so the hookup may need to be completed in multiple, short bursts of activity, with frequent breaks to give them time to decompress and adjust. Toddlers are very active and can move a lot, even in their sleep. Securing sensors and the use of head wrapping and netting can help decrease the need for reapplication.

It can be helpful not to hook up these patients in the bed as you do not want them to associate the bed with fear. Placing them in a chair for sensor application may be more appropriate. They could also benefit from role play such as using a toy or doll to demonstrate what you are going to do, and giving them extra sensors to touch and explore can help ease their fears. Guardians can be very helpful during the hookup to soothe and assist in distraction. Be sure to discuss these things with them either before the study or at arrival. Normal bedtime routines should be encouraged.

Preschool (3-5 Years)

By the time they are preschool-aged, most children have the ability to tell you what fears they have, allowing you to address them and more easily move on. This can include assurance that their guardian will be with them the entire time and that there is nothing that you will be doing that will cause pain. It is also possible to explain rules and set boundaries with preschoolers such as not touching wires or that they are allowed to play in a certain part of the room but not on the bed, for example. Play is very important at this age and can assist you in your work. Giving patients sensors and "jobs" to do as you prepare them for the study can be very distracting and make them feel like they are doing important work to help you. Offering choices and rewards can also be helpful as it will allow them to gain a slight sense of control and set expectations but also reward proper behavior. Keeping a normal bedtime routine is still important for preschoolers, and setting time expectations so that they know what to expect can be helpful. For example, "we are going to go to sleep after one episode of (insert favorite show)." Comfort items and favorite snacks from home can be helpful in soothing a preschooler, but new toys and games can also be a great distraction from what you are doing.

Specific safety concerns for toddlers and preschoolers include making sure that there are bedrails on the beds and that they are up and secured if they are too big for a crib. Typically, co-sleeping is acceptable, and possibly preferred, depending on the situation, for guardians of some children over the age of 2. These children are very mobile, and sometimes overly active but still a little clumsy. Be sure to have nonskid socks available for them to wear while in the room and shoes are removed as regular socks and bare feet can be hazardous.

School Age (6-12 Years)

Once children reach school age, they are able to understand much more and can be reasoned with more readily. With this age group, it is important to pay attention to and address fears but understand that you can explain the process and ensure that their questions are addressed. Children of this age group can vary widely in their autonomy and maturity. They may also swing widely between being overly interested in what you are doing, thinking it is very fascinating, and acting as if they are completely uninterested in the process. Typical school-age children will need fewer safety precautions than toddlers and preschoolers, but an abundance of safety should still be exercised to prevent accidental injuries. It may also be easier to get patients of this age group to cooperate in helping you set them up for the study, adhere to study initiation, and be more self-sufficient throughout the night.

Privacy may be of increased importance to these children. By this age, the technologist should ask permission to place leads in somewhat private places, such as the chest or legs. Involving the patient in the process, asking them questions, and allowing them to be part of the decision-making, such as agreeing to a time for electronics to be put away, can help build trust and rapport. Some children may also have developed a negative reaction to medical procedures by this time. It is important to reassure them that you will do nothing to them that will hurt and that they are not in your lab as a punishment for having bad sleep.

Adolescents (12-19 Years)

Typically, PSGs in adolescents are very similar to those in adults. However, there are still some slight differences to keep in mind. The level of maturity of this age group can vary widely, even for two children of the same age. Usually, they will understand the purpose of the sleep study, but it is still a good idea to explain it to them, as well as how the entire process will go so that they have a clear understanding and can ask any questions that they may have. They may also have questions or need help that they do not want to ask for, so giving them that opportunity will help them feel less uncomfortable about any potential fears. This age group typically craves control, so it may be helpful to ask questions directly to them, rather than the guardian, to give them more autonomy over their own testing process.

Keep in mind that children of this age typically require more sleep than adults but rarely get it consistently. A glorification of decreased sleep and later bedtimes, plus the added complication of increased use of electronic devices, particularly late at night, creates poor sleep habits for many adolescents. It is important to set firm ground rules about the expectations of these things when the patient arrives but also to emphasize how important good sleep hygiene is to their overall well-being. The use of electronics may be unavoidable, but it may be a good idea to have them moved to somewhere out of reach once you set "lights out" so the temptation to return to the device is eliminated until the study is complete.

Other Potentially Complicating Factors

Some children may also have movement or mobility abnormalities that make it difficult to apply sensors or keep them affixed. Close teamwork with the patient's accompanying guardian or health worker will be very important as they can help you navigate any issues that may complicate your ability to successfully complete the study. Being proactive in asking the guardian and the patient what you can do to help them may also give you good clues as to how to work with the patient to achieve the best possible outcomes.

Some children have communication barriers that can make working with them more difficult. In these cases, you may find it tempting to communicate only with the guardian. However, depending on the patient's age, communication barrier, and cognition, it is also important to appropriately address the patient, as well. Include them in the conversation and be sure to address them as they are able to receive and reciprocate. Some children may also be more or less comfortable with eye contact, and that should never be forced if they cannot or are not comfortable in engaging with you in this way. You may find it helpful to have communication tools such as translation devices for both verbal and sign language, picture cards with common terms that can be pointed to, and simply understanding the patient's preferred communication methods can be the difference between a frustrating and a highly enjoyable experience for everyone.

De-Escalating Troubling Behaviors

Children of any age or developmental capacity may reach certain points where they need a break. If a patient has escalating behaviors of aggression or is not cooperating, it is important to recognize when those behaviors are becoming a potentially volatile or even dangerous situation for the technologist, the patient, or both. At the beginning stages of disobedience, the patient may be able to readjust to the process at hand by simply redirecting their attention in a different way. When things continue to escalate, it may be necessary to take a break and rely on the guardian to help get the situation better under control using strategies based on their own past personal experience with the child. If situations become violent, as they can with combative children or those with developmental disabilities, the staff needs to be continuously aware of and remove anything in the environment that could cause injury. Children, particularly at the school-age or adolescent ages, sometimes may be stronger and faster than may be anticipated and should not be underestimated. Because of this, the staff must also know the emergency protocols for situations of the highest escalation that require assistance from facility security or for situations of the patient potentially self-harming and work diligently to de-escalate the situation as quickly as possible, followed by appropriate measures such as providing patients and guardians with resources for help with these kinds of situations. Just as with any emergency situation, preparation for behavioral escalations is the key to keeping the environment safe and the situation calm and productive for everyone. Knowing about potential behavioral or sensory problems before the patient arrives can help the staff prepare and have discussions with the guardians to plan for how to best work with the patient if these kinds of situations begin to arise.

DESENSITIZATION

For any children, but particularly those with excessive fears, cognitive disabilities, or behavioral issues, a desensitization appointment before the PSG may be beneficial to the success of the study. If available, behavioral health specialists, which many pediatric labs now have as part of their medical staff, can be very helpful in these desensitization processes. In-person desensitization provides a brief practice session with some sensations the child would be exposed to during the study. A simple prestudy tour of the sleep center is helpful for all pediatric patients and their guardians. This can be done in person or virtually through a website or posted video online. The family should be given information explaining the PSG procedure, preparation for the study, and follow-up information. The prestudy tour will help reduce anxiety (for both the child and the caregiver) and assist the caregiver in recognizing the proper necessities to bring on the night of the study (medications, bedclothes, tablet, favorite toy or blanket, etc). Conducting the desensitization session in one of the rooms used for sleep studies will also help the child become more comfortable with the surroundings and the procedure. During the setup, allowing the child to apply sensors to the guardian or to the doll may diminish apprehension or fascination with the unusual objects being presented.

Desensitization for patients is especially important before a PAP titration. The PAP desensitization process will assist the technologist performing the study to be prepared in advance with helpful techniques. Daytime lab staff can be very helpful in assisting with these types of PAP desensitization visits beginning the process of fitting patients with PAP masks during these visits to help reduce the number of tasks that would need to be completed during the night of the study.

Begin desensitization for sleep study preparation starting with the child's feet and working up to the head because most children seem to have the hardest time with head/face sensations. Let them feel the sensation of having an electrode site prepped and how it feels to have the electrode applied to their skin. It can be helpful to prep a site on their hand so they can see what you will be doing to their head. Allow the child to feel and hold the nasal cannula before placing it in their nose. When fitting the PAP mask, give them the mask to touch and hold so they know it will not harm them. Guide the patient's hand, while holding the mask, up over their nose and involve the guardian by having them assist with this process. Allow the child to become comfortable with the mask before turning on the air pressure. Try to apply the head straps as the last step so the child has some sense of control while adapting to the air pressure. The family can assist in the desensitization process by practicing at home, particularly with the nasal cannula and PAP mask, which seem to be the most difficult items for children to tolerate. The desensitization process must remain flexible depending on the child's progress.

Children with sensory processing disorders may need additional care and time to adjust to the PSG process. It is important to limit the patient's exposure to irritants or triggers such as sound, textures, or other people. Speaking with the guardians before the study about the specific triggers and needs of the patient is a very important step in planning for their arrival and study. Some ways to do this are to get them settled in their own room as quickly as possible and to give them time to adjust to their surroundings. Depending on their age, you may also be able to acclimate them to the sensors and other monitors by explaining it to them and letting them explore them, if appropriate. If this method does not work, then you may need to just work very quickly while the patient is distracted by something or someone else.

DAYTIME STUDIES

Nap Studies

Infants younger than 3 months have a cyclic sleeping pattern of 3 to 4 hours asleep with wakefulness for 1 to 2 hours. As the infant matures, the sleep cycles lengthen, with less sleep occurring during the daytime, usually around 6 months of age (12).

For evaluation of infants, a daytime nap study could be appropriate to evaluate breathing and oxygen saturation as long as they sleep sufficiently. An adequate nap study will typically include about 4 hours of sleep with consolidated sleep and observation of REM sleep.

ESSENTIAL RECORDING ELEMENTS

Pediatric Considerations

As previously discussed, the sleep center environment, guardians, and the child should be prepared appropriately to obtain a successful pediatric PSG. Efforts should be made to meet the needs of the guardian and child. Anticipating the child's needs can reduce stress and anxiety for everyone involved. Although the primary purpose of the room should be to afford the ability to complete the necessary testing in the safest possible environment, it should also be considered that a room with a sterile appearance can produce fear in many children. Efforts should be made to make the room more inviting for children such as child-appropriate art on the walls or having age-appropriate prizes, toys, or items to assist with distraction to help make the experience more enjoyable for the children.

Before the patient arrives, prepare the room and determine the type of bed the patient needs, either a crib for infants and toddlers or a bed with side rails for young children or those with special needs. It is important to have a bed or recliner in the same room for the guardian throughout the study. A rocking chair is also useful for guardians of infants and toddlers who may need to be held during the hookup, comforted, or fed during the night.

Application of Sensors

Electrodes and sensors should be applied in a position that is comfortable for the child and technologist. Usually, the ideal position for an older pediatric patient is sitting up. Sitting allows the child to maintain a sense of control and security, whereas laying a child down creates a sense of vulnerability. It is imperative that the setup position is ergonomically comfortable for the technologist and may require raising the bed or having a taller chair available for the child and/or caregiver to sit on. Sensor application for an infant is normally performed with the infant lying in a crib or being held by the guardian.

The order in which electrodes are placed may also lower the child's anxiety and improve the level of cooperation by earning the patient's trust. It can be helpful to start with the least threatening sensors like leg leads and respiratory effort belts. This allows the child to see and touch the equipment and can satisfy their curiosity. Some children realize that nothing will hurt them after touching or holding the electrodes. Sensors that are poorly tolerated, like the EEG, EMG, EOG leads, nasal pressure/Etco$_2$ cannula, and thermistor, should be placed at the end of the setup process, placed last, or placed when the child falls asleep.

Properly positioned sensors with optimal contact to the skin are essential for obtaining artifact-free signals. Correct electrode placement also minimizes the need for adjusting filters unnecessarily or re-referencing channels. Skin oils, as well as dead or dry skin cells, can act as barriers to electrical conduction. If a patient has lotion or baby oil on their skin, or an infant with cradle cap, it may interfere with electrical conduction and electrode adherence. It is important to let caregivers know to refrain from applying such substances to the child's skin on the day of the study, if at all possible. In cases where application of such materials cannot be avoided, sensor sites should be prepped using a fine-particle mild abrasive skin preparation product. Gentle scrubbing in one direction will avoid possible irritation of the skin. After preparation, the skin should be dried with a gauze pad before placing the electrode. A nontoxic water-soluble colored marker or wax pencil is typically used for marking the scalp when measuring the head. Allowing the child to participate by choosing a color will engage the child and create a sense of control, keeping the process fun. EEG electrodes should be applied to the scalp using a conduction paste, which has both adhesive and conductive qualities. The conduction paste should be hypoallergenic and water soluble. To secure the electrode to the scalp, a small square of gauze with a dab of conduction paste can be used to cover and adhere the electrode to the patient's scalp. The use of collodion is usually not advised for the pediatric population. Collodion has a strong odor, is highly flammable, and must be used in a well-ventilated room. Because children often move a lot, there is a risk of accidents and spills. Collodion should especially be avoided in children diagnosed with respiratory illnesses like asthma.

Once the technologist has completed the setup, securing the electrode wires will reduce the possibility of leads being removed throughout the night. Infants and toddlers can be active sleepers. Proactively securing electrodes and sensors anticipating possible movements, such as rolling or standing in a crib, is time well spent. Guardians handling their child during diaper changes, bottle feeding, and burping can affect electrode placement and increase the likelihood of electrodes coming off. Electrode wires should be gathered together in ponytail fashion at the base of the neck and bundled with tape or wire covers. Socks or mittens can be used to cover the hands of infants, allowing them to move freely and not grab the electrode wires. Wrapping the child's head with gauze or stretch mesh netting is another way to secure the EEG electrodes, which makes the wires less accessible to curious fingers. Wrapping of the head should not be excessive, because undesirable effects such as sweat artifact and electrode popping may result. Excessive wrapping of the head may also make it difficult to reach the scalp in the event that a sensor should need to be replaced at any point during the study. Alternatively, a piece of tubular elastic retainer net dressing can be placed over the scalp area of the child's head. The mesh material permits better air circulation, keeps the head cooler, and allows easier access to the electrodes.

Airflow Sensors

The *AASM Manual for the Scoring of Sleep and Associated Events* clearly describes the technical requirements for pediatric PSG. Oronasal and thermal airflow sensors are sufficient to monitor airflow in pediatric patients during diagnostic studies; however, when this sensor is not functioning properly, or when the identification of hypopneas is required, a nasal pressure transducer is recommended for monitoring airflow in pediatric patients. Likewise, if the nasal pressure transducer is not properly functioning or is producing an unreliable signal, the RIPsum, RIPflow, or dual thoracoabdominal respiratory inductance plethysmography (RIP) belts are appropriate to use for the detection of hypopneas in a diagnostic study (3).

Capnography

For patients younger than 13 years, carbon dioxide (CO_2) monitoring, either transcutaneous or end-tidal, is recommended by the AASM. Capnography is a noninvasive way to measure the adequacy of ventilation during sleep. Both methods are acceptable noninvasive methods for assessing alveolar hypoventilation. Measuring CO_2 is a useful assessment tool in children with chronic lung disease, those on ventilatory support, or when initiating supplemental oxygen during a PSG. Some patients may be dependent on their hypoxic respiratory drive, and the initiation of oxygen without monitoring CO_2 may lead to worsening hypoventilation. Sleep is normally associated with an increased transcutaneous CO_2 ($tcco_2$) level of approximately 4 to 6 mm Hg (13).

End-Tidal CO2

End-tidal CO_2 ($Etco_2$) can be measured using a side stream nasal cannula or directly from a tracheostomy or an endotracheal tube. $Etco_2$ measurements are subject to breath-to-breath fluctuations and may be affected by varying respiratory patterns such as tachypnea, sighs, or mouth breathing. Measurement of end-tidal fluctuations can also be used as an "alternative" channel for scoring respiratory events according to the AASM scoring manual. For mouth-breathers, signals may be obtained by placing the sampling cannula over the patient's mouth. The technologist should be vigilant to keep the sampling lines open as these lines may become occluded on account of humidity and patient secretions, which may affect accuracy.

Because of breath-to-breath variability, $Etco_2$ values should be assessed as a percentage of total sleep time with hypercapnia rather than isolated peak values during the night. The values obtained using $Etco_2$ monitoring must be evaluated very carefully and require a good signal plateau to be accurate. A poor-quality signal plateau will show a lower than actual CO_2 reading, which may occur in patients with nasal obstruction, mouth breathing, nasal cannula delivery of supplemental oxygen, technical issues with placement of $Etco_2$ cannula, and severe chronic obstructive lung disease (14).

Transcutaneous CO2

Monitoring of $tcco_2$ is accomplished using a CO_2 measurement obtained through the skin, and it closely mimics arterial CO_2. The transcutaneous electrode warms the skin surface, increasing local capillary perfusion, and measures the CO_2 as it diffuses from the dermis across a gas-permeable membrane. End-tidal monitoring provides breath-to-breath variability, transcutaneous measurements tend to respond more slowly (2 minutes or more) and demonstrate a trending pattern. Transcutaneous CO_2 ($tcco_2$) monitoring is valuable in patients who have interstitial lung disease (a group of rare lung diseases) where $Etco_2$ is not accurate (15). $tcco_2$ monitoring is also beneficial during PAP titration. With children using continuous positive airway pressure (CPAP), the use of $tcco_2$ monitoring is preferred because the end-tidal sampling cannula is typically removed during a PAP titration.

Care must be taken to prevent possible skin burns caused by the heat emitted by the electrode. Most $tcco_2$ monitors allow for variable temperature settings, which impacts the duration that the sensor can be safely left on one skin site and makes it less likely to cause harm. It is essential to follow the manufacturer's safety recommendations regarding temperature settings, particularly when testing young children. Adherence to the manufacturer's instructions for proper calibration and electrode maintenance will maximize optimal electrode performance, accuracy, and safety.

Audio and Video Recordings

The ability to record high-quality audio and video recordings during an acquisition is essential for observation of sleep behaviors and accurate evaluation of the child's activity. For the safety of the child and protection of the staff, the lab may want to consider a policy that the video recording begins as soon as the patient arrives and does not end until they leave. An infrared light source is essential when viewing and recording the patient inside a dark room. There are several behavioral parameters that can be monitored via video during a PSG, which include body position, respiratory patterns, breathing sounds (eg, snoring, stridor, catathrenia), possible seizure activity, bruxism, and other parasomnias. The technologist must remain attentive and ready to adjust the camera as needed to capture the patient's behavior. The technologist must also document their observations to further assist the physician in making a diagnosis. Recording unusual interactions between the child and the person accompanying them to their study may also present opportunities for education, particularly in relation to inappropriate practices (eg, placing the infant in a prone position and bottle propping).

Video data must be synchronized with the PSG data in accordance with the AASM standards. Most acquisition systems have the ability to record the video digitally and at a high sampling rate for a better-quality recording. Cameras with pan-tilt-zoom capability (as opposed to a single, fixed focal point) enable the technologist to frame the patient for a better recording image and follow active sleepers as they move in the bed or crib. Zooming in can be useful for highlighting the respiratory patterns and observing nasal flaring, retractions, mouth breathing, or paradoxical respiratory effort. High-resolution video should be used to record the child's behavior, but keep in mind high-resolution recording will result in larger electronic file size and increase data storage requirements.

Electrode and Sensor Placement Adjustments

It is imperative that all technologists clearly understand the use of the 10-20 method of measuring patients' heads for electrode placement. This is of particular importance for infants and children as they may have extreme variations in shapes and sizes, even for children of similar ages. Because of their small sizes, infants may require slight adjustments when placing specific electrodes. It may be acceptable to do so but should always be accompanied with proper documentation of any modifications. Smaller head size often requires slight modifications when placing electrodes on the scalp and face. The distance between the chin electromyogram (EMG) leads in small children should be reduced from 2 to 1 cm. Electrooculographic (EOG) leads may need to be placed 0.5 cm from the outer canthus instead of 1 cm as recommended in adults (3).

Standard 10-mm electroencephalogram (EEG) electrodes may also be too large for neonates; therefore, using 6-mm electrodes is recommended. A poorly positioned effort belt may lead to positional artifact because of slippage or may miss paradoxical breathing if the belts are too loose or too tight.

Pediatric Recording Parameters

The physiologic parameters measured during a pediatric PSG are similar to those of adult studies with a few exceptions. The elements of a pediatric montage are outlined in Table 59-2. In addition to the *recommended* EEG derivations F4-M1, C4-M1, and O2-M1, the contralateral electrodes, F3, C3, and O1, are referenced to M2 and added as backup sites in the event a *recommended* electrode becomes dislodged during the study. The extra electrodes provide the technologist with the flexibility to re-reference electrodes and often prevent having to enter the child's room unnecessarily. Similarly, redundancy is seen when measuring airflow. Airflow sensors include nasal pressure transducer, oronasal thermal airflow, RIPsum and RIPflow, and $Etco_2$. The technologist may not need to immediately replace a sensor that comes off when utilizing alternative respiratory sensors.

Table 59-2 Suggested Polysomnography Montage

Signal	Measured Parameters
EEG derivations	F4-M1, F3-M2
	C4-M1, C3-M2
	O2-M1, O1-M2
EOG derivations	E1-M2
	E2-M2
ECG	Lead II
Chin EMG	Mentalis and submentalis muscles
Leg EMG	Anterior tibialis muscle
Nasal pressure	Nasal air pressure transducer
Oronasal airflow	Oronasal thermal sensor
Respiratory effort: chest and abdominal wall motion	Dual thoracoabdominal RIP belts or esophageal manometry
Capnography	End-tidal and/or transcutaneous
Snore	Snore sensor
Oxygen saturation	Spo_2
Body position	Body position sensor
Audio and video recordings	Time synchronized with polysomnography data

ECG, electrocardiogram; EEG, electroencephalogram; EMG, electromyogram; EOG, electrooculography; RIP, respiratory inductance plethysmography.

Equipment Adjustments Based on the Age of Child

Sleep centers performing pediatric sleep studies must have various types and sizes of equipment readily available. Sensors should be specifically designed for pediatric patients rather than modified adult sensors. Ill-fitting sensors may be poorly tolerated and produce a lesser-quality signal. Adult cannulas for measuring nasal pressure or $Etco_2$ monitoring may have prongs that are too long and wide to accurately sample lower pressure or CO_2 fluctuations sometimes seen in pediatric patients. Adult respiratory effort belts are usually wider than pediatric belts and may yield dampened signals. Pediatric oximeter sensors are designed specifically for a child's small finger or toe to provide a "snug" fit. Proper use and fit of pediatric oximetry sensors will reduce motion artifact and the chance of the sensor falling off.

Similar to adult PSG, having a well-thought-out plan with deliberate application of electrodes ensures a high-quality acquisition. Making recording parameter changes to clean up recording artifacts is not recommended. For example, increasing the low-frequency filter to 1 Hz will reduce slow-wave artifact and respiratory sway artifact that degrades slow-wave EEG signals, but this is not recommended. Excellent electrode and sensor application is the best approach. The PSG system should have the ability to adjust sensitivity/gain settings to accommodate the high-amplitude EEG signals characteristic of pediatric waveforms. This is an acceptable, often necessary, setting change to record a readable EEG in infants and young children.

The AASM recommends a minimum sampling rate of 200 Hz and, ideally, 500 Hz for EEG. For more detailed EEG analysis, higher sampling rates and high-frequency filter (HFF) settings are desirable. For accurate EEG representation, the sampling rate should be at least 3 times the frequency of the fastest signal to be recorded. For recording seizure activity, higher sampling rates of 500 to 1,000 Hz are recommended in conjunction with HFF settings of 70 to 75 Hz.

The frequency of waveforms often increases as the child grows and develops. From infancy to childhood, EEG patterns will vary at different growth phases. Differentiating age-related morphology makes scoring pediatric sleep more challenging. Primarily, the background rhythms in pediatric EEGs are of higher amplitude than those seen in adults and are prone to waveform blocking and signal channel overlap. Reducing sensitivity settings may be necessary to preserve waveform reconstruction.

Expanded Montage

A sleep EEG montage corresponds to the underlying area of the cerebral cortex specific to sleep stage activity. Although it is common to capture seizure activity during a PSG, the modified EEG montage used in a PSG is often missing channels helpful in differentiating seizures versus nonepileptic events (16). The addition of temporal leads T3 and T4 improves the accuracy of detecting temporal lobe seizure, and using 7 and 18 channels of EEG has the best sensitivity for seizure detection. However, frontal lobe seizure detection is not affected by the number of channels used (17).

As a minimal testing requirement, the American Clinical Neurophysiology Society guidelines require all 21 electrodes of the International 10-20 system and standard adult montages be used (18,19). PSG equipment should be able to record the expanded EEG montage as well as standard channels for the detection of sleep apnea, periodic limb movements, and parasomnias. A qualified neurologist should determine the appropriate seizure montage to be used and ideally interpret the EEG.

Biocalibrations

Before lights out, biocalibrations should be performed to confirm accurate sensor responsiveness. Table 59-3 shows the recommended biocalibration commands and corresponding sensors.

Cooperation will vary greatly depending on the child's level of comprehension, temperament, and mental and physical development. Some children may not be able to complete all or any of the biocalibrations. Creativity and use of age-appropriate terminology may be needed to elicit the desired biocalibration response. For example, a few rounds of "peek-a-boo" can produce open and closed eyes. Moving a penlight or flashlight beam on the ceiling or a toy in the child's vision field can help track their eyes in the desired direction. Biting down like you are chewing gum may simulate jaw-clenching. With pediatric patients, the usual adult biocalibrations are used; however, infants require a thorough documentation of observations because they are incapable of following biocalibration instructions.

Recording Duration

As mentioned earlier, within the pediatric age group, recommended sleep duration ranges from 12 to 16 hours/d for infants, 10 to 12 hours for children, and 8 to 10 hours for teenagers. "Lights out" for a pediatric

Table 59-3 Biocalibration Commands and Affected Sensors

Command	Sensor
Eyes open, eyes closed	O1 and O2
Eyes up, eyes down	REOG and LEOG
Eyes left, eyes right	REOG and LEOG
Jaw clench or smile	Chin EMG
Count aloud or snore	Snore microphone
Nose breathe, mouth breathe	Thermistor and nasal pressure
Big breath and hold	Respiratory effort belts Thermistor and nasal pressure
Move left foot, move right foot	Left and right leg EMG

EMG, electromyogram; LEOG, left electrooculography; REOG, right electrooculography.

polysomnogram should start at or as close to the child's normal bedtime as possible. Because the pediatric patient goes to bed earlier and sometimes sleeps later, it is common for the PSG to last more than 7 hours, and the child's last REM cycle should be captured before ending the study.

Behavior Observations and Documentation

As with all other aspects of pediatric PSG, sleep behaviors may vary as the child grows and develops. Behavioral observations are an important aspect of the PSG and provide additional information about the child's sleep quality and respiratory patterns. Observations and time of occurrence should be documented by the technologist and captured on video. Observations commonly include respiratory changes (paradoxical breathing, mouth breathing, snoring, wheezing, gasping), positional changes, and parasomnias. Behavioral characteristics are used in determining infant wake and sleep cycles because their brain waves are not fully developed. For example, wakefulness is identified when the eyes are open or there is obvious crying; scanning eye movements and brief eye closure may occur with crying. Sleep is identified when the eyes are closed, fewer body movements are occurring, and possibly sucking or snoring sounds are present. It is important to be vigilant with infant observations and thoroughly document all behaviors such as grimacing, hiccups, and startle jerk.

SUMMARY

Pediatric overnight PSG is a common procedure and remains the gold standard for identifying sleep-disordered breathing and other sleep disorders in children. Although challenges often occur with either the patient or the caregiver, the pediatric PSG can be successfully performed with minimal stress when the technologist is properly prepared for the unexpected. Keys to success are (1) anticipation and advance preparation for the child and caregiver's basic needs based on the child's age, development, and any special needs; (2) attention to the specific safety needs of each individual patient; (3) a family-centered approach: engaging the child and caregiver in the process, including prestudy education, a sleep center tour, the hookup process, and using age-appropriate distractors; (4) extra attention to securing sensors; and (5) a high level of vigilance and responsiveness to recognize and replace sensors when appropriate and accurately documenting behavioral observations.

REFERENCES

1. Kryger MH. Differential diagnosis of pediatric sleep disorders. In: Sheldon SH, Ferber R, Kryger MH, et al, eds. *Principles and Practice of Pediatric Sleep Medicine*. 2nd ed. Elsevier Saunders; 2014:13-16.
2. DelRosso LM. Overview of pediatric polysomnography: a newborn infant with snoring and witnessed apnea. In: DelRosso LM, Berry RB, Beck SE, et al, eds. *Pediatric Sleep Pearls*. Elsevier; 2017:10-11.
3. Troester MM, Stuart FQ, Berry RB, et al. *The AASM Manual for the Scoring of Sleep and Associated Events: Rules, Terminology and Technical Specifications (Version 3)*. American Academy of Sleep Medicine; 2023.
4. Bhattacharjee R, Kheirandish-Gozal L, Spruyt K, et al. Adenotonsillectomy outcomes in treatment of obstructive sleep apnea in children: a multicenter retrospective study. *Am J Respir Crit Care Med*. 2010; 182(5):676-683.
5. Moon RY; Task Force on Sudden Infant Death Syndrome. SIDS and other sleep-related infant deaths 2016 updated recommendations for a safe infant sleeping environment. *Pediatrics*. 2016;138(5): e20162940. doi:10.1542/peds.2016-2940
6. Batra EK, Midgett JD, Moon RY. Hazards associated with sitting and carrying devices for children two years and younger. *J Pediatr*. 2015;167(1):183-187.
7. Paruthi S, Brooks LJ, D'Ambrosio C, et al. Recommended amount of sleep for pediatric populations: a consensus statement of the American Academy of Sleep Medicine. *J Clin Sleep Med*. 2016; 12(6):785-786.
8. American Association of Sleep Technologists. *Sleep Technology: Core Competency*. American Association of Sleep Technologists; 2017.
9. Beck SE, Marcus CM. Pediatric polysomnography. *Clin Sleep Med*. 2009;4(3):393-406.
10. Zaremba EK, Barkey ME, Mesa C, et al. Making polysomnography more "child friendly:" a family-centered care approach. *Clin Sleep Med*. 2005;1(2):189-198.
11. Larsen PD, Stensaas SS. Pediatric neurologic exam—6 months. Updated August 2016. Accessed November 22, 2018. http://library.med.utah.edu/pedineurologicexam/html/06month.html
12. Wagner MH. A 2-month-old infant with sleep-onset REM period on polysomnography. In: DelRosso LM, Berry RB, Beck SE, et al, eds. *Pediatric Sleep Pearls*. Elsevier; 2017:27-28.
13. Siobal MS. Analysis and monitoring of gas exchange. In: Kacmarek RM, Stoller JK, Heuer AJ, eds. *Egan's Fundamentals of Respiratory Care*. 10th ed. Elsevier; 2013:381.

14. DelRosso LM. A 14-year-old with an abnormal end-trial CO2 waveform during polysomnography. In: DelRosso LM, Berry RB, Beck SE, et al, eds. *Pediatric Sleep Pearls*. Elsevier; 2017:16-19.
15. Katz ES, Marcus CL. Diagnosis of obstructive sleep apnea. In: Sheldon SH, Ferber R, Kryger MH, et al, eds. *Principles and Practice of Pediatric Sleep Medicine*. 2nd ed. Elsevier Saunders; 2014:225.
16. Foldvary-Schaefer N, De Ocampo J, Mascha E, et al. Accuracy of seizure detection using abbreviated EEG during polysomnography. *J Clin Neurophysiol*. 2006;23(1):68-71.
17. Foldvary N, Caruso AC, Mascha E, et al. Identifying montages that best detect electrographic seizure activity during polysomnography. *Sleep*. 2000;23(2): 221-229.
18. Jasper HH The ten-twenty electrode system of the International Federation. *Electroencephalogr Clin Neurophysiol*. 1958;10:371-375.
19. Kuratani J, Pearl PL, Sullivan L, et al. American Clinical Neurophysiology Society guideline 5: minimum technical standards for pediatric electroencephalography. *J Clin Neurophysiol*. 2016; 33:320-323.

Chapter 60
Pediatric Scoring

JEREMY JAMES ROY

KEY CONCEPTS/LEARNING OBJECTIVES

On completion of this chapter, the reader should be able to describe the stages of sleep seen in infants and children, recognize the differing characteristics in polysomnogram tracings between an infant, a child, and an adult study, and state the age criteria for infant and pediatric scoring rules, as well as explain the importance of technologist notes during pediatric studies. They should also be able to recognize respiratory events in the pediatric patient, identify cardiac dysrhythmias common to the pediatric patient, and describe common artifacts in pediatric sleep studies, describe common challenges in scoring pediatric studies, know what to look for in pediatric patients when marking arousals, and list the elements of the summary report in pediatric polysomnograms, and explain the limitations of limited channel sleep studies in children.

KEY TERMS

Dominant posterior rhythm (DPR)
Dysrhythmias
Hypnagogic hypersynchrony
Stage N (NREM)
Stage R (REM)
Stage T (Transitional)
Stage W (Wakefulness)
Supraventricular tachycardia
Tracé alternant
Tracé discontinue

Sleep disorders are extremely common during childhood. Unfortunately, even with the prevalence of sleep problems and despite being either preventable or treatable, childhood sleep disorders often go underrecognized and undiagnosed. There are many reasons for this, but the fact remains that children are not receiving the attention they need when it comes to sleeping. Proper restorative sleep for children is critical for their development, and quality sleep for a child is just as important as, if not more so than, it is for adults. Even though sleep disorders are prevalent in children, the majority of the literature regarding sleep testing primarily covers adult disorders. Despite the massive amount of research on pediatric sleep disorders, which grows by the day, the pediatric content in most sleep medicine textbooks receives very limited coverage. Published in 1968, *A Manual of Standardized Terminology, Techniques, and Scoring System for Sleep Stages of Human Subjects* standardized sleep stage scoring in adults; pediatrics was not addressed in the manual. In 1971, a committee cochaired by Drs. Anders, Emde, and Parmelee authored *A Manual for Standardized Techniques and Criteria for Scoring of States of Sleep and Wakefulness in Newborn Infants*. Not addressed in that publication were standards for evaluating sleep in older infants, toddlers, children, and preadolescents.

In the last few decades, standards for pediatric sleep testing have received increased attention. In 2007, the American Academy of Sleep Medicine (AASM) published *The AASM Manual for the Scoring of Sleep and Associated Events: Rules, Terminology, and Technical Specifications*. This manual includes sections on sleep staging and respiratory rules for pediatric patients. In 2011, the AASM published *Respiratory Indications for Polysomnography in Children: An Evidence-Based Review* to help sleep specialists determine the appropriateness of ordering a sleep study in children. Standards for staging and scoring pediatric studies have evolved since 2007. With several revisions in the last few years and regular updates, the *AASM Scoring Manual* is frequently redefining and issuing improved rules for pediatrics.

Sleep architecture changes significantly over the first two decades of life. Sleep patterns and sleep behaviors evolve and are modified by both "intrinsic" (eg, normal development) and "extrinsic" (eg, environment and parenting practices) processes as we progress from infancy to childhood and through adolescence. This chapter will discuss the developmental issues inherent when performing pediatric sleep studies as related to both sleep staging and respiratory event scoring. It will review the current scoring rules implemented by the AASM and how to apply these rules for pediatric patients. This chapter will focus on differences between adults and children as they apply to performing and scoring pediatric polysomnography. Techniques used to identify staging and events specific to children will be included. The goal is to provide an overall enhanced appreciation regarding the complexities involved with pediatric sleep scoring.

THE PEDIATRIC DIFFERENCE

Even though most of what is written about sleep medicine concerns adults and their disorders, children experience the same broad range of sleep disorders encountered in adults, including sleep apnea, insomnia, parasomnias, movement disorders, circadian sleep-wake syndromes, narcolepsy, and restless legs syndrome. In fact, a pediatric sleep center will encounter a diverse population of disorders on a more regular basis than the typical breathing and arrhythmia disorders seen in an adult sleep center. Sometimes labeled the same in adults and children, the clinical presentation, evaluation, and management of some disorders may differ significantly. For example, an adult with obstructive sleep apnea (OSA) may present with excessive sleepiness and lethargy, whereas a child with OSA could present with hyperactivity and restlessness, sometimes labeled incorrectly as attention-deficit hyperactivity disorder (ADHD). Although snoring and sleep apnea are common indications for referral to a sleep specialist, many children also have a behavioral or nonrespiratory sleep disorder either as another comorbid diagnosis or as a primary sleep disorder. In addition, and similar to adults, children are increasingly prescribed medications that affect their sleep, making treatment more complicated (1).

Scoring pediatric sleep studies is a challenging experience but so can be performing sleep studies on pediatric patients. Adult sleep centers might not be properly suited to treating young children. A pediatric sleep center needs an atmosphere designed with the child's acceptance, comfort, and safety in mind. There should be child-pleasing surroundings and decorations that help soothe and distract. Well-trained sleep center staff are necessary to care for the pediatric population. To be prepared, staff must be well informed regarding the variances in development, not only physically but also mentally, with the age and medical condition of each patient. Competent pediatric sleep technologists understand proper distraction techniques, and they are provided the tools needed to perform this function well for each patient. It is also helpful to have the parent or caregiver involved to make the testing go smoothly. There should be accommodations for the parent or caregiver to stay in the room with the child. Furthermore, consider the testing equipment. It is best if the monitoring equipment is contained outside the bedroom or in a cabinet hidden from view, as it can seem intimidating to a child. As much as possible, keep equipment and supplies away from the reach of the curious child.

The physical and anatomic differences between younger children and older adults are obvious, but also consider mental development before performing a sleep study. It is best practice to have the child seen by a clinician familiar with pediatric sleep who can review the history and symptoms in a clinical setting. The sleep specialist has the opportunity to assess for and prioritize the various sleep concerns before ordering appropriate testing. Pediatric sleep studies can be "customized" on the basis of the child's symptoms. An enuresis alarm, esophageal pressure monitoring, pH recording, capnography, and seizure montage are some of the additional monitoring tools often added for pediatric testing. At this time, it may be determined that a sleep diary or actigraphy monitoring is essential to collect additional information on sleep behavior. Some children and their families find it helpful to visit the sleep center before the actual study. This is often possible during the clinic visit and should be encouraged. Making the surroundings friendly and familiar to the child increases compliance during the night of the study.

It is best practice to have a prescreening tool in place to assess the child's needs and developmental level. Information gathered at the clinic visit and during the scheduling portion is helpful in predicting what to expect on the night of the study. By the day of the study, staff should be aware of the patient's needs for testing and preparation in staffing adjusted so it is appropriate for difficult or medically complex children. On the night of the study, schedule the family to arrive at the sleep center early enough so that the study begins as close as possible to the child's normal bedtime. If clinically appropriate, children may be encouraged to bring any favorite toys, pillows, and even videos that will make their stay in the sleep center more comfortable. To help children and parents feel more comfortable, show them the area where the parent or caregiver is to stay overnight. During the stay, involving the parent or caregiver as much as possible will enhance the experience of the child and create a more peaceful experience.

Many adult sleep centers have a protocol of performing a split-night test, in which the first part of the night is diagnostic to determine if the patient has sleep-disordered breathing or other events affecting sleep. If the study uncovers events that warrant positive airway pressure (PAP) treatment, then a titration study is performed in the second part of the night. In pediatrics, there is a concern that a shortened study may underestimate the degree of sleep-disordered breathing in children. Most often, respiratory events increase in frequency or become more severe as the night progresses and the child spends more time in rapid eye movement (REM) sleep. It is highly recommended to perform a baseline study for an entire night to get a full appreciation of the child's sleep-disordered breathing. In addition, from a practical standpoint, many children with OSA do not require PAP treatment. Instead, children with sleep apnea typically receive referrals to an otolaryngologist for consideration of an adenotonsillectomy. If it is decided that a titration study is needed, it will be performed on another night, preferably after the child has undergone a desensitization period with the PAP mask. Then, when the child returns for their PAP study, it will allow the technologist a full night to properly titrate the patient and find the correct pressure.

Proper application of the electroencephalogram (EEG) electrodes and other monitoring leads is critical to acquiring a quality sleep study in children and lays the foundation for quality scoring. There are many techniques available to help the child feel comfortable and to cooperate while applying electrodes. In spite of this, if the child adamantly refuses to allow the sensors to be applied, the technologist may, depending on the type of study to be performed, allow the child to first fall asleep without applying the full montage. At times, adding the additional electrodes and sensors after the child has entered deep delta sleep results in better impedances, improving the quality of the study collected for scoring.

Performing patient calibrations is another important step in performing quality sleep studies and aids the technologist in proper scoring. Because of their lack of a clear alpha pattern, it is especially important to obtain a lengthy sample baseline of wake EEG in children. This recording portion is helpful during staging of the study as a reference to aid in determining wake versus sleep. Calibrations can be difficult, if not impossible, in the noncompliant or very young child. There are a variety of methods that can be used depending on the situation. One technique to obtain calibrations in this population is with the assistance of another technologist or parent. For instance, to check electrooculogram (EOG) waveforms, the assistant or parent can move an object back and forth for the child to track with the eyes, and leg movement calibrations can be done with the assistant flexing the child's foot when instructed.

One important respiratory measurement collected routinely in pediatric studies and not always recorded in adult studies is carbon dioxide (CO_2) monitoring obtained through either end-tidal CO_2 nasal cannula or placement of a transcutaneous CO_2 monitor. Because of airflow concerns, using transcutaneous CO_2 monitoring at times may be more beneficial, especially with infants or children on positive pressure ventilation. In addition to providing another assessment of air exchange, end-tidal CO_2 measurements allow for the detection and quantification of hypoventilation, often more commonly seen in children than in adults.

IDENTIFYING SLEEP STAGES IN INFANTS AND CHILDREN

Newborn infants or neonates do not have fully developed sleep stages, as those seen in adults. Infants have a *dominant posterior rhythm* (DPR) EEG pattern slower than that seen with adults, who have an 8- to 13-Hz alpha rhythm (Figure 60-1). The DPR in most normal children develops as they grow, changing from a 3.5- to

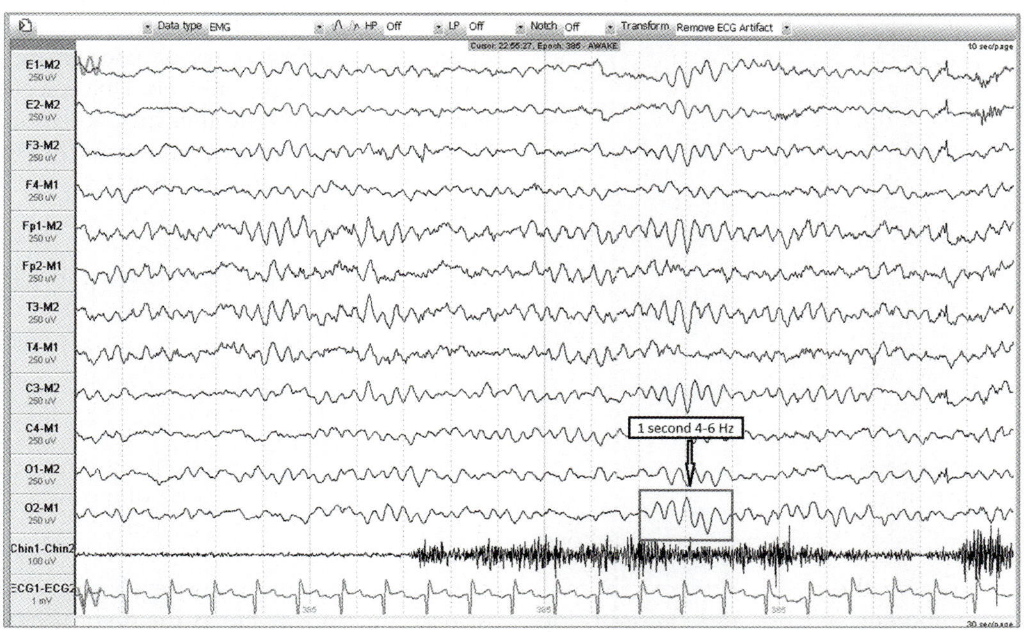

Figure 60-1 Dominant posterior rhythm in a 3-month-old.

Table 60-1 Pediatric Sleep Stages
Stage W (Wakefulness)
Stage N1 (NREM1)
Stage N2 (NREM2)
Stage N3 (NREM3)
Stage N (NREM)
Stage R (REM)

NREM, nonrapid eye movement; REM, rapid eye movement.

4.5-Hz rhythmic activity at 3 to 4 months postterm to a 5- to 6-Hz activity by 5 to 6 months of age, and 7.5 to 9.5 Hz by 3 years of age and amplitude usually greater than 50 uV. Vertex sharp waves are sharply contoured waves with duration less than 0.5 seconds (as measured from the base of the wave), maximal over the central region and distinguishable from background activity. Typically, these waveforms first appear 4 to 6 months postterm. Sleep spindles can be seen by 6 weeks postterm. K-complexes seen as early as 3 months are usually present by 6 months of age, as is slow-wave activity. Sleep spindles are usually first seen in infants 4 to 6 weeks postterm maximal over the vertex region and are usually well-developed and present in infants 8 to 9 weeks. K-complexes are usually present 3 to 6 months postterm and are maximal over the prefrontal and frontal regions and appear similar to those seen in adults. Infants 2 months or older postterm typically can be staged using W, N1, N2, N3, and R stages (Table 60-1) (2,3).

There is a period when some infants will not have developed all the well-defined characteristics of nonrapid eye movement (NREM) sleep stages as seen in N1, N2, and N3. Sleep spindles, K-complexes, or slow-wave sleep may not be easily recognizable in the EEG waveform for these infants. During this time, the epochs that do not meet the criteria for stages W, N1, N2, or N3 are scored as stage N (NREM). The rules state that if all the epochs of NREM sleep in an infant study show no sign of sleep spindles, K-complexes, or high-amplitude slow-wave sleep, then score all these epochs as stage N. If there are any epochs that have sleep spindles and K-complexes, score these epochs as stage N2. If some epochs contain more than 20% slow-wave activity, score these as stage N3, and otherwise score the NREM sleep as stage N (4).

Scoring Sleep Stages

Although EEG characteristics will be different because of the age of the patient, sleep staging in pediatrics follows the adult rules for stages N2, N3, and R. One difference in children will be the greater amount of high-amplitude slow-wave sleep, especially in younger children. Slow-wave sleep decreases as we age. Compared with the preteen child, there will be a noticeable reduction in slow-wave activity as the child ages into their late teenage years and beyond. Younger children entering sleep will show a slowing of their DPR and will often have *hypnagogic hypersynchrony*. Hypnagogic hypersynchrony (HH) appears as paroxysmal bursts or runs of diffuse, high-amplitude, sinusoidal, 75 to 350 uV, 3 to 4.5 Hz waves that begin abruptly, are usually widely distributed but often maximal over the central, frontal, or frontocentral scalp regions. HH is a distinctive EEG pattern of drowsiness and stage N1 that often disappears with deeper stages of NREM sleep. HH is seen in approximately 30% of infants at 3 months postterm and in 95% of children ages 6 to 8 months and is less prevalent after age 4 to 5 years. Unless there are events causing disturbances either from the patient or externally, children do not stay in stage N1 for long periods. Within minutes, they progress into deeper stages of sleep. The younger the child, the sooner this tends to happen.

Sleep staging in children is similar to that of adults, except that the younger child will have a slower DPR or baseline pattern. The DPR indicates wakefulness, and it varies from child to child because of the wide range of maturity levels seen in a pediatric sleep center. Again, for this reason, patient calibrations used as a reference can be extremely helpful in determining what pattern of EEG is predominant in the wakeful child.

Once you are comfortable with recognizing the DPR wakefulness EEG pattern in your patient, look for a slowing and attenuation or lowering of amplitude in the EEG waveform to detect sleep onset. If you see this change in waveform pattern for more than 50% of the epoch, then score that epoch as stage N1. To further help recognize the beginning of stage N1 or sleep onset, watch closely for the EEG waveform to become clearer and sharper as artifact is decreased or drops out as the child relaxes on entering sleep. This is seen more noticeably in infant polysomnography and, along with other signs, can indicate relaxation into sleep (see Figure 60-2 that determines sleep and sleep HH).

SLEEP IN INFANTS UNDER 2 MONTHS POSTTERM

Pediatric sleep staging rules can be applied to infants 2 months postterm or older. For infants less than 2 months postterm who have not yet developed recognizable sleep spindles, there is another set of sleep staging criteria created by Anders et al. and detailed in their publication from 1971, *A Manual of Standardized Terminology, Techniques and Criteria for Scoring of States of Sleep and Wakefulness in Newborn Infants*. This guide was developed over 40 years ago and until recently, was still acceptable to use in practice for scoring infant studies.

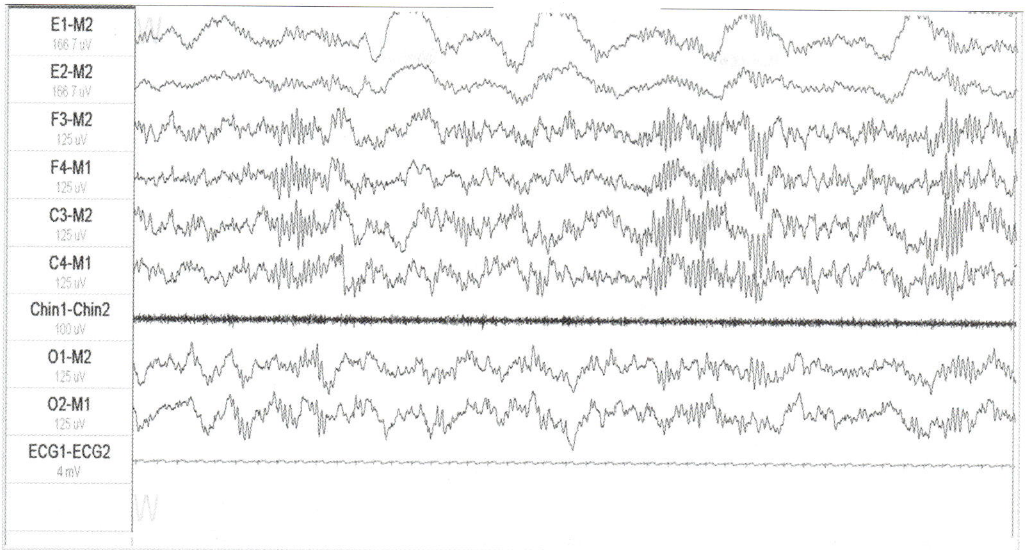

Figure 60-2 Hypnagogic hypersynchrony occurs normally in infants and children. Hypnagogic hypersynchrony are paroxysmal bursts or runs of diffuse, high-amplitude, sinusoidal, 75 to 350 uV, 3 to 4.5 Hz waves that begin abruptly, are usually widely distributed, but often maximal over the central, frontal, or frontocentral scalp regions.

It described sleep staging in infants using the terminology *quiet*, *active*, and *indeterminate* sleep. Today, these terms are replaced with stage *W (Wakefulness)*, stage *N (NREM)*, *stage R (REM)*, and *stage T (Transitional)*, and rules for infants are now covered in the *AASM Scoring Manual.*

Infant Patterns of Electroencephalogram

Sleep staging is based on five criteria: eye movements, EEG, body movements, submental electromyogram (EMG), and cardiorespiratory pattern (Table 60-2). Newborn infants manifest four general EEG patterns. These include *low-voltage irregular* (LVI), *tracé alternant* (TA), *high-voltage slow waves* (HVS), and *mixed* (M). LVI is mostly theta activity (5-8 Hz) and slow activity (1-5 Hz) and can range between 14 and 35 μV in amplitude. TA is 3 to 8 seconds of high-voltage (0.5-3 Hz) slow waves separated by 4 to 8 seconds of lower-voltage mixed-frequency waves (see Figure 60-3 for an example of stage N with a TA EEG). HVS is continuous rhythmic 50 to 150 μV waves at a frequency of 0.5 to 4 Hz. M contains both HVS and LVI waves (5). Infants born prematurely often have a pattern of EEG called *tracé discontinue*. This waveform is similar to TA; however, it shows longer periods of very low-amplitude activity in between HVS (see Figure 60-4 for an example of *tracé discontinue*).

Wakefulness

Body movements, crying, or quiet awake when the infant is inactive and the eyes are open and alert can distinguish wakefulness in the newborn infant. Body movements, vocalizations, and facial or limb twitches can also occur during sleep, so it is important to know if the eyes are closed and for how long. Infants will not close their eyes and remain awake, although brief eye closure can occur with crying. Synchronized digital video

Table 60-2 Infant Sleep Scoring

	Stage R (REM) Sleep	Stage N (NREM) Sleep
Behavior	Movements, smiles, grimaces, squirming, sucking	Movements rare, sucking can occur
Respirations	Irregular, some central pauses (may or may not meet criteria for apnea)	Regular
Eye movements	Present, eyes closed, REM seen under closed eyelids	Absent, eyes closed
Electroencephalogram	Low voltage, mixed frequency	High-voltage slow waves or TA
Electromyogram	Suppressed	High

NREM, nonrapid eye movement; REM, rapid eye movement; TA, tracé alternant.

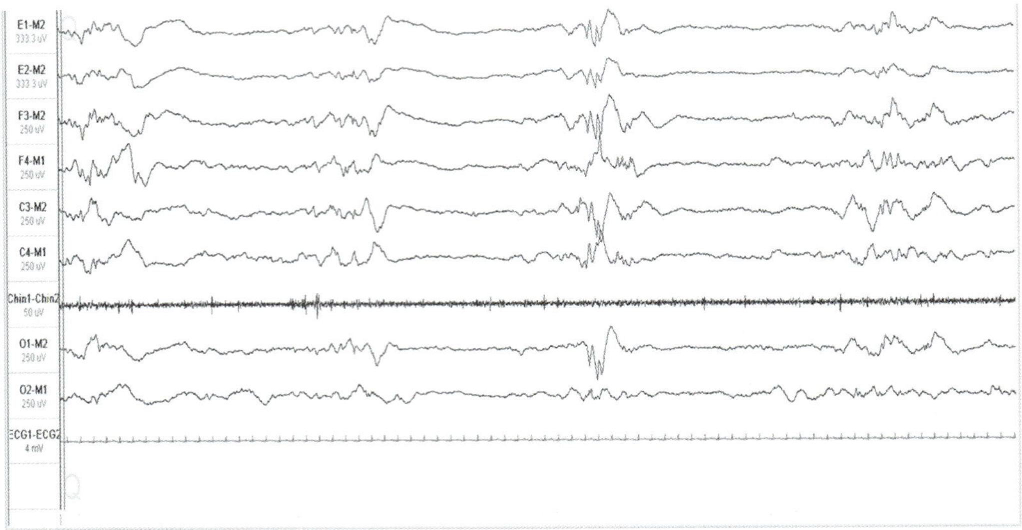

Figure 60-3 Electroencephalogram waveform showing immaturity and tracé discontinue pattern in a 7-week premature infant. This tracing shows short bursts of high-amplitude waves separated by long periods of very low-amplitude activity.

is helpful in determining whether the infant is awake or asleep, although video recording is not the only method of documenting patient activity. Technologist notations regarding patient activity, along with documentation of any other issues, are important for accurate scoring.

Upon review of the completed study, there may be problems with the video or sound not discovered or corrected during the actual recording, such as a broken microphone, reduced lighting, poor camera angle, or something obstructing the camera view. It is imperative that the technologist monitoring the study frequently observe and note whether the infant's eyes are open or closed; the level of any snoring, vocalizations, and body movements; along with any other details specific to the study, such as whether the infant is receiving oxygen or settings of a ventilation device. Because it may be impossible to distinguish sleep from quiet wakefulness, without the technologist's documentation, determining sleep is often difficult (Figure 60-5). The EEG pattern of the infant in quiet wakefulness will not show the alpha rhythm seen in older children and adults. Instead, it will be a low-amplitude, mixed-frequency waveform with no delta waves. The voltage is usually less than 75 μV. The chin EMG is usually high, and the EOG will show REMs

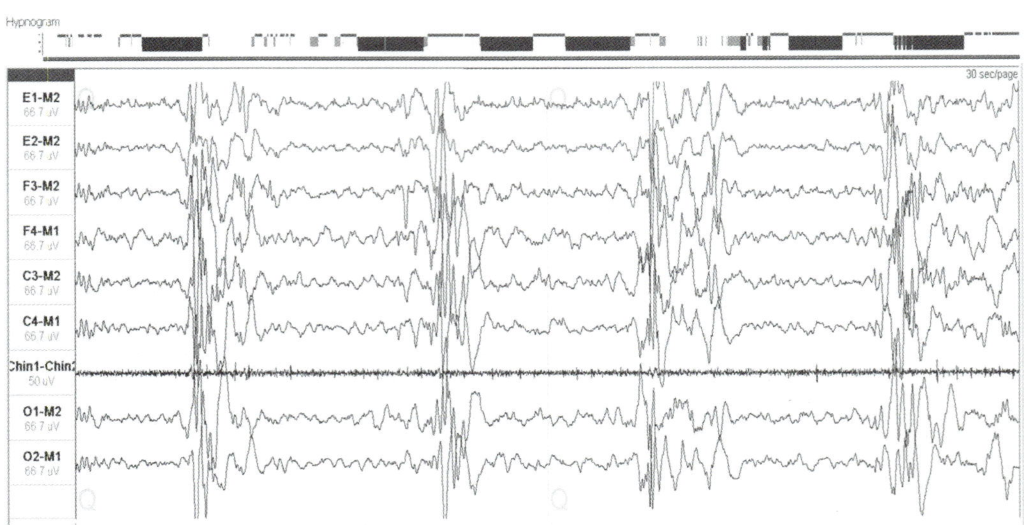

Figure 60-4 Maturation of the electroencephalogram waveform showing the development of tracé alternant pattern in a 4-week-old postterm infant. This tracing shows short bursts of high-amplitude delta waves interrupted by periods of low-amplitude mixed-frequency activity.

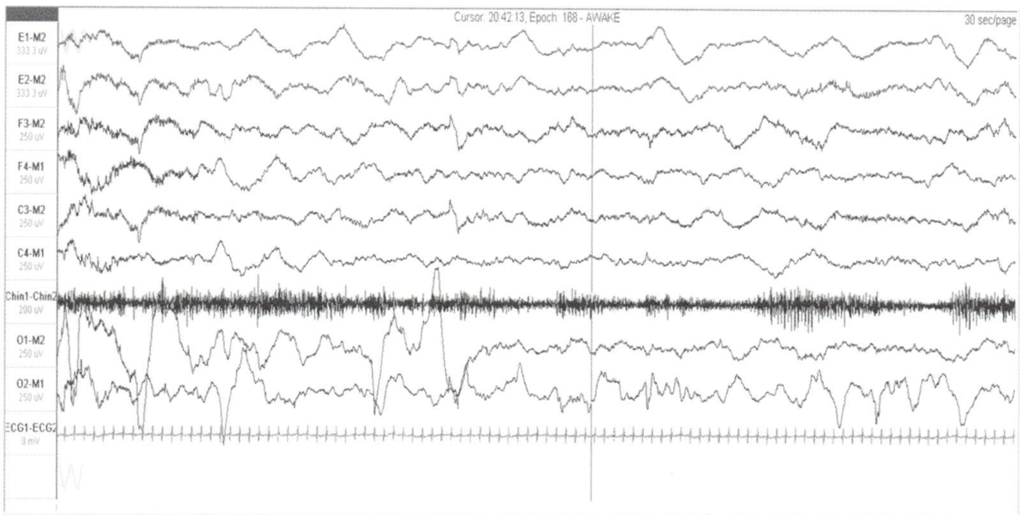

Figure 60-5 Awake movement and increased electrical activity seen in electroencephalogram. Awake waveforms are darker and thicker than seen in a sleep state. Utilize video to determine quiescence.

or scanning eye movements. Eyes will open intermittently, and irregular respirations are noticeable. When more than 50% of the epoch displays all of the aforementioned nonsleep characteristics, eyes wide open, vocalization (whimpering, crying, etc), or actively feeding, it is scored as *wake* (6).

Infant Stage R (Rapid Eye Movement)

Sleep onset is often very difficult to establish because of the variable DPR among newborns (Figure 60-6). When infants become drowsy, they become inactive, and the eyes become unfocused, blinking and closing for longer periods until they fall asleep. Most infants will enter sleep in *stage R (REM)*, characterized by eye movements, along with other facial movements in the way of smiles, frowns, and sucking. The EEG channels show theta waves of low voltage in an irregular mixed pattern. The eyes are closed, although sometimes not completely, and the EOG channels will show out-of-phase movement similar to the REM period seen in an adult study. The chin EMG is usually reduced but can be variable. Respirations will become irregular, and short central pauses are common with short, rapid breathing at other times. Body movement is present at times throughout this stage, most commonly, twitches or brief head movements.

When an epoch has four or more of the following criteria present in the EEG, EOG, EMG, and respiratory

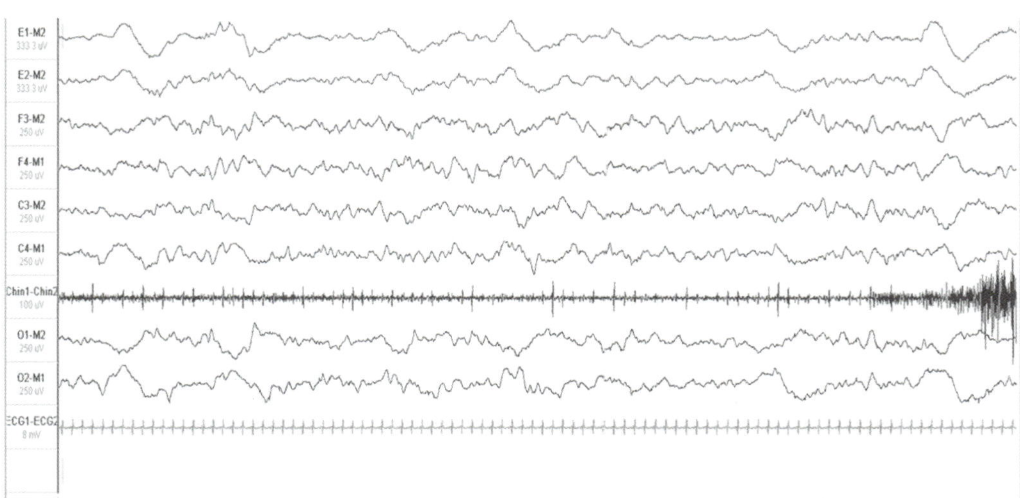

Figure 60-6 Sleep-onset electroencephalogram electrical activity quiets down and waveform clears, becoming thinner and less dark. Waveform frequency slows. Infant has eyes closed.

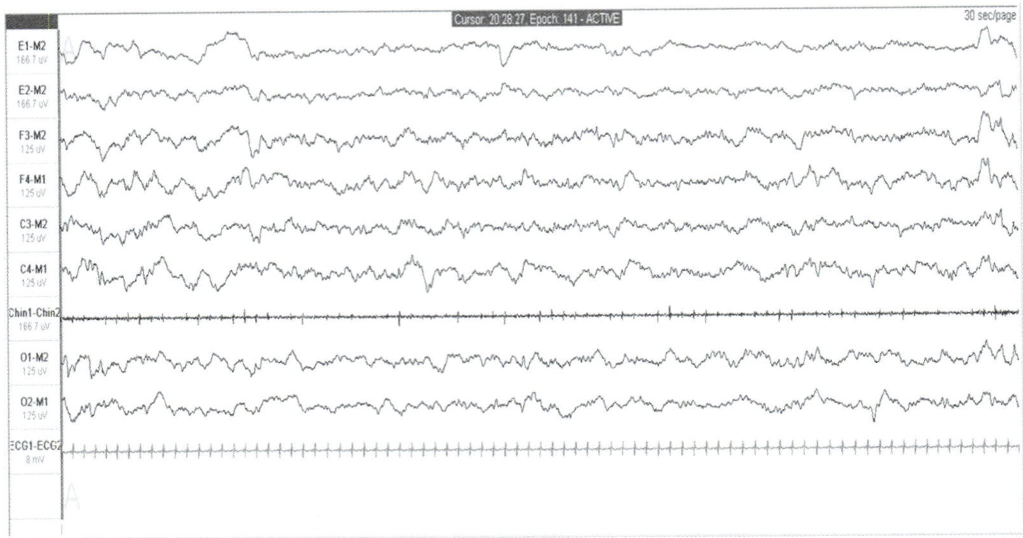

Figure 60-7 This polysomnographic tracing of stage R sleep in a 5-week postterm infant shows electroencephalogram—low-voltage mixed-frequency waves, electrooculogram—rapid eye movements, and electromyogram—(chin) low muscle tone.

channels for more than 50% of the epoch, it is scored as *stage R* sleep (see Figure 60-7, which demonstrates the eye movements, low-voltage mixed-frequency EEG, and reduced EMG tone seen in stage R).

A. Low-chin EMG
B. Eyes closed with at least one REM
C. Irregular respiration
D. Mouthing, sucking twitches or brief head movements
E. EEG exhibits a continuous pattern without sleep spindles

Irregular respirations AND rapid eye movements must be present to score REM.

In the absence of rapid eye movements, you may score stage R if all the following are present:

a. The EEG shows low or medium amplitude mixed-frequency activity without TA or sleep spindles.
b. The chin tone is low for the majority of the epoch.
c. There is no intervening arousal.

This stage will make up approximately 50% of a newborn's sleep time. After about 3 months of age, an infant begins to enter into sleep in an NREM state, similarly to what is seen in older children and adults (4).

Infant Stage N (Nonrapid Eye Movement)

An EEG pattern with HVS, TA, M waveforms, or sleep spindles categorizes *stage N (NREM)*, with one of these patterns primarily present depending on the maturity of the newborn. The EOG will show no REMs. The chin EMG is higher in tone than during *stage R* sleep. The breathing pattern is regular and cyclical, much like the breathing pattern seen in deep sleep in an adult study. There are no body movements, outside of respiration, except for phasic activity such as startles or sucking (6). When an epoch has four or more of the following present in the EEG, EOG, EMG, and respiratory channels for more than 50% of the epoch, one of which must be regular respiration, it is scored as stage N (NREM) (see Figure 60-8) (4).

a. Eyes closed with no eye movements
b. Chin EMG tone present
c. Regular respiration (post sigh respiratory pauses may occur)
d. TA, HVS, or sleep spindles present
e. Reduced movement relative to wake

Notice that during this time there is a lack of eye movement and slower higher voltage EEG.

Infant Stage T (Transitional)

Epochs that do not meet the criteria for one of the two sleep states, R or N sleep, are scored as *stage T (transitional sleep)*. This is a transitional sleep state more likely to be seen when the infant is alternating between stages R and N sleep, at sleep onset, or during arousals. Stage T can also be scored when a combination of different sleep states is seen in one epoch, with none being the dominant state (see Figure 60-9 for an example of transitional sleep) (4).

For a technologist inexperienced with scoring infant studies, it is best to start with determining sleep and wake activity, staging as much sleep time as possible. Next, try to recognize stage R versus stage N activity. It is normal to sometimes not realize what stage R or REM

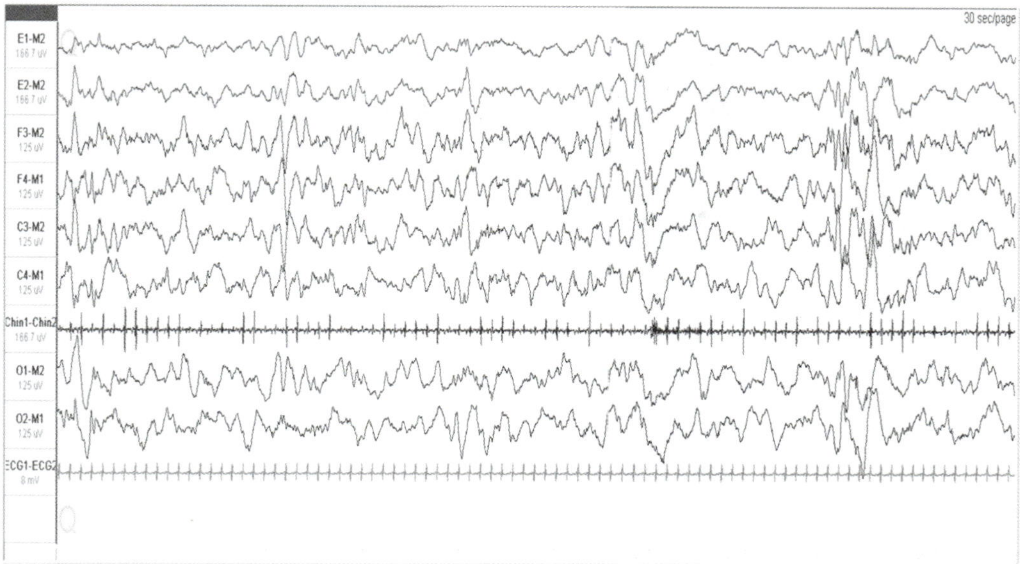

Figure 60-8 Stage N sleep in a 5-week postterm infant, which includes absence of eye movements, sustained muscle tone, and regular breathing and heart rate patterns. Few body movements are noted in this state. The electroencephalogram pattern evolves from tracé discontinue to tracé alternant and then into mature nonrapid eye movement sleep by age 6 months postterm.

looks like for that particular patient until the later part of the study. As with any study, if this happens, go back to the beginning to look for any possible missed REM periods. Once comfortable with finding wake, stage N, and stage R, look to mark *stage T* during the epochs just before each stage change. If the epoch contains either 3 NREM and 2 REM characteristics or 2 NREM and 3 REM characteristics, it should be changed to *stage T*. When staging infant sleep, it is important to determine wake and sleep states, while keeping in mind that the infant is most likely having the study performed to check for a breathing disorder. Therefore, respiratory events are extremely important, and proper staging is needed to recognize and score events correctly.

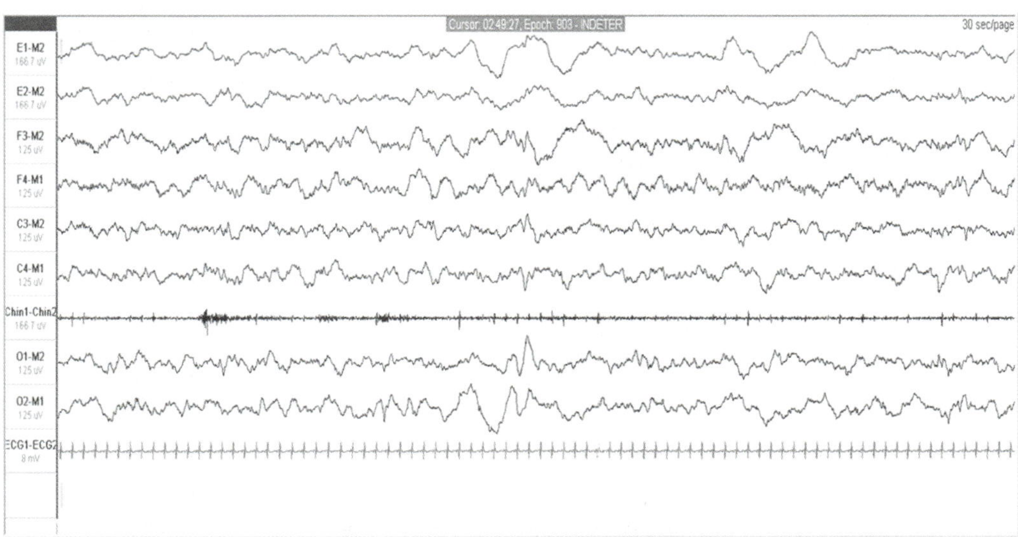

Figure 60-9 Example of transitional sleep. Electroencephalogram is disorganized, and the epoch cannot be classified as stage R or stage N sleep. Commonly seen in a transition period, such as from stage N to stage R sleep.

SCORING PEDIATRIC RESPIRATORY EVENTS

When scoring respiratory events in children, it is necessary to know the developmental level of the child and apply the appropriate rules for pediatrics. The AASM defines an abnormal respiratory event in the adult patient as one lasting greater than 10 seconds. In that period, the adult may miss two or three respiratory cycles, whereas young children have a higher respiratory rate and can easily have missed four to six or more breaths in the same 10-second period. This is one reason why respiratory events in children, and especially in infants, have different standards. Because young infants have a more compliant chest wall than do older children or adults, paradoxical movements of the chest wall and abdomen may be normal. Therefore, constantly maintaining good airflow signals is important during the study.

Respiratory event scoring rules from *The AASM Manual for the Scoring of Sleep and Associated Events* have been established for infants and children under 18 years. However, at the discretion of the sleep specialist, children 13 years and older can be scored using the established adult standards.

Apnea

Many pediatric laboratories enhance their ability to detect deficits of airflow and respiration by applying several different sensors, including thermistors, nasal pressure transducers, capnography, and esophageal pressure monometers, and use the sum channel of respiratory inductance plethysmography. Oronasal thermal sensors are recommended for use in detecting and classifying apneas, and a nasal pressure signal is used if the thermal sensor is unreliable. In pediatrics, score a respiratory event as an apnea when ALL of the following criteria are met:

a. There is a drop in the peak signal excursion by greater than or equal to 90% of pre-event baseline using an oronasal thermal sensor (diagnostic study), PAP device flow (titration study), or an *alternative* apnea sensor (diagnostic study).
b. The duration of the drop in sensor signal greater than or equal to 90% lasts at least the minimum duration as specified by obstructive, mixed, or central apnea duration criteria.
c. The event meets respiratory effort criteria for obstructive, central, or mixed apnea.

If airflow is absent for the duration of two baseline breaths and is associated with the presence of respiratory effort throughout the entire period of absent airflow, then the event is considered to be an *obstructive apnea*. A central apnea is marked if apnea criteria are met, respiratory efforts are absent, and one of the following criteria are met:

a. The event lasts greater than/equal to 20 seconds.
b. The event lasts for the duration of two breaths during baseline and is associated with an arousal or a greater than/equal to 3% arterial desaturation.
c. The event lasts at least the duration of two breaths during baseline breathing and is associated with a decrease in heart rate to less than 50 beats per minute for at least 5 seconds. For infants less than 1 year of age, the decrease in heart rate requirement adjusts to less than 60 beats per minute for 15 seconds due to higher baseline heart rates.

Central apneas associated with movement or a sigh should not be marked. Central apneas less than 20 seconds are considered normal in children and are *not* scored unless they cause an associated arousal or a greater than or equal to 3% desaturation. *Mixed apnea* is scored if the event meets apnea criteria and contains a portion with no respiratory effort and a portion with respiratory effort, regardless of which occurs first.

Hypopneas

Ideally, the waveform from a nasal air pressure transducer signal detects hypopneas; however, the waveform from an oronasal thermal sensor is used if the nasal pressure signal is unreliable. A respiratory event where there is a reduction in the waveform of greater than or equal to 30% for a period of two baseline breaths or more accompanied by an arousal, or a desaturation equal to or greater than 3% should be scored as a hypopnea. Some centers distinguish between obstructive and central hypopneas. Generally, if the respiratory efforts remain in phase (assuming good belt position), score a hypopnea as obstructive if *any* of the following criteria are met:

a. There is snoring during the event.
b. There is increased inspiratory flattening of the nasal pressure or PAP device flow signal compared to baseline breathing.
c. There is an associated thoracoabdominal paradox that occurs during the event but not during pre-event breathing.

Score the *hypopnea* as central if *none* of the aforementioned criteria are met.

In contrast to adults, children may sleep through respiratory events and, therefore, may not have an arousal associated with a respiratory event (7). Children tend to have a higher threshold for arousal. Another important difference is that children have a more compliant respiratory system, allowing them to maintain their oxyhemoglobin status without the oxygen desaturations or arousals seen more prominently with adults.

Respiratory Effort–Related Arousal

Perhaps because their need for sleep is greater than their need to wake up to breathe, younger children do not arouse from sleep as easily as from respiratory events. Unlike with adults, respiratory effort–related arousal (RERA) events in childhood are less common. For the child to have a scorable arousal from sleep, the respiratory event is usually significant enough to meet the criteria for either apnea or hypopnea. The AASM scoring rules for a RERA include the requirement of a respiratory sequence that does not meet the scoring rules for apnea or hypopnea. In pediatrics, scoring RERAs differs from that for adults in duration requirement. In children, events are a sequence of greater than or equal to two breaths, instead of 10 seconds for adults (4). The important aspect in scoring a RERA is that the event, although not an apnea or a hypopnea, still involves an associated arousal. One or more of the following should be present during the breathing sequence:

a. Increasing respiratory effort
b. Flattening of the inspiratory portion of the nasal pressure (diagnostic study) or PAP device flow (titration study) waveform
c. Snoring
d. An elevation in the end-tidal P_{CO_2} above pre-event baseline

In children younger than teenage, RERA events are less likely.

Younger children more frequently have periods of nonarousal respiratory episodes that do not meet the criteria to be scored as a RERA, apnea, or hypopnea (see Figure 60-10 for an example of a nonarousal respiratory episode). Often seen in pediatric patients are periods of increased work of breathing with substernal retractions, snoring, an increase in end-tidal CO_2, and a flattening in the nasal pressure waveform for a period of at least two breaths. There is no scorable cortical arousal seen in the EEG waveform, and desaturations are less than 3%. By AASM rules, these episodes do not meet the criteria for an apnea, hypopnea, or RERA and cannot be scored as a respiratory event. During these episodes, careful review using the data from sensors such as pulse oximeter, nasal pressure transducer, esophageal monometer, and respiratory inductance plethysmography can identify subtle events that could possibly be scored as hypopneas in these periods.

Partial airway obstruction, characterized by an increasing respiratory effort similar to obstructive events, but without a significant drop in oxygen saturation or a 30% drop in airflow, may signify upper airway resistance. Even without a desaturation, these occurrences may be fragmenting the patient's sleep, resulting in hypersomnolence, difficulty attending school, or other daytime sequelae. These episodes, although not scorable as a RERA, may be contributing to the child's symptoms, and therefore the epochs should be noted and brought to the attention of the sleep specialist for careful analysis.

Sleep-Related Hypoventilation

Distinct extended periods of sleep where CO_2 level is increased and/or respiratory effort is lower in amplitude than resting wakefulness baseline can indicate sleep-related hypoventilation in pediatric studies. Neuromuscular weakness and other congenital disorders such as

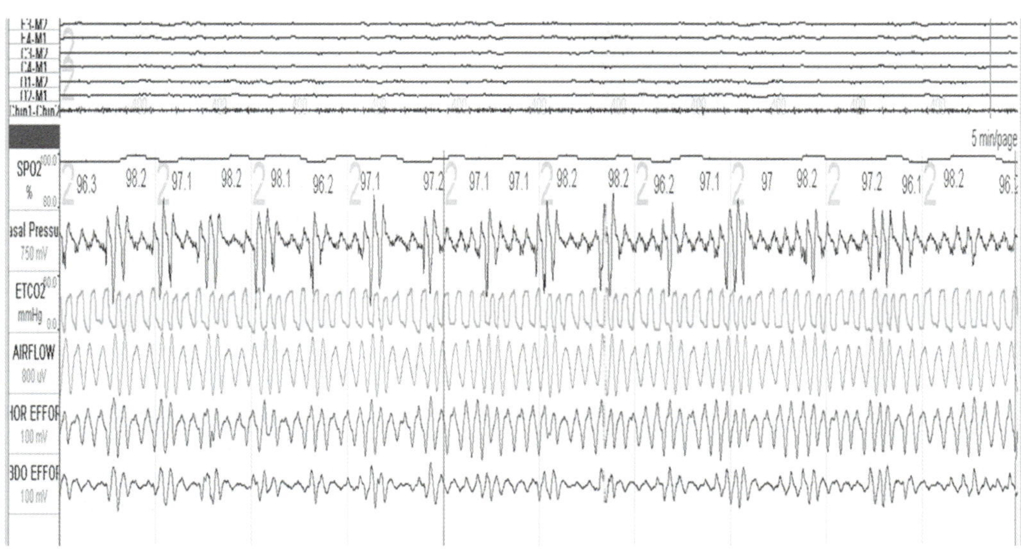

Figure 60-10 Nonarousal-related episode. Periods of reduction in nasal pressure waveform. Patient has increased work of breathing with snoring, and desaturations of only 1% to 2% with no scorable electroencephalogram arousal.

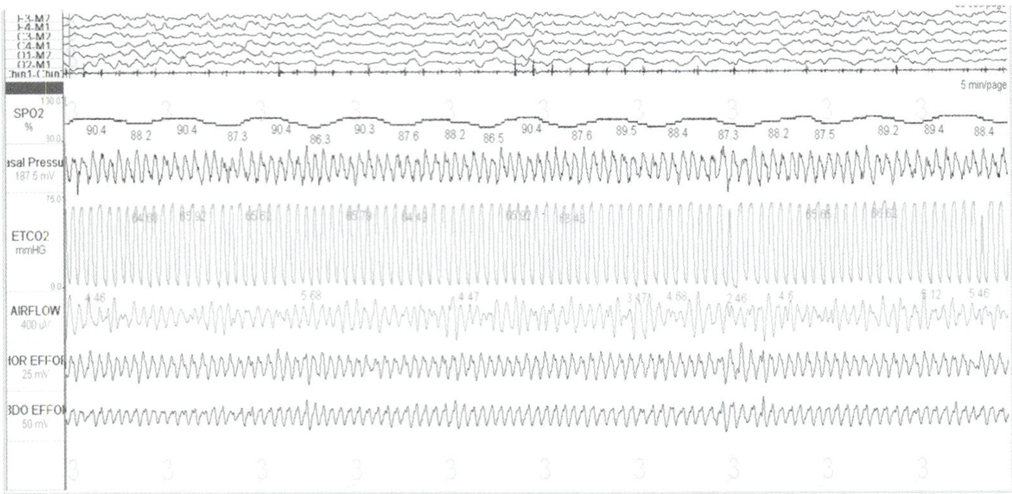

Figure 60-11 Central congenital hypoventilation syndrome showing increased CO_2 and cyclic desaturations.

chronic lung disease can contribute to hypoventilation. This is one of the reasons pediatric studies utilize end-tidal CO_2 monitoring (see Figure 60-11 for an example of hypoventilation). When the PCO_2 is greater than 50 mm Hg for more than 25% of the total sleep time, it is considered hypoventilation.

- For detection of hypoventilation during a diagnostic study, use arterial PCO_2, transcutaneous PCO_2, or end- tidal PCO_2.
- For detection of hypoventilation during PAP titration, use arterial PCO_2 or transcutaneous PCO_2.

Mark epochs from the start of these periods to the end and submit for further evaluation by the interpreting physician.

APNEA OF PREMATURITY, APNEA OF INFANCY, AND PERIODIC BREATHING

Short central apneas are common in children of all ages during REM sleep, during transitions between sleep stages, or following an arousal. Children can have central apneas after a sigh or movement that last more than 10 seconds without a related oxygen desaturation.

Distinguished by central apneas lasting 20 seconds or longer, shorter central apneas associated with bradycardia, significant oxygen desaturation, and/or neurologic sequelae, *apnea of prematurity,* as its name suggests, occurs in premature infants and is quite common. These respiratory events usually resolve when the infant reaches full-term gestational age. If the infant is not premature, the condition is then called *apnea of infancy*. These events can be very frightening to parents and can be very serious when associated with frequent bradycardia or oxygen desaturations.

Another breathing disorder commonly seen in newborns is *periodic breathing*. Characterized by three or more central respiratory pauses of 3 seconds or more each and with less than 20 seconds of regular respiration between each apnea, periodic breathing can occur in normal newborns, particularly during active sleep. It is more likely in premature infants and usually decreases as the infant's respiratory control system matures. Depending on the age and development of the infant, periodic breathing episodes during sleep are considered normal if they occur only for a small percentage of the total sleep time. Higher percentages of periodic breathing during sleep time or those causing desaturations and/or arousals may require treatment. Begin scoring periodic breathing events starting from the beginning of the first apneic event and continuing until the end of the last event that meets the criteria (Figure 60-12 shows an episode of periodic breathing).

Arousals

Subcortical arousals may occur more often than we capture with scalp EEG electrodes, yet arousals are extremely important in discovering the cause of poor-quality sleep. In pediatrics, there is no rule difference in scoring arousals; therefore, score them following the same criteria as for adults. The rules state that the duration of the EEG waveform shift must be a minimum of 3 seconds. The variation observed in children having arousals is that they will often have subtle events with periods of EEG shifts less than 3 seconds in length. By AASM rules, these do not count to be scored as an arousal.

An arousal can be caused by a respiratory or movement disorder. Careful examination utilizing all EEG channels is best to score arousals in pediatric patients. Respiratory events, leg movements, video, and additional

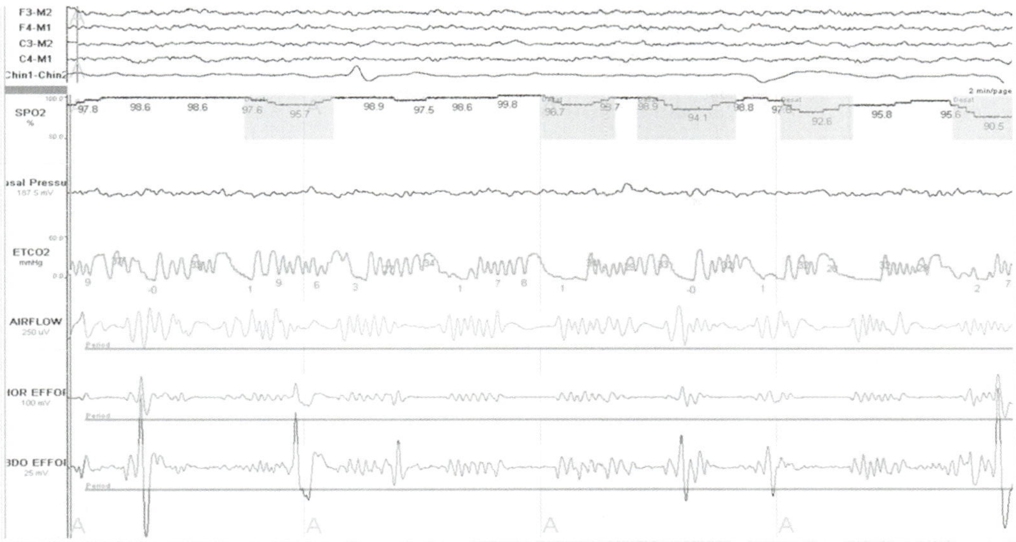

Figure 60-12 Periodic breathing in a full-term infant at 4 weeks of age.

channels are important indicators of the presence of an arousal. If you suspect arousal events, use the video and waveforms to identify what is occurring. Then look closely at the EEG waveform for the earliest increase in artifact or an increased frequency within alpha range of 8 to 13 Hz in the EEG waveform. In an infant, darkening or thickening of the waveform can indicate arousal from sleep. Mark the event from the point of the EEG change until the end, when the EEG waveform returns to its previous sleep pattern. If this period in the waveform meets the criteria, then score it as an arousal.

Cardiac Dysrhythmias in Children

Cardiac dysrhythmias are uncommon in children, but as in adults, the technologist monitoring the sleep study should be familiar with the different types and their electrocardiogram (ECG) characteristics. The technologist must be able to recognize life-threatening conditions and must feel comfortable with responding appropriately according to their specific sleep center protocols.

Dysrhythmias are conditions where the heart rhythm is irregular, too fast (tachycardia), or too slow (bradycardia). A heart rate of less than 80 bpm for the first month of life, less than 70 bpm in an infant 1 to 2 months of age, or less than 60 bpm for an older infant is considered bradycardia. A brief period of sinus bradycardia is common following a respiratory event. Tachycardia is defined as a heart rate of more than 190 bpm for a newborn or more than 160 bpm for an infant. Both of these conditions occur commonly for brief periods during phasic REM sleep, when the heart rate increases and then decreases before recovering to normal baseline (8). They can also occur during apnea episodes or arousals, as the heart slows down and then works harder to recover. Cardiac decelerations can also occur and are defined as a drop in heart rate from baseline, where the rate does not achieve the minimum level necessary to be considered bradycardia. These are usually of sinus origin seen in association with a respiratory event.

Other dysrhythmias in children are similar but less common than those witnessed in adults. Children can have premature ventricular contractions (PVCs) occurring during the night. PVCs, where the heart produces an extra ectopic beat that originates in the ventricles rather than the sinus node, are common in normal children and adults. However, PVCs that occur in series or appear to have more than one focus (different appearances to the waveform) should be brought to the attention of the physician.

One dysrhythmia that occurs more commonly in children is supraventricular tachycardia. It produces a heart rate greater than 220 bpm and can produce increased respiratory rate, anxiety, fussiness in the infant, or discomfort. Most episodes last only a few seconds and should be noted by the technologist. Prolonged or frequent episodes indicate the need for intervention, and the technologist should treat this condition as indicated in their protocols.

MOVEMENT, ARTIFACT RECOGNITION, AND BEHAVIORAL NOTATION

Bruxism, rhythmic movement disorder, myoclonus, and other movement disorders are all seen in pediatric sleep studies. Movement disorders are not specific to pediatric polysomnography and are scored using the same rules as in adult studies. These are mentioned here because the main difference is that in children, there is the potential for seeing more of them. These events can and will occur anytime during studies performed in a pediatric sleep center. Expect to see them and know how to differentiate between a movement disorder and other causes of artifact. For specifics on the variety of disorders, their characteristics, and scoring of these events, turn to the chapters on movement disorders and adult scoring. Also, refer to the *AASM Scoring Manual* for rules on how to mark each event accordingly.

As displayed in the sleep study waveforms, artifacts seen in the pediatric study are similar to those associated with adults. Sweat, movement, muscle contraction, and 50/60-Hz artifacts are as common in pediatric sleep studies as they are in adult studies. Along with these artifact types, children generate artifacts from crying, rocking, sucking, and feeding that will appear at different times throughout the study. Although it is often helpful during a study to have a parent stay in the room with the child, the parent can cause artifact by touching or rubbing the child to provide comfort. Sometimes, the snoring of a parent can be mistaken as coming from the child. Artifact from laptop computers and cell phones and noise from TVs used by the parents can also interfere with the recording. Not only can the noise and light cause problems, but the devices can also cause artifact. Some parents arrive at the sleep center expecting to talk on their phone during the night or wanting to use their laptop. It is important to address this before the night of the study and while scheduling so that the parent or guardian is aware of the sleep center policy.

Children find it very difficult to get back to sleep, and correcting artifacts during the recording usually means disrupting their sleep and potentially awakening them. Some artifacts do not need immediate attention and can wait until the child is in deep sleep to avoid waking the child. It takes an experienced, knowledgeable technologist who has reviewed the child's history and symptoms to determine when to correct the artifact. For instance, a leg lead that has fallen off a sleeping patient with suspected narcolepsy does not require replacement immediately if it has fallen off just after lights out. In that case, it is best to wait and capture sleep and REM latencies. The redundancy built into the studies with several EEG channels collecting brain waves and a thermistor, capnography, and nasal pressure, all assessing the presence of airflow, allows the technologist to use their best discretion in regard to when it is appropriate to disturb the patient in order to correct artifact. It is essential that the technologist document patient movements and parental actions that may indicate the source of the artifact. Children are often restless during a sleep study, making application of the electrodes challenging. If the electrodes are not attached properly, it will lead to a long night of adjusting or reattaching to try to correct the artifacts that occur when the child moves, pulls, or touches the electrodes. Properly applying electrodes and achieving low impedances from the start is the best way to reduce artifacts throughout the study.

LIMITED CHANNEL STUDIES

Although there are some pediatric patients who could benefit from home sleep apnea testing or pneumograms, these limited channel studies are not as useful in the pediatric population as they are in adults. Generally, these devices measure airflow by thermistor, chest wall movement by impedance, ECG, heart rate, and oximetry, with additional channels sometimes added such as snore, EMG, or EEG. Without a technologist present to correct artifacts and document activities such as feeding, movement, or breath sounds, quality can be variable in children. Video, sound, extended EEG, EMG, or EOG are often not collected, making it difficult to assess arousals and sleep.

The data obtained from these studies is quite limited (9). Sleep latency is approximated, and an activity log documented by a parent may be helpful in some cases; however, the limited number of channels does not offer a comprehensive view of sleep cycles or assessment of sleep stages, and REM latency cannot be determined with any certainty. Generally, home sleep apnea testing is not recommended in the pediatric population. The AASM position paper for the use of a Home Sleep Apnea Test (HSAT) for the Diagnosis of OSA in Children specifically states that the use of a HSAT is not recommended for the diagnosis of obstructive sleep apnea in children. The ultimate judgment regarding any specific care must be made by the clinician (9).

PREPARING THE SUMMARY REPORT

Report Values

The content of any sleep study report can change from center to center. It is up to each center to decide what criteria are useful and how it wants to display data in its reports. The report generated for the interpreting physician should include any specific equipment used and variables collected during the study. It should state and define the center's criteria for scoring events. Documentation should include detailed technologist notes explaining procedures during the testing along with all interventions made during the study such as adding or adjusting oxygen, initiation or adjustment of PAP, ventilator adjustments, or any other changes made, along with an explanation for the change. For the duration of their stay in the sleep center, patient behaviors such as crying, screaming, talking, feeding, parent comforting, intensity of any snoring, and any other interventions before, during, and after the study should be included in the technologist documentation along with the report for interpretation. Any comment the technologist makes regarding breathing effort, respiratory rate, or heart rate, along with deviations from their norm, should include the time of occurrence and epoch numbers.

Final reports for infant studies will include some of the same data parameters as older child and adult reports. Apnea and hypopnea indexes, along with low, average, and high heart rates and oxygen saturations, as well as the patient's body position status during the study, are incorporated. Include total recording time, together with a breakdown of total and percentage of stage R, N, and T sleep times (10). In the report of an infant study, the total number of periodic breathing episodes, percentage, and index are calculated. The number and duration of bradycardia and desaturation events should be reported. Baseline, low, average, high, and the amount of time spent in certain heart rate and oxygen level ranges are also important. As with adult studies, report events by position and in what state of sleep they occurred.

Any additional data points should be included in the report and presented in a digestible manner. These are often represented in custom tables. Examples include capnography, use of oxygen, oral appliance titration, and Inspire therapy.

A carefully performed, documented, scored, and interpreted study can provide invaluable data for diagnosing and treating sleep disorders in infants and children. Review the parameters to be reported for polysomnography contained in the AASM *Scoring Manual* to decide what other information to include in a computer-generated report. Given that there are a great deal of data to present, it may be a good idea to have several report templates customized for different types of studies. In this way, the report is concentrated on the data collected for that type of patient, and useful for diagnoses, leaving unnecessary information out of the report.

REFERENCES

1. Wise MS, Nichols CD, Grigg-Damberger MM, et al. Executive summary of respiratory indications for polysomnography in children: an evidence based review. *Sleep*. 2011;34(3):389-398.
2. Sheldon S, Riter S, Detrojan M. *Atlas of Sleep Medicine in Infants and Children*. Futura Publishing; 1999: 99-135.
3. Grigg-Damberger MM, Gozal D, Marcus CL, et al. The visual scoring of sleep and arousal in infants and children. *J Clin Sleep Med*. 2007;3(2):201-240.
4. Berry RB, Albertario CL, Harding SM, et al; for the American Academy of Sleep Medicine. *The AASM Manual for the Scoring of Sleep and Associated Events: Rules, Terminology and Technical Specifications [Version 3.0]*. American Academy of Sleep Medicine; 2023.
5. Anders T, Emde R, Parmelee A, eds. *A Manual of Standardized Terminology, Techniques and Criteria for Scoring of States of Sleep and Wakefulness in Newborn Infants*. Brain Information Service/Brain Research Institute; 1971.
6. Crowell DH; the CHIME Study Group. *An Atlas of Infant Polysomnography*. Parthenon Publishing; 2003:63-77.
7. Marcus CL. Sleep-disordered breathing in children. *Am J Respir Crit Care Med*. 2001;164:16-30.
8. American Thoracic Society. Standards and indications for cardiopulmonary sleep studies in children. *Am J Respir Crit Care Med*. 1996;153:866-878.
9. Ramanathan R, Corwin MJ, Hunt CE, et al; The CHIME Study Group. Cardiorespiratory events recorded on home monitors: comparison of healthy infants with those at increased risk for SIDS. *JAMA*. 2001;285: 2199-2207.
10. Iber C, Ancoli-Israel S, Chesson A, et al. *The AASM Manual for the Scoring of Sleep and Associated Events: Rules, Terminology and Technical Specifications*. American Academy of Sleep Medicine; 2007.

Chapter 61
Sleep-Related Breathing Disorders in Children

JORDAN E. RUSK

KEY CONCEPTS/LEARNING OBJECTIVES

The key concepts for this chapter include describing sleep-related breathing disorders in children; reviewing existing, current treatment options; and discussing the relationship between sleep-related breathing disorders and comorbidities and the effects of sleep-related breathing disorders on quality of life.

KEY TERMS

Adenotonsillectomy
Apnea of prematurity (AOP)
Apparent life-threatening event (ALTE)
Brief resolved unexplained event (BRUE)
Congenital central hypoventilation syndrome (CCHS)
Obstructive sleep apnea syndrome (OSAS)
Sleep-related breathing disorder (SRBD)
Sudden infant death syndrome (SIDS)

Sleep is essential for a child's growth, development, and overall well-being. However, for some children, sleep is disrupted by breathing difficulties that can have serious health consequences. Sleep-related breathing disorders (SRBDs) encompass a range of conditions in which abnormal breathing patterns occur during sleep, leading to fragmented rest, oxygen desaturation, and increased cardiovascular strain. These disorders can vary in severity from primary snoring to obstructive sleep apnea (OSA) and central sleep apnea (CSA). Without proper diagnosis and treatment, SRBDs can negatively affect cognitive function, behavior, and physical health, making early recognition critical (1).

DEFINITION OF SLEEP-RELATED BREATHING DISORDERS

SRBDs refer to a group of conditions characterized by disordered respiration during sleep, ranging from mild airflow limitations to complete airway obstruction. The most common pediatric SRBD is OSA, in which intermittent upper airway collapse leads to disrupted sleep and decreased oxygen levels (2). Other forms include CSA, where the brain fails to send proper signals to the muscles that control breathing, and hypoventilation syndromes, which result in inadequate air exchange. While some children may experience only mild disturbances, others may suffer from significant daytime fatigue, neurocognitive impairments, and increased cardiovascular risk if left untreated (3).

IMPORTANCE OF RECOGNIZING AND MANAGING SLEEP-RELATED BREATHING DISORDERS IN CHILDREN

Early detection of SRBDs is essential because these conditions can profoundly impact a child's cognitive, behavioral, and physical development. Studies have linked untreated SRBDs to attention-deficit/hyperactivity disorder (ADHD)–like symptoms, learning difficulties, and poor academic performance (4). Additionally, children with untreated OSA are at higher risk for hypertension, metabolic dysfunction, and cardiovascular complications (5). Given that symptoms such as snoring, restless sleep, and behavioral changes may be subtle, parents and health care providers must remain vigilant in recognizing the signs. Prompt diagnosis and intervention—whether through adenotonsillectomy, continuous positive airway pressure (CPAP) therapy, or lifestyle modifications—can significantly improve a child's quality of life (QOL) (6).

PREVALENCE AND DEMOGRAPHIC CONSIDERATIONS

SRBDs are more common in children than previously thought, with estimates suggesting that 1% to 5% of children have OSA, while habitual snoring affects up to 27% of the pediatric population (7). Certain risk factors increase a child's likelihood of developing an SRBD, including:

- Enlarged tonsils and adenoids (a leading cause of pediatric OSA)
- Obesity (associated with increased airway collapsibility)
- Craniofacial abnormalities (such as micrognathia or midface hypoplasia)
- Neuromuscular disorders (which can impair airway tone)
- Prematurity (higher incidence of central apnea and immature respiratory control)

SRBDs are common yet frequently underdiagnosed in children, with significant consequences if left untreated. By recognizing the symptoms and risk factors early, health care providers, educators, and caregivers can play a vital role in improving health outcomes and ensuring children receive the necessary interventions to thrive.

APNEA OF PREMATURITY

Apnea of prematurity (AOP) is a condition commonly observed in preterm infants (born before 33 weeks of gestation), characterized by pauses in breathing lasting 20 seconds or more. These episodes are primarily due to the underdevelopment of the central respiratory centers in the brain, leading to central apnea. Obstructive and mixed apneas can also occur when there is a blockage in the airway or a combination of central and obstructive factors. The incidence and severity of AOP are inversely related to gestational age; the more premature the infant, the higher the likelihood and severity of apnea episodes (8). These infants often exhibit exaggerated responses to hypoxia and hypercarbia, along with impaired ventilatory reflexes (9). Even full-term newborns can experience occasional respiratory pauses lasting 30 seconds or more (10). Premature infants are at an even greater risk, with more frequent and prolonged pauses, often accompanied by bradycardia, hypoxemia, and/or hypercarbia. Their rapid respiratory rate and limited oxygen reserves further exacerbate these issues (11).

If apnea is well-documented in the neonatal intensive care unit (NICU), treatment is usually initiated without a sleep study. A full polysomnography (PSG) is required to assess obstructive events, while a pneumogram—measuring chest wall movement, airflow, heart rate, oxygen saturation, and, possibly, esophageal pH—can help evaluate central apneas and their potential link to gastroesophageal reflux (GER) (10).

Methylxanthine therapy, using caffeine or theophylline, is a common treatment for AOP (12). Caffeine can significantly reduce apnea episodes within the first week of treatment, while theophylline improves periodic breathing and central apneas in both rapid eye movement (REM) and nonrapid eye movement (NREM) sleep, although it does not affect bradycardia or obstructive events (10). If significant obstructive events persist, positive airway pressure therapy (CPAP or BPAP) may be necessary (13). CPAP has been shown to decrease obstructive apneas and reduce the severity of desaturations. Combining caffeine with CPAP therapy may shorten the duration of respiratory support and offer neurodevelopmental benefits (12). While caffeine use in newborns has not been linked to an increased risk of OSA, it may contribute to periodic limb movements during sleep (14).

Sleeping position can influence the frequency and severity of cardiorespiratory events. Preterm infants in the supine position tend to have higher respiratory rates, lower oxygen saturation, and a diminished ventilatory response to hypercapnia compared to those sleeping prone. While supine sleep is associated with nearly twice the number of obstructive events, prone sleeping leads to deeper, quieter sleep with fewer arousals but an increased risk of central apnea (15). However, due to the heightened risk of sudden infant death syndrome (SIDS) in the prone position, it is recommended that healthy term newborns sleep on their backs (11).

BRIEF RESOLVED UNEXPLAINED EVENT AND APPARENT LIFE-THREATENING EVENT

A brief resolved unexplained event (BRUE) is defined by the American Academy of Pediatrics (AAP) as "a sudden, brief, and now resolved episode in an infant younger than 1 year involving one or more of the following: (1) cyanosis or pallor; (2) absent, decreased, or irregular breathing; (3) a marked change in tone (hypertonia or hypotonia); and (4) altered level of responsiveness" (8). BRUEs are classified as either low risk or high risk, based on the patient's history, physical examination, and risk factors.

For low-risk infants, AAP guidelines recommend minimal diagnostic testing and focus on caregiver education and reassurance rather than hospitalization (8). Suggested interventions may include pulse oximetry monitoring during observation, pertussis testing if clinically indicated, and an electrocardiogram to rule out cardiac arrhythmias. A child abuse evaluation should be considered if concerning historical features are present. Families should receive education on BRUEs and cardiopulmonary resuscitation (CPR) training resources (16).

For high-risk BRUEs, there are no specific universal treatment recommendations, as management depends on the underlying etiology, if identified. High-risk factors include recurrent episodes, a history of prematurity, significant medical conditions, and concerning findings on physical examination. Hospital admission, continuous monitoring, and further investigations such as a PSG or pneumogram may be warranted (16,17).

Previously, some BRUEs were classified as apparent life-threatening events (ALTEs), a term that is now largely replaced by BRUE. An ALTE was described as "an episode that is frightening to the observer and involves apnea (central or obstructive), color change (cyanosis or pallor), significant change in muscle tone, choking, or gagging" (8). Unlike BRUE, ALTE placed greater emphasis on caregiver perception, rather than objective criteria. ALTEs often prompted extensive testing and hospitalization, even in cases where no serious medical condition was identified (16).

Common conditions associated with BRUEs and ALTEs include seizures, GER, cardiac arrhythmias, laryngomalacia, tracheomalacia, and child abuse (16). If obstructive events are suspected, an overnight PSG should be conducted to evaluate for sleep-disordered breathing. A pneumogram—which assesses chest wall movement, airflow, heart rate, and oximetry—may be used to differentiate central apnea from GER-related events. If GER is suspected, esophageal pH or impedance monitoring can help establish a correlation between reflux events and respiratory symptoms (16).

SUDDEN INFANT DEATH SYNDROME AND SLEEP POSITIONING

A relationship between ALTE and SIDS has not been definitively established. According to the Centers for Disease Control and Prevention (CDC), SIDS is defined as "the sudden death of an infant under 11 years of age that remains unexplained after a complete autopsy, death scene investigation, and clinical history review" (18). The prevalence of SIDS in the United States is approximately 0.35/1,000 live births, with the highest risk occurring between 1 and 4 months of age (19).

The risk of SIDS is significantly increased in infants placed in the prone sleeping position (19). Since the introduction of the "Back to Sleep" campaign in 1992, which promoted supine sleeping, the incidence of SIDS has decreased by more than 50% (19). However, some studies suggest an increase in GER and ALTE cases, potentially related to the supine sleep position (16). Despite this, the AAP continues to recommend supine sleep as the safest position for infants, as the risk of SIDS outweighs concerns about reflux (19).

Additional safe sleep recommendations include using a firm sleep surface; avoiding soft bedding; room-sharing without bed-sharing; and eliminating exposure to smoke, alcohol, and overheating (19). Caregivers should also be educated on the dangers of inclined sleepers, commercial sleep positioners, and other non-recommended sleep products that have been linked to airway obstruction and suffocation (16).

CHILDHOOD OBSTRUCTIVE SLEEP APNEA

The majority of children referred to a sleep center are evaluated for suspected obstructive sleep-disordered breathing (SDB), which, in pediatrics, encompasses a spectrum ranging from primary snoring to OSA. Approximately 10% to 12% of children snore regularly, with pediatric OSA affecting 1% to 5% of children, particularly in the preschool and early school-age years (5). Pediatric OSA is defined by prolonged partial upper airway obstruction (hypopnea) and/or intermittent complete obstruction (apnea), leading to disruptions in ventilation and sleep architecture (1).

Risk Factors and Symptoms

Key risk factors for snoring and OSA include conditions that reduce pharyngeal airway size or alter airway compliance, such as adenotonsillar hypertrophy, obesity, neuromuscular disorders, and craniofacial abnormalities (eg, Down syndrome or Pierre Robin Syndrome) (20). Parents often report snoring, gasping, choking, frequent nighttime awakenings, enuresis, diaphoresis, and observed apneic events. In contrast to adults, children with OSA may present with daytime hyperactivity rather than excessive sleepiness, along with irritability, poor academic performance, mouth breathing, and morning headaches (5).

Neurocognitive and Developmental Impact

Even primary snoring, previously considered benign, has been linked to neurocognitive deficits and academic difficulties, particularly in math, science, and reading comprehension (21). Pediatric SDB has been associated with impaired memory, attention deficits, and reduced executive function, highlighting the importance of early identification and treatment (20).

Considerations in Infants

Newborns evaluated for apnea of infancy may initially appear to have severe obstructive events on PSG, partly due to their higher baseline respiratory rate and periodic breathing patterns (1). However, respiratory stability improves with maturation, and true OSA in infants is less common outside of underlying medical conditions such as laryngomalacia, bronchopulmonary dysplasia, or central nervous system disorders (16).

CLINICAL EVALUATION

The clinical evaluation of OSA in children involves a comprehensive assessment of risk factors, symptoms, and physical examination findings. Clinicians should maintain a high index of suspicion for OSA in children presenting with risk factors such as obesity, enuresis, or attention difficulties in school. A thorough history should include inquiries about snoring, labored or obstructed breathing during sleep, and restless or nonrestorative sleep (22). Physical examination should assess tonsil size, as adenotonsillar hypertrophy is a common contributor to pediatric OSA.

However, clinical evaluation alone may not be sufficient to accurately diagnose OSA. Studies have shown that only about half of children with suggestive history and physical examination findings have OSA confirmed through objective assessment. PSG is considered the gold standard for diagnosing OSA in children, as it provides a definitive evaluation of SRBDs. While clinical evaluation is essential in identifying children at risk for OSA, objective testing with PSG is often necessary to confirm the diagnosis and guide appropriate management (2).

POLYSOMNOGRAPHY

PSG remains the gold standard for diagnosing OSA in children. An overnight, in-laboratory PSG is essential not only for confirming the presence of OSA but also for assessing its severity, which guides subsequent treatment decisions. Nap studies are generally inadequate for this purpose, as they often fail to capture sufficient REM sleep, leading to an underestimation of OSA severity (2).

Home-based or abbreviated sleep studies are not recommended for pediatric populations due to concerns about their accuracy in predicting the severity of the disorder. Children present unique challenges during PSG, such as noncooperation and increased movement during sleep, which can compromise signal quality. Therefore, it is crucial that PSGs in children are conducted by staff experienced in pediatric sleep medicine. In addition to the standard adult PSG montage, monitoring of end-tidal or transcutaneous carbon dioxide levels is recommended to assess for hypoventilation. For children who are medically or developmentally complex, a higher level of staffing, potentially on a one-to-one basis, may be necessary to ensure a successful study.

There are home sleep testing devices that are Food and Drug Administration (FDA) approved for pediatric populations. For example, the Nox T3 is FDA approved for children two and over. The Itamar WatchPAT is approved for children 12 and over. Home sleep testing can be used in children when in-lab testing is not possible for geographic, financial, or complex health reasons. It is an option when children are unable to tolerate a full PSG due to developmental or sensory issues. The choice to use a home testing device over an in-lab study should be made carefully by the provider ordering the study based on the patient's history and surrounding situations.

Current guidelines emphasize the importance of overnight, in-laboratory PSG for the accurate diagnosis and assessment of OSA in children, highlighting the need for specialized pediatric expertise and appropriate monitoring techniques during the study (23).

SEQUELAE OF OBSTRUCTIVE SLEEP APNEA SYNDROME

Pediatric OSA can lead to a range of adverse health outcomes if left untreated. Cardiovascular consequences include hypertension and endothelial dysfunction, which may persist even after accounting for obesity. Metabolic disturbances are also observed, with untreated OSA contributing to insulin resistance and alterations in glucose metabolism, increasing the risk of metabolic syndrome. Neurocognitive and behavioral issues are prevalent, manifesting as attention deficits, hyperactivity, and learning difficulties, which can significantly impact academic performance and QOL. Early diagnosis and appropriate management of pediatric OSA are crucial to mitigate these sequelae and promote optimal health outcomes.

Pediatric OSA is associated with significant health consequences to multiple organ systems, including cardiovascular, metabolic, neurocognitive, and psychological domains (18).

Cardiovascular Consequences

Children with OSA are at increased risk for developing systemic hypertension, endothelial dysfunction, and left ventricular hypertrophy. These cardiovascular effects may persist even after controlling for obesity, indicating an independent relationship between OSA and cardiovascular morbidity. Recurrent episodes of hypoxia and sleep fragmentation contribute to sympathetic nervous system activation, oxidative stress, and inflammation, all of which contribute to long-term cardiovascular risk (24).

Treatment of OSA, particularly adenotonsillectomy, has been associated with improvements in blood pressure regulation and overall cardiac function.

Metabolic and Growth Implications

OSA in children is linked to metabolic dysregulation, including insulin resistance and increased risk for metabolic syndrome. Studies suggest that OSA contributes to dysregulated glucose metabolism, even in the absence of obesity, potentially mediated through alterations in adipokines such as leptin and adiponectin. Additionally, failure to thrive can be an initial presentation of pediatric OSA, as increased work of breathing during sleep may lead to increased energy expenditure. Following adenotonsillectomy, improvements in growth parameters have been observed, likely due to enhanced secretion of growth hormone, which occurs predominantly during slow-wave sleep (24).

Neurocognitive and Behavioral Effects

Children with OSA frequently exhibit symptoms such as hyperactivity, aggression, emotional dysregulation, and difficulty concentrating. These behavioral manifestations can mimic ADHD, leading to misdiagnosis. Moreover, neurocognitive impairments related to verbal fluency, memory, and executive function have been reported, with evidence suggesting that untreated OSA may negatively impact academic performance. While adenotonsillectomy often results in improvements in behavior and attention, it remains unclear whether neurocognitive deficits fully resolve posttreatment (24).

Quality of Life and Sleep Disturbances

Pediatric SDB is associated with reduced QOL metrics, including excessive daytime sleepiness, decreased alertness, and impaired social and emotional functioning. QOL measures have been shown to improve significantly after adenotonsillectomy, even in cases where polysomnographic parameters do not completely normalize (5).

Nocturnal Enuresis

Children with OSA have a higher prevalence of nocturnal enuresis, with mechanisms likely related to increased nighttime urine production, altered arousal responses, and disruptions in antidiuretic hormone secretion. Studies indicate that adenotonsillectomy leads to a substantial reduction in bed-wetting episodes, suggesting that OSA contributes to enuresis through sleep fragmentation and autonomic dysregulation (18).

In summary, untreated pediatric OSA can have profound and widespread consequences. Early recognition and appropriate intervention, primarily through adenotonsillectomy or positive airway pressure therapy in select cases, are critical in mitigating long-term health risks and improving overall well-being.

TREATMENT

Unlike adults, for whom positive airway pressure (PAP) therapy is the primary treatment for OSA, children typically respond well to adenotonsillectomy as the first-line intervention. This surgical procedure significantly reduces the apnea-hypopnea index (AHI), although complete normalization may not always occur, particularly in cases of severe OSA or obesity. In addition to improving respiratory parameters, adenotonsillectomy has been shown to enhance cardiovascular function and alleviate behavioral symptoms associated with pediatric OSA.

Surgery

AAP clinical practice guidelines for management of obstructive sleep apnea (2012):

1. Adenotonsillectomy is recommended as the first-line treatment of patients with adenotonsillar hypertrophy. High-risk patients should be monitored as inpatients postoperatively.
2. Patients should be reevaluated postoperatively to determine whether further treatment is required. Objective testing should be performed in patients who are high risk or who have persistent symptoms/signs of OSAS after therapy.
3. CPAP is recommended as treatment if adenotonsillectomy is not performed or if OSAS persists postoperatively.
4. Weight loss is recommended in addition to other therapy in patients who are overweight or obese.
5. Intranasal corticosteroids are an option for children with mild OSAS in whom adenotonsillectomy is contraindicated or for mild postoperative OSAS (25).

Maxillomandibular advancement surgery should be considered for those children with craniofacial defects, including midfacial or mandibular hypoplasia and for some with severe OSAS (25).

Oral Appliance Therapy

Dental devices that reposition the jaw and/or tongue may be useful in children with mild OSA. These should be initiated and followed by a dentist/orthodontist with training and experience using these devices in children. Before beginning treatment, a comprehensive clinical assessment of the pediatric patient with OSA is essential. In otherwise healthy children with OSA, cephalometric studies have indicated a narrower posterior airway space, along with abnormalities in mandibular occlusion and vertical alignment. When adenoid hypertrophy is present, children often extend their heads to enlarge the posterior airway space, which affects mandibular positioning, leading to mouth breathing and transverse maxillary constriction. In children with genetic syndromes, craniofacial abnormalities are more pronounced, making OSA more common and potentially more severe. Follow-up is especially important in view of the growing teeth and jaw. Rapid maxillary expansion has also been successfully used in select groups of children, including newborns with micrognathia (26).

Positive Airway Pressure Therapy

Adenotonsillectomy is often the first-line treatment but may not be suitable or effective for all pediatric patients. Obesity, craniofacial anomalies, recurrent idiopathic OSAS post adenotonsillectomy, Down syndrome and Prader-Willi syndrome are common indications for CPAP therapy. In such cases, PAP therapy serves as a noninvasive alternative, delivering pressurized air through a mask to maintain airway patency during sleep. PAP therapy has demonstrated efficacy in alleviating upper airway obstruction and improving ventilation in children with OSA (27).

Implementing PAP therapy in pediatric populations requires careful consideration of various factors to ensure safety and effectiveness. Challenges include selecting appropriate pressure settings, ensuring mask fit and comfort, and addressing adherence issues, as consistent use is crucial for therapeutic success. Studies have shown that adherence can be influenced by family dynamics; for instance, children with a family member already using PAP therapy often exhibit better compliance. Additionally, improvements in neurobehavioral functions have been observed in children adhering to PAP therapy, even with suboptimal usage. Active management, including patient and family education, regular follow-ups, and support, is essential to optimize outcomes and address barriers to adherence in pediatric PAP therapy (27).

BPAP, or bilevel positive airway pressure, is a form of PAP therapy that delivers two distinct pressure levels: a higher-pressure during inhalation (inspiratory positive airway pressure, or IPAP) and a lower pressure during exhalation (expiratory positive airway pressure, or EPAP). This dual-pressure approach is particularly beneficial for patients who require higher pressures, struggle with CPAP intolerance due to discomfort at high pressures, or experience significant hypoventilation. Additionally, auto-adjusting BPAP is available for individuals whose SDB varies based on sleep stage or body position, ensuring more personalized and effective treatment.

For patients with more complex respiratory needs, advanced BPAP modes provide enhanced support. BPAP spontaneous-timed (ST) mode includes a set respiratory rate to maintain a minimum number of breaths per minute, making it useful for those with CSA or complex sleep apnea syndromes. Another advanced option, volume-assured pressure support (VAPS) mode, automatically adjusts pressure support to achieve a target tidal volume. This feature is particularly advantageous for patients with restrictive lung disease due to conditions such as obesity or neuromuscular disorders, ensuring adequate ventilation while minimizing discomfort (27).

Weight Loss

Weight loss should be encouraged in all obese patients but can be difficult to achieve. School-aged children with obesity and OSA are more likely to eat fast food, consume fewer fruits and vegetables, and be less active in organized sports compared with healthy children (28).

Medications

Adenotonsillectomy is the treatment of choice for OSAS in children, but alternative choices to treat residual or mild apnea have shown some promise. Topical nasal steroids may help alleviate sleep apnea symptoms in children with mild OSA. Common medications in this category include fluticasone (Flovent HFA, Xhance, and others) and budesonide (Rhinocort, Pulmicort Flexhaler, and others). For children with allergies, montelukast (Singulair) can be beneficial in managing symptoms, either on its own or in combination with nasal steroids (25).

Oxygen

Oxygen therapy can be used as a treatment option for pediatric patients with SDB, particularly in cases where significant nocturnal hypoxemia occurs and other treatments like CPAP are not tolerated, serving as a temporary measure to improve oxygen saturation levels while awaiting definitive treatment like surgery or other interventions; however, it is crucial to closely monitor patients for potential complications like hypercapnia and to consult with a specialist before initiating oxygen therapy in children with SDB. Studies have shown the benefit of supplemental oxygen on central apnea, periodic breathing, and sleep architecture in infants with AOP. The safety and efficacy of supplemental oxygen administration to infants with OSA, however, is not well studied (29).

Congenital Central Hypoventilation Syndrome

Congenital central hypoventilation syndrome (CCHS), also knowns as "Ondine's curse," is a rare pediatric disorder characterized by impaired autonomic control of breathing, leading to alveolar hypoventilation that is more pronounced during sleep. This condition is caused primarily by mutations in the PHOX2B gene, which plays a crucial role in the development of the autonomic nervous system. Children with CCHS often present with symptoms such as central apneas, periodic breathing, and hypoventilation, typically manifesting in the neonatal period, although some cases may present later. Unlike other SRBDs, CCHS is distinguished by a diminished or absent ventilatory response to hypercapnia and hypoxemia, particularly during sleep. Some patients may do well with noninvasive ventilation, for example, BPAP during sleep, with supplemental oxygen or even room air during wakefulness. Management of CCHS requires lifelong ventilatory support, especially during sleep, and continuous monitoring to prevent complications arising from hypoventilation. Early diagnosis and intervention are critical to optimize outcomes and reduce morbidity associated with this condition (30).

Rapid-Onset Obesity With Hypothalamic Dysfunction, Hypoventilation, and Autonomic Dysregulation

Rapid-onset obesity with hypothalamic dysfunction, hypoventilation, and autonomic dysregulation (ROHHAD) is a rare pediatric disorder that significantly impacts respiratory function during sleep. Typically manifesting after the age of 1.5 years, children with ROHHAD experience rapid-onset obesity, often gaining 20 to 30 lb within 3 to 12 months, followed by hypothalamic dysfunction and central hypoventilation. This central hypoventilation leads to SDB, characterized by inadequate ventilation and diminished responsiveness to hypercapnia and hypoxemia during sleep. Consequently, affected children are at risk for severe hypoventilation during sleep, which may progress to respiratory failure if not promptly addressed. Management of SDB in patients with ROHHAD often necessitates ventilatory support during sleep, such as noninvasive positive pressure ventilation or, in severe cases, tracheostomy with mechanical ventilation. Early recognition and intervention are crucial to mitigate the respiratory complications associated with this syndrome (30).

SUMMARY

Respiratory issues, particularly apnea, are the leading reason children are referred to sleep centers. SDB in children differs from adults in its presentation, consequences, and treatment. Premature infants are more prone to central apneas, while obstructive events are more prevalent in children and adolescents. Those with neurologic, neuromuscular, craniofacial, or genetic conditions face a higher risk of respiratory compromise and may require ventilatory support through CPAP or BPAP. SDB in children can impact neurocognitive function, behavior, cardiovascular health, growth, metabolism, and overall QOL. However, many of these effects can be mitigated with proper clinical management. Caring for children in the sleep center requires a friendly environment and good rapport between the sleep technologist, the child, and the family.

REFERENCES

1. Marcus CL, Brooks LJ, Draper KA, et al; American Academy of Pediatrics. Diagnosis and management of childhood obstructive sleep apnea syndrome. *Pediatrics*. 2012;130(3): e714-e755.
2. Aurora RN, Zak RS, Karippot A, et al. Practice parameters for the respiratory indications for polysomnography in children. *Sleep*. 2011;34(3):379-388.
3. Kaditis AG, Alonso-Alvarez ML, Boudewyns A, et al. Obstructive sleep disordered breathing in children: a European Respiratory Society clinical practice guideline. *Eur Respir J*. 2016;47(1):69-94.
4. Beebe DW, Rausch J, Byars KC, Lanphear B, Yolton K. Persistent snoring in preschool children: predictors and behavioral and developmental correlates. *Pediatrics*. 2010;126(2):e558-e566.
5. Brockmann PE, Urschitz MS, Schlaud M, Poets CF. Primary snoring in school children: prevalence and neurocognitive impairments. *Sleep Breath*. 2012;16(1): 23-29. doi:10.1007/s11325-011-0480-6
6. Mitchell RB, Kelly J. Adenotonsillectomy for obstructive sleep apnea in children: outcome evidence. *Laryngoscope*. 2019;129(2):510-516.
7. Lumeng JC, Chervin RD. Epidemiology of pediatric obstructive sleep apnea. *Proc Am Thorac Soc*. 2008; 5(2):242-252.
8. Moon RY, Carlin RF, Hand I; American Academy of Pediatrics. Sleep-related infant deaths: updated 2022 recommendations for reducing infant deaths in the sleep environment. *Pediatrics*. 2022;150(1): e2022057990. doi:10.1542/peds.2022-057990
9. Martin RJ, Abu-Shaweesh JM, Baird TM. Apnea of prematurity. In: Denny FH, Martin RJ, eds. *Fanaroff and Martin's Neonatal-Perinatal Medicine*. Elsevier; 2011: 1091-1106.
10. Dobson NR, Hunt CE, Lipps TM. Apnea of prematurity: pathogenesis and management strategies. *Curr Pediatr Rep*. 2017;5(3):161-170.
11. Eichenwald EC. Apnea of prematurity. *Pediatrics*. 2016;137(1):e20153757.
12. Schmidt B, Roberts RS, Davis P, et al. Caffeine therapy for apnea of prematurity. *N Engl J Med*. 2007;357(19):1893-1902.

13. Kumar VK, Lipshultz SE, Chikkabyrappa SM. Noninvasive respiratory support for neonates: current practices and future directions. *Front Pediatr.* 2020; 8:293.
14. Henderson-Smart DJ, Davis PG. Methylxanthine treatment for apnea in preterm infants. *Cochrane Database Syst Rev.* 2010;2010(12):CD000140.
15. Ramanathan R. Sleep position and apnea in premature infants: balancing benefits and risks. *Pediatr Pulmonol.* 2017;52(4):493-501.
16. Graham CJ, Kinane TB, Katz ES. Brief resolved unexplained events (BRUE): Evaluation and management. *UpToDate.* 2021. https://www.uptodate.com/contents/acute-events-in-infancy-including-brief-resolved-unexplained-event-brue
17. Centers for Disease Control and Prevention. Sudden unexpected infant death and sudden infant death syndrome. 2022. Accessed November 22, 2025. https://www.cdc.gov/sids/
18. Jönson Ring I, Markström A, Bazargani F, Nevéus T. Sleep disordered breathing in enuretic children and controls. *J Pediatr Urol.* 2017;13(6):620.e1-620.e6. doi:10.1016/j.jpurol.2017.05.012
19. Moon RY; Task Force on Sudden Infant Death Syndrome. SIDS and other sleep-related infant deaths: updated 2016 recommendations for a safe infant sleeping environment. 2016. Accessed November 22, 2025. https://pubmed.ncbi.nlm.nih.gov/27940805/
20. Kirk V, Baughn J, D'Andrea L, et al. American Academy of Sleep Medicine position paper for the use of a home sleep apnea test for the diagnosis of OSA in children. *J Clin Sleep Med.* 2017;13(10):1199-1203. doi:10.5664/jcsm.6772
21. Menzies B, Teng A, Burns M, Lah S. Neurocognitive outcomes of children with sleep disordered breathing: A systematic review with meta-analysis. *Sleep Med. Rev.* 2022;63:101629. doi:10.1016/j.smrv.2022.101629
22. Spilsbury JC, Storfer-Isser A, Drotar D, et al. Effects of the home environment on school-aged children's sleep. *J Clin Sleep Med.* 2006;2(4):403-407.
23. American Academy of Family Physicians. Diagnosis and management of obstructive sleep apnea syndrome in children. *Am Fam Physician.* 2012;85(3): 290-296.
24. Witmans M, Young R. Update on pediatric sleep-disordered breathing. *Pediatr Clin North Am.* 2011;58(3):571-589. doi:10.1016/j.pcl.2011.03.013
25. Thomas RJ, Rosen CL, Roux F, Marcus CL, Morgenthaler TI. Pediatric obstructive sleep apnea: mechanisms, evaluation, and management. *J Clin Sleep Med.* 2022;18(2):445-460.
26. Marciuc D, Morarasu S, Morarasu BC, et al. Dental appliances for the treatment of obstructive sleep apnea in children: a systematic review and meta-analysis. *Medicina.* 2023;59(8):1447. doi:10.3390/medicina 59081447
27. Hady KK, Okorie CUA. Positive airway pressure therapy for pediatric obstructive sleep apnea. *Children.* 2021;8(11):979. doi:10.3390/children8110979
28. Spruyt K, Sans Capdevila O, Serpero LD, et al. Dietary and physical activity patterns in children with obstructive sleep apnea. *J Pediatr.* 2010;156(5):724-730.
29. Brockbank J, Astudillo CL, Che D, et al. Supplemental oxygen for treatment of infants with obstructive sleep apnea. *J Clin Sleep Med.* 2019;15(8):1115-1123. doi:10.5664/jcsm.7802
30. Ghosh R, Malik M, Daley TC, Kasi AS. Images: sleep-disordered breathing and hypoventilation in a child with obesity and hypothalamic dysfunction. *J Clin Sleep Med.* 2022;18(1):339-342. doi:10.5664/jcsm.9636

Chapter 62
Non-respiratory Pediatric Sleep Disorders

ELIZABETH Y. WIESEMANN

KEY CONCEPTS/LEARNING OBJECTIVES

The key concepts for this chapter include a review of the essential features of nonrespiratory sleep disorders in children, examples of how nonrespiratory sleep disorders manifest differently in children at various age ranges, the uses and limitations of polysomnography in the evaluation of pediatric sleep disorders other than sleep apnea, and the role that clinical observations play in the diagnosis of nonrespiratory sleep disorders in children.

KEY TERMS

Enuresis
Insomnia
Narcolepsy
Sleep

Approximately 25% of all children experience some type of sleep problem during childhood (1). Although some pediatric sleep disorders are treatable, many become chronic if left untreated (1). Chronic insufficient sleep is increasing because of competing priorities such as homework, television, social activities, and poor sleep hygiene (1). Sleep disorders are preventable through education regarding normal sleep behavior, routines, self-soothing techniques, and sleep hygiene. Sleep problems in children have a direct effect on parents' sleep, stress levels, and family interactions. Most importantly, sleep is necessary for children to function optimally (1).

Although insufficient quantity and quality of sleep in children usually result in excessive daytime sleepiness, children may not exhibit the same symptoms as adults. Sleepiness in children often manifests as mood disturbances, hyperactivity, poor impulse control, and neurocognitive dysfunction. Mood disturbances such as irritability, temper tantrums, and poor emotional regulation are some of the many signs of insufficient sleep. Cognitive dysfunction may appear as inattention, poor concentration, decreased reaction time, impaired vigilance, poor decision-making and problem-solving, learning problems, and poor academic performance. Behaviorally, the child may be overactive, noncompliant, have poor impulse control, and demonstrate oppositional behavior, and increased risk taking (2).

Sleep disturbances in children are most often reported by the parents or caregivers because of the negative impact that they have on the family. It makes sense that pediatricians are often the first to hear a complaint regarding pediatric sleep disorder. Pediatricians, in collaboration with the Sleep Disorders Center, should take an aggressive approach to the early detection and treatment of sleep disorders.

AGE-RELATED FEATURES OF NONRESPIRATORY PEDIATRIC SLEEP DISORDERS

Depending on the child's age and maturity, nonrespiratory sleep disorders can manifest themselves in different ways. Some sleep disorders are more frequent at certain ages, and it is helpful for the sleep technologist to be aware of the signs and symptoms of common nonrespiratory sleep disorders seen in each age range. The technologist must also have an understanding of normal sleep patterns for each of the age groups to understand the impact that a sleep disorder can have on the individual's sleep requirements.

Normal Sleep Patterns for Newborns and Infants

Newborns (0-2 Months)

Hours of sleep: 16 to 20 hours per 24 hours. No nocturnal/diurnal pattern in the first few weeks; sleep is distributed throughout the day and night (1).

Infants (2-12 Months)

Hours of sleep: nighttime 9 to 12 hours and daytime naps 2 to 4.5 hours. Regular rhythm of periods of sleepiness and alertness will emerge by 2 to 4 months.

Common sleep disorders in this age group include the following:

- Colic
- Body rocking and headbanging
- Sleep-onset association disorder

Colic is one of the most common causes of sleep disturbance in the 3- to 6-month-old infant. Colic appears to be related to digestion and is an often-misunderstood condition. The most common form of colic is circadian in nature and begins at approximately 2 to 3 months, resolving spontaneously at approximately 5 to 6 months.

The pediatrician must distinguish colic from milk intolerance or gastroesophageal reflux disease. An important feature of the differential diagnosis is that in colic, the crying has a clear circadian rhythm. The baby does not cry after daytime feedings but becomes irritable in the evening and fusses inconsolably until around the same time in the late evening or night (2). Parents will often misperceive the "vomiting" that occurs because of swallowing air while crying to be a symptom of a stomach upset. Infants with central or obstructive sleep apnea syndrome may also have frequent arousals with crying, but this occurs during all sleep periods, day or night (1).

CASE EXAMPLE Severe Colic in a 4-Month-Old Infant

A 4-month-old baby girl is accompanied by her parents to the sleep center. The baby appears content, but the parents complain of fatigue and lack of sleep. They report that at approximately 9 PM every day, their usually good-natured baby becomes a different child. She begins fussing, squirming, and drawing her legs up in pain. The parents have tried medication for possible reflux, medication for allergies, changing the formula from milk to soy, all to no avail. They take turns walking and patting her, which often leads to more crying and screaming. The only thing that seems to calm her is a drive around the neighborhood with her in the car seat. She falls asleep at about midnight and is fine for the rest of the night. The next morning, she is back to her usual happy self. The sleep physician ordered a polysomnogram to rule out apnea and reflux.

Normal Sleep Patterns for Toddlers and Preschool Children

Toddlers (12 Months-3 Years)

Hours of sleep: 12 to 13 hours per 24 hours. Daytime naps: from two to one nap by age 18 months lasting 30 minutes to 2 hours.

Preschool-Age Children (3-5 Years)

Hours of sleep: 11 to 12 hours per 24 hours. Daytime naps: from 1 to none.

Sleep problems occur in 25% to 30% of children in the preschool-age group. This is a time when many developmental changes occur. Naps decrease from two to one by 3 years of age and then to none by age 5. Timing and duration of naps can affect nighttime sleep. The child gives up the bottle and moves to a big bed. At around 3 years, the child develops imagination and fantasy, which can lead to increased night fears. Bedtime routines need to be consistent with a progression toward relaxation. Transitional objects such as blankets, dolls, and stuffed animals help the child learn to self-soothe for sleep onset and after arousals. Parental reassurance that the child is safe is more effective than actions, which reinforce the idea that a "monster" exists (1).

Common sleep disorders in the preschool-age group include the following:

- Sleep-onset association disorder/nighttime waking
- Limit-setting sleep disorder/bedtime resistance
- Rhythmic movement disorders like headbanging, body rocking, and body rolling
- Nighttime fears and nightmares

Normal Sleep Pattern for School-Age Children (5-11 Years)

Hours of sleep: 10 to 11 hours per 24 hours.

School-age children may not obtain sufficient sleep, and this can lead to behavioral and learning problems. The child may be misdiagnosed with attention-deficit disorder or learning disabilities, particularly in classroom subjects that require complex problem-solving or sustained attention (2).

Some of the more common nonrespiratory sleep disorders in the school-age child are as follows:

- Sleepwalking and sleep terrors
- Bruxism
- Insufficient sleep
- Inadequate sleep hygiene
- Periodic limb movement disorder (PLMD)

Disorders of arousal parasomnias are more frequent in childhood than in adolescence. Estimates of sleep terrors range from 1% to 6%, sleepwalking up to 17% with a peak at 8 to 12 years, and confusional arousals up to 17.3% (1). School-age children with chronic sleep deprivation rarely articulate the need to nap or rest because they do not know what it feels to be adequately rested.

Bruxism is a movement-type sleep disorder characterized by repetitive grinding or clenching of the teeth during sleep. It is accompanied by scraping and clicking sounds. Bruxism has two distinct patterns, diurnal and nocturnal. Although bruxism is closely related to stress, the two etiologies appear to be different (1). Allergies, cerebral palsy, intellectual disability, alcohol, stimulant medications, and seizure can contribute to bruxism. Adult-type bruxism usually begins in childhood or adolescence; however, most cases of bruxism are self-limiting and may even disappear with the eruption of secondary teeth. Diagnosis rarely involves a sleep study. Bruxism can lead to excessive wear of the teeth, periodontal tissue damage, jaw pain, and headache. Dental appliances, sleeping position, pharmacotherapy, or psychological treatment may be used to alleviate the symptoms (2).

Inadequate sleep hygiene is caused by activities that increase arousal, like caffeinated soda, stimulating television, and play. Napping during the day, nighttime awakenings from periodic limb movements (PLMs), loud noises, and bright lights lead to disorganized and often insufficient sleep for the youngster.

Normal Sleep Pattern for Adolescents (Ages 12-18)

Hours of sleep: 9 to 9.5 hours needed but 7 to 7.25 hours obtained.

Sleep disorders seen in this age group include the following:

- Insufficient sleep
- Inadequate sleep
- Insomnia
- Delayed sleep phase syndrome
- Restless legs syndrome (RLS)/PLMD
- Narcolepsy
- Kleine-Levin syndrome

Around puberty, hormonal changes cause a daily delay in melatonin secretion. This delay results in a delayed sleep onset of approximately 2 hours. Despite the circadian rhythm delay, the adolescent still needs 9 to 9.25 hours of sleep. With early school start times, extracurricular activities, more independence, part-time jobs, and increasing socialization, adolescents manage an average of 7 to 7.5 hours of sleep, causing them to be chronically sleep deprived. Insomnia may be caused by new social pressures, academic pressures, increased responsibilities, or a bedtime too early for the adolescent's circadian rhythm (3). Parents and adolescents may attribute the symptoms of RLS or PLMD to growing pains or sports injuries. A polysomnogram is useful in identifying the movements and the extent of related arousals.

Chronic sleep restriction can cause mood disturbances, depression, poor academic performance, attention or memory deficits, risk-taking behavior, and increased involvement in traffic accidents (3). All the previously listed sleep disorders lead to excessive daytime sleepiness. However, narcolepsy has more complex symptomatology.

Narcolepsy is caused by impaired sleep-wake regulation of the central nervous system (CNS). The patient complains of excessive daytime sleepiness, cataplexy (the abrupt loss of muscle tone provoked by strong emotion), hypnagogic hallucinations (vivid auditory or visual "dreams" that are often frightening), and sleep paralysis (inability to move or speak for a few seconds at sleep onset or offset). Although narcolepsy is reported for all age groups, it is most often reported by teenagers and young adults (2).

Kleine-Levin syndrome (4), or recurrent hypersomnia, is characterized by acute episodes of excessive sleepiness, hyperphagia, and hypersexuality lasting up to several weeks at a time. Kleine-Levin syndrome usually occurs during adolescence and is more common in males. Sleep and behavior are normal between episodes (4).

TECHNICAL CONSIDERATIONS

Technical considerations related to polysomnographic (PSG) testing in the child begin with a consideration of the environment in the sleep center. The sleeping environment should provide separate beds for parent, baby, child, or adolescent. Keep in mind that the parent is usually suffering from sleep deprivation because of the child's problem.

1. A foldaway bed, not a recliner, must be provided to ensure that the parent is rested well enough to take the child home after the polysomnogram.
2. Room temperature should be comfortable for an average adult.
3. The crib slats should be no greater than 23/8 in (6.03 cm) apart.
4. The crib mattress should be firm and tight fitting in the crib, and no comforters or pillows should be used.
5. The American Academy of Pediatrics recommends that the baby be placed on the back, during sleep, to reduce the risk of sudden infant death syndrome (4).
6. Infants can be swaddled or wear mittens, during setup, to prevent them from inadvertently pulling off leads.
7. Place belts under pajama top, bring wires and leads to the side of the infant, and bind them together.

Point head leads toward the top of the head and bind together. This placement will allow the infant or child to sleep supine or on one side without lying on wires.

8. Toddlers and children enjoy participating in the setup with the support of a parent. Props, such as flashlights, music, dolls, and stickers, can be used to make the "sleepover event" into a game. Have the toddler sit on the parent(s') lap during setup to help reduce anxiety.
9. Adolescents need to feel informed regarding the purpose of each lead.
10. The sleep technologist should observe parent-child interactions and document them in the log. An audiovisual recording should be made during setup, polysomnogram recording, and takedown to document all interactions for the sleep specialist.

CLINICAL OBSERVATIONS

The clinical observations made by the technologist during the PSG recording are extremely valuable in the diagnosis of pediatric sleep disorders. The technologist serves as the eyes and ears of the sleep physician, and, therefore, thorough documentation is essential.

The initial assessment of a pediatric sleep disturbance will include the following:

- Detailed sleep history from the parents, a home video, if possible, and a sleep diary
- Medical history, with a developmental assessment of school functioning
- Family history, a psychosocial history, and a behavioral assessment
- Physical examination

This information will direct the sleep technologist to focus on the observations most valuable to the sleep physician. The use of video recordings during PSG is important in documenting both parent and child behavior. However, the technologist's written observations can provide the sleep physician with information regarding how the child feels, what they believe is happening, what they need, and whether the family can support their needs.

The technologist should document anything out of the ordinary such as the following:

- Unusual behavior of the child
- Headbanging or rocking
- Sleepwalking
- Prolonged crying
- Hypersomnolence
- Hypersexuality
- Hallucinations
- Sleep paralysis or cataplexy
- Unusual behavior of a family member (swearing, yelling, and rough handling)
- Unusual eating habits (eating during sleep time and overeating)
- Unusual sleeping positions (arched back and sitting up)
- Unusual verbalization (screaming, prolonged crying, and words inappropriate for age)
- Signs of abuse; bruises (black eyes)
- Bed-wetting (sleep stage and parents' and child's reactions)
- Numerous visits to the bathroom or resistance to bedtime

Clinical Observations in the Infant to Preschool Population (Ages 0-5)

Bedtime in the sleep center should be identical to the bedtime in the child's home, and the nighttime routine should approximate the routine at home as closely as possible. Although the environment is obviously different, the parent should nevertheless be encouraged to attempt to simulate the environment and bedtime routine. Have the child bring their favorite blanket, pillow, pajamas, bedtime snack, and snuggle toy. Document the bedtime routine, use of a night light, bedtime stalling, and the interaction between the parent(s) and the child at or around sleep onset. Some of the most common sleep disorders in this age group are sleep-onset association disorders in which the child's innate self-quieting skills are replaced by a need for the physical presence of the parent and/or some parental bedtime behavior in order to initiate sleep. The best course in documentation is to describe an observed activity quoting the dialogue between parent and the child. The technologist should not write an opinion or make any judgment regarding the activity or event.

Clinical Observations in the School-Age Child

While scheduling the sleep study, the technologist should identify and document any special needs the child may have during the test. Based on the child's normal bedtime, plan the setup to allow for a night's sleep that is as representative as possible. The child should be offered a tour of the lab and given an overview of the procedure. The technologist should involve the parent or caregiver in the study setup and explain the procedure. The child's nightly routine should be followed as closely as the situation will allow, and the technologist should take careful and elaborate notes. The parent or caregiver must spend the night in the lab, either in a separate bed or in another bedroom.

Following the onset of sleep, it is important for the technologist to be especially vigilant at the beginning of the night when slow-wave sleep ensues. Many of the disorders seen during this stage of development occur in stage N3 sleep. Any awakening from slow-wave sleep should be carefully observed and thoroughly described. The primary disorders that may occur at this age during deep sleep include confusional arousals, sleepwalking, and sleep terrors. As is the case with any partial arousal disorder, it is the responsibility of the technologist to provide for the safety of the child. Review the electroencephalogram (EEG) before the episode and after the episode for epileptiform and/or postictal activity, and document the activity on the study log (4).

It is important to remember that the technologist's responsibility to observe the patient continues after the polysomnogram is completed. The behaviors observed following lights on might be a crucial component in the evaluation of the patient. Before lights on, determine roughly the amount of sleep the child actually obtained during the night, and compare this with the normative value for the child's age. The technologist should observe and record at lights on to document paralysis, automatic behaviors, confusion, or amnesia. This documentation should include the reaction of the child and any behaviors that might be seen up to the time when the child leaves the facility.

Clinical Observations in the Adolescent

When the sleep study is being scheduled, the teen should be asked if they have any special needs or prefer a technologist of the same sex. The teen should be offered a tour of the lab and given an overview of the procedure. Privacy is very important to the adolescent patient, and this need must be respected. The patient may also have concerns and misperceptions about the polysomnogram procedure but may not always express these concerns directly. The technologist should explain the purpose of each measurement device during the setup. The technologist can ask if the adolescent has any questions and answer them with patience. The principles of behavioral observations in adolescents are similar to those in other children as well as adults (3).

SLEEP DISORDERS

The *International Classification of Sleep Disorders*, third edition, divides sleep disorders into seven categories as follows: (5)

1. Insomnia
2. Sleep-related breathing disorders
3. Central disorders of hypersomnolence
4. Circadian rhythm sleep-wake disorders
5. Parasomnias
6. Sleep-related movement disorders
7. Narcolepsy

Although the neurobiology of sleep is a constant, psychosocial and cultural practices, such as co-sleeping, can change the natural sleep behavior of a developing brain. Other variables, like the child's temperament and medical problems, can affect their response to zeitgebers (ie, environmental cues) for signaling circadian rhythms. For example, the easygoing child may adapt to varying bedtimes, whereas the more anxious child may need a consistent bedtime to foster a more predictable and secure environment. A child who is blind may not respond to the light versus dark zeitgeber. Parenting styles, education levels, mental health issues, family stress, and lifestyle also have an effect on both the real and the perceived pediatric sleep pattern. Sleep habits are influenced by normal developmental changes. For example, toddlers experience separation anxiety, which may lead to bedtime resistance. The pediatric sleep technologist observes the family dynamics and behaviors for the sleep physician and must therefore be knowledgeable in all the disorders listed earlier (6).

Sleep-related breathing disorders and parasomnias are discussed in other chapters in this textbook. Nonrespiratory sleep problems most frequently studied by the pediatric sleep technologist are hypersomnia, circadian rhythm disorders, and epilepsy. Insomnia, per se, is relatively rare in the pediatric population (7).

INSOMNIA

Insomnia is defined as a persistent difficulty with sleep initiation, duration, consolidation, or quality that occurs despite adequate opportunity to sleep and results in some form of daytime impairment (1). Because the child cannot articulate the sleep complaint, the pediatrician often makes a referral to a sleep specialist when the parent or caregiver voices concern over the child's sleeplessness (1). A polysomnogram may be ordered to evaluate the duration of sleep and the underlying causes for the sleep complaint. Some of the most frequently encountered causes of sleep-onset insomnia and prolonged nocturnal awakenings in children are as follows:

1. Sleep-onset association disorder
2. Circadian rhythm disorders
3. Inadequate sleep hygiene
4. PLMS and RLS
5. Limit-setting behaviors
6. Obstructive sleep apnea syndrome

Sleep-Onset Association Disorder

Approximately 25% to 50% of 6- to 12-month-olds and 30% of 1-year-olds experience sleep-onset association disorder. The child cannot fall asleep without a habituated set of conditions that require parental intervention to initiate sleep. Parental interventions include the following: being held, rocked, breastfed; watching television; or listening to music. When the condition is present, sleep onset is normal. When the association is absent, sleep latency is increased at sleep onset and after nocturnal arousals. The child has no underlying medical or mental disorder, and the symptoms do not meet the criteria for any other sleep disorder. Transitional objects such as a pacifier, special blanket, or stuffed animal allow the child to self-soothe and fall asleep without parental response (1).

CASE EXAMPLE **Feeding as a Sleep-Onset Association in an Infant**

A 9-month-old breastfed baby boy is referred to the sleep center for numerous arousals and excessive crying at night. His mother nurses him until he falls asleep. She puts him in the crib, next to her bed, and goes to sleep. The baby's father sleeps in another room to obtain adequate sleep. The baby boy wakes up every 2 to 3 hours and cries until his mother gets up and nurses him back to sleep.

CASE EXAMPLE **Use of the DVD Player as a Sleep Aid in a Preschool Child**

A 4-year-old boy is being evaluated in the sleep center for daytime sleepiness. He has a regular bedtime and rise time, respectively, of 9 PM and 6 AM. He states that he cannot fall asleep without the movie, *Toy Story*, playing on his bedroom television. If he wakes up during the night, his mother starts the movie again, and he returns to sleep, after watching for 20 to 30 minutes. This pattern may repeat itself several times during the night. The patient went to his grandmother's house for the summer. But the grandmother did not have the movie. The 4-year-old hardly slept for the first week, but during the second week, he slept very well and felt great during the day. When he returned home, he resumed his Toy Story movie habit and his daytime sleepiness returned. The sleep physician ordered a sleep diary and behavioral therapy.

CASE EXAMPLE **Pet Dog Presence With Physical Contact as a Sleep Aid for an Adolescent**

A 14-year-old boy insists on having his pet collie sleep in his bed every night. He tosses and turns until the dog is lying firmly against his side. If the dog gets out of bed to drink or go outside, the boy wakes up. He cannot return to sleep until the dog comes back and gets into her usual place, beside the boy. When the collie was hospitalized, the boy was unable to fall asleep until past 3 AM and was late for school. This pattern continued until the adolescent's dog was returned home.

Inadequate Sleep Hygiene

Inadequate sleep hygiene, which frequently results in insufficient sleep, can be divided into two sleep-related behaviors.

1. Practices that increase arousal
2. Practices that reduce sleep organization

Practices that increase arousal before bedtime are stimulating TV or movies, games, team sports, and excessive caffeine intake. Practices that reduce sleep organization are afternoon napping, inconsistent sleep schedule, light, noise, bed type, co-sleeping, and use of the bedroom for activities other than sleep.

Inadequate sleep hygiene is the most common cause of difficulty initiating and maintaining sleep (5). The patient has a complaint of excessive sleepiness, delayed sleep onset, and nighttime awakenings for at least 3 months. The patient's usual sleep episode is shorter than expected for their age. A therapeutic trial of a longer sleep episode eliminates the symptoms (8). The sleep physician will request that the parent complete a sleep diary, which can identify the aforementioned behaviors. Generally, a polysomnogram is not ordered. Behavioral therapy is the typical treatment.

CASE EXAMPLE **Irregular Sleep Schedule With No Bedtime Routine in a Toddler**

A 2-year-old boy and his parents are in the sleep clinic for evaluation of problem behaviors occurring both day and night. The child falls asleep in his car seat. When his mother wakes him to go into the grocery store, he has temper tantrums in the store. He often falls down screaming and kicking when his mother refuses him a treat. He kicks strangers in the legs when they approach him. His height, weight, and head circumference are, respectively, in the 60%, 50%, and 50%, for his age. The parents state that he eats well but is a very restless sleeper. He often gets out of the family bed and plays for hours until a parent takes him back to bed. The child falls asleep when he is sleepy and is placed in the family bed when the parents go to bed. He has never had a regular bedtime because the father works rotating shifts. The parents estimate that he sleeps 6 to 7 hours each day. After a complete physical workup, the sleep physician ordered a sleep diary and PSG to rule out other causes for his sleep problems, such as sleep apnea, seizure, and restless legs. When the PSG revealed no pathology, family behavioral therapy was suggested.

CASE EXAMPLE **Insomnia Caused by Inadequate Sleep Hygiene**

A 17-year-old female who is obese is referred to the sleep center for difficulty initiating and maintaining sleep. She complains that it often takes her 30 to 45 minutes to fall asleep, and she awakens frequently. She is an A-B student, active in drama, math club, and band. She gets up at 6 AM to attend band practice at 7 AM. She drinks a caffeinated power drink as she leaves home. School starts at 8 AM, so she has another caffeinated soft drink and some breakfast bars at school. From 4 to 6 PM, she has drama and math club. The family has dinner, with iced tea, at 7 PM. The 17-year-old makes phone calls until 9 PM, then has a caffeinated power drink, and does homework until 11 PM. She showers and does her hair before going to bed at midnight. She rarely sleeps in on the weekends because she is participating in one or more of her extracurricular activities. She feels tired in the morning, but the power drinks perk her up. Lately, she has been falling asleep at lunch break. The sleep physician ordered a sleep diary and a PSG to rule out sleep apnea and seizures. The PSG revealed a prolonged sleep onset but no pathology. The study was allowed to continue past her normal wake-up time and she slept until 9:00 AM. Sleep hygiene training was recommended for the family.

Limit-Setting Type

Limit-setting sleep disorder is characterized by difficulty initiating sleep. The child stalls or refuses to go to sleep at the set bedtime. After lights out, the child will get up for a drink, another kiss, or to ask "one last question." Once the child is asleep, sleep quality and duration are normal.

When limits are not set or enforced consistently, the child's sleep is delayed, and the sleep period may be insufficient for their needs. Bedtime resistance occurs in 10% to 30% of toddlers and preschoolers and 15% of 4- to 10-year-old children (1). Permissive or conflicting parenting styles, environment (such as co-sleeping with parents or grandparents), and circadian cycles can contribute to limit-setting sleep disorder.

CASE EXAMPLE **Insomnia Caused by Limit-Setting Sleep Disorder**

A 2-year-old girl is brought to the clinic for what the parents describe as refusing to go to bed on time. Her mother says she began fighting sleep when they got her a "big girl bed." She has a nap around 1 to 2 PM and dinner around 5 PM. She then has her bath and bedtime stories until around 8 PM, which is lights out time. She climbs out of bed several times for the next 2 hours asking for a drink, another hug, or an "important question." She had surgery for a hernia at the age of 6 months, and her mother has a fear of upsetting the child. Limit-setting therapy was recommended.

HYPERSOMNIA

- Insufficient sleep quantity
- Fragmentation or poor sleep quality
- Inappropriate timing of the sleep period
- Narcolepsy and idiopathic hypersomnia

Insufficient Sleep

Insufficient sleep quantity may be the result of difficulty in initiating sleep, prolonged periods of wake time during the night, or the need to terminate the sleep period early. Ultimately, the child obtains less sleep than needed and experiences excessive daytime sleepiness (3).

Sleep Fragmentation

Sleep fragmentation is usually the result of repetitive brief arousals. Practices such as caffeine use before bedtime and bright light and loud noises in the bedroom frequently lead to arousal during sleep. Sleep fragmentation can also be caused by disorders of arousal such as sleepwalking, confusional arousals, and sleep terrors. These arousals occur most often during slow-wave (N3) sleep, which is most prominent in the first third of the night. The child's transition from N3 to a lighter stage appears to be incomplete, and phenomena such as automatic behavior, altered perception of the environment, and amnesia regarding the event result in disturbed sleep (4).

Delayed Sleep-Wake Phase Disorder

Inappropriate timing of the sleep period is often the result of delayed sleep phase disorder (DSPD). The adolescent or child has a persistent shift in the sleep-wake schedule, which conflicts with school, or lifestyle. Sleep onset may be delayed, causing the adolescent to complain of insomnia. This delay is seen in combination with difficulty waking in the morning to participate in the daily routine. Typically, DSPD begins during adolescence, when the "night owl" preference becomes exaggerated by social, academic, or work demands. It affects about 5% to 10% of adolescents (1). It may show up on sleep tracking software from a smart watch or ring health tracking device. The sleep physician will request a sleep diary, and actigraphy may be utilized to confirm a phase delay. A polysomnogram may be appropriate in some patients to rule out other pathology. Behavior modification may be used to move bedtime forward until a more desirable circadian rhythm can be established.

CASE EXAMPLE **Insomnia Caused by Delayed Sleep Phase Disorder**

A 15-year-old male came to the sleep clinic accompanied by his father. The patient says that he avoids all caffeine, does not nap in the day, and still cannot fall asleep at night. Bedtime is 10 PM every night. He waits for his parents to go to bed at 11 PM, then gets up and plays on the computer for a couple of hours. He tries to go back to bed but cannot sleep, so he gets up again. He has been prescribed various sedative-hypnotic medications. He was also prescribed medication to improve his daytime alertness but developed headaches, so this was discontinued. He feels that the sedating medications do not help him fall asleep and that he has even more difficulty getting out of bed in the morning when he takes his medications. He likes school but is in constant trouble for falling asleep in class, losing his temper when the kids tease him for being sleepy or sneaking into the library for a nap. He frequently misses morning classes and has missed so many classes that he will have to repeat the ninth grade. During summer break, the adolescent is allowed to stay up until he feels sleepy. He generally falls asleep around 3 AM and gets up at 11 AM, feeling refreshed, and has no need for naps.

Narcolepsy

Primary disorders of excessive daytime sleepiness involve more complex pathophysiology, which presents as excessive daytime sleepiness. A salient feature of narcolepsy is hypersomnia (2). Type I narcolepsy is primarily characterized by excessive daytime sleepiness and cataplexy and is associated with a deficiency in hypothalamic hypocretin (orexin) signaling (6). Type II narcolepsy is characterized by excessive daytime sleepiness and abnormal manifestations of rapid eye movement (REM) sleep without cataplexy (5).

The four hallmark clinical features of narcolepsy (also called the "narcoleptic tetrad") are as follows:

1. Excessive daytime sleepiness
2. Cataplexy
3. Sleep paralysis
4. Hypnagogic hallucinations

Excessive daytime sleepiness is the irresistible urge to fall asleep when environmental stimulus is relatively reduced. Children may appear inattentive, lazy, sleepy, or hyperactive. Narcolepsy-cataplexy is most commonly caused by a loss of hypocretin (Hcrt-1)-producing cells in the hypothalamus. Low cerebral spinal fluid Hcrt-1 levels can be used to diagnose the condition. Whether narcolepsy is an autoimmune disorder is still unclear, but the evidence of autoimmune destruction of Hcrt-1-producing cell is documented (6). Children of persons with narcolepsy have a 40 times greater risk for developing narcolepsy than the general population. Narcolepsy is also associated with head trauma, brain tumors, and demyelinating disease. Narcolepsy onset is most common in the second decade of life, and the incidence of onset falls with each subsequent decade (4).

Nighttime symptoms of narcolepsy may include sleep disruption, sleep paralysis, and hallucinations. Daytime symptoms may include falling asleep at school, inattentiveness, poor concentration, distractibility, academic problems, and automatic behavior. Children may report that daytime naps help in maintaining alertness. Narcolepsy symptoms in children are frequently misdiagnosed as psychiatric or behavioral disorders, including attention-deficit/hyperactivity disorder (ADHD), depression, conversion reaction, and psychosis.

Other symptoms of narcolepsy include *hypnagogic/hypnopompic hallucinations*, which are often described as "dreams," but are actually vivid auditory or visual hallucinations. They occur during transitions from wakefulness to sleep (hypnagogic) and from sleep to wakefulness (hypnopompic). It is reported that 50% to 70% of people with narcolepsy experience these hallucinations during both day and nighttime sleep periods.

Sleep-onset REM is defined as stage R occurring within the first 15 minutes of sleep. However, neonates enter sleep through stage R about 50% of the time. Sleep-onset REM periods can occur in children who are sleep deprived or who have sleep apnea; therefore, the interpretation of sleep-onset REM periods during the multiple sleep latency test (MSLT) in the pediatric population can be deceiving. Because of this phenomenon, it is particularly important to assess sleep patterns and perform a polysomnogram the night before performing an MSLT in children (2).

Cataplexy is defined as the loss of muscle tone provoked by strong emotion such as laughter, surprise, anger, or sadness. During cataplexy, the individual is conscious and remembers the event. Loss of muscle tone can be localized to the face, eyes, and jaw or can cause complete body collapse. Cataplexy usually develops within a year of the excessive daytime sleepiness symptom. In children with narcolepsy, cataplexy is uncommon.

After a thorough medical history and tests to rule out underlying medical conditions, alcohol, and drug use, the sleep physician will order an overnight sleep study, followed by the MSLT to evaluate symptoms of narcolepsy. In children with narcolepsy, the polysomnogram should indicate a sleep latency of less than 10 minutes and a sleep efficiency of greater than 90%. The MSLT begins 1½ to 2 hours after awakening. The test consists of five 20-minute nap opportunities spaced at 2-hour intervals during the day. An MSLT with a mean sleep latency for all naps of less than 8 minutes, and with at least two sleep-onset REM periods, is consistent with narcolepsy (5). A sleep-onset REM period (SOREMP) occurring during the preceding PSG can replace one of the required SOREMPs on the MSLT.

CASE EXAMPLE **Narcolepsy in an Adolescent**

A 16-year-old male was seen in the clinic for what his parents reported as severe sleepiness to the point of falling down. They reported that the young man "falls asleep any time he is not eating or walking around." At first, the parents thought the adolescent was not sleeping well because of a history of bad dreams. They monitored his nighttime routine and found that he was consistently falling asleep by about 10 PM and waking up at 7 AM, with the alarm clock. He would stare at the ceiling for a few minutes and then get out of bed. Nevertheless, he falls asleep doing homework, watching television, and texting his friends. When his friends tease him about his clumsiness, he does not laugh. He closes his eyes and makes a face. After a physical workup, the sleep physician ordered a polysomnogram, followed by an MSLT.

Idiopathic Hypersomnia

Idiopathic hypersomnia can be differentiated from narcolepsy by the lack of refreshment from napping, the absence of cataplexy, and sleep-onset REM periods, however, some patients with idiopathic hypersomnia may experience sleep paralysis and hallucinations, although less frequently than those with narcolepsy. After a rigorous evaluation to rule out organic causes, encephalopathy or a CNS space-occupying lesion, substance misuse, and psychiatric conditions, a polysomnogram is generally ordered to rule out apnea, PLMD, seizure activity, or a phase delay syndrome. An MSLT is necessary to rule out narcolepsy. The underlying cause of idiopathic hypersomnia is unknown (1).

PARASOMNIAS

Parasomnias are generally classified as follows:

1. Disorders of arousal from non-REM sleep
2. Parasomnias usually associated with REM (R) sleep
3. Other parasomnias

Common characteristics of these disorders include an incomplete transition from stage N3 to a lighter stage of sleep, automatic behavior, altered perception of the environment, and amnesia for the event. Disorders of arousal tend to occur in the first third of the night when stage N3 is most prominent. Essentially, parasomnias occur in the transition between stage N3 and stage R sleep and wakefulness. The EEG presents a mixture of theta, delta, and alpha frequencies. Additional information on the parasomnias can be found in other chapters in this textbook.

Sleep Enuresis (Bed-Wetting)

Enuresis is the involuntary voiding of urine during sleep that occurs at least twice a month in a child age

5 or older. If the child has never been dry for a period of 1 year, the condition is called "primary enuresis." Primary enuresis constitutes 80% of all bed wetters. Secondary enuresis is the recurrence of bed-wetting after at least a year of being dry. The child wets during the first third of the night, which coincides with the longest period of stage N3 sleep. The child has no recollection of the event. Enuresis is slightly more common in boys than in girls (2).

A number of factors may contribute to enuresis:

- A family history of enuresis
- Delayed maturation
- A stressful life event such as divorce or the birth of a sibling
- Delayed arousal from sleep
- Small functional bladder capacity
- Some organic causes for enuresis are as follows:
- Chronic constipation, which can irritate the bladder
- Sleep apnea
- Urinary tract infection
- Diabetes causing excess urine production
- Seizure causing loss of bladder control

After the pediatrician has ruled out organic causes of bed-wetting, a polysomnogram may be useful to determine the phase of sleep during which the enuresis occurs and whether it is related to sleep apnea or nocturnal seizures. Every year, about 15% of bed wetters become dry without treatment. The pediatrician can treat persistent enuresis using both medication and behavioral therapy (1).

Sleep-Related Seizure Disorders

PSG performed with an expanded EEG montage is very useful in the evaluation of nocturnal seizures. Sleep deprivation, illness, fever, irregular sleep schedules, obstructive sleep apnea, and medications used for the treatment of behavioral or psychiatric problems can exacerbate seizures. A nocturnal seizure can occur at any time during a polysomnogram, but seizures are more commonly seen at the beginning or end of slow-wave sleep and just after awakening in the morning (9).

Acute or chronic sleep deprivation increases the probability of a seizure in susceptible individuals. The most frequently seen EEG abnormality, in children with seizure disorders, is isolated spikes prominent in the temporal and central EEG placements and 3-Hz spike-wave discharges. Sleep-related seizure disorder is part of the differential diagnosis for primary enuresis and non-REM parasomnias (2). Seizures can be isolated to either sleep or waking. However, seizures can occur in both states (9).

CASE EXAMPLE **Status Epilepticus of Sleep in an Adolescent With a History of Frequent Generalized Tonic-Clonic Seizures After Awakening for School in the Mornings**

A 15-year-old male with a long history of generalized tonic-clonic seizures is referred to the sleep center by his neurologist for evaluation of nonrestorative sleep. He has approximately one generalized tonic-clonic seizure per month, always in the morning within the first few minutes after his dad awakens him for school. These seizures do not seem to be related to the adolescent's sleep schedule, which is highly regular. He goes to bed at 9:30 PM and is awakened for school at 7 AM. He never resists going to bed. He admits to feeling sleepy in class almost every day but had always thought this was due to his anticonvulsant medications. The polysomnogram revealed electrical status epilepticus throughout 90% of non-REM sleep, but the patient's EEG was essentially normal during REM sleep.

SLEEP-RELATED MOVEMENT DISORDERS

Restless Legs Syndrome

RLS (also known as Willis-Ekbom disease) is diagnosed based on the clinical history of the child. The child may describe the symptoms as creepy/crawly, itchy bones, spiders in my legs, or growing pains. The symptoms are usually worse in the evening or during the night and can be relieved by movement or rubbing the legs. Primary RLS is idiopathic in nature. Secondary RLS can be related to a number of factors such as iron deficiency anemia, neurologic disorders, medical disorders (uremia, diabetes, cancer, etc) drugs, or chemicals. RLS is usually worse in the evening and during the night, which may lead to difficulty falling asleep and maintaining sleep. All these symptoms can reduce sleep time and be associated with mood, behavioral, and academic problems. RLS is found in 5% to 15% of the general adult population, and first-degree relatives are 6 to 7 times more likely to have early-onset RLS. The technologist should make note of leg movements before sleep onset or during wake time in the sleep study log.

The essential diagnostic features of RLS in pediatric patients include additional criteria over and above the criteria used to diagnose adults. In adults or children older than 12 years, specific criteria are used to diagnose RLS. They include a reported urge to move the legs accompanied by an uncomfortable or unpleasant sensation in the legs, worsening of the urge to move or unpleasant sensations during periods of inactivity; the urge to move or unpleasant sensation is relieved by movement, and symptoms are worse or occur only in the evening or at night (1).

In pediatric patients under age 13 years, the child must meet all the essential criteria and relate a description that is consistent with leg discomfort. If the child is unable to relate a description that is consistent with leg discomfort, they must meet all the essential criteria and meet two of three additional criteria. The additional criteria include a sleep disturbance for age, a biologic parent or sibling with definite RLS, or PSG-documented PLMS (Periodic Limb Movements in Sleep) index of 5 or more per hour of sleep.

Periodic Limb Movement Disorder

PLMD should be diagnosed by a polysomnogram identifying five or more periodic limb movements (PLMs) per hour of sleep. A PLM is defined as lasting 0.5 to 5 seconds, separated by 4- to 90-second intervals. PLMs often do not disturb sleep; however, limb movements that occur within 3 seconds of an arousal or an awakening are associated with a sleep disturbance. Because about 80% of patients with RLS also have PLMD, these findings support the diagnosis of RLS. It is believed that central dopamine may be involved in the pathophysiology of primary PLMD. Secondary PLMD can be the result of the same factors that cause secondary RLS (6).

CASE EXAMPLE **Insomnia Caused by Restless Legs Syndrome**

A pleasant, outgoing 12-year-old girl came to the sleep clinic with her parents. She cannot fall asleep until after midnight and has to be out of bed for school by 6:30 AM. On weekends, she sleeps until about 8:30 AM and awakens spontaneously. She has a long history of behavioral problems and hyperactivity, fairly well controlled on a moderate dosage of a long-acting stimulant plus an additional dose of a short-acting stimulant after school. She has been a very restless sleeper who has complained about leg discomfort at night since she was about 3 years old. She often asks her mom for a leg rub at night, and this helps a little bit. The leg discomfort was thought to be related to "growing pains." She does not consume any caffeine. Her parents describe a clear circadian pattern to the restless legs, with increased restlessness in the evening. She also admits that she has difficulty keeping her legs still in class, reporting that she "just has to move." This was one of the symptoms leading to the diagnosis of ADHD. She also has learning disabilities and mild speech impairment. She did not start on stimulant medication until she was 7 years old. She has had drug holidays from the stimulant medication during the summer, with little to no change in her restless legs. Ferritin level was 52 (within normal limits). There is a prominent family history of restless legs, in the patient's mother, mother's sister, and maternal grandmother.

Headbanging and Body Rocking

Studies indicate that approximately two-thirds of 9-month-old infants use body rocking to self-soothe at sleep onset and after nighttime arousals. Half of all babies continue this rhythmic behavior to 18 months (1). Headbanging usually begins at around 9 months of age (2). The child may be lying prone and lifting the head and banging it down on the bed, on hands and knees rocking and banging the head against the crib, or sitting upright and banging the head against the crib. Other rhythmic movements include head rolling and body rolling side to side. PSG findings indicate that these movements can occur in all stages of sleep or in wakefulness. There is no seizure activity involved. In the absence of underlying medical problems, this behavior is normal, common, and is outgrown by 2 or 3 years of age (6).

SUMMARY

Performing a polysomnogram on a pediatric patient is a team process. It begins with the sleep specialist identifying issues, building trust with the parents, and communicating carefully. Acquiring an adequate study necessitates the involvement and support of both child and caregiver. The technologist should involve the parents in all aspects of the sleep study to maintain their trust and cooperation. The technologist should exercise patience and tact when performing the setup and answer questions from both parents and child. An understanding of the signs, symptoms, and characteristic clinical presentation of children with sleep disorders helps the technologist to be alert for specific behaviors that should be documented. This documentation can aid substantially in the identification of sleep disorders in the pediatric population that are nonrespiratory in origin.

REFERENCES

1. Mindell J, Owens J. Sleep in infancy, childhood and adolescence. In: *A Clinical Guide to Pediatric Sleep*. 3rd ed. Wolters Kluwer; 2015:15-36.
2. Sheldon S, Kryger M, Gozal D, et al, eds. *Principles and Practice of Pediatric Sleep Medicine*. Elsevier Saunders; 2024.
3. Carskadon M, ed. *Adolescent Sleep Patterns: Biological, Social, and Psychological Influences*. Cambridge University Press; 2002.
4. Kryger M, Avidan A, Berry R. *Atlas of Clinical Sleep Medicine*. 2nd ed. Lippincott, Williams & Wilkins; 2014.
5. American Academy of Sleep Medicine. *International Classification of Sleep Disorders: Diagnostic and Coding Manual*. 3rd ed. American Academy of Sleep Medicine; 2014.
6. Chokroverty S. *100 Questions and Answers About Sleep and Sleep Disorders*. 2nd ed. Jones and Bartlett; 2008.
7. Loughlin G, Carroll J, Marcus C, eds. *Sleep and Breathing in Children*. Marcel Dekker; 2000:347-362.
8. Jenni O, Bourgeois M. Understanding sleep-wake behaviour and sleep disorders in children: the value of a model. *Curr Opin Psychiatry*. 2005;19:282-287.
9. Eisermann M, Kaminska A, Moutard M. Normal EEG in childhood from neonates to adolescents. *Neurophysiol Clin*. 2013;43:35-36.

Chapter 63
Parasomnias and Movement Disorders in Children

MATTHEW J. BALOG AND DARIUS LOGHMANEE

KEY CONCEPTS/LEARNING OBJECTIVES

The key concepts for this chapter include describing the evaluation of children with suspected parasomnias and movement disorders and explaining the differences between sleep-wake transition disorders, parasomnias associated with nonrapid eye movement (NREM) sleep, parasomnias associated with REM sleep, and movement disorders common in children.

KEY TERMS

Children
Parasomnias
Sleep

Parasomnias are dysfunctions associated with transitions into sleep, partial arousals during sleep, or following arousals from sleep (1). Exclusive to sleep and wake-to-sleep transitions, these phenomena include arousals with abnormal motor, behavioral, autonomic, or sensory symptoms. Parasomnias can be noticeably dissimilar in clinical manifestations, but most share biologic characteristics. Symptoms typically begin early in childhood, gradually transform, and resolve themselves, which suggest a maturation etiology. Although often benign, these sleep disorders can be disruptive and even dangerous to the patient (2). In some cases, psychopathology plays a crucial role in sleep disorders; however, in other cases, recurrent parasomnia episodes induce psychopathology (2). Few pathologic abnormalities or objective diagnostic criteria can be identified, despite the presence of intense and often striking symptoms. Although symptoms are significant, spontaneous remission is typical.

Transitional parasomnias, partial arousals during sleep, or undesirable events or experiences following arousals from sleep may gradually appear or have a sudden and unexpected onset. Frequency can vary from a single episode to multinightly events. In the case of multinightly events, these parasomnias typically occur at 60-to-90-minute intervals, which correspond to transitions out of slow-wave sleep (SWS) (2). Patients appear medically and developmentally normal, with no obvious clinical abnormalities present during wakefulness, although unusual motor activity, behavior, or undesirable events or experiences occur during or immediately surrounding the sleep period.

ETIOLOGY

The etiology of arousal disorders, partial arousal disorders, and transitional parasomnias is unknown; however, it is generally thought to be multifactorial, with both predisposing and precipitating factors contributing to parasomnia appearance (2,3). Classification of these disorders in the child and adolescent separates them into three broad categories: (1) nonrapid eye movement (NREM)–related parasomnias, (2) REM-related parasomnias, and (3) other parasomnias. Classification is based on observable behaviors (Table 63-1) (1).

EVALUATION

Evaluation begins with a comprehensive medical history and physical examination. These are essential and usually result in an accurate diagnosis without elaborate testing. Emphasis should be placed on a detailed description of the abnormal sleep behaviors. A comprehensive history should include, but not be limited to, the following:

- Time of occurrence
- Symptoms manifested

Table 63-1 Comparison of Parasomnias

Parasomnia	Characteristics	Sleep Period	Polysomnography
Somniloquy	• Not associated with any pathologic states • May be related to other parasomnias	Any sleep stage	• Increased activity in the snore mic and chin EMG • Artifact in the EEG may be present
Confusional arousals	• Partial awakenings from SWS • Confusion and disorientation are prominent	Usually seen in the first half of the sleep period but may occur at any time during the night	• EEG shift from N3 sleep to wake rhythm • Vocalization post arousal may occur
Somnambulism	• Abrupt arousal from SWS, which can produce sitting up in bed to a full ambulatory session	• First third to first half of the sleep period	• EEG shift from N3 • Significant body movement • Muscle artifact in EEG
Isolated sleep paralysis	• Inability to move skeletal muscles, but the patient is fully awake	• Beginning of a sleep period, or upon awakening	• Reduction in general EMG activity with wake EEG rhythm • EOG movements may be present
REM sleep behavior disorder	• Considerable motor activity • Elaborate, purposeful movements, which may be accompanied by vocalizations	• REM sleep	• Increased muscle tone and movements while exhibiting REM sleep in other aspects (EEG, EOG)
Sleep-related enuresis	• Involuntary and repeated voiding of urine	• Any sleep stage, but usually in the first few hours of sleep	• Arousals may be more prevalent before the voiding event
Bruxism	• Forceful clenching or grinding of teeth, which produces an unmistakable sound • EEG arousals may or may not be present	• Generally, N1 and N2 sleep	• Increased activity in chin or masseter EMG • Muscle artifact in EEG, typically in the temporal region, but may be found in other channels

EEG, electroencephalogram; EMG, electromyogram; EOG, electrooculogram; REM, rapid eye movement; SWS, slow-wave sleep.

- Discussion of results of caretaker's intervention
  - Do symptoms quickly improve with intervention?
  - Do symptoms worsen with intervention?
- Length of episode
- Intensity of autonomic nervous system discharge
- Presence or absence of agitation during the episode
- Symptoms following waking
- Presence or absence of stereotypic activity

It is important to begin by assessing neurodevelopmental landmarks. The presence of daytime waking behavioral or developmental abnormalities may suggest other underlying disorders. Sleep-wake schedules, habits, and the typical pattern of the appearance of these sleep behaviors require delineation. Morning wake time, evening bedtime, and nap time rituals require description. Sleep logs or sleep diaries are frequently helpful. Video recordings of the episodes often reveal identifiable characteristics and can be very helpful in understanding the nature of the episodes. Evaluating for the presence of excessive daytime sleepiness, unintentional sleep episodes/sleep attacks, restless sleep, limb movements during sleep, and/or snoring may assist in determining precipitating factors (2). A careful evaluation of family history is also quite important as many parasomnias demonstrate a familiar pattern.

Comprehensive physical examination with emphasis placed on neurologic function and developmental assessment is required. Developmental delays, chronic medical or surgical history, or symptoms suggestive of neurologic disorders might indicate an organic basis for symptoms. Comorbid states are often present. Primary sleep disorders such as obstructive sleep apnea (OSA) or periodic limb movement disorder (PLMD) must be first addressed, and treatment may often result in symptom resolution.

Home video recording of the episodes may provide important diagnostic information. Under certain circumstances, video polysomnography (PSG) is indicated (2). Using an expanded electroencephalogram (EEG) electrode array during PSG provides additional information and increases sensitivity for identifying neurologic pathology. Concurrent video recording of the patient during PSG may demonstrate symptoms and document movements.

Analysis of the PSG should place special emphasis on the identification of primary sleep-related pathology that may be a factor in the precipitation of spells or fragmentation of sleep (eg, OSA, PLMD). Increased amplitude of slow waves, synchronization of slow-wave activity (Figure 63-1) occurring sporadically or just before a spell, as well as arousal rhythms occurring during SWS, and intrusion of 4 to 7 Hz EEG activity may be noted in older patients (2).

Other common PSG findings include movement arousals without state change, frequent arousal rhythms on EEG without state change (Figure 63-2), and theta-delta sleep pattern (hypersynchronous theta activity intruding into SWS at an age where this hypersynchrony should not still be present; Figure 63-3). Another common finding is the presence of *cyclic alternating pattern* (CAP), a marker of sleep instability. These findings are associated with, but not diagnostic of, disorders of arousal from NREM sleep (2).

Sleep-Wake Transition Disorders

Sleep-wake transition disorders are classified in the ICSD-3 as movement disorders. They are most common in children. Most commonly noted at the beginning of the major nocturnal sleep period, sleep-wake transition disorders may also occur following arousals, awakenings, or during naps. They may involve stereotypic movements, including, but not limited to, hypnic jerks, or "sleep starts," body rocking, head rolling, or head banging. Movements may persist into NREM sleep and may occur following arousals or during waking from sleep. The etiology of these movements is unknown.

Sleep-related rhythmic movement disorder (SRRMD), classified as a movement disorder in the ICSD-3, is very common and predominantly seen in infants and young children. Rhythmic movements generally have a frequency of 0.5 to 2 seconds with episodes lasting less than 15 minutes. Prevalence is especially high in infants with a 59% incidence rate, which drops to 6% by 5 years of age (2,4). A strong bidirectional relationship between SRRMD and attention-deficit/hyperactivity disorder has been noticed (2,4). Children with neurologic sequelae from brain injury, children with autism, and children with developmental delay show an affinity for SRRMDs even into adulthood (4). Rhythmic movements typically resolve spontaneously by 4 years of age; however, sleep-disordered breathing (SDB) may act as a trigger for the reemergence of these episodes in adults who experienced rhythmic movements as children (2,5). Most sleep-related rhythmic movements are benign. If, however, a child's head banging continues for a prolonged period, steps should be taken to protect the child from causing any injury to themself. At the same time, efforts should be made to help the child fall asleep without relying on rhythmic movements to calm down. PSG is generally not indicated, because diagnosis can be made by history and physical examination alone; however, when associated with other symptoms that might suggest a primary sleep or neurologic disorder, a polysomnogram with an expanded EEG array may reveal

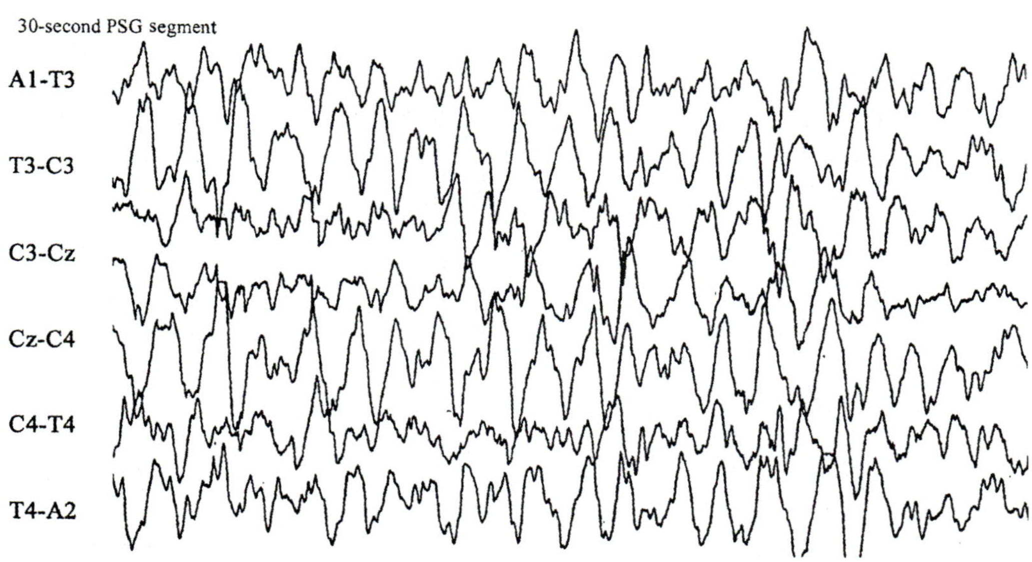

Figure 63-1 Hypersynchronous delta activity. This segment demonstrates an episode of hypersynchronous delta activity during slow-wave sleep. This delta hypersynchrony occurred immediately before a partial arousal with agitation and confusion. PSG, polysomnography.

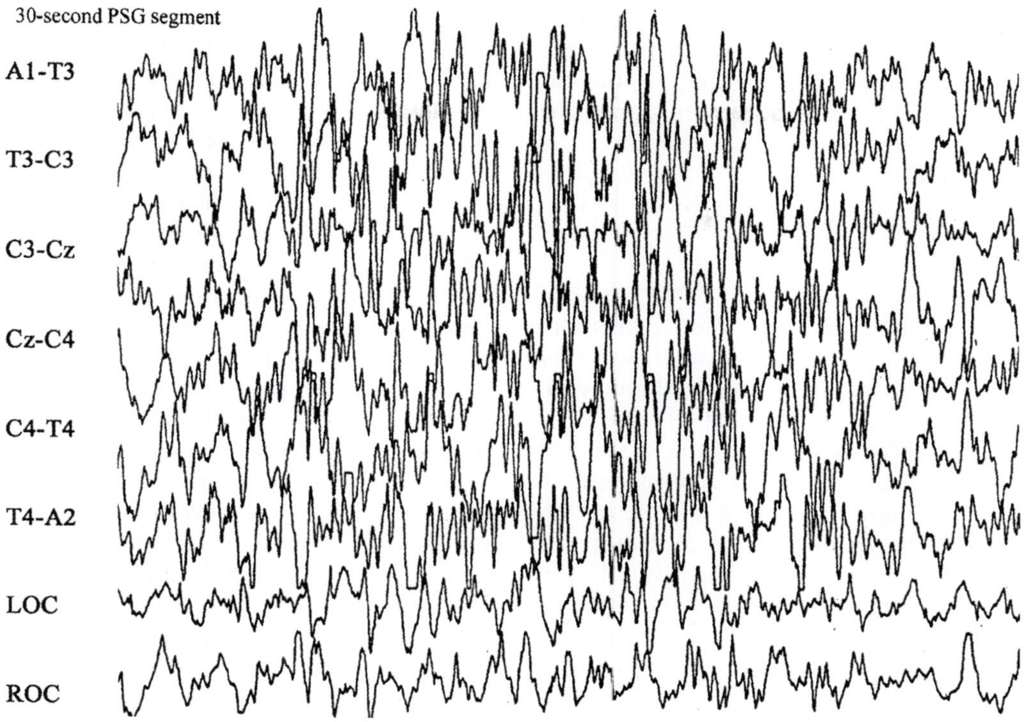

Figure 63-2 Arousal rhythm in slow-wave sleep (SWS). This segment is from the same patient as depicted in Figure 63-1. There is an arousal rhythm lasting about 10 seconds, occurring without state change during SWS. PSG, polysomnography.

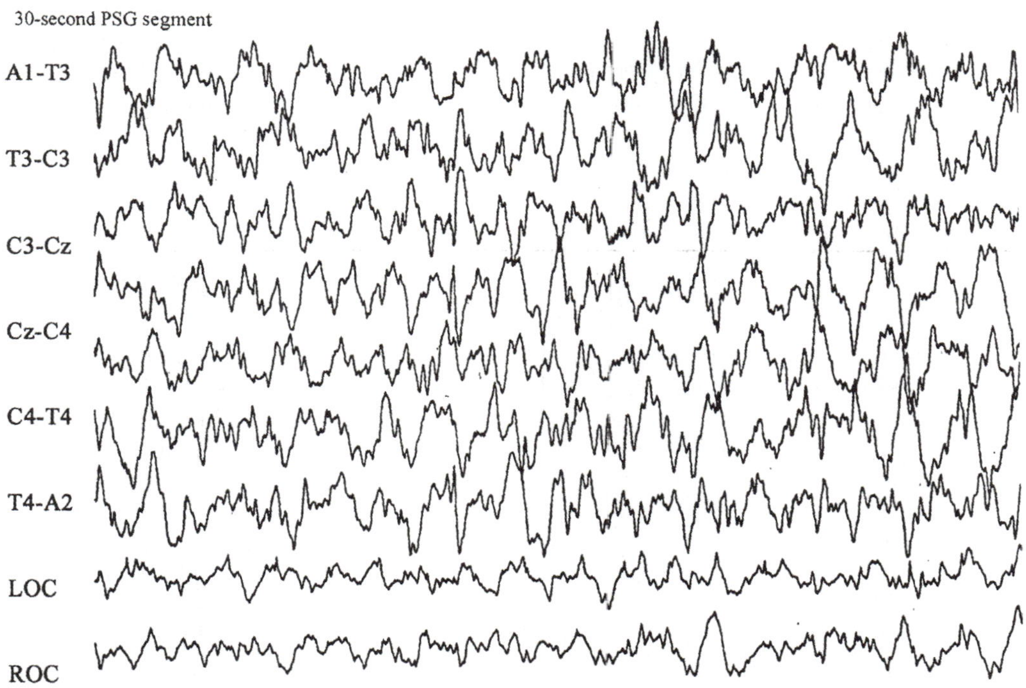

Figure 63-3 Theta-delta sleep. This segment of a 30-second polysomnography (PSG) epoch was recorded from an 8-year-old child with a history of agitated sleepwalking. There is considerable 4 to 7 Hz activity superimposed on 0.5 to 1 Hz activity.

typical rhythmic movements (2). Focal, paroxysmal, or epileptiform activity is notably absent. Rarely, prolonged EEG recording may be required to rule out a seizure disorder. Sleep architecture, progression of states, and state percentages as proportions of the total sleep time are generally normal for age.

SOMNILOQUY

Somniloquy (sleep talking) is a common occurrence that often happens in conjunction with other parasomnias and is a frequent occurrence during childhood with studies suggesting a prevalence between 7% and 60% (6). Somniloquy is most frequently of little concern to parents or health care practitioners, but rare episodes of vocal outbursts, loud talking, or unintelligible speech may occasionally be significant enough to disturb the sleep of other family members. Somniloquy is not associated with pathology but can occur during sleep terrors, confusional arousals, sleepwalking, or other NREM- or REM-related parasomnias (2).

Diagnosis is based on typical manifestations of either apparent coherent speech or incoherent mumbling during sleep. The child is typically amnestic for the event, and somniloquy is most often self-limited. PSG is rarely indicated unless other clinical manifestations are present. When noted outside of the context of a primary sleep disorder, treatment is unnecessary.

PARASOMNIAS ASSOCIATED WITH NONRAPID EYE MOVEMENT SLEEP

Parasomnias during NREM sleep (typically, SWS) are considered part of a continuum of undesirable manifestations of arousal or partial arousal that occur during sleep. Symptoms typically begin in childhood and resolve spontaneously. Rarely do they persist into adolescence or adulthood. Manifestations can be alarming, and, in certain circumstances, injury might occur. Spontaneous resolution and benignity of most signs and symptoms suggest a maturational etiology. Stereotypic movements characteristic of some parasomnias most likely arise from disinhibition of subcortical central pattern generators. Genetic predisposition, inherent instability of NREM sleep, and underlying sleep disturbances such as OSA may predispose to the activation of confusional arousals, sleepwalking, or sleep terrors. Inherited anatomic risk factors, present at birth, and even subtle SDB can lead to sleep disruption, instability of NREM sleep, and an increase in the number of parasomnia activities (2). Many of these parasomnias can be recognized by history alone, but some require nocturnal PSG to guide further evaluation and treatment (2).

Arousal and partial arousal disorders can cause simple symptoms, such as briefly sitting up in bed with rapid return to sleep or bizarre, dramatic symptoms. Nonetheless, these phenomena share several common features, which seem to occur during or following abrupt arousals from SWS. Confusion, disorientation, and amnesia for the event are common.

Arousal disorders occur more frequently during periods of anxiety or stress, with bladder distension, following periods of sleep deprivation, in the context of fever, or with hypersomnolence due to sleep deprivation or prolonged sleep fragmentation. Stress can increase the number and frequency of brief partial arousals in normal children. SWS rebound (increased time spent in SWS following sleep deprivation) can exacerbate partial arousals. These events may also be precipitated by external environmental stimuli. Computer-assisted identification of nonvisible arousals, CAPs, or respiratory cycle-related EEG changes may complement what can be accomplished by human scorers. Addition of autonomic arousal measures, such as heart rate variability, pulse transit time, and peripheral arterial tonometry, into standard reports may help discover more subtle sleep fragmentation (7).

CONFUSIONAL AROUSALS

Confusional arousals consist of partial awakenings from SWS usually occurring in the first half of the sleep period but may happen at any time during the night (2). Episodes are sudden, startling, and may be precipitated by environmentally induced awakenings. Children may appear fully awake during the episode but may not respond appropriately to commands or may resist being consoled. Confusion and disorientation are prominent. Attempts to abort the episode may make the symptoms more severe. These differ from agitated sleepwalking in that the patient is more aware of the environment, and the EEG may progress abruptly from SWS to wake following a very brief period of partial arousal.

Factors that increase SWS, such as rebound from sleep deprivation, or those that impair arousal may result in confusional arousals. Hypersomnia secondary to narcolepsy, OSA, PLMD, or idiopathic hypersomnia may exacerbate symptoms. Confusional arousals are often seen in patients with narcolepsy syndrome following prolonged daytime naps with resultant sleep inertia. As with other parasomnias, stress, anxiety, and fever may precipitate attacks. Organic pathology is rarely present. Injuries during confusional arousals may occur if the youngster leaves the bed or if dangerous objects are left within reach.

The prevalence of confusional arousals has been noted to be as high as 56.2% for children between 1.5

and 13 years of age, with the yearly incidence decreasing as the child ages (2). There appears to be an equal distribution between males and females. Although clear genetic mechanisms for transmission are unknown, a strong familial pattern has been noted.

Symptom onset is between 3 and 10 years old for 85% of children who report confusional arousals, with only 6.7% of children experiencing these arousals after the age of 13 years (2). Patients may thrash about or fall from the bed. Combativeness may occur, and attempts at consolation may result in the worsening of symptoms. Episodes are usually brief, lasting for only a few minutes; however, on rare occasions, they may be prolonged and last for several hours (8). As with other NREM parasomnias, patients are amnestic for the spell.

Diagnosis is based on the identification of classical symptoms of confusion, disorientation, agitation, and/or combativeness upon arousal, typically occurring during the first third to first half of the sleep period. Comorbid medical or psychiatric disorders are typically absent. Occasionally, the description of a confusional arousal may require differentiation from partial complex seizures with automatisms.

PSG, although rarely indicated, might reveal sudden arousal from SWS, brief episodes of hypersynchronous delta activity, theta-delta sleep, recurrent microsleep episodes, or poorly reactive alpha activity. Focal, paroxysmal, or epileptiform activity is absent in the EEG.

The presence of obstructive SDB or periodic limb movements might precipitate a spell. Symptoms are most frequent during middle childhood and then undergo spontaneous remission. Clinical course is usually benign. Physical injury might occur, and the child must be protected from trauma during the episode.

SOMNAMBULISM

Somnambulism, or sleepwalking, may vary in presentation from simple sitting up in bed to agitated running during sleep (2). A complex series of automatic behaviors are present and may seem purposeful. As with other NREM parasomnias, sleepwalking episodes occur following an abrupt arousal from SWS during the first third to first half of the sleep period. When accompanied by agitation, spells may be quite alarming, and injuries may occur. Because of the possibility of injury, agitated sleepwalking should be addressed quickly to protect the child from harm.

Somnambulism has been reported to occur in 15% to 29% of children with a yearly prevalence of between 2.6% and 13.4% (9). Symptoms are most common during childhood and reduce significantly during adolescence, usually disappearing by age 13 years (2). Episodes can vary broadly in frequency, intensity, and length. Parental reports may be quite inaccurate, and the true incidence is unknown. There appears to be an equal sex distribution, as well as a significant familial pattern. The genetic locus for sleepwalking is identified at chromosome 20q12-q12.12 in a multiplex family (10). There is a 60% incidence when both parents were affected as children, 45% when one parent was affected, and 22% when there was no family history of sleepwalking (2).

Sleepwalking typically has its onset between 4 and 8 years of age, although onset may occur at any time after the child develops the ability to walk. Symptoms range from quietly walking around the home to extremely agitated, semi-purposeful automatisms and frantic running. Performance of complex tasks, such as unlocking doors, taking food from the refrigerator, and eating, is common. Children have been noted to leave the house and wander around the neighborhood. Despite the apparent purposeful movement, these behaviors are often meaningless and unusual. Vocalizations may occur. Eyes are typically open, and the youngster may appear awake. Choreiform movements (repetitive and rapid, jerky, involuntary movements that appear well coordinated) may occur during spells. Enuretic episodes may occur, and the child may urinate (or attempt to urinate) at unusual places around the house. During a somnambulistic episode, the child is extremely difficult to wake, although complete arousal is possible. If awakened, confusion and disorientation are often present.

Motor activity can quickly cease, and the child may lie down on the floor or return to sleep at unusual places around the home. On the other hand, the child may return to bed without ever becoming alert.

Many factors similar to those previously mentioned may expedite sleepwalking spells. Fever, sleep deprivation, and sudden changes in environment are notable for increasing the frequency of spells. Any disorder that can produce significant disruption of SWS may precipitate events. In addition, sleepwalking can often be precipitated by urinary bladder distension in the susceptible patient. Environmental noise may also trigger an event. Several medications can exacerbate the disorder, including thioridazine, fluphenazine, perphenazine, desipramine, and chloral hydrate.

PSG typically reveals an arousal from stage N3 sleep, most commonly seen during the first half of the sleep period. Most of the background EEG activity is obscured by muscle artifact; however, seizure activity is notably absent.

Clinically, somnambulism can be differentiated from other disorders of arousal, such as confusional arousals and night terrors. Leaving the bed and calm nocturnal wanderings are less common with confusional arousals. Sleep terrors are more typically associated with the appearance of intense fear and panic and are less likely to be associated with the child leaving the bed.

Intense autonomic discharges and an initial scream herald a sleep terror and are usually not present in sleepwalking. Nocturnal seizure disorders typically reveal epileptiform discharges during spells; however, the interictal EEG may be normal. REM sleep behavior disorder (RBD) has been rarely described in children. It characteristically occurs during REM sleep in adults and is associated with clear verbalizations, more purposeful movements, and dream reenactment.

SLEEP TERRORS

Sleep terrors are often confused with nightmares as the nighttime appearance, initially, may look similar to parents, yet nightmares are drastically different from sleep terrors in etiology and presentation. The onset of a sleep terror is sudden, abrupt, striking, and frightening. These arousals are associated with profound autonomic discharges and behavioral manifestations of intense fear, with parental intervention generally leading to an escalation of the episode (2). In contrast, parental intervention can aid in calming the child having a nightmare.

The prevalence of sleep terrors is 1% to 6% of children 1 to 12 years of age (11). Males are typically affected more frequently than females, and there appears to be a clear familial pattern. Onset of symptoms is usually between 5 and 7 years of age, with sleep terrors typically occurring between 4 and 12 years old. Sleep terrors seldom occur past puberty (11). Precipitating factors are similar to other NREM parasomnias and include fever, bladder distension, sleep deprivation, and central nervous system (CNS) depressant medication. Symptoms tend to decrease during puberty and rarely persist into adolescence. Psychopathology can be associated with sleep terrors in adolescents and adults but is unusual in children.

Sleep terror episodes usually begin suddenly as the child sits upright in bed and emits a powerful, piercing scream. Severe autonomic discharge occurs, manifested as eyes opening widely and pupils dilating, tachycardia, tachypnea, diaphoresis, and increased muscle tone. During the sleep terror, the child is unresponsive, and efforts to restrain the child or console the youngster might exacerbate autonomic and motor activity. If awakened, the child is confused and disoriented, and there is amnesia for the event. In contrast to confusional arousals, episodes of sleep terrors are usually brief, lasting only a few minutes, and subside spontaneously.

Diagnosis is based on identification of the aforementioned symptoms and exclusion of organic pathology. PSG is rarely indicated, but if conducted, it may reveal sudden arousal from SWS during the first third to first half of the major nocturnal sleep period. Sleep terrors, however, can occur at any time during the night. Partial arousals without motor manifestation occur more frequently in children with sleep terrors compared with normal children. Autonomic discharge, in the form of tachycardia, can be seen during these partial arousals without full-blown symptoms.

Sleep terrors are clinically differentiated from partial complex seizures by their characteristic history and clinical course. Epileptic events may also be distinguished from disorders of partial arousal by the presence of a combination of clinical features and stereotypic behaviors and the fact that they may occur during wakefulness. Identification of epileptiform activity, however, does not completely rule out the presence of a partial arousal, because they may occur concomitantly in the same patient. Patients should also be evaluated for causes of sleep fragmentation, such as SDB or PLMD, as the arousals associated with these disorders can trigger episodes.

THERAPEUTIC CONSIDERATIONS

Symptoms of NREM parasomnias and childhood movement disorders are most often mild, occur less than once per month, and typically do not result in injury to the child or parents. In these *mild* cases, reassurance may be all that is necessary. A comprehensive explanation of the nature of these events and reassurance that the child is normal mentally and developmentally should be provided. Parents should be encouraged to let the event run its course. Interventions, if needed, should be focused on preventing injury and guiding the child back to bed. Vigorous intervention may prolong and exacerbate the episode. Discussions surrounding sleep hygiene and proper bedtime routines should occur, even in mild cases, as sleep deprivation and fragmentation are precipitating factors in these events.

Parents can be warned of a sleepwalking episode by a simple alarm system, such as fixing a bell to a door. Sleep deprivation should be avoided, and regular sleep-wake schedules should be maintained. Brief daytime naps might be attempted, and a period of quiet activity or relaxation techniques should be instituted before bedtime. Excessive fluids after the evening meal should be avoided, and the child should be encouraged to void before bedtime. If episodes of sleepwalking occur at the same time every night, waking the child 20 to 30 minutes before the regular time of occurrence can often prevent sleepwalking episodes from occurring. Fever, if present, should be appropriately treated; the cause of the fever should be identified and appropriately handled.

Severity of partial arousals is considered *moderate* when symptoms occur more than once a month but less than once per week and do not result in harm to the patient or to others. In these cases, reassurance and a behavioral approach (including behavior training, sleep hygiene, psychotherapy, and/or hypnosis) have been successful (2).

In *severe* cases, when episodes occur almost nightly or are associated with injury, nondrug approaches are considered first. Drug treatment, when used, should be prescribed for a short period and should be used in conjunction with a behavioral approach. Medications should be discontinued when behavior therapy begins to take effect (2,12).

PARASOMNIAS ASSOCIATED WITH RAPID EYE MOVEMENT SLEEP

Manifestations of REM sleep parasomnias are dissimilar to those occurring during NREM sleep. Most of these disorders can be differentiated by clinical evaluation alone. Frequency of REM sleep parasomnias varies considerably in children, ranging from common (nightmares) to rare (RBD).

NIGHTMARES

A nightmare occurs during REM sleep and is manifested by a frightening dream, followed by a prolonged period of wakefulness (2). Clear recall of the dream with varying degrees of anxiety may be present. Nightmares are characterized by a sudden arousal from REM sleep to a fully awake state. The child is fully oriented to the environment and sensorium is clear. Mild autonomic nervous system discharges may occur.

Nightmares most commonly occur during the last half to last third of the sleep period, although they may occur at any time during the night. A vivid story is often present, there is often complex mentation, and recall is appropriate for the child's developmental level. Nightmares are associated primarily with an emotional response rather than the intense autonomic activity exhibited with sleep terrors. Children are usually easily comforted following a nightmare, but return to sleep is delayed. Nearly all children experience a nightmare at one time or another. According to some studies, approximately 75% of children have experienced at least one nightmare (2,8). Prevalence of nightmares is increased in children who experienced a severe traumatic event with rates between 50% and 80% (2). Prevalence data for the general population is not consistent, with studies varying between 17% and 81% (13). Peak nightmare prevalence is also not clear but thought to be between 6 and 13 years of age, declining steadily with advancing age (8,13).

Movements, other than phasic twitches and/or other phasic activity, are rare. Arousal from sleep with vivid dream recall is typical. Clinical symptoms are generally mild. Diagnosis is based on identification of the milder characteristics, such as time of occurrence, vivid story line, and prolonged return to sleep. PSG is rarely necessary because nightmares and sleep terrors can usually be differentiated on clinical grounds alone.

PSG findings associated with nightmares typically depict an abrupt waking from REM sleep, followed by a somewhat prolonged period of wake after sleep onset. Mild tachycardia may be present, associated with a degree of anxiety. Increased eye movement density and increased phasic muscle twitches may be present during REM sleep but are not diagnostic. Focal, paroxysmal, and epileptiform activity are notably absent.

Occasional nightmares during childhood are common; however, if they are frequent, persist for prolonged periods, or associated with daytime behavioral problems, underlying medical or psychological causes should be sought.

Treatment is based on reassurance and identification of stressors. Maintenance of appropriate sleep hygiene is important. Relaxation before bedtime and identification and elimination of stressors are very helpful. Occasionally, further psychological and/or psychiatric evaluations are needed if symptoms are frequent, severe, or associated with other clinical manifestations. As a suspected correlation between anxiety and nightmares is present, cognitive-behavioral therapy (CBT) with image rehearsal therapy (IRT) and reduction in viewing graphic material is generally helpful. Most medication-focused studies on treating nightmares reside within the adult population. The few studies that focused on children targeted adolescents with posttraumatic experiences and showed that the use of Prazosin decreased the frequency of trauma-related nightmares (2,14).

ISOLATED SLEEP PARALYSIS

Isolated sleep paralysis is characterized by a period of inability to voluntarily move skeletal muscles at the beginning of a sleep period (hypnagogic) or immediately after awakening (hypnopompic) in the absence of a narcolepsy diagnosis (3). Consciousness is maintained, but the child feels paralyzed and is unable to open the eyes or speak. This phenomenon is typically due to persistent active inhibition of alpha motor neurons that persist after cortical waking. A sensation of difficulty breathing may occur, and episodes are typically frightening. Episodes of sleep paralysis may be prolonged or brief and subside spontaneously. Isolated infrequent episodes of sleep paralysis can occur in normal individuals. Frequent events are present in patients with narcolepsy and in familial sleep paralysis.

Onset of isolated sleep paralysis typically occurs during adolescence, but symptoms may begin before the onset of puberty. Children have difficulty describing the event. They may appear asleep during the spell and are often anxious or frightened on waking. Complaints may center on difficulty waking. Parents may be unaware of their occurrence, and symptoms can be mistaken for resistance to waking. Typically, children who resist waking arouse cranky and may pull away from the parent trying to wake them; conversely, during a spell of sleep paralysis, children appear "floppy" and cannot resist parental interventions.

The clinical course varies. Most episodes are isolated and are provoked by sleep deprivation, excessive sleepiness, stress, irregular sleep-wake schedules, or acute changes in sleep phase (15,16). Sleep paralysis might run a more chronic course in patients with narcolepsy syndrome or in the familial form of the disorder.

Diagnosis is based on the identification of presenting symptoms; however, symptoms may be nonspecific. Prevalence data vary, with studies suggesting that 15% to 40% of the population have experienced at least one episode of sleep paralysis (15). Sleep paralysis associated with narcolepsy can be differentiated from the isolated form by the absence of chronic excessive daytime sleepiness, sleep attacks, cataplexy precipitated by emotions, and hypnagogic hallucinations. Atonic generalized seizures or "drop attacks" occur during wakefulness and may or may not be associated with changes in levels of consciousness. Syncope occurs during wakefulness as well and is commonly associated with altered levels of consciousness.

PSG is typically not indicated, but if a spell occurs in the sleep center, it might reveal decreased skeletal muscle tone in the presence of a normal waking EEG pattern and conjugate eye movements.

Due to the self-limiting nature of isolated sleep paralysis, treatment is not necessary. Establishing good sleep hygiene and bedtime routines to achieve adequate nighttime sleep is generally all that is needed. Treatment of other sleep disorders that fragment sleep will aid in limiting episodes of paralysis.

RAPID EYE MOVEMENT SLEEP BEHAVIOR DISORDER

RBD differs from sleep terrors and NREM parasomnias by considerable motor activity and state dissociation during REM sleep. RBD may be characterized by elaborate, purposeful movements accompanied by vocalizations. There is a paradoxical increase in muscle tone and frequent limb movements during REM sleep, which has been considered a form of state dissociation. Occasionally, violent behaviors occur, with patients punching, kicking, and/or leaping out of bed. This motor activity is associated with dream recall as patients seem to be acting out their dreams (2). An injury to the patient or bed partner may occur in adults with RBD.

RBD usually begins during late adulthood and progresses over a variable period. Children may also be affected, but little is known of its prevalence, frequency, or natural history. Much of the pediatric literature is comprised of small case studies (2). Many cases are idiopathic in nature. RBD, although rare in the pediatric population, can be seen in children who have narcolepsy with cataplexy (17). RBD has a direct association with neurologic disorders, especially neurodegenerative diseases, in the adult population (2). Signs and symptoms of RBD and REM sleep without atonia (RSWA) have also been reported in posttraumatic stress disorder.

PSG reveals increased muscle tone and frequent limb movements that persist throughout sleep, especially in REM sleep. There is increased phasic muscle activity and excessive limb movements. No epileptiform activity is noted on the EEG. Medication use can be helpful in treating persistent RBD. Symptoms of RBD in both children and adults may respond to benzodiazepines. Sodium oxybate (SO) usage has been shown to reduce complex movements during REM sleep and improve clinical complaints in children (17).

OTHER PARASOMNIAS

Sleep-Related Enuresis

Sleep-related enuresis (SRE), or bed-wetting, is separated into two categories (primary and secondary) and is characterized by recurrent and involuntary voiding of urine during sleep that occurs in children older than 5 years old for at least 3 months (18).

- Primary enuresis diagnostic criteria include: the patient is older than 5 years, bed-wetting occurs at least twice per week, bed-wetting has been present for at least 3 months, and the child has not been consistently dry during sleep for at least 6 months (18).
- Secondary enuresis diagnostic criteria are the same with the exception that the child has been consistently dry during sleep for at least 6 months (18).

Bed-wetting is common during childhood and affects between 4% and 16% of schoolchildren and 5 to 7 million children in the United States (2,18). These episodes can occur during any stage of sleep but usually occur during the first third of the night (18). OSA is present in up to 47% of SRE cases (18). Children with snoring and OSA have been shown to have elevated brain natriuretic peptide levels that cause increased urine production during sleep (19).

As children age, the incidence of bed-wetting diminishes (2,18). The underlying causes vary between primary and secondary SRE. Primary SRE has a strong familial component as SRE occurs in 77% of children who have both parents with a history of SRE and 44% of children who have one parent with an SRE history (18). SRE has been linked to chromosomes 8, 12, 13, and 22 with a predominantly autosomal dominant inheritance (2,18). Primary SRE is usually not associated with daytime accidents (18). Etiology of primary SRE is unknown, but proposed mechanisms include the following: polyuria leading to nocturia, reduced bladder functional capacity, increased nocturnal bladder activity, decreased secretion of vasopressin causing increased urine production during sleep, difficulty arousing from sleep, and a hindrance to development of portions of the CNS required for maintenance of continence (2,18). In childhood, primary SRE is seen more commonly in boys than girls at a rate of 3:1; however in adults, primary SRE is seen more commonly in women than in men (2,18).

Primary SRE can be further separated into two subgroups: diuresis-dependent enuresis and detrusor-dependent enuresis (2).

- The diuresis-dependent enuresis children may or may not have vasopressin deficiency, usually do not experience daytime bladder issues, and wet their beds due to the nocturnal urine output exceeding the bladder capacity and do not wake to bladder distention due to deep sleeping (2).
- The detrusor-dependent enuresis children usually have daytime urinary urgency or constipation symptoms and usually wet their beds due to uninhibited detrusor contractions that fail to awaken the child during sleep (2).

As no methodology fully explains why children with SRE do not arouse from sleep to void, SRE is thought to be multifactorial (2).

Secondary SRE is a result of an acquired factor or underlying comorbid condition (18). This may include increased liquid intake prior to bed, diabetes mellitus/insipidus, anatomic anomalies in the genitourinary tract, constipation, chronic bladder or urinary tract infections, ADHD, developmental delay, OSA, epilepsy, spinal cord lesions, and diuretic use (18).

PSG is not indicated in diagnosing SRE as patient history and physical examination are all that is needed, but a sleep study may be helpful in ruling out contributory primary sleep disorders, including OSA and seizure disorders (2). If PSG is conducted, it may show an increased number of arousals (18).

Treatment options start with the diagnosis and management of any organic or pathologic condition. Treatment of SDB and sleep fragmentation often alleviates the enuretic episodes as OSA has been shown to contribute greatly to SRE episodes (2). Initial treatment should include behavioral modifications in conjunction with fluid reduction 2 hours prior to bedtime, dairy restrictions at least 4 hours prior to bedtime, and voiding prior to bedtime (2). Scheduled night wakings, outside of enuresis alarms, to void are generally not effective (18). Medications, such as desmopressin or imipramine, may be used in severe cases (2,18). It should be noted that only enuresis alarms, desmopressin, and imipramine have had randomized, placebo-controlled trials conducted (2). Currently, only enuresis alarms and desmopressin therapy can be recommended for routine treatment of SRE (2). Success rates of enuresis alarms are reported to be between 60% and 70%, with relapse occurring in 5% to 30% of children. Desmopressin therapy success rates vary at a wider range, between 40% and 80%; however, most children relapse after treatment (2). Because the spontaneous cure rate for children aged 5 to 16 is roughly 15% per year, treatment options are often not aggressively pursued; however, once SRE has been identified in children at least 5 years old, treatment should be started and tailored to the patient's underlying cause, especially in the context of OSA (2). Patience and vigilance are required, as initial changes in the model of bed-wetting take time. Parents should be understanding and avoid showing disappointment or disciplining the child for any relapse as some bed-wetting will continue throughout the course of treatment.

Sleep-Related Bruxism

Sleep-related bruxism, which is also a movement disorder, is characterized by rhythmic jaw movements, which produce grinding or clenching of teeth during sleep and which may or may not cause arousals (2). These movements are caused by involuntary contractions of the masseter, temporalis, and pterygoid muscles. Recent thinking has suggested that bruxism is regulated centrally by several neurotransmitters. When grinding occurs, there is generally an unmistakable noise produced. This noise is a reliable means of making a diagnosis.

Predisposing factors have been reported to include minor abnormalities of the teeth, malocclusion, stress, anxiety, SDB, and comorbid sleep disorders, which cause arousal from sleep (2,18).

Although the exact prevalence is unclear, bruxism is a common occurrence, with an approximate prevalence of 13%. (2). Bruxism is most prevalent in children. The condition seems to have an equal sex distribution as well as a familial pattern without clear genetic transmission (2,18).

Episodes of rhythmic jaw movements occur either periodically or paroxysmally in bursts, in varying durations but most commonly, 5 to 15 seconds. These movements are generally repeated throughout the night. Daytime complaints are common and include jaw pain, craniofacial pain, painful teeth, morning headaches, chronic wear to the crowns of the teeth, periodontal tissue damage, and bleeding from the gums. Resorption of the alveolar bone, hypertrophy of the masseter and temporalis muscles, and dysfunction of the temporomandibular joint can occur. Bruxism can occur in any stage of sleep; however, it is most common in stages N1 and N2 (2).

PSG shows paroxysmal, rhythmic muscle activity manifested by about 1 Hz muscle artifact over the temporalis muscle. This rhythmic activity may also be seen in the chin muscle electromyogram or masseter muscle groups. If it is associated with occlusive SDB, the muscle activity occurs during the arousal immediately after the obstructive respiratory event.

The most important therapeutic measure is appropriate dental management to minimize damage to teeth, especially in young adults (2). A mouth guard may be worn at night, which will not alleviate the symptoms but serve as more of a preventive dental intervention. If stress, anxiety, or other pressures are prominent, efforts should be taken to alleviate or minimize the causes of these troubles as this may prove helpful. Treatment of dental and/or other anatomic abnormalities through surgical intervention may not alter the bruxing behavior. If bruxism is associated with a comorbid sleep disorder of any kind, this should be managed. Benzodiazepines and muscle relaxants have been shown to decrease bruxism (2). Due to the vast nature of the treatment plan for bruxism, a collaborative approach involving sleep medicine, dentistry, psychology, and psychiatry specialties is warranted (2).

SUMMARY

Despite the broad spectrum of clinical manifestations of pediatric parasomnias and movement disorders, most of these occurrences share some biologic and etiologic characteristics. Children experiencing these disorders will tend to show no obvious clinical or developmental abnormalities when awake despite having disrupted sleep patterns. Parental accounts of the child's sleeping habits may or may not be accurate or helpful in some instances, yet PSG is not always the best clinical course in making a diagnosis, primarily because parasomnias may not be consistently noted in the sleep laboratory. As is the case for most pediatric sleep disorders, children with parasomnias require a thorough history and a physical examination by a health practitioner with experience in sleep disorders so that the most appropriate plan for evaluation and treatment could be determined.

REFERENCES

1. American Academy of Sleep Medicine. *International Classification of Sleep Disorders* 3rd ed. American Academy of Sleep Medicine; 2014.
2. Sheldon SH, Kryger M, Gozal D, Canapari C, Oyegbile-Chidi TO. *Principles and Practice of Pediatric Sleep Medicine*. 3rd ed. Elsevier; 2025.
3. IsHak WW. *Atlas of Psychiatry*. Sringer; 2023.
4. Lam N, Veeravigrom M. Sleep-related rhythmic movement disorder in children: a mini-review. *Front Neurol*. 2023;14:1165130. doi:10.3389/fneur.2023.1165130
5. Chiaro G, Maestri M, Riccardi S, et al. Sleep-related rhythmic movement disorder and obstructive sleep apnea in five adult patients. *J Clin Sleep Med*. 2017;13(10):1213-1217. doi:10.5664/jcsm.6778
6. Alfonsi V, D'Atri A, Scarpelli S, Mangiaruga A, De Gennaro L. Sleep talking: a viable access to mental processes during sleep. *Sleep Med Rev*. 2019;44:12-22.
7. Paruthi S, Chervin RD. Approaches to the assessment of arousals and sleep disturbances in children. *Sleep Med*. 2010;11(7):622-627.
8. Mindel JA, Owens JA. *A Clinical Guide to Pediatric Sleep: Diagnosis and Management of Sleep Problems*. 3rd ed. Wolters Kluwer; 2015.
9. Stallman HM, Kohler M. Prevalence of sleepwalking: a systematic review and meta-analysis. *PLoS One*. 2016;11(11):e0164769. doi:10.1371/journal.pone.0164769
10. Licis A, Desruisseau D, Yamada K, et al. Novel genetic findings in an extended family pedigree with sleepwalking. *Neurology*. 2011;76:49-52.
11. Leung AKC, Leung AAM, Wong AHC, Hon KL. Sleep terrors: an updated review. *Curr Pediatr Rev*. 2020;16(3):176-182. doi:10.2174/1573396315666191014152136
12. Mainieri G, Loddo G, Provini F, Nobili L, Manconi M, Castelnovo A. Diagnosis and management of NREM sleep parasomnias in children and adults. *Diagnostics (Basel)*. 2023;13(7):1261. doi:10.3390/diagnostics13071261
13. Sabbagh EE, Johns AN, Mather CE, Cromer LD. A systematic review of nightmare prevalence in children. *Sleep Med Rev*. 2023;71:101834.
14. Keeshin BR, Ding Q, Presson AP, Berkowitz SJ, Strawn JR. Use of prazosin for pediatric PTSD-associated nightmares and sleep disturbances: a retrospective chart review. *Neurol Ther*. 2017;6(2):247-257. doi:10.1007/s40120-017-0078-4
15. Stefani A, Högl B. Nightmare disorder and isolated sleep paralysis. *Neurotherapeutics*. 2021;18(1):100-106. doi:10.1007/s13311-020-00966-8

16. Hefnawy MT, Amer BE, Amer SA, et al. Prevalence and clinical characteristics of sleeping paralysis: a systematic review and meta-analysis. *Cureus*. 2024;16(1):e53212. doi:10.7759/cureus.53212
17. Antelmi E, Filardi M, Pizza F, et al. REM sleep behavior disorder in children with type 1 Narcolepsy treated with sodium oxybate. *Neurology*. 2021;96(2):e250-e254. doi:10.1212/WNL.0000000000011157
18. Kryger M, Roth T, Goldstein CA, Dement WC. *Principles and Practice of Sleep Medicine*. 7th ed. Elsevier; 2022.
19. Sans Capdevila OS, Crabtree VM, Kheirandish-Gozal L, Gozal D. Increased morning brain natriuretic peptide levels in children with nocturnal enuresis and sleep-disordered breathing: a community-based study. *Pediatrics*. 2008;121(5):e1208-e1214. doi:10.1542/peds.2007-2049

Chapter 64
Interventions in the Pediatric Sleep Center

ELIZABETH Y. WIESEMANN

KEY CONCEPTS/LEARNING OBJECTIVES

The key concepts for this chapter include the nuances of positive airway pressure titration in children, the importance of monitoring carbon dioxide when titrating oxygen in children, and when and how to initiate noninvasive ventilation in children.

KEY TERMS

Continuous positive airway pressure
Hypoventilation
Invasive ventilation
Noninvasive ventilation
Oxygen
Sleep apnea

This chapter reviews interventions relevant to sleep-disordered breathing (SDB) in children. All these disorders can be diagnosed in the sleep laboratory and can be simply grouped as disorders of:

1. upper airway obstruction (ie, obstructive sleep apnea [OSA]),
2. restrictive lung function and/or poor muscle tone (ie, hypoventilation), and
3. impaired respiratory drive (ie, central sleep apnea [CSA] or hypoventilation).

Interventions that will be discussed include continuous positive airway pressure (CPAP), bilevel positive airway pressure (BPAP), supplemental oxygen, and noninvasive and invasive ventilation. All forms of respiratory support therapy need to be adjusted to suit the patient's requirements, and regular reviews and titrations are to be performed in the sleep laboratory to accommodate for growth and monitoring of disease progression.

DETERMINING WHICH RESPIRATORY SUPPORT TREATMENT TO USE

Optimal gas exchange is dependent on three variables: brain and central nervous system (CNS) function, the structural design of the airways, and muscle tone. If there is a fault with any one of these variables, then a child is at risk for developing SDB. On the basis of the child's clinical history and physical examination, one can hypothesize the nature of the SDB the child will develop. Diagnostic polysomnography and blood gas testing allow clinicians to diagnose the problem and to determine the treatment to be initiated. Treatment recommendations may include CPAP, oxygen therapy, and/or ventilation (Figure 64-1).

Central Respiratory Control

A number of conditions interfere with normal regulation of breathing by the brain and the CNS. Respiration is initiated in the pre-Bötzinger complex in the pons and medulla oblongata in the brainstem and further regulated by the carotid and aortic bodies. These areas submit electrical pulses to the diaphragm through the phrenic and thoracic nerves in the spinal column. Conditions associated with the spinal column or head, such as trauma, tumors, or malformations (eg, an Arnold-Chiari malformation), can interfere with respiratory drive, respiratory rhythm, or respiratory regulation. The hypoxic response is driven primarily by the carotid bodies, whereas the response to carbon dioxide (CO_2) is driven primarily by brainstem structures. These combined abnormalities result in susceptibility to CSA and/or hypoventilation and a need for the child to be treated with positive pressure or volume ventilation in order to regulate the respiratory rate and/or tidal volume. If a child requires only nocturnal support, then noninvasive ventilation (NIV) is the optimal treatment. On the basis of modern technology, NIV is predominately positive pressure ventilation. If the individual requires assistance during wake and sleep and has a chronic condition, then invasive ventilation should be considered. Depending on the severity of the lack of respiratory drive, invasive ventilation can be pressure or volume ventilation.

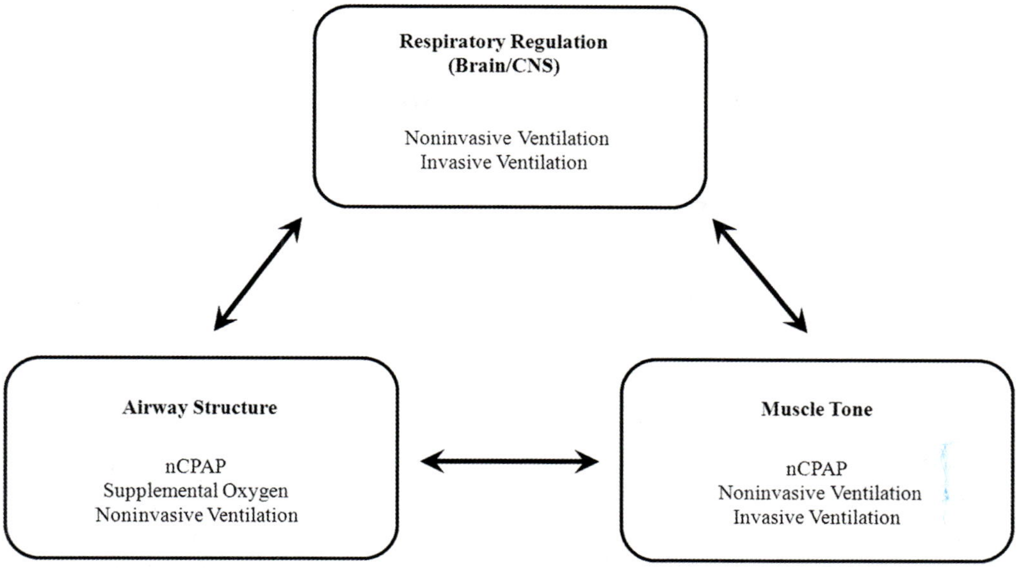

Figure 64-1 The pathophysiology of sleep-disordered breathing. On the basis of the origin of the sleep-disordered breathing, the appropriate respiratory therapy can be determined. CNS, central nervous system; nCPAP, nasal continuous positive airway pressure.

Structural Compromise of the Airway

Structural abnormalities in the airway can interfere with optimal gas exchange by predisposing to narrowing or collapse. Obstruction to airflow can occur at any point along the airway from the nares to the alveoli. Examples of the physical obstruction in the upper airway include adenoid and/or tonsil hypertrophy, choanal atresia/stenosis, a cleft palate, or an enlarged tongue (macroglossia). These may be identified on physical examination or through more invasive testing procedures, including nasal endoscopy. Children at risk for upper airway obstruction may also be assessed using the Mallampati score. Other causes of structural narrowing include micrognathia, a congenitally narrow airway, or childhood obesity whereby increased adipose tissue surrounds the muscular soft tissue of the upper airway. The primary example of a congenital floppy airway is laryngomalacia in infants, usually presenting soon after birth.

Surgical interventions can often alleviate these problems, but positive airway pressure (PAP) may be required for stabilization or long-term therapy when surgery is either contraindicated or not curative. The most easily corrected cause of obstruction is adenotonsillar enlargement, but other commonly performed surgical procedures include mandibular distraction and supraglottoplasty.

Gas exchange abnormalities can also be caused by structural abnormalities in the lower airway such as restrictive lung disease and/or chest wall abnormalities (ie, kyphoscoliosis, cystic fibrosis, and bronchiectasis). It is important to note that morbidly obese children (particularly adolescents) may be at an increased risk of nocturnal hypoventilation because of the excessive adipose tissue deposited on the trunk and abdomen restricting pulmonary function. If hypoventilation is present, treatment with NIV (with or without oxygen therapy) should be considered. It is common for children with lung disease (ie, neonatal lung disease and cystic fibrosis) to be treated with supplemental oxygen, but in some cases, PAP or NIV is also required because of associated conditions such as OSA or airway malacia.

Poor Muscle Tone

Gas exchange is also influenced by the effectiveness of respiratory muscle function. Many congenital myopathies are associated with progressive muscle weakness; the classic example is Duchenne muscular dystrophy. Mild loss of muscle tone can also affect the upper airway and predispose to upper airway obstruction, and treatment with PAP therapy may be sufficient in these cases.

More severe loss of muscle power, such as in spinal muscular atrophy or at the later stages of Duchenne muscular dystrophy, requires ventilation because of loss of diaphragmatic and/or intercostal muscles, with additional compromise in sleep due to loss of respiratory accessory muscle activity.

Congenital Heart Disease

The use of PAP or NIV for patients with congenital heart disease (CHD) is often for the management of respiratory issues occurring secondary to the underlying cardiac condition. CHD can affect the respiratory system by causing obstructive and/or diffusion defects.

Direct anatomic compression of the airway can occur in association with cardiac abnormalities, secondary to the enlargement of cardiac structures or abnormal vascular structures (such as vascular rings). As an example, tetralogy of Fallot is associated with the narrowing of the pulmonary artery as well as ventricular septal defect and leads to the deviation of the aorta to the right and thickening of the right ventricle. This, in turn, can lead to pulmonary artery dilation, bronchial or tracheal compression, and atelectasis, resulting in respiratory distress.

In terms of diffusion defects, ventricular or atrial septal defects can result in increased pulmonary blood flow because of left to right shunts. The increase in pulmonary blood flow can result in loss of elasticity in pulmonary vessels and increase the resistance in the pulmonary bed, thus impacting gas exchange.

The use of PAP therapy or NIV should be aimed at relieving airway compression, increasing lung volume, equalizing transalveolar pressures (in addition to cardiac medications), and expanding surface area available for gas exchange to occur in the pulmonary bed.

POSITIVE AIRWAY PRESSURE THERAPY FOR CHILDREN

The most common reason for initiating PAP therapy in a child is to treat upper airway obstruction, predominantly OSA. But under what circumstances and how severe does the upper airway obstruction have to be before PAP therapy is warranted? There is no consensus on this matter, but from clinical experience, a number of factors can be evaluated to help with this decision. From diagnostic polysomnography, the main variables used include the following:

1. The obstructive apnea-hypopnea index (AHI)
2. Oxygen desaturation index and oxygen saturation nadir (Spo_2)
3. Evidence of CO_2 retention
4. Increased arousal frequency and fragmentation of sleep architecture
5. Increased work of breathing

OSA in children is diagnosed as an AHI greater than or equal to one event per hour (1,2); however, PAP therapy is generally commenced only on children who have at least a moderate OSA or who have a mild OSA with at least one comorbidity. A symptomatic child with mild OSA may be recommended PAP therapy if they have poor sleep quality, that is, an inability to fall asleep due to the obstruction, an elevated arousal index ($>$10 events per hour), and/or poor sleep architecture. Clinically, if the child has a high work of breathing, failure to thrive (3), poor development (4), poor daytime performance and/or behavior, and/or respiratory distress, then PAP therapy may also be considered. Using PAP therapy alleviates the high work of breathing, thus conserving calorie consumption and allowing weight gain (5), and improves sleep quality and thus daytime function and behavior (6). Nasal steroids, body positioning, and surgical intervention (ie, adenotonsillectomy) may be used without PAP therapy for milder cases of OSA or in conjunction with PAP therapy to help alleviate OSA in more severe cases (7).

The most common correctable pathologies underlying OSA in children are adenoid and/or tonsil hypertrophy and obesity. The most common age for presentation with adenoid and tonsil hypertrophy as the cause of OSA is 2 to 5 years, and this subsequently declines with age. Conversely, the risk of OSA associated with obesity increases with age. Although most children with mild-to-moderate OSA respond to adenotonsillectomy (8), a proportion of children fail to respond to this surgery. Persistence of disease in a number of these children is reflected by the fact that a history of past adenotonsillectomy increases the risk of current OSA more than 2-fold, whether or not there is an underlying abnormality such as myelomeningocele (9). Clinical practice has demonstrated that treatment with PAP therapy is a viable option for the majority of children who fail surgery. Treatment with PAP therapy is also increasingly recognized as effective for the management of perioperative airway obstruction (10). Criteria for such intervention are becoming clearer as the predictors for perioperative problems are clarified (11).

A number of syndromes and conditions increase the risk and severity of OSA and therefore increase the likelihood of requiring PAP therapy. These include Trisomy 21, achondroplasia, Pierre Robin sequence, Prader-Willi syndrome, cerebral palsy, and obesity. In these instances, although surgical intervention remains appropriate, it is likely to alleviate but not "cure" the OSA, and PAP therapy may still be required for effective long-term management of the upper airway obstruction. Nonetheless, it is important to note that a proportion of children who present with OSA, particularly those presenting during infancy, show improvement as they get older. Experience suggests that if we can provide respiratory support during early development, many of these children are able to cease treatment. The caveat in this circumstance is that the presence of disease during childhood may be an indicator of small central and upper airways that will persist throughout life and into adulthood (12). At the more severe end of the spectrum or where the diagnosis of upper airway obstruction is made in later childhood, the prognosis for cure appears to be poor.

Beginning Positive Airway Pressure Therapy

The data presented here regarding the commencement of PAP therapy in children are derived largely from clinical practice and experience. An intervention that can be specific for children includes behavioral strategies to assist with compliance. If hospital or home nursing resources are available, another strategy can be PAP acclimatization in a clinical setting. This provides family support, aids with adherence, and optimizes PAP pressure. Otherwise, many of the other steps for commencing PAP therapy follow adult practice (13). A few published studies address the issues surrounding PAP initiation and adherence for children, and there has been limited formal evaluation of the acceptance by pediatric patients of different devices (14). However, what is known is that with proper training, good adherence can be achieved in children (15,16) and that it can be maintained with careful follow-up.

The strategies to commencing PAP therapy vary according to the age and development of the child. For infants (less than ~6 months old), the therapy can generally begin immediately, with no need for prior behavioral programs. Instead, intervention strategies and education should be geared primarily toward the parents/primary caregiver because of their primary role in achieving adherence with therapy. The adaptation process for PAP therapy is approximately 3 to 7 days; however, in some cases, infants take to the therapy almost immediately.

For older children, success in implementing PAP therapy is improved if it is commenced in a graduated manner. To maximize adherence, the children must first become adapted to the nasal mask. This takes approximately a week and is done in the home environment. Role-playing with the child (eg, acting as an elephant, scuba diver, "Buzz Lightyear," or an astronaut) assists with this. Allowing the child to wear the mask for 10 to 15 minutes when awake minimizes the "scare factor." Once the mask is accepted, the child is admitted to hospital, and a PAP pressure is introduced. Others report successful introduction of PAP therapy in an immediate manner, with or without the addition of behavioral intervention programs.

In adolescents, the process is broadly the same as for adult patients. Reports now suggest that adults utilizing PAP therapy also benefit from access to a multidisciplinary approach to aid adherence with therapy (17). Practice guidelines derived from evidence in the literature suggest that once a diagnostic study has demonstrated the presence of OSA, the patient is fitted with the mask interface, and the process is explained to the patient. A trial of PAP therapy can be undertaken with the patient awake and participating. An overnight sleep study for pressure titration can be undertaken almost immediately. Pressures are adjusted during the study, and the patient is discharged the next day on the pressure setting deemed optimal on the basis of a single night of determination. Although this may be appropriate for the older adolescent, a hospital admission to commence therapy may still be appropriate for younger or developmentally delayed teenagers.

In all age categories, PAP therapy is commenced on a low pressure (eg, 5 cm H_2O CPAP) to allow the child to get used to the sensation of the therapy and therefore maximize the likelihood of adherence. The first stage is to achieve overnight adherence with low-pressure therapy. A clinical review permits appropriate pressure changes to follow, for example, in the presence of ongoing snoring, pressures need to be increased. It is also important to note, depending on the age and complexity of a child's condition, that commencing PAP therapy at home with the assistance of a community nurse may also help the child and parents adjust to using PAP therapy as part of their bedtime routine.

PRINCIPLES OF TITRATION

For disorders with upper airway obstruction, the goal of pressure support is to splint the airway open in order to relieve the obstruction and achieve normal ventilation. When performing polysomnography for PAP pressure determination, the channels that should be closely monitored in order to achieve an optimum PAP pressure are nasal airflow, respiratory effort, oxygenation (Spo_2), and CO_2. Monitoring of CO_2 during titration studies requires the use of transcutaneous ($Tcco_2$) rather than end-tidal measurements ($Etco_2$). With the exception of children with lung or cardiac disease, the aim of a PAP pressure titration study is to achieve a normal oxygen saturation (ie, $Spo_2 \geq 95\%$) and CO_2 concentration (ie, $35 \leq Tcco_2 \leq 45$ mm Hg). The pulmonologist and/or cardiologist should set discretionary guidelines for children with underlying/associated lung and/or cardiac disease.

Titrating Continuous Positive Airway Pressure During Polysomnography

Once the patient has adapted to the use of the pressure support, a full PAP titration polysomnogram is undertaken in the sleep center. It is recommended that titration studies follow the American Academy of Sleep Medicine (AASM) guidelines (18). In general, pressure titration studies commence with minimal CPAP of 4 cm H_2O and do not exceed 15 cm H_2O CPAP for children less than 12 years old. The priorities for pressure adjustment are to eliminate discrete obstructive respiratory events, eliminate signs of increased work of breathing, and eliminate signs of airflow limitation.

Discrete obstructive events and labored breathing on the polysomnogram are seen as a loss of nasal airflow and increased respiratory effort with, or without, oxygen desaturations and/or arousals. The general practice is to increase the CPAP in 1 cm H_2O increments if at least one obstructive apnea or two hypopneas are seen in children aged 12 or less or at least two apneas or three hypopneas are present in children greater than age 12. Each pressure change should be separated by at least 5 minutes of recording.

Once discrete obstructive events are eliminated, the next step is to put an end to nasal airflow limitation, residual snoring, and respiratory effort–related arousals (RERAs). CPAP pressure for children aged less than 12 years is to be increased if there are at least three RERAs or 1 minute of loud or unambiguous snoring. CPAP is to be titrated higher for children 12 years or older who experience at least five RERAs or 3 minutes of loud or unambiguous snoring. CPAP is increased in approximately 1 cm H_2O increments until this is achieved.

Once optimal pressure is achieved, there should be no snoring or stridor, and there should be normal nasal airflow and respiratory effort, stable oxygenation without intermittent desaturations, and normal CO_2. Allowing 30 to 60 minutes before additional incremental increases in CPAP will provide sufficient time for the patient to blow off any excess CO_2 and allow adequate sleep for analysis by the assessing physician. To allow the sleep physician to assess and confirm the optimal pressure, an ideal study includes pressure adjustments to a level slightly above the optimal CPAP. Acute signs that the CPAP has been increased too high include increased frequency of arousals, recurrence of the use of accessory muscles, fall in baseline oxygenation and CO_2 retention, and the occurrence of central (rather than obstructive) respiratory events (4). AASM standards indicate that an optimal CPAP is achieved when the respiratory disturbance index (RDI) is less than five events per hour for at least 15 minutes, Spo_2 is above 90%, and a rapid eye movement (REM) period in the supine position is recorded. The titration is considered good when the RDI remains greater than 10 events per hour and Spo_2 is above 90%. The titration may be adequate if the RDI has been reduced by 75% from diagnosis or titration was not assessed during supine REM sleep. AASM standards indicate that a titration is unacceptable when any of the aforementioned criteria remain unmet.

Titrating Bilevel Positive Airway Pressure During Polysomnography

If CPAP is not well tolerated or a pressure higher than the recommended CPAP of 15 cm H_2O is needed, consider switching the patient to BPAP therapy. The starting pressure should be an inspiratory positive airway pressure (IPAP) of 8 cm H_2O and an expiratory positive airway pressure (EPAP) of 4 cm H_2O. If the patient is to be switched from CPAP to BPAP, the minimum EPAP should be 4 cm H_2O or the CPAP level at which obstructive events were eliminated. The highest IPAP for patients younger than 12 years should be 20 cm H_2O and for patients aged 12 and older 30 cm H_2O. The minimum IPAP-EPAP differential should be 4 cm H_2O and the maximum 10 cm H_2O. The IPAP and/or EPAP should be increased by a minimum of 1 cm H_2O every 5 minutes, as warranted by the applicable titration algorithm for the age group. For patients less than 12 years of age the IPAP and EPAP should be brought up by 1 cm H_2O if one obstructive apnea is observed. For children 12 years and older, the IPAP and EPAP should be raised by 1 cm H_2O if two obstructive apneas are observed. IPAP should be increased by 1 cm H_2O if one hypopnea is observed in children less than 12 years of age or if three hypopneas are observed in patients 12 years of age and older. IPAP should be increased by 1 cm H_2O if three RERAs are observed in children less than 12 years of age or if at least five RERAs are observed in children 12 years of age or older. IPAP should be increased by 1 cm H_2O if 1 minute of loud and unambiguous snoring is observed in children less than 12 years of age or if 5 minutes of loud and unambiguous snoring is observed in children 12 years and older.

For long-term users of PAP therapy, the prescribed pressure requires regular review to ensure that ongoing optimal therapy is maintained (19). This is particularly true in children where growth increases the likelihood of change in airway structure, muscle tone, and tidal volume. Infancy, in particular, is a period of rapid growth and may therefore require more frequent review, for example, repeating a sleep study at the age of 3 months, 6 months, and 1 year. As children become older, these can be spaced further apart, until annual reviews are undertaken. However, in other practices, retitrations are undertaken only as clinically indicated, by growth, weight changes, or changes in nocturnal or diurnal symptoms.

Advancements in PAP technology continue to refine how pressure is delivered. PAP devices come with expiratory pressure relief options or can be set to automatically adjust pressure to optimize airflow. Care must be taken in the selection of devices used in young or small children to ensure that tidal volume and flow rates generated are detected by the device. Some model devices are generally produced with adult specifications, and children may not trigger them, so care is required to ensure that their specifications and functions will translate to pediatric patients.

Common Problems and Solutions Experienced With Children on Continuous Positive Airway Pressure

The most common problems experienced are pressure sores generated by the PAP mask, air leak, and drying of the nasopharynx. The range of pediatric masks is increasing, but one of the most common difficulties in children is finding an appropriately sized nasal mask. The criteria for usage vary by manufacturer and are set primarily by patient age or weight. Masks designed for adults may be used off-label on pediatric patients under the guidance of a physician. The following table lists the FDA-approved pediatric mask as of August 2025.

Mask Name	Age Restrictions	Weight Restrictions
Respironics Wisp Nasal	none	>22 lb
ResMed Pixi Nasal	2-7 y only	none
ResMed Kidsta Nasal	>7 y	>40 lb
SleepNet MiniMe 2 Nasal	2-12 y only	none
Circadiance Sleep Weaver Nasal	2-7 y only	none

These are the age and/or weight restrictions for pediatric PAP masks with FDA approval. These values are from the manufacturer's instructions for use.

Caregivers, including technologists and parents, must be vigilant to assure there is no facial skin breakdown. Careful observation of the face when the mask is removed every day is essential, just as with mask care for NIV. Rotating among two or more commercially available mask types can help minimize the risk of pressure sore. It is helpful to allow the child to choose their own mask from a suitable group. This implied consent gives the patient some control over their own care and improves cooperation.

Pressure sores generated from masks are a common problem in pediatrics, whether for long periods of acute treatment or for regular nocturnal support. They occur more often because of either the straps being adjusted too tightly onto the face and/or an ill-fitting mask. Suggestions to alleviate pressure sores include adding padding and/or applying a dressing to the affected area at night. Massaging the facial areas improves circulation when the mask is removed every morning.

A poorly fitting mask can also be associated with a mask leak. It is important to correct any leaks during the pressure titration polysomnogram as these lead to loss of pressure and, in turn, affect the optimum pressure settings. No air should escape around the perimeter of the mask. Mask leaks can also cause eye irritation and reduced user adherence.

Pressure loss can be generated by a mouth leak. Nasal masks are often the primary mask type used in pediatrics, and full-face masks are used only after careful evaluation by the sleep team. An adult full-face PAP mask or chin strap can be used off-label in pediatric populations under the guidance of a physician. Pediatric sleep physicians can be hesitant to use full-face masks in young, developmentally delayed, or physically impaired children because of the risk of vomiting into the mask as well as the inability of the child to remove the mask themself.

There are no FDA-approved pediatric full-face PAP masks or pediatric chin straps. Alternate solutions to full-face masks and chin straps are alleviating mouth leaks in children include using a pacifier, wedging a rolled washcloth between the chin and the chest, and/or adding humidification.

The delivery of dry and/or cold air can precipitate or exacerbate nasal mucosal swelling and/or inflammation. Humidification is useful as it keeps the nasopharynx warm and humidified, preventing drying of the nasal passages. Maintaining humidification of the nasal passages minimizes the likelihood the user will open their mouth on inspiration. Humidification also minimizes inflammation of the nasal epithelium and consequent nose bleeds. For young children, the impact of CPAP without humidification can be significant in fluid balance, and for this reason, we never use CPAP without humidification in children aged less than 24 months.

Other problems that may be associated with CPAP are gastrointestinal wind and excessive salivation. Children, particularly infants, often swallow air when CPAP is commenced, perhaps exacerbated by sucking on a pacifier, poor tone in the lower esophageal sphincter, or if the pressure is set too high. Infants can develop abdominal distention, but this is usually a temporary problem that settles over the first 7 to 10 days of CPAP use. Children may also experience increased drooling, and occasionally, this becomes excessive. Finally, removal of the mask during sleep times is a common problem that may be helped by adding mittens to the hands or using infant sleeping bags, making it difficult for the infant to grasp at the mask or head strap.

Equipment for infants should be soft, with minimum capacity for causing pressure sores. In infants, it is especially important to ensure that the fit of the mask and head strap does not lead to air leak into the eyes. Infants should always be placed supine or in a lateral position to permit direct visualization and to ensure that the nostrils do not become occluded by the mask. It is also important that the tubing does not pull the mask up or off the face; in infants, the weight of the tubing can displace small masks and head straps upward; one way to alleviate this problem is to slacken the weight of the tubing by anchoring it to the side of the crib.

Acute and chronic pressure effects have been described in children, including the potential for midface hypoplasia (20). The concern is that during body development, the nasal mask can push on the midface, altering the growth patterns to affect the shape of the face. It is, therefore, important to monitor the development of the face for long-term users of CPAP or NIV and consider alternating between different masks so that points of maximum pressure vary.

If leaks or other problems associated with PAP are evident during the polysomnogram, it is important for the sleep technologist to document and report this to the physician so appropriate steps can be taken to alleviate the problems and maximize user adherence.

NASAL INSUFFLATION

Klein et al (1986) suggested the use of insufflation (passage of warm humidified air through a thin nasopharyngeal tube at 2-10 lpm; mean 3.5 lpm) to treat upper airway obstruction in children. They pointed out that airway obstruction in children commonly presents with prolonged periods of partial upper airway obstruction, rather than the longer discrete obstructive events seen in adults, and demonstrated a marked reduction in the work of breathing in children treated with this modality (21). One significant benefit of transnasal insufflation is that it is better tolerated than CPAP, with 23.5% to 63.2% reductions in the AHIs in studies of adults. The flow rates used in studies of adults and children were 15 to 20 lpm (22). At these flow rates, the insufflation increases nasal pressure by approximately 2 cm H_2O and inspiratory airflow by approximately 100 mL/s. Airway obstruction may not be completely eliminated with this technique, but it is particularly useful for patients who have trouble tolerating CPAP and may be more effective in treating children because it is most effective for those with partial obstruction or hypopneas rather than discrete apneic events. The use of insufflation is effective with flow rates of 7 to 10 lpm in infants and children where CPAP is not tolerated and/or where upper airway obstruction is moderate, rather than severe.

NONINVASIVE VENTILATION FOR CHILDREN

Noninvasive therapy is recommended for children with nocturnal hypoventilation or CSA. Unlike children with OSA, surgical procedures are rarely an option for treatment of hypoventilation or CSA. A range of disorders can underlie hypoventilation and vary from congenital disorders affecting the CNS control of breathing to progressive or acquired disorders affecting the heart, lungs, and/or respiratory musculature. Children may suffer from severe restrictive lung disease, chest wall deformities, myopathies, and congenital or acquired abnormalities of the CNS. An increasing number of children are also being commenced on NIV because of the long-term adverse effects of chemotherapy on the lungs for treatment of oncologic diseases and as a support mechanism for children waiting for lung transplantation. Whether the condition affects tidal volume, respiratory rate, and/or gas exchange in the lower airway, if the end result is inadequate minute ventilation, then NIV may assist lung inflation and/or produce an artificial breath rate to normalize gas exchange.

Sleep-associated changes in respiratory control and respiratory dynamics mean that hypoventilation will usually manifest first during sleep and only later progress to include daytime respiratory compromise. Broadly speaking, NIV is commenced when respiratory failure is demonstrated during sleep. A number of factors determine the time to commence NIV. Children with CSA will start on NIV if the polysomnography shows the following:

1. Bradypnea sufficient to compromise ventilation
2. Pathologic or extreme central apneic events
3. Evidence of respiratory failure—usually nocturnal

The changes occurring in blood gases are usually progressive, rather than being related to frank respiratory events. The common definition of acute respiratory failure is a CO_2 greater than 50 mm Hg and a PaO_2 lesser than 50 mm Hg, thus acknowledging that hypoxia and hypercapnia occur simultaneously in disorders that compromise ventilation.

NIV can be started in the intensive care unit if children are acutely unwell but can also be commenced in a ward environment following a planned admission. It is recognized that children presenting with recurrent respiratory failure, or respiratory failure in the presence of an underlying (especially progressive) disorder, have frequently experienced acute or chronic respiratory failure (23). That is, they regularly experience respiratory deterioration during sleep times, but acute respiratory failure can develop rapidly during a superimposed respiratory infection or with acute deterioration in their underlying condition. Recognition of the risk of sleep-associated respiratory deterioration has led to more proactive screening and identification of the disorder before these florid deteriorations occur. Children who are recommended NIV following polysomnography generally require NIV long term. Polysomnography can also be undertaken to screen children before surgery for scoliosis and, if required, NIV commenced to maximize their lung health before the scheduled surgery. Children who commence NIV in an acute setting may have a newly identified disorder and require only short-term therapy or may need to continue on to long-term therapy after review in the period of recovery.

Hypoventilation of central origin leads to maximum blood gas abnormalities during slow-wave sleep when ventilation is almost exclusively under automatic control (no cortical influences). Congenital central hypoventilation syndrome (CCHS) may be attributable to a Phox2B gene mutation or to other CNS disorders that affect ventilatory control, such as a hypoxic insult or a brainstem pathology, including the Arnold-Chiari malformation with or without syringomyelia, hypoxic insults, spinal cord trauma, or tumors. At best, the absence of CO_2 sensitivity results in a dependence on hypoxic ventilatory drive.

Peripheral hypoventilation describes failure of the respiratory pump to allow adequate gas exchange (ie, chest wall and/or respiratory musculature movement). Conditions that pose a risk of peripheral hypoventilation are often linked with restrictive lung disease and include kyphoscoliosis, cystic fibrosis, bronchiectasis, myopathies, and morbid obesity. Peripheral hypoventilation results in both hypoxia and hypercapnia that are most apparent during REM sleep when there is skeletal muscle atonia, particularly affecting activity of the respiratory accessory muscles. Such loss of accessory muscle activity can shift marginal respiratory function to respiratory failure in children who can otherwise maintain adequate respiratory function while awake or in slow-wave sleep by recruiting respiratory accessory muscles.

One major advantage of NIV is fewer and shorter hospital admissions and maintenance of a better quality of life in children with neuromuscular disorders (24). Follow-up of a group of patients, the majority of whom had neuromuscular disease, suggested that the commencement of NIV for nocturnal hypoventilation arrests deterioration rather than improving the underlying disease processes, with gains attributable to reversal of respiratory failure and improvement in sleep.

Commencing Noninvasive Ventilation Therapy

Although it is clear that NIV can reverse alveolar hypoventilation, the criteria for establishing ventilation are not universal. It is generally agreed that NIV should commence in the presence of daytime hypercapnia or during an acute or chronic exacerbation. Nocturnal hypoventilation likely heralds imminent daytime hypoventilation, but currently, there is no consensus about when to start screening children with progressive disorders. Further studies will need to determine what level of nocturnal dysfunction will be associated with improvement if nocturnal ventilation is established.

Our processes for commencing NIV therapy in children follow the same strategies as those for PAP outlined earlier. Although NIV may be commenced in the intensive care unit, elective treatment can also start in a general medical ward with overnight monitoring of Spo_2 and CO_2. Unlike CPAP or BPAP, there are multiple settings (ie, IPAP, EPAP, and backup rate) that may require adjusting and fine-tuning when a child is commenced on NIV. Therefore, it would not be practical to commence NIV within the home setting. In the hospital setting, adjustments to ventilation can take place in a closely supervised environment, with titration sleep studies performed only after the child has adapted to the therapy and shows stability of blood gases. Noninvasive therapy requires more frequent adjustments during periods of growth, especially puberty.

Principles of Titration

The primary principle for titrating NIV is to achieve normal gas exchange, indicated by normal oxygenation, CO_2, pH, and bicarbonate measures on blood gases. A number of primary settings are utilized in NIV in order to achieve normal gas exchange and user comfort (Figure 64-2). The first setting to be considered is the "mode"; this dictates how the respiratory rate is regulated. The "mode" determines if the respiratory rate is regulated solely by the user, the device, or a combination of both. The "spontaneous" mode allows the user to have a spontaneous respiratory rate 100% of the time. "Timed" mode allows the NIV device to regulate the respiratory rate at all times and overrides the user's spontaneous respiratory rate. Because of user discomfort and asynchrony between the user and the device, in our clinic, this setting is rarely used. The final, but the most commonly used mode is "spontaneous/timed," which allows the user to breathe spontaneously but delivers breaths to meet a fixed, minimum rate if the patient does not trigger the machine within a prescribed time period.

EPAP is a positive airway pressure delivered on expiration. It can act as CPAP, providing an air splint to prevent collapse of upper and/or lower airways. EPAP is also termed "positive-end expiratory pressure" or PEEP. IPAP is the positive inspiratory pressure being delivered. To deliver ventilation, not CPAP, the IPAP should be at least 4 cm H_2O higher than the EPAP. This pressure difference between IPAP and EPAP is termed "the delta (Δ) swing" or "pressure support." The larger the delta swing, the greater the lung expansion and collapse. Increased pressure support increases pulmonary expansion and can increase CO_2 clearance.

The "backup respiratory rate" setting is activated only on "spontaneous/timed" and "timed" modes to control the minimum respiratory breath allowed by the user.

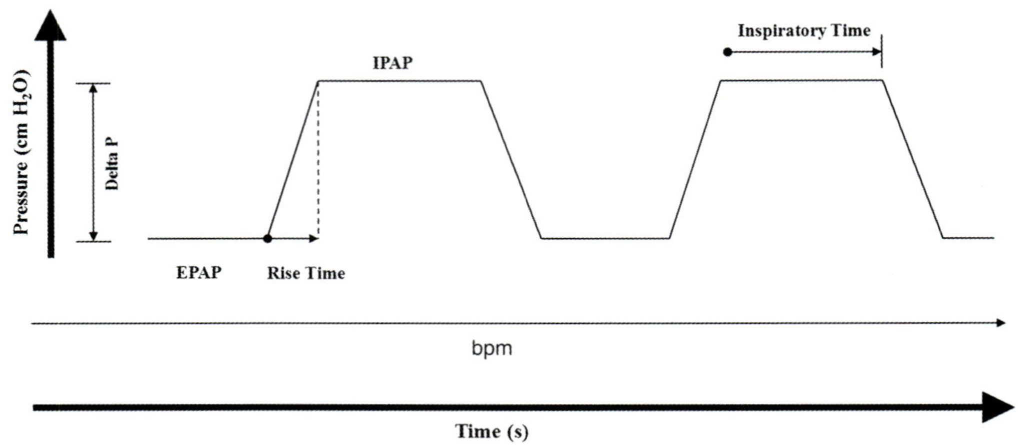

Figure 64-2 Fundamental settings of noninvasive ventilation. bpm, beats per minute; EPAP, expiratory positive airway pressure; IPAP, inspiratory positive airway pressure.

The "inspiratory time" (alternatively known as "IPAP max") is a setting that works in parallel with the backup respiratory rate. This determines the maximum inspiratory time and the maximum duration of IPAP delivery before the pressures return to EPAP. The "rise time" setting is used for comfort and is the time taken to increase the pressure from EPAP to IPAP. Our clinical experience suggests that small infants and patients with stiff lungs tolerate a shorter rise time, whereas children with muscle weakness prefer a longer rise time.

AVAPS (average volume–assured pressure support, also known as iVAPS) is another form of NIV but delivers a set tidal volume rather than fixed pressures. It helps patients maintain a fixed tidal volume by controlling the pressure support. In AVAPS, a minimum and maximum IPAP are set, and the device fluctuates within this range to deliver a set tidal volume. EPAP is a set pressure. This mode allows for improvement in synchrony between the patient and the device. As the patient's effort reduces, the device will deliver higher pressure to ensure that the prescribed volume is delivered. AVAPS is becoming increasingly used in children (25).

In order to correctly commence NIV, one must first identify the cause of the hypoventilation/CSA. If the pathophysiology is caused by impaired brain/CNS function, whereby the CNS fails to regulate respiratory rate and blood gases, then a backup rate is mandatory to ensure that the patient breathes at the minimum prescribed rate. Backup respiratory rates are also required for patients with hypoventilation caused by myopathies and/or kyphoscoliosis, where the patient may not be able to generate sufficient negative pressure to trigger the device.

If hypoventilation and poor gas exchange are related to restrictive lung disease, then NIV titration focuses on correct titration of the IPAP and EPAP settings. In the majority of cases, a backup respiratory rate is also used to help regulate CO_2. Earlier generations of devices were designed for adults who weighed at least 25 kg, and if a child cannot trigger the device, then a mandatory respiratory rate may need to be used to deliver adequate support. Obese adolescents diagnosed with nocturnal hypoventilation and patients with cystic fibrosis tend to be the only instances in pediatric practice where a backup respiratory rate is not routinely required.

Titrating Noninvasive Ventilation Pressures During Polysomnography

In the context of our protocols, which aim to optimize ventilation before the pressure determination sleep study, monitoring in the sleep center generally results in only small additional changes. This minimizes the number of changes required in the course of a single study while still aiming to achieve the following: (1) Spo_2 greater than or equal to 95% and (2) $Tcco_2$ between 35 and 45 mm Hg and maximize synchrony between the user and the device (Figure 64-3). Titrating NIV pressures should be in keeping with the AASM guidelines (18).

Ideally, the recording should include a period of quiet wakefulness off NIV to document the respiratory rate, Spo_2, and $Tcco_2$ during wakefulness. Once this is achieved and the patient has fallen asleep, the first step is to normalize oxygen saturation, which is usually achievable by adjusting EPAP. Changes in oxygenation can be seen almost immediately. If upper airway obstruction is seen, the EPAP is adjusted to overcome this, in the same manner as for CPAP.

Once the desired oxygen saturation is achieved, the next step is to eliminate CO_2 retention. This can be achieved by two methods: (1) increase IPAP to increase the delta swing and/or (2) increase the respiratory rate. After each adjustment to improve CO_2 clearance, approximately 30 minutes should be allowed for the changes to have an effect before the next pressure change or adjustment in respiratory rate.

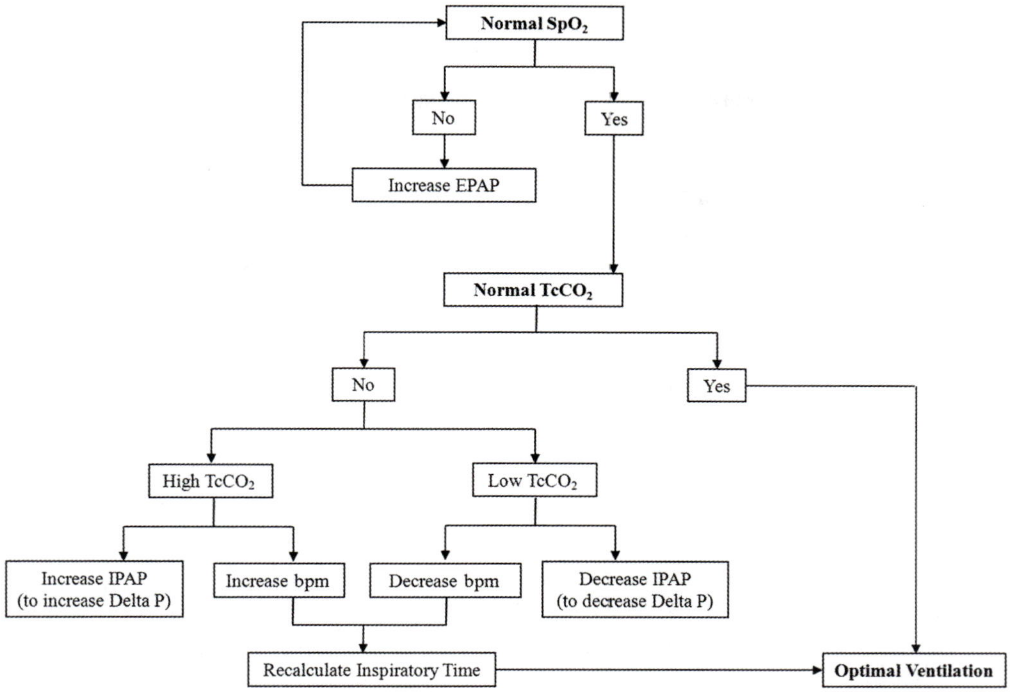

Figure 64-3 Titrating noninvasive ventilation settings to optimize blood gases. bpm, beats per minute; EPAP, expiratory positive airway pressure; IPAP, inspiratory positive airway pressure; Spo_2, oxygen saturation; $Tcco_2$, transcutaneous CO_2.

As a rule, setting the backup respiratory rate 1 to 2 bpm slower than the child's spontaneous respiratory rate during sleep regulates CO_2 while maximizing synchrony. As children grow, their spontaneous respiratory rate decreases with age, and backup respiratory rates need to be reviewed. Any alterations to respiratory rates should be accompanied by adjustment of the "inspiratory time" setting. The "inspiratory time" setting can be calculated using the following steps:

α (seconds) = 60 seconds/backup respiratory rate

β (seconds) = $\alpha \times 1/3$

Inspiratory time (seconds) = $\beta + 0.2$ seconds

The rationale for this formula is based on (1) the number of breaths per minute (ie, 60 seconds), (2) the inspiratory to expiratory ratio (I:E ratio) of 1:2; thus, for every respiratory cycle, one-third of that time is spent on inspiration, and (3) to assist with comfort and compliance, 0.2 seconds is added to allow extra time for the patient to breathe spontaneously before the machine initiates premature expiration.

The primary cause(s) of asynchrony during the polysomnogram are an incorrect backup respiratory rate and/or incorrect inspiratory time (usually too long). Asynchrony can also occur if the child fails to trigger either inspiration or expiration.

Common Problems and Solutions Experienced With Children on Noninvasive Ventilation Therapy

Children on NIV therapy can experience the same or additional problems as those on CPAP. Other than the common problems with mask interfaces seen in children on CPAP therapy, as outlined previously, the major issues we confront are due to limitations of the technology relative to the requirements of children. In particular, these include sensitivities that are not appropriate for the smaller sized patients, lack of alarms for caregivers, and limited portability of the devices; young children are frequently required to sleep in transit or away from the family home.

The limited number of products suitable for children that are currently being manufactured can require compromise in the mode of ventilation being used or desired respiratory rates due to lack of flexibility in the technology, rather than the child. Poor alarm systems may limit the ability of caregivers to determine when the child is experiencing problems—whether on account of their limited mobility or young age. Many current alarms are designed to only be loud enough to wake the user, who would then troubleshoot and correct the problem themself. The need for internal batteries ensures safety by providing continued support in the event of an AC power failure and during transport. Travel demands occur in several ways. Infants sleep for long periods, and family demands may limit the ability of parents to stay home whenever the child sleeps.

With increasing numbers of children being supported with NIV in the community, we regularly see these children present with respiratory failure during acute illnesses. During these acute exacerbations, many children can be managed with a short-term increase in either pressure settings or the duration of their NIV (in each 24-hour period) and therefore avoid admission to the intensive care unit and intubation (26). In general, once a child commences therapy with nocturnal ventilation, their need is ongoing, although some disorders improve over time. Adults who commence nocturnal ventilation have reduced annual mortality, but equivalent information is not available for children.

The domains in which we are required to support the delivery of NIV therapy continue to expand. During acute illnesses, patients who live long distances from hospitals may be faced with the need to provide support while seeking medical assistance and ambulance transport. Traditionally, our medical transportation services intubate children in order to secure their airway for transport, but there are increasing demands to provide NIV during transport. Finally, as quality of life improves and these children actively participate in a broad range of family activities, we have increasingly frequent requests for NIV therapy during travel for leisure. One exciting development has been the need to oversee the transition of children who receive respiratory care, including ventilatory support, into adult services.

SUPPLEMENTAL OXYGEN THERAPY FOR CHILDREN

Disorders affecting lung diffusion include abnormalities of the small airway structure or function and abnormalities of the alveolar wall or its components. In children, this includes various disorders, but the most common disorders leading to a need for oxygen include neonatal lung disease, cystic fibrosis, and chronic lung disease associated with aspiration secondary to neurologic conditions. Other examples include a selection of "orphan" lung diseases, which are rare individually, but together comprise a group of chronic lung diseases, such as abnormalities of surfactant proteins, and infiltrations or abnormalities of the alveolar wall, such as interstitial fibrosis or lymphangiectasis. For these disorders, where children are unable to maintain appropriate oxygen saturations, oxygen therapy is commonly recommended. Cardiac problems are the most common nonpulmonary disorders that lead to a need for oxygen, particularly those associated with pulmonary hypertension, where the pulmonary vasculature is (and therefore pulmonary pressures are) responsive to oxygen. The use of oxygen therapy in children under palliative care is becoming more common to alleviate symptoms toward the end of life. Occasionally, children with OSA who do not tolerate CPAP are recommended oxygen to alleviate the oxygen desaturations associated with the respiratory events.

High-Flow Oxygen Use in Children

Traditionally, oxygen therapy is delivered only at low flows less than 2 L/min via nasal prongs or 4 L/min via Hudson mask. The drying effect of the higher flows of the oxygen can irritate the nasal mucosa and cause distress and discomfort to the children as well as effecting secretion clearance and mucociliary functions. Recent technical advancements have led to the development of devices that deliver high-flow oxygen/air mix (26,27). Adding heated humidification to the circuits allows for enhanced patient comfort, and this is used in a variety of settings, including palliative care and periods of acute respiratory distress.

The underlying diagnosis is the major determinant of whether the disorder is progressive or will improve with growth and development. For example, during infancy, chronic neonatal lung disease requiring oxygen supplementation tends to improve with age. In contrast, adolescents requiring oxygen because of a progressive lung disorder, such as cystic fibrosis, will inevitably deteriorate over time. Ideally, oxygen therapy should be utilized only to maintain oxygen saturation (as clinically appropriate). In all cases where oxygen therapy is being provided, care should be taken to ensure that CO_2 retention is not precipitated in patients who are reliant on their hypoxic drive to maintain their ventilation. If this cannot be achieved, then NIV may be required, whether oxygen is required in addition or not.

Commencing Oxygen Therapy

The goal of oxygen therapy is to maintain adequate oxygenation without precipitating hypoventilation by removing hypoxic ventilatory drive. A diagnostic study (eg, oximetry, $Tcco_2$ monitoring, or polysomnography) should be undertaken to evaluate the degree of hypoxia that is anticipated and to confirm a need for oxygen supplementation. The most common indicators of a need for oxygen supplementation are low baseline oxygen saturation levels. Other indicators may include tachypnea, deterioration in oxygen saturation levels during REM sleep, or the absence of REM sleep.

For infants who were transferred out of an intensive care unit, it is often helpful to "recommence" treatment by undertaking a diagnostic study and reviewing their absolute need for oxygen supplementation as well as to ensure that there is no accompanying evidence of CO_2

retention indicating hypoventilation. Passive hypercapnia is used in some of these infants on the basis that they will drive their CO_2 down as their lung function improves. The purpose of the review is to ensure that the hypercapnia is not unstable and that there is no additional CO_2 retention during REM sleep.

The signals in the sleep study, which provide most information, are sleep stages, airflow, respiratory rate, respiratory effort, oxygenation (Spo_2), and CO_2 ($Etco_2$ or $Tcco_2$ monitoring). It is important to monitor these children with full polysomnography as hypoxia is often accompanied by fragmented sleep with arousals, and adequate oxygenation may lead to an increase in REM sleep.

Principles of Titration

Oxygen therapy is a very common therapy in hospital environments, so detailed titration of oxygen requirements is necessary only in situations where oxygen use is expected to continue in the home environment. The supplemental oxygen concentration should be titrated with simultaneous oximetry and CO_2 monitoring to document when specified oxygen saturation is achieved and to determine if there is any CO_2 retention. Hypoventilation resulting from the removal of the hypoxic drive is relatively common in infancy and childhood. This makes it imperative for CO_2 monitoring when supplemental oxygen therapy is commenced, especially in children with chronic conditions. Children with potentially progressive disorders require regular review to ensure that hypoventilation is detected and treated should their disease progress.

Children requiring less than 2 liters per minute (lpm) supplemental oxygen can use a nasal cannula. Higher oxygen concentrations require the use of a face mask, although, as mentioned earlier, there is increasing use of high-flow mixtures of air and oxygen up to 60 lpm delivered via nasal cannula. An oxygen concentrator is often used to deliver oxygen therapy for patients who require up to 5 lpm in the home. Children who require very small flow rates (<0.5 lpm) can use oxygen cylinders. Children with daytime oxygen requirements are also provided oxygen cylinders to permit mobility. It is helpful to use the appropriate mechanism during the sleep study (ie, wall oxygen or a concentrator, with a low-flow regulator if required), so that monitoring is undertaken at an equivalent flow as achieved in the home environment.

Titrating Oxygen During Polysomnography

Our protocols for monitoring during an overnight sleep study begin with the infant/child breathing room air to record baseline ventilation. Oxygen flow rates are then increased at timed intervals (usually 2-hour increments), although, ideally, each period of monitoring should include both nonrapid eye movement (NREM) and REM sleep. Depending on the age of the child and any observations of prior oxygen requirements, titration can follow low-flow or high-flow regimes: (1) for infants, increments of 0.25, 0.5, 0.75, and 1.0 lpm (2) for older children, 0.5, 1.0, and 2.0 lpm. However, a physician may also specify certain flow rates on the basis of individual patient needs. Ideally, 2 hours of recording should be achieved at each flow rate in order to capture a full sleep cycle and the presence of CO_2 retention, changes in oxygenation saturation between NREM and REM sleep, and/or ongoing sleep fragmentation. Where there is any question about hypoventilation, it is extremely helpful to have a period of monitoring with saturation in the high 90% range to allow exclusion of hypoventilation secondary to loss of a hypoxic ventilatory drive.

Common Problems and Solutions Experienced With Children on Oxygen Therapy

In children, the most common problems associated with oxygen therapy are noncompliance with the nasal cannula, skin breakdown associated with the use of adhesive tape, and/or drying of the nasal passages and mouth. For skin problems, we apply a "second skin" type of adhesive tape to the cheeks to minimize direct contact with the adhesive tape. With an oxygen flow rate greater than 4 lpm, patients can experience symptoms of a dry mouth and nasal airways, and to alleviate these symptoms, the oxygen can be delivered through a heated humidification device.

TRACHEOSTOMY AND INVASIVE VENTILATION

When to Consider Tracheostomy

Deciding to proceed to tracheostomy requires input from the patient, parents, and a multidisciplinary health care team. This should include the practicalities of other therapies, including whether alternative surgery can help avoid this outcome (28). Initial clinical responses to mask treatments are very favorable, but treatment failures do occur and tracheostomy remains an important clinical treatment option. Episodes of life-threatening obstruction can mean that despite the recognized morbidity and mortality related to the procedure, tracheostomy is required for safe management of the airway. Children who require greater than 16 hours' respiratory support per day on a long-term basis should be considered for insertion of tracheostomy to facilitate safer delivery of the pressure and reduce the impact (pressure area skin breakdown) of wearing a nasal/face mask for that period, as well as permitting normal developmental activities such as eating.

When to Consider Invasive Ventilation

Our usual first line of treatment is nocturnal pressure support ventilation through a mask interface. In disorders where respiratory failure is secondary to a lung (rather than a systemic) disorder, nocturnal ventilation is regularly used as a bridge to lung transplantation. Once full-time ventilation is required, then a tracheostomy is often required for the ventilatory interface. This may be from the outset, for example, traumatic quadriplegia or CCHS with full-time ventilation requirements or may evolve over time in a child with progressive lung disease. Commencing full-time ventilation through a tracheostomy inevitably requires the involvement of a multidisciplinary team. Discharging children on full-time ventilation requires recruitment and training of overnight caregivers, modifications to the home environment, and the ongoing maintenance of equipment and supplies of consumables. The availability of such resources can vary among states and countries, and establishing the capability and proficiency in coordinating such care has proven to be the ambit of centers of expertise, where experienced staff can support and train the families and their caregivers in a way that will prepare and support the children as they are discharged into the community.

Children on ventilation are reviewed, at a minimum, annually, with more frequent review during times of rapid growth, the first year of life and puberty, when scoliosis and restrictive lung disease may show rapid progress. The main goal is to ensure that the treatment is matching their requirements as they change with growth and development. Changes to ventilation often comprise only a minor part of comprehensive medical care. Monitor with blood gases as well as overnight sleep studies, again taking the approach that any adjustments made in the sleep center are for fine-tuning.

For children with progressive underlying disorders, the transition from nocturnal to full-time ventilation may need to be accompanied by evaluation for lung transplant. Although the initial progression may only be during acute lower respiratory tract infections, frank discussions regarding long-term prognoses often need to be held repeatedly. Eventually, a decision may need to be made about the introduction of tracheostomy. In some cases, prospective medical management requires that the devices be utilized in the palliative care setting, and our preference for palliative care is to use noninvasive respiratory support through a nasal interface. The benefits are that ventilatory support can permit ongoing care in the home, providing parents with a means to intervene and reduce respiratory distress as needed.

SUMMARY

The overarching goal of these therapies is to maximize children's participation in the community despite their underlying respiratory problems. Concrete outcomes include reduced hospital admissions, improved quality of life, and the encouragement of social and emotional development. Continuing advances in the technology available to assist these children have enabled us to steadily improve our capacity to achieve these goals.

REFERENCES

1. Redline S, Tishler PV, Schluchter M, et al. Risk factors for sleep-disordered breathing in children. *Am J Respir Crit Care Med*. 1999;159(5):1527-1532.
2. Goodwin JL, Kaemingk KL, Fregosi RF, et al. Clinical outcomes associated with sleep-disordered breathing in Caucasian and Hispanic children—the Tucson Children's Assessment of Sleep Apnea study (TuCASA). *Sleep*. 2003;26(5):587-591.
3. Witmans M, Young R. Update on pediatric sleep-disordered breathing. *Pediatr Clin North Am*. 2011; 58(3):571-589.
4. Amin RS, Kimball TR, Bean JA, et al. Left ventricular hypertrophy and abnormal ventricular geometry in children and adolescents with obstructive sleep apnea. *Am J Respir Crit Care Med*. 2002;165(10):1395-1399.
5. Marcus CL, Carroll JL, Koerner CB, et al. Determinants of growth in children with the obstructive sleep apnea syndrome. *J Pediatr*. 1994;125(4):556-562.
6. Blunden SL, Beebe DW. The contribution of intermittent hypoxia, sleep debt and sleep disruption to daytime performance deficits in children: consideration of respiratory and non-respiratory sleep disorders. *Sleep Med Rev*. 2006;10(2):109-118.
7. Georgalas C, Thomas K, Owens C, et al. Medical treatment for rhinosinusitis associated with adenoidal hypertrophy in children: an evaluation of clinical response and changes on magnetic resonance imaging. *Ann Otol Rhinol Laryngol*. 2005;114(8):638-644.
8. Brietzke SE, Gallagher D. The effectiveness of tonsillectomy and adenoidectomy in the treatment of pediatric obstructive sleep apnea/hypopnea syndrome: a meta-analysis. *Otolaryngol Head Neck Surg*. 2006;134(6):979-984.
9. Waters KA, Forbes P, Morielli A, et al. Sleep-disordered breathing in children with myelomeningocele. *J Pediatr*. 1998;132(4):672-681.
10. Carroll JL. Obstructive sleep-disordered breathing in children: new controversies, new directions. *Clin Chest Med*. 2003;24(2):261-282.
11. Jaryszak EM, Shah RK, Vanison CC, et al. Polysomnographic variables predictive of adverse

respiratory events after pediatric adenotonsillectomy. *Arch Otolaryngol Head Neck Surg*. 2011;137(1):15-18.
12. Tasker C, Crosby JH, Stradling JR. Evidence for persistence of upper airway narrowing during sleep, 12 years after adenotonsillectomy. *Arch Dis Child*. 2002;86(1):34-37.
13. O'Donnell AR, Bjornson CL, Bohn SG, et al. Compliance rates in children using noninvasive continuous positive airway pressure. *Sleep*. 2006;29(5): 651-658.
14. Marcus CL, Rosen G, Ward SLD, et al. Adherence to and effectiveness of positive airway pressure therapy in children with obstructive sleep apnea. *Pediatrics*. 2006;117(3):e442-e451.
15. Rains JC. Treatment of obstructive sleep apnea in pediatric patients. *Clin Pediatr*. 1995;34(10):535-541.
16. Koontz KL, Slifer KJ, Cataldo MD, et al. Improving pediatric compliance with positive airway pressure therapy: the impact of behavioral intervention. *Sleep*. 2003;26(8):1010-1015.
17. Engleman HM, Wild MR. Improving CPAP use by patients with the sleep apnoea/hypopnoea syndrome (SAHS). *Sleep Med Rev*. 2003;7(1):81-99.
18. Kushida CA, Chediak A, Berry RB, et al. Clinical guidelines for the manual titration of positive airway pressure in patients with obstructive sleep apnea. *J Clin Sleep Med*. 2008;4(2):157-171.
19. Tan E, Nixon GM, Edwards EA. Sleep studies frequently lead to changes in respiratory support in children. *J Paediatr Child Health*. 2007;43(7/8):560-563.
20. Villa MP, Pagani J, Ambrosio R, et al. Mid-face hypoplasia after long-term nasal ventilation. *Am J Respir Crit Care Med*. 2002;166(8):1142-1143.
21. Klein M, Reynolds L. Relief of sleep-related oropharyngeal airway obstruction by continuous insufflation of the pharynx. *Lancet*. 1986;327(8487):935-939.
22. McGinley B, Halbower A, Schwartz AR, et al. Effect of a high-flow open nasal cannula system on obstructive sleep apnea in children. *Pediatrics*. 2009;124(1):179-188.
23. Ward S, Chatwin M, Heather S, et al. Randomised controlled trial of non-invasive ventilation (NIV) for nocturnal hypoventilation in neuromuscular and chest wall disease patients with daytime normocapnia. *Thorax*. 2005;60(12):1019-1024.
24. Fauroux B, Lofaso F. Non-invasive mechanical ventilation: when to start for what benefit? *Thorax*. 2005;60(12):979-980.
25. Johnson KG, Johnson DC. Treatment of sleep-disordered breathing with positive airway pressure devices: technology update. *Med Devices (Auckl)*. 2015;8:425-437.
26. Ramnarayan P, Lister P, Dominguez T, et al. FIRST-line support for Assistance in Breathing in Children (FIRST-ABC): protocol for a multicentre randomised feasibility trial of non-invasive respiratory support in critically ill children. *BMJ Open*. 2017;7(6):e016181.
27. Hernández G, Roca O, Colinas L. High-flow nasal cannula support therapy: new insights and improving performance. *Crit Care*. 2017;21(1):62.
28. Cohen SR, Simms C, Burstein FD, et al. Alternatives to tracheostomy in infants and children with obstructive sleep apnea. *J Pediatr Surg*. 1999;34(1):182-186; discussion 187.

Chapter 65
Infant Polysomnography

PATRICK SORENSON

KEY CONCEPTS/LEARNING OBJECTIVES

On completion of this chapter, the reader should be able to identify the indications for infant polysomnography (PSG), describe electrode and sensor application techniques to achieve an optimal PSG in the infant patient population, disorders found in medically complex infant patients, essential documentation during a polysomnogram, how to assess for central apnea and periodic breathing, methods for working with an infant's caregiver, and performing studies in the neonatal intensive care unit.

KEY TERMS

Apnea
Central nervous system (CNS)
Chronologic age (CA)—age since birth
Corrected age—GA + CA
Gestational age (GA)—age since end of last menstrual cycle
Home cardiorespiratory monitors
Serotonin
Treatment

The polysomnographic (PSG) technologist performing studies on an infant population in no small measure provides this service not only with prior extensive experience in the field of PSG, in general, but also with expertise specifically in pediatric PSG with a knowledge base of the factors that can positively and negatively affect the scoring and interpretation of a polysomnogram on an infant. The consequences of both positive and negative production aspects can be significant in the diagnosis of the infant. This chapter seeks to provide the biologic, environmental, interpersonal, logical, and technical underpinnings necessary to provide the technologist performing PSG on an infant population with the information necessary to achieve and maintain a positive and rewarding experience not only for the technologist themselves but as a critical member of a team of infant specialists providing other medical providers and caregivers accurate and helpful information most expeditiously.

Chapter 59 (Pediatric Polysomnography) also addresses aspects of infant PSG such as age classifications that can determine how and when an infant's PSG can and should be done and interpreted, as well as general PSG knowledge. Some of these areas are addressed only tangentially within this chapter, and the reader is encouraged to seek additional information to gain a comprehensive understanding of infant PSG. Also recommended is that a new technologist seek a mentoring relationship with a provider well versed in infant PSG. Although the sleep of infants can be more challenging to study than that of an adult, working with infants can be a highly rewarding aspect of one's career.

INDICATIONS FOR INFANT POLYSOMNOGRAPHY

An understanding of why most infants undergo PSG testing is critical to the technologist's approach to the study. Infants being tested belong to the following two main categories:

1. To assess for sleep-related breathing problems because of concerns following observations by caregivers, referred to as symptoms, or medically documented evidence causing concerns for the infant's medical providers, referred to as signs. There may also be signs that central nervous system (CNS) abnormalities or immaturity may play a part in the signs and symptoms of concern. Symptoms are often confirmed by signs before the physician orders the PSG.
2. To confirm signs and/or symptoms of improvement or worsening or to assess changes, if any, following treatment referred to as efficacy of treatment. PSG evaluation to assess improvement may also simply include maturation of the infant, and worsening may include a progression of a disease process or syndrome that may or may not yet be confirmed by genetic or other types of testing.

STAFFING AND SPECIAL CONCERNS FOR INFANT POLYSOMNOGRAPHY

Technologists working with the infant population should *want* to work with this population. Many PSG technologists enjoy working with this population and seek out these younger patients. However, technologists who, for whatever reason, clearly do not desire to work with this population should not be forced to. The results of an infant sleep study are directly dependent on the technologist's role and effort. The technologist should be thoroughly dedicated to working with this potentially challenging population and should possess the knowledge necessary to produce an optimal PSG on an infant as well as the desire and ability to work diligently to produce an artifact-free recording. Just imagine trying to accurately evaluate a PSG on an infant with artifactual oxyhemoglobin saturation data and/or no airflow signal. Without the technologist's full dedication to ensuring the integrity of each channel, the recording will be considered suboptimal, and the scoring and interpretation may not be accurate.

Infants are not a population where guesswork should be employed. For an accurate diagnosis, only a PSG technologist invested in the study can consistently perform at this level of expertise. PSG technologists working with this age group must be certified in infant and pediatric cardiopulmonary resuscitation (CPR). This kind of work is not for all PSG technologists, an aspect that should be recognized by management—even as early as when the hiring process begins.

TECHNOLOGISTS' ROLE—WORKING OPTIMALLY WITH CAREGIVERS

Producing PSGs on the infant population certainly has its own challenges, and working with the infant's parent or parents can, at times, be challenging. Caregivers often bring a level of stress to the situation, which can manifest itself in difficult interactions with the technologist. However, with a few simple strategies, these stressors can be minimized or eliminated. Most, if not all, of these difficult interactions result from occurrences that have little or nothing to do with the technologist but that are related to other aspects of care of their infant. Emotions can be heightened for many reasons; some of these include complications during the birth, fear, and alarm following the witnessing of an apparent life-threatening event (ALTE) or a brief resolved unexplained event (BRUE) that may or may not have the required contacting emergency medical professionals; the loss of some control over the care of their newborn by medical staff; and the birth order of the infant where the first-born infant can elicit additional anxiety. The PSG may be seen by a caregiver as a stressful medical procedure caused by unfamiliarity with the process and the perceived or real consequences of a positive study.

Although there can be many more reasons for heightened anxiety of the caregiver, the PSG technologist can work to reduce it by clearly understanding the patient's history and what is to be ruled out with a sleep study and exhibiting sensitivity to the caregiver's state of mind. To address the caregiver's anxiety, it is important to thoroughly review with the caregivers the exact procedures that will occur during the study and the technologist's role. Explaining the procedures and function before touching the infant and checking the caregivers' complete understanding is essential. Keep the initial explanation on a basic level unless the caregivers ask for a more in-depth explanation, which the technologist can provide if requested. Remember that results are not available until the study is completely scored and evaluated by the medical staff and that the technologist cannot make any statements about whether the findings are abnormal or normal. Remind caregivers that your primary purpose is to obtain an optimal study according to the protocols set forth by the medical director of the sleep center.

Technologists should be knowledgeable regarding the clinic's policies and procedures so that they can be cited quickly and with confidence. For example, if your laboratory has a co-sleeping policy for infants, the caregivers should be informed about it during the initial instructions and not at the time of lights out. Another example is a policy about when and how to feed the infant during the study. In this regard, the technologist should retain sensitivity to the mother and infant while still being able to describe the clinical picture for the clinicians and scoring personnel.

Technologists' Role—Assuring Accurate Documentation

Staging an infant's sleep may be difficult, particularly during the infants' transitions to and from sleep, which often includes entering the sleep state in rapid eye movement (REM). This may appear as wakefulness due to respiratory rate and eye movements. The technologist must provide a clear description of what is happening with the infant and, particularly, be sure to include comments of whether the eyes are open or closed because an infant usually cannot maintain wakefulness with eyes closed; even brief eye closure indicates drowsiness. In this regard, it is helpful to perform modified patient calibrations, ideally, *before* the child falls asleep to aid in sleep-state determination later during the study.

Additional comments on the recording should indicate the technologist's clinical impressions using comments such as "looks awake," "looks asleep," "feeding," "burping infant," "bouncing infant," and *anything else* that can help identify the sleep state more clearly.

HELPFUL TIPS

While video recording an infant, focus the video camera on the closed eyelids to show eye movements under the closed or partially closed eyelids during REM sleep. This helps confirm that the infant is in REM. Be sure to zoom out and readjust the view to include the infant's entire body and head after the close-up of the face.

Try to make the caregivers a part of the study by questioning them regarding the infant's history and their approach to initiating sleep in the home for their infant. An infant-specific pre- and postsleep questionnaire can yield a great deal of information—especially at this age. The presleep questionnaire should address information such as sleep habits, medications, exposure to nicotine in utero or postnatally in the home, and the infant's age. A postsleep questionnaire assesses the caregiver's impression of the typicality of the infant's sleep and breathing in the laboratory as compared to in the home if the infant is old enough to have established recognizable patterns. The infant's respiratory pattern, both when awake and when asleep, may be the sole reason the sleep study was ordered. At times, color changes during feeding may also be the reason for the referral, and close observation during both sleep and wakefulness is important in this population. Medical personnel caring for the infant on an inpatient unit are an excellent additional source for this information because parental caregivers may not be present during an inpatient study or might not have noticed something the medical staff observed.

NORMAL SLEEP DEVELOPMENT

An infant is defined as a child from birth to 2 years of age. Age difference from birth to 2 years, although comparatively short over the lifespan, shows many differences within a matter of a few months or even weeks or days. Therefore, it is important for the technologist to report the gestational age (GA) along with chronologic age (CA) to derive the infant's corrected age. The infant's GA is the age of the child at birth expressed in weeks from the first day of the mother's last normal menstrual period to the day of birth. The CA is the amount of time since the birth. From the GA and CA, the corrected age is derived. Obtaining the corrected age of the infant assists the clinician in determining the maturity of the CNS, and this maturity is linked to the electroencephalogram (EEG) waveforms obtained during the polysomnogram.

Since EEG features, both normal and abnormal, are closely linked to the corrected age of the infant, reporting the corrected age will affect the production and interpretation of the infant polysomnogram. The age of the infant can influence many facets of the study. An infant born at less than 36 weeks GA is considered preterm, between 36 and 40 weeks CA is considered term, and at 40 weeks is considered full-term. Since infants at less than 4 months corrected age sleep (<53 weeks corrected age) demonstrate an ultradian rhythm (repeated cycles across a 24-hour period) rather than a circadian rhythm (cycles driven by environmental cues), a sleep study on an infant can be performed at any time, day or night. After 4 months corrected age, the infant begins to have more consolidated night sleep with a series of naps during the day, and environmental cues begin to have an effect.

Neonates cycle through REM and non-REM (NREM) sleep differently than an older child or adult (1). In the first few months of life, they have not yet become fully entrained on a day-night cycle, and more of the control of sleep is internal. Full-term infants can spend as much as 50% of their total sleep time in REM sleep. At this age, this is often referred to as "active sleep" (1). The infant often enters the sleep cycle in REM. By about 4 months of age, as the infant approaches the adult mode of sleep-state cyclicity, sleep-state progression matures, and NREM sleep typically precedes REM sleep. Breathing abnormalities, including obstructive sleep apnea syndrome (OSAS), may be exacerbated or only seen in REM sleep. For this reason, sleep staging is an important aspect of infant PSG evaluation to assess the sleep-state dependence of breathing abnormalities and to ensure that all stages have been documented during the study (2).

Normally, brief arousals occur as the sleeper transitions between each stage of sleep, usually without a return to full wakefulness (1). These endogenous transitional arousals are common as sleep begins to differentiate in the REM and NREM progression of the infant both quantitatively and qualitatively as the infant matures. As an individual transitions to REM through the lighter phases of NREM sleep during the night, a continuum of behaviors, including stretching, brief vocalizing, crying, or changing of position, are common. Cortical arousals during infant PSG are scored because these may also be the consequences of abnormal breathing events during sleep, but the significance of cortical arousals in infants remains uncertain because there is the suggestion that apnea in children may not always be terminated with frank cortical arousal (2).

POLYSOMNOGRAPHY PARAMETERS

The data used for the staging of infant sleep include the combined measurement of the EEG to record brain activity, the electrooculogram (EOG) to record bilateral eye movements, and the electromyogram (EMG) to record facial and intercostal muscle tone. The placement of the EEG leads should always be on the basis of the International "10–20" system of electrode placement so that the clinician can determine the maturity of the CNS as well as the exact location of any abnormalities. EEG placement for scoring sleep in infants is similar to that used in an adult population. For a sleep study, electrodes are placed at M1, M2, F3, F4, C3, C4, O1, and O2 for ease of sleep staging due to the increased amplitude obtained in referential lead derivations. The exploratory leads are referenced to the opposite mastoid. The central leads show activity at the vertex such as vertex sharp waves and sleep spindles, which develop by about 2 to 3 months post term and K-complexes that do not start to develop until about 5 to 6 months post term and are usually not fully formed until around 2 years of age. In infants, sleep spindles migrate to the vertex where they generally start more anteriorly and are often asymmetric until they are seen consistently centrally and become symmetric to both hemispheres. Activity in both hemispheres changes rapidly in the first few months of life until around 4.5 to 6 months, when the infant approaches the adult pattern of sleep-state cyclicity.

Even infants have a posterior dominant rhythm (PDR) seen mainly in the occipital channels, which in younger children starts at about 4 Hz and gradually increases as the child ages. The PDR in infants typically contains intermixed slower EEG activity (3). This frequency provides information to the clinician to help determine wakefulness versus sleep. Children with developmental delays may retain a slower PDR longer than typically developing children. Because of the special criteria used to define sleep states in infants younger than 6 months and the unique EEG features for this population, an extended EEG montage, or PSG channel derivation, is preferred. This extended montage should include bilateral EEG electrodes, utilizing the addition of bipolar channels to more accurately evaluate the EEG of the two hemispheres of the brain. EEG features specific to infants, such as tracé alternant and "delta brushes," as well as certain epileptiform activity can provide useful information regarding the maturity of the brain and alert clinicians to potential problems in brain activity.

Certain normal features of the infant EEG, such as rudimentary sleep spindles, are better seen using an extended EEG montage that includes some derivation referencing frontal to central to parietal to occipital leads in a bipolar array. The addition of T3-T5 and T4-T6 can provide more complete information regarding the maturity and function of the temporal lobes. This is referred to as a bilateral parasagittal montage with the addition of the temporal leads bilaterally and should be considered the minimum number of EEG leads. Other options would include a transverse EEG montage or the more inclusive "double banana" used more often during formal EEG evaluation. Because developing sleep spindles may not be symmetric and begin to develop more anteriorly migrating to the vertex as the infant matures, the bilateral parasagittal with the midtemporal leads derivation provides a more comprehensive monitoring of both hemispheres of the brain. Two more aspects in monitoring the EEG of infants are that the lead placement should be precise, and the head accurately measured, and that EEG lead placement should not be "estimated" or "eyeballed." In an infant, imprecise placements can and often do yield erroneous information. Additionally, no matter how young and fragile the infant appears, gentle prep of each site, using a mild abrasive, and avoiding the more abrasive preps that are commercially available, the technologist can and should obtain balanced impedances of less than 5 kΩ (3). To expect an accurate representation of the infant's EEG, without performing these two critical functions, is tantamount to doing a disservice to the patient.

The accurate scoring of sleep stages also requires the proper application of EOG sensors bilaterally to monitor REMs that normally occur during the phasic portion of REM sleep, as well as the slow eye movements that occur with the onset of sleep seen even at younger ages. The REMs of an infant appear more pronounced than those of older children or adults, and the placement of both leads at the outer canthi bilaterally rather than offsetting them is left to the discretion of the technologist. The placement of eye leads should be as close to the sclera as possible, as long as the tape used does not encroach on the sclera or the lashes of the eye. The EOG leads are referenced to the same mastoid to more easily discern true eye movements from the higher voltages produced by the CNS and picked up in the EOG leads and the mastoid, a site felt to be electrically neutral but known to produce signal voltages sufficient to have an effect on the recording channel once amplified. The impedances for these leads should be at or below 5 kΩ, and the more abrasive skin preps should certainly be avoided around this sensitive area (3).

An EMG recording of facial muscle tone assists the clinician in more accurately determining the presence of REM sleep when skeletal muscle tone, particularly the muscles of the face, is normally inhibited. For infants, chin EMG leads should be placed adjacently and close together on the anterior aspect of each cleft of the chin following sufficient prep. In this manner, the channel will accurately represent the atonia of REM sleep in this population. Since oral and nasal secretions are common in this age group, covering the chin EMG leads with a moisture-resistant tape will usually assure the integrity of the channel and is removed easily following the study.

To comprehensively assess the adequacy of respirations and ventilation and identify and differentiate between central and obstructive apnea and its severity, the recording should also include effort movements of the chest wall and abdomen, ideally, with a summation channel output, airflow at the nose and mouth, transcutaneous oxygen saturation data with a validating plethysmograph waveform from the monitor (also known as a "pleth wave" or pulse wave), and end-tidal carbon dioxide ($Etco_2$) or transcutaneous CO_2 ($Tcco_2$) monitoring measures (3).

A summation channel is simply an output representing the combination of the chest and abdominal effort channels and acts as a fourth airflow signal should airflow or $Etco_2$ sensors become dislodged during the study. A pulse waveform assists to assess the reliability of oxygenation data because oxygen saturation monitors can yield artifactual data at times usually when the infant is feeding or moving. It may be difficult to attach an oxyhemoglobin probe to infant digits, and this recording can be difficult to obtain. On small infants, the oxyhemoglobin probe may be placed on the side of the foot. If the technologist notices a poor output from the oxyhemoglobin sensor, a second probe may be added, allowing the technologist to choose the signal that is most optimal without waking the infant. Capnography, a graphic representation of $Etco_2$, is recommended for infant PSG because it can assess airflow and ventilation simultaneously. It detects the retention of CO_2 associated with sleep-related breathing abnormalities in this population (3). Calibrated CO_2 measurements can effectively detect CO_2 retention associated with apnea or prolonged hypoventilation.

CO_2 retention can also be seen following the administration of exogenous supplemental oxygen as the hypoxic drive is suppressed. In this regard, and as in the adult population, supplemental oxygen can blunt the desaturations that the ordering physician is asking to document and make the determination of respiratory impairments more difficult. The medical director in consultation with the ordering physician should determine how supplemental oxygen is to be administered for each study with the goal of treating sustained hypoxia rather than individual desaturations. The definition of sustained hypoxia is determined by the medical director of the laboratory and is dependent on the clinical presentation of the child. Usually, a sustained baseline of 88% or below for 5 or 10 minutes is indicative for the administration of supplemental O_2. At this age, small amounts of O_2 in quarter-liter increments are delivered until baseline saturations are maintained at 94% to 96%. Thus, a low-flow oxygen meter should be used to more precisely titrate exogenous O_2 in this population. Consultation with the medical director during the study will likely be necessary, particularly if the child's CO_2 values begin to climb significantly above baseline CO_2 values as documented prior to O_2 administration. Finally, if the child has a standing O_2 order at baseline, consultation with the medical director, the medical team managing the patient, and the nursing staff caring for the patient should occur *prior* to the study to avoid any miscommunication between team members. Ideally, all sleep studies, depending on the clinical presentation of the child, should begin on room air to make an accurate determination of the need and optimal level for supplemental O_2.

Standard PSG also includes additional parameters that can provide important information relevant to the patient's electrophysiologic status. An electrocardiogram (ECG) monitors cardiac rate and rhythm and is useful in evaluating the consequences of breathing disorders on the heart. An EMG recording of the intercostal muscles detects expansion of the chest wall to assess for the presence of respiratory effort to help differentiate between central versus obstructive apnea. An infant PSG could include EMG of the anterior tibialis muscles to identify periodic limb movement disorders, although these disorders are rare in infants and leg EMG channels are not routinely monitored in children younger than about 2 years unless specified by the medical director or ordering physician. Limb movements in infants are generally a startle response to exogenous or endogenous stimuli and usually unrelated to low ferritin levels or known nervous conditions seen in older populations. Further, treatment modalities used for these disorders in the adult populations may be inappropriate for infants.

To assess for the presence of gastroesophageal reflux, and its potential cardiorespiratory consequences, continuous esophageal pH measurement can be performed in conjunction with PSG to assess the temporal relationship, if any, to reflux and apneic events. A pH probe is placed either just above the gastroesophageal junction or, using the newer pH probes that detect acidity in both the liquid and the aerosol states, anywhere in the aerodigestive tract (from the esophagus to the nasopharynx) by the clinician and is normally less invasive.

Video recording with highly sensitive sound assessment is essential because it provides invaluable information on sleep behavior, snoring, respiratory effort, and sleep positions associated with a particular respiratory pattern. PSG on infants must be attended by a trained technologist who ensures the integrity of the recording, provides descriptions regarding unusual events or behaviors, and makes notations on the recording regarding physiologic changes such as snoring and color changes such as cyanosis, pallor, and erythema.

The foregoing sensors suggest that infant PSG performed outside of a center or on an in-home basis is contraindicated and that polysomnographic studies on infants should always be attended by a technologist.

ASSOCIATED CONDITIONS FOR POLYSOMNOGRAPHY IN INFANT POPULATIONS

Sudden Infant Death Syndrome

Sudden infant death syndrome (SIDS), previously referred to as "crib death," is a major disorder associated with sleep during the first year of life. It is the leading cause of death in infants between 1 week and 1 year of age. In the United States, mortality rates have steadily declined from more than 5,000 infant deaths per year in the early 1990s to just over 2,500 deaths per year by 1999. This decline is largely attributed to avoidance of placing infants prone or on their sides to sleep. By the year 2000, the incidence of SIDS around the world varied from about 0.1 to 1 case per 1,000 live births (4). According to the Centers for Disease Control and Prevention, the incidence of SIDS (see Figure 65-1) in the United States as of 2016 was 38.0 deaths per 100,000 live births, which is greatly reduced from a rate of 130.3 per 100,000 live births in 1990. SIDS is best defined as the sudden and unexpected death of an infant for which sufficient cause cannot be found by a death scene investigation, review of the history, and a postmortem examination. As this definition implies, it is a diagnosis of exclusion; there are no findings on autopsy that are entirely specific for SIDS. Because of the breadth of the definition and the lack of specific postmortem lesions, it is probable that SIDS has multiple causes (4).

Closely linked to any discussion of SIDS is that of ALTEs. An ALTE is defined by the American Thoracic Society (ATS) as "an episode of apnea, color change (pallor, cyanosis or erythema), and hypotonia that the observer believes to be life-threatening to the infant and for which some intervention (stimulation, shaking, and/or cardiorespiratory resuscitation) is felt to be required" (5). Recently, the American Academy of Pediatrics recommended the replacement of the term ALTE with BRUE. Although the relationship between ALTE and SIDS is poorly understood, many believe that ALTE may indicate a risk of cardiorespiratory instability, which could lead to death.

SIDS almost always takes place when the infant is presumed to have been asleep, either during the day or during the night. However, more than 70% of its victims are found in the early morning hours after nighttime sleep (4). SIDS is widely considered to have a developmental component because infants in the first month of life are generally spared. The incidence then peaks in infants from 2 to 4 months of life, which coincides with significant changes known to occur in sleep

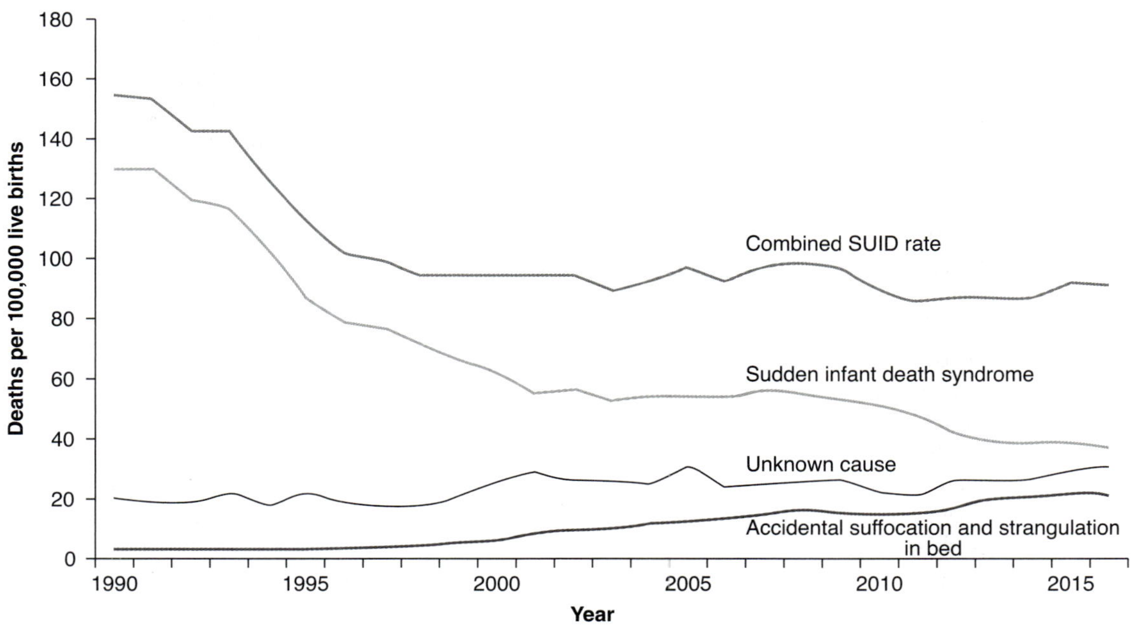

Figure 65-1 This graph shows the trends in sudden unexpected infant death (SUID) rates in the United States from 1990 through 2016. Sudden infant death syndrome rates declined considerably from 130.3 deaths per 100,000 live births in 1990 to 38.0 deaths per 100,000 live births in 2016. (Source: Centers for Disease Control and Prevention, US Department of Health and Human Services, National Vital Statistics System, Compressed Mortality File. Retrieved from https://www.cdc.gov/sids/data.htm)

BOX 65-1: Risk Factors for Sudden Infant Death Syndrome

Male sex
African-American race
Teenaged mother
Exposure to opioids and cocaine in utero
Anemia during pregnancy
Late or no prenatal care
Bottle-feeding
Prematurity
Low birth weight
Prone position
Winter season

organization and in the modulation of brainstem centers involved in respiratory and arousal state control by the forebrain (6). Crib death is uncommon after infants are 6 months old, with 90% of SIDS victims affected in the first 6 months of life. It is rare after the first birthday. This particular pattern of incidence is unique to SIDS.

There are many risk factors for SIDS, most of which cannot be easily eliminated. However, there are several risk factors that lend themselves to intervention. They are (1) prone positioning, (2) maternal smoking, and (3) bottle-feeding (see Box 65-1).

Historically, numerous international epidemiologic studies pointed to an increased risk of SIDS when infants are put to sleep in the prone position (7-9). A US study confirmed this relationship, although the relative risk of prone versus supine posture in this study was lower than it had been in the foreign studies. Many mechanisms have been proposed to explain the relationship to sleep position, but most have not been tested or have not withstood critical examination. One hypothesis is that a subgroup of prone-positioned infants actually "burrow" their faces into their bedding rather than keep their heads turned to one side. These infants are theorized to die because of suffocation or rebreathing of CO_2 (10). An analysis of one supine-sleeping campaign in Norway published in 1998 showed that the SIDS rate dropped from 3.5 deaths per 1,000 live births to 0.3 deaths per 1,000 live births 4 years after an intervention program designed to avoid prone sleeping (7). Similar public education campaigns to inform parents about the risk factors associated with SIDS in the United States have yielded a clear decline in the incidence of SIDS. Other risk factors besides prone and side infant sleeping positions include exposure of infants to cigarette smoke (11), potentially hazardous crib-related sleeping environments, infant feeding, and perhaps the absence of a pacifier (9).

Maternal cigarette smoking during pregnancy is associated with increased risk in a dose-dependent manner: the more cigarettes smoked, the greater the risk (11). This dose dependency suggests a relationship between a factor that may be causing SIDS and prenatal maternal cigarette smoking. In addition, there is evidence that postnatal exposure to cigarette smoke (passive smoking) further increases the risk. Some studies have found breastfeeding to be partly protective against SIDS, but other studies have found no effect. Any beneficial effect may be related to the fact that breastfed babies have fewer infections than do bottle-fed babies because infections may increase the risk of SIDS.

Normal Control of Breathing and Heart Rate

Much of the control of breathing resides in the most primitive part of the brain, the brainstem. It is there that the central rhythm generator (CRG) is postulated to exist, and information flows from the peripheral chemoreceptors and the mechanoreceptors to the brainstem, modulating the output from the CRG. The presence of an "off switch" mechanism is also postulated because phrenic nerve output to the diaphragm is absent during expiration. The off switch terminates inspiration by inhibition of the CRG. Input from higher centers of the brain, such as the cortex, is also integrated within the brainstem. Hence, the ability to voluntarily control breathing also exists.

Control of the heart rate occurs primarily through the autonomic nervous system, which is divided into sympathetic and parasympathetic branches. Sympathetic stimulation of the heart increases the heart rate, whereas parasympathetic stimulation acts to decrease the heart rate. The vagus nerve is the parasympathetic conduit from nuclei (ambiguous nuclei and tractus solitarius) in the brainstem to the heart. "Vagal" stimuli, such as coughing, choking, or expiring against a closed glottis (the Valsalva maneuver), can induce bradycardia. The bradycardia that follows obstructive apnea may also be vagally mediated.

Sudden Infant Death Syndrome and Control of Breathing

The importance of the brainstem in the control of breathing and, possibly, SIDS is further supported by the fact that apnea in premature infants is associated with immaturity of the brainstem. Premature infants with apnea have prolonged brainstem conduction times for auditory-evoked responses compared with premature infants without apnea. Also, some SIDS victims have gliosis (representing scarring) of cellular bodies in the medulla oblongata, specifically in the area of the arcuate nucleus that controls respiratory and cardiac function (11,12). Finally, newer research on the etiology of SIDS indicates that the syndrome likely comprises heterogeneous disorders that lead to death that is not explained following a thorough postmortem investigation and review of the child's history. It has been reported by Kinney et al (12) that approximately 40% of SIDS deaths were associated with serotonergic abnormalities in brainstem regions with homeostatic regulation where there were elevated serotonin (5-hydroxytryptamine) levels. This finding suggests that SIDS may be associated with peripheral abnormalities in the pathway for transportation of serotonin. Serotonin is one of the most important neurotransmitters in the regulation of the sleep-wake cycle, and its expression is related to the maintenance of wakefulness. The deficit in serotonin suggests that abnormalities in this pathway prevent the sleeper from awakening under certain conditions and is a compelling explanation for the infant's inability to arouse from sleep despite conditions such as elevated CO_2 levels requiring the infant to arouse to resolve the adverse condition (12).

Although the specific neuronal dysfunction that leads to both central apnea and periodic breathing has yet to be determined, it appears as though factors in the maturation of central chemoreceptors and mechanoreceptors play a pivotal role in the alterations of respiratory drive in preterm infants. Some preterm infants exhibit an unexpected and paradoxical decrease in ventilatory response to increases in CO_2 values. Also, preterm infants often respond to a fall in inspired oxygen concentrations with a transient increase in ventilation, followed by a return to baseline or even a depression of ventilation. The diminution of respiratory drive during hypercarbia and the biphasic response to hypoxia can potentially predispose a vulnerable child to apnea and its sequelae (13).

As intriguing as these hypotheses may be, the precise cause of SIDS is still unknown. SIDS may have several causes, but all are likely to be related to a developmental immaturity or malfunction of the brain, leading to either cardiac or respiratory death.

There is no test that accurately predicts the risk of SIDS, perhaps because it has multiple causes and because most tests are performed weeks or months before death, during a period of life in which the infant is undergoing rapid change. Some laboratories may assess an infant with a pneumocardiogram consisting of a two- to four-channel recording usually consisting of transthoracic impedance (chest movements) and heart rate, as well as oxygen saturation data and an airflow channel in the more sophisticated models. The pneumocardiogram is usually performed overnight in a controlled but unattended setting. Its value is markedly diminished because it provides limited ability to differentiate between central and obstructive apnea and does not provide thorough information regarding the severity and physiologic consequences of the breathing disturbance. It is widely accepted that the pneumocardiogram is not effective at screening for the risk of SIDS (14). In this regard, home sleep apnea testing (HSAT) fares no better, despite the addition of effort and electrocardiograph channels.

PSG performed according to the standards accepted by the ATS (5) and the AASM (3) provides the clinician with a more thorough evaluation of pediatric sleep and breathing disorders than a pneumocardiogram or HSAT. PSG for cardiopulmonary indications includes simultaneous recording of physiologic variables, including sleep state, respiration, cardiac rhythm, muscle activity, gas exchange, and snoring data. The technologist, in attendance during PSG, is trained to evaluate and document behavioral and physiologic changes as well as quality of sleep. Thus, a more accurate diagnosis of obstructive sleep apnea (OSA) is possible with PSG, in contrast to the lack of this capability in the limited-channel sleep apnea studies.

Although PSG is not always indicated after an uncomplicated ALTE or BRUE, it may be helpful to define the frequency of the type of apnea and the extent of cardiac, blood gas, and sleep alterations in certain infants with apnea or an ALTE. PSG is especially useful for the detection of occult hypoxemia by the child's caregivers in a controlled environment. Test results may also suggest the further direction of the workup; for example, if abnormal amounts of obstructive apnea are noted, consultation with an otolaryngologist may be indicated. In addition, data acquired from these studies are often helpful in the later interpretation of waveforms from home monitors. However, the major concern after an ALTE episode is the related risk of recurrent events or death.

THE PEDIATRIC SLEEP FACILITY

Laboratory Supervision

A pediatrician with training and experience in pediatric respiratory disorders and/or sleep medicine should be responsible for the supervision of a sleep laboratory whose primary activity is performing PSG in infants and children with cardiorespiratory disorders. If this is not possible, because of limited medical staff resources, it is recommended that a pediatrician with expertise in pediatric pulmonology, neonatology, neurology, or pediatric sleep medicine oversee laboratory operations in studying children in sleep centers. A pediatric specialist can ensure that the PSG is performed, scored, and interpreted appropriately for the age and condition of the child.

Setting

Infants should be studied in a dedicated pediatric facility with a laboratory decor that is both age-appropriate and nonthreatening. If a separate pediatric laboratory is not available, an area of the laboratory should be dedicated for infants. Accommodations for a parent to sleep near the infant are recommended because immediate parental access to the infant is often necessary to reduce fear and anxiety and provide ordinary child care while the study is in progress. Safe and comfortable bedding is necessary when performing PSG on infants and children, and the technologist should be aware that they may be modeling appropriate or inappropriate sleeping practices. Mattresses should be made of material that is easy to clean and disinfect if soiled.

Personnel

A pediatric sleep laboratory should be staffed with personnel trained to deal with infants and their caregivers. Because PSG evaluation can be seen as stressful, particularly in this age group, laboratory personnel should have knowledge of infant behavior and developmental stages to effectively deal with children and provide medical information in a nonthreatening manner. Because of the differences in the sleep characteristics of children when compared with adolescents and adults, only qualified individuals who know the unique characteristics of sleep breathing in children of different ages should evaluate the PSG (3).

INFANT BREATHING DISORDERS

Apnea

Apnea is best defined as the absence of airflow at the nostrils and mouth. The three main categories of apnea are central, obstructive, and mixed. Central apnea occurs when respiratory effort ceases; there is no chest movement and hence no airflow. Diagnosis of central apnea must take into account a multitude of factors. It is ordinarily significant when it exceeds 20 seconds in duration. Because infants normally have a more rapid baseline respiratory rate and a reduced respiratory reserve, and, therefore, less protection from hypoxia, shorter central events can be more clinically significant in this age group. Central apnea can yield significant physiologic compromise such as bradycardia or color change associated with declining oxyhemoglobin levels.

For infants, central sleep apnea must be distinguished from other causes of respiratory pauses, including the more common periodic breathing pattern and the obligatory respiratory pauses that often follow a deep yawn or sigh. Although a rare cause of central apnea, seizures will also change the respiratory pattern seen on a recording. In the more severe cases, central apneas can be treated with medication. The presence of frequent central sleep apnea is a usual cause for respiratory monitoring during sleep. Premature infants are at increased risk for central apneas. Central apnea accounts for 10% to 25% of all apneas in premature infants (15).

Obstructive Sleep Apnea Syndrome

In children, OSAS is a disorder of breathing during sleep that is characterized by prolonged partial upper airway obstruction (hypopnea) and/or intermittent complete obstruction (apnea) that disrupts normal ventilation during sleep and normal sleep patterns. Clinically, obstructive apnea is the lack or diminution of airflow, despite the continuation of respiratory efforts. The obstruction can be functional or anatomic. When obstruction is present, respiratory efforts continue, and tugging or retraction of the chest wall can be seen. OSAS accounts for only 10% to 20% of all apneas in preterm infants (2). It has been estimated that 7% to 9% of children snore regularly, with an estimated prevalence of OSAS of 0.7% in 4- to 5-year-old children. Most affected children breathe normally while awake. However, a minority with marked upper airway obstruction also have noisy, mildly labored breathing while awake.

Obstruction lasting the length of two missed breaths or longer is regarded as significant in infants. In some infants with clinically significant OSAS, little or no snoring may be heard by the caregiver, unlike the clinical manifestations of OSAS in older children and adults (3). To accurately diagnose OSAS in an infant, clinical descriptions of the infant's noises by the technologist doing the study are critical because of the consistent presence of paradoxical breathing in the infant related to the way the infant breathes. Infant breathing is primarily costal in nature, and the chest wall at this age is pliable, yielding paradoxical efforts seen mainly in REM sleep. The clinician needs to rely on the airflow channels, the intercostal EMG channels, and the technologist's descriptions to accurately classify sleep-related breathing abnormalities as obstructive.

Obstructions can be caused by the presence of an anatomic abnormality, neurologic condition, or medical condition. Reduction of the airway size leads to increased respiratory effort, which can create negative airway pressure and, paradoxically, worsen the obstruction. The most common anatomic factors leading to OSAS include large tonsils or adenoids, obesity, micrognathia (small jaw), or other anatomic anomalies. Muscular hypotonia is one of the most common neurologic factors contributing to OSAS in infancy. Normal muscle tone inhibition during REM sleep can change respiratory patterns, with more breath-to-breath variability increasing the risk of full or partial airway obstruction. Hypotonia can be commonly seen in Down syndrome, muscular dystrophy, and other genetic disorders. Allergies or even mild upper respiratory tract infections can serve to swell mucous membranes and thereby contribute to obstruction. Some of the less common risk factors include laryngomalacia, pharyngeal flap surgery, sickle cell disease, structural malformations of the brainstem, and certain metabolic and genetic disorders.

Apneas and hypopneas lead to a drop in oxygen saturations and an increase in blood CO and will often cause a full or partial arousal pattern in sleep EEG recordings. When these events occur multiple times at night, there are several anticipated effects. The presence of frequent arousals leads to fragmented and inefficient sleep as yet not clearly defined for infants. This can lead to increased daytime sleepiness.

Adenoid and tonsillar removal is contraindicated for most cases of infant OSA. Other ways to relieve the obstructed breathing could include a tongue-lip adhesion, continuous positive airway pressure using a large cannula that does not create a seal but stimulates breathing, or perhaps tracheostomy may be necessary.

Mixed sleep apnea is the combination of central and obstructive apnea, with the central component usually followed by obstruction. Because of this, therapies that are effective for central apnea are also effective in treating mixed apnea. For example, during infancy, medications can be used to treat both forms of apnea.

Periodic Breathing

In the normal neonate, particularly the premature infant, breathing can be irregular. Periodic breathing is defined as episodic pauses in respiratory movements, each lasting 4 to 10 seconds alternating with several appropriate breaths. Periodic breathing is most easily seen by reviewing the breathing pattern in compressed view. Figure 65-2A-E provides examples of periodic breathing at increasingly compressed views. Apnea is considered a more serious condition because the respiratory pause is long lasting and frequently associated with more significant decreases in heart rate below 80 bpm and declining oxyhemoglobin values. Although periodic breathing is usually considered benign, for very small infants, even short apneic pauses can cause significant bradycardia and oxygen desaturations.

Periodic breathing can occur during wakefulness, active sleep (REM), and quiet sleep (NREM), but its prevalence is increased in active sleep. In quiet sleep, periodic breathing becomes regular, that is, breathing and apneic intervals are of similar duration. In active sleep, the frequency of respirations and, subsequently, periodic breathing becomes irregular. The most well-defined periodic breathing observable in small infants

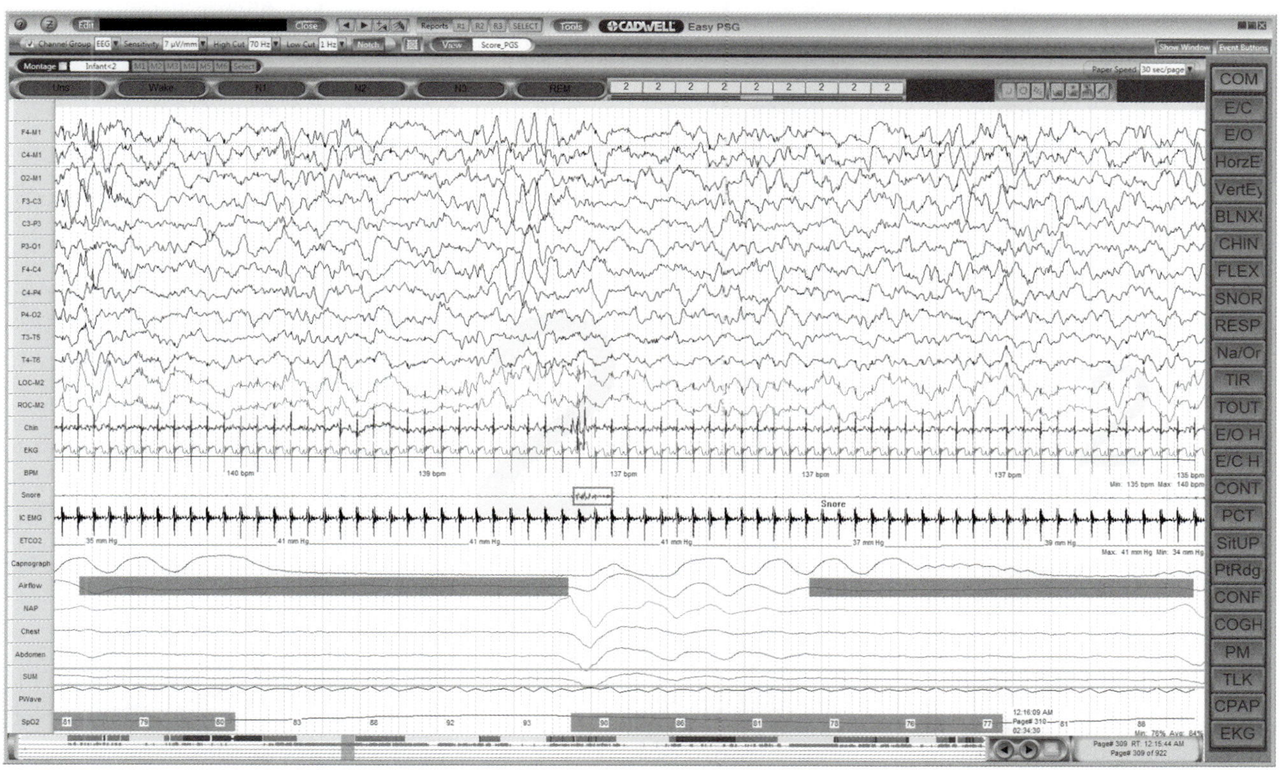

Figure 65-2 The following are examples of periodic breathing in an infant at increasing epoch time spans. Note the difficulty in making this determination using a shorter window. A: 30-second epoch.

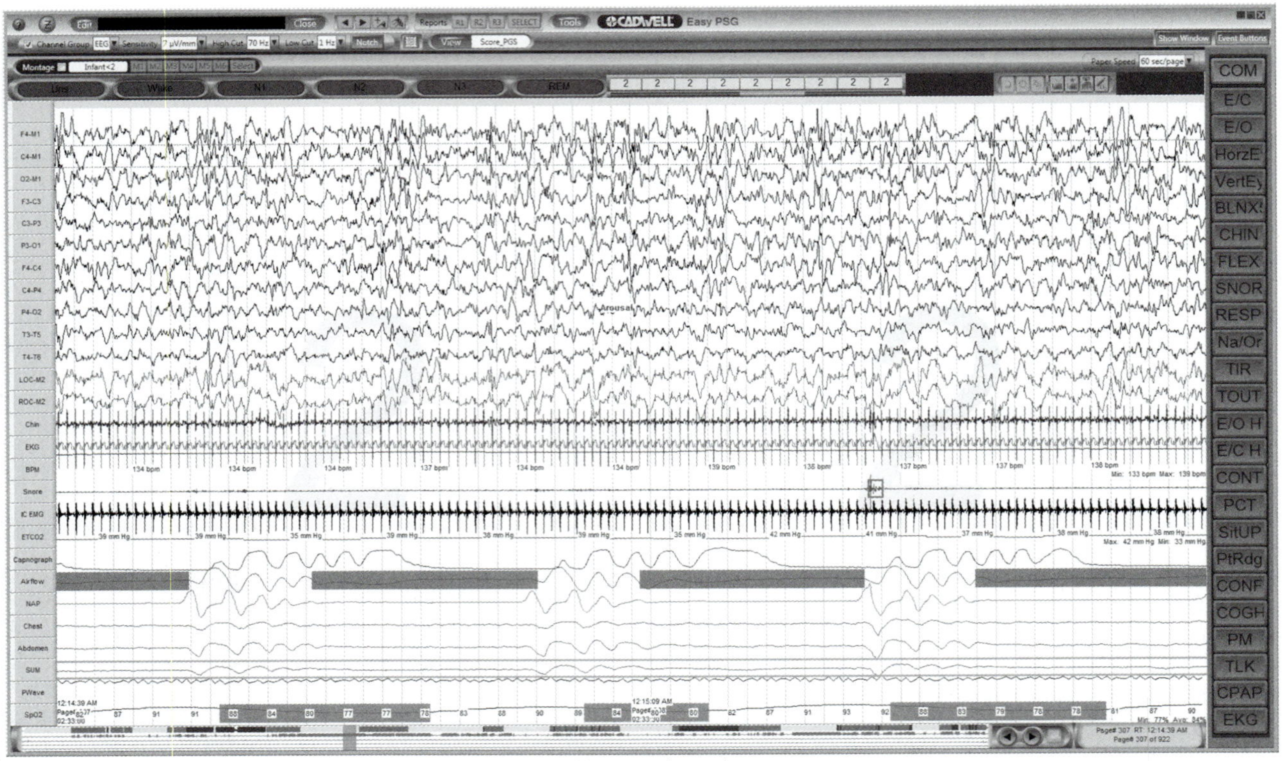

B

60-second epoch

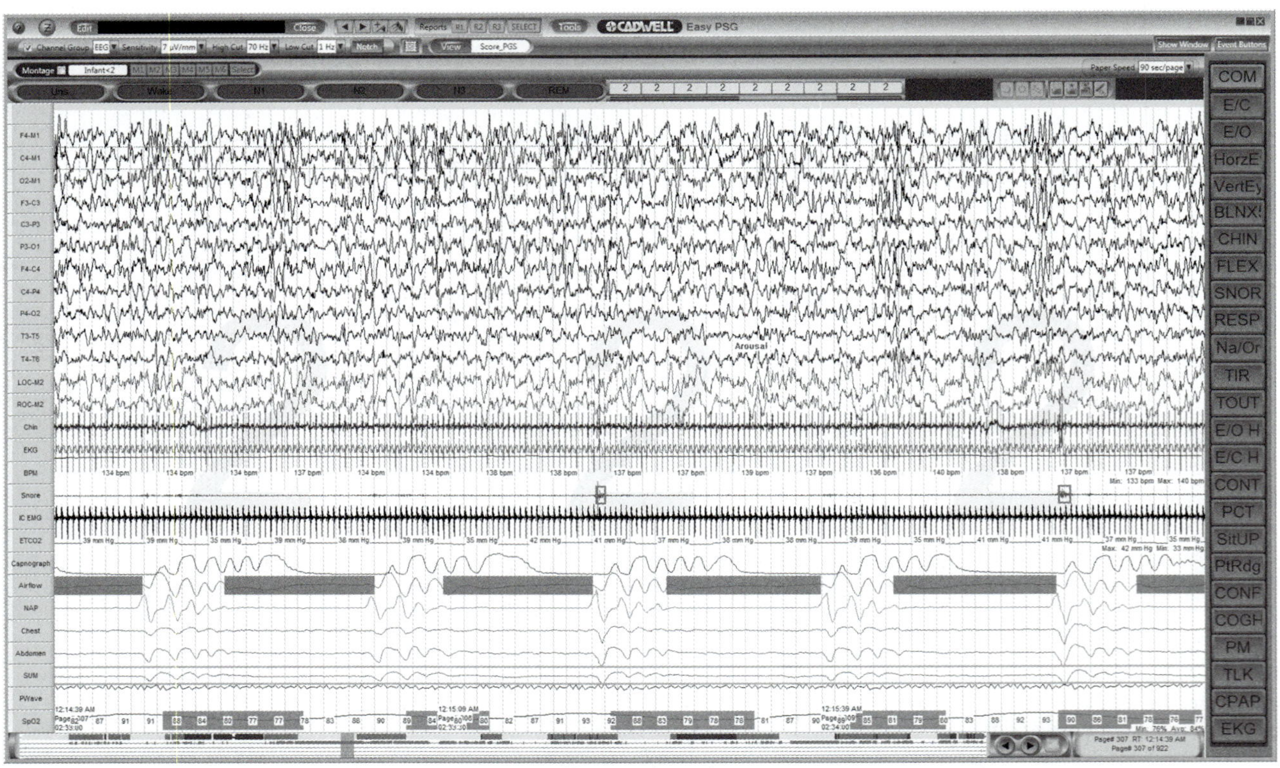

C

90-second epoch

Figure 65-2 (*continued*) B: 60-second epoch. C: 90-second epoch.

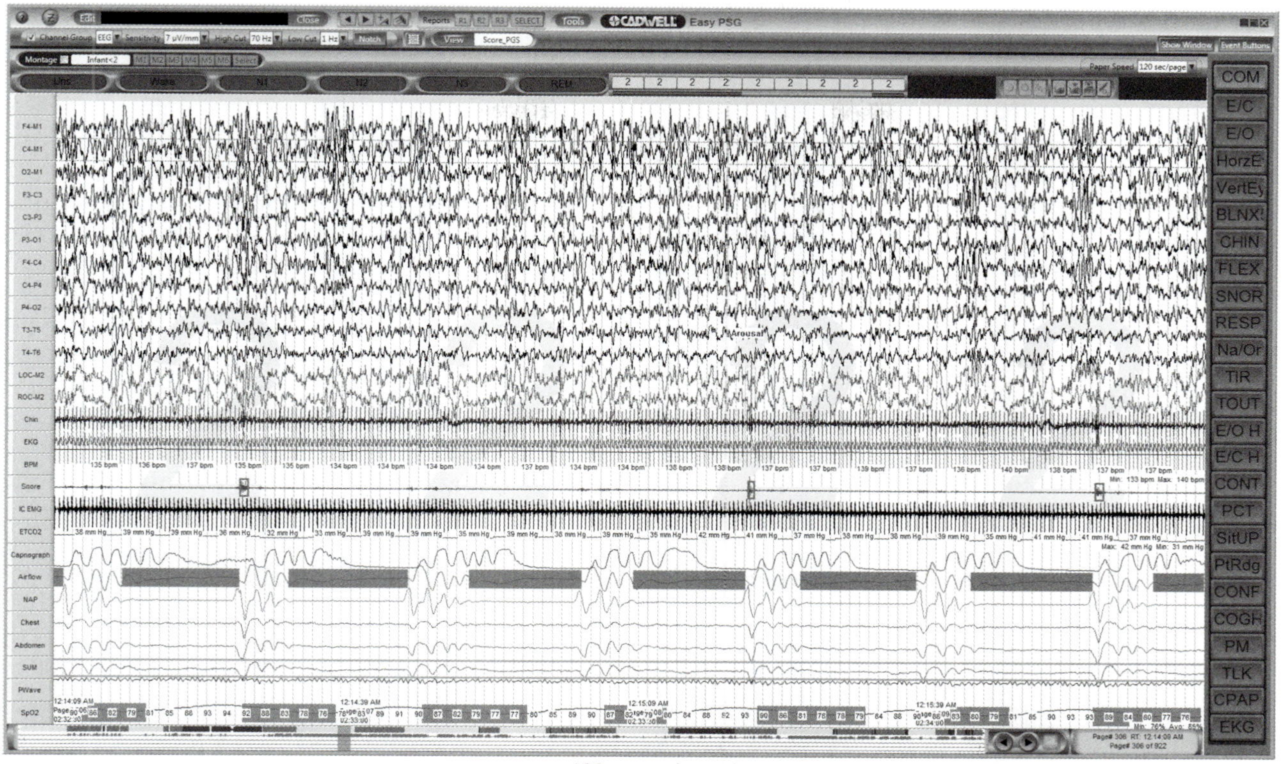

D

120-second epoch

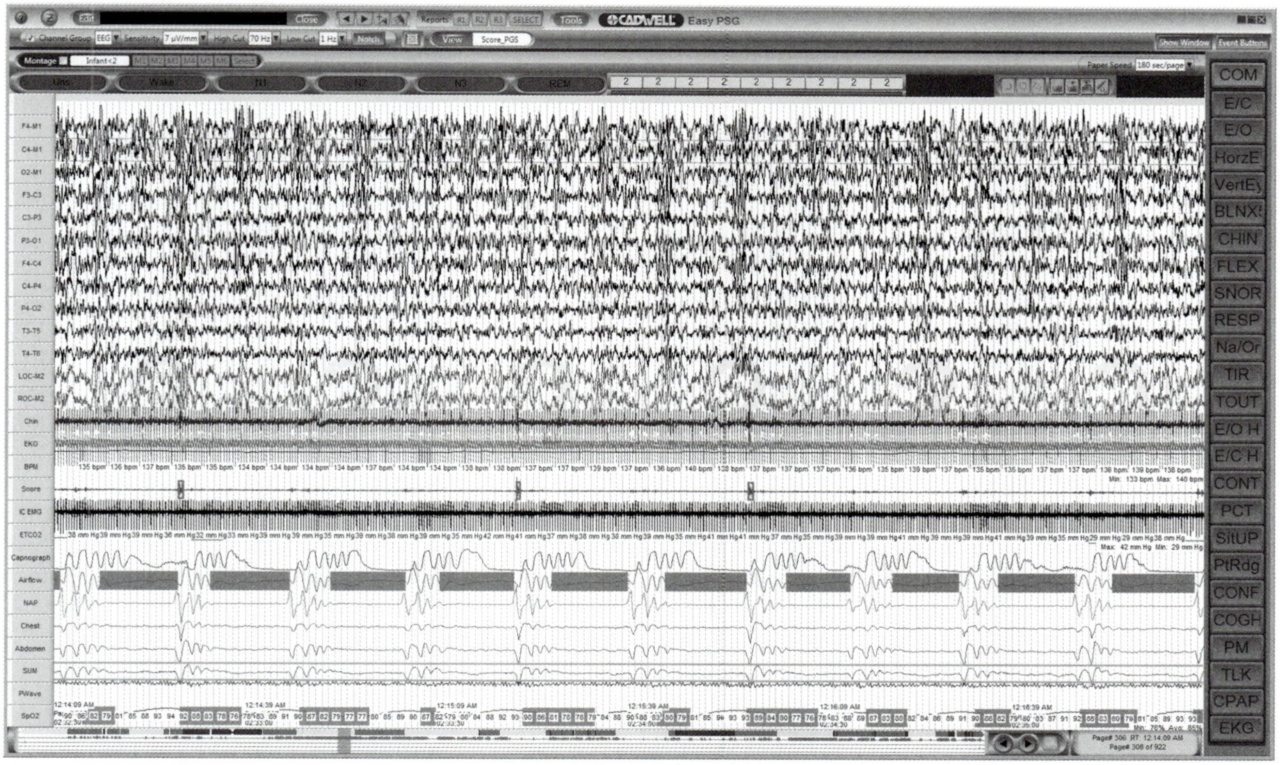

E

180-second epoch

Figure 65-2 *(continued)* D: 120-second epoch. E: 180-second epoch.

is in quiet sleep during the EEG pattern known as tracé alternant, commonly seen in infants younger than 44 weeks' conceptional age (16). Tracé alternant is an episodic EEG pattern in which complex bursts of moderate- to high-amplitude slow waves are superimposed on a continuous background of polymorphic theta and faster rhythms (16).

All types of apneas are seen in the neonatal intensive care unit (NICU) and at home during the first year of life, although obstructive apnea is less common in infants. The causes of apnea in the NICU are numerous. The most important include apnea of prematurity (idiopathic), gastroesophageal reflux, hypoxia, anemia, and intraventricular hemorrhage. Sedative drugs passed to the infant during labor and delivery, or later through breast milk, can also lead to apnea.

Apnea during infancy at home can be a component of an ALTE. These episodes were often referred to as "near miss" SIDS in the past. Those that require vigorous stimulation or CPR are severe ALTEs and demand special attention because there is an increased risk of subsequent death. Episodes that occur while the infant is awake are more likely to be associated with gastroesophageal reflux, seizures, incoordination of swallowing and breathing during feedings, and crying with breath holding (17). In contrast to the neonate in the NICU and the infant at home, the older child is predominately affected by OSAS.

HOME CARDIORESPIRATORY MONITORS

Because apnea and/or respiratory instability has been the most prominent hypothesis for several decades, cardiorespiratory monitors (also called apnea monitors) are frequently prescribed for high-risk infants. Recordings of a small number of SIDS deaths, however, show that bradycardia is present for several minutes before the advent of central apnea (18). The cause of this bradycardia then becomes the crucial issue. It may be secondary to hypoxemia after apnea.

One of the consequences of our uncertainty about the cause or causes of SIDS is that a rational approach to prevention is difficult. Cardiorespiratory monitors should theoretically be useful in the prevention of either cardiac or respiratory death, but the efficacy of these devices has not been scientifically proved or disproved, and monitored infants have died despite quick parental response to the alarm (14). Conversely, there are hundreds of anecdotal reports that infants have been saved after a caregiver is alerted by a monitor alarm.

Cardiorespiratory monitors for use at home provide two immediate purposes: (1) to alert the caregiver to a cardiorespiratory abnormality and (2) to serve as diagnostic devices (19). Ultimately, they are intended to prevent death. The standard monitor in the United States is an impedance-type monitor that detects chest movements and ECG tracings through electrodes placed on the chest. The monitors contain alarms for conditions such as apnea, tachypnea, bradycardia, tachycardia, and, sometimes, oxygen desaturation. The settings at which each alarm may ring are typically adjustable. Because the monitors detect chest wall movement, they are not very sensitive for obstructive apneas, since chest wall movements may continue through the apnea (20).

Many monitors can record data in memory for later downloading and analysis. In this manner, the conditions leading up to an alarm can be evaluated for clinical significance and "false alarms" eliminated. Often, alarms will be programmed to save data recorded just before, during, and after an alarm. However, the alarm memory will also indicate the total recording time, which is a useful gauge of parental compliance with monitoring. Ensuring compliance may be important because some studies suggest that the majority of infant deaths with prescribed monitors occur during periods of noncompliance or inappropriate use (21,22). Hence, encouraging parents to use the monitor is vital.

False alarms are often apnea alarms for which the monitor fails to detect the breathing movements that are actually present or shallow. Inspection of the recorded waveforms may show a complete lack of breathing movements but without any associated change in the heart rate or oxygen saturation. The presence of the ECG allows confirmation of bradycardia and recognition of some arrhythmias. This is how the monitor functions as a diagnostic device.

Several studies have shown that false apnea alarms and loose lead alarms can be frequent and can substantially outnumber true alarms (20,21). False alarms can be reduced by attention to electrode placement so that the electrodes "see" maximal chest or abdominal wall movements. This often means that parents must be properly trained in lead placement. However, there will always be some false alarms. Some PSG studies may be ordered to help differentiate alarms in the home from false alarms by running the home monitor concurrently with the PSG. If an alarm sounds, the parent is asked if the occurrence was typical as in the home. Appropriate attention to the monitor settings can help eliminate false alarms set off by patient crying or movement.

Discharge and Parents' and Caregivers' Training

It is essential that parents and other caretakers be fully trained in how to respond to an alarm. This includes being able to distinguish a false alarm from a true event and to be prepared to administer CPR if necessary. CPR is a complex skill that we expect parents to be able to perform effectively at a time when they are worried or panicked. In fact, there is evidence that parents forget CPR training within a matter of weeks (23). Affording the parents the opportunity to have repeated CPR training sessions may be lifesaving because many repeat ALTEs occur within weeks after discharge from the hospital on a home monitor.

Monitors are traditionally intended only for infants in various high-risk groups, which include those with severe ALTEs and preterm infants who continue to have apneas and bradycardias as discharge from the NICU approaches. As monitoring is begun, it is often helpful to have clear clinical criteria for the discontinuation of monitoring at a later date. Monitoring is often perceived by families as an important safety net, and it can often be difficult to stop monitoring even when the clinical indications for monitoring are no longer present. Because parents are understandably often incorrect in their assessment of alarms, it follows that discontinuation is much easier and surer when the infant is on a memory-equipped monitor.

The time of hospital discharge is an emotionally taxing time for parents. The anxiety produced by having a child on a monitor at home is magnified by the likelihood that parents' sleep will be more disrupted to attend to false alarms during the night. A support system comprising personnel from the monitor supply company and medical professionals responsible for the infant's care can lessen this burden (21). The most important criterion for the discontinuation of a home apnea monitor is the absence of any significant events for two consecutive months. A significant real event is a real alarm for which the infant, in the judgment of the clinician, required stimulation.

REFERENCES

1. Anders T, Keener M. Developmental course of nighttime sleep-wake patterns in full-term and premature infants during the first year of life. *Sleep.* 1985;8:173-192.
2. Kelmanson IA. *Sleep and Breathing in Infants and Young Children (Chaps. XIV–XVII)*. Nova Biomedical Books; 2006.
3. Troester MM, Quan SF, Berry RB, et al; for the American Academy of Sleep Medicine. *The AASM Manual for the Scoring of Sleep and Associated Events: Rules, Terminology and Technical Specifications. Version 3.* American Academy of Sleep Medicine; 2023.
4. Glotzbach S, Ariagno R, Harper R. Sleep and the sudden infant death syndrome. In: Ferber R, Kryger M, eds. *Principles and Practice of Sleep Medicine in the Child.* W. B. Saunders; 1995:231.
5. American Thoracic Society. Standards and indications for cardiopulmonary sleep studies in children. *Am J Respir Crit Care Med.* 1996;153:866-878.
6. Tildon JT, Meny RG, O'Brien J. Sudden infant death syndrome. In: Dulbecco R, ed. *Encyclopedia of Human Biology*. Academic Press; 1991:315-322.
7. Skadberg BT, Morild I, Markstad T. Abandoning prone sleeping: effect on the risk of sudden infant death syndrome. *J Pediatr.* 1998;132(2):340-343.
8. Mitchell EA, Thach BT, Thompson JMD, et al; for the New Zealand Cot Death Study. Changing infant's sleep position increases risk of sudden infant death syndrome. *Arch Pediatr Adolesc Med.* 1999;153:1136-1141.
9. Oyen N, Markestad T, Skaerven R, et al. Combined effects of sleeping position and prenatal risk factors in sudden infant death syndrome: the Nordic epidemiological SIDS study. *Pediatrics.* 1997;100:613-621.
10. Kemp JS, Kowalski RM, Graham MA, et al. Positional ventilatory impairment in a serial study of 23 SIDS cases. *Pediatr Res.* 1992;31:360A.
11. Haglund B, Cnattingius S. Cigarette smoking as a risk factor for sudden infant death syndrome: a population-based study. *Am J Public Health.* 1990;80:29-32.
12. Kinney HC, Burger PC, Harrell FE Jr, et al. Reactive gliosis in the medulla oblongata of victims of the sudden infant death syndrome. *Pediatrics.* 1983;72:181-187.
13. Rigatto H. Control of breathing during sleep in the fetus and neonate. In: Ferber R, Kryger M, eds. *Principles and Practice of Sleep Medicine in the Child.* W. B. Saunders; 1995:35.
14. Meny RG, Blackmon L, Fleischmann D, et al. Sudden infant death and home monitors. *Am J Dis Child.* 1988;142:1037-1040.
15. Miller MJ, Martin RJ. Pathophysiology of apnea of prematurity. In: Polin RA, Fox WW, eds. *Fetal and Neonatal Physiology*. W.B. Saunders; 1998:1129-1143.
16. Pedley TA, Lombroso C, Hanley R. Introduction to neonatal electroencephalography: interpretation. *Am J EEG Technol.* 1981;21:15-29.
17. Spitzer AR, Boyle JT, Tuchman DN, et al. Awake apnea associated with gastroesophageal reflux: a specific clinical syndrome. *J Pediatr.* 1984;104:200-205.
18. Kelly DH, Pathak A, Meny R. Sudden severe bradycardia in infancy. *Pediatr Pulmonol.* 1991;10:199-204.
19. Weese-Mayer DE, Brouillette RT, Morrow AS, et al. Assessing validity of infant monitor alarms with event recording. *J Pediatr.* 1989;115:701-708.
20. Nathanson I, O'Donnell J, Commins MF. Cardiorespiratory patterns during alarms in infants using apnea/bradycardia monitors. *Am J Dis Child.* 1989;143:476-480.
21. Ahmann E, Wulff L, Meny RG. Home apnea monitoring and disruptions in family life: a multidimensional controlled study. *Am J Public Health.* 1992;82:719-722.
22. Carroll JL, Siska ES. SIDS: counseling parents to reduce the risk. *Am Fam Physician.* 1998;57:1566-1572.
23. Dracup K, Doering LV, Moser DK, Evangelista L. Retention and use of cardiopulmonary resuscitation skills in parents of infants at risk for cardiopulmonary arrest. *Pediatr Nurs.* 1998;24(3):219-225.

SECTION VIII

Sleep Center Management

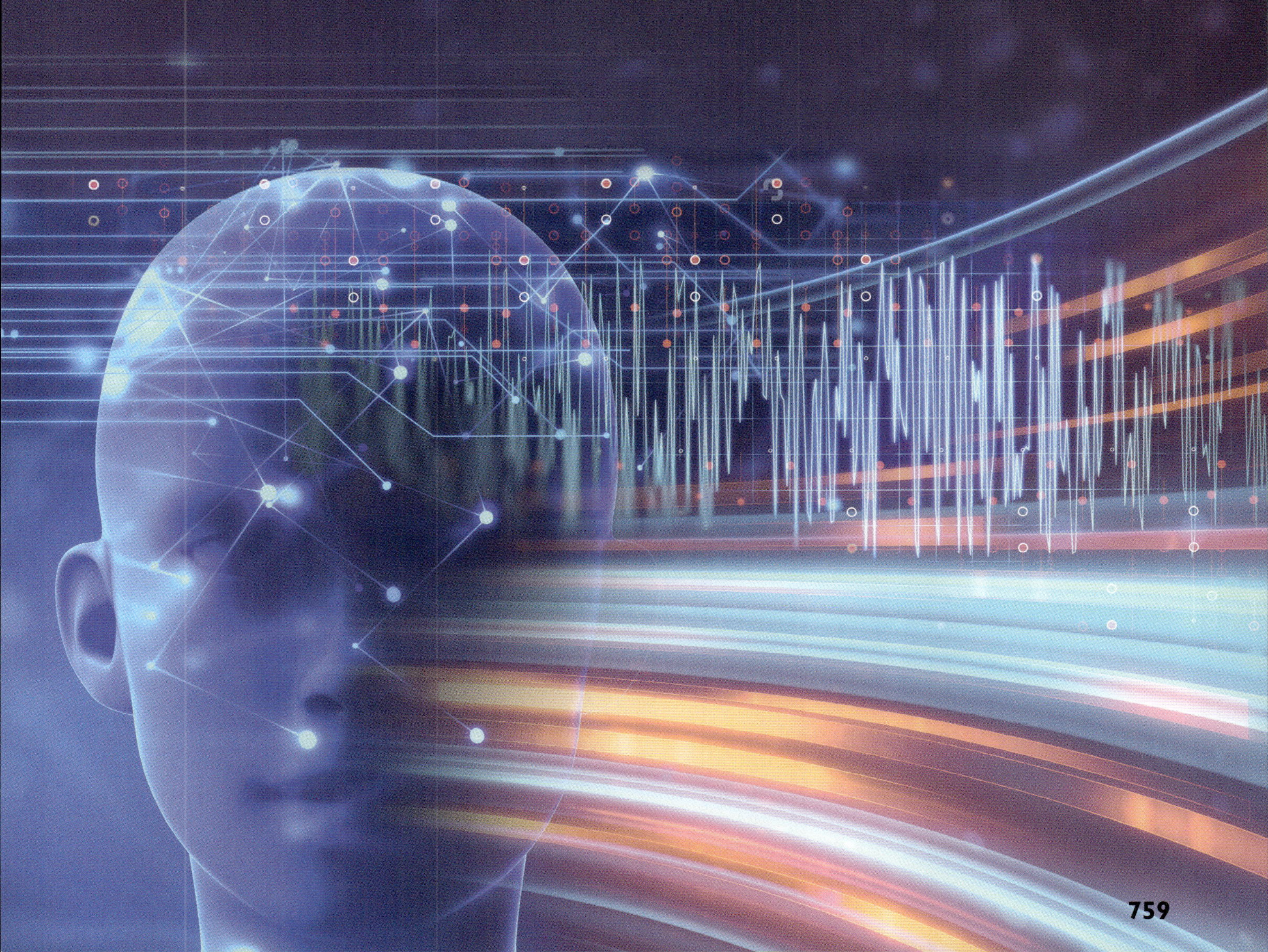

Chapter 66
Sleep Center Facilities and Equipment

TODD EIKEN

KEY CONCEPTS/LEARNING OBJECTIVES

The key concepts for this chapter include describing the key components of a conventional sleep center facility, reviewing the advantages and disadvantages of converting traditional hospital rooms to patient rooms for sleep testing as against facility renovation, and explaining the importance of ensuring patient privacy and confidentiality through facility design.

This chapter will describe the general applications of video/audio recording in the sleep center; outline the available options for camera, lighting, microphone, and sound processing equipment; describe data archiving options available for polysomnographic (PSG) data files; and list the general categories of instrumentation, the primary options and variables associated with PSG acquisition systems, and the sensor options available for each common PSG physiologic parameter.

KEY TERMS

Analog
Ancillary equipment
Data acquisition
Data analysis
Digital
Omnidirectional
PSG time synch
Screen resolution
Unidirectional

THE SLEEP CENTER PHYSICAL PLANT

The primary components of a sleep center facility consist of designated areas intended to separate patients from each other, separate patients from employee areas, and allow for designated activities to take place, such as patient setup, equipment cleaning and storage, continuous positive airway pressure (CPAP) patient education and data download, and polysomnographic (PSG) data acquisition, analysis, and review (Figure 66-1).

Current Trends in Sleep Center Construction

As awareness of sleep disorders, obstructive sleep apnea, in particular, continues to grow within the medical community, an increasing number of sleep centers are being established. This great demand for testing has resulted in sleep centers being established outside of the conventional hospital setting. Facilities such as professional/medical office buildings, bed and breakfast inns, hotels, and even condominiums have been converted for use as sleep disorder testing facilities. This departure from the conventional hospital setting does not always allow the inclusion of all the previously described primary components of a conventional full-service sleep disorders facility.

The use of computer networking within and among sleep testing facilities allows increased efficiency for analysis and interpretation tasks utilizing remote connectivity. PSG data files can be moved between computers; and scoring as well as interpretation tasks can be performed outside of the sleep center. Network cabling must be installed within the facilities between patient rooms and control rooms, and servers must be stored and powered. Wireless network communications can considerably reduce the network cabling requirements within a sleep center facility, but attention must be given to data encryption and security.

As the number of sleep testing beds increases within a particular community, competition among facilities can often become an ongoing operational factor. Facility design considerations, particularly features intended to increase patient comfort, can become a pivotal marketing point within advertising strategies and can significantly impact a center's testing volumes, as well as the facility's reputation within the local community.

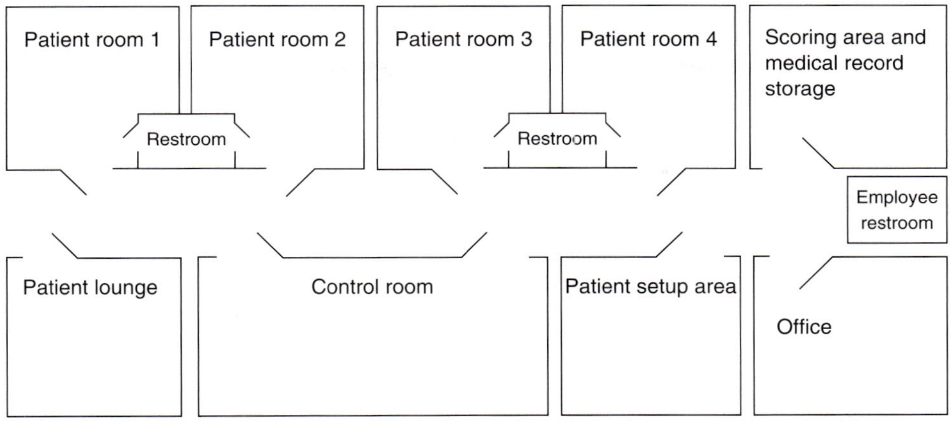

Figure 66-1 Efficient, cost-effective layout for a first-stage sleep center facility. Two of these four rooms could be eliminated from the design, thereby reducing costs even further.

General Location Considerations

The first step in converting existing space into a functional sleep center is to determine the benefits of using existing space as against renovating the space. Within a hospital setting, the most common "first-stage" design for a sleep testing area involves three adjacent standard hospital rooms. The two outside rooms are furnished with a variety of home furnishings intended to reduce the sterile hospital environment, such as a TV, bedside stand, and perhaps a recliner and wall art. The room in the middle of the two outside patient rooms serves as the control area. This area houses the diagnostic equipment for the two beds and provides storage for supplies, a desk for the technologists, filing cabinets, and chart storage. This scenario is a very efficient and quick way to establish a sleep testing program with very little, if any, facility renovation. However, only two patients can be monitored per night, and the many other primary components described, which could enhance patient satisfaction and testing quality, cannot be utilized in this scenario because of space limitations.

Environmental noise is a very important factor to consider when choosing an area to establish a sleep center facility. Noise can play a major role in prolonging sleep latency and disrupting the patient's sleep during a PSG. When identifying a space within the community for a freestanding facility, one should consider the proximity of the facility to highways and freeways, which produce significant noise. Proximity to an airport should also be considered. When identifying space within an existing facility such as a hospital, environmental noise should also be considered. Common sources of undesirable noise within a hospital facility include the following:

- Emergency room areas
- Helicopter landing areas
- Psychiatric ward
- Heating and cooling room
- Outside trash dumpsters

Occasionally, during a sleep study, oxygen may need to be administered to the patient. Within a hospital setting, oxygen, as well as room air and suction, is typically supplied to each patient room throughout the facility through a complex system of piped medical gases. If a center is to be established within an existing hospital facility, it is likely that existing medical gases can be delivered to patient rooms within a sleep center and accessed through wall-mounted regulators. However, in a nonhospital facility, consideration should be given to the method of providing supplemental oxygen to patients. If renovating the facility for piped gases is determined to be cost prohibitive, oxygen can be delivered to most patients through the use of an oxygen concentrator. When an oxygen concentrator is utilized, backup oxygen tanks should be available in the sleep center in case of a power failure. It is important to be aware that the maximum liter flow of an oxygen concentrator is typically lower than that available from a piped gas flow regulator system. In addition, portable suction devices may be used outside of a conventional hospital setting.

The issue of cabling is certainly a very important consideration when designing a sleep center space. Cabling is required to transfer the physiologic PSG signals from the patient room to the control room. Some sleep testing–related hardware items have maximum cable length specifications that need to be considered. Clinical CPAP systems that incorporate a flow generator unit in the patient room and a remote pressure control in the control room will require cabling between the two locations. Intercom systems and closed-circuit video/audio systems may also require cabling between the patient and the control room. Extraordinarily long cables can occasionally result in a reduction of signal strength as well as the introduction of electrical interference into the signal.

Common sources of electrical interference include fluorescent light fixtures and elevator areas. The type of cable, as well as maximum cable length requirements for the mentioned devices, may differ among manufacturers. Advances in technology allow many computer-based monitoring instruments in a sleep center facility to communicate using a wireless networking method, thereby eliminating the need for physical cabling. This may be advantageous and cost-effective for some facility designs.

When evaluating existing space for a sleep center, future expansion potential should be considered as well. In light of the prevalence of sleep disorders, particularly sleep apnea, once a sleep center has been established and is operational, the number of patients referred for testing will usually increase to the point of a scheduling backlog. In established sleep center facilities, expansion of the number of testing beds will be the only option to reduce the scheduling backlog. Therefore, the presence of nearby space that could be renovated in the future for patient room expansion will definitely be advantageous. Also, additional space within the control room to house additional diagnostic equipment should be considered.

Consideration should be given to handicapped and disabled patients when identifying areas within a sleep center facility that will be used by patients. This includes reasonable accommodations for wheelchair access within the patient rooms, hallways, and doorways; support bars within restroom and shower facilities; and patient beds equipped for raising and lowering the head and foot sections.

Many cities and towns require facilities to be built in a manner that allows for fast evacuation of people in case of fire and incorporates specific building materials that are either fire retardant or capable of slowing the spread of fire, such as a door. When establishing a sleep center within an existing space, local fire codes should be reviewed to ensure that the space meets the specific code requirements, such as location of fire sprinklers. Building codes will specify the requirements for lighted exit signs and backup lighting necessary in case of a power failure or an emergency.

As a sleep center is typically open for operations 24 hours a day, security for patients as well as the staff is important, especially in freestanding facilities. Security personnel employed within a hospital facility will usually address these issues for hospital-based sleep centers. In the case of freestanding facilities, issues including door locks, security systems, intercoms, and a communication protocol with law enforcement must be considered.

If initial startup capital expenses are of concern, utilizing existing space within a facility is certainly the least expensive route. However, if absolutely no facility renovation can be performed, many of the described primary components of a conventional full-service sleep center will, in most cases, need to be sacrificed. This may impact a program's ability to meet the standards defined by various sleep center certification or accreditation entities. Some programs that exist today choose to "specialize" in diagnosing and treating only a portion of the many sleep disorders that have been identified to date, such as sleep apnea and periodic movements of sleep. This scenario may reduce not only costs as well as reliance on some of the primary sleep center facility components but also the number of patients a sleep center can accept for testing. Utilizing existing space and performing a moderate amount of facility renovation to meet instrumentation and environmental requirements and to allow for the inclusion of primary sleep center facility components will result in the most cost-efficient startup scenario and will allow the program to meet all of the patient's diagnostic and treatment needs. Building an entirely new facility is, of course, the most expensive scenario but allows the facility to be so designed as to meet all possible facility and patient population needs and considerations, as well as allowing for the incorporation of unique facility features that can be marketed to the community.

Functional Considerations and Descriptions of Sleep Center Facility Components

Patient Room

The patient room is one of the most important components of the sleep center. Its design and construction can affect not only the quality of data acquired during a PSG procedure but also the facility's reputation within a community. Design considerations should facilitate not only the night testing procedures but daytime testing procedures as well. In addition, patients will most likely occupy the room for those periods when no testing is being performed, and ensuring patient satisfaction within a room during this time is just as important as during testing periods. Facility design should include analysis of the type of patients evaluated at the sleep center.

As a general rule, there is no minimum size requirement for a patient room, although 140 ft^2 is often recommended. The preeminent considerations relating to room size include the ability of a medical emergency team to have easy access to the patient from either side of the bed and the ability of the patient to move safely in the space available. The American Academy of Sleep Medicine (AASM) accreditation standards require that the room be of sufficient size to accommodate emergency personnel access, with a minimum of 24 inches (60.96 cm) of available clear space on three sides of the bed (1). Consider the need for a code cart, often referred to as a "crash cart," that is readily accessible to health care workers and strategically placed in a hospital sleep center.

An important goal in designing a patient room is to eliminate a sterile, hospital-based atmosphere and have the room look and feel like either a hotel or a home bedroom. One of the most effective ways to accomplish this is through the selection of bedroom furnishings. A patient room should include a bed, preferably a full-size bed that has an adjustable head and foot section (Figure 66-2A). A headboard and footboard made of finished wood is also effective in providing a home-like feel. In addition, in the interest of minimizing patient injury, the bed should have side rails that can be used for patient safety during testing conducted for parasomnia disorders or abnormal behaviors during sleep.

Bedside stands are an important furniture component of the patient room. Aside from selecting a more home-style designed stand, the stands should have enough room to store any diagnostic or treatment devices required during testing such as a CPAP flow generator. Some bedside stands incorporate a small drawer that can be very useful for storing commonly used disposable supplies in the room for easy access by the technologist during the night. Other common items placed on a bedside table include a telephone, reading lamp, and tissues. If space permits, it can be useful to add a bedside stand on each side of the bed to accommodate all of the possible items commonly placed on one (Figure 66-2B).

Seating for the patient and guests should be available in each patient room. Some obese patients and visitors may be hesitant to sit on a chair that they perceive may collapse beneath them. Furniture may need to be able to withstand weight of 500 lb (227.27 kg) to 800 lb (363.64 kg). Because the patient will be seated in the chair during hookup, the design of the chair should allow the technologist ease in applying the sensors and electrodes. When selecting patient seating, consider the patient's comfort and dignity.

It is certainly desirable to have windows in a patient room. If a patient is undergoing a multiple sleep latency test (MSLT) during the day, it is often useful to allow daylight into the room between nap trials to aid the patient in staying awake. However, windows can be a problem during daytime testing, because it can be difficult to totally eliminate the daylight from the room during MSLT nap trials. A type of blind often referred to as a blackout blind should be considered for better control of daylight within the patient room. This blind incorporates tracks on the bottom and sides of the window, thereby blocking out all light coming in through the window. It can be useful during the night as well, because it will block moonlight or streetlights in the same manner.

It will be important for the patient to have a closet or armoire available in the room to store and hang daytime clothing. In addition, this space can be used to store extra blankets or pillows that the patient may request during an all-night test.

Other optional furnishings to consider that add to the home-style setting include wall art, waste receptacles, and remote-controlled televisions. If you choose to allow patients to watch television, pay special attention to designing the sleep center patient room with acoustic/sound attenuation in mind. One of the easiest things that can be done in this regard is to construct each wall of a patient room to extend up to, and connect with, the ceiling. This method greatly reduces the amount of noise that can travel above typical hanging or suspended ceiling tiles. Placing insulation in the ceiling can provide some noise reduction. Some of the more expensive commercially available ceiling tiles have sound attenuation ratings. Disregarding this construction consideration can lead to noise from one patient room disturbing another patient, or even control room noise traveling to patient rooms. Floor carpeting is certainly advantageous

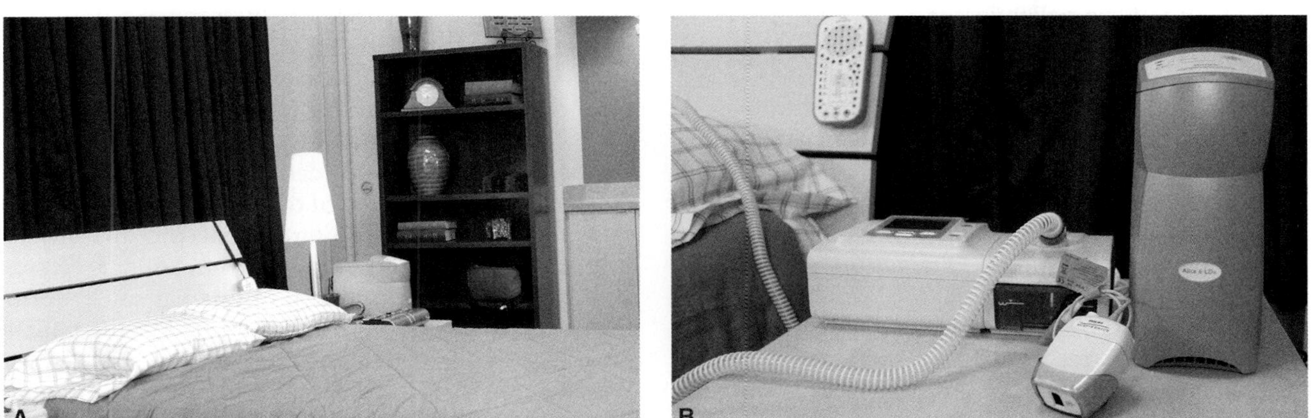

Figure 66-2 A: Patient bedroom. B: Two bedside stands provide room for the positive airway pressure device and acquisition system amplifier and also a lamp.

in reducing environmental noise, as is the use of inner wall insulation. A thick fire door for the patient room entrance can also reduce noise.

A number of electrical lighting options should be considered for the patient room. Certainly, a general ceiling-mounted light, which illuminates the entire room, should be in place and controlled at the room entrance. A reading lamp located on a bedside stand can also be used. However, many existing sleep centers shy away from allowing patients the opportunity to control any aspect of the environment such as light, as they may inadvertently disrupt testing procedures by turning the lights on and off during the test. Some patients are unable to tolerate total darkness. In such cases, a small night-light plugged into a wall receptacle can be useful. Also, connecting the general ceiling-mounted light to a dimmer control will allow only minimal light to illuminate the room for certain patient needs. Incandescent black light illumination is an additional lighting option that can significantly enhance coexisting infrared illumination for video recording. A light fixture with a blacklight bulb, installed somewhere near the patient and connected to a dimmer control, will work quite well to accomplish this method of increasing video display quality.

One of the most important facility considerations related to a patient room is temperature control. A patient's comfort relative to room temperature can, in many cases, make or break the ability to perform a quality sleep study. In order to most effectively control this aspect of the testing environment, individual thermostat controls assigned to each patient room are the most advantageous. This method will allow one patient's room to be set much cooler than a nearby patient's room, thereby allowing both patients a degree of comfort to facilitate a quality test. However, this method can be rather expensive. In cases where individual temperature controls are not an option, every effort should be made to assign the fewest patient rooms to each thermostat control. More than three patient rooms assigned to one temperature control will most certainly result in conflicting patient temperature preferences from time to time, resulting in one or more patients experiencing disrupted, poor-quality sleep during the test. Consideration should also be given to the placement of the thermostat control. If possible, mounting a control outside of a patient room is most desirable. Otherwise, a technologist may be required to enter one patient's room to adjust the temperature of a different patient's room, potentially disrupting both patients' sleep. Making sure that any ceiling or wall-mounted vent used for heating or cooling is not near, or directed specifically toward, the patient can minimize the impact of room temperature on the patients.

Alternatively, placement of fans in the patient rooms allows a degree of flexibility in cooling the room when individual controls are not an option. Many patients sleep at home with a fan, and one should be available on request.

The technologist should also be cognizant of technical considerations for the integrity of the PSG such as sweat artifact caused by overly warm room temperatures and carefully monitor the room temperature. In addition, thought should be given to maintaining an adequate supply of blankets to accommodate the needs of individual patients when individual thermostat controls are not available.

Restrooms

Restrooms for patients and staff are an obvious necessity in a sleep center facility. The most desirable and comfortable design for patients and staff allows for multiple restrooms designated for both patients and staff. This design eliminates the potential scenario of a patient interrupting a PSG procedure to use the restroom but being unable to do so because it is being occupied by a staff member, thereby increasing the duration of the test interruption. The AASM accreditation standards require that the sleep facility have clean bathrooms with a minimum ratio of one bathroom for every three testing rooms; these bathrooms must each contain a toilet and a sink. Toilet fixtures can be floor mounted or wall mounted. A floor-mounted toilet can support up to 800 lb (363.64 kg) and toilet-to-floor supports can be added as required. Patients often lean on a sink, and floor-mounting the sink helps distribute weight. Each bathroom must have a working privacy door. Sole access to a shared bathroom cannot be through a testing bedroom. All restrooms should be minimally furnished with a toilet, sink, hand soap dispenser, paper towel dispenser, wall-mounted mirror, ceiling light, ceiling vent, and an electrical outlet (1).

An ideal sleep center design relative to restroom facilities allows for a private restroom for each patient room. This provides patient privacy, reduces the duration of restroom breaks during the PSG, and allows patients the option of preparing for and departing directly from the sleep center to their daytime job, following the conclusion of the test in the morning. The option of departing directly to work is certainly desirable and convenient for most patients who are tested during weeknights and can be a pivotal marketing point for a sleep center located within a town or city that offers competing sleep center facilities. A fully functional private patient restroom should be designed for access from within the patient room and should include shower facilities.

The provision of shower facilities will introduce patient expectations for personal items such as soap, shampoo, and appropriate towels and linen to be provided, as would commonly be found in a hotel. It will also demand increased housekeeping and/or environmental services involvement, which may increase a facility's operating expenses.

In situations where private restrooms are not possible, a common solution is to use a shared patient restroom design. This can be advantageous from a facility design perspective but may result in patient dissatisfaction. The single shared patient restroom not only limits a patient's morning personal hygiene options, but during the night, there may be patients who leave the restroom soiled or in an undesirable condition for the next patient. This scenario may require staff members to clean the restroom, which can result in staff dissatisfaction and interrupt the PSG procedure.

Private patient restrooms can be constructed without shower facilities for cases in which construction cost restraints are an issue. A single shower area can then be shared by patients, which will most likely be better tolerated relative to patient satisfaction.

If the sleep center facility will include a patient reception or waiting area used during the day to process physician office or clinic appointments, consideration should be given to the facility's proximity to the nearest public restroom, as waiting patients or family members will most likely require this. Construction of a public restroom may be required if a nearby access does not exist.

Reasonable accommodations for disabled persons should be made in all patient, public, and staff restrooms. This would include adequate space for patients using wheelchairs and walkers to access and utilize the area, wall-mounted support bars near the toilet and within the shower area, optional sitting stool for use within the shower area, and a mechanism for patients to activate a call for assistance such as a wall-mounted help button or pull chain. The AASM accreditation standards require that at least one testing bedroom and bathroom be handicap accessible as defined either by local building regulations or by sections 6.3 and 6.4 of the Americans with Disabilities Act (1).

Control Room

A control room must be large enough to comfortably house working space for the PSG technologist staff and required equipment. The control room is the hub of activity within the sleep center, and technologists spend most of their work time within this area. Therefore, it is important to design the control area to be as comfortable as possible for the technical staff, taking into consideration the amount of general traffic projected for the area, equipment placement, and individual staff member workstations and related furniture. The AASM accreditation standards require that the dimensions of the control room be not less than 40 ft^2 in total or 20 ft^2 per testing bedroom, whichever is larger (1).

Ideally, the control room should be centrally located a relatively short distance away from patient rooms. As patients will commonly call for assistance from technologists during a sleep study, a short distance between the control room and the patient room will reduce the amount of time it takes for the technologist to enter the patient room in response to the call. This is also an important consideration with regard to technologist reaction time in emergencies such as cardiac arrhythmias or seizure events. In addition, some of the monitoring devices used during a PSG that incorporate connected components in both the control area and the patient room specify maximum cabling lengths that are important for proper equipment operation. These specifications may impact the distance requirements between the control room and the patient rooms as well.

Despite the importance of maintaining a relatively short distance between the patient rooms and the control room, noted previously, it is important to maintain strict boundaries between employee areas and patient areas. Patient privacy and confidentiality should be considered when designing the control room. Patients should at no time be allowed to physically enter, or visually observe, the control room. Video monitors should be so placed and located as to be visually unobservable from patient areas. Patients should not see documents containing another patient's information within the control room. Patients should neither hear telephone conversations within the control room relating to other patients nor be able to hear audio sounds that originate from a patient room. Succeeding in maintaining patient privacy and confidentiality within the control room may result in unique construction or facility renovation requirements (Figure 66-3).

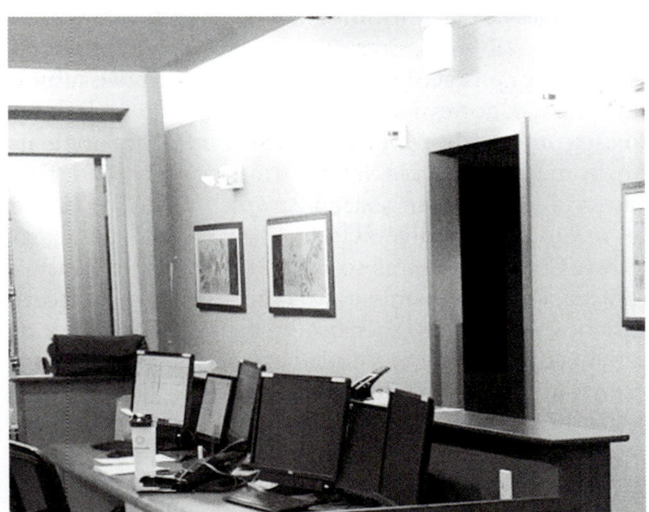

Figure 66-3 Technologist control room for four-bed acquisition.

Once the area of the control room that will house the monitoring equipment has been identified, adequate access to electricity will need to be established in that area. Multiple wall outlets will most likely be required in order to furnish sufficient power to all of the varying monitoring instruments. An ideal wiring design allows for multiple instruments assigned to a particular patient room to be powered by outlets, utilizing a separate independent ground. By providing separate grounds for each patient room, the potential for electrical interference originating in one patient room to travel to the next patient room is significantly reduced. In facilities where emergency auxiliary power is available, such as in a hospital, connecting the primary PSG unit or computer processing unit to an outlet with automatic auxiliary power switching can be advantageous during periods of power outages in order to minimize the amount of data lost during a power failure. If facility-furnished emergency auxiliary power is not available, the use of an uninterrupted battery power supply with surge protection is recommended for the previously mentioned units. If intermittent power outages are common in the facility, then an uninterrupted battery power supply with surge protection is recommended regardless of the presence of emergency auxiliary power.

Cabling is an important consideration in designing the control room area. Many of the monitoring devices housed within the control room are interfaced through cabling to components housed in the patient room. In addition, sleep center entrance security video signals and audio intercom signals may also require a cabled connection to related devices in the control room. The control room design should allow for a designated space, chute, or conduit intended to introduce these multiple cables from above the ceiling, inside the wall, and into the control room near the floor. This design allows for quick access to all incoming and outgoing cables; can improve troubleshooting efficiency; and makes it easier for outside contractors to locate, add, or remove cables. Importantly, however, when placing multiple cables next to each other as described, electrical interference originating from within a cable can transmit to other cables. This can be a problem for some instruments that are prone to receive extraneous AC electrical interference such as a PSG system. In this scenario, using shielded cables can reduce the transmission of this interference. In the case of PSG systems, specifically, the use of network or serial cabling is recommended, because it is much less prone to receive extraneous interference. Network or serial cabling is commonly used with PSG systems.

Patient Setup Area

An area specifically used for patient setup procedures can be advantageous for the patients as well as the staff. It allows for all of the required sensors and application chemicals to be stored and easily accessed during the setup procedure, saving time for the technologist performing the procedure. Some of the chemicals used to apply electrodes and sensors to patients have strong odors. Maintaining a specific setup area when these chemicals are in use will keep the odors away from patient rooms, thereby avoiding the potential for patient irritation and disruption of a PSG test. Also, it can be advantageous to remove electrodes and sensors the morning following a test within the patient setup area. Reusable sensors can be more easily cleaned and returned to their respective storage area, ready to be used for the next patient.

The size requirements of the room will vary depending on the amount and size of furnishings used and the number of patients being set up simultaneously. A common list of furnishings for a single-patient setup area consists of a chair, a cart with drawers to store disposable supplies, a standard sink used for cleaning sensors, hooks to hang and store sensors and electrodes, a flammable storage container for collodion and acetone if used, and a waste receptacle. A television for the patient to watch during the setup procedure or a radio in this area can often be useful. A reasonable single-patient setup area would require to be at least 6 × 8 ft. In sleep centers where collodion and acetone are not utilized may plan and effectively use a setup area with a bright overhead light within the patient room, if space allows. The use of movable setup carts facilitates this scenario.

Areas used for multiple simultaneous setup procedures will need to be designed and constructed in a much larger space. Patient setup areas should be constructed and placed within a sleep center facility with patient privacy in mind. Patients or visitors should not be able to view other patients being set up for a PSG, especially as the procedure will commonly require the patient to remove specific parts of clothing. If more than one patient will be set up simultaneously within the area, care should be taken to partition the individual areas to maintain patient privacy.

An extremely important design consideration is a ventilation system when collodion or acetone is used. A patient setup area ventilation system that will actively remove odors should be located in the ceiling. Ideally, the air should be entirely removed from the area and transferred to the outside of the building, as opposed to filtered and recycled within the area. A variety of ventilation systems are commercially available. The size of the setup area will dictate how many individual ventilation intakes will be required. Issues such as general noise level, electrical power requirements, filtering options, and cleaning requirements should be reviewed before purchasing a system.

Lighting preferences within a control area may vary depending on the time of day or the type of job task being performed. Common fluorescent ceiling units can be used in a control room to illuminate the work area. It can be advantageous to wire segments of the ceiling units within the control area to different on/off switches. This gives staff members the ability to alter the amount of illumination in a particular area of the control room. Higher amounts of work area illumination are usually preferred when staff are performing job tasks such as daytime PSG scoring and analysis and reading or writing patient chart information. When performing PSG procedures during the night, many technologists prefer a lower or softer degree of illumination within the control area. Conversely, in the interest of reinforcing and maintaining the sleep-wake cycle of nightshift technologists, high-intensity fluorescent lights can be used in a control room during the nighttime hours to simulate sunlight. Some research shows this can be of benefit to the nightshift staff, as it can increase employees' total sleep time as well as the quality of sleep during the daytime hours.

As both the patient setup procedure and the sensor removal procedure result in numerous waste items, it is important to provide adequate waste receptacles. The area should facilitate adherence to conventional policies and procedures relating to proper labeling and disposal of contaminated waste. A "sharps" disposal system should be in place for the disposal of blunt tip needles and other sharp objects. Arrangements should be made for the routine removal of waste from the setup area on a daily basis.

Patients who are studied for a variety of neurologic disorders will occasionally display symptoms or behaviors such as seizures or cataplexy. Unfortunately, these events can occasionally occur before the start of the recording phase of a PSG test, often during the setup procedure. Activating a video camera within the patient setup area can be useful for at least capturing the event on video, despite the lack of PSG data. In addition, it is becoming increasingly common for sleep centers to video-record all tech-patient interactions. Some patients may choose to take legal action against a particular sleep facility or sleep technologist, claiming inappropriate contact or communication. Placing a video camera in the setup area and recording the procedure provides video documentation that could become critical evidence in defending one's actions with a patient if brought to litigation.

Scoring/Record Review Room

There can be advantages to creating a room with the sole purpose of conducting PSG scoring and interpretation activities. Although scoring can usually be performed in most control rooms on the computer where the data were acquired, the level of control room traffic and noise during the day, daytime testing activities, and general clerical activities can be a distraction to those scoring and interpreting the data in the control room.

In order to review digital PSG recordings within a scoring/record review room, computer workstations often referred to as review stations are required. PSG data are transferred from the acquisition computer in the control room to the review station or to a central server for scoring and interpretation. Data are usually transferred through a local area network (LAN). The sleep center LAN allows PSG data files located on any computer within the network to be accessed, viewed, and scored on a review station. Special consideration for a network-cabling pathway should be included in the construction design of the scoring/record review room for LAN connectivity.

A scoring/record review room can serve quite well for a PSG archive storage area as well. PSG files can be managed and moved through a LAN, allowing files to be archived to a variety of digital storage devices and stored within the room. This allows for convenient access to past archived PSG files for review as needed.

Other optional uses for a scoring/record review room include conducting PSG scoring education and training, physician dictation stations, Internet research activities, and patient database management.

Patient Lounge

A patient lounge area can be used for a variety of patient needs during the night, as well as daytime operations. A common recommended method for dealing with patients who experience insomnia during an all-night PSG is to have the patient leave the room for a period. A patient lounge provides a comfortable change of environment for these patients away from their room. The room can contain features such as comfortable chairs and sofas and small food/snack items. If a television will be installed, consideration for cabling should be included in the facility design.

Often, parents of younger patients, or personal care attendants of disabled patients who are required to accompany the patient while they are being tested in the sleep center, may utilize this area to nap during the night while the patient is undergoing testing.

Depending on the location of the patient lounge within the sleep center facility, the area can also serve as a reception area during daytime operations. For this functionality, the area should, ideally, be located at the point of entrance into the sleep center, and clerical/reception staff should be present within or adjacent to the area.

Utility Room

An area designated for equipment repair and maintenance can be beneficial in a sleep center facility. It provides a location for broken sensors and electrodes to be placed for subsequent repair. Diagnostic/repair instruments such as a volt ohm meter and replacement batteries can be utilized and stored within the area as well.

Cleaning and cold sterilization can also take place in this area. Reusable items such as electroencephalogram (EEG) electrodes and humidifier canisters can be soaked in this area during cold sterilization procedures.

Facility construction considerations for this area specifically relating to the building and repair of electrical sensors and sterilization procedures would include a counter with electrical wall outlets, a deep sink for cold sterilization, adequate lighting, and ceiling ventilation.

Office Space

It is useful to have office space designated for management personnel. Confidential employee meetings and interviews can take place in this area, as well as storage of confidential employee files, policy and procedures documents, and equipment purchase records. The construction considerations for this area should be similar to those of most conventional offices, including telephone and LAN access; electrical wall outlets; and sufficient space for a desk, chairs, and file storage. A locked door is required to ensure the security of confidential documents.

Of all the primary components of a sleep center facility mentioned earlier, the absolute minimum functional requirements are a control and patient room. Many sleep programs begin very small until a reliable referral base has been established. The three adjacent standard hospital rooms' design mentioned earlier in this chapter is a common first-stage scenario implemented within an existing hospital facility. However, with first-stage freestanding facilities, more facility design options will often be available at reasonably low cost.

An additional method of reducing construction costs when establishing or expanding a sleep center facility is to utilize wireless connections between the control room and the patient room, which is available with some digital PSG systems. Labor costs associated with running conventional cables; the cost of the cables themselves; and later labor costs associated with repairing, removing, or adding cables can be eliminated by using wireless technology.

POLYSOMNOGRAPHY EQUIPMENT

The task of evaluating and replacing diagnostic equipment in a sleep lab is essential not only to ensure a sleep center's diagnostic capabilities when establishing operations but also to maintain and expand a center's diagnostic capabilities and efficiencies as the patient population varies over time. Certainly, the PSG system is the most significant equipment item to evaluate, because it can dictate a center's diagnostic capabilities, and the cost of the system can significantly impact a center's financial condition. However, limitations and/or unique operational requirements of other instrumentation items commonly used in a sleep center can also impact a center's ability to meet the dynamic diagnostic demands of a full-service sleep center. In general, commercially available PSG systems should incorporate the following features as recommended by the AASM (1):

- A toggle switch permitting visual (on-screen) standard negative 50 μV DC calibration signal for all channels to demonstrate polarity, amplitude, and time constant settings for each recorded parameter
- A separate 50/60 Hz filter control for each channel
- The capability of selecting sampling rates for each channels
- A method of measuring actual individual electrode impedance against a reference (the latter may be the sum of all other applied electrodes)
- The capability of retaining and viewing the data exactly in the manner in which it was recorded by the attending technologist (ie, retain and display all derivation changes, sensitivity adjustments, filter settings, temporal resolution)
- A filter design for data collection, which functionally simulates or replicates conventional (analog-style) frequency response curves rather than removing all activity and harmonics within the specified bandwidth

Understanding the general categories of instrumentation in the sleep lab, as well as the primary options and variables associated with PSG systems and ancillary equipment, will be extremely beneficial when evaluating and replacing PSG-related equipment.

Polysomnography Instrumentation

Data Acquisition Hardware

Until the mid-to-late 1990s, conventional PSG acquisition hardware consisted of racks of analog physiologic amplifiers, paper chart drives, and mechanical ink pen systems. More current digital PSG acquisition systems incorporate computer-based hardware, typically consisting of a desktop configuration computer, miniaturized amplifiers with analog-to-digital conversion circuits, and an electrode/sensor signal input box.

When evaluating the hardware components of a PSG system, the number of channels available for physiologic recording is an important consideration. In order to meet all of the diagnostic needs of a full-service sleep center, the number of channels available should meet the channel capacity requirements ranging from the more simple procedures such as an MSLT to the more extensive procedures such as those required for diagnosing parasomnias that include an extended EEG montage and multiple extremity electromyographic (EMG) channels. Depending on the usage frequency and amount of ancillary equipment used in the center, the number of analog DC input channels available for interfacing ancillary devices is also an important consideration. As a general rule, a PSG system with a channel capacity that exceeds the number of channels used during routine procedures not only is of potential benefit for the expanded recording requirements mentioned earlier but also allows for channel redundancy, which can help deal with amplifier failure during a recording.

The distance between the control room and the patient room is an important consideration in an evaluation of PSG hardware. Some PSG systems have maximum cable length specifications between the patient sensors and the amplifiers. This particular portion of the signal path is most prone to receive extraneous electrical interference.

PSG systems incorporate a sensor input box with input jacks designed to receive a wide variety of sensors, including electroencephalographic (EEG) electrodes, airflow monitoring devices, and respiratory effort sensors. Many PSG system manufacturers also manufacture sensors that are designed with unique connectors that will only fit into their proprietary system's sensor input box. A wide variety of sensors are manufactured by companies specializing exclusively in sensors. Although sensor manufacturers commonly provide sensors with a variety of optional connectors designed to interface with a variety of sensor input boxes, compatibility with every system may not always be possible. In addition, the signal strength produced by some third-party sensors may not be compatible with some PSG system amplifiers. Therefore, if there are specific sensor preferences within a center, or if unique sensors are used in a center such as in a research protocol, it is important to consider these compatibility issues when evaluating amplifier and sensor input box hardware.

When performing a PSG, it is often necessary to interface signals provided by ancillary equipment to the PSG system for simultaneous display with physiologic data and to analyze and report the data. These ancillary devices may include oximeters, CPAP units, and CO_2 monitors. The typical output signals provided by these devices are analog in nature and range from 1 to 10 V DC. When evaluating and selecting PSG hardware, consideration should be given to the number of DC inputs available and the range of acceptable voltage allowed to ensure compatibility with a center's specific ancillary equipment.

PSG systems allow sleep centers the ability to store and archive PSG data very efficiently. The PSG data acquisition procedure results in a number of digital computer files ranging in total size from 50 to 150 MB per recording, depending on the duration of the recording, number of channels being recorded, and the varying sampling rates used for each parameter. The AASM accreditation standards specify minimum sampling rates of 1 to 200 Hz, depending on the type of data being recorded (1,2).

The ability to share and move data between computers within a sleep center can be very advantageous. Technologists or physicians may wish to review data in an area separate from the control room or simply on a different computer than what was used during the acquisition. This can be accomplished through a LAN. Almost any computer can be networked, but certain hardware is required. The most significant hardware requirement for networking is an Ethernet port. This port or jack provides the computer with the ability to receive a special cable that interconnects the computers within the network. Digital communication technology also allows the option of wireless (WiFi) networking. This method incorporates a router that receives and transmits wireless data between computers. If networking of hardware is desired in a sleep center, the computer hardware being evaluated should either include an Ethernet port or have integrated WiFi capabilities.

Data Analysis Software

Once physiologic data have been acquired and digitized, software is required to view and manipulate the data. Most data analysis software programs are proprietary and are included as a component of a PSG system. The analysis program provides users with the ability to view, score, and generate reports that communicate analysis values and results.

Although there are a number of stand-alone PSG data analysis programs available, the majority of PSG systems include a proprietary data analysis program. Data acquired using a particular PSG system's acquisition program are commonly so formatted as to allow only that PSG system's analysis program to read and interact with the data. As these analysis programs are proprietary, the functionality may vary. According to the AASM standards (1,2), when evaluating PSG data analysis programs, the following common functions should be included at a minimum:

- Ability to provide a digital screen resolution of at least 1,600 × 1,200 for display and scoring of raw PSG data
- Ability to display a histogram with stage, respiratory events, leg movement events, O_2 saturation and arousals, with cursor positioning on histogram and ability to jump to the page
- Ability to view a screen on a time scale ranging from the entire night to windows as small as 5 seconds
- Recorded video data synchronized with PSG data with an accuracy of at least one video frame per second.

There is a growing trend to utilize third-party services that provide automated scoring and analysis of PSG data. A PSG system should be able to export recorded PSG data into a data format that is acceptable by an automated sleep scoring service provider should be chosen.

The ability to set a variety of filter settings, background colors, and other features specific to a particular parameter can be accomplished through the use of user-defined display templates. Once all of the display and filtering options available for each parameter have been set to a user's preference, the user can save the settings as a template. Then, as the user accesses different patient data in the future, rather than having to repeatedly adjust the display and filtering options for each individual parameter, the user can simply apply their template to the recording. This is clearly a time-saving tool for technologists and physicians and should be considered when evaluating analysis software.

A very significant function that analysis software provides is the generation of the PSG analysis report. Most sleep centers will require the ability to configure this report according to the preferences of either their medical staff or their referring physicians. Configurable features within a report will typically include the following:

- Report layouts and templates
- Analysis values
- Graphic summaries
- Color or B/W graphs
- Ability for consolidated split-night reporting
- MSLT reporting
- Configurable analysis start and end times

The PSG analysis report represents the sleep center's entire PSG end product and communicates the test results to the sleep center's customers, whether that is the patient or referring physician. From a marketing perspective, the PSG analysis report is the most visible and effective marketing tool a center has and is certainly critical to its image and customer satisfaction. Therefore, the configurability of presentation options, and the number and categories of available reporting values calculated, is an important consideration when evaluating PSG analysis software.

Ancillary Equipment

A variety of optional instruments are sometimes not included in a PSG system that require interfacing with the PSG system. Some of the more commonly used devices include pulse oximeters, end-tidal or transcutaneous CO_2 monitors, and clinical CPAP systems.

When evaluating a patient to rule out sleep apnea, the pulse oximeter is a critical tool used to determine the severity of sleep-disordered breathing. Most PSG systems are manufactured with oximetry technology built into the hardware, thereby eliminating the requirement for a stand-alone oximeter device to be interfaced with the PSG system. In addition, some sleep centers prefer the ability to incorporate pulse rate data provided by an oximeter into the PSG data. If this signal is not available from oximetry circuitry, which is built into a PSG system, then a stand-alone unit will need to be interfaced to the PSG system as described. If it is determined that a stand-alone oximetry unit will be required, the unit should have user-configurable alarm limits, because alarms can disrupt patient sleep.

Monitoring a patient's CO_2 levels is often required during PSG procedures. The most noninvasive method of accomplishing this is through the use of an end-tidal CO_2 monitor or a transcutaneous CO_2 monitor. Many of these devices allow recorded data to be integrated into the recording. When this is not possible, printouts should be able to be downloaded, stored, and/or sent to a printer to display trend data. As with oximetry or pulse rate data, it is important to incorporate real-time CO_2 information into the PSG tracing. The CO_2 monitoring device should provide a DC analog output that can be interfaced with the PSG system hardware. In addition, alarms should be configurable to adjust limits and avoid awakening patients during testing.

To titrate nasal CPAP during a PSG procedure without disrupting the patient by entering the room to change pressures, a CPAP unit that incorporates a remote pressure control is required. Most CPAP manufacturers provide clinical CPAP units that are designed to be used in a sleep center setting and to provide a variety of unique functions, including a remote pressure control. Remote pressure controls are typically connected to the CPAP flow generator unit via a cable, or the controls are software based and installed on the PSG computer. Consideration should be given to the manufacturer's maximum cable length specification and the distance between the patient room and the control area.

Clinical CPAP units commonly allow for a variety of positive airway pressure modes. These modes often consist of standard CPAP, auto-adjust, spontaneous bilevel positive airway pressure, bilevel positive airway pressure with backup rate, and auto-servo ventilation. An evaluation of clinical CPAP systems should include a review of the positive airway pressure modes available and the type of pressure mode requirements the center's patients and physician staff require.

Many clinical CPAP systems also provide a variety of analog output signals intended to be interfaced into the PSG system. These signals are usually DC in nature and commonly include flow, machine pressure, mask leak, estimated tidal volume, and nasal pressure–based airflow. The location of these signal outputs may vary between designs, and the signal outputs are usually incorporated into either the flow generator unit or the remote control unit. These signals are typically interfaced to the PSG system through a cable that plugs into the system's DC input hardware. Consideration should be given to the location of a particular clinical CPAP system's output ports and the location of the PSG system's DC input hardware. If output ports are to be located in the patient room, such as those that are incorporated into a flow generator, then the PSG system's DC input hardware must also be located in the patient room. Conversely, if the output ports are located in the control room, as those that are incorporated into the remote pressure control, then the PSG system's DC input hardware must also be located in the control room.

Most clinical CPAP systems incorporate an internal pressure transducer designed to measure intramask pressure changes, detect mask leaks, and provide pressure data for auto-adjusting algorithms. The manufacturer typically calibrates the pressure transducer component of a clinical CPAP unit during production of the unit. The calibration process will usually incorporate the use of a specific nasal mask, most likely a mask produced by the same manufacturer. Given the wide variety of mask designs available, many aspects of the varying designs, particularly the degree of leak allowed for a CO_2 exhaust port, may conflict with a clinical PSG manufacturer's pressure transducer calibration settings and result in flow generator malfunction. Evaluation of clinical CPAP systems should include the manufacturer's supported nasal mask designs.

The ability to communicate with a patient located in the bedroom from the control room is essential. In particular, the sequence of physiologic calibrations performed before beginning a study and ending it requires verbal commands to be communicated to the patient while the technologist is interacting with the acquisition computer in the control room. This is most easily accomplished through an intercom system. Wireless intercom systems that are commercially available are often subject to signal interference. However, depending on the amount of extraneous electrical noise in a particular sleep center environment, a wireless intercom system may be a very efficient, cost-effective solution. Otherwise, a wired intercom system can be used for this purpose. As with most devices that interconnect with cabling, attention must be given to the device manufacturer's maximum cable length specifications. Some intercom systems incorporate a hub that could be located in a control room, which transmits to and receives audio from a number of patient rooms. This is a common intercom configuration found in hospital nursing stations or building security offices. Some may find this configuration useful in a sleep center setting, but others may find that it is more advantageous to have a separate receiver and transmitter for each room located near each computer workstation in the control room. If the patient room component of the intercom system is placed within reach of the patient's bed, then potential benefits of a patient call button feature, which is available in some intercom system designs, should be considered.

Audiovisual recording of patient activities is an essential component of a PSG test. In many ways, audio/video information acquired during a PSG plays as significant a role in diagnosing sleep disorders as the physiologic PSG data recorded. A wide variety of equipment options are available relating to digital versus analog video data, wireless versus closed-circuit video, color versus black and white, and digital video formatting and editing. Many PSG systems provide recommended video hardware and software as a feature of the PSG system. Careful review of the key components of a video/audio system is essential when evaluating devices for a new sleep center or when upgrading existing equipment.

Sensors/Electrodes

Many digital PSG systems come with a sensor pack when the equipment is initially purchased. However, a host of manufacturers provide disposable and reusable electrodes and sensors for use in PSG. These sensors include EEG electrodes, airflow monitoring devices, leg movement sensors, and respiratory effort sensors. Some PSG system manufacturers also use proprietary sensors that are manufactured exclusively for use with their PSG system.

Although many PSG systems may provide a starter kit containing the various sensors and electrodes required to perform a PSG, there are typically a wide variety of sensors and electrodes to choose from. Scalp electrodes are used to record EEG activity. Many are made from either gold or silver-silver chloride material and formed into a cup. An electroconductive material is placed in the cup, the outer portion of which is either glued or pasted to the patient's head. Scalp electrode evaluation should include the preferred length of the electrode lead wire, compatibility of the lead wire jack with the PSG system hardware, the potential for dissimilar metal artifact occurring from the simultaneous use of different electrodes made with different metals, cost, reusable or disposable options, ease of application, and ease of cleaning.

In addition to scalp electrodes, adhesive electrodes are often used to record electrocardiogram (ECG), electrooculography, and other parameters. When evaluating adhesive electrodes, the following should be considered: the length of time the adhesive bond remains strong, the ease of attaining and maintaining acceptable electrode impedances, length of the lead wires, cost, and the general size of the electrode relative to the placement area on the patient.

In the evaluation of patients for obstructive sleep apnea, the airflow signal is a critical parameter. This is accomplished through the use of an airflow sensor. The most common types of airflow monitoring methods include thermal sensing devices such as a thermistor or thermocouple, polyvinylidene fluoride (PVDF) film, which is thermal and pressure based, and a nonthermal method of nasal pressure monitoring. The AASM specifies that identification of a hypopnea event or flow limitation pattern must be accomplished using the nasal pressure method, whereas the identification of an apnea episode is accomplished using a thermal method (2). Many PSG systems incorporate amplifiers that are especially designed for specific airflow monitoring devices, often produced by the PSG system manufacturer. However, there are many airflow monitoring devices to choose from.

Nasal pressure monitoring incorporates an air pressure transducer connected to a nasal cannula or oral/nasal cannula. This technology has a faster response time than thermistors and thermocouples. The nasal cannula can easily be modified and connected to a standard supplemental oxygen port found on a conventional CPAP mask, which provides an easy method of in-line airflow monitoring during CPAP titration in the lab, without the patient discomfort and mask leaks sometimes experienced with a thermocouple or thermistor placed under a CPAP mask. Nasal pressure monitors are commonly nonlinear. This results in the device exaggerating both apnea and hypopnea waveform changes. Specific filter settings must be incorporated in order to record or display nasal pressure data accurately.

PVDF is a treated plastic film that is polarized with an electric charge, which is used as an airflow monitoring sensor. The sensor has the fast response time (0.005 seconds) of the nasal pressure monitors, while retaining the linear flow measurement of other thermal sensing methods. It is usually smaller than other thermal devices and can be manufactured in a disposable or reusable option.

When evaluating airflow monitoring devices, the following issues should be considered:

- Do the devices meet the requirements of the AASM for recommended or acceptable sensors for each event type?
- Are the device connectors compatible with the PSG system input hardware?
- Are there external power source requirements (batteries)?
- Can the device provide a combined oral/nasal signal?
- Is the device affordable, and how often will it require replacement?

Monitoring respiratory effort during a PSG is essential in determining whether or not a patient's sleep-disordered breathing is obstructive or central in nature. A number of methods are available to detect and record respiratory effort. The easiest and most cost-effective way is to monitor intercostal EMG activity. This simply requires many electrodes to be placed in the correct locations, with the signal amplified and filtered through a conventional differential AC amplifier. Common drawbacks of this method include excessive ECG artifact and the inability to capture the EMG activity as a result of excessive tissue in obese patients.

A number of respiratory effort devices are available that incorporate the method of impedance pneumography. This also requires many electrodes to be placed on the patient's chest and abdomen areas and is a relatively cost-effective method. Common disadvantages of this technology include poor signal quality resulting from limited respiration-related surface area changes in obese patients, as well as cardiogenic pulse artifact. An external power source is typically required with these devices as well.

Another method available for monitoring respiratory effort utilizes belts with PVDF sensors, which are wrapped around the patient's thorax and abdomen. As the patient breathes and the chest or abdomen surface area changes, the belt stretches, causing the PVDF sensor to emit a voltage change. The device is easy to apply to the patient and does not typically require an external power source but is typically more expensive than the methods previously described. Common drawbacks of this method include poor signal caused by limited respiration-related surface area changes in obese patients and the designated abdominal or thoracic belt sliding on the patient into the other belt's source area, resulting in both belts displaying the same effort source.

The AASM standards specify that the detection of respiratory effort be performed using either esophageal manometry, which is fairly invasive, calibrated or uncalibrated inductance plethysmography, or PVDF sensors (2). Respiratory inductance plethysmography technology uses two sinusoid wire coils insulated and placed within two 2.5 cm (about 1 inch) wide, lightweight elastic and adhesive bands. The transducer bands are placed around the rib cage under the armpits and around the abdomen at the level of the umbilicus (belly button). During inspiration, the cross-sectional area of the rib cage and abdomen increases, altering the self-inductance of the coils and the frequency of their oscillation, with an increase in cross-sectional area proportional to lung volumes. The electronics convert this change in frequency to a digital respiration waveform where the amplitude of the waveform is proportional to the inspired breath volume. Additionally, the AASM allows the use of respiratory effort sensors that use PVDF technology for the detection of respiratory effort. These effort monitors are also acceptable for monitoring effort during a home sleep apnea test (HSAT). When evaluating respiratory effort devices, the following issues should be considered:

- Is the device able to detect minimal effort signals when used on obese patients?
- Is the device able to adequately reject ECG or pulse artifact?
- Are the device connectors compatible with the PSG system input hardware?
- Are there external power source requirements (batteries)?
- Is the device affordable, and how often will it require replacement?

Recording the movement of a patient's extremities is a very important part of studying a patient to rule out periodic limb movements of sleep or other abnormal sleep-related behaviors categorized as parasomnias. Since the advent of clinical sleep centers, monitoring of limb movements has been accomplished by monitoring the EMG activity of specific muscles located in the patient's legs and arms using surface electrodes. This is a very cost-effective method and is usually very reliable. The AASM recommends that surface electrodes be placed longitudinally and symmetrically around the middle of the muscle so that they are 2 cm apart. Both legs should be monitored for the presence of leg movements. Separate channels for each leg are strongly preferred (2). A number of limb movement sensors are available that incorporate piezoelectric materials to generate an electrical response during limb movements. These devices typically tape onto the patient's limbs, thereby greatly reducing the application time when compared with applying EMG surface electrodes. The limb movement sensors are more expensive than the EMG method and are not acceptable alternatives for monitoring EMG during PSG.

It is advantageous to graphically record snoring sounds generated by a patient during a PSG. A common method used to achieve this is to attach a small audio microphone element to the patient's neck and connect the microphone to a standard PSG differential amplifier. The microphone will detect and display not only snoring but also subtle breathing sounds. However, this method will also result in the detection and display of audio signals generated from extraneous environmental noise, position adjustments, and CPAP mask exhaust port sounds that can be mistaken for snoring. An alternate method of recording snoring sounds is to utilize a commercially available piezoelectric sensor designed specifically for snoring detection. It produces a signal by detecting the movement and vibrations in the patient's neck tissue that are associated with snoring. The device is relatively inexpensive and eliminates the potential artifact mentioned previously.

Identifying and recording the body position of a patient during a PSG is essential in order to document the existence of positional sleep-disordered breathing. A wide variety of body position sensors are commercially available, and they are all based on similar technology. The sensor is typically attached to the midline, anterior chest area of the patient. As the patient changes to a lateral, supine, or prone position, the device changes its output voltage by a small degree. The device is calibrated to the PSG system before the beginning of the test, identifying each voltage output with a particular position. This is a convenient device, especially for the technologist performing the study, because the change in position is recorded automatically. Drawbacks of this method include the internal battery within the device losing power and ultimately failing and the inability of the device to move enough to trigger the voltage change when it is used with very obese patients. An alternate method of recording body position is for the technologist to manually enter the position changes. This is obviously a much more cost-effective method but eliminates the automated function of the sensor. Not all PSG systems allow manual entry of body position changes, and this is an important feature to consider when evaluating PSG systems.

Audiovisual Equipment

Since the advent of clinical sleep disorders medicine, simultaneous video and audio monitoring of the patient during a PSG has been a standard data parameter. The interpreting physician or analyzing technologist most often uses these data to correlate questionable physiologic data in the PSG with patient or environmental activity that occurred during the test.

For patients suspected of sleeping disorders categorized as parasomnias, video and audio information can be critical for diagnosis. Many parasomnias involve unusual behaviors that occur during sleep and that can only be confirmed visually through video monitoring. These parasomnias include somnambulism, REM sleep behavior disorder, and abnormal movement disorders. In addition, suspected epileptiform activity seen in the EEG can be correlated with seizure-related motor activity displayed within the video information to assist in diagnosing nocturnal seizures.

Many patients with sleep disorders, particularly those whose disorders result in very mild daytime sleepiness or fatigue, have difficulty being convinced of their condition. Many patients who demonstrate mild-to-moderate obstructive sleep apnea during a sleep study will not believe the physician's interpretation or report and are unwilling to comply with the prescribed treatment. In these cases, the physician may choose to play back the video/audio information for the patient to convince them of the condition.

Many sleep centers maintain a library of video clips taken from routine PSGs comprising patient behaviors indicative of a wide range of sleep disorders. This information can be used for training new employees as well as for educational presentations, with a signed consent from each patient that allows recordings to be used for teaching purposes.

More recently, the video recording of the patient-technologist interaction in the sleep center has become an essential means of liability protection. Some patients may choose to take legal action against a particular sleep center facility or sleep technologist, claiming inappropriate contact or communication. In light of the fact that sleep studies are lengthy, occur in bedrooms, and are often conducted in isolated situations, it is wise for the sleep technologist to video-record all interactions with patients, including sensor hookup. This video documentation can become critical evidence in defending one's actions with a patient if brought to litigation.

Most commercially available PSG data acquisition systems incorporate digital video/audio functionality. During a PSG, digital PSG systems allow the user to view a small video window on the computer screen simultaneously with scrolling physiologic data. The user can easily identify specific video clips of interest for the reviewer the next day. In addition, the reviewers can very easily and quickly locate video data associated with a point in time on the PSG, as the video and PSG data are linked.

General Equipment Considerations

The most important component of the video/audio system in a sleep center facility is the camera. Selecting a camera for use in a sleep center should include considerations within a number of areas. The AASM accreditation standards require that each testing bedroom in the facility have a mechanism for visual monitoring and video recording of patients during testing. Time-delayed photographs are not considered compliant with this standard (1).

The camera must be able to function in low-light environments. Many cameras designed and intended for use within an outdoor security system meet these low-level lighting requirements. When a camera such as this is operating in a low-light environment, its iris adjustment is typically set wide open. If light were suddenly to be introduced into the environment being recorded by the camera, this wide-open iris setting would "white out" the video display, and the user would not be able to recognize objects within the display until the iris was adjusted to a smaller opening. This scenario occurs frequently within a sleep center when the light within a patient's room is turned on and off during the course of a study. Therefore, only cameras with an auto-adjusting iris function should be considered for use in a sleep center. Otherwise, the iris will need to be adjusted manually to view and record events in both lighted and low-light conditions, which is not practical within a sleep center setting.

Because of the general low-light environment of patient rooms in a sleep center, as well as the high cost of color video cameras, video information acquired during a PSG has historically been black and white. As technology has evolved and costs have decreased, color cameras have found a place in the sleep center. Activities such as patient hookup procedures and monitoring patient activity between daytime MSLT trials can be videotaped in color. Ideally, color cameras used for both low-light PSG recording and normal light activities should be able to automatically switch from black and white mode during low-light recording to color mode during normal light recording.

A wide variety of options are available for mounting a camera within a sleep center patient room. The camera should be mounted in a location that will allow the entire patient bed to be viewed in the video display. A fixed camera mount is the most inexpensive method for mounting a camera. This hardware allows for manipulating the angle of the camera and then tightening a number of screws, thereby obtaining a fixed camera angle. In addition, there are mounting systems available that enclose the camera, usually within a plastic mirrored dome. This enclosed mounting method will typically require that the camera be mounted on the ceiling of the room, as opposed to the wall. This can be advantageous in some circumstances involving patients who are overly conscious of a camera in the room and hence unable to sleep.

If cost is not a significant issue, a camera mounting system that incorporates pan and tilt functions is ideal in a sleep center patient room. This allows the technologist to move the camera vertically and laterally to capture specific activity or behaviors of the patient during the sleep study. The camera that is typically used with a pan and tilt mounting system will incorporate a zoom lens. The zoom, pan, and tilt functions are all controlled by the user via a remote console typically placed within the sleep center control room or may be integrated into the user interface of the PSG system computer (Figure 66-4A).

In order to video-record patient activity in a room that is totally dark, the most common type of lighting system used is infrared illumination. An infrared illuminator manufactured as a stand-alone unit can be mounted on the wall or ceiling of the patient room, ideally, near the patient (Figure 66-4B). There are also cameras designed for low-light conditions that have built-in infrared illuminators. This can be a convenient feature, but in this scenario, placement of the camera relative to the patient is critical to ensure that the infrared illumination reaches the patient.

A less costly way to light a patient room for video recording utilizes an incandescent blacklight bulb. The bulb can be placed in a portable or permanent light fixture within the room. A disadvantage of this method is

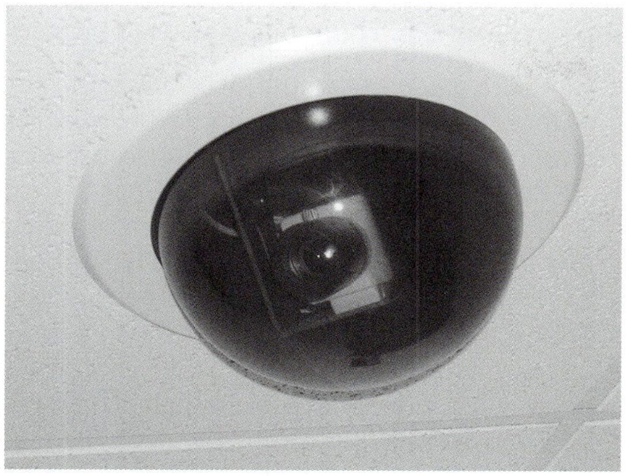

A

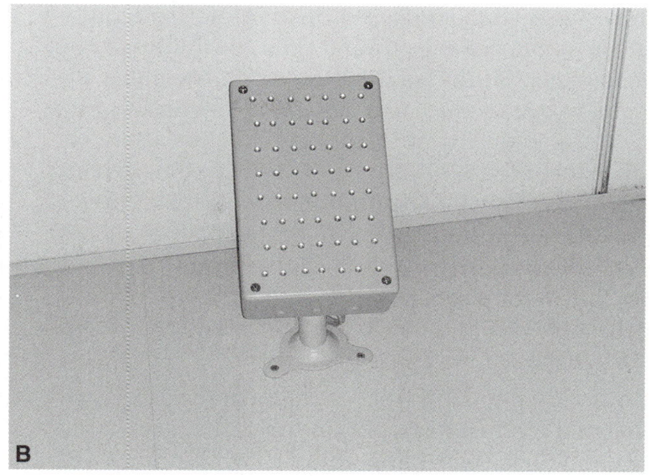

B

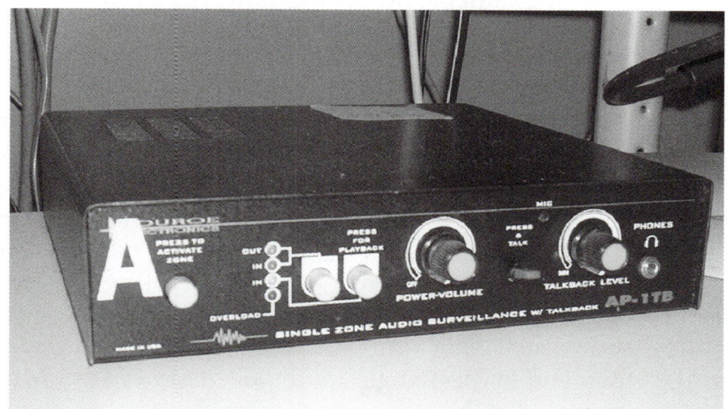

C

Figure 66-4 The most common analog video components. A: Pan-tilt camera. B: Wall-mounted infrared light source. C: Audio monitoring base station with listen and talkback.

that the black light creates a degree of light within the room that is noticeable to the patient, as opposed to the infrared illuminator, which produces no visible light within the room. Some sleep centers have incorporated both methods in patient rooms, using a conventional dimmer control with the black light to fine-tune the amount of blacklight illumination, ultimately optimizing the overall illumination within the room without disturbing the patient.

The audio portion of the video data is most often used to detect and assess a patient's breathing sounds such as snoring, as well as facilitate communication between the patient and the technologist during a PSG test. The audio data are acquired through a microphone placed in the room. Some cameras have a microphone built into the camera. Also, a number of intercom systems designed specifically for sleep centers provide an audio output signal that can be introduced into the audio recording device. However, to effectively sample the more subtle breathing sounds from a patient, a microphone mounted close to the patient is ideal. Microphones can be omnidirectional or unidirectional. An omnidirectional microphone will receive audio information from a broad 360° angle. A unidirectional microphone will receive audio data from a more focused angle, usually directed through the top of the microphone. If the primary interest in the audio data is to hear and analyze a patient's breathing sounds, a unidirectional microphone will perform best, as extraneous noise within the patient's room will not be sampled. To focus the microphone on the patient, the microphone should be mounted on the wall directly above the head of the patient's bed or on the ceiling directly above the patient's bed. An omnidirectional microphone can be placed practically anywhere, as it will be sampling all sounds within the room.

Just as physiologic data recorded during a sleep study can be processed through the use of frequency filters and amplifier gain, so can the audio data. The easiest way to accomplish audio processing is through the use of an audio mixer, which provides processing functions of signal gain or volume, and frequency equalization typically characterized as bass, midrange, and treble controls (Figure 66-4C). Signal gain or volume controls can be very useful for boosting subtle patient breathing sounds of interest, as well as compensating for low-signal strength caused by long cabling requirements from the patient's room to the control room. Extraneous noise in the patient's room that remains at a constant frequency such as a heating or air-conditioning unit can be filtered out of the audio signal using the equalization controls. Fifty or 60 Hz line interference can be filtered as well. In addition, specific breathing or snoring sounds of particular interest can be focused and boosted using the equalization controls.

Fundamentals of Analog Video/Audio Recording

A conventional analog video system configuration will consist of a camera, microphone, videocassette recorder (VCR), date/time generator, and display monitor. With the exception of the camera and microphone, which are source devices, all other components within the interface chain have signal input and output connections. Analog video/audio systems are rarely used today, as almost all PSG systems currently on the market have built-in digital audiovisual capabilities.

Fundamentals of Digital Video/Audio Recording

Most PSG systems incorporate digital video. Rather than acquiring audiovisual data onto a magnetic tape cassette, the video and audio signals are digitized either at the camera source or at the computer, displayed within a window on a PSG system's computer screen simultaneously with scrolling physiologic data, and stored on digital media such as a hard drive or CD-ROM disc. Using a digital camera that converts the images to digital information within the camera eliminates entirely the analog VCR and monitor requirements and interfaces directly into the computer. However, interfacing the video and audio output signals of a VCR to a computer equipped with a video A/D conversion card can easily digitize an analog video system as well.

In order to adequately acquire and play back digital audio/video data during a PSG, the following minimum computer hardware requirements need to be considered.

1. *Hard disk space:* Minimum of 500 GB. Ideally, 1 TB or more. The minimum space will require relatively frequent archiving of video data because these files are large and will use up the disk space.
2. *RAM:* Minimum of 1 GB (2-3 GB recommended)
3. *Processor speed:* Minimum of 1 GHz. Although audiovisual acquisition has been performed during PSG with slower processors, this minimum recommendation will resolve the "choppy" or fragmented video playback, which is commonly experienced with slower processors.
4. *Monitor resolution:* 15" screen; minimum 1,600 × 1,050 or higher recommended
5. *Analog-to-digital conversion:* This video card will convert incoming video and audio signals from an analog source such as a VCR to digital information to be displayed and stored within the computer.

In general, digitized video in its raw form will utilize a large amount of hard disk space as well as archiving media. For this reason, there are a wide variety of video formats that incorporate degrees of data compression, thereby minimizing disk space requirements. In most cases, digital PSG system manufacturers will determine which format the system will utilize. A specific format will affect not only disk space usage, but also playback quality and editing capabilities. The most common formats are listed in Table 66-1. At the time of this writing, the MPEG-4 format continues to be very popular for its ability to significantly compress the size of raw video files without causing any noticeable effect during playback.

In most cases, digital video acquired during a PSG is viewed in real time on the computer screen and is unaffected by file compression algorithms. It is only during subsequent playback that the compression scheme may be noticeable.

Table 66-1 Common Digital Video File Formats

Suffix	File Type	Features and Limitations
.mov	QuickTime movie	An industry standard developed as part of an entire multimedia architecture by Apple, the QuickTime movie is an open multimedia format, which has multiplatform, multibrowser support.
.asf	ASF	Developed by Microsoft as a multimedia successor to AVI and other individual media file formats, ASF files can contain up to seven media types, including streaming video. ASF is optimized for network distribution and desktop playback.
.avi	AVI (video for Windows)	The precursor to ASF, AVI files are limited to audio and video only.
.mpg	MPEG	MPEG-4 is the latest standard for video compression and file format developed by an industry group.

ASF, advanced streaming format; AVI, audio-video interleave; MPEG, motion picture experts group.

The use of digital video allows significantly more efficient utilization of PSG time synchronization features. Unlike the analog method, which requires time for the VCR to rewind or fast-forward to a point in time identified within the PSG data, a digital system allows very fast seek and playback functionality within the video data.

The PSG time synch feature can also complement the functions of digital video editing. Once a particular video segment of interest is identified, the segment can be removed from the entire raw video file and saved as a separate file, manipulated for contrast and color, or text can be superimposed into the video display. Not only can this be useful for educational presentations, but the segments of interest can be archived for medicolegal purposes, and the rest of the large raw video file can be discarded, significantly reducing the archive media space required.

Comparison of Digital and Analog Methods

There are clear advantages and disadvantages to both digital and analog video methods if only one is used exclusively. As mentioned previously, the user may benefit from using both methods (converting analog signals to digital signals through an A/D conversion card) and therefore enjoy the best of both worlds. However, some features are available only through a commitment to either analog or digital hardware.

Many of the commercially available digital video cameras connect to a computer through a universal serial bus (USB) connection. Since the digital camera actually converts and creates digital information as it is being acquired, there is no need for an A/D or video capture card in the computer. Therefore, the camera can be connected directly to the USB port. A USB connection facilitates very fast data communication, which is beneficial for real-time monitoring during a PSG. In addition, some digital cameras can receive power from the computer via the USB cable, thereby eliminating the external power supply requirement for the camera.

Some digital cameras can connect to a computer via an Ethernet connection. An Ethernet connection is typically used within a LAN to connect different computers and peripheral devices to a network. A digital camera that is designed for Ethernet connectivity will transmit its own IP address to other devices. An IP address is a set of numbers that identifies the device to other computers within a network. This can be beneficial in a sleep center setting, because the camera does not need to be interfaced directly to a specific computer but can be interfaced to any Ethernet entrance into the network (hub, switch, etc). In addition, any other computer connected to the LAN can view the digital video images.

Clearly, one of the more extraordinary differences between analog and video cameras is size. Digital cameras have progressively downsized to where they can very easily be placed in a variety of locations within a sleep center's patient bedroom. This can be advantageous in terms of not only minimizing construction or facility renovation but also "hiding" the camera by mounting it in an inconspicuous location to minimize the patient's awareness of being on camera, which can make sleeping difficult for some patients.

Digital video systems are clearly beneficial in that they lower not only the initial hardware purchase expense but also expenses related to archiving the data. S-VHS videocassettes and video recorders are obsolete. A recordable DVD will hold from 1.46 to 4.7 GB of data, which will allow a large number of video segments to be archived on a single disc. There is clearly a cost advantage to using digital video as opposed to analog. If the PSG system computers are networked to a LAN server, a larger-capacity storage disk (1 TB or greater) available via the network can be used for data archiving, thereby eliminating the requirement for data storage disks.

In many ways, audio/video information acquired during a PSG plays as significant a role in diagnosing sleep disorders as the physiologic PSG data recorded. Video information can assist clinicians with treatment as well, by convincing patients of their symptoms during sleep. Considering the local patient population, referral patterns, facility issues, and physician preferences, the type of video camera, digital hardware, and archiving methods used should be tailored to best meet a particular sleep center's requirements. Digital video acquisition is the current standard. Lower capital costs, lower archiving media and storage space costs, efficient PSG/video time synchronization functionality, and video editing can all be realized through a digital video system. Video equipment used in the sleep center has become smaller and less costly and has become standard in the field of sleep disorders medicine.

Data Storage and Archiving Equipment

Once digital PSG files have been accessed and modified during the analysis, and scoring and report generation procedures completed, the files will continue to reside on the computer's hard drive until they are removed to make space for future recordings. When evaluating computer hardware, consideration should be given to archiving capabilities. Archiving is most commonly accomplished with secure cloud storage for long-term data storage, and many sleep management software systems utilize this method. In addition, the data can also be saved to a portable medium such as a recordable CD (CD-R), DVD (DVD-R), optical disc, or external hard drive. To accomplish this task, the computer tower must have access to drives designed to read and write digital information to varying types of portable media or network access to a server and storage space.

Sleep center PSG computers connected via a LAN to a server that contains a drive with the capacity to store large amounts of data are ideal for archiving PSG and video data. PSG files can simply be moved with a click of a computer mouse to a storage location on the LAN. This archive method eliminates the physical storage space required for portable media and allows a more efficient way to retrieve the files when required.

A number of commercially available digital PSG systems incorporate a software function relating to sleep center operational management that includes patient information database features. Archiving digital PSG files through the system's patient database function can facilitate very efficient and quick retrieval of the data when needed.

SUMMARY

Clearly, the process of establishing a new sleep center or upgrading the instrumentation within an existing sleep center requires careful study and consideration of the sleep center's needs and currently available technology before purchasing equipment. Strategies such as upgrading hardware versus purchasing new, as well as combining new and old technology, can often be utilized to reduce costs. It is essential to understand the general components of the sleep center physical plant, categories of instrumentation used within a sleep center, sensor options, and features common to, or expected to be found in, PSG-related software applications. Attention to the requirements outlined in accreditation standards is also essential in order to perform an accurate assessment of the sleep center's physical layout requirements and hardware and software needs and to adequately evaluate the equipment available.

REFERENCES

1. American Academy of Sleep Medicine. Standards for accreditation. 2025. https://aasm.org/wp-content/uploads/2025/01/Standards-for-Accreditation-1.1.2025-New-Model_Final_Updated11.21.2024-1.pdf
2. Troester MM, Quan SF, Berry RB, et al; for the American Academy of Sleep Medicine. *The AASM Manual for the Scoring of Sleep and Associated Events: Rules, Terminology and Technical Specifications. Version 3*. American Academy of Sleep Medicine; 2023.

Chapter 67
The Manager's Role in a Sleep Center

GERALD GEORGE MANNIKAROTE

KEY CONCEPTS/LEARNING OBJECTIVES

The key concepts for this chapter include an introduction to sleep center management, its importance, and the processes related to effective sleep center management.

KEY TERMS

ADA
Compliance
DOT
Safety

INTRODUCTION

What Is Sleep Center Management?

Management and leadership are similar but different. We will explore both of these topics within this chapter. There will be an emphasis on center management and a short discussion on leadership later on.

What Is Center Management?

Center management can be defined as ensuring the day-to-day functions of the center are moving as smoothly as possible. This means that as a center manager, your job is to ensure the functions of the center are running smoothly.

Why Is Center Management Important?

What is the end goal of a center? It is to complete a sleep study of a patient and get those results to the physician that ordered the study. In order to make this happen, a center must be managed well. Center management is important because it ensures that the end goal of the center is attained without hiccups or at least with the fewest possible issues.

What Are Some of the Goals of Effective Center Management?

Ultimately, the goals of the sleep center are to ensure patient safety and privacy, first and foremost, providing deliverables to all stakeholders (referral sources, investors, management), and a safe and equitable work environment for all team members. Further breakdown of these goals could include:

- Receive and process physician's orders for sleep studies.
- Safely complete the patient's sleep study.
- Get the results of the sleep study to the ordering physician's office.
- Ensure the center maintains compliance with regulatory and accreditation parameters.
- Ensure the center follows proper policies and protocols.
- Ensure the center is properly stocked with all required supplies and materials.
- Maintain a hygienic environment for teammates and, most importantly, patients.
- Follow and maintain proper billing practices.
- Sales, marketing, and promotion of the center

What Are the Various Types of Sleep Centers?

There can be many different types of sleep centers. Each of them has their own individual and nuanced challenges. Overall, however, they are managed in a similar fashion. Some of the different types of centers include:

- Research focused
- Academic
- Mainstream commercial
- DOT (Department of Transportation) focused
- Corporate focused
- Hospital focused

SETTING UP THE SLEEP CENTER

You may, at times, as a manager, be required to develop a sleep center from scratch. When doing so, consider the layout. At times, you may be required to upgrade the current center. Consider the layout in those situations as well. Some things to consider include developing an efficient workflow design. This should accommodate easy movement between patient rooms and the tech areas. Additionally, considerations for Americans with Disabilities Act (ADA) and emergency personnel need to be kept in mind.

Develop areas for specific activities within the center. These could include:

- Area within bedroom/test room for setup
- Clean up area
  - Wet
  - Dry
- Storage area
- Reception
  - Front office
  - Waiting area
- Tech room
- Physician room
- Bathrooms/showers

Equipment Maintenance

You will also encounter times when you will be in charge of acquiring and organizing equipment. When setting up the center from scratch, or upgrading an existing center, you will have to choose the right types of equipment. There will be multiple types of equipment you may be charged to make decisions on. These will include but not be limited to:

- Diagnostic equipment
  - Software/hardware
  - Leads
  - Disposable connecting equipment
    - Conductive paste
    - Preparation scrubs
    - Tape
    - Adhesive remover
- Furniture
  - Murphy bed
  - Standard beds
  - Place for patients to store their personal effects
  - Chairs for patients to sit in during setup
  - Standard office equipment (chairs, desks, filing solutions) for different stations
- Fax and copier logistics
- Linen and linen service
- Maintenance and calibration schedules
- Linen service
- Annual maintenance of center equipment
- Maintenance of accreditation standards
- Equipment maintenance and replacement
  - Regular replacement of leads
  - Updates on diagnostic software
  - Updates on diagnostic hardware

SAFETY AWARENESS AND PROMOTION

You will also need to develop, understand, and maintain a safety plan. Follow the guidelines provided by the accrediting body you choose to follow as well as the local laws and codes. Some of the components of the safety plan may include developing ways to identify hazards and train your teams to identify and address them. The following is a short list of hazards to consider. It is not a comprehensive list but a starting point. Follow local and accreditation body guidelines. If you are affiliated with a larger entity, they may offer guidelines as well.

- Cross contamination
- Trip hazards
- Pathway clearance
- Chemical isolation
- Fire hazard

You must also develop emergency protocols. Follow local and accreditation body guidelines. If you are affiliated with a larger entity, they may offer guidelines as well. Here are some points to consider when developing emergency protocols.

- What to do when there is a patient emergency
- What to do in case of fire or fire alarm
- Overall patient safety
- Overall employee safety
- Accident prevention
- Eye wash station

General safety training is essential for all staff. Follow local and accreditation body guidelines. If you are affiliated with a larger entity, they may offer guidelines as well. Here are some points to consider when developing emergency protocols. The following is a limited example of some of the safety training points for your center.

- Review of fire exits
- Review what to do in various patient situations
  - Unruly patient
  - Patient emergency
- CPR certification
- Activating the emergency system

BUILDING AND DEVELOPING A STRONG TEAM

In order to develop a strong team, it is important to understand the roles and responsibilities. This will directly impact how you develop your team. Once you understand this piece, it will help you identify the right people for the right positions. This will ultimately put you on the road of developing a strong team.

What is the center manager's role in the team? It is vital to remember that the center manager is the team lead. They need to provide direction and guidance to the team to ultimately ensure a smooth flow of daily functions. This does not mean ruling with an iron fist but motivating teams to complete their duties and jobs at their fullest. If you keep this point in mind, you will build a world class team that delivers excellent patient outcomes while achieving goals and objectives as developed by leadership.

Roles can include technicians and technologists, researchers, and support staff roles. The typical team would include the following:

- Front desk
  - This team member will answer phone calls and basic inquiries, schedule patients, and welcome patients and others during the day shift.
- Billing staff
  - These team members would manage the billing of insurance, working with payers, and ensuring revenue cycle. Oftentimes, this is outsourced or completed by another department within the hospital/institution.
- Home sleep test technologist
  - This technologist is responsible for the preparation, cleaning, and distribution of home sleep tests. In most cases they also provide education to the patient regarding the use of the device.
- Daytime technologist
  - This team member typically scores the nighttime studies, builds reports to send to referral sources, follows up with referral sources, answers clinical questions to those inquiring on the phone, and runs daytime studies.
- Night technologist
  - These team members set up patients for nighttime studies, run studies, score, and maintain equipment.
- Salesperson/Marketer
  - This team member will liaison with referral sources to request them to send orders for studies to the center.
- Medical director
  - This team member maintains the medical direction of the center. This includes providing clinical direction and guidance, particularly with policies and procedures.

All of these team members would need to be increased or decreased depending on the volume of business you are dealing with.

Hiring and onboarding is an important part of a manager's role. As a manager, one must ensure that those that are employed in the facility have not only the necessary skills to do the job (or be coachable) but also the right fit for the center. Additionally, you must have people available as backup in case of emergent situations, such as illness, leave of absence, resignation of employees, or termination of employment.

Although skills and qualifications for individual team members are beyond the scope of this chapter, it must be noted that each new hire should interact well with all other team members. They should enhance the culture of the center and not detract from it. If possible, have potential candidates meet current team members to get an idea of how they interact with each other as well as discern how they will fit within the center culture.

The onus of training new hires effectively is on the center manager. Onboarding for each position is vital. Developing onboarding plans for each position should be part of the manager's role. This will ensure there is consistency in processes for anyone that takes on a role within the center. The manager should establish a system, both digital and traditional, of onboarding materials for each position. Develop timelines, objectives, and goals for each role to ensure the new hire is able to perform per the center's standards.

The center manager should encourage collaboration and communication within the teams. Without this, you will have a very disjointed center. Regular communication is vital to the smooth functioning of the center. The manager must be the point person for this. There is a bit of a challenge for the manager as the sleep center is operational both night and day. The manager must be the bridge between multiple shifts. Regular meetings and updates are important. Monthly in-person meetings are a great way to foster good relations among all team members and between the two shifts. These monthly meetings should have center updates, clinical education, any general (not individual) issues, and celebrations of efforts of team members.

ENSURING COMPLIANCE AND SAFETY

A large part of the sleep center manager's responsibility is understanding and adhering to all regulatory requirements. These policies and procedures must follow the regulatory requirements of the governing body that you have chosen to work with (eg, AASM, JACHO, CMS). Additionally, you must be aware of the local, state, and federal regulations for your facility. An example of this would be following local fire safety guidelines.

Be sure to maintain the standards of the accrediting body you are following. Weekly and monthly check-ins are recommended for this. Schedule time in your week and month to ensure you are following accreditation standards. This will also help prepare for reaccreditation.

Record keeping and maintenance is integral to successful center management. Here are some of the records that must be kept in mind for proper center management. This is not a comprehensive list. The list may vary depending on your facility, accrediting bodies, and affiliated entities.

- Patient records are by far the most important part of the records within a center. Proper patient privacy must be maintained for these records. Protocols must be in place for storage and maintenance of both electronic and physical patient records. Accessibility and retrieval must also be kept in mind.
- Recorded studies must be stored and archived. Electronic and physical solutions must be developed for them. Accessibility and retrieval of studies must also be kept in mind.
- There will be quite a bit of inventory for an active center. A regular log must be kept and par levels developed. This will not only ensure that materials are used properly but also facilitate ease of ordering more supplies.
- Medical devices will need to be periodically checked for safety and functionality. Hospital-based facilities have bio-med departments that typically maintain these records. It would still be a good idea to maintain the center's equipment calibration records separately. If not a hospital-based sleep center, be sure to maintain equipment records to ensure that you are following accreditation standards.

Earlier in the chapter, regular compliance check-ins were recommended. This point is reinforced here. Conduct regular compliance and safety check-ins and audits. Let your team know of the importance of maintaining compliance and standards.

MANAGING INVENTORY AND RESOURCES

Tracking and reordering of supplies will be part and parcel of the role of the center manager. An inventory management system needs to be developed. This will help prevent shortages and overstocking. Involve staff on both shifts, day and night, with inventory management. Develop par levels and educate the teams to use them and maintain those logs.

Budgeting and cost control may also come under the purview of the sleep center manager. This would include allocating funds for supplies and maintenance and developing cost-saving strategies. Proper budgeting leads to economic and financial success of this center. And that will ensure the longevity of the center and its ability to serve patients.

Waste management is an important part of center management. As a result, it is part of the sleep center manager's role. As with most facilities, maintain a hazardous waste disposal system. Do not mix hazardous waste with standard waste. Generally speaking, there is very little hazardous waste within a sleep center. However, there are occasions where it may occur. Follow guidelines provided by your accrediting bodies, local authorities, as well as affiliated entities.

MAINTAINING WORKFLOWS AND PRODUCTIVITY

Maintaining workflows and productivity is an essential part of any manager's day-to-day function. It is no different for a sleep center manager. As a leader, setting goals and priorities is a must. If you don't know where you're going, how will you know if you've arrived? This is the reason for developing goals and priorities. In order to maintain good workflows and productivity, it is important to develop goals and priorities. Develop daily, weekly, monthly, and long-term goals. The following is a list of some goals you could use within your center. Consider using these or developing your own.

- Time to have completed reports ready and delivered to referral sources
- Minimum inventory par levels
- Education credits for clinical staff
- Minimum time to return patient calls
- Inter-scorer reliability expectations

Time management techniques are something a manager needs to consider. A center manager will quickly find that they are stretched thin with all the work that is required of them. Good time management practices are required to ensure the manager is able to not only address daily tasks and issues but also maintain good mental and physical health and prevent burnout. It is advisable to refer to one of the various time management books or consider attending a time management course to make the most of your day.

Think about how you can optimize your center's processes. For example, do not overlook technology! The field of sleep technology should embrace all technology. Leverage technology to your advantage. Look at automation tools and software to help you achieve efficiency. Consider the latest developments in artificial intelligence to assist with repetitive tasks. The latest technologies will help you develop a better and more efficient center.

In order to maintain productivity and efficiencies, monitoring progress and performance will be part of the job. Develop key performance indicators (KPIs) for all staff members. This will help you not only measure each team member's performance but also better run the facility efficiently and thereby provide a pleasant experience for your referral sources and, ultimately, the patients you serve.

HANDLING DATA AND TECHNOLOGY

As mentioned earlier, patient data and privacy are of utmost importance. Follow all practices to ensure security of patient data. Be sure to install firewalls for all data systems within the center. Install other security measures to reduce the chances of a security breach. For physical files, maintain a locked filing system. This should be fireproof and difficult to breach.

There are various health care appropriate information management systems available these days. Consider leveraging these technologies for data collection, storage, and protection.

Develop backup protocols for all data, particularly patient data. Cloud services that are compliant with local and federal regulations can be leveraged for this. Explore various backup and security options before settling on a particular system. This will help the center protect sensitive information.

Keep in mind that no system is 100% secure. Be prepared for security breaches and develop protocols for such situations. This is why backup protocols and redundancies are important.

MANAGING RELATIONSHIPS

Earlier in the chapter, we discussed the importance of communication. Keep in mind that open lines will ensure a smooth running of your sleep center. Regular communication will allow all parties to feel they are an integral part of the center. Owners and other parties that may have a financial stake in the center must be communicated with regularly as well.

Consider collaborations with other centers and institutions. If these other institutions have backlogs, overflows, etc, they could leverage your facility and vice versa. Additionally, you can learn from other centers on their practices, education sources, etc.

It is important to engage regularly with clients and, ultimately, patients. Once again, communication is key. Build trust and transparency with your referral sources and your patients. Let them know how your center operates within the standards of your accrediting body of choice. Consider holding an open house for your referral sources.

Address feedback and concerns of both referral sources and patients. Maintain a log of all feedback, good and bad. Include how you have addressed the feedback within the log.

Relationships within your center are very important. This is true whether the team member is seasoned or new to the industry. Extra care must be considered for a newcomer to the field. Different considerations must be kept for those aspiring for growth in the industry.

Be sure to let new or inexperienced team members know that you are there for support when they join your team. As discussed in the onboarding section, set clear objectives and goals. This is the first step in letting new team members know that there is a clear support system in place. Check in with new team members regularly during the onboarding process to provide any additional support needed. Also, consider developing a buddy or mentoring system for new hires.

A good manager encourages professional growth. Monthly meetings, as mentioned before, should have an educational component. Regularly discuss educational opportunities. If there are opportunities for higher level positions, encourage team members to look into them. Identify team members that want growth. Groom them for their next position. At times, growth may be outside your center. Be supportive of your team member's choice to leave the facility to pursue other options.

ADDRESSING CHALLENGES IN SLEEP CENTER MANAGEMENT

Issues are expected to come up in any business or clinic. It is no different in a sleep center. The center manager would be the key person to resolve issues in the sleep center. Develop contingency plans for issues that crop up. It is beyond the scope of this chapter to list all challenges, but a few are listed in what follows.

Be prepared for staff turnover. There is already a known shortage of sleep technologists. As discussed earlier, keep staffing available for such situations. Team members working as needed are great for this.

Illness and emergencies are a part of life. Be sure to have redundancies for these situations. PRN staff, cross training of team members, etc., will help with these situations. A center manager should be able to jump in where needed as well. Do not ever think that any station or role is beneath that of a manager.

Be prepared to face budget constraints from time to time. Based on how the center is funded, a manager is expected to budget funds for procurement of materials and payroll. At times, leadership may change the budget. During those times, crucial decisions must be made. Be prepared for such situations.

At times, the sleep center will come across uncooperative or unruly patients. Protocols must be developed for such situations. Sometimes, these situations must be escalated to the center medical director or other higher level of management, requiring them to deal with the situations directly.

THE CHANGING ROLE OF A SLEEP CENTER MANAGER

In the past, the center manager did many of the tasks that were described earlier: day technologist, front desk, marketer, etc. These days, with the help of technology, the manager has a more specialized role. There is more of a need to understand the role of a leader: developing their center into an example of clinical, economical, and productive excellence. This goes beyond simple day-to-day task management. This calls for vision and some amount of dreaming.

SUMMARY

A Final Word on Leadership

Management and leadership are two different concepts. They are, however, intertwined. To quote two of the most respected names in management and leadership, Peter Drucker and Warren Bennis, "Leadership is doing the right things; management is doing things right."

Let this be your guiding light for your role as a center manager. Don't just be a manager to make sure things are done right. Be a leader and do the right things.

SUGGESTED READINGS

American Association of Sleep Technologists. Sleep center manager/director. Accessed February 15, 2025. https://www.aastweb.org/Career/Sleep-Center-Manager-Director

Bobinski D. The difference between management & leadership. Management-Issues.com. Published February 17, 2004. Accessed February 15, 2025. https://www.management-issues.com/opinion/1125/the-difference-between-management-leadership/

Peek S. P.F. Drucker (Peter Drucker): modern management theory & MBO. Business.com. Accessed February 15, 2025. https://www.business.com/articles/management-theory-of-peter-drucker/

Chapter 68
Sleep Center Policies and Procedures

DOTTIE COVEY-ELLEBY

KEY CONCEPTS/LEARNING OBJECTIVES

The key concepts for this chapter include recognizing the regulatory bodies that require policies and procedures, the difference between a policy and a procedure, describing an alignment continuum, identifying core processes, policies and procedure manuals needed and the relative content, and guidelines for when a policy needs to be written as well as the value of policies and procedures.

KEY TERMS

Accreditation
Accreditation Commission for Health Care
Alignment continuum
American Academy of Sleep Medicine (AASM)
American Association of Sleep Technologists (AAST)
Joint Commission (JC)
Mission statement
Occupational Safety and Health Administration (OSHA)
Strategic plan
Vision

Policies and procedures are essential to management and fundamental to the operation of a sleep center. They are the handbook of operations for managers and employees. They convey the correct work processes for a sleep center that lead to quality services. Everyone needs to know what to do and how to do it. Policies and procedures provide this knowledge for all members of the staff. They include a wide array of applications and vary in degree of specificity. Applications may range from acquisition of supplies to following emergency protocols. Good policies and procedures provide insight into what management believes is important. They define expectations of employees, purpose of these expectations, and consequences of failure to abide by them (1). Consequently, they are used as a measure of employee performance.

Policies and procedures are critical to the evaluation of regulatory compliance because regulatory standards and subsequent levels of compliance are often measured against policies and procedures. The American Academy of Sleep Medicine (AASM) requires specific policies and procedures to be in place for accreditation as do other accrediting organizations such as the Joint Commission (JC) and the Accreditation Commission for Health Care. These organizations set standards for operations and assess compliance for accreditation. When a sleep center is accredited by one of these health care agencies, it is because they have met or exceeded standards of quality imposed on them by these organizations. Reimbursement for services rendered by sleep centers also depends on accreditation, especially Medicare.

There is a difference between policies and procedures, but they go hand in hand. Policies define the standards employed for the strategic direction of operations in order to reach goals. They state management's position on a situation, action, or behavior. They are a set of guidelines and rules. Procedures are the specific processes employed to express policies in action for day-to-day operations and to achieve the standards of an organization, resulting in the highest quality of patient care (2). For the most part, a procedure will serve as an adjunct to policy; however, not every policy will require a written procedure. These documents provide direction, guidance, and accountability and are a reflection of the organization's culture. By utilizing policies and procedures, the sleep center will operate with greater efficiency, and staff members will have a defined sense of purpose.

ALIGNMENT CONTINUUM

Every organization has a reason for its existence, a sense of purpose. When such a purpose is put on paper, it is iterated as a mission statement. Because goals and objectives progress naturally from the knowledge of why an organization exists, a mission statement provides a sense of direction. In the absence of this direction, decisions and their consequences can drive an organization down the road to failure.

A mission statement is the beginning of a policy and procedure manual and serves as a reference to determine the core processes within the written policy. It is the essence of an organization's vision, values, and strategic goals. Writing effective policies and procedures can be challenging if these elements of business have not been defined because the direction of the organization is vague and subsequent management expectations are undefined. The mission of the American Association of Sleep Technologists (AAST), "AAST provides education, resources and advocacy, and leads sleep-care professionals to be the most knowledgeable in the field resulting in the highest quality of care for patients," illustrates this nicely.

Alignment continuum is a term used to describe the relationship between the mission, vision, values, and strategic goals and subsequent core processes. The individual(s) responsible for developing the policy and procedure documents should work to understand the elements of the alignment continuum to ensure continuity with the policies and procedures.

The purpose of the *vision* is to determine whether the direction of the sleep center and its current scope of practice accurately reflect the direction of the organization. The vision captures an organization's purpose and values and embodies the future of the organization. The vision of the AAST, "AAST will play a key role in setting the standard for professional excellence in the evolving practice of sleep healthcare," illustrates this focus on direction.

The *strategic plan* outlines the goals and priorities of the sleep center and assures they are consistent with the direction and focus of the organization. The strategic plan is the road map to accomplish the vision.

Core processes are essential business functions for the organization. There are two types of core processes: operational and clinical. In a sleep center, operational processes establish rules for running the center. Clinical processes regulate patient care. Core processes require a definite course of action or policy. Policies and procedures support these processes and provide a framework for planning, action, and decision-making for management and employees. Many core processes for sleep centers have already been identified, so much so that defined supporting policies and procedures are required for accreditation. For instances where there is no precedent, the process of identifying core processes or essential business functions is necessary.

DEVELOPING POLICY AND PROCEDURE MANUALS

Essential business functions can be determined from areas of management that are included in an organizational chart. The manual title represents one of the organization's essential functions (eg, human resources). If the sleep center is a hospital-based facility, the sleep professional may need to be concerned only with the development of a single manual specific to the operations and core processes of the department. Conversely, a freestanding sleep center typically operates independently, and the sleep professional will need to ensure that manuals for all the essential business functions are developed. Careful consideration needs to be given to the number of business functions identified. The fewer manuals that exist, the easier it will be to manage the set of policies and procedures developed to create a desired outcome. The process of development begins the moment a policy topic is selected and is complete only after the document has been distributed and employees have been trained.

References and resources for developing policy and procedure manuals for a sleep center are available online. They include generic templates and downloadable word documents. There are businesses that assist with or develop policies and procedures for sleep centers, as well as online policy and procedures available from established institutions. The JC provides a "standards sampler" pertaining to sleep centers (3). The more specific resources are those available from the AAST and AASM. The AAST offers a manual of policy and procedure templates for sleep centers and a policy and procedure manual for home sleep apnea testing programs (4). The AASM *Accreditation Reference Manual* (5) was created to assist sleep centers in the development of a policy and procedure manual in conjunction with their accreditation.

Another very important regulatory reference and resource for developing policies and procedures is the United States Department of Labor Occupational Health and Safety (OSH) Act (6). Under the Occupational Safety and Health Administration (OSHA) law, employers are responsible for providing a safe and healthy work environment. No manual is complete without established policies and procedures that are in compliance with the employer responsibilities established by the OSHA.

The format for a manual does not have to be printed paper in three-ring binders. Technology has opened the door to online policy and procedure manuals. An electronic format facilitates management of updating and revising content. It also makes it easier for employees to access information by entering key words (7). Whatever format is used, it must be kept up-to-date and readily available.

Policies

Policies should be written in plain English, without legal jargon, and in sync with the concepts of the mission statement. When properly aligned with the mission statement, policies will enable the vision and direction of the organization. They are more focused than the mission statement and provide the basis for the code of conduct employed internally within the organization and externally with entities outside the organization.

Policies focus on the rules and regulations of the organization. There are operational and clinical policies. In a sleep center, operational policies regulate the manner of functioning of the sleep center. Consider personnel policies as an example, specifically, a policy pertaining to paid time off (PTO). The policy may indicate the criteria necessary to approve PTO requests. It may also specify how PTO hours are accrued, the maximum PTO hours allowed, and/or whether or not PTO hours could be carried over subsequent years. Other operational policies can include:

- Patient acceptance criteria
- Method for tracking direct referrals
- Verification of insurance
- Protecting the privacy and security of patient information
- Scheduling of patients
- Organization of medical charts
- Establishing a quality assurance program and means for monitoring outcomes
- Establishing and maintaining a database
- Dress code for employees
- Recording required employee continuing education
- Requirements for attendance at staff meetings
- Maintenance of equipment and electrical safety

Clinical policies regulate patient care. Examples of clinical policies are:

- Patient education
- Practice parameters for all test protocols
- Administration of oxygen
- When to contact the physician during a sleep study
- Interscorer reliability
- Documentation of patient evaluation/management and positive airway pressure assessments.

Without policy, a recurring situation can take on a life of its own and become "company policy" by virtue of its recurrence; or worse, it may take a life of its own with the refrain, "That's not our policy." Policies are written to clarify the rules of an organization and to ensure a safe, organized, convivial, empowering, and nondiscriminatory workplace for employees and safe, clinically sound environment for patients.

The following guidelines indicate when a policy is needed:

- If the actions of the employees indicate confusion about the most appropriate way to behave (dress codes, e-mail and Internet policies, and cell phone use)
- If guidance is needed about the most suitable way to handle various situations (standards of conduct, travel expenditures, and purchase of sleep center merchandise)
- When needed to protect the sleep center legally (consistent investigation of charges of harassment, nondiscriminatory hiring, and promotion)
- To keep the sleep center in compliance with government policies and laws (eg, American Disabilities Act, Minimum Wage Act, Affordable Care Act)
- To establish consistent work standards, rules, and regulations (progressive discipline, safety rules, break rules, and smoking rules)
- To provide consistent and fair treatment for employees (benefits eligibility, PTO, bereavement time, and jury duty)

There are additional reasons to develop a policy. Remember, one employee's poor behavior does not require a policy that will affect all employees.

Identifying the appropriate individuals to write and approve policy is crucial. In a hospital setting, the human resources department writes the policies that define appropriate behavior of hospital employees and hospital benefits for employees. The department manager writes operational and clinical policies and procedures specifically for the sleep center. Input from the staff members in this process is invaluable. Their involvement assists management in ensuring that all policies needed exist and increases employee compliance. These policies are approved by hospital administration and the medical director. In a freestanding sleep center, the manager writes the policy and the medical director approves it.

Procedures

A procedure details the implementation of a policy. It is a series of steps with a specific order that are sufficiently detailed to guide the performance of the policy.

Figure 68-1 outlines the technologist's role in the process for creating and maintaining a policy and procedure manual.

Sleep Facility Policy and Procedure	
TITLE: Split-Night Study Guidelines	
ORIGINAL DATE:	EFFECTIVE DATE:
REVIEW DATE(s):	REVISION DATE(s):
APPROVAL(s):	
SIGNATURE:	TITLE: Medical Director
SIGNATURE:	TITLE: Sleep Facility Manager
SIGNATURE:	TITLE:

To provide a process to combine the diagnostic and positive airway pressure (PAP) titration portions of the evaluation process. A split-night titration encompasses both continuous PAP and bilevel PAP titration processes.

Split-night studies require that specific requirements are met during the diagnostic portion of the study in order to initiate PAP therapy. Technologists must fit the PAP interface and perform patient teaching prior to lights out, explaining to the patient that PAP therapy may be instituted during the night if the requirements for a split-night study procedure are met.

This policy provides the American Academy of Sleep Medicine (AASM) guidelines for initiating PAP during a diagnostic study and Centers for Medicare and Medicaid Services (CMS) requirement for initiating PAP for home use. The sleep facility medical director may designate adjustments in criteria indicated below.

AASM criteria for initiating PAP during a diagnostic study:
A minimum of 2 hours of diagnostic recording is required.
A minimum of 3 hours of titration time is required.
The titration procedure should be identical to the full night titration protocol.
PAP may be increased at larger increments (2 to 2.5 cm H_2O) during a split-night titration.
Initiate PAP when an apnea–hypopnea index (AHI) >40 per hour is documented during 2 hours of diagnostic recording time OR when an AHI of 20 to 40 per hour is documented and is accompanied by clinical symptoms.

CMS criteria for initiating PAP for home use:
AHI or respiratory disturbance index is >15 events per hour, with a minimum of 2 hours for sleep time OR
AHI is <14 accompanied by clinical symptoms including:

• Excessive daytime sleepiness		
• Impaired cognition	OR	• Hypertension
• Mood disorder		• Ischemic heart disease
• Insomnia		• History of stroke

References
1. Department of Health and Human Services & Centers for Medicare & Medicaid Services. (2016, October). *Positive airway pressure (PAP) devices: Complying with documentation & coverage requirements*.
2. Kapur VK, Auckley DH, Chowdhuri S, et al. (2017). Clinical practice guideline for diagnostic testing for adult sleep obstructive apnea: An American Academy of Sleep Medicine clinical practice guideline. *Journal of Clinical Sleep Medicine, 13*(3), 479–504.
3. Medicare Coverage with Evidence Development 1/240.4/ Continuous Positive Airway Pressure (CPAP) Therapy of Obstructive Sleep Apnea (OSA) (March 18, 2015).

Figure 68-1 Sample policy and procedure.

Policies and procedures provide specific instructions for employees. Well-written procedure documents state explicitly who is supposed to do what and how it is to be done. Consequently, there is less room for misunderstanding and subsequent discord. When misunderstandings occur, and disparity exists between employees or between an employer and employee, policies and procedures provide a reference for clarification and problem-solving. Sometimes, legal resolution of a situation is needed. The first course of action to be pursued by legal counsel in a labor dispute is a review of the policies and procedures. Employees are required to read the entire policy and procedure manual and sign a statement saying they have done so, which will avoid confusion later.

A policy and procedure manual is a reference manual that answers employees' questions. In the sleep center environment, a staff technologist is responsible for data acquisition, patient titrations, and data analysis (scoring). When procedures are communicated to those involved, processes can begin to ensure compliance and accountability for assigned responsibilities.

Policies and procedures define roles and responsibilities and complement the performance expectations outlined in a program's job descriptions. The role of management becomes more efficient when written guidance and direction are established and communicated for operations that occur on an ongoing basis. They give employees defined expectations of their employer.

SUMMARY

Great sleep centers do not just happen, nor do they just stay great. The successful sleep center is made up of individually successful people who do the right things at the right time under the right circumstances. Policies and procedures provide direction for decisions that are made by management and the parameters within which employees can make appropriate judgments. They are a set of documents that establish guidelines for operations, facilitate training of employees, provide a resource for decision-making, and promote consistency in delivery of services. Effective policies and procedures are critical to developing competent technical staff, building professionalism, and creating and maintaining a successful sleep center.

REFERENCES

1. Bizfluent. What is the difference between a policy & a procedure? Published 2018. Accessed April 26, 2025. https://bizfluent.com/about-5100532-difference-between-policy-procedure.html
2. University of Wisconsin-Madison Policy Library. Is it a policy, procedure, or guideline. Published 2024. Accessed April 26, 2025. https://development.policy.wisc.edu/2022/06/01/is-it-a-policy-procedure-or-guideline/
3. The Joint Commission. Applicable standards for diagnostic sleep centers. Published 2025. Accessed April 26, 2025. https://digitalassets.jointcommission.org/api/public/content/2834e716c8c943f381ef3e6d7001d249?v=210a55ce
4. American Association of Sleep Technologists. Published 2018. Accessed January 18, 2019. https://members.aastweb.org/page/online-store
5. American Academy of Sleep Medicine. Standards for accreditation. Published 2018. Accessed April 26, 2025. https://aasm.org/wp-content/uploads/2025/01/Standards-for-Accreditation-1.1.2025-New-Model_Final_Updated11.21.2024-1.pdf
6. Occupational Safety and Health Administration. Employer responsibilities. Published 2018 Accessed April 26, 2025. https://www.osha.gov/as/opa/worker/employer-responsibility.html
7. Hamlett C. How to write an office procedures manual. Bizfluent. Published 2017. Accessed April 26, 2025. https://bizfluent.com/how-6241242-write-office-procedures-manual.html

Chapter 69

Ethics and Professionalism for Sleep Health Professionals

ROBYN V. WOIDTKE

KEY CONCEPTS/LEARNING OBJECTIVES

The key concepts for this chapter include a review of the concepts of professionalism and how the sleep professional is viewed in the field of allied health, discusses the contributions of the sleep professional and the educational aspects of a profession, and assesses the implications of social media use for the sleep professional.

KEY TERMS

Competency
Ethics
Professionalism
Social media

The field of sleep technology is constantly evolving. Technological advances in home sleep testing, wearables, nearables (consumer sleep technology), artificial intelligence, and machine learning provide new possibilities for scoring sleep-related data, and new treatment options are emerging. Patient personal health information uploads may create vulnerability to data breaches and cybersecurity concerns. Social media has the potential to distribute misinformation regarding sleep health. Also, changes in health care delivery models and insurance may create a conundrum of difficult choices that might conflict with putting the patient first, which is the health care provider's role.

The complexity of these new advances in our field and elsewhere can impact professional conduct and ethical standards, including social media posts. Although the landscape has changed, the need for professionalism and ethical behavior has not. For those working in this field, the main focus remains unwavering: we watch and monitor individuals while they sleep in the sleep laboratory or view data from home sleep testing, and we provide patient-centered care, education, and support throughout the patient journey. Professionalism and ethical conduct must be considered the highest priority at each encounter.

PROFESSIONALISM IN HEALTH CARE

Professionalism—the term is rather generic; however, professionalism encompasses an array of concepts. Professionalism and behavior go hand in hand, whether at work or otherwise. The health care professional has a societal responsibility and a "contract" with the public to do no harm and treat patients with humanity, grace, respect, and kindness.

Professionalism is not exclusive to an individual, and organizational professionalism can directly impact patient care and staff's ability to act professionally and ethically (1). In 2017, the Association of American Medical Colleges published its charter on organizational professionalism. The committee comprised of nurses, physicians, organizational leaders, and others. This document provides a path for organizations to follow and considers the impact of organizations on individual professionalism. In short, organizations have a duty to provide a structure to promote and secure professionalism for those under their auspices. Additionally, the document states that organizations also have a responsibility to patients and the communities in which they provide care. Although there are barriers to achieving this standard, organizations would do well to embody the recommendations of this charter (1).

Many words and concepts can be used to define professionalism within a health profession; however, a common thread of words is found across the literature, as summarized in Figure 69-1. The American Medical Association also highlights that a care provider must also care for themselves to provide the most competent service to their patients (2).

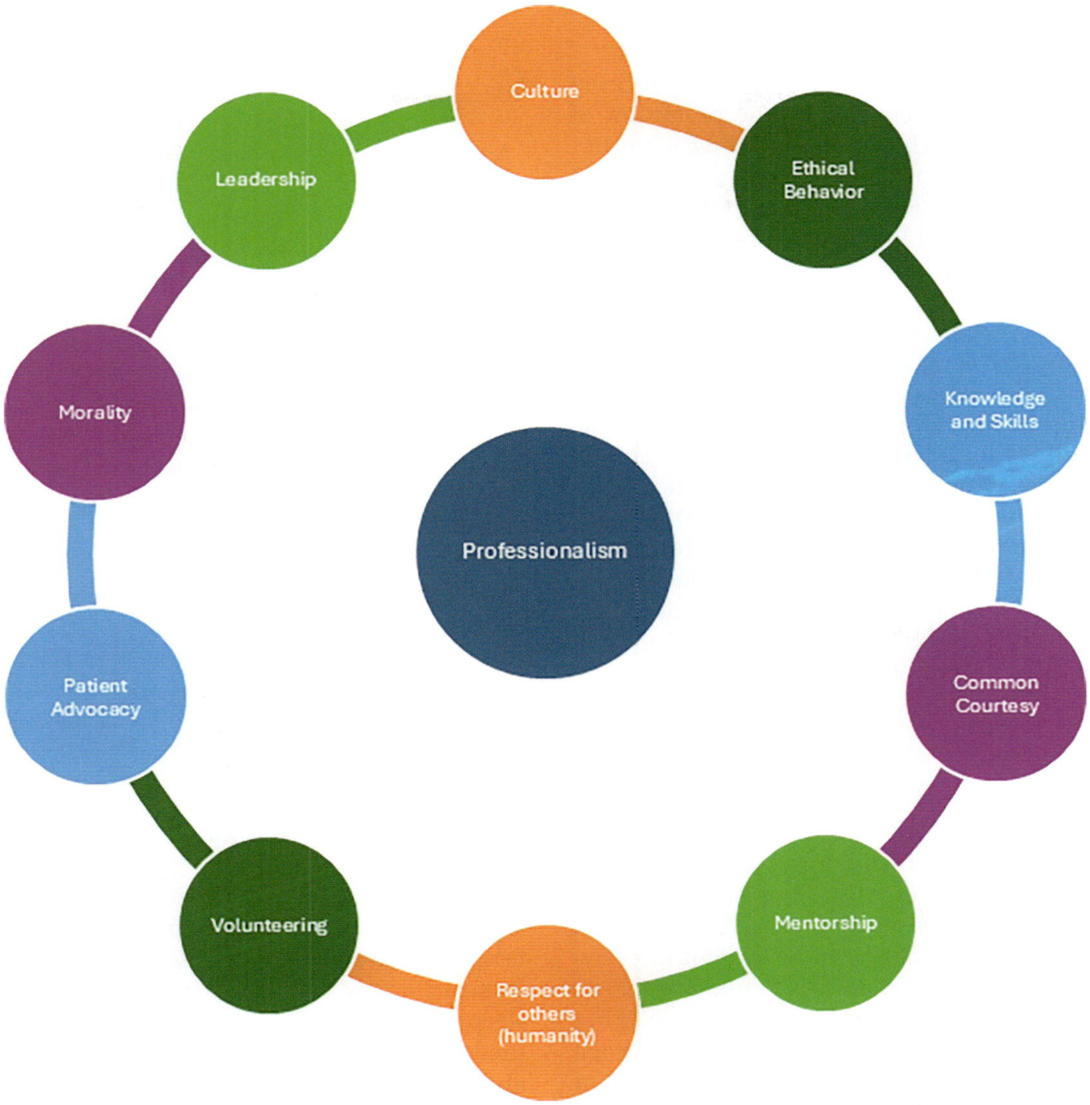

Figure 69-1 Components of professionalism.

COLLABORATION

As professionals in roles such as sleep technology, nursing, respiratory therapy, and other allied health fields working with patients with sleep-related problems, we experience a unique perspective on patients' lives. The professionals in sleep health roles are trained to look at a component of life that is often forgotten—sleep! (3). This fact is essential as many medical specialties address a variety of medical disorders but may not include sleep in their assessments. Sleep health and associated disorders in other medical specialty areas are vital to good health care, and sleep health professionals can be a wonderful resource in collaborative care. This is just one component of professionalism. Collaboration is one form of high ethical patient care (4).

PUBLIC HEALTH

In 2006, the Institute of Medicine (5), published their seminal book on sleep disorders and sleep deprivation. This publication points out that sleep and associated disorders are considered a public health issue. Almost 20 years later, this continues to be the case as is substantiated by increased research and practice. In addition to the provision of clinical care, sleep professionals must also not only understand and recognize professionalism from a personal perspective but also need to have an appreciation of how their professionalism is encompassed within the field of sleep medicine as part of a health care team and organization and the public at large. Professionalism is a foundation of patient care, community, and professional relationships.

ETHICS IN HEALTH CARE

Although the Belmont Report (6) was initially focused on ethical practices for research for the protection of human subjects and specifically defines clinical practice as differing from research, the principles of this document can be applied to everyday practice. The primary constructs of the Belmont Report are respect for persons, beneficence, and justice. As part of respect for persons, the individual has autonomy to make their own decisions and individuals who lack capacity are protected from undue harm. The term beneficence essentially means doing no harm, but, additionally, the provider should strive to maximize the benefits of treatment. The last is justice. The concept of justice includes the idea that people should be treated equally. Applying these principles such as informed consent and autonomy in everyday work means that patients should be treated with appropriate care and treatment. They should be offered understandable information, enabling them to make decisions regarding their health care, including risks and benefits, and be allowed to evaluate if the recommended care is the right option for them and their circumstances (7).

SUM OF MANY PARTS

Professionalism is the sum of many parts—personal experience, culture, religion, education, skills, ethics and morality, and a sense of altruism. Professional behaviors extend beyond the job; they must be evident in everything we do and conduct ourselves (Table 69-1). The American Association of Sleep Technologists (AAST) has provided the sleep professional community with a scope of practice position statement. Although professionalism is not explicitly mentioned, the document provides the sleep technologist with a foundation of behaviors and skills that form the profession (see additional resources).

Professionalism can also lead to improved patient satisfaction. This is important on many levels. When patients have a good experience, they are more likely to feel confident and more trustful of the people who care for them; thus, when a technologist embodies professionalism and greets a patient, educates them, and treats them with respect and dignity, the patient and facility both reap the rewards (8).

The professional conduct practiced by thousands of sleep professionals is ongoing proof that, as individuals and an organization of allied health care workers, they have endorsed a high level of ethical and responsible conduct and understand what that means to how they practice daily.

Being a professional also means contributing to your field by volunteering, patient advocacy, leading, and engaging in educational and organizational pursuits and scholarship (9). The contributions that sleep professionals have made to the field of sleep medicine are incalculable and should not be discounted. Without the sleep technologist, many of the techniques that are now used would not exist, and our knowledge about sleep and its many disorders would not be as complete. Together with physicians and scientific teams, technologists have made significant inroads into understanding sleep and its disorders.

Sleep technologists have determinedly participated in grassroots efforts, including obtaining funding and initiating legislative activities, to ensure their right to practice as sleep professionals is preserved. Outside of the sleep laboratory, sleep professionals have continued to contribute to the education of legislators, teachers, and those in other health-related fields. Some of these activities include organizing and participating in local, state, and national efforts toward the recognition of sleep disorders as a significant health problem. Sleep professionals are ongoing advocates of patient education and awareness. Patient advocacy by technologists' continuing commitment is demonstrated by the numerous local activities in education and awareness of sleep-related topics in their respective communities.

Our activities and those of our professional associations demonstrate that the field of sleep technology

Table 69-1 Categories of Professional Behavior With Examples

Altruism	**Contributes to the profession; helps others in the workplace**
Honor and integrity	Forthcoming with information; does not withhold information for power; admits errors
Responsibility and accountability	Accountable for deadlines; arrives on time; takes responsibility for their share of the workload
Excellence in scholarship	Masters techniques and technologies in learning; has internal focus and direction; setting own goals
Respect	Respects patients and staff; demonstrates tolerance for a range of behaviors and beliefs
Leadership	Teaches others; perpetuates a culture of professionalism
Caring and compassion	Treats the patient as an individual; supports a balance between work and home with peers and subordinates

Used with permission from NBME.

is indeed a profession whose members meet high standards of behavior and competence and are indeed professionals. We are bound together by our skills and abilities to watch while others sleep, to make appropriate clinical decisions, and to conduct ourselves appropriately. Sleep technologists possess the skills required of professionals, including clinical competence, effective communication skills, and ethical decision-making regarding the patients' best interest. Their ongoing desire for excellence, ensuring the utmost in quality, and compassionate and knowledgeable care of the patients they serve will enhance the ability of the profession of sleep technology to mature and remain sustainable into the future. Professionalism is not stagnant; we must continue to learn from our successes and mistakes and put into action the lessons we have learned.

Standards of Conduct for Registered Polysomnographic Technologists

The standards of conduct for registered polysomnographic technologists are located on the Board of Registered Polysomnographic Technologists' (BRPT) website and consist of five sections (10). These standards focus on ethics, customs, competency, and the law and include sections that address responsibilities to the patient and responsibilities of the technologist to their profession, including dignity, solicitation, and examination. The code of conduct also addresses the relationship of the technologist to other caregivers to include working collegially and ensuring that care is given appropriately and ethically. The final section of the standards discusses the technologist's appropriate use of their credential. The standards of conduct apply to the range of certifications the BRPT offers.

Although the BRPT is not a membership organization, it still provides the foundation for maturing and the ongoing development and sustainability of the profession. Nevertheless, the organization offers an infrastructure that defines the profession; however, it is up to the individual to exercise professional competence, which is a component of professionalism. A commitment to the field is accomplished through continuing education, recertification, and ongoing demonstration of competency and daily on-the-job conduct.

Social Media Use

As sleep professionals, we are all aware of the possibility that untrained and misguided individuals may cause health misinformation to be disseminated on the internet. This fact was demonstrated during the COVID pandemic, when misinformation was rampant (1). Such misinformation can cause undue harm to people. The article by Nelson et al (11) explains that social media contributed to increased death and morbidity because of misleading claims. It is important for the sleep professional to discover between truth and fiction and be a voice of reason regarding sleep health should that conundrum present itself. A good resource from the United States Health and Human Services entitled *Confronting Health Misinformation* can be a useful tool for patients and sleep professionals alike (2). In addition, there must be a clear distinction between personal and professional content and treating colleagues with respect and care (Table 69-2).

Table 69-2 Common Guidelines for the Use of Social Media by Health Care Professionals

Context	Concept
Content credibility	Share only information from credible sources. Refute any inaccurate information you encounter.
Legal concerns	Remember that the content you author may be discoverable. Comply with federal and state privacy laws. Respect copyright laws.
Licensing concerns	Know professional licensure requirements for your state.
Networking practices	Do not contact patients with requests to join your network. Direct patients who want to join your personal network to a more secure means of communication or to your professional site.
Patient care	Avoid providing specific medical advice to nonpatients. Make appropriate disclosures and disclaimers regarding the accuracy, timeliness, and privacy of electronic communications.

Table 69-2 Common Guidelines for the Use of Social Media by Health Care Professionals (*continued*)

Context	Concept
Patient privacy	Avoid writing about specific patients. Make sure you are in compliance with state and federal privacy laws. Obtain patient consent when required. Protect patient information through "deidentification." Use a respectful tone when discussing patients.
Personal privacy	Use the most secure privacy settings available. Keep personal and professional profiles separate.
Professional ethics	Disclose any in-kind or financial compensation received. Do not make false or misleading claims.
Self-identification	Identify yourself on professional sites. Make sure that your credentials are correctly stated. Specify whether or not you are representing an employer.

Reprinted with permission from Ventola CL. Social media and health care professionals: benefits, risks, and best practices. *P T*. 2014;39(7):491-499.

THE TEACHING OF PROFESSIONALISM

The American Board of Pediatrics provides an excellent resource for individuals in teaching and leadership roles in health care regarding professionalism (3). Although the focus is on pediatricians, the lessons apply to all and are readily accessible at the time of this writing. The various chapters touch on these topics. The chapter on professionalism and patient care was particularly insightful for the sleep professional and discussed commitments and competencies. Tables 69-3 and 69-4 provide a list of these topics (see additional resources).

SUMMARY

In summary, the importance of professionalism for individuals working in the sleep health profession cannot be overstated. Since professionalism is not just one idea or component, including behavior, it is essential to realize how they intertwine. It is good, from time to time, to review and make individual assessments of how we conduct ourselves professionally and personally. The ultimate goal is to be a patient servant and do the best we can to achieve the best health and well-being for the patients and their families ethically and professionally.

Table 69-3 Commitments for Professionalism

Commitments	Summary
Commitment to professional competence	Lifelong learning, maintaining clinical acumen and working team skills
Commitment to honesty with patients	Being truthful with patients and providing them with information to be able to understand their condition and treatment as prescribed
Commitment to patient confidentiality	Safeguarding patient personal information and understanding the laws surrounding the public good
Commitment to maintaining appropriate relations with patients	Sleep technologists take care of patients when they are most vulnerable and should be of the utmost concern.
Commitment to improving quality of care	Staying up to date with the literature and working with organizations and colleagues to provide patient safety should include the public health arena.

From American Board of Pediatrics. Education and Training Committee. Teaching, promoting and assessing professionalism across the continuum: a medical educator's guide. https://www.abp.org/professionalism-guide Used with permission.

Table 69-4 Competencies for Professionalism

Patient care	**Provide education, supporting guidance and understanding of the social determinants of health regarding sleep and associated disorders.**
Practice-based learning	Identify strengths and areas for improvement in practice, partake in personal and professional development, and participate in education regarding sleep health, including other health care providers and patients and their families.
Interpersonal and communication skills	Develop insight into the human response, learn communication techniques such as TeachBack and motivational interviewing.
Professionalism	Cultural competency, humanism, and professional conduct
Systems-based practice and improvement	Continuous quality enhancement, assessing current practices, maintain cost effectiveness
Personal and professional development	Demonstrate self-confidence regarding your skills and knowledge and exhibit trustworthiness to patients and colleagues.

From American Board of Pediatrics. Education and Training Committee. Teaching, promoting and assessing professionalism across the continuum: a medical educator's guide. https://www.abp.org/professionalism-guide Used with permission.

ADDITIONAL RESOURCES

Office of the Surgeon General. *Confronting Health Misinformation*. U.S. Department of Health and Human Services. https://www.hhs.gov/surgeongeneral/reports-and-publications/health-misinformation/index.html

The American Board of Pediatrics. Teaching, promoting, and assessing professionalism across the continuum: a medical educator's guide. https://www.abp.org/professionalism-guide/toc

REFERENCES

1. Egener BE, Mason DJ, McDonald WJ, et al. The charter on professionalism for health care organizations. *Acad Med*. 2017;92(8):1091-1099. doi:10.1097/ACM.0000000000001561
2. Staff News Writer. The top 10 ethical issues medical students should be taught. American Medical Association. Accessed February 8, 2025. https://www.ama-assn.org/education/changemeded-initiative/top-10-ethical-issues-medical-students-should-be-taught
3. Kurtz MJ, Starbird LE. Interprofessional clinical ethics education: the promise of cross-disciplinary problem-based learning. *AMA J Ethics*. 2016;18(9):917-924. doi:10.1001/journalofethics.2016.18.9.nlit1-1609
4. Grandner MA, Malhotra A. Sleep as a vital sign: why medical practitioners need to routinely ask their patients about sleep. *Sleep Health*. 2015;1(1):11-12. doi:10.1016/j.sleh.2014.12.011
5. Colten HR, Altevogt BM, Institute of Medicine (US) Committee on Sleep Medicine and Research, eds. *Sleep Disorders and Sleep Deprivation: An Unmet Public Health Problem*. National Academies Press (US); 2006.
6. U.S. Department of Health and Human Services. The Belmont Report. 1979. https://www.hhs.gov/ohrp/regulations-and-policy/belmont-report/read-the-belmont-report/index.html
7. Varkey B. Principles of clinical ethics and their application to practice. *Med Princ Pract*. 2021;30(1):17-28. doi:10.1159/000509119
8. Brennan MD, Monson V. Professionalism: good for patients and health care organizations. *Mayo Clin Proc*. 2014;89(5):644-652. doi:10.1016/j.mayocp.2014.01.011
9. Strkljevic I, Tiedemann A, Souza de Oliveira J, Haynes A, Sherrington C. Health professionals' involvement in volunteering their professional skills: a scoping review. *Front Med (Lausanne)*. 2024;11:1368661. doi:10.3389/fmed.2024.1368661
10. Board of Registered Polysomnographic Technologists. Standards of conduct. Accessed February 9, 2025. https://www.brpt.org/ethics/standards-of-conduct/
11. Nelson T, Kagan N, Critchlow C, Hillard A, Hsu A. The danger of misinformation in the COVID-19 crisis. *Mo Med*. 2020;117(6):510-512.

Chapter 70
Coding, Billing, and Regulatory Compliance

KATHRYN HANSEN

KEY CONCEPTS/LEARNING OBJECTIVES

The key concepts for this chapter include defining regulatory compliance as it applies to billing and coding of procedures performed in the sleep center, reviewing coding guidelines used for billing sleep diagnostic procedures, and describing preauthorization requirements that impact sleep center approval processes. Case studies are presented to demonstrate the implementation of regulatory compliance, and coding and billing constructs that impact revenue integrity.

KEY TERMS

Common procedural technology (CPT)
Conditions of Participation (CoP)
Diagnostic related grouping (DRG)
Financial responsibility
Healthcare Common Procedure Coding System (HCPCS)
Informed consent
Insurance contracts
International Classification of Diseases 10th Revision Clinical Modifications (ICD-10 CM)
International Classification of Sleep Disorders, third edition (*ICSD-3TR*)
Modifiers

Medical insurance plays an important role in the financial well-being of every health care business. The regulatory environment of medical insurance is evolving faster than ever because of the introduction of Benefits Management Programs, which are mandated to keep control over escalating health care costs through the preauthorization and preapproval processes that have become a normal operational requirement in recent years. These changes have introduced more challenges to maintaining our volume and revenue. As a result, health care professionals must be familiar with the rules and guidelines of each health plan in order to submit proper documentation to assure payment. Always refer to the most current policies and regulatory guidelines related to coding and billing for each geographic region or country. This familiarity begins with the knowledge of insurance basics.

WHAT IS MEDICAL CODING?

Medical coding is a system of number and letter labels that are unique for each diagnosis, symptom, or symptom set, which is used to track prevalence of diseases and associated diagnoses. Additionally, codes are used for standard communication of procedures used in the treatment of diseases with subsequent treatments. Therefore, accurate medical coding is important for submission of billing claims and in tracking statistics for disease and medical treatment.

Correct coding of the medical claim is essential to obtain insurance reimbursement as well as maintain patient records. Coding claims accurately convey to the insurance payer and other health care entities a standardized reporting of the patient illness or injury and the method of diagnosis and/or treatment.

Medical coding involves using one or more of the following types of codes:

1. International Classification of Diseases (ICD) codes are used to standardize the reporting of diagnoses, symptoms, and causes of health condition in humans into specific categories with approved code sets using numbers and letters to characterize the diseases. Currently, the manual is the 10th revision for clinical modification.
   The World Health Organization (WHO) creates, copyrights, and oversees these classifications, which are recognized by every medical facility and practitioner worldwide. In the United States,

the National Center for Health Statistics, which is a part of the Centers for Medicare and Medicaid Services (CMS), manages any amendments to the ICD codes alongside the WHO (1).

2. *International Classification of Sleep Disorders*, third edition (*ICSD-3*) codes provide specific information on sleep disorders, including diagnostic criteria, essential features, and objective findings. The American Academy of Sleep Medicine (AASM) creates, copyrights, and maintains these classifications, which are used primarily by sleep specialists. The *ICSD-3* references appropriate *ICD-10* codes for the sleep disorders identified in this manual (2).
3. Common Procedural Technology (CPT) codes are a five-digit number or a four-digit number with one alpha character assigned to every procedure and service, which medical practitioners include in documentation to designate a medical, surgical, or diagnostic service. These codes are used by third-party payers to determine the amount of reimbursement that a practitioner will receive from the payer for the service. They are standardized to define the specific elements of the procedure to describe the same procedure across all providers with the intent of creating uniformity in billing (3).
4. CPT codes are developed, maintained, and copyrighted by the American Medical Association (AMA). They are Level I codes, which means they are used for procedures and services usually provided by physicians or other approved licensed clinical providers, such as nurse practitioners, physician assistants, and doctors of osteopathy. As the practice of health care changes, new codes are developed for new services; current codes may be revised; and old, unused codes are retired. Thousands of codes are in use and are updated annually (3).
   To search for a CPT code and its description, these options are available:
   a. Purchase the CPT manual from the AMA, which is a comprehensive listing of all CPT and Level I codes.
   b. Perform a CPT code search on the AMA website by registering (for free) for five searches per day. This allows a limited search for a CPT code or the use of a keyword to identify the associated CPT code description.
   c. Contact the referring doctor's office to request the CPT codes and services requested for the patient.
   d. Contact the payer's billing manual or benefits specialists to obtain clarification of the code and description associated with the procedure.
5. Healthcare Common Procedure Coding System (HCPCS) is a set of codes used and maintained by the CMS and used for billing Medicare, Medicaid, and many other third-party payers. If you are billing a Medicare claim, an HCPCS code will be reported in your paperwork. These are considered Level II codes, which cover health care services and procedures that are not provided by physicians. Examples of items billed with Level II codes are medical equipment, supplies, and home sleep apnea testing (HSAT) for Medicare beneficiaries such as G0399. HCPCS Level II codes start with a letter and have four numbers. A modifier attached to the code, consisting of either two letters or a letter and a number, may be required for coding integrity. The coding guidelines will reflect the need for an additional modifier, which is generally cross-referenced in the description of the code, or in a paragraph preceding the specific coding chapter or section in the manual (4).
   To search for an HCPCS Level II code and its description, these options are available:
   a. Purchase the current HCPCS manual
   b. Search the CMS website: https://www.cms.gov/Medicare/Coding/HCPCSReleaseCodeSets/Alpha-Numeric-HCPCS.html
   c. Complete a web search online.
6. Diagnostic Related Grouping (DRG) codes are used by Medicare and some other third-party payers to categorize hospitalization costs and determine how much to pay for a patient's hospital stay. Rather than paying the hospital for what it spent caring for a hospitalized patient, Medicare pays the hospital a fixed amount based on the patient's DRG or diagnosis. Essentially, the DRG-based payment means that if a patient admitted to the hospital is treated for less money than the DRG payment, a profit is associated with that admission. Likewise, the opposite is true: if the patient care expenses for the same admission are more than the DRG payment, the facility loses money.
   Therefore, instead of paying for each day the patient is hospitalized and each procedure completed, Medicare pays a single amount based on the DRG, which is based on the diagnosis(es), age, and gender of the patient. Each DRG is grouped into a category of clinically similar diagnoses, which require similar resources and care to treat.
7. Modifiers are additional two-digit numbers, two-letter numbers, or alphanumeric characters used with the CPT and HCPCS codes to convey additional information about the procedure being billed. They may be used to identify a change in the procedure or multiple procedures completed

in the same patient encounter. For instance, if a procedure is discontinued before the completion of the required monitoring time, a modifier is appended to the CPT code to describe reduced services.

KEY MODIFIER FACTS

a. Inappropriate use of modifiers can cause a delay or reduction in payment in the same manner as use of an inappropriate CPT code.
b. For a complete list of modifiers, turn to Appendix A of the CPT manual.
c. Append modifiers only according to individual insurance payer guidelines.
d. Modifier use is different for services provided by licensed providers as opposed to the technical services.
e. Modifier use may be different for services provided in the physician practice compared with those provided in the hospital. These requirements are included in the insurance agreement, a document called the Conditions of Participation (CoP).

Knowledge of these coding tools is important for communication and billing purposes. The use of coding in all types of medical practice is not only important but also imperative because commercial insurance payers, Medicare, Tricare, and Medicaid, will not pay a claim if it is not properly submitted with acceptable diagnosis(es) and procedure codes.

CODES FOR BILLING PROCEDURES PERFORMED

It is time to define the details associated with coding for procedures performed in all monitoring settings.

CPT procedure codes 95800 through 95811 are utilized for diagnostic sleep testing services, which include coding for both sleep studies and polysomnography (PSG). The respective definitions of these two levels of service are provided in the introduction to the Medicine Chapter of the CPT manual.

They are defined as continuous and simultaneous monitoring and recording of multiple physiologic and pathophysiologic parameters for a minimum of 6 hours of monitoring, which includes the physician's review, interpretation, and reporting of the findings. The monitoring time starts with "lights out" and ends with "lights on." It does not include the time spent completing questionnaires or the time to apply and remove all monitoring sensors (3).

In 2013, two monitoring codes were added to expand coding and differentiate coding for adult and pediatric sleep monitoring:

1. 95782—younger than 6 years; diagnostic study that requires a documentation of greater than or equal to 7 hours' monitoring time
2. 95783—younger than 6 years; positive airway pressure study that requires a documentation of greater than or equal to 7 hours' monitoring time (3)

Table 70-1 provides a summary of the CPT codes and their respective descriptions for polysomnograms and sleep studies completed in the sleep center as well as those used for HSAT (5). A more detailed discussion on HSAT is available in Chapter 40.

For appropriate billing, these codes must include documentation of the required hours of monitoring time. If less time is reported on the scoring summary sheet, a modifier 52 should be appended to the procedure code to indicate that a reduced service was provided and that the reason for the shortened study is unrelated to the patient's clinical condition or a physician's decision to terminate the study. Appending a 52 modifier will result in the study being paid at a reduced reimbursement. Typically, the reimbursement in this case is one-half of the customary payment. Documentation on the technologist's notes as to the reason for the reduced services is important, because this is to be correlated in the interpretation of the study.

On occasion, during a study, the patient develops a clinical change such as shortness of breath, cardiac arrhythmia, severe headache, or unilateral numbness or weakness. These signs and symptoms may represent an emergency condition, which requires transfer to another level of care and hence a termination of the study before the required monitoring time. Confirmation with a provider supports the need for transfer to another service such as the emergency room. These clinical changes may require initiation of cardiopulmonary resuscitation. In this situation, a modifier 53 is appended to the procedure code, indicating that the study was terminated early because of the patient's condition, as ordered by a licensed clinical provider. Again, documentation in the technologist's notes is critical for inclusion in the interpretation.

In 2008, CMS created HCPCS codes or G-codes (G0398, G0399, and G0400) to describe HSAT services. These codes can be found in the HCPCS Level II codebook and on the CMS website.

Some Medicare contractors and third-party payers will require the use of G-codes and will not accept CPT codes when reporting HSAT. The criteria for use of the appropriate codes for non-Medicare claims may be found in the insurance company's Internet Only Manual or in the CoP associated with the insurance contract for the respective insurance companies.

Table 70-1 Common Procedural Technology Codes for Sleep Studies

Codes Associated With Type of Monitoring	Description of CMS Classification for Type of Monitoring
95810 95811	Type I PSG is an adult-attended study performed in a sleep center using sleep staging in addition to EEG, EOG, ECG/heart rate, chin EMG, limb EMG, respiratory effort at thorax and abdomen, nasal and oral airflow and positive airway pressure as indicated, which requires at least 6 h of monitoring.
95782 95783	Type I PSG is an attended study performed in a sleep center using sleep staging in addition to EEG, EOG, ECG/heart rate, chin EMG, limb EMG, respiratory effort at thorax and abdomen, nasal and oral airflow in a patient younger than 6 y, which requires at least 7 h of monitoring.
95805	Multiple sleep latency or maintenance of wakefulness testing, recording, analyzing, and interpreting physiologic measurements of sleep during multiple trials to assess a degree of sleepiness when compared with the ability to remain alert
G0398	HSAT with type II portable monitor, unattended; minimum of seven channels: EEG, EOG, EMG, ECG/heart rate, airflow, respiratory effort, and oxygen saturation
G0399 95806	HSAT with type III portable monitor, unattended; minimum of four channels: two respiratory movements/airflow, one ECG/heart rate, and one oxygen saturation
95800	HSAT with type III portable monitor, unattended; minimum of four channels: respiratory analysis, one ECG/heart rate, and one oxygen saturation with measurement of sleep time
95801	HSAT with type III portable monitor, unattended; minimum of four channels: respiratory movement/ airflow, one ECG/heart rate, and one oxygen saturation
G0400	HSAT with type IV portable monitor, unattended; minimum of three channels

CMS, Centers for Medicare and Medicaid Services; ECG, electrocardiogram; EEG, electroencephalogram; EMG, electromyogram; EOG, electrooculogram; HSAT, home sleep apnea test; PSG, polysomnography.

Be certain to understand the carrier's requirement when submitting the claim. Typically, the code that best describes the procedure is reported. However, in the absence of definitive requirements stipulated by the insurance company, and when services are similar, reporting the CPT code is preferentially accepted rather than using the G-code (3).

Additional definitions of the respective studies completed in the sleep center may be referenced in the CPT coding manuals or online at www.cms.gov.

COMPLIANT BILLING

Understanding the difference between the technical, professional, and global codes is necessary for accurate billing and, in return, getting paid for your work.

If the facility performs the testing and a separate credentialed provider is interpreting the procedure, two modifiers are used on the billing claim: the facility providing the technical services attaches a technical component (TC) modifier to the CPT code, and the interpreting medical director (MD) attaches a 26 modifier to the same code. If the procedure is recorded in a facility where the doctor owns the equipment to record the procedure *and* interprets the recording, then the claim is submitted as a global charge, meaning it does not use any modifiers. If the procedure is recorded in a facility and the interpreting doctor is employed by the facility, it is necessary to confirm with the Revenue Integrity Team or Coding Department how to submit a charge because it may still use a modifier, depending on the financial relationship of the employed provider.

The following example demonstrates the use of two of the most common modifiers used by the sleep center, "TC" to designate the technical component of a procedure and "26" to designate the professional component of a study:

- 95810-TC—PSG—Code for the diagnostic PSG to bill the technical component, which includes the equipment, space supplies, and personnel
- 95810-26—PSG—Used to code for the diagnostic PSG for the interpreting physician
- 95810—PSG—A "global" code to bill both the professional and technical services together in one code. Used for billing a PSG with sleep staging and four or *more* additional parameters of sleep, attended by a technologist, and the review of the study and the interpretation

To be compliant with coding for a split-night study, use code 95811 for either a continuous positive airway pressure (CPAP) or bilevel titration. If a split-night study is performed, the interpretation should include both the diagnostic and the treatment information in one report. This is how to document it on the billing claim:

- 95811-TC—PSG (CPAP/Bilevel Titration Study) or split-night studies—Code for the PSG to bill the technical component, which includes the equipment, space supplies, and personnel
- 95811-26—PSG (CPAP/Bilevel Titration Study) or split-night studies—Used to code for the interpreting physician
- 95811—PSG (CPAP/Bilevel Titration Study) or split-night studies being billed for both the technical and the professional components using a global billing code to include the interpretation

Coding and billing for the multiple sleep latency test (MSLT) and the maintenance of wakefulness test (MWT) is completed using CPT 95805:

- 95805-TC—MSLT or MWT to bill for the technical component
- 95805-26—MSLT or MWT to bill for the professional component, which is the interpretation of the study
- 95805—MSLT or MWT to bill globally for both the technical and professional services

Alert: If a full study is not recorded and is less than the required hours as stated in the CPT code, then a modifier of 52 (reduced services) on that specific claim for the respective date of service is added to the CPT code. For example, note how to bill only the technical services of a titration study that was monitored for 4 hours: to append the modifier for reduced services and to bill for only the technical services, the documentation on the billing claim will be entered as 95811-TC-52. The insurance company will process this claim for only the titration technical services for less than 6 hours of monitoring.

DISCOVERING THE DIAGNOSIS

It is important to use the correct *ICD-10-CM* code for billing any diagnosis associated with the diagnostic testing, because this describes the reason for completing the procedure. In addition, the correct diagnosis code must be reported to describe the patient's condition. To obtain the most appropriate diagnosis code, take the following steps:

a. Review the medical record to determine what medical conditions or symptoms are described by the documentation to support the medical necessity for performing the procedure.
b. Cross-reference the disease, signs, symptoms, or condition in the front of the *ICD-10-CM* manual, volume II, and locate the corresponding code.
c. To verify the specificity of the code, locate the corresponding code in the volume I tabular list within the *ICD-10-CM* manual and further analyze the most appropriate code that correlates with the documentation.
d. Routinely refer to the tabular list to locate the most specific code.
e. Coding conventions will reference other diagnoses, which describe in greater detail the information needed to convey to the third-party payer additional information to justify the medical reason for the procedure.

It is important to review the approved diagnoses codes for associated CPT codes, which are defined by individual insurance payers. Examples of the approved codes accepted by CMS for PSG are listed in the region's Local Coverage Determination (LCD) for PSG. An example of an LCD (6) and these approved codes in one region may be reviewed online.

Compliance with coding and billing requires systematic review of all diagnoses codes commonly used for submitting claims in the sleep center. Ideally, this review is completed semiannually to remain informed of changes to the covered diagnostic codes and to prevent denial of claims.

BILLING AND CODING GUIDELINES

Most insurance payers require that the polysomnogram be performed to include the titration with positive airway pressure, that is, CPT code 95811, when clinical criteria support the need for a split-night study. The CPT code 95810 is allowable only when the sleep study does not demonstrate events consistent with sleep apnea and when the PAP titration cannot be completed for unforeseen reasons as documented in the physician's interpretation. Examples include, but are not limited to, the following:

- Insufficient total sleep time
- Criteria for obstructive sleep apnea (OSA) met late in study with insufficient sleep time left for PAP titration
- PAP trial attempted but not tolerated by patient

At this time, many third-party payers will approve only one polysomnogram for a defined number of years, unless there is a significant change in patient status. A repeat polysomnogram will be reviewed for medical necessity with documentation of the following clinical findings:

- Weight gain or loss of a prescribed percentage, with required documentation of body weight;
- After surgical or oral appliance treatment of patients with moderate-to-severe OSA;

- When clinical response is insufficient or when symptoms return despite a good initial response to treatment with PAP device.

For a complete list of the criteria for repeat testing, consult the respective insurance company's CoP for polysomnograms.

Other measurements performed during a sleep study (eg, vital signs, muscular activity, oximetry, airflow, blood gases, electrocardiogram analyses, gastroesophageal reflux) are also included in the coding for the respective polysomnogram and will not be paid separately. It is important to note that billing for extended electroencephalogram monitoring in addition to the PSG base code is not acceptable practice. The CPT manual does not provide guidelines at this time to support the additional code.

Actigraphy as a stand-alone test (CPT code 95803) is not medically necessary as a routine diagnostic procedure done in the sleep center and requires the insurance company MD's review before completion of the testing.

When seeking preauthorization for a PSG, most commercial insurance companies expect to review clinical information to differentiate between the need for a facility-based test versus HSAT. The following are general contraindications for HSAT:

- Moderate or severe chronic obstructive pulmonary disease—forced expiratory volume in 1 second (FEV1)/forced vital capacity less than or equal to 0.7 and FEV1 less than 80% of predicted
- Moderate or severe congestive heart failure—New York Heart Association Class III or IV
- Cognitive impairment (inability to follow simple instructions)
- Neuromuscular impairment
- Suspicion of a sleep disorder other than OSA (such as central sleep apnea, narcolepsy, restless legs syndrome, circadian rhythm disorder, parasomnias, periodic limb movement disorder)
- Previous technically suboptimal HSAT (two nights of study attempted)
- Previous two-night HSAT that did not diagnose OSA in a patient with ongoing clinical suspicion of OSA
- Patient has demonstrated oxygen desaturation for a defined period of time for any reason
- History of cerebrovascular accident within the preceding 30 days
- History of ventricular fibrillation or sustained ventricular tachycardia
- Pediatric patient under age 18

Documentation of these clinical findings must be included in the history and physical examination from the referring provider and available for the individual completing the preauthorization for the study, if required by the insurance company. The history and physical examination are also required for review by the billing entity because it provides the medical necessity required for payment for the procedure.

REGULATIONS AND COMPLIANCE

All personnel representing your sleep center and respective health care providers are required to adhere to a high level of personal and professional conduct. Inherent in this conduct is the need to maintain clinical competence and core knowledge of the regulatory standards that govern this changing health care industry. It includes the intent to maintain and protect the confidentiality of patient and organizational information, as well as to ensure the practice of legal and ethical standards in all dealings and transactions. The intent is to observe all laws and regulations that govern the sleep industry.

Therefore, to stay abreast of the changes, continuing education is a must. What exactly does this mean? Knowing the regulations for your respective insurance providers and the state insurance statutes is the first place to start.

FINANCIAL REGULATORY REQUIREMENTS

Clinical personnel are being asked to perform more of the comprehensive tasks that are associated with medical testing, such as documenting the procedure billing code (CPT code) on the practice's encounter or billing form. As a result, it is important to have an understanding of regulatory requirements concerning financial practices.

Follow these steps to embark on getting paid for your work.

a. The process starts with preauthorization or a predetermination for completing the procedure, which is the third-party payers' preliminary commitment to pay for the procedure.
   Precertification, preauthorization, or predetermination should be obtained quickly so that the patient's procedure may be carried out without delay. To do this, you need to have the medical history and physical examination from the referring physician, or one that has been completed by the clinic's board-certified sleep specialist. This document must include a chief complaint, which states in the patient's words why they are seeking medical care. The chief complaint links to the medical necessity for the procedure and for treatment to be approved for payment.

Staff may be asked to assist and instruct the patient to complete a patient information form, as a way of documenting accurate and complete demographic data and a clinical history.

Information that is needed to complete a preauthorization for a procedure includes the sleep history and symptoms including, but not limited to, snoring, daytime sleepiness, observed apneas, choking or gasping during sleep, morning headaches; the Epworth Sleepiness Scale; the physical examination that documents body mass index, neck circumference, and a focused cardiopulmonary and upper airway system evaluation. Additional detail to have available before calling for preauthorization is listed in the section Billing and Coding Guidelines.

Currently, for Medicare patients to qualify for PAP therapy, they must meet either of the following criteria: the apnea-hypopnea index (AHI) is greater than or equal to 15 events per hour with a minimum of 30 events; or the AHI is greater than or equal to 5 and less than or equal to 14 events per hour with a minimum of 10 events and documentation of excessive daytime sleepiness, impaired cognition, mood disorders, or insomnia; or hypertension, ischemic heart disease, or history of stroke.

b. Take time to explain to the patient the sleep center's Notice of Privacy Practices and the Patient Rights and Responsibilities, making sure you are familiar with both notices and are competent in explaining the form accurately. A third form, the Notice of Financial Responsibility, conveys to the patient their consent to submit a claim for payment on their behalf. It also confers the patient's responsibility for payment of their portion of the bill. The facility has the responsibility to inform the patient of the charge, the expected reimbursement for the procedure, and their financial responsibility before receipt of the services. To attest to all three of these regulations, written documentation that the patient was informed of the discussion must be in the patient's permanent chart as evidence of adherence to the federal regulations.

c. Informed consent

This is a process in which the patient authorizes medical treatment after a discussion with a physician or a licensed clinical provider that includes the plan of care. During this interview, the assessment, risks, and recommendations are discussed with the patient and documented in the patient's record.

The informed consent is required in advance of any testing. It is witnessed by the clinical provider and signed and dated at the time of discussion.

The Consent for Testing and Treatment, generally a requirement for all procedures, is completed in accordance with state and federal requirements.

Consent forms also include the permission for release of patient information as required by the Health Insurance Portability and Accountability Act of 1996 (HIPAA).

Under the HIPAA Privacy Rule, providers do not need specific authorization to release patients' personal health information if used for treatment, payment, and health care operations (TPO).

Examples of TPO are as follows:

a. Treatment: discussion of the patient's clinical information with other providers
b. Payment: submission of the billing claim on behalf of the patient
c. Operations: activities related to staff training and quality improvement

SUBMISSION OF THE BILLING CLAIM

Promptly transmit an accurate insurance claim data to the third-party payer so that reimbursement is timely received. This is usually completed through an electronic data interface. Several areas of complexity with submission of billing claims for sleep studies include the following:

1. An order with diagnosis code(s) is required from the referring physician. Neither the sleep center nor its supervising physicians can prescribe a sleep test for patients they do not treat. If the physician serving as the supervising physician or the MD of the sleep center orders the procedure, the supervising physician/MD must be the patient's treating physician. Therefore, this same provider must have had a relationship with the patient before the performance of the testing and is now managing the care of the patient for their specific medical problem.
2. The PSG/sleep study must be performed by appropriately credentialed technologists. Each insurance plan defines required credentialing. Traditionally, CMS qualifies the required credentials at a minimum as Registered Sleep Technologist (RST), Registered Respiratory Therapist (RRT), Registered Respiratory Therapist–Sleep Disorders Specialist (RRT-SDS), Certified Respiratory Therapist (CRT), Certified Pulmonary Function Technologist (CPFT), Registered Pulmonary Function Technologist (RPFT), Certified Respiratory Therapist–Sleep Disorders Specialist (CRT-SDS), Registered Polysomnographic Technologist (RPSGT). Technologists working in states with state licensure requirements governed by a state practice act are required to demonstrate evidence of meeting all credentialing and licensure requirements by possessing both credentials before working as a direct care provider.

3. Another important credentialing requirement that requires attention concerns direct care providers who work in one state and provide services to a patient living in another state. That provider is required to have a license to work both in the state where the patient resides and in the state where the patient is receiving the care and services. Insurance contracts routinely reinforce this expectation as a condition of participation with their plans.
4. The sleep study is completed in accordance with the criteria defined by the respective CPT code. Focus on the parameters required to support the appropriate CPT code and document the duration of the study. This is discussed in additional detail in other sections of this chapter.
5. The sleep study is interpreted by an appropriately credentialed physician. This is defined in each insurance plan and typically requires a board-certified sleep medicine specialist. Evidence of a face-to-face medical interview is required to process the claim. Notes or proof of the physical examination must be placed in the patient's chart. The treating physician is the one who furnishes a consultation or treats a patient for a specific medical problem and uses the results of the test to treat and manage the patient's medical problem.
6. The names of the ordering physician with credentials, interpreting physician with credentials, supervising technologist with credentials, when applicable, and the actual technologist with credentials performing the study must be documented in the patient file and on the interpretation of the procedure to demonstrate compliance with the credentialing regulations.
7. The need for accreditation of the facility must be addressed before submission of billing claims. All CMS regions are rapidly moving toward mandating accreditation through one of the following accrediting entities: Accreditation Commission for Health Care (ACHC) (7), AASM (8), or The Joint Commission. These entities have established standards that must be in place before the sleep center is awarded an accreditation required by the CMS. This has led the charge for other commercial insurances, who are also changing their CoP to require accreditation of the sleep center. A point of note: if sleep services, including HSAT, are contracted out to another company, both the billing facility and the contracted service must fulfill the standards as written in the accreditation guidelines.
8. Clinicians who complete the insurance claim need to be able to explain complex billing requirements and answer insurance questions to patients. Take time to explain billing parameters to all business and clinical team members associated with your program so that they have a general understanding of the insurance and billing process and are able to address patient questions correctly.

Tests ordered by physicians who are not treating the patient are rendered medically unnecessary and are not reimbursable in the eyes of the insurance company. When receiving a referral from the attending physician, the sleep center must maintain a record of the attending physician's orders and any test results that may impact the interpretation of the procedure. The interpreting physician must indicate a final diagnosis from the sleep study on the interpretation that correlates with the diagnosis for billing. The diagnosis code for the symptoms or the reason for testing the patient is not to be used on the billing claim.

When billing for a diagnostic test, the ordering physician's National Provider Identifier number must be indicated on the claim form, and the order must be kept on record. If more than two nights of testing are performed, documentation justifying the medical necessity for the additional test(s) must be provided to the insurance company on request.

Ideally, to remain competent, billing and coding staff will need to obtain training in CPT, *ICD-10-CM*, and HCPCS coding and have access to the annually updated coding resources. The billing encounter forms, billing software, and any cheat sheets used need to be updated every year with any changes as defined in the standard coding resources. It is beneficial to subscribe to newsletters or other website resources to keep abreast of coding changes. Use an official source such as CMS or the AMA to verify any changes or updates received. Ask for information from other third-party payers in writing or verify changes on the payer's online resources page to keep abreast of contracted coding changes. Each quarter, check the CMS National Coverage Determination and LCD requirements for any changes made by the designated regional Medicare Administrative Contractor who administers the LCD. The responsibilities for knowing what changes are integrated that may affect your practice rests with the sleep center billing and coding experts.

INSURANCE CONTRACTS

Many health insurance companies provide different types of individual and group plans, which many employers offer to their employees. These plans have different coverage, referral restrictions, and payment schedules. They have clinical exclusions, which may be implemented midway in the contract period, in addition to the annual edits. As a result, health insurance plans are always changing, and the patient often has a difficult time understanding what their health plans cover.

To obtain a better understanding of the insurance contracts, investigate the following issues when evaluating coverage to ensure correct billing and coding:

a. Medical conditions establish the medical necessity for services.
   Documenting the clinical symptoms or reasons for the procedure justifies the medical necessity, which is required to be noted in the medical record, a legal document. Complete and comprehensive documentation is important to show that clinicians have appropriately assessed medical need indicated by medical standards of care.
   Services are medically necessary when they are reasonable and essential for the diagnosis or treatment of illness or injury or to improve the functioning of an individual's health status. Such services must also be consistent with generally accepted standards of care. Normally, these standards of care are published practice parameters by national professional organizations, such as the AASM, and other professional organizations such as The American College of Physicians. Practice parameters are peer-reviewed, clinically based protocols that have been tested and validated to elicit effective outcomes in care.
b. Evidence of certification requirements by approved accreditation agency
   All CMS claims and many other commercial insurances now have certification requirements to obtain payment for diagnostic and therapeutic testing performed in a hospital-based lab, a freestanding facility (includes sleep clinics that are a part of a physician's office), independent diagnostic testing facilities, and all other non–hospital-based facilities where sleep studies are performed. This includes the requirement for the facility to have on file, and available on request, evidence that they are credentialed by one of the approved accreditation agencies.
c. Requirements for patient encounter are documented.
   Documentation is expected to be generated during a face-to-face encounter with the patient. Insurance contracts have defined criteria for how the encounter occurs: face-to-face is the norm today either in person or using telemedicine, and reimbursement is linked to the direct discussion with the patient. If information is not available at the time of this direct discussion, there are requirements for amending the patient encounter. Delayed entries, documented within a time frame, generally not to exceed 48 hours, are acceptable for purposes of clarification, error correction, addition of information not initially available, and when certain unusual circumstances prevented the generation of the documentation at the time of service.
   The medical record cannot be altered or redacted, and amendments must be legibly added so the clinician can draw an inference to confirm, clarify, or support the initial entry. Corrections or additions must be dated, timed, and legibly signed or initialed. Delayed written explanations will be considered for clarification only. This explanation is not used for the purpose of increasing the services billed, because of a lack of documentation at the time of service, or retrospectively substantiating medical necessity. All entries must be legible to another person reading the chart signed by the original author. If the signature is not legible and does not identify the clinician, a printed example of the name should be included under the signature with the appropriate credentials to support the required scope of practice.
d. Claim is audited for excluded services prior to submission.
   Billing federal insurance providers for a noncovered service constitutes fraud. Under Medicare, if a patient elects to have a procedure and it is not covered under the Medicare health plan, an Advanced Beneficiary Notice is required *before* providing services. This form is obtained from the Medicare website. Knowledge of the patient's insurance plan is a must to reduce the potential for billing fraud.
e. Health plan billing requirements are met.
   This may include completion of certain activities before testing, such as preauthorization, completion of a medical questionnaire before approval for the procedure, or a face-to-face interview with the treating physician. Payment for certain treatment devices, such as an oral appliance, may require a failure of PAP therapy before submission of the claim for the device, depending on the insurance plan.
f. Patient financial responsibility education
   Discussing the practice's financial policy with the patient and/or their guardian is critical to receiving payment for services. To have a constructive proactive discussion, it is necessary to be educated about the sleep center's financial policies. It means one also needs to be in tune with the patient's way of thinking, conveying information in a compassionate positive manner, in an effort to share with the patient that payment of their bill is the patient's responsibility. Medical providers are expected to devote time to verifying and understanding each patient's particular insurance coverage to increase collections and cash flow. The first step toward gaining an understanding of the claim management and reimbursement processes is to review the insurance plan contract and clarify the definitions and terminology listed in each insurance plan.
   This makes a discussion with the patient about the sleep center's payment options more beneficial. Ideally, the copayment is collected at the time of service and, if not paid then, subsequent evidence of the attempt to collect the copayment is documented in the patient's medical chart.

SUMMARY

Understanding how to accurately code and bill for clinical encounters is critical to getting paid for services rendered, reducing risk for fraud and abuse, and making a profit. Regulatory standards expect the integration of financial requirements and statutes that are the basis for compliance with coding and billing requirements. Competency with these financial practices establishes credibility with peers, third-party payers, and the community, because providing services is based on integrity and honesty. When we add the expectation for appropriate documentation, it becomes necessary to have a core structure to coordinate the many facets of sleep center billing. Therefore, completing an annual review of all billing contract requirements will contribute to the financial success of the sleep center. Taking time every year to attend a presentation on the recent coding and billing updates will help to maximize the potential for increased revenue. Completing this education is worth the time and energy required to be successful and sustain a profitable venture.

REFERENCES

1. American Academy of Professional Coders. *ICD-10-CM Expert for Providers and Facilities*. American Academy of Professional Coders; 2025.
2. American Academy of Sleep Medicine. *International Classification of Sleep Disorders*. 3rd ed. American Academy of Sleep Medicine; 2023. https://aasm.org/wp-content/uploads/2023/05/ICSD-3-Text-Revision-Refs.pdf
3. American Medical Association. *CPT® 2025 Professional Edition*. American Medical Association; 2025.
4. Optum360. *HCPCS Level II Expert Codebook*. Optum360; 2025.
5. Aronsky AJ. 4 Steps to correct coding for home sleep apnea testing. Published April 19, 2015. Accessed August 6, 2018. https://sleepreviewmag.com/practice-management/money/coding/4-steps-correct-coding-home-sleep-apnea-testing/
6. Centers for Medicare & Medicaid Services. Local coverage determination: polysomnography and other sleep studies (L36839). Accessed February 2025. https://www.cms.gov/medicare-coverage-database/view/lcd.aspx?LCDId=36839
7. Sleep Accreditation Commission for Health Care. ACHC sleep accreditation standards. Accessed February 2025. https://achc.org/wp-content/uploads/2025/08/SLP-Standards-Update-Guide-Aug-2025.pdf
8. American Academy of Sleep Medicine. Standards for accreditation. Accessed February 2025. https://aasm.org/resources/standards-for-accreditation/

Chapter 71
Quality Assurance and Quality Improvement

RITA J. BROOKS

KEY CONCEPTS/LEARNING OBJECTIVES

The key concepts reviewed in this chapter include describing the basis for quality assurance and quality improvement defining structural, process, and outcome measures, discussing the process for measuring data (what, how, and when), and describing the process for analyzing data and reporting outcomes.

KEY TERMS

Continuous quality improvement
Data
Epworth Sleepiness Scale
Multiple Sleep Latency Test
Quality assurance
Quality improvement
Reliability
Sentinel event
Validity

"I think we can do better." This quote from an Australian comedian is, in six words, the basis for quality assurance and, its close cousin, continuous quality improvement. There are a variety of elements in the process, beginning with measurement and manipulation. The process requires reliability and validity. Constructs are examined and operationalized. Data are collected and analyzed. Hypotheses are tested. Theories are developed and supported, modified, or abandoned. Does this sound like scientific method? Most definitely.

A variety of businesses have benefited from a quality assurance (QA) process. This process relies on standards of performance, whether in manufacturing screws to exacting specifications or inserting those screws into luxury automobiles with precise torque. An acceptable range of performance is defined. When the range is not met for a certain predetermined percentage of products, an attempt is made to define the problem and propose a solution. QA is critical when the product has safety implications. If the screw holds the brakes in place, failing to meet the acceptable range of performance can have disastrous consequences. Therefore, the percentage of products meeting specifications must be extremely high, if not 100%. On the contrary, a burnt potato chip may irritate some consumers but is unlikely to have serious consequences.

Quality improvement does not have an end goal and works in a more continuous fashion. When used in customer service, surveys may be used to obtain satisfaction scores. No matter what the score, an intervention is proposed to try and improve it. When the score is at the top of the range, a new measure of satisfaction is developed that leaves room for improvement.

QA and improvement processes are both important in medicine, specifically in sleep medicine. There are some areas where the goal should be a total absence of events. For example, patient deaths in the sleep center should not merely be infrequent but should never happen. These "sentinel events" should result in an immediate change in policies to ensure that they do not happen again. Improving care in sleep medicine is an imperative that benefits sleep centers and patients. The goals are to improve the quality of care, improve the health of populations, and reduce the costs of health care (1).

Measures can be divided into structural, process, and outcomes (1). For example, if you want to know if the number of patients visiting your sleep center is higher today than it was a year ago, you can review billing data or procedure logs. This is considered a structural measure. If you want to know if visiting the sleep center results in reduced blood pressure on the next clinic visit, you can review vital signs from the patient's chart. This would be a process measure. It is nice to have blood pressure in the normal range, but in itself, this conveys no specific benefit. The benefit to the patient would be a reduction in the risk of stroke or heart attack, and the number of these events is considered an outcome measure. Outcome measures often require an extended period of time to collect, and, as a result, may suffer from lower reliability.

> *Measure that which can be measured and make measurable what cannot be measured.*
>
> *Galileo Galilei*

The first step in QA or improvement is to measure. The first question is "What am I interested in?" and the second question is "How can I measure it?" The first question asks for a construct and the second for an operational definition. This can range from a simple question with obvious measures to more complex constructs that require more complicated measurement tools.

Here's an example from home sleep apnea testing (HSAT) that starts with a simple question and ends with a more complex question. The simple question is "How many studies do I need to repeat?" The simple measure is to count the number of studies that were considered inadequate and required retesting and divide by the total number of studies run per month. Setting a goal for a small percentage of inadequate studies has implications for patient satisfaction and profit margin. Patients do not want to be told that they need to repeat a study. This delays determination of the results of the study and requires additional work, causing discomfort to the patient. In addition, current reimbursement rates provide a small margin between the cost of the HSAT and the revenue produced. A few inadequate studies per week might make HSAT unprofitable, leading to discontinuation of the service and an increase in patients who are not diagnosed. A high percentage of inadequate tests tells you there is a problem but gives no insight into how to correct the problem. In our fictional sleep center, more than 20% of our HSATs are rejected by the physicians. Something must be done. But what?

The more complex question is "Why were the studies considered inadequate?" The idea of an inadequate study is a construct that needs to be defined operationally. That is, we need to make it measurable. This typically starts with observation. We could put a box on the interpretation form that asks the physician, "Why was this study inadequate?" These open-ended questions are difficult to quantify because similar responses can be provided with slightly different language, making it difficult to decide if the causes are actually the same. One physician writes, "oxygen problem," and another physician writes, "saturation measurement lost." Can we offer the physicians some options with check boxes? The American Academy of Sleep Medicine (AASM) Scoring Manual (2) provides a starting point. The features of an acceptable HSAT device must be met in order to provide an adequate study. These features include oxygen saturation and heart rate as well as a measure that allows for the calculation of a surrogate of the apnea-hypopnea index (typically airflow for the numerator and recording time for the denominator). Of the 20% of recordings rejected by the physicians in our fictional center, 75% are identified as oxygen saturation problems.

Now we are back to a simple measure: How often were HSATs inadequate because of an oxygen saturation problem? During the monthly conference, we find that Dr Copperfield rejects studies if the oximeter fails for more than 10% of the study but that Dr Kepler is willing to accept studies with up to 50% oximeter data lost. In order to be a reliable indicator, the criteria for inadequate must be the same for all of our physicians. After a vigorous discussion, a compromise is reached, and inadequate oximetry is defined as more than 30% of the recording without adequate oximetry data. It is important to document this criterion in the center's Policy and Procedures Manual. This way, everyone can create data that can be used for comparisons in later stages of the quality improvement process.

All aspects of the sleep center's activity can be assessed using quality improvement measures. The AASM helpfully provides starting points in a series of articles in the *Journal of Clinical Sleep Medicine*. A range of sleep disorders are covered, but for most centers, the majority of patients have sleep apnea. In an article devoted to obstructive sleep apnea quality measures (3), the AASM recommends 10 process measures and 3 outcome measures that can be incorporated into a center's quality improvement process. These measures were developed through literature review, evaluation of physician burden, and a consensus meeting.

Process measure #5, for example, assesses sleepiness in patients. The center is required to determine the "Proportion of patients aged 18 years and older diagnosed and treated for obstructive sleep apnea that had sleepiness assessed annually" (3). Sleepiness is a construct, and it needs to be operationalized. Some centers use the Epworth Sleepiness Scale (ESS), whereas others prefer the Multiple Sleep Latency Test (MSLT). The AASM does not specify what measure is used but only that a measure is obtained. The outcome measure that is associated with this process measure is to improve quality of life. Again, the AASM does not specify a measure, and a wide variety of instruments can be debated by the center staff.

"Sleepiness" and "quality of life" are constructs, and some may say they are difficult to measure, but valid and reliable methods for operationalizing these constructs are available. It is important that the measures provide construct validity—that is, they measure the range and breadth of the construct. It would be inadequate to ask, "Do you fall asleep watching television?" as the only measure of sleepiness. Sleepiness involves falling asleep while driving, during conversations, after a heavy lunch, and even feeling sleepy without any actual loss of consciousness.

The next step in our quality improvement process is to compare our measures with those of other similar entities. Everything is relative. We will need to set a minimum criterion for triggering of an intervention. From a purely business standpoint, this could be based on practical measures such as profit. But patient satisfaction will also be relevant as patients will fail to return to the center or recommend the center to family and friends if they are not satisfied with the treatment they receive. Establishing criteria that are, as much as possible, objective and consistent among staff will improve the validity of measures as they are compared over time.

Equally importantly, using measures that are the same as the measures that other centers are using will allow comparisons with "industry standards." Unfortunately, there is little consensus among sleep centers in regard to how to measure quality indicators. For example, the AASM deems acceptable measures of quality of life to include the SF-36, SF-12, Nottingham Health Profile, EuroQoL, EQ-5D, FOSQ, and SAQLI (3).

In our fictional sleep center, 20% of HSATs were inadequate. A study comparing laboratory testing and HSAT (4) found that 147 of 180 patients had acceptable home studies the first time, resulting in 18.3% of studies scored as inadequate. This means our fictional sleep center is in the same ballpark as the centers participating in the research study. But a failure rate of one in five is high, and improving this would result in both higher patient satisfaction and profit margins. In a competitive market, a 2% difference might be significant, and patients may gravitate away from our center to the competition.

However, the problem remains that your measurement is based on the standard criteria you have established for your center. The research study did not define "inadequate study," and therefore your comparison may be flawed. Fortunately, this does not invalidate the quality improvement process.

There are no big problems, there are just a lot of little problems.

Henry Ford

When analyzing the data that have been collected, it's often necessary to examine the component parts of the construct. A center may record low scores on a patient satisfaction survey. That's a big problem. What are the little problems that could contribute to the low satisfaction score? Patients may report long wait times, grumpy staff, uncomfortable beds, and a lack of privacy or have a variety of other complaints. As we work through the quality improvement process, we will try to identify areas of concern and seek to investigate changes that can influence our measures.

In our fictional sleep center, 20% of HSATs were inadequate. Of these, 75% were due to oximeter failure. This means we can reduce our percentage of inadequate studies to only 5% if we can eliminate the oxygen saturation problems. Can we break this problem down into something we can work on?

A review of the technologist notes finds that for 10% of the studies that were inadequate, the patient reported being unable to plug in the oximeter. For another 20% of studies, the signal was inadequate from the start, with evidence that the probe was not attached properly. And for 70% of the studies, the patient reported waking up with the probe not attached to the finger. You measure the duration of valid oximetry readings for your patients and find that the average is only 4.5 hours. From these data, it is clear that we can achieve the largest effect on our measure by improving the way the oximeter probe is attached to the patient's finger. What could be done to keep the probe in place?

A brainstorming session at the sleep center leads to a list of possible interventions: buy a different probe, use stronger tape, educate patients to use a pressure relief loop in the probe cable, or have the technologist attach the probe to the patient when they come to pick up the home-testing device. Some of these methods can be eliminated because of cost or logistics. Settling on a method to try can be the result of a consensus.

Because quality improvement is an experiment, it is important to manipulate only one independent variable at a time. This provides experimental control and supports a cause-and-effect conclusion. In other words, keep the conditions as similar as possible and change only one thing at a time. If you buy a new probe, change to a stickier tape, and modify your patient education strategy, you may reduce the number of inadequate home sleep apnea tests. But what caused the reduction? It would be impossible to know. A more effective strategy may be to use different tape that is known to work well for studies done in the sleep center. If this change causes a significant reduction in inadequate tests, you have determined an effective intervention; if not, you can change something else and see if it works.

You must take your place in the Circle of Life.

Mufasa, the Lion King

Quality improvement is a circular process. First, you measure. Compare your measure with others. Then you analyze. Finally, make a change. But to close the circle you must measure again and follow the circle of life for another cycle. First, you measure. It is important to use the same measures and the same criteria the second time around. This allows for a valid comparison.

Compare your measure with others. Now that you have completed a cycle, you can compare the new results with the results you measured the first time. There are three possible outcomes: things got better, things got worse, or things didn't change. The outcome will determine what you do next.

If things got better, did they exceed what would be expected by chance? You will need to compare your measure before and after the change. Slight variations in your measures are to be expected. The best way to know if you have exceeded those slight variations is to run a statistical test, such as an independent samples *t*-test. It's not hard, and it will let you know if moving forward is worth the effort. If possible, do more of what you did to cause the improvement.

If things get worse, stop the change and start over. Again, make sure the difference between before and after is statistically significant before you give up on the change.

The tricky outcome is that things didn't change. This can happen for several reasons. One reason is that there really is an improvement, but your statistical comparison lacks power. The best way to get more power is to keep going and add more patients to your comparison. If your statistical test is close to showing an improvement, this is the best option. A second option is that your manipulation wasn't powerful enough. You can use a stronger manipulation and see if that makes a difference. The third option is that your change really didn't work. If your measure did not change, you will need to analyze your problem again.

At our fictional sleep center, the staff agreed to buy a higher-priced tape for patients in an attempt to better secure the oximeter probe. Data were collected for 3 months. This improved the number of hours of valid oximetry to 4.8 hours, but this was not statistically different from the 4.5 hours recorded before the change. In addition, the number of inadequate studies did not change. One staff person related that another sleep center across town uses tape from a different supplier and that it works fine for them. Another suggested that two rolls of tape should be provided to each patient instead of one. Dr Kepler recommended trying forehead reflective oximetry. Dr Kepler won the debate, and they all agreed to continue the quality improvement process with new technology.

It is important to remember that quality improvement is a circular process and therefore has no end. Even when one change results in a significant improvement, other aspects of job performance, equipment efficacy, and patient satisfaction will present themselves. And in the end, we can all do better.

AASM Sleep Center Accreditation standards require quality improvement measurements. All sleep centers should be involved in quality measurement and improvement. There are a variety of quality measures available on the AASM website for review and adoption in your sleep center (5). This is a good place to begin to determine what quality improvement measures are meaningful in the field of sleep medicine and may assist you to develop these measures for your sleep center.

REFERENCES

1. Morgenthaler TI, Aronsky AJ, Carden KA, et al. Measurement of quality to improve care in sleep medicine. *J Clin Sleep Med.* 2015;11(3):279-291.
2. Troester MM, Quan SF, Berry RB, et al; for the American Academy of Sleep Medicine. *The AASM Manual for the Scoring of Sleep and Associated Events: Rules, Terminology and Technical Specifications* (Version 3). American Academy of Sleep Medicine; 2023.
3. Aurora RN, Collop NA, Jacobowitz O, et al. Quality measures for the care of adult patients with obstructive sleep apnea. *J Clin Sleep Med.* 2015;11(3):357-383.
4. Rosen CL, Auckley D, Benca R, et al. A multisite randomized trial of portable sleep studies and positive airway pressure autotitration versus laboratory-based polysomnography for the diagnosis and treatment of obstructive sleep apnea: the HomePAP study. *Sleep.* 2012;35(6):757-767.
5. American Academy of Sleep Medicine. Quality measures. Accessed March 9, 2025. https://aasm.org/clinical-resources/practice-standards/quality-measures/

Chapter 72
Research in the Sleep Center

CHRISTINA SAULYS

KEY CONCEPTS/LEARNING OBJECTIVES

The key concepts for this chapter include describing the purpose of research and types of research commonly performed in a sleep center and defining research, drug development, and regulations pertaining to clinical research trials. The author describes the drug development process, phases of research and key stakeholder roles, defines the methods of data collection and processing for sleep research, describes the regulatory governance of clinical research, and discusses how clinical sleep research is evolving.

KEY TERMS

Contract research organization (CRO)
Decision-making capacity
Delegation of Authority log
In vitro
In vivo
Institutional Review Board (IRB)
Investigational new drug (IND) process
Investigational product (IP)
Investigator's brochure (IB)
New drug application (NDA)
Preclinical research
Principal investigator (PI)

If sleep does not serve an absolutely vital function, then it is the biggest mistake the evolutionary process has ever made.

—*Prof. Emeritus Allan Rechtschaffen*

Sleep is a fundamental biologic process that affects nearly every aspect of human health, making the study of sleep disorders and sleep-related health issues an essential area of research. Early sleep research and investigation centered on discovering and quantifying the stages and cycles occurring during sleep and how these cycles relate to sleep and wake circadian rhythms. A host of distinguished sleep researchers, including Nathaniel Kleitman, Eugene Aserinsky, Alan Rechtschaffen, and many others, championed early experiments and discoveries (1). This and other detailed research set the foundations from which impaired or disrupted sleep and wake functions were evaluated.

As the developing field of sleep medicine progressed, research began shifting from scientific curiosities and inquiries needed to define the physiologic functions of sleep toward the pathologies and disorders associated with disrupted, excessive, or insufficient sleep. As eloquently described in the 2005 publication of the History of the Development of Sleep Medicine in the United States (2), the science-based foundation paved the way for detailed quantifications of disorders such as narcolepsy, restless legs syndrome, and rapid eye movement (REM) behavior disorder.

Interest in the research of sleep and wake has expanded exponentially over the last decade. Today's sleep research environment is considerably different from that of earlier years. More medical sites are available to conduct research, and rather than being only academically or scientifically focused, some research centers have clinical research units or clinic sites that specialize in scientific sleep research. Although there will always be the need for basic science, the majority of clinical trials involve pharmaceuticals or device manufacturers who seek to prove the clinical effectiveness of their devices, algorithms, or services. Sleep research centers are vital in clinical trials related to sleep disorders, medications, and sleep-related medical devices. These centers serve as specialized sites for researching how sleep impacts health, testing new treatments and diagnostic tools, and evaluating the effectiveness of therapies. They are a critical hub for clinical trials involving sleep disorders, new treatments, and innovative medical devices. The following are some types and examples of research in a sleep center. Research on sleep also includes the use of in vitro testing, animal models, and big data. Artificial intelligence is now playing an increasingly important role in sleep-related research.

- Clinical Sleep Research: Focuses on diagnosing and treating sleep disorders like insomnia, sleep apnea,

narcolepsy, and restless legs syndrome. This structured research investigates new treatments, medications, and behavioral therapies.
Examples: Studies on continuous positive airway pressure (CPAP) adherence, new insomnia medications, and cognitive-behavioral therapy (CBT) for sleep disorders.

- Neuroscientific Sleep Research: Examines brain activity during sleep using electroencephalography (EEG), functional MRI (fMRI), and other neuroimaging and analytic techniques such as spectral analysis, quantitative EEG (qEEG), and other signal processing metrics (REM density, spindle analysis). This research may explore sleep's role in memory consolidation, emotional regulation, and neural plasticity.
  Example: Studying changes in how EEG spectra during REM sleep affects emotional processing.
- Genetic and Molecular Sleep Research: Investigates genetic factors influencing sleep patterns and disorders. This type of research may look at molecular mechanisms, including circadian rhythm regulation.
  Example: Identifying genes linked to insomnia or narcolepsy.
- Sleep and Mental Health Research: Studies the connection between sleep and psychiatric conditions like depression, anxiety, and posttraumatic stress disorder (PTSD). Studies may include how sleep deprivation affects mood, cognition, and stress response.
  Example: Research on sleep interventions for patients with PTSD.
- Technology and Sleep Research: This area evaluates the impact of devices, wearables, mobile apps, and artificial intelligence (AI) on monitoring and improving sleep. This may include using algorithms to assess sleep, movement, and automated scoring techniques.
  Example: Validating the accuracy of consumer sleep tracking devices.
- Sleep and Public Health Research: Investigates the societal effects of sleep deprivation, shift work, and chronic sleep loss. This research may examine interventions for improving sleep hygiene at population levels.
  Example: Studying school start times and their impact on adolescent sleep and function.

DEFINITION OF RESEARCH

To better understand the evolution of sleep research, we must first understand the definition, categorization, and regulations pertaining to research and clinical trials. The U.S. Department of Health and Human Services (HHS), Office for Human Research Protections (OHRP), defines research in 45 CFR 46.102(l) (Revised Common Rule, 2018) as "[a] systematic investigation, including research development, testing, and evaluation, designed to develop or contribute to generalizable knowledge." This definition emphasizes that research must be systematic (following an organized method), involve investigation (gathering and analyzing data), and aim to produce generalizable knowledge (findings that extend beyond a specific study population).

A sleep research center is a critical hub for clinical trials involving sleep disorders, new treatments, and innovative medical devices. Sleep centers and staff conducting research must also ensure that new diagnostic and therapeutic interventions are scientifically validated, safe, and effective before reaching the public.

Clinical trials follow a predefined and preapproved systematic process (organized method) in the form of a protocol that is intended to find out the safety and efficacy of a drug (Interventional Product/IP), device, or behavioral intervention in treating, preventing, and/or diagnosing a disease or medical condition. Trials involve research participants, often referred to as "subjects." Participation in clinical trials not only increases participants' role in their health care but also plays a critical role in increasing the generalizable knowledge gained during the investigation. Participants have the potential opportunity to access experimental treatments, to which their outcomes can directly contribute to medical research.

Four main types of clinical studies are widely recognized. These include human pharmacology, exploratory, confirmatory, and postapproval studies (3).

There is other clinical research involving the validation and verification of medical devices. According to the Food and Drug Administration (FDA), the goal of human factors engineering is to reduce or eliminate errors that occur during use of a device that could cause harm or degrade medical treatment to the greatest extent possible (4). This involves assessments at one or more stages during the device development process to identify strengths, weaknesses, or deficiencies that could possibly harm the user. The assessment process utilizes market research, competitor research, failure mode and effects analysis (5), formative and summative in small groups, and well-designed protocols for clinical trials. Device manufacturers developing new or improved positive airway pressure (PAP) machines, hoses, and interfaces are reliant on this process, and they frequently utilize sleep centers, personnel, and patients as trial participants during the usability segments of development. The results of these trials are then used to make improvements on current designs or validate user acceptance criteria.

For the purposes of discussion, this chapter will focus primarily on pharmacologically related clinical trials. Device trials, such as those investigated for premarket release trials (nasal PAP and other sleep-related equipment), are governed by 21 CFR 821 (6).

DRUG DEVELOPMENT PROCESS

The drug development process in the United States is regulated by the FDA (7). This development process consists of several stages, each designed to ensure a new drug is safe, effective, and suitable for human use before it reaches the market. The first step in the process is discovery and development. Researchers discover new drugs using several methods that include:

- Newly revealed knowledge or insights within a disease that allow researchers to formulate a product that will, at the minimum, stop the disease progress or possibly reverse the effects of the disease.
- Testing multiple molecular compounds with the intent of identifying beneficial effects when applied to any of a large number of diseases.
- Investigating already existing compounds or treatments that have effects that were not anticipated in the original design.
- Technologic developments that provide new methods or pathways that were not previously available as a means to assist treatment. Examples of this include new surgical devices that allow access within specific areas of the body or genetic coding or AI-driven drug discovery.

The identification of a promising compound leads to further experiments in order to gather information on items like absorption, distribution, metabolization, and excretion. Other information collected includes dosage, delivery route, side effects or adverse reactions, and intractability with other drugs. All of these results are gathered to serve as the basis for what will become the Investigator's Brochure (IB). This document summarizes the body of knowledge gained through testing and experimentation throughout the development of the IP or study drug.

The second step in the drug development process is preclinical research. Researchers must find out if the newly discovered compound has the potential to cause serious harm before testing is conducted in humans. Specifically, the effort is to identify its toxicity, conducted through two types of preclinical research areas: in vitro and in vivo. An in vitro test is conducted with glass or plastic laboratory vessels ("petri dishes"), whereas in vivo testing is conducted within the body of a living organism.

Types of preclinical testing evaluations:

- Safety (toxicity studies)
- Pharmacodynamics (PD)—how the drug affects the body
- Pharmacokinetics (PK)—how the body absorbs, distributes, metabolizes, and excretes the drug

Following the successful conclusion of preclinical testing, the IP is ready for human application. Preclinical research, as thorough as it is at answering basic safety questions, is no substitute for actual IP applications in humans. Clinical trials reveal a wealth of information when the IP interacts with the human body in ways bench testing cannot. However, before ever making the first human application, the developers carefully design the overall clinical study (or study plan). They consider what is to be accomplished at each phase. This begins the investigational new drug (IND) process, in which an IND application is submitted to the FDA before clinical research begins (8). This application includes data from animal studies, toxicity, and any prior human research. Additionally, information about the investigator, manufacturing information, and the clinical protocols (study plan) are included in the submission. Only after FDA approval can the development move to clinical trials and into the next step of the drug development process, clinical research.

Clinical drug research typically has four phases (I-IV) of trials, which may overlap or be combined. A basic overview of these phases is set out as follows (3):

1. Phase 1 Trials—Early-stage trials that assess the safety, dosage range, and side effects of a drug or treatment in a small group (typically 50 or less) of healthy volunteers or patients. These trials are often conducted at a single center.
2. Phase 2 Trials—Focused on evaluating the efficacy of a treatment in a group of patients with a specific condition while continuing to assess safety. The primary goal is to determine if the drug works for the intended condition, evaluate short-term side effects, and target optimal dosage.
3. Phase 3 Trials—Large-scale trials (hundreds to thousands of subjects) that compare the new treatment to standard treatments or a placebo, determining effectiveness, monitoring side effects, and gathering data for regulatory approval. These trials are often conducted across multiple research sites in multiple countries to ensure diverse patient populations.
4. Phase 4 Trials (Postmarketing Studies)—Conducted after FDA approval to monitor long-term effects, safety, and effectiveness in the general population. Even after approval, drugs undergo ongoing monitoring to detect long-term side effects, rare adverse reactions in a larger patient population, and new uses or formulations for the drug. If safety concerns arise, the FDA may issue warnings or restrictions, require additional clinical trials, or even withdraw the drug from the market if necessary (9).

There are advantages and disadvantages of the many different types of clinical trial designs conducted in phases of clinical research. Trial designs may be controlled or noncontrolled; randomized or nonrandomized; open label or blinded; and parallel, crossover, or factorial. The International Council for Harmonisation (2022), the guidance for General Considerations for Clinical Studies (ICH E8 R1) specifically reviews the clinical trial design, with an utmost focus on designing quality into clinical research trials.

Some recent changes in drug development that are of importance to the sleep research community include:

- AI and Machine Learning are expediting drug discovery and clinical trial analysis. Researchers have developed AI algorithms that analyze data from wearables like smartwatches, rings, and wireless patches to detect obstructive sleep apnea (OSA) in real time. Patients at high risk for OSA can be flagged for further clinical evaluation and potentially faster treatment.
- Adaptive Clinical Trials allow modifications to studies based on interim data. For example, adaptive Bayesian design has been used in sleep medicine trials, particularly when studying OSA treatments, insomnia therapies, and narcolepsy drug trials. Researchers start with multiple interventions, such as PAP therapy, oral appliances, weight loss programs, or pharmacologic treatments. Interim data analyses are conducted at prespecified intervals to assess treatment efficacy and patient adherence. Based on interim results, the study adapts by dropping ineffective treatments (eg, if oral appliances are found ineffective, they may be removed from the trial). They may also adjust randomization to assign more patients to the most promising interventions or modify dosage or duration for a particular treatment based on patient response.
- Real-World Evidence (RWE) is increasingly used for drug approvals. For example, wearable sleep trackers collect RWE on sleep duration, efficiency, and disturbances. Online surveys and sleep diaries are used to track changes in insomnia symptoms with cognitive-behavioral therapy for insomnia (CBT-I) (10).
- Emergency Use Authorizations (EUAs), like those seen during COVID-19, have sped up drug and device availability for urgent needs. For example, the FDA issued EUAs to expand the use of CPAP and BiPAP (bilevel positive airway pressure) devices for respiratory support, including for patients experiencing sleep-disordered breathing and COVID-related breathing issues. This helped address ventilator shortages.

KEY PERSONNEL IN CLINICAL RESEARCH

There are a variety of key personnel involved in clinical research.

Sponsor. According to regulation 21 CFR 312.3(b), the sponsor is defined as "a person who takes responsibility for and initiates a clinical investigation. The sponsor may be an individual or pharmaceutical company, governmental agency, academic institution, private organization, or other organization." This is the individual or group that initiates the development of the IP or device. Regulatory requirements are detailed in 21 CFR 312, subpart D, Responsibilities of Sponsors and Investigators.

CONTRACT RESEARCH ORGANIZATION

According to regulation 21 CFR 312.3(b), a CRO is "a person that assumes, as an independent contractor with the sponsor, one or more of the obligations of a sponsor, for example, design of a protocol, selection or monitoring of investigations, evaluation of reports, and preparation of materials to be submitted to the Food and Drug Administration."

The term CRO is broad by definition and can be extended to those individuals or organizations that are assigned the responsibility of performing even the smallest of tasks by the sponsor. More commonly, CROs are contracted to provide project oversight of clinical trials. They are often the intermediary for contract and budget negotiations, but more commonly, the CRO oversees the trial-related performance of the clinical sites.

The CRO can be assigned a spectrum of responsibilities by the sponsor. However, a participating site must be aware of the scope of the CRO's responsibilities in order to properly address various trial functions and communications to the most appropriate party. This is particularly true in the event the sponsor has transferred a limited number of responsibilities to the CRO. The site will not want to communicate information inappropriately to the wrong party.

PRIMARY INVESTIGATOR

In clinical research, the investigator is defined as the person who actually conducts a clinical investigation and is responsible for the research subjects. This is the person who specifically agrees to all of the requirements in Section 9, Commitments of the FDA Form 1572. In this section, the investigator agrees to protect the rights, safety, and welfare of participants; follow the rules of the protocol; control the IP; and obtain informed consent (IC) from all participants. Additionally, it is the investigator's responsibility to ensure trained, licensed, or certified personnel are appropriately selected for inclusion on the Delegation of Authority form for each specific trial. Moreover, the investigator is responsible for ensuring all trial-related staff are familiar with the purpose of the trial and the protocol (11).

The investigator should ensure that any individual to whom a task is delegated is qualified by education, training, and experience (and state licensure where relevant) to perform the delegated task. Appropriate delegation is primarily an issue for tasks considered to be clinical or medical in nature, such as evaluating study subjects to assess clinical response to an investigational therapy (eg, global assessment scales, vital signs) or providing medical care to subjects during the course of the study. Most clinical/medical tasks require formal medical training and may also have licensing or certification requirements (eg, Registered and/or licensed sleep technologists). Licensing requirements may vary by jurisdiction (eg, states, countries). Investigators should take such qualifications/licensing requirements into account when considering delegation of specific tasks.

In the event there is more than one investigator on the research project, one person is designated as the principal or primary investigator (PI). All others are recognized as subinvestigators or "sub-I's."

The PI role is most commonly filled by a physician, but it is not uncommon to see a PharmD or PhD as the PI. In the case where IP is being investigated, a physician should be included as a sub-I on the trial. As this pertains to sleep/wake-related clinical trial activity, the PIs have extensive clinical training and experience not only in their own subspecialties (ie, neurology, pulmonology, psychiatry and otolaryngology) but also in clinical research. Although many subjects are recruited from within active medical practices, the practice of medicine is not always the same as clinical trial oversight.

CLINICAL RESEARCH ASSOCIATE

A clinical research associate (CRA) (also often referred to as a monitor) is the representative of either the sponsor or the CRO and is assigned the task of assuring the clinical site is performing to the expected standards of the protocol. This is a partial list of the many tasks they perform:

- Assess the site initially for ability to perform as needed for an upcoming trial: in a sleep research center, this may include tasks such as checking relevant sleep tech credentials, equipment bio-med and maintenance records, and equipment ability to record the required data.
- Train the site to the protocol and its associated procedures.
- Activate the site as a trial becomes open to accepting new subjects.
- Routinely monitor activity and document for completeness and accuracy: in a sleep research center, this may include tasks such as checking any documentation sources for accuracy against any recorded data and audit trails and verifying the data was collected properly based on the protocol and study manuals provided.
- Assist the site in developing or improving recruitment plans.
- Perform the close-out visits.

Although the majority of CRAs have a clinical background, there are very rare circumstances in which they interact with subjects during a trial.

CLINICAL RESEARCH COORDINATOR

The clinical research coordinator (CRC) represents the principal investigator (PI) at the clinical site. They are directly responsible for direct subject interaction under the direction of the PI. However, the CRC can perform only the tasks they have been assigned and trained to do. The Delegation of Authority log for the site outlines the specific tasks each of the site's personnel has been assigned to perform, and it is the PI's responsibility to ensure all personnel remain within their own scope of performance.

It is possible for a sleep technologist to be a CRC and vice versa. In many clinical sleep research sites, it is necessary for the coordinator to have a strong understanding of sleep medicine and related technology. However, the requirements for sitting for the sleep technologist registry examinations are insufficient to adequately prepare one for clinical research work. Additional research-specific training, trainee-mentorship guidance, and work experience are minimum requirements for a sleep technologist to either augment or transition to a career in clinical research.

SLEEP RESEARCH CENTER REGULATORY RESPONSIBILITIES

A sleep research facility involved in a clinical trial must comply with many regulatory, ethical, and operational guidelines to ensure patient safety, data integrity, and legal compliance. They must navigate FDA (in the United States), IRB, Good Clinical Practice (GCP),

Health Insurance Portability and Accountability Act (HIPAA), and increasing data security regulations while ensuring high-quality sleep data collection, protocol adherence and participant safety. Here are the key regulatory considerations:

1. Compliance With FDA Regulations. The U.S. Food and Drug Administration (FDA) regulates clinical trials involving drugs, biologics, and medical devices (12). Sleep research facilities must adhere to:
   - 21 CFR Part 50—Informed Consent: Patients must be fully informed about risks, benefits, and trial protocols before participation.
   - 21 CFR Part 56—Institutional Review Board (IRB) Oversight: An IRB must approve and monitor all sleep-related clinical trials.
   - 21 CFR Part 812—Investigational Device Exemptions (IDE): If testing medical devices (eg, CPAP, neurostimulation implants), an IDE may be required to ensure safe testing.
   - 21 CFR Part 11—Electronic Records and Signatures: If electronic systems are used for data collection or patient monitoring, they must comply with FDA standards for data security and data integrity.
2. IRB Approval
   Before conducting a clinical trial, a registered IRB must review the study protocol for ethical concerns, ensure participant safety and IC, and monitor ongoing research for adverse events and protocol deviations. IRB approval must be obtained and maintained for each participating site.
3. GCP Compliance
   Among the myriad guidelines established by the ICH, the GCP guidelines (Code E6) stand out as a fundamental pillar in clinical trial conduct. These guidelines outline the ethical and scientific standards for designing, conducting, recording, and reporting clinical trials involving human subjects. The overall objective is to provide a unified standard to facilitate the mutual acceptance of clinical trial data for ICH member countries and regions by applicable regulatory authorities. GCP guidelines apply to all clinical trials (13). Sleep research sites must ensure proper training of all staff, sleep technologists and investigators, maintain high-quality data collection through adherence to protocol-specific standardized procedures, and ensure the highest data integrity and security standards are maintained. While polysomnography (PSG) is generally a low-risk, noninvasive test, adverse events can still occur, and it is important that all sleep technologists understand what adverse and serious adverse events are and how to respond to and document them.
4. HIPAA and Data Privacy Regulations
   Since sleep studies involve sensitive health data, sleep research centers must have a good understanding of Protected Health Information (PHI) as well as comply with:
   - HIPAA—Protects patient confidentiality and requires secure handling of electronic medical records.
   - GDPR (General Data Protection Regulation) (for international studies)—If data is collected from European patients, GDPR rules apply. Other countries may have other specific regulatory guidelines.
5. Investigational Product (IP) Handling and Storage
   If the trial involves a new sleep medication or device, research facilities must maintain proper drug storage conditions (temperature, expiration tracking), keep a detailed log of drug/device distribution to participants, and ensure trained personnel handle IPs following regulatory guidelines.
6. Clinical Trial Registration and Reporting
   Clinical trials in the United States must be registered on ClinicalTrials.gov before recruitment begins. All results, including adverse events and final trial outcomes, must be reported per FDA and National Institutes of Health (NIH) guidelines.
7. Site Inspections and Audits
   The FDA (or other international regulatory authority), sponsors, or IRBs may conduct site inspections to ensure compliance. Facilities should be audit-ready, maintaining all required documents, including study protocols and IRB approvals, IC forms, adverse event reports, all applicable sleep study data, and related documentation (PSG and/or other collected data in native and any converted formats, reports, documentation/logs, CPAP compliance data, etc).

GOVERNANCE OF CLINICAL RESEARCH

Research involving human subjects is highly regulated by national and international bodies. It is the responsibility of all clinical research professionals to know and abide by all applicable regulations, policies, guidelines, and standards to protect the health and welfare of human subjects involved in clinical research. Failure to maintain strict adherence can put trial participants in risky conditions that could have catastrophic consequences as well as legal and civil consequences for the professionals conducting the trial.

BELMONT REPORT

The Belmont Report (14) is considered to be one of the most important works on ethics and health care research. Like its predecessors that addressed ethics, the

Belmont Report's primary purpose is to protect subjects who participate in clinical trials or research studies. The report focused on three specific areas: first was defining the differences between practice and research. This was followed by a section on Basic Ethical Principles; Respect for Persons, Beneficence, and Justice. Finally, the committee concluded with a third section on Application, IC, Assessment of Risks and Benefits, and then Selection of Subjects.

DECLARATION OF HELSINKI

The World Medical Association, in 1964, released a document containing a set of ethical principles regarding human experimentation. The Declaration of Helsinki has been updated regularly over the years (15). Its purpose was to outline defining ethical principles for the protection of participants in experimentation. The document contains 37 articles relating to the following principles:

- General principles
- Risks, burdens, and benefits
- Vulnerable groups and individuals
- Scientific requirements and research protocols
- Research ethics committees
- Privacy and confidentiality
- Informed consent
- Use of placebo
- Posttrial provisions
- Research registration and publication and dissemination of results
- Unproven interventions in clinical practice

The Declaration of Helsinki is considered to be the cornerstone statement of research in medical investigations. Nevertheless, the NIH released its own statement of Ethical Guidelines (16), which include:

- Social and clinical value
- Scientific validity
- Fair subject selection
- Favorable risk-benefit ratio
- Independent review
- Informed consent
- Respect for potential and enrolled subjects

NUREMBERG CODE

From 1946 to 1947, three judges and one alternate of the International Military Tribunal heard the case presented against 23 defendants (20 of whom were physicians) who were accused of murder and torture in the conduct of medical experiments on concentration camp inmates. At the conclusion of "The Doctors' Trial," the judges compiled a set of 10 research principles for the protection of human subjects. Where the Hippocratic Oath focused on the physician, The Nuremberg Code focused on the subjects who were participating in research (17).

Widely recognized for its influence on global human rights law and medical ethics, the basic requirement of IC has been accepted as the first step in protecting research subjects. Along with the other nine principles, the Nuremberg Code indicates:

1. The voluntary consent of the human subject is absolutely essential.
2. The experiment should be such as to yield fruitful results for the good of society, unprocurable by other methods or means of study, and not random and unnecessary in nature.
3. The experiment should be so designed and based on the results of animal experimentation and a knowledge of the natural history of the disease or other problem under study that the anticipated results will justify the performance of the experiment.
4. The experiment should be so conducted as to avoid all unnecessary physical and mental suffering and injury.
5. No experiment should be conducted, where there is an a priori reason to believe that death or disabling injury will occur, except, perhaps, in those experiments where the experimental physicians also serve as subjects.
6. The degree of risk to be taken should never exceed that determined by the humanitarian importance of the problem to be solved by the experiment.
7. Proper preparations should be made and adequate facilities provided to protect the experimental subject against even remote possibilities of injury, disability, or death.
8. The experiment should be conducted only by scientifically qualified persons. The highest degree of skill and care should be required through all stages of the experiment of those who conduct or engage in the experiment.
9. During the course of the experiment, the human subject should be at liberty to bring the experiment to an end, if they have reached the physical or mental state where continuation of the experiment seems to be impossible to them.
10. During the course of the experiment, the scientist in charge must be prepared to terminate the experiment at any stage, if they have probable cause to believe, in the exercise of the good faith, superior skill, and careful judgment required of them, that a continuation of the experiment is likely to result in injury, disability, or death to the experimental subject.

INTERNATIONAL COUNCIL FOR HARMONIZATION

The International Council for Harmonization (ICH) Technical Requirements for Pharmaceuticals for Human Use (18) was formed in 1990 as a global entity to address and create the Guidelines on Safety, Quality, and Efficacy. It later added the subcategory of Multidisciplinary Guidelines. As the organization reports,

The resulting ICH association establishes an Assembly as the overarching governing body with the aim of focusing global pharmaceutical regulatory harmonization work in one venue that allows pharmaceutical regulatory authorities and notably concerned industry organizations to be more actively involved in ICH's harmonization work.

On 6 January 2025, the GCP E6 (R3) reached Step 4 of the ICH process, adopting the principles and Annex 1. The overall objective is to provide a unified standard to facilitate the mutual acceptance of clinical trial data for ICH member countries and regions by applicable regulatory authorities. Specific areas of ICH that cover clinical research can be found in the Efficacy Guidelines section. For those working in a clinical research site, the following have the greatest influence in the conduct of a trial:

E6(R3): Guideline for Good Clinical Practice
E2A: Definitions and Standards for Expedited Reporting
E8 (R1): General Considerations for Clinical Trials
E9: Statistical Principles for Clinical Trials
E11(R1): Clinical Investigation of Medicinal Products in the Pediatric Population
E19: Optimization of Safety Data Collection

Clinical trials with origins in non-US countries focus on similar rigorous regulatory standards rooted in ICH guidelines.

U.S. FOOD AND DRUG ADMINISTRATION

An agency within the U.S. Department of HHS, it is the FDA's responsibility to protect public health by making sure that human and veterinary drugs; vaccines and other biologic products; medical devices; the nation's food supply; cosmetics; dietary supplements; and products that give off radiation are safe, effective, and secure.

Specific sections of the Code of Federal Regulations (19) that apply to clinical research are:

45 CFR 46: Protection of Human Subjects
Subpart A: Basic HHS Policy for Protection of Human Research Subjects ("Common Rule")
Subpart B: Additional Protections for Pregnant Women, Human Fetuses and Neonates Involved in Research
Subpart C: Additional Protections Pertaining to Biomedical and Behavioral Research Involving Prisoners as Subjects
Subpart D: Additional Protections for Children Involved as Subjects in Research
Subpart E: Registration of Institutional Review Boards
21 CFR Part 11 Electronic Records, Electronic Signature
21 CFR Part 50 Protection of Human Subjects
21 CFR Part 54 Financial Disclosure by Clinical Investigators
21 CFR Part 56 Institutional Review Boards
21 CFR Part 312 Investigational New Drug Application
21 CFR Part 812 Investigational Device Exemptions

The FDA recognizes the ICH guidelines and has adopted various sections within the agency (ie, Good Clinical Practices). But in specific areas of overlap, the FDA sets U.S. CFR as precedent.

HEALTH INSURANCE PORTABILITY AND ACCOUNTABILITY ACT

The *Health Insurance Portability and Accountability Act*, known as HIPAA, originated in the Office of Civil Rights. Although it is not specific to research, it impacts research with the section called the "privacy rule." The "privacy rule" protects the use and disclosure of patient information, also known as Protected Health Information (PHI) or Personally Identifiable Information (PII). It refers to any information that is related to a person's health, health care, or payment for health care services that can be used to identify that individual. These "personal data" include, but are not limited to:

- Personal identifiers: Names, addresses, dates of birth, Social Security numbers, and other identifiers that can be used to trace an individual's identity.
- Health information: Medical records, diagnoses, treatment information, and health conditions, including both physical and mental health information.
- Health care services information: Any data about a person's health care history, current care, or future treatment plans.
- Billing and payment information: Insurance information, billing records, and payment details.

Personal data can exist in any form, including paper, electronic, or oral communication. The key is that the information can be linked to an individual and is used for health care-related purposes. Under HIPAA, health care providers, health plans, and health care clearinghouses are required to safeguard PHI to maintain patient privacy and confidentiality. What is considered personal data depends on the context as well as which country a research participant lives in and has data. Different parts of the world have factored in definitions of what it is in their laws. It is advisable to read up on the laws relevant to your part of the world. For those recording sleep research studies, the person entering patient information must also be aware of these identifiers.

PROTOCOL

According to *Merriam-Webster*, one of the four definitions of "protocol" is "a detailed plan of a scientific or medical experiment, treatment, or procedure." In clinical research, the protocol is a road map under which the trial is to be conducted. A very detailed document provides the reader with an IP's background, the intention of the trial and its anticipated outcomes, the intended subject population, and the analysis process.

For a sleep research site, the protocol can be viewed as the "Rule Book." The protocol and any protocol-specific supplemental manuals for sleep or wake recordings must be followed as closely as possible. Failure to follow the rules may be minor, or more serious deviations could result in serious consequences and regulatory impacts.

A deviation is a lesser situation that may occur without significant consequences. For example, if a subject missed a PSG within the protocol-specified time frame (or window) because they were traveling, this is a deviation. On the other hand, a violation is a much more serious event. These can range from events that have an impact on data collection completeness to making IC inaccurate or impacting the subject's health, safety, and welfare. Examples of a violation include incomplete or inaccurate record keeping or intentional deviation from protocol requirements.

Protocol deviations are sometimes unavoidable, but all attempts should be made to minimize these occurrences. On the other hand, violations (especially those that affect safety, health, and welfare) can have dire consequences. Willfully putting the subject in a compromising position can result in legal actions for the individual who perpetrated the action. This can include removal from the trial, loss of clinical licensure, and criminal prosecution if the infraction warrants. To this end, compliance with the protocol is paramount only to the subjects' welfare.

INFORMED CONSENT

IC is a process, not just a form. The IC is a document recorded and signed by the PI and the subject. Moreover, it must occur before any subject participation can occur. There are three critical areas and essential elements of an IC: voluntarism, information disclosure, and decision-making capacity.

The subject retains the right to withdraw consent without repercussion at any time during a clinical trial. The PI is obliged to give the subject all relevant new information concerning the trial as it occurs during the subject's time of participation. And lastly, it is the subject who retains the final say in the decision to participate or not. The subject has the right to refuse.

CLINICAL RESEARCH IN SLEEP

There are many avenues of clinical investigations in today's sleep research community. Newer trials are diversifying from primarily pharmaceutical IP investigations to newer technology involving a variety of devices, wearables, techniques (eg, algorithmic analysis or assessments), and treatments. Whereas it was once a matter of giving an IP treatment, recording the sleeping subject, and then analyzing the data to measure the effects (or not), today's trials may include indirect or inferred measures of sleep.

Early clinical sleep research trials involving the measurement of sleep on analog polygraphs involved two different methods for analysis. The first method was to produce the recording and then ship it to a site where it was scored (using a paper case report form (CRF) to report results) by either one person or a select few scorers. Reducing the number of scorers meant there would be a potential reduction in interscorer differences; thus, quality control was easier to maintain. However, this method of centralizing analysis was expensive and slow. In addition, bulky boxes of irreplaceable participant data were subject to shipping losses. Another popular method of the time was to have each site score their own PSGs. This reduced the analysis time as well as shipping costs. Rather than shipping the records, the "scoresheets" could be faxed to the sponsor. This too had its shortfalls when sponsors pressed the CROs to provide proof of scorer competency and interrater reliability from the sites. In order to provide evidence, CROs produced an oversight process by which select personnel at the site would become "certified scorers" for that specific protocol.

As technology evolved and the industry shifted to digital PSG, the problem of assembling data from multiple sites that may have produced the records from many manufacturers prompted additional regulatory requirements placed by the European Union (EU). Consequently, EU regulators made a condition of sale of polysomnographic and electroencephalographic digital recording systems requiring a data output whereby a third-party independent software reader could import the recording and correctly display the attributes.

First published in 1992, European Data Format (EDF) became the de facto standard for the manufacturers to incorporate as a means of record sharing (20). Using EDF, the records could be imported into an EDF reader software, and the manufacturers' native software remained proprietary, including their algorithms for exporting from native to EDF. Nevertheless, this advance allowed for the electronic transmittal of records from the site to a central reader. As with previous methods of certifying scorers, sponsors required the central readers to provide proof of site competency by producing a recording capable of being imported to an EDF reader. Many central readers require sites to produce sample recordings made to the protocol requirements, and if successfully and accurately produced, the central readers certify the sites as ready to begin enrolling participants. Early digital sleep research recordings were converted to EDF, then burned to a CD and shipped to a central scoring facility. Instead of taking days for shipping and additional time for analysis, time frames could be drastically reduced to, in some cases, a day or two for reporting results. For modern sleep research trials, it is typically a requirement for sleep sites to have internet capabilities so they can upload recorded research data to a secure portal as soon as the recordings are complete.

Most device recording manufacturers incorporated EDF as a standard data output or export option. Instead of creating a proprietary digital output no other system software could decipher, emphasis was placed on developing analysis packages and creating robust reporting analytics in order to gain a market advantage. They have validated their analysis programs to EDF standards, thus paving the way for large, multisite trials to transmit their records to a centralized site for scoring and analysis.

Not all clinical trials involving sleep parameters require a participant to have an in-lab PSG. Depending on the focus of the trial, it can be more advantageous to use a "home sleep test" or other device or wearable (eg, actigraphy) to collect participant data. But this is strictly dependent on the data needs of the trial and compliance with the protocol requirements.

In the course of clinical trials, there are many measures of sleep and wake that can indicate the effects of treatment (Table 72-1). These are referred to as "end points," and they can be the primary focus of the trial or secondary measures of trial outcomes.

Table 72-1 Sleep and Wake Measurement Endpoints

Sleep efficiency	How well or how poorly a participant sleeps during the PSG recording can be correlated as an effect of the treatment, whether it is better, worse, or the same. This can apply to both IP and device trials.
SL	Sleep latency is captured during PSG, MSLT, and MWT and may be defined in multiple ways. SL captures how quickly sleep onset is achieved, typically from the point of lights out. This measure can be used to gauge treatment effect and is a primary factor in determining mean sleep latency values in MSLT and MWT end points.
LPS	By definition, LPS (latency to persistent sleep) occurs at the beginning of the first 10 min of sleep after lights out. This measure can be used to gauge treatment effect in relation to sleep-onset arousals that prevent consolidated sleep early in the recording.
WASO	"WASO" (wake after sleep onset) is frequently used as a treatment efficacy measure in IP and device trials. As an end point, it reveals how well treatment has impacted the participants' ability to sleep all the way through the recording after initially falling asleep. It is frequently used in insomnia treatment trials.
Arousals	In large part, arousals during sleep occur secondarily to other disrupting factors, such as apnea or periodic limb movements. However, arousals in narcolepsy appear to occur spontaneously and without provocation. Hence, the frequency of arousals is an important treatment indication for these related trials.
REM latency	REM latency during the PSG and/or MSLT can reveal the effects of untreated or undertreated sleep pathologies, whether a circadian rhythm disorder or narcolepsy. Hence, its measurement indicates treatment efficacy.
Sleep stages	Increases in percentages of certain sleep stages with decreases in others when measured in baseline and treatment nights can indicate the effectiveness of the intended treatment. To reduce the chances of bias, IP trials may use a randomized double-blind, crossover pattern of IP and placebo. As such, the sleep stage percentages (or time duration) from baseline (no treatment), Night 1 (treatment or placebo), and Night 2 (switch from Night 1) are compared for differences.

(continued)

Table 72-1 Sleep and Wake Measurement Endpoints (*continued*)

LM/PLMA	Reduction of LM (limb movement) or periodic limb movement arousals (PLMA) during sleep in one IP trial may be the intended result, whereas an increase in another IP trial may be indicative of an unanticipated adverse event. Therefore, although the first trial may use the reduction as a primary end point, the second trial might use LM/PLMA as a secondary end point because this would be an unintended result of treatment.
Respiratory events	Results of respiratory measures can be end point data for both device and IP trials. Clearly, the goal in breathing-related sleep disorders device trials is to reduce the occurrence of events, which is a primary end point of investigation. It may be the same during an IP trial, but it may also be the unintended effect of the IP treatment. In this case, the outcome of respiratory event changes can become a secondary end point with an emphasis on safety.
PROs or ePRO	PROMs (patient-reported outcomes) or ePRO (electronic patient-reported outcome) are used as a means of corroboration of the participants' perspective in relation to trial activities. They are often evaluated immediately after a diagnostic (ie, PSG, MWT) or treatment evaluation or during the period between measures. Common PROs include: • Epworth Sleepiness Scale (ESS) • SF-36 Health Survey; Short Form 36 (captures participants' perceptions of their health-related quality of life). • Karolinska Sleepiness Scale (KSS)

IP, investigational product; LM, limb movements; LPS, latency to persistent sleep; MSLT, multiple sleep latency test; MWT, maintenance of wakefulness test; PROs, patient-reported outcomes; PSG, polysomnography; REM, rapid eye movement; WASO, wake after sleep onset.

SPECIFICS FOR SLEEP RESEARCH

In order to produce all the sleep- and wake-related end points that are required for a research protocol, standardization at every level is paramount. Even though sleep centers around the world may use the same basic set of rules, references and guidance principles, in practice, there are often inherent biases and differences across sites. These differences may be attributed to types of recording equipment, shift schedules, recording montages, settings, monitoring and troubleshooting, emergency procedures, sleep lab focus (academic vs hospital-based lab), PI specialty (pulmonary, neurology, pediatrics, or psychiatry), and regional practice (sleep labs in the United States may have differences from research sites in other countries). For this reason, in most clinical research trials involving sleep research sites, it is customary to use a central processing/reading center. The central processing vendor is typically responsible for a number of tasks, such as creating standardized specific procedures for recording and monitoring the related data to support the protocol and end points the sponsor defines. This may include establishing certification and training requirements for site staff that will be recording or processing data and/or an operations manual for all protocol-specific and technical data acquisition settings. Research recordings may have different requirements from typical clinical practice. If the specific research criteria are not followed by the recording staff, data end points may be unevaluable or lost.

A few examples:

For research PSGs, there are often specific schedule requirements for when to complete specific assessments that need to be done in a standard order using a standard method (eg, each PSG recorded may need to be scheduled based on a participant's recorded mean habitual bedtime). This may relate to when to start the PSG recording, perform calibrations, and have a scheduled lights off and lights on (eg, if protocol specifies 8-hour recordings: PSGs from lights off to lights on should be 8 hours/960 epochs/480 minutes). The recording montage may require different settings, or recordings may have restrictions based on EDF conversion requirements.

A protocol may call for maintenance of wakefulness test (MWT) recordings, and instead of a clinical standard of four MWT trials, the research protocol may call for six trials, run overnight, and may have different recording/stopping criteria.

Standardizing recording, monitoring, and documentation procedures across research sites helps to control variability and homogenize the dataset across all sites collecting all data. One central processing site then allows for an unbiased central team to use the same standardized methods to verify, assess quality, and process all data and documentation per sponsor and protocol definitions. This minimizes variability and collates all data in one location for reporting, review, and audit.

Pharmacologic developments and investigations will continue as long as the need remains, and there are many opportunities for sleep technologists to expand their careers in the clinical research arena.

REFERENCES

1. Wood M. Allan Rechtschaffen, sleep research pioneer, 1927-2021. Accessed March 6, 2025. https://news.uchicago.edu/story/allan-rechtschaffen-sleep-research-pioneer-1927-2021
2. Quan SF. The Journal of Clinical Sleep Medicine—a decade of progress: looking backward and forward. *J Clin Sleep Med*. 2014;10(1):5-6. doi:10.5664/jcsm.3344
3. International Council for Harmonisation of Technical Requirements for Pharmaceuticals for Human Use. E8(R1) general considerations for clinical studies. 2022. Accessed December 7, 2025. https://www.federalregister.gov/documents/2022/04/11/2022-07690/e8r1-general-considerations-for-clinical-studies-international-council-for-harmonisation-guidance
4. U.S. Department of Health and Human Services, Food and Drug Administration, Center for Devices and Radiological Health, & Office of Device Evaluation. Applying human factors and usability engineering to medical devices: guidance for industry and Food and Drug Administration staff. Published 2016. Accessed March 7, 2025. https://www.fda.gov/regulatory-information/search-fda-guidance-documents/applying-human-factors-and-usability-engineering-medical-devices
5. American Society for Quality. FMEA. Accessed March 7, 2025. https://asq.org/quality-resources/fmea
6. U.S. Department of Health and Human Services. Medical device tracking requirements (21 C.F.R. § 821). U.S. Government Publishing Office. Published 2025. Accessed March 7, 2025. https://www.ecfr.gov/current/title-21/chapter-I/subchapter-H/part-821
7. U.S. Food and Drug Administration. Development & approval process: drugs. Published 2022. Accessed March 7, 2025. https://www.fda.gov/drugs/development-approval-process-drugs
8. U.S. Food and Drug Administration. Investigational new drug applications (21 C.F.R. § 312.21). U.S. Government Publishing Office. Published 2025. Accessed March 7, 2025. https://www.ecfr.gov/current/title-21/chapter-I/subchapter-D/part-312/subpart-B/section-312.21
9. U.S. Department of Health and Human Services. Investigational new drug application: phase 4 studies (21 C.F.R. § 312.85). Published 2025. Accessed March 7, 2025. https://www.ecfr.gov/current/title-21/chapter-I/subchapter-D/part-312/subpart-E/section-312.85
10. U.S. Food and Drug Administration. Designing sound clinical trials to incorporate real-world data. Published 2022. Accessed March 7, 2025. https://www.fda.gov/science-research/real-world-evidence/fda-use-real-world-evidence-regulatory-decision-making
11. U.S. Department of Health and Human Services. 21 C.F.R. § 312.53(c)—Selection of investigators. Accessed March 8, 2025. https://www.ecfr.gov/current/title-21/chapter-I/subchapter-D/part-312/subpart-D/section-312.53
12. U.S. Food and Drug Administration. Regulations: good clinical practice, and clinical trials. Accessed March 8, 2025. https://www.fda.gov/science-research/clinical-trials-and-human-subject-protection/regulations-good-clinical-practice-and-clinical-trials
13. U.S. Food and Drug Administration. Good clinical practice (GCP) inspection collaboration with international regulators for drug development. Accessed March 8, 2025. https://www.fda.gov/science-research/clinical-trials-and-human-subject-protection/good-clinical-practice-gcp-inspection-collaboration-international-regulators-drug-development
14. National Commission for the Protection of Human Subjects of Biomedical and Behavioral Research. The Belmont report: ethical principles and guidelines for the protection of human subjects of research. Published 1979. Accessed December 7, 2025. https://www.hhs.gov/ohrp/regulations-and-policy/belmont-report/read-the-belmont-report/index.html
15. World Medical Association. WMA declaration of Helsinki: ethical principles for medical research involving human participants. World Medical Association. Published 2024. Accessed March 8, 2025. https://www.wma.net/policies-post/wma-declaration-of-helsinki/
16. National Institutes of Health. Guiding principles for ethical research. National Institutes of Health. Accessed March 8, 2025. https://www.nih.gov/health-information/nih-clinical-research-trials-you/guiding-principles-ethical-research
17. Trials of War Criminals before the Nuremberg Military Tribunals, Volume 2. Nuremberg Code. U.S. Government Printing Office. 1949. Accessed December 7, 2025. https://collections.nlm.nih.gov/catalog/nlm:nlmuid-01130400RX2-mvpart
18. International Council for Harmonisation of Technical Requirements for Pharmaceuticals for Human Use. International Council for Harmonisation (ICH). Accessed March 8, 2025. https://www.ich.org/
19. U.S. Department of Health and Human Services, Office for Human Research Protections. About OHRP. Accessed March 8, 2025. https://www.hhs.gov/ohrp/regulations-and-policy/index.html
20. Alvarez-Estevez D. European data format. Accessed March 8, 2025. https://www.edfplus.info/

Chapter 73
The Sleep Technologist in the Medical Office

SARAH WAHHAB

KEY CONCEPTS/LEARNING OBJECTIVES

The key concepts for this chapter include defining how home sleep apnea testing is influencing the various functions and expanding roles for the sleep technologist discussing the comprehensive sleep program models and the use of technology to support patients and describing how to grow an expanded sleep program.

KEY TERMS

Alternative therapy
Comprehensive sleep program
HSAT
Integration systems
Team-based practice
Technology
Utilization management

CHANGES IN SLEEP CENTER FUNCTION

The Effect of Home Sleep Apnea Testing on Sleep Centers

Health care reforms are bringing changes to health insurance plans and pushing providers to improve the continuity and coordination of care in an effort to improve patient outcomes and provide cost-effective and efficient care. A significant impact of these measures in sleep medicine is the shift toward home sleep apnea testing (HSAT) for diagnosing obstructive sleep apnea (OSA) and increasing attention to developing practices for improving positive airway pressure (PAP) therapy delivery and compliance. The sleep center is moving from a fee-for-service reimbursement model to an outcomes-based model. The purpose is to reduce costs and optimize patient care.

Sleep testing is trending more and more toward HSAT, rather than in-laboratory overnight testing, and this is directly related to the payer policies. Sleep centers have seen different degrees of adoption of HSAT; however, the trend is shifting away from overnight in-laboratory testing because of changes in reimbursement, as well as patient preference for the convenience of testing in the home. This trend is affecting the growth of sleep centers and altering the necessary skill level and knowledge base of technologists (1).

Historically, the majority of patients referred for overnight testing were being evaluated for suspected OSA. With the huge impact of HSAT as the primary diagnostic tool for diagnosing these patients, the dynamics of in-laboratory overnight testing needs to focus on evaluating complex patients with multiple comorbidities or in some instances to validate the findings of the HSAT (2). These patients include those with hypoventilation, cardiac patients with low ejection fraction, chronic respiratory failure, and premature infants with complex breathing problems.

Technologist Involvement

To manage overnight testing for complex patients, sleep technologists require proper education and strong critical thinking skills. Technologists need to perform patient assessments and be familiar with looking at patient test results (eg, pulmonary function tests, routine blood work, echocardiograms). It is critical that technologists have a good understanding of the underlying pathophysiology of particular disease processes. Complex patients require close monitoring of ventilatory patterns while they are sleeping. Technologists also require the knowledge to manage complex ventilatory devices like volume-assured pressure support and adaptive servo-ventilation.

The changes occurring represent an opportunity for technologists to utilize their skills in an ambulatory sleep center or office-based sleep program. This necessitates that sleep laboratories become comprehensive sleep centers and that physicians educate and work with technologists to integrate their skills into the patient care process. Services that can benefit from technologist knowledge and skills and reduce physician workload may include a PAP follow-up program, a PAP walk-in clinic, an alternative therapy program, remote patient monitoring (RPM), a hypersomnolence program for patients that were not diagnosed with OSA during their HSAT, or an insomnia program. Expansion of sleep center services could also include neonatal and pediatric inpatient testing and a perioperative screening program. The technologist/clinician's role includes utilizing clinical judgment by making clinical assessments, providing patient education, communicating test results to the patient, and communicating with non–sleep department medical staff.

Insurance Authorization

Another function that can benefit from technologist knowledge and experience is management of the testing and treatment authorization processes. With the introduction of HSAT, the majority of patients with basic OSA are being referred for a daytime educational instruction and sent home with a cardiorespiratory device for overnight testing. HSAT is much less expensive than in-laboratory testing and can accurately assess the patient suspected to have moderate-to-severe obstructive apnea (3). Patients requiring differential diagnoses, those with complex comorbidities, and pediatric patients will still require overnight polysomnography (PSG).

The insurance type (eg, Preferred Provider Organization, Health Maintenance Organization, Medicare, Medicaid) will determine how an authorization is obtained. Multiple private insurers not only require preauthorization but also regularly make use of utilization management companies to review preauthorization documents. Utilization management incorporates devices and methods for determining if the testing is medically necessary and if the patient can be tested using HSAT versus in-laboratory overnight testing. The utilization management companies' purpose is to assist the insurer to form authorization processes. The downside of utilization management is clinical decision limitations to the physician. In many cases, the need for an in-laboratory assessment requires additional effort by the provider to obtain preauthorization.

Some sleep facilities require the physician's office to obtain the insurance authorization before sending the referral to the sleep center; however, sleep center personnel may have the responsibility for obtaining preauthorization. When a referral is received, it should specify the type of study ordered or if a sleep physician consult is necessary before testing. Some facilities consider the referral as the prescription; otherwise, a prescription stating the type of study needs to be provided. A history and physical that includes a sleep history, along with patient demographics, signed and dated office visit notes explaining what medical history is prompting the sleep study referral, and insurance billing information, will need to accompany the referral. The sleep history should include documentation of body mass index, height, weight, and neck size.

Depending on the insurance company and type of insurance plan, it may take several days to a couple of weeks to obtain authorization. To obtain insurance authorization, the appropriate *International Classification of Diseases (ICD)-10* diagnosis codes will need to be listed to identify the patient's symptoms. An appropriate procedure code like the Current Procedural Terminology (CPT) is also required for authorization of the type of study to be conducted. It is important to know which procedure codes a particular insurer accepts. For example, for HSAT testing, some insurers accept a G-code procedure code, whereas others accept the corresponding CPT procedure code. There are also specific procedure codes for pediatric patients less than 6 years of age. It is the provider's responsibility to contact the insurance company to identify which codes are accepted for testing and to understand the requirements specified by the institution billing the charges as per their referral acceptance policy.

In some cases, hospitals may interpret billing requirements more stringently to ensure compliance with their accreditation body. As a result, even if the insurance does not mandate that the CPT code appear on the referral, the institution billing the charges might require it.

It is recommended to have a list of procedural codes available for reference. Be mindful to contact the insurance company if the study conducted fell under a different CPT code than what was authorized (eg, code 95811—PSG with PAP was authorized but 95810—PSG was completed due to the patient not meeting the lab's apnea-hypopnea index (AHI) policy to convert to the treatment portion of testing). Sleep center personnel are often also required to verify the patient's insurance benefits and determine any deductible or copayment that may be required. This information should be available to review with the patient at the time of scheduling or, at a minimum, prior to presenting for testing as stated by the No Surprises Act, so that they are informed of payment due before the sleep study date.

These functions are often most easily accomplished by a sleep technologist with a knowledge of sleep disorders and their symptoms as well as comorbidities that might influence the decision to approve in-laboratory testing, as opposed to HSAT.

A COMPREHENSIVE SLEEP PROGRAM MODEL

A comprehensive sleep center expands patient services to make the center prosper and provides a wide spectrum of clinical patient care activities. An expanded ambulatory program in a comprehensive program may include services such as PAP trials, a PAP follow-up program, management of non-PAP therapies for OSA, a weekly PAP walk-in clinic, RPM, a hypersomnolence program for patients that were not diagnosed with OSA during their HSAT, and an insomnia program. Other methods of extending services include working with in-hospital partners. A perioperative screening program can be developed by partnering with anesthesia and surgeons. Inpatient testing or screening programs can be developed by partnering with pulmonologists and neonatologists to identify patients in need of diagnosis, treatment, and continued follow-up after discharge. All of these services include the need for experienced sleep personnel—a natural fit for the sleep technologist.

A comprehensive care model requires a close-knit multidisciplinary team to manage program growth and the use of protocols to drive patient care. Telemedicine and technologies such as video and telephone visits, remote monitoring, and automated care mechanisms will improve efficiency and effectiveness of patient care and workflow. In this care model, the medical director leads a team of case managers comprising respiratory therapists with formal sleep training and sleep technologists. This type of sleep care program will not only alter a physician's role but also enhance the role of the sleep technologist and ensure the future of sleep centers.

Technology to Support Patients and Treatment

Advancements in technology have significantly enhanced the ability of sleep technologists to support patient compliance with therapy. By providing accessible data for patients, technology serves as a valuable tool to encourage adherence to PAP therapy. The increasing use of HSAT technology has made a substantial impact in this area.

Additionally, a variety of wearable devices enable motivated patients to monitor their caloric intake, exercise, weight management, and even estimate their sleep patterns. These devices are often integrated into RPM programs, which allow clinicians to work closely with patients during the initial compliance period. This collaboration ensures that patients not only adhere to therapy but also experience meaningful benefits. Furthermore, RPM programs create additional billing opportunities for physicians while simultaneously improving therapeutic outcomes.

PAP devices have wireless modems either built in or attached to the device. This permits patient adherence checks and adjustment of PAPs remotely. Utilizing wireless modems enables the sleep center staff to track patient adherence while decreasing the number of patient office visits required, thereby increasing patient satisfaction. Sleep technologists typically manage this type of therapy monitoring program in either an office-based or a comprehensive sleep program.

Much of the work of monitoring patient PAP adherence can benefit from technology. A PAP modem attached to an automated platform can send feedback to the clinician and a message to the patient for any issues detected or be used to motivate the patient who is doing well with treatment. This type of patient feedback has been shown to improve PAP adherence by 66% (4). The automated platform assists clinicians to focus on patients who are struggling and make more efficient use of their time in daily operations.

The integration of automated mechanisms and the creation of a closed-loop system in the sleep program can reduce primary care physician (PCP) visits, improve PAP therapy adherence, and reduce the need for PCPs to manage sleep disorders. A closed-loop system enhances and streamlines the end-to-end patient care continuum. In a closed-loop system, the sleep team works together to provide optimal patient care and continuous long-term management. A closed-loop system means the sleep specialist is responsible not just for diagnosis and study interpretation but for long-term follow-up care as well and can also provide inpatient program support.

Internet-based patient education programs are available that can ease the anxiety of patients and help them understand how to prepare for a sleep study, what to expect when they go to a sleep center, educate them on OSA and PAP therapy, and explain the difference between an HSAT study and a polysomnogram. These programs have soothing voices, animated graphics, and easy-to-read text, and patients are able to watch the program as many times as they wish. They are a helpful adjunct to technologist-provided education and support.

EXTERNAL INTEGRATION SYSTEMS

Traditionally, sleep centers have focused on diagnostic testing, providing PAP therapy, and patient follow-up. Comprehensive care under an end-to-end workflow model begins with population management using risk identification screening, patient preassessment using web-based education, sleep history intake questionnaires, and wearable sensors. However, managing all of these components can be very problematic as each is independent of the other. The results are not attached to the electronic health record (EHR), and a provider has to "hunt and peck" to find and compile all the information. An external integration system incorporates mechanisms that connect the entire health care team and improve workflow. The system is the core, connecting all aspects of patient care, including self-directed care platforms, automated care processes, and other remote technologies. This approach creates a seamless connection between the patient and provider team, with the EHR serving as the central hub to facilitate effective team-based care.

INTERNAL INTEGRATION SYSTEMS

Integrated care involves creating a team-based practice, protocols to drive patient care, and utilizing individual and group patient appointments and technology to enable patient engagement and improve efficiencies.

The physicians create clinical care pathways and protocols for the staff to follow. They provide training material and case studies for staff education, check and assure quality, and conduct chart reviews. The physicians not only read and interpret sleep studies but also provide patient consults and conduct research projects. They function as the leaders within the sleep medicine program and partner with other specialists to create care pathways and improve the management of patients.

In this model, the technologists/clinicians are using clinical judgment and collaborating with the physicians in the diagnosis and treatment of patients by reviewing the preliminary sleep testing results and initiating treatment. They make appropriate referrals from HSAT testing to in-laboratory testing or to other specialties as indicated by protocols or the physician. Integration and automated mechanisms with the sleep technologist at the forefront facilitate efficiency and provide the patient with effective care.

TEAM-BASED CARE

Team-based care structures sleep center programs and services to utilize specific levels of care for a patient's situation. Although all team members should be informed and kept updated with all aspects of the sleep services available, a multidisciplinary team approach allows a sleep program to provide specific levels of care on the basis of patient needs.

There are numerous potential areas of growth for sleep technologists and clinicians within a focused team-based care approach. Opportunities include supporting specialized programs such as a commercial driver program, a durable medical equipment (DME) program for dispensing PAP devices, or an insomnia program integrated with Internet-based cognitive behavioral therapy.

With sufficient training, technologists can also play a vital role in managing complex sleep patients—such as those with respiratory failure or muscular dystrophy—under the supervision of a physician.

RPM presents another significant opportunity, enabling care providers to track patient progress more closely. This not only enhances patient care but also creates various billing opportunities for providers, tailored to the specific comorbidities they are managing in relation to the patient's PAP therapy compliance and usage.

Creating an alternative therapy program is another avenue for sleep centers to offer options for nonadherent PAP patients. Technologists/clinicians trained in this specialty area can evaluate the patient for the appropriate pathway to alternative therapy, such as oral appliance therapy (OAT), positional therapy, or, when appropriate, implantable devices.

Workflows need to be developed for each specialty area and team to care for these patients. Patients with complex sleep disorder are fragile and require very close, timely, and consistent follow-up and encouragement. In this model, the technologist/clinician centrally coordinates the patient's care; close and thorough management will steer the direction of care that the patient requires.

With the appropriate training and education, the technologist/clinician can review and monitor diagnostic tests, which may include pulmonary function studies, arterial blood gas results, echocardiograms, and chest x-rays. It is important to know and understand such physiologic information as the patient's vital capacity, oxygen and carbon dioxide levels, and cardiac function, including ejection fraction percentage. The technologist/clinician may also monitor the patient's adherence to noninvasive ventilation and make adjustments to PAP as needed for comfort and acclimation. Utilization of transcutaneous carbon dioxide monitoring can indicate how well the patient is ventilating. Overnight oximetry is often useful to determine the need for supplemental oxygen during sleep.

PATIENT ENGAGEMENT

All patient care providers need certain skills in order to build a rapport with patients. The ability to demonstrate compassion, confidence, patience, and understanding are skill sets that will assist the technologist to gain the patient's trust and assist them to successfully implement their treatment plan. As providers, we perform a routine of day-to-day procedures, and we do not necessarily think from a patient's perspective. We need to remember that this is a new experience for patients and sometimes not a pleasant one. It is important to realize that every patient is unique and needs to be treated as an individual.

Routine medical procedures can often feel intimidating to patients. Before beginning any medical task during a visit, it is crucial to first establish a personal connection. Start by introducing yourself, positioning yourself at eye level with the patient, and engaging them with open-ended questions. Actively listening is key—not just with your ears but also with your eyes and heart.

Throughout the visit, pay attention to both the patient's body language and your own. A small investment of extra time to build rapport can lead to a deeper trust in you and the care plan you are proposing. Studies reveal that only 7% of communication is verbal, while 38% comes from tone and pitch, and 55% is conveyed through body language and facial expressions.

By taking these steps, you can create a supportive environment where patients feel heard, valued, and confident in their care journey.

To effectively communicate the impact of sleep apnea to patients, take the time to explain how it directly affects their health and quality of life. Begin by thoroughly reviewing their chart before the visit or conversation. This enables you to connect their specific symptoms and concerns with the comorbidities documented in their medical history, steering the discussion away from generalized terms and making it personally relevant.

By personalizing the conversation, you empower patients to understand the significance of their condition and the potential benefits of treatment. For example, ask "What would it mean to you if you woke up feeling more refreshed and energized?" This approach encourages them to see how treatment could improve their daily life, making the conversation more impactful.

Finally, consider what might motivate the patient to remain adherent to therapy. Tailoring the conversation to their goals and priorities will help them feel more engaged and committed to their care plan.

Will patients have the perception that they are going to stop breathing and die in their sleep, or might they think that they are having some pauses in their breathing and that this machine will help them sleep better? Their perception is based on the technologist's approach to explaining the disorder and treatment options to the patient. When terms like heart attack, stroke, and diabetes are used, it instills fear in the mind of a patient and can sometimes result in resistance. Inform the patient, but keep it simple so they can understand the information and be less fearful. Communicating using language at a third-grade level improves patient understanding. The use of visual cues and graphics, avoiding the use of technical jargon, and speaking in layman's terms increase the patient's acceptance of information. As a technologist, it is imperative to connect with patients at their level to ensure that they understand the information. Utilize open-ended questions when reviewing information with patients to further strengthen their knowledge and gauge their level of understanding. Keeping patients motivated increases the probability of starting, continuing, and adhering to therapy. Inform patients you are there for them, provide contact information, and educate them regarding additional resources available for support.

CHALLENGES

Growth and a shift to a comprehensive sleep center or program from a testing-based sleep laboratory present many challenges. There must be a change in culture and focus to a new global perspective. People may be very resistant and fearful of change. However, the change will create growth, and with utilization of new technology, the sleep technologist can have a significant role in the medical office or expanded sleep program. Sleep medicine has become extremely specialized, and, therefore, innovation helps improve efficiency by utilizing new technologies.

Employee engagement and performance excellence require continuous education. Learning new methods and understanding current technology are critical to successfully working with patients. The field of sleep medicine is rapidly changing and evolving into a complex specialty. Weekly staff education time should be scheduled for physicians and staff to present patient case studies and participate in learning new technology and programs. This will keep the technologist involved and using critical thinking skills.

The expansion of sleep center services requires a quality improvement tracking system to analyze the many different types of encounters. Quality improvement is not just a regulatory exercise or a program that is required to perform services but a living, dynamic process that drives the procedures in the sleep program. When data show poor outcomes, the workflow will need to change, providing another challenge that sleep programs face.

ALTERNATIVE THERAPY

The sleep technologist in the medical office or expanded sleep program is likely to interact with and educate patients undergoing PAP and other alternative therapies. This requires an expanded view of patient therapies. Alternative therapy is multifaceted and includes many different forms of therapy. Even positional therapy, that is, assisting a patient with positional OSA to avoid the supine position during sleep, is considered an alternative therapy.

ORAL APPLIANCE THERAPY

An oral appliance is a device that may be utilized for the treatment of OSA and snoring. The technologist should be familiar with oral appliances, which primarily comprise tongue retaining and mandibular advancement devices (MADs). These devices are small, easy to use, portable, and designed to pull the tongue forward or hold the jaw in a forward position to keep the airway open during sleep. The most common device is the MAD.

Indications for an oral appliance include OSA of all severities, although efficacy may be limited in those with severe OSA. Contraindications include central sleep apnea, dentures, loose teeth, or a significant number of missing teeth and extensive gum disease. A specialized dentist trained in sleep dentistry and oral appliances works with the sleep team to customize OAT for patients with OSA.

A temporary MAD device is a short-term type of therapy to identify responders before prescribing a custom oral appliance. This device is a boil-and-bite apparatus that provides horizontal and vertical adjustments to the mandible. A temporary oral appliance has been shown to predict success of a custom oral appliance (5). The technologist instructs the patient how to use the device and also makes necessary adjustments. The patient should have follow-up sleep testing to check the efficacy of the oral appliance (6). If the patient is successful with the temporary oral appliance, the sleep specialist will refer the patient for a custom device consultation. The dentist recommends the style and type of device best suited to the patient. The technologist educates and works with the patient to ensure proper follow-up with the dentist and the sleep physician.

EXPIRATORY POSITIVE AIRWAY PRESSURE

This therapy may be prescribed for patients with OSA. The technologist must be familiar with the therapy and contraindications, which include severe breathing disorders such as hypercapnic respiratory failure, respiratory muscle weakness, severe heart disease, and acute upper respiratory infections.

The device provides positive expiratory pressure when a patient breathes out, as a means to keep the airway open. It consists of a pair of oval-shaped devices that fit over the nares. The patient will use one set per night as they are disposable. The technologist should instruct the patient on the use of the device and discuss possible complications before the patient starts therapy.

Explain to the patient that discomfort during wake time is possible, as it can be challenging to exhale through the nose while using the device; however, the effort to breathe out activates the airway, helping it remain "splinted" open. It is important for the technologist/clinician to instruct the patient to breathe through the mouth while they are awake and adjusting to the device. Coach the patient to breathe normally and not force the air out through the nose because this can damage the ear drum. Upon falling asleep, there will be a natural shift to nasal breathing, and the patient will not be aware of the expiratory pressure created.

The patient should have a follow-up HSAT study approximately 2 weeks after the start of therapy to validate the effectiveness of this therapy.

SURGICAL OPTIONS

Patients who are nonadherent to other forms of sleep apnea therapy may have surgical options; however, this is dependent on whether surgery will be beneficial for them. There are multiple sites within the upper airway that may contribute to OSA and the severity of the apnea. The technologist's role in patients undergoing surgical therapies for sleep-disordered breathing is providing education and postprocedure support if needed. All complications or continuing symptoms must be brought to the attention of the surgeon and/or sleep physician. Surgical patients should be retested once healing from surgery is complete to ensure that their sleep-disordered breathing has resolved.

TONSILLECTOMY/ADENOIDECTOMY

In nonobese children, surgery is usually the first line of treatment in the form of tonsillectomy/adenoidectomy. Craniofacial surgeries are helpful for correcting deformities but are not usually considered in otherwise normal children whose facial structure is still growing. If surgery is performed because of OSA, follow-up PSG is highly recommended, particularly in obese children.

UPPER AIRWAY SURGERY

Traditionally, uvulopalatopharyngoplasty (UPPP) was at 1 time one of the most common surgical procedures performed for OSA. New emerging therapies such as hypoglossal nerve stimulation are promising, although additional evidence regarding long-term impact is needed (7).

Nasal obstruction and nighttime nasal congestion are known risk factors for sleep-related breathing disorders. Common areas of the nasal passage that may contribute to sleep apnea prevalence are deviated septum, enlarged turbinates, and nasal valve collapse. The medical specialist will evaluate the patient to determine the type of procedure that will be most effective for that patient (eg, septoplasty, turbinate reduction, cartilage graft). Patients with a deviated nasal septum might be corrected simultaneously with UPPP for moderate-to-severe OSA; however, UPPP is not considered to be a primary therapy in itself.

MAXILLOMANDIBULAR ADVANCEMENT AND GENIOGLOSSUS ADVANCEMENT

This surgical procedure moves the jaw forward to enlarge the upper airway. It is normally performed after other forms of surgical treatment have failed. A genioglossus advancement may be done concurrently to pull the tongue forward and prevent it from blocking the airway. Patients with high residual apnea-hypopnea index and respiratory disturbance index after other types of unsuccessful surgical procedures may benefit from maxillomandibular advancement as a subsequent step after UPPP (8).

POSITIVE AIRWAY PRESSURE THERAPY

Positive Airway Pressure Trial

A continuous positive airway pressure (CPAP) therapy trial program allows patients to try PAP therapy for approximately 7 days. The patient returns to the sleep center for a follow-up adherence check at the end of the trial to assess the efficacy of therapy. If the patient's OSA is well controlled with PAP therapy, home equipment can then be ordered through a DME company. This is an excellent way to assess the likelihood of adherence to therapy in patients who are hesitant to use PAP.

New Positive Airway Pressure User Class (or Peer-to-Peer Support)

Another service that sleep programs can provide is a new PAP user class. This is a group setting in which a sleep technologist instructs the patients on the use of PAP therapy and care of their equipment and provides information on an approximate timeline for replacement of supplies. In many cases, the group setting is appropriate as a peer-to-peer support mechanism, but keep in mind that some patients may not be comfortable in a group setting.

Troubleshooting Appointments and Follow-Up

Patients often experience anxiety and difficulty with initiation of PAP therapy. Offering support programs assures the patient that there are options and other modalities to help them become and remain adherent with therapy.

PAP therapy troubleshooting and desensitization appointments are a valuable service for patients. The technologist is an integral component—assessing the patient, working out issues with equipment or therapy, and assisting the patient to achieve long-term success with PAP therapy. Technologists must assess the patient's anatomy, sleeping position, air pressure leaks, any disabilities that may hinder application of the mask, and check PAP adherence. Desensitization appointments are useful as a means to assist patients who are struggling with PAP therapy. They may need a different form of treatment for their OSA (eg, CPAP vs auto-PAP or a different type of equipment).

Another useful tool to assist the patient having difficulty using PAP is breathing exercises. Breathing exercises can be a valuable tool for patients experiencing difficulty with PAP therapy. Technologists can teach these exercises to help patients relax and adapt to using their device. Practicing these techniques prior to initiating sleep with PAP may be particularly beneficial. Additionally, technologists can encourage patients to wear their PAP device at a low-pressure setting, such as while watching television in the living room. This practice not only helps patients become accustomed to fitting their interface and using the device but also allows them to accrue compliance hours without the immediate stress of trying to fall asleep.

To monitor and evaluate treatment effectiveness, schedule a 90-day follow-up appointment. This is reassuring to patients and indicates you will continue to support the patient to succeed with therapy.

Growing an Extended Sleep Program

The sleep technologist/clinician is well positioned to be a major part of sleep center and program growth. There are many opportunities for the technologist to develop and utilize their clinical skills. With the multiple changes occurring in the health care industry and the direct impact to sleep centers, it is critical for the technologist in any setting to be open to change and utilize the many tools that are already available to grow and enhance sleep program services. HSAT offers additional avenues for innovation and to support a successful sleep program. Technology is a key factor that can be used to provide support to patients and to the sleep program. Utilizing all of these tools changes how we deliver care and manage patients with sleep disorders. A program that utilizes all of these modalities together will successfully provide the patient with long-term continuous care and assure sustainability as a comprehensive sleep center or program.

REFERENCES

1. Brooks R, Trimble M. The future of sleep technology: report from an American Association of Sleep Technologists summit meeting. *J Clin Sleep Med*. 2014;10(5):589-593.
2. Parish JM, Freedman NS, Manaker S. Evolution in reimbursement for sleep studies and sleep centers. *Chest*. 2015;147(3):600-606.
3. Collop NA, Anderson WM, Boehlecke B, et al. Clinical guidelines for the use of unattended portable monitors in the diagnosis of obstructive sleep apnea in adult patients. *J Clin Sleep Med*. 2007;3(7):737-747.
4. Hwang D, Chang JW, Benjafield AV, et al. Effect of telemedicine education and telemonitoring on CPAP adherence: the tele-OSA randomized trial. *Am J Respir Crit Care Med*. 2018;197(1):117-126.
5. Hwang D. Evaluating the use of a titratable prefabricated mandibular advancement device to predict response to a custom device. Abstract Presented at: Associated Professional Sleep Societies, 2018; Baltimore, MD.
6. Ramar K, Dort LC, Katz SG, et al. Clinical practice guideline for the treatment of obstructive sleep apnea and snoring with oral appliance therapy: an update for 2015. *J Clin Sleep Med*. 2015;11(7):773-827.
7. Strollo PJ Jr, Soose RJ, Maurer JT, et al; STAR Trial Group. Upper-airway stimulation for obstructive sleep apnea. *N Engl J Med*. 2014;370(2):139-149.
8. Zaghi S, Holty JE, Certal V, et al. Maxillomandibular advancement for treatment of obstructive sleep apnea: a meta-analysis. *JAMA Otolaryngol Head Neck Surg*. 2016;142(1):58-66. doi:10.1001/jamaoto.2015.2678

Chapter 74
The Sleep Technologist in Home Health

ROBERT MILLER

KEY CONCEPTS/LEARNING OBJECTIVES

The key concepts for this chapter include educational pathways and credentialing for the technologist in a home health care role involving patient care and/or leadership roles.

KEY TERMS

Adherence
CCSH
Coaching
DME
Outcomes

As the health care landscape undergoes a significant transformation, there's a growing emphasis on providing medical services in the home rather than in traditional hospital settings. This shift is driven by advancements in technology, patient preferences for more convenient care, and the need to reduce health care costs. These changes are especially evident in the realm of sleep medicine.

Innovations in sleep technology are enabling more patients to be diagnosed and treated for sleep disorders from the comfort of their homes. This transition from in-lab sleep studies to home-based studies, with some home tests now capable of performing full polysomnography, presents a significant opportunity for sleep technologists.

Sleep technologists, or polysomnographic technologists, are essential health care professionals specializing in the diagnosis and treatment of sleep disorders. As the demand for home-based sleep studies grows, so does the need for skilled technologists who can facilitate these studies and interpret the complex data they generate.

By working in home health, sleep technologists have the chance to make a substantial impact on patient care. They can provide personalized education and support to patients, helping them understand their sleep disorders and treatment options. Additionally, they can ensure that the technology used for home-based sleep studies is accurately set up and functions correctly, guaranteeing reliable results.

The role of sleep technologists in home health is not only expanding but also evolving. As technology continues to advance, these professionals will need to stay updated on the latest developments in sleep medicine and home-based diagnostic tools. This ongoing learning and adaptation make the field both challenging and rewarding.

CLINICAL EDUCATION BACKGROUND AND CERTIFICATE IN CLINICAL SLEEP HEALTH CREDENTIAL

The clinical education background of sleep technologists is comprehensive and prepares them for various roles in sleep medicine. Key aspects include:

- **Educational Pathways:** Sleep technologists typically pursue education through vocational schools, community colleges, or universities. Programs may offer certificates, associate degrees, or bachelor's degrees in sleep technology or related fields. Accredited programs ensure that technologists receive quality education and hands-on training.
- **Certification:** The Registered Polysomnographic Technologist (RPSGT) certification is a common credential for sleep technologists. This certification requires passing an exam that assesses knowledge and skills in sleep technology.
- **CCSH Credential:** The Certification in Clinical Sleep Health (CCSH) is an advanced credential that emphasizes the role of sleep technologists as sleep coaches. The CCSH credential requires a combination of educational and clinical experience, as well

as passing a comprehensive exam. This certification validates the technologist's ability to provide sleep health education, coordinate patient care, and improve patient outcomes.

Positive Airway Pressure Education, Setup, and Sleep Coaching Support

Sleep technologists are integral to the successful implementation of Continuous Positive Airway Pressure (CPAP) therapy, a common treatment for obstructive sleep apnea (OSA). Their responsibilities in this area include:

Positive Airway Pressure Setup

Sleep technologists are responsible for setting up home positive airway pressure (PAP) equipment such as CPAP machines for patients. This involves several key steps:

- Equipment Selection: Choosing the appropriate CPAP machine and mask based on the patient's specific needs and preferences
- Mask Fitting: Ensuring the mask fits comfortably and securely to prevent air leaks and maximize therapy effectiveness
- Device Configuration: Setting the CPAP machine to the prescribed pressure settings and adjusting other features such as ramp time and humidification
- Patient Education: Providing detailed instructions on how to use and maintain the CPAP equipment, including cleaning and troubleshooting tips

Positive Airway Pressure Adherence

Ensuring patients adhere to CPAP therapy is a critical aspect of the sleep technologist's role. This involves:

- Sleep Coaching Support: Beyond the technical setup, sleep technologists offer ongoing support and coaching to patients. This includes educating patients about sleep hygiene, troubleshooting equipment issues, and providing encouragement to ensure adherence to therapy. Effective sleep coaching can significantly improve patient outcomes by enhancing compliance with CPAP therapy.
- Initial Assessment: Conducting a thorough assessment to understand the patient's needs, preferences, and potential barriers to adherence
- Personalized Care Plan: Developing a tailored plan of care that addresses the patient's specific challenges and promotes adherence. This may include regular follow-ups, adjustments to equipment, and behavioral interventions.
- Monitoring and Support: Continuously monitoring the patient's progress and providing ongoing support to address any issues that arise. This proactive approach helps identify and resolve problems early, improving long-term adherence.

Challenges

- Patient Adherence: Ensuring patients consistently use their CPAP machines can be difficult due to discomfort, claustrophobia, or inconvenience.
- Technical Issues: Troubleshooting equipment malfunctions and addressing mask fit problems can be time-consuming and require ongoing support.

Benefits

- Improved Patient Outcomes: Effective CPAP setup and coaching can lead to better sleep quality, reduced symptoms of sleep apnea, and overall improved health.
- Patient Satisfaction: Personalized support and education can enhance patient satisfaction and adherence to therapy.

Impact

- Patients: Successful PAP setup and coaching result in higher adherence rates, leading to better health outcomes and improved quality of life.
- Referral Sources: Positive patient experiences can lead to increased referrals from health care providers who trust the sleep technologist's expertise.

Tactics Supporting Sleep Technologists as Sleep Coaches

- Motivational Interviewing: This technique helps assess a patient's readiness for change and supports them in setting and achieving sleep-related goals.
- Patient Education: Educating patients about the importance of sleep, sleep hygiene practices, and the benefits of CPAP therapy can enhance adherence and outcomes.
- Behavioral Interventions: Implementing strategies to address behavioral sleep issues, such as cognitive-behavioral therapy for insomnia (CBT-I), can be part of the sleep technologist's role.

Challenges

- Keeping Up with Advances: Staying current with the latest developments in sleep medicine and technology can be demanding.
- Patient Engagement: Effectively engaging patients and encouraging adherence to treatment plans can be challenging.

Benefits

- Enhanced Patient Care: Advanced credentials and education enable sleep technologists to provide higher quality care and support to patients.
- Professional Recognition: Credentials like the CCSH enhance professional credibility and recognition within the field.

Impact

- Patients: Well-educated and credentialed sleep technologists can provide superior care, leading to better patient outcomes and satisfaction.
- Referral Sources: Health care providers are more likely to refer patients to sleep technologists with advanced credentials, knowing they will receive high-quality care.

Disclaimer: It is important to note that some state regulations may prohibit CPAP setups by anyone other than a licensed respiratory therapist. Sleep technologists should be aware of and comply with their state's specific regulations regarding the provision of CPAP therapy.

OPERATIONAL LEADERSHIP ROLES

Sleep technologists can advance into various operational leadership roles within durable medical equipment (DME) companies and sleep clinics. These roles require a blend of clinical expertise and managerial skills:

General Manager of a Branch Location

In this role, sleep technologists oversee the daily operations of a sleep clinic or DME branch. Responsibilities include managing staff schedules, coordinating patient appointments, maintaining medical records, and ensuring compliance with health care regulations. They also handle budgeting, procurement of supplies, and equipment maintenance.

Preparation for Durable Medical Equipment Operational Roles

Experience as a manager of a sleep lab or sleep clinic can be invaluable for sleep technologists aspiring to take on operational roles in the DME space. Key responsibilities in these managerial roles include:

- Staff Management: Overseeing the recruitment, training, and performance of clinical and administrative staff
- Operational Efficiency: Implementing policies and procedures to ensure smooth clinic operations, including patient scheduling, equipment maintenance, and inventory management
- Financial Oversight: Managing budgets, billing processes, and financial reporting to ensure the clinic's financial health
- Quality Assurance: Ensuring compliance with health care regulations and accreditation standards and maintaining high-quality patient care
- Patient Interaction: Directly engaging with patients to address their concerns, provide education, and ensure satisfaction with services

These experiences equip sleep technologists with the skills needed to manage DME operations, such as overseeing the distribution of medical equipment, ensuring regulatory compliance, and maintaining high standards of patient care.

Challenges

- Balancing Clinical and Managerial Duties: Managing both clinical responsibilities and administrative tasks can be challenging and may require strong time management skills.
- Regulatory Compliance: Ensuring compliance with health care regulations and accreditation standards can be complex and demanding.

Benefits

- Career Advancement: Operational leadership roles offer significant opportunities for career growth and professional development.
- Impact on Patient Care: Effective management can lead to improved patient care and operational efficiency, benefiting both patients and the organization.

Impact

- Employees: Successful operational leadership fosters a positive work environment, enhances team performance, and boosts employee morale.
- Patients: Efficient clinical operations result in better patient care, reduced wait times, and higher patient satisfaction.
- Referral Sources: Reliable and well-managed clinics attract more referrals from health care providers who value consistent and high-quality patient care.

Entry-Level Sales and Sales Leadership Roles

The sales aspect of DME offers sleep technologists opportunities to leverage their clinical knowledge in a commercial setting. Career progression in sales typically follows a path from entry-level positions to leadership roles:

- Entry-Level Sales Roles: Sleep technologists can start their sales careers in roles such as Sales Development Representatives (SDRs) or Inside Sales Associates. These positions involve generating leads, engaging with potential clients, and understanding customer needs. Entry-level sales roles provide a foundation in the sales process and customer relationship management.
- Sales Leadership Roles: With experience, sleep technologists can advance to sales leadership positions such as Sales Manager or Director of Sales. These roles involve overseeing sales teams,

developing sales strategies, and driving revenue growth. Sales leaders are responsible for setting sales targets, mentoring junior sales staff, and building strong client relationships.

Challenges

- High Turnover Rates: Sales roles often experience high turnover due to the pressure to meet targets and the competitive nature of the field.
- Maintaining Team Morale: Keeping the sales team motivated and engaged can be challenging, especially during periods of low performance.

Benefits

- Financial Rewards: Sales roles often come with performance-based incentives, offering significant earning potential.
- Skill Development: Sales positions provide valuable skills in communication, negotiation, and customer relationship management, which are beneficial for career advancement.

Impact

- Referral Sources: Effective sales strategies and strong client relationships can lead to increased referrals from satisfied customers and health care providers.
- Employees: Successful sales leadership fosters a motivated and high-performing sales team, leading to better sales outcomes and career growth opportunities.
- Patients: Knowledgeable sales representatives can ensure patients receive the right equipment and support, improving their overall experience and satisfaction.

SUMMARY

In conclusion, the shift toward home-based medical services is transforming the health care landscape, particularly in sleep medicine. Innovations in sleep technology are enabling more patients to receive diagnosis and treatment for sleep disorders from the comfort of their homes. Sleep technologists play a pivotal role in this transition, facilitating home-based sleep studies and ensuring accurate data interpretation. Their expertise is crucial in the successful implementation of CPAP therapy for OSA. By setting up CPAP machines, educating patients, and providing ongoing support, sleep technologists help improve patient adherence and outcomes.

Operational leadership roles in DME companies and sleep clinics offer significant career advancement opportunities for sleep technologists. These roles require a combination of clinical knowledge and managerial skills, focusing on staff management, operational efficiency, and quality assurance.

Additionally, sales roles in the DME sector allow sleep technologists to leverage their clinical expertise in a commercial setting, with opportunities for career progression from entry-level positions to leadership roles.

The comprehensive education and certification of sleep technologists, including credentials like the Registered Polysomnographic Technologist (RPSGT) and the CCSH, prepare them for diverse roles in sleep medicine. Advanced credentials enable sleep technologists to provide high-quality care, enhance patient outcomes, and gain professional recognition.

Overall, the evolving role of sleep technologists in home health, operational leadership, and sales underscores the growing importance of their expertise in the health care industry. Their contributions are vital to the success of home-based medical services and the improvement of patient care.

Chapter 75
The Sleep Technologist Working in Industry

ANDREA RAMBERG, KIMI CLARK RODAHAFFER, JESSICA MOORE, AND LACEY ADAMS

KEY CONCEPTS/LEARNING OBJECTIVES

The key concepts for this chapter include defining the opportunities in industry for the sleep technologist and describing the role of continuing education for technologists seeking work in the sleep industry.

KEY TERMS

Computer networking
Digital
Electronic medical record (EMR)
HTML
Positive airway pressure
Registered polysomnographic technologist

The landscape for sleep technologists has drastically changed compared to decades past. Entering the rapidly expanding field was considerably more accessible, with entry-level positions readily available across various settings. Even individuals without prior allied health experience could often find sleep laboratories willing to provide in-house training or orientation programs to facilitate their transition into the profession.

Today, the scope of the field extends well beyond performing overnight studies; sleep technologists are increasingly embracing roles as patient educators, sleep coaches, and industry consultants. By working closely with physicians and developers, they are helping to integrate advanced technologies—such as artificial intelligence (AI), digital platforms, and innovative home testing devices—into everyday practice. Whether collaborating on product development, driving sales and marketing strategies, or enhancing installation and technical support processes, sleep technologists are now at the forefront of shaping the future of sleep medicine. In the following sections, we will explore these diverse opportunities in detail, highlighting how expanding educational roles and emerging technologies create a more dynamic and impactful career landscape for sleep professionals.

EDUCATION

As the sleep industry expanded, sleep laboratories faced a challenge in hiring individuals. Recognizing the need for knowledgeable staff, these facilities sought personnel proficient in essential medical areas, such as terminology, physiology, cardiology, neurology, and pulmonary function, as well as computer skills. In response, a network of educational programs, from sleep technologist training companies to colleges and accredited schools, sprang up to equip aspiring sleep technologists with the necessary expertise.

This matrix of educational opportunities allowed those already trained in sleep technology to share their knowledge with newcomers eager to join the field. Although the number of sleep education programs has recently declined, the role of the educator remains a reliable path to advancement in this dynamic industry. The American Association of Sleep Technologists (AAST), American Academy of Sleep Medicine (AASM), the Board of Registered Polysomnographic Technologists (BRPT), and other institutions continue to provide comprehensive training, ensuring a lasting presence for sleep technology educators.

Today, continued education remains a cornerstone of career advancement, allowing sleep technologists to enhance and optimize their patient care and technological skills and explore emerging roles beyond the sleep laboratory. Professionals in sleep medicine also leverage their extensive clinical expertise to drive product innovation, technology implementation, and field progression all through education to their clinical and nonclinical peers.

THE CERTIFICATION IN CLINICAL SLEEP HEALTH AND SLEEP EDUCATOR

One of the most significant career advancements for sleep technologists is the opportunity to earn their Certification in Clinical Sleep Health (CCSH) credential. Unlike traditional sleep technologists focused on diagnostic testing, CCSH credentialed-professionals specialize in patient education, therapy adherence, holistic sleep health strategies, and a myriad of other roles. This role extends the impact of sleep technologists beyond the laboratory, emphasizing education and long-term patient engagement. Sleep technologists who pursue the CCSH certification are well positioned for roles in hospital-based sleep navigation, remote patient monitoring, and corporate wellness programs, reflecting the growing recognition of sleep health across diverse industries. With the expansion of telemedicine, remote sleep coaching has emerged as a critical avenue for patient engagement. This allows patients to receive real-time support, reducing geographical, mobility, or scheduling barriers.

Sleep educators help with patient education and therapy adherence support in several ways. This can help patients understand their sleep disorders and prescribed therapies, such as positive airway pressure (PAP) therapy, oral appliances, or cognitive behavioral therapy for insomnia (CBT-I). They also play a pivotal role in helping patients overcome barriers to therapy adherence, ensuring long-term success. Sleep educators contribute to peer and interdisciplinary education by training and mentoring new sleep technologists. They can foster professional development within the field by collaborating with dentists, primary care physicians, and respiratory therapists to promote an integrated approach to sleep health.

REMOTE SLEEP COACHING AND TELEHEALTH

Remote sleep coaching offers a unique opportunity for sleep technologists to expand their impact beyond the laboratory. These roles focus on patient education, adherence support, and lifestyle counseling. Technologists can guide patients in managing sleep apnea, adopting behavioral interventions for insomnia, or optimizing their sleep hygiene.

Remote sleep coaching for a technologist or sleep educator can look like conducting virtual consultations for patients, helping them optimize their sleep hygiene and lifestyle under the supervision of a physician. It can also look like supporting employers, athletes, and executives in managing their sleep health for peak performance in a nonclinical setting.

In telehealth consultations, technologists play a critical role in:

- Educating patients about PAP therapy setup, usage, and troubleshooting.
- Reviewing data to identify trends and address therapy nonadherence early.
- Providing real-time coaching during home sleep apnea testing (HSAT) or wearable device monitoring.

To thrive in these roles, technologists must develop:

- Strong Communication Skills: Building rapport through virtual platforms is essential to ensure patients feel supported and engaged.
- Proficiency in Telehealth Platforms: Familiarity with videoconferencing software, remote monitoring tools, and electronic health records (EHRs) is crucial.
- Understanding of Privacy Laws: Ensuring compliance with Health Insurance Portability and Accountability Act (HIPAA) and other data protection regulations is a key responsibility.

Integrating Technology into Sleep Coaching

Advancements in wearable devices and mobile apps have enhanced remote coaching capabilities. Sleep technologists can use these tools to monitor patient progress, provide actionable feedback, and adjust interventions based on real-time data. These technologies also empower patients to take an active role in their sleep health, fostering long-term success.

Future Trends

The telehealth landscape is expected to grow, with increasing integration of AI. AI-driven chatbots may supplement coaching by providing 24/7 support for common patient questions, but there are still limitations that require the clinician's expertise and intervention. Sleep technologists who adapt to these technologies will remain at the forefront of patient care.

PRODUCT DEVELOPMENT AND MANAGEMENT

During the rapid expansion of the sleep medicine industry, new career opportunities have emerged to address the growing need to develop and manage diagnostic and therapeutic products. These include devices such as HSAT devices, PAP devices and masks, as well as polysomnography hardware and software. Many manufacturers are designing innovative, improved equipment, creating demand for professionals with expertise not only in sleep diagnostics and therapy but also in product development and industry-specific needs.

This convergence of skills has opened pathways for sleep technologists to move beyond traditional clinical or educational roles into engineering, manufacturing, product development, and sales. As technology continues to evolve rapidly, the demand for experienced sleep technologists in research, product development, and management roles is growing. Emerging trends such as wearable health devices, AI in data analysis, and remote monitoring systems are driving further innovation in the field, creating opportunities for technologists to play an integral role in shaping the future of sleep medicine and technology.

The Role of Sleep Technologists in Artificial Intelligence Integration

The integration of AI is revolutionizing the medical industry as a whole, and this includes sleep technology—offering automation, precision, and personalized patient care. AI-powered tools now assist in automating data analysis, such as scoring sleep studies and identifying patterns that may indicate sleep disorders. To maximize the benefits of AI, sleep technologists must develop complementary skills:

- Data Interpretation: Technologists must understand and verify AI-generated reports, ensuring accuracy and clinical relevance.
- Collaboration: Working closely with AI developers, technologists can provide clinical insights to improve algorithms and software design.
- Troubleshooting: Understanding the underlying systems allows technologists to address technical issues quickly and effectively.

Personalized Sleep Solutions/Wearables

AI enables the development of personalized sleep solutions tailored to individual patients. Wearable devices and mobile apps are leveraging AI to monitor sleep patterns in real time, offering actionable insights directly to users. Sleep technologists can guide patients in using these tools effectively while interpreting the data for clinical decisions.

SOFTWARE DEVELOPMENT AND INFORMATION TECHNOLOGY

With the shift to digital equipment in the late 1990s and early 2000s came a growing demand for information technology (IT) professionals. The next two decades saw immense development in the digital landscape, especially in acquisition and therapy equipment, as well as software solutions, including advances in in-lab and networking. Today, sleep diagnostic systems are integrated through facility networks, cloud-based platforms, and electronic medical records (EMR) software, allowing for seamless review, storage, and sharing of data across multiple platforms.

To effectively collaborate with IT professionals and software developers, sleep technologists need a basic understanding of software, software development, HTML, and computer networking. Technologists with IT knowledge are in a unique position to help bridge the gap between clinical needs and technical solutions. Their expertise allows them to work with developers and engineers to shape the future of sleep medicine by providing valuable input on the design and functionality of software and products tailored to the field.

Today, the opportunities for sleep technologists extend well beyond traditional clinical roles. Social media, mobile apps, websites, and other digital platforms are becoming increasingly important in promoting and supporting sleep medicine products. With the rise of telemedicine, at-home sleep studies, and digital health tools, sleep technologists can leverage their knowledge of sleep disorders and technology to create content and digital solutions that enhance patient care and drive industry innovation. The tools available today make it easier for sleep technologists with moderate software development skills to merge their clinical expertise with digital platforms, allowing them to contribute to the marketing, promotion, and functionality of sleep products. Whether it is designing user-friendly mobile apps for sleep monitoring, creating educational content for social media, or developing online resources for sleep apnea treatment, sleep technologists are becoming key players in the intersection of sleep medicine, technology, and digital marketing.

SALES

The equipment and software industry is highly competitive, and vendors often seek sleep technologists who bring clinical expertise and a knack for communication to sales roles. These roles may fall into two primary categories: inside sales and outside sales.

Inside Sales

Inside sales positions typically involve engaging with clients remotely within a defined territory. These accounts can include government agencies, hospitals, or private sleep labs. A key advantage of inside sales is the ability to work primarily from a home or office setting, as most client interactions are conducted via phone, email, or virtual meetings. This allows for greater stability and flexibility, making it an appealing option for those who prefer minimal travel or have significant home responsibilities.

Outside Sales

Outside sales roles, on the other hand, emphasize in-person client interactions. Representatives may visit accounts several times a year, often within an assigned domestic or international territory. Travel in these roles can range from day trips to multiweek engagements, depending on the nature of the accounts and opportunities. These positions are ideal for individuals who thrive on building personal connections, enjoy travel, and have a solid support system to accommodate the demands of being on the road. Both inside and outside sales roles frequently include attending trade shows and conferences, offering opportunities to network, showcase products, and stay updated on industry trends.

Supporting the Sales Team

Providing clinical expertise to nonclinicians on the sales team can be a rewarding way to facilitate knowledge transfer. Clinical expertise fosters understanding, ensuring product solutions address workflow challenges. Extensive product knowledge and clinical inputs enable seamless process efficiency, strengthening the connection between users and the tools designed to support them.

Challenges and Rewards

While sales can be an exciting and lucrative career path, it is not without challenges. Compensation often includes commission-based earnings, which can fluctuate depending on performance and market conditions. The competitive nature of the industry means that success depends not only on the quality and pricing of the software or equipment but also on the salesperson's ability to foster relationships and build trust. This requires persistence, adaptability, and a strong personal brand.

For individuals with an outgoing personality, excellent communication skills, and a passion for problem-solving, a sales career offers immense potential. The financial rewards can be substantial, and the opportunity to travel and connect with professionals across the industry adds an enriching dimension to the role.

Ultimately, whether pursuing an inside or outside sales position, success hinges on a combination of technical knowledge, interpersonal skills, and a genuine commitment to understanding and addressing customer needs.

MARKETING

For those with a creative side and a meticulous attention to detail, marketing can be a fascinating and rewarding career path. Marketing is the bridge between product development and sales, where strategies and tools are crafted to help the sales team generate interest and close deals. These products can range from entirely new platforms or designs to upgrades or revamps of existing systems. Marketing is where the tactics are developed that make the product stand out and connect with its target audience.

The marketing team is responsible for designing and developing a variety of sales resources, including high-quality photographs, promotional videos, brochures, press releases, social media campaigns, sales sheets, technical manuals, and product guides. They also organize promotional events and develop incentives, campaigns, and promotional items to generate buzz around the product. Furthermore, they often identify and attend industry trade shows and conferences to network and promote the product directly to potential buyers.

Today, social media has become an essential tool for marketing, allowing companies to instantly reach a global audience with just a few clicks. Information such as product releases, updates, and marketing materials can be shared across digital platforms, from Instagram and TikTok to YouTube and LinkedIn, often going viral within hours. This fast-paced digital landscape presents an exciting opportunity for sleep technologists with an interest in marketing and social media. With their expertise in sleep disorders, technology, and health care, sleep techs are increasingly being called upon to contribute to marketing campaigns, creating engaging content that educates and informs consumers. Whether it is hosting live Q&A sessions about sleep health, creating educational videos about sleep apnea treatments, or sharing patient success stories, sleep techs have the chance to make a significant impact in promoting products and services in the digital age. Their unique combination of clinical knowledge and digital savvy can help bridge the gap between health care professionals and a broader audience, making them valuable assets to any marketing team.

PRODUCT INSTALLATION AND TRAINING

Another important and growing role for sleep technologists is in the installation of purchased products or product upgrades. This role requires not only a deep understanding of the product but also the technical skills to both install the product and act as the educator for its proper use. The process typically involves an extended on-site visit to the customer's facility to install the equipment and provide hands-on training, often for both day and night shift staff, including physicians.

Given the complexity of integrating new equipment with an existing EMR system or facility firewall, collaboration with the biomed and IT departments is usually necessary. The physical installation, such as running cables and setting up audio and video equipment, is often contracted out and may or may not be completed before the actual product installation. The bulk of the time during an installation is spent positioning the equipment, setting up the internal network interfaces, and configuring the system for optimal operation, like user preferences.

The sleep technologist dedicates significant time to training the staff on the new or upgraded product. A growing trend in installation and training is using virtual and hybrid methods to supplement or even replace in-person training sessions. For example, remote training through videoconferencing tools, online webinars, and on-demand instructional content allows sleep technologists to train staff more efficiently, especially in cases where multiple locations are involved or the laboratory must remain operational during installation. The preferred method for training is still often "train the trainer," where a select group of technologists, providers, or other key staff receive detailed training and are responsible for sharing that knowledge with the rest of the team. This method helps reduce confusion and ensures staff members receive consistent, in-depth training.

As remote work and digital tools continue to play a larger role in health care, even in installation and training, sleep technologists will likely find more opportunities to incorporate these tools into their work, enhancing their ability to support both the technical and educational needs of a facility.

CLINICAL, TECHNICAL, AND CUSTOMER SUPPORT

Once any product is installed and put into actual use, there is a need for ongoing product support. This can range from providing a simple refresher on best practices for maximizing efficiency to assisting with product upgrades and repairs. In cases where a product component or process fails, customers typically reach out to the vendor or manufacturer for technical assistance. Product support has always been a critical area where experienced professionals can showcase their expertise—not only in the clinical or operational spaces but also across hardware, software, and educational domains.

In the post-COVID world, technical support is more flexible and accessible than ever before. Advances in technology, coupled with a shift toward remote work, have enabled support to be delivered from corporate headquarters, designated support centers, or increasingly from remote locations, including the support technologist's home. The pandemic accelerated the adoption of remote work across many industries, and this trend is continuing to grow. Increased internet speeds, cloud-based platforms, and collaborative tools have made it possible to offer comprehensive, seamless support from virtually anywhere.

For home sleep testing (HST) companies, remote technical support has become especially crucial. With the growing trend of at-home sleep studies, which allow patients to conduct tests in the comfort of their homes, support needs have become more complex and urgent. These companies rely heavily on efficient technical assistance to ensure devices are functioning correctly, troubleshoot any issues remotely, and provide guidance for both patients and health care professionals. The ability to offer seamless remote support not only improves patient satisfaction but also helps to maintain the accuracy and reliability of these diagnostic tools, which are critical for effective sleep apnea treatment and management.

Ensuring ongoing customer success often requires clinical and operational knowledge. This person works with existing customers to optimize their product use, liaises with prospective users of the product user training, and provides ongoing input to the Product Development team. The person in this role applies sleep medicine and informatics knowledge to assist in the product's design, development, and ongoing modification for overall customer satisfaction. The role of customer support can also be strategic, working with customers to ensure goals have been met with implementation and long-term success.

SUMMARY

In recent years, the skill sets required for professionals in all facets of sleep medicine and technology have expanded to keep pace with the technological advancements. Entry-level roles now demand a stronger educational foundation. Fewer positions are available that do not necessitate a certain level of advanced training or education prior to commencing a career as a sleep technologist. Obtaining a Certification in Clinical Sleep Health credential (CCSH) has been a positive step forward. Transformations have occurred in both the clinical environment and the industries supplying products to meet patients' clinical needs. Today's and tomorrow's sleep technologists must possess a diverse range of knowledge encompassing electroneurodiagnostics, respiratory therapy, pulmonary function, cardiology, computer technology, customer service, and education. Moreover, industry opportunities are boundless for those willing to continue their education, stay current with medical and industry trends, and acquire the requisite skill sets to fulfill these demands.

Diverse industry prospects await sleep technologists, offering vast potential for growth and advancement. Dedicated skill development and knowledge expansion equip professionals to seize emerging opportunities, shaping rewarding career trajectories within the dynamic sleep medicine and technology landscape.

SECTION IX
Scoring Atlas

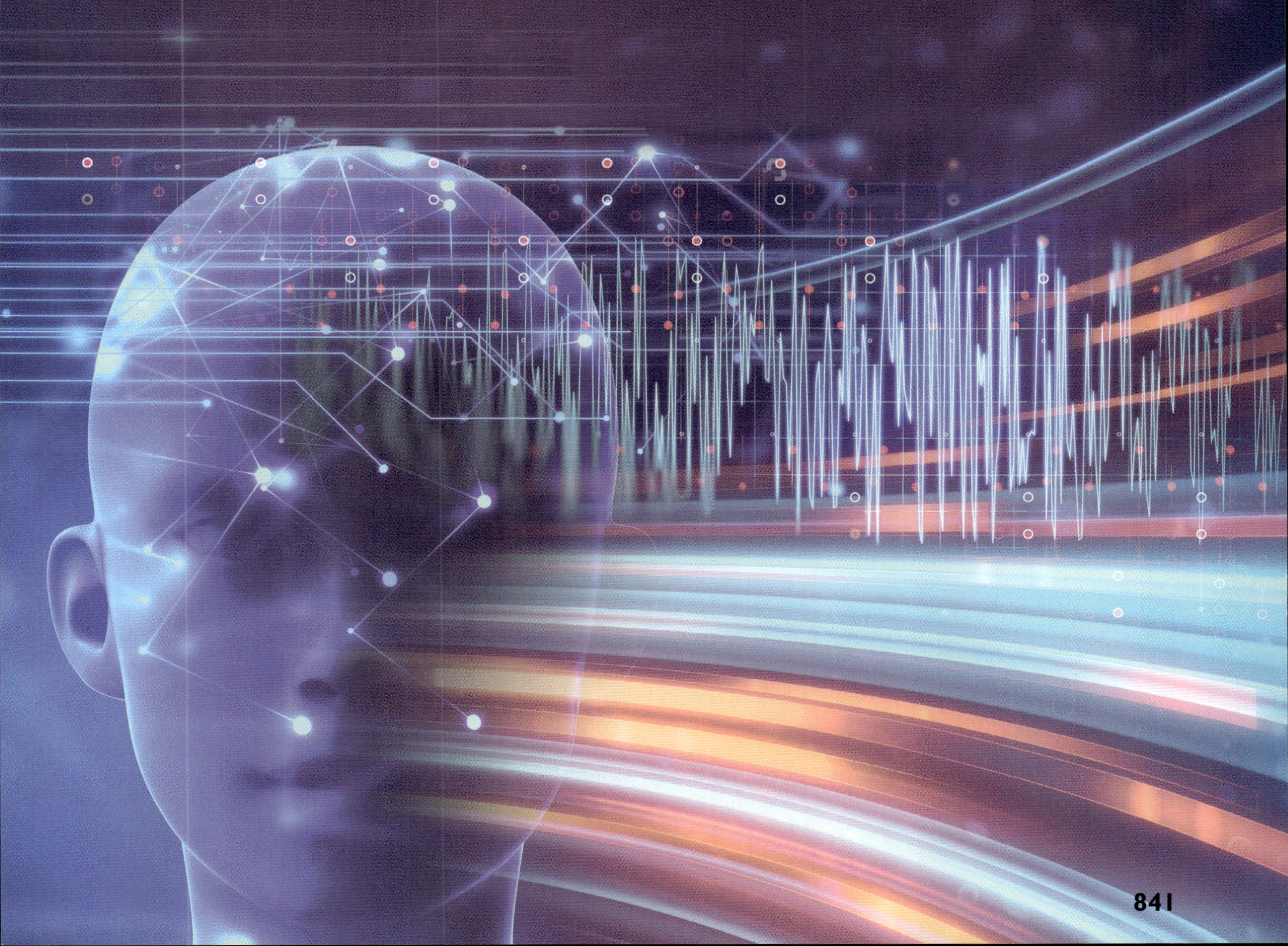

Chapter 76
Adult Sleep Scoring

LAREE J. FORDYCE

KEY CONCEPTS/LEARNING OBJECTIVES

The key concepts for this chapter include recognizing electroencephalogram waveforms of wakefulness and sleep and defining and implementing the rules for staging sleep and scoring events in adults.

KEY TERMS

Alpha rhythm
Central apnea
Hypopnea
K complexes
Low-amplitude mixed-frequency activity
Mixed apnea
Obstructive apnea
Rapid eye movements
Respiratory effort-related arousals
Sleep spindles
Slow-wave activity
Vertex sharp waves

The scoring of sleep and its events represents at least half of what the technologist must do on a nightly basis, whether the technologist is doing hookups at night, running multiple sleep latency tests (MSLTs) during the day, or scoring records as a scoring technologist. Although the scoring technologist might spend most of the day scoring polysomnograms (PSGs), the technologist working at night must understand and implement the scoring rules to run a PSG well. Similarly, the technologist working during the day running MSLTs and maintenance of wakefulness tests (MWT) must also understand and implement the scoring rules to execute the respective procedure properly. As AI scoring is on the rise in our field, it is not replacing technologists. It is helping create efficiencies. In short, all technologists must understand and be able to implement the scoring rules.

Scoring is usually performed using a two-pass method, meaning that the entire recording is looked through at least twice. In the first pass, the recording is viewed in 30-second epochs, and a sleep stage is assigned to each epoch between lights out and lights on. Arousals are also generally scored during sleep staging. In the second pass, the resolution of the display is changed to 60 seconds, 120 seconds, or even 5 minutes, and events are marked. The summary data that result from this process are then tabulated and reported according to the current version of the *AASM Manual for the Scoring of Sleep and Associated Events* (1).

HISTORICAL PERSPECTIVE

The history of how we describe and quantify sleep is the story of how technology has helped us observe the rhythms of the human in a relatively nonintrusive manner. The first person to report recording the electrical biopotentials of the brain in mammals was Richard Caton, who recorded brain waves from the exposed brains of dogs and rabbits in 1875 (2). It was not until brain waves could be recorded through the skin and scalp that the field of electroencephalogram (EEG) was born. Hans Berger reported the presence of what he called the *alpha rhythm* using electrodes attached to his own scalp and his son's in 1929 (Figures 76-1 and 76-2).

Loomis and others at Harvard adopted this technology and were the first to describe sleep stages using features of the EEG in 1937. They classified five different stages of what we would now call nonrapid eye movement (NREM) sleep (stages A through E). Several other investigators added to this early work in EEG, but it was not until the landmark article in 1953 by Eugene Aserinsky and Nathaniel Kleitman that described regularly occurring bouts of rapid eye movements (REMs) during sleep that the standard of the recording montage including more than simply the EEG was recognized.

Eugene Aserinsky adopted Jacobson's technique of monitoring eye movements using EEG electrodes to study infants. It should be noted that he spent many hours collecting the data himself, much like the sleep technologist does today. He noticed regularly occurring periods of "jerky eye movements" in more than 50

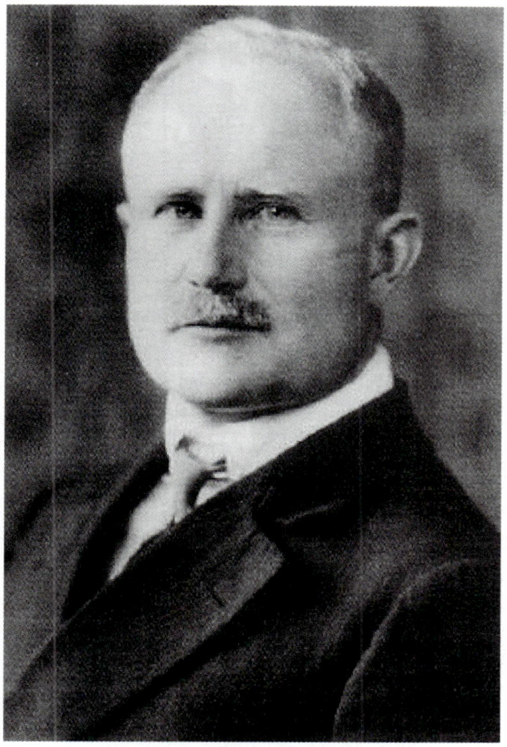

Figure 76-1 German psychiatrist Hans Berger (1873-1942) is best known as the inventor of electroencephalography and is the discoverer of the alpha wave rhythm.

recordings by 1952. This added the electrooculogram (EOG) to what we now know as the PSG.

A few years later, a young medical doctor named William Dement joined the Kleitman group at the University of Chicago. In 1957, Dement and Kleitman published a landmark article entitled *Cyclic Variations in EEG During and Their Relation to Eye Movements, Body Motility, and Dreaming*. This article outlined four stages of what we now call NREM sleep as well as REM sleep.

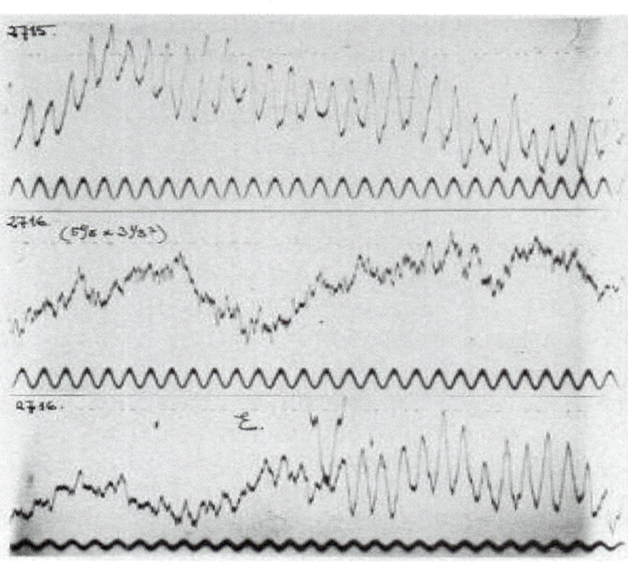

Figure 76-2 Hans Berger reported the presence of what he called the *alpha rhythm* using electrodes attached to his own scalp and his son's in 1929.

In 1968, *A Manual of Standardized Terminology, Techniques and Scoring for Sleep Stages of Human Subjects* was published (2). This manual was the result of the efforts of a committee led by Allan Rechtschaffen and Anthony Kales and represents the first consensus-based set of rules for the scoring of sleep in humans. Its intended application was for the sleep research community to aid in the standardization and compatibility of research data in adults. This R&K manual, as it has become known, was the most widely used set of rules in scoring sleep until 2007, when the American Academy of Sleep Medicine (AASM) put together a task force to compose a new set of rules that would address its shortcomings.

Although the R&K manual was the most widely used scoring system for 39 years, it was not the only scoring system in use. Several years later, in 1971, a similar set of scoring rules was published by a committee led by Anders, Emde, and Parmelee. *A Manual for Standardized Terminology, Techniques, and Criteria for Scoring of States of Sleep and Wakefulness in Newborn Infants* was intended to serve much the same purpose as the R&K manual: a set of rules by which increased comparability of research results might be achieved, albeit for PSG data from newborns and infants instead of adults.

A group from the University of Florida also published a scoring system at about the same time as the R&K manual was being developed. The scoring rules put forth by Williams, Karacan, and Hursch used 1-minute epochs instead of the 20- or 30-second epochs suggested in the R&K manual, as well as slightly different frequency bands and amplitude requirements. Although not widely used, the group did publish an impressive summary of normative PSG data using their guidelines in 1974 (3).

The R&K manual has several significant drawbacks that have been described in detail elsewhere (4,5). Many of these drawbacks stem from the fact that the manual ended up being used for purposes other than its intended original purpose: to aid in the standardization of sleep research data between laboratories. The clarity and economy of its rules made it easy to use, and thus, with no other clear alternative in existence, clinicians began to use the scoring rules for sleep studies in the clinical setting. In the clinical setting, several additional channels were added: channels to monitor respiratory airflow and effort, an electrocardiogram (ECG) channel, and electromyogram (EMG) channels to monitor limb movements (LMs). There are no definitions for respiratory events, arousals, or rules for the scoring of LMs in the R&K manual. To address these other features of sleep, additional guidelines were developed (6-8).

A second drawback of the R&K manual is that it was intended only for adults and thus does not address the effect of age on sleep. Although a separate manual was developed for the scoring of sleep in newborns and infants (9), the changes in sleep due to advancing age are not addressed in the R&K manual. For example, the 75 mV criteria for the scoring of slow-wave sleep has been questioned (5).

A third issue not addressed in the R&K manual is the absence of digital specifications for the acquisition and scoring of PSG data. The R&K manual was developed in the late 1960s, before the use of computers became the norm for recording sleep. Thus, R&K only provides guidelines for the use of paper machines, and many of the choices for the number of channels to be recorded were determined by the use of eight-channel recorders. As such, only one central EEG signal was required as a minimum EEG channel because all of the waveforms of sleep can be seen from this derivation. Two EOG leads were suggested, as well as a single chin EMG channel. This allowed two participants to be recorded on a single machine. The advancement of digital technologies now allows for as many as 256 channels to be recorded and analyzed with relative ease.

Taken together, these many drawbacks led to the re-evaluation of the R&K manual. To this end, the AASM board approved the development of a new scoring manual. Over the course of 2 years, a steering committee and eight task forces were brought together with members of the AASM board and content experts in various aspects of sleep. Six of the eight task forces were developed to investigate and report on major content areas of the new manual: visual scoring, digital scoring, arousal, movement, respiratory issues, and cardiac issues. The issue of age effects was addressed by the two remaining task forces, one for pediatrics and the other for geriatrics.

Each task force followed the same process for the development of the new manual. They performed a literature search and review, from which they produced evidence tables and a review article, which served to provide transparency about the decisions made in the new manual. Each of these articles was published in a single issue of the *Journal of Clinical Sleep Medicine* in 2007 and provides a thorough review for the curious reader.

Since 2007, there have been eleven versions of the *AASM Manual for the Scoring of Sleep and Associated Events*, the most recent of which, version 3.0, was released in early 2023. The reader is encouraged to read page 83 of version 3.0 for a brief review of the committee-recommended changes made since the 2007 manual was written. Some of the changes introduced in these eleven updates to the manual have been minor, such as to the terms to be used, while other changes were more substantive, including the addition of home sleep apnea testing (HSAT) and infant rules for scoring sleep and associated events. These substantive changes have been examined in detail in other chapters.

TECHNICAL SPECIFICATIONS

The AASM Manual for the Scoring of Sleep and Associated Events contains important technical specifications for the collection of PSG data. These rules represent the first consensus-based set of rules for the use of digital technology in polysomnography.

The maximum impedance allowed for EEG and EOG is 5 kΩ. The minimum digital resolution is 12 bits per sample. The sampling rates and filter settings for each channel are detailed in (1).

The minimal sampling rate for the EEG, EOG, EMG, and ECG channels is 200 samples per second; the preferred sampling rate is 500 samples per second for these parameters. The sampling rate is chosen on the basis of what the frequency of interest is in the signal being viewed. The AASM Scoring Manual suggests that the sampling rate and high filter settings may be increased if needed to more accurately display EEG spikes. In this case, the sampling rate should be "at least five times the high frequency of interest" (1).

Usually, a sleep study is scored in two passes. The scorer will first view the sleep study in 30-second epochs to determine the appropriate sleep stage. After determining sleep and wakefulness, the scorer will do a second pass in a more compressed view, usually a 60- to 120-second epoch, to determine sleep-related events.

RECOGNIZING WAVEFORMS

There are four features of the EEG signal that are informative to the categorization of the signal as a distinct waveform (Table 76-1). They are the *amplitude*, *frequency*, *morphology*, and *distribution* of the waveform. We use these four features of the EEG signal to identify the waveforms that are a part of the definition of sleep stages. The *amplitude* of the signal refers to its vertical distance from the isoelectric baseline, measured in microvolts (μV). The *frequency* refers to the number of waves per second, measured in Hertz (Hz) or the number of cycles per second. The *morphology* of the waveform refers to its shape. The *distribution* of the waveform is the source of the signal, or the region in which the amplitude is the highest.

Alpha Rhythm

The first waveform that we must recognize is the *alpha rhythm* or Berger rhythm. As with several waveforms, the alpha rhythm is defined by its frequency, which is between 8 and 13 Hz (Figure 76-3). Different people have slightly different alpha frequencies, and some people

Table 76-1 Summary of Waveforms Used in Scoring Sleep and Wakefulness

	Alpha Activity	Low-Amplitude Mixed Frequency	Vertex Sharp Wave	Spindle	K Complex	Slow Wave
Amplitude	Not defined	"Low"	Not defined	Not defined	Not defined	75 μV
Frequency	8-13 Hz	4-7 Hz	≥2 Hz	11-16 Hz	<2 Hz	0.5-2 Hz
Waveform	Sinusoidal	Mixed	Sharp	"Distinct"	Negative followed by positive	Not defined
Distribution	Occipital	Not defined	Central	Central	Frontal	Frontal

have no alpha frequency at all. Some people display alpha that cycles at about 11 Hz, whereas others may have an alpha rhythm that cycles at around 9 Hz. Although they are different frequencies, both are considered alpha since they fall between 8 and 13 Hz.

Another helpful feature of alpha is its occipital distribution (Figure 76-4). Although alpha can usually be seen in each of the three EEG channels, its amplitude is the highest in the occipital channel.

Low-Amplitude Mixed-Frequency Activity (Theta)

The second waveform to recognize is theta activity, also known as *low-amplitude mixed-frequency (LAMF) activity* (Figure 76-5). The frequency of LAMF activity is 4 to 7 Hz. The amplitude is quite loosely defined as "low." In the R&K manual, the term "low-voltage mixed frequency" was used, and the frequency range was from 2 to 7 Hz, a slightly larger frequency range. This overlapped with what is referred to as *theta* activity by the International Federation of Clinical Neurophysiology (10). The amplitude is quite loosely defined as "low." The distribution of the activity is diffuse, meaning it occurs in all channels.

Vertex Sharp Waves

The third waveform to recognize is the *vertex sharp wave* (Figure 76-6). The AASM Scoring Manual defines vertex sharp waves as "sharply contoured waves with duration <0.5 seconds maximal over the central region and distinguished from the background activity" (1). There is no amplitude criterion for a vertex sharp wave. The distribution is central, meaning that the vertex sharp wave will usually have its highest amplitude in the central channels. The most recognizable feature of the vertex sharp wave is its characteristic morphology.

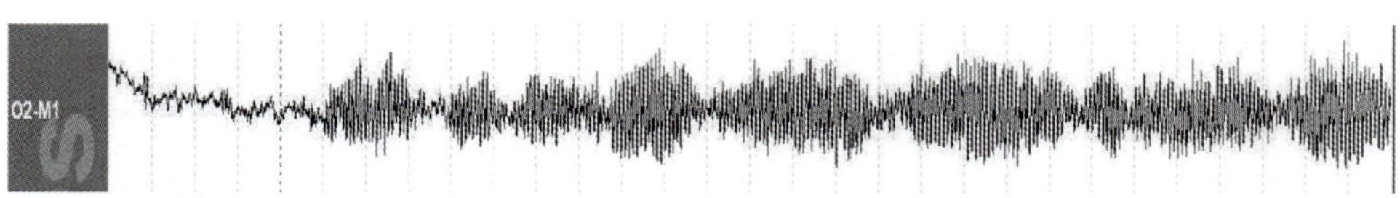

High-amplitude alpha of a 27-year old female (Vertical dotted line is an "eyes closed" instruction).

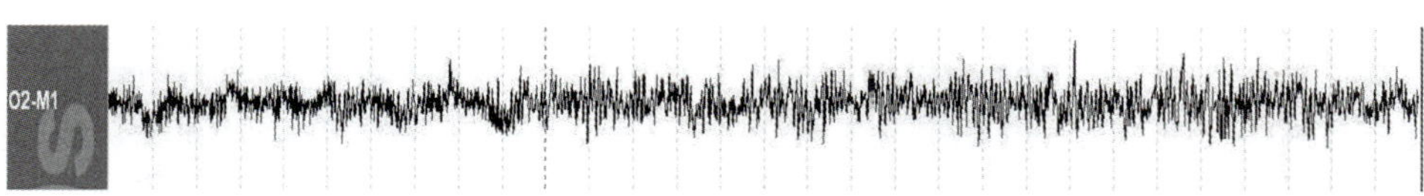

Moderate-amplitude alpha of a 20-year old male (Vertical dotted line is an "eyes closed" instruction).

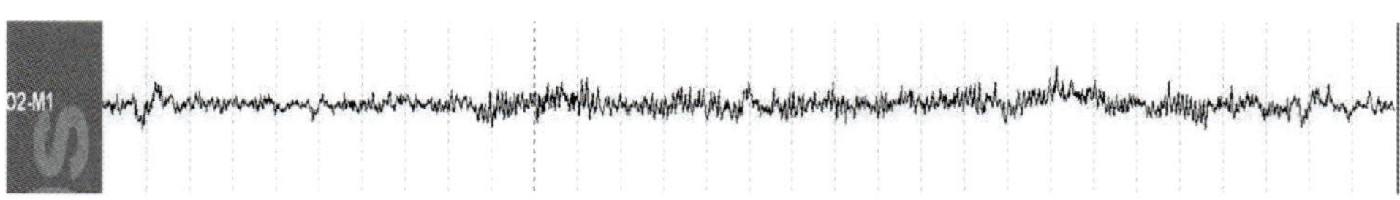

Low-amplitude alpha of a 20-year old male (Vertical dotted line is an "eyes closed" instruction).

Figure 76-3 Varying amplitudes of the alpha rhythm.

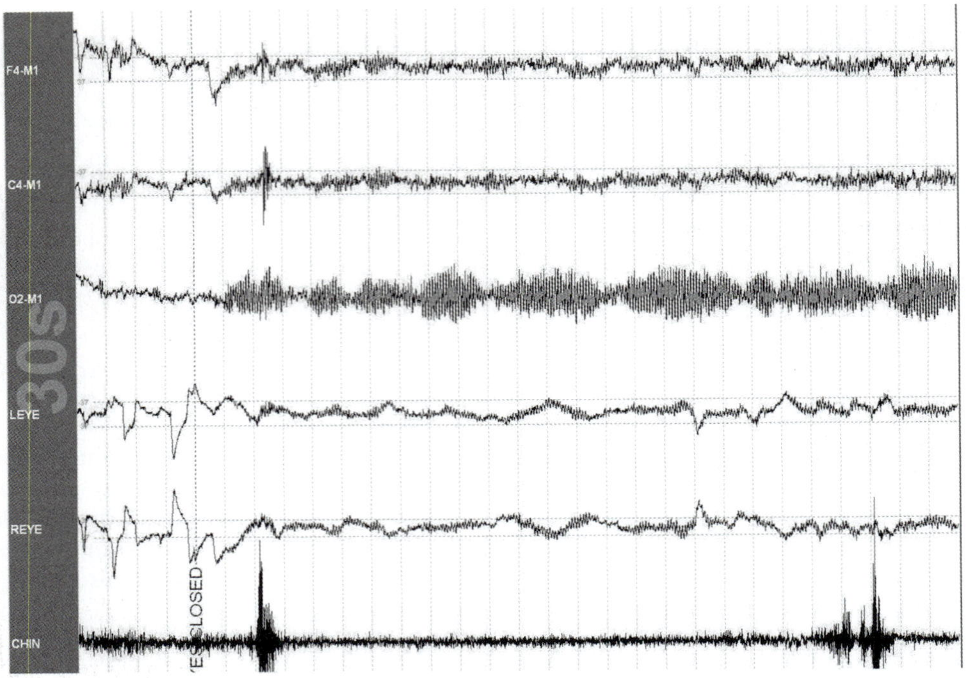

Figure 76-4 Maximal alpha amplitude in the occipital region of a 27-year-old female (horizontal dotted line is an "eyes closed" instruction).

K Complex

The fourth waveform to recognize is the K complex (Figure 76-7). The AASM Scoring Manual defines a K complex as "a well delineated negative sharp wave immediately followed by a positive component standing out from the background EEG, with a total duration ≥0.5 seconds, usually maximal in amplitude when recorded using the frontal derivations" (1). K complexes may or may not be associated with arousals. When a K complex is part of an arousal (Figure 76-8), it is not used as evidence of stage N2 sleep. A common misconception of K complexes is that they must have a spindle immediately following them, thus making them a complex. This is not the case.

Sleep Spindle

The fifth waveform to recognize is the sleep spindle (Figure 76-9). The AASM Scoring Manual defines a sleep spindle as "a train of distinctive waves with a frequency

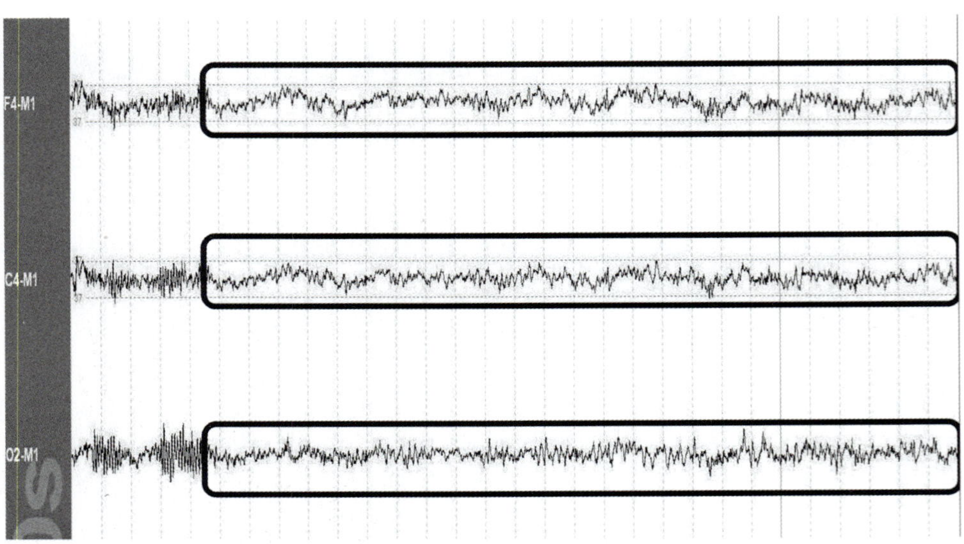

Figure 76-5 Alpha in the first 4½ seconds is replaced by low-amplitude mixed-frequency electroencephalography activity in a 27-year-old female.

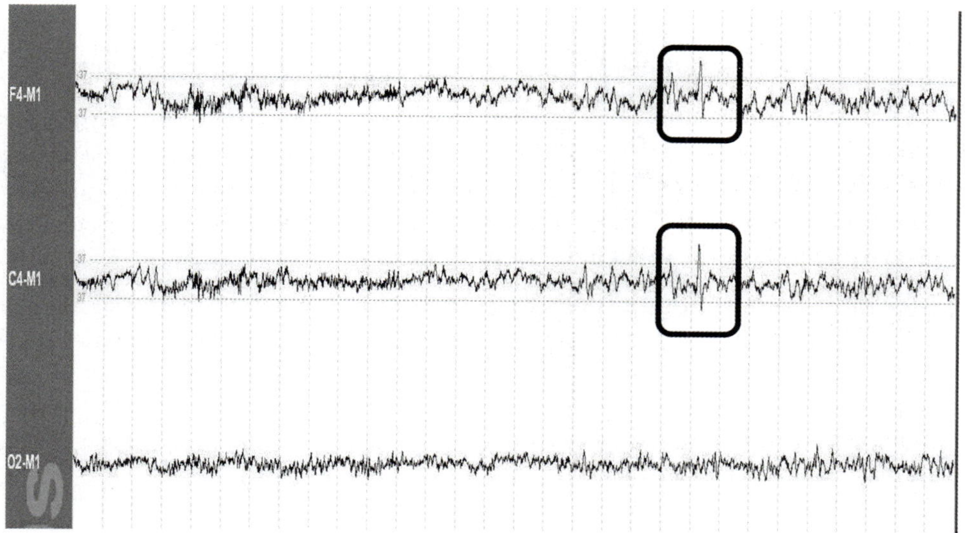

Figure 76-6 An example of a vertex sharp wave in a 26-year-old male.

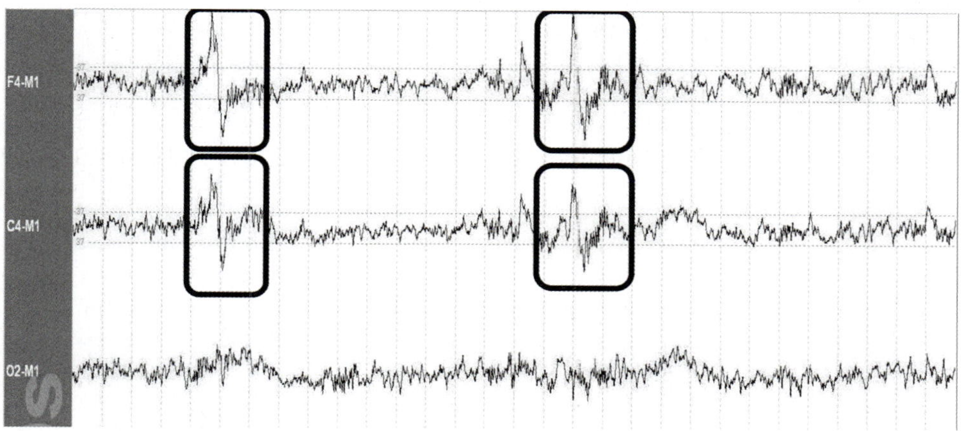

Figure 76-7 Two K complexes in a 27-year-old female. The first at the 4th second of the epoch has no spindle associated with it, while the second at the 16th second does. Both are considered K complexes. Note also the higher amplitude in the frontal derivations.

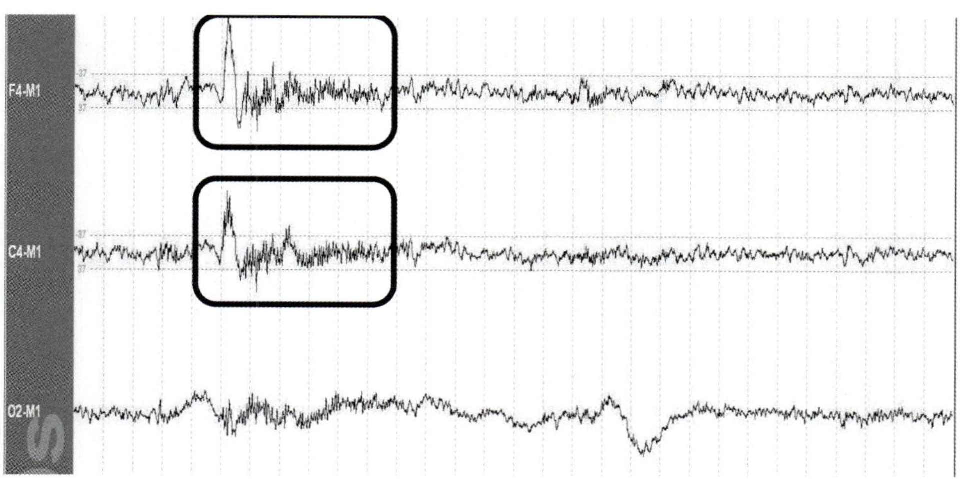

Figure 76-8 A K complex associated with an arousal. Although a K complex, we would not use it to score N2 sleep in this example.

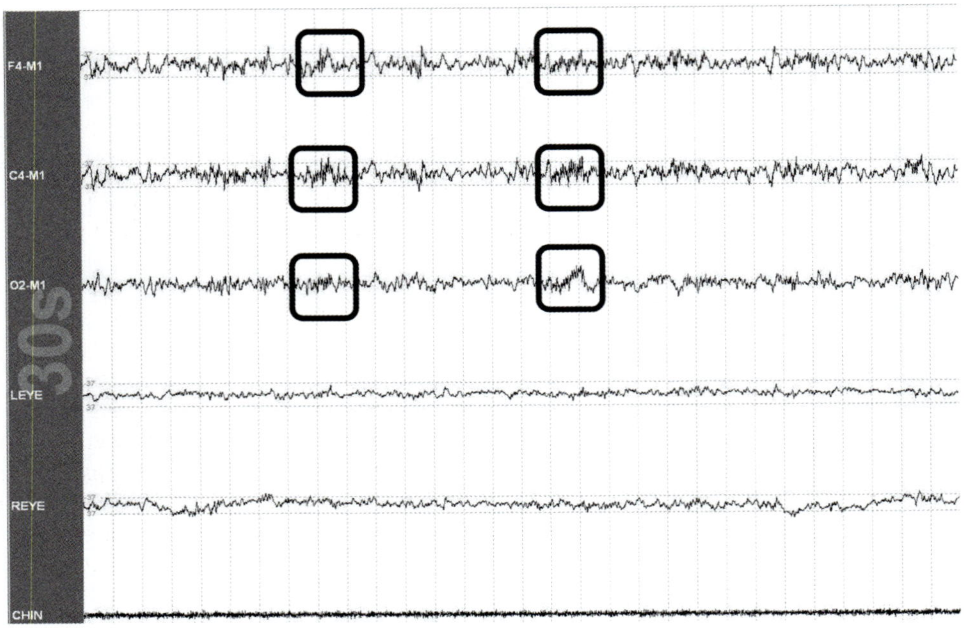

Figure 76-9 Sleep spindles in a 25-year-old male; note the maximal amplitude in the central derivation.

11 to 16 Hz (most commonly 12-14 Hz) with a duration ≥0.5 seconds, usually maximal in amplitude in the central regions" (1).

Slow-Wave Activity

The sixth waveform to recognize is slow-wave activity (Figure 76-10). Slow-wave activity consists of waves with a frequency of 0.5 to 2 Hz and a peak-to-peak amplitude greater than 75 μV. This wave activity is measured over the frontal region. This definition can be difficult to apply to the EEG signal in practice. Although we know we are to measure the "peak-to-peak" amplitude, the current definition does not tell us whether to begin counting at the most negative part of the wave or the most positive part. In addition, some K complexes may fit the definition of slow-wave activity. Although several automated algorithms have been developed, none have

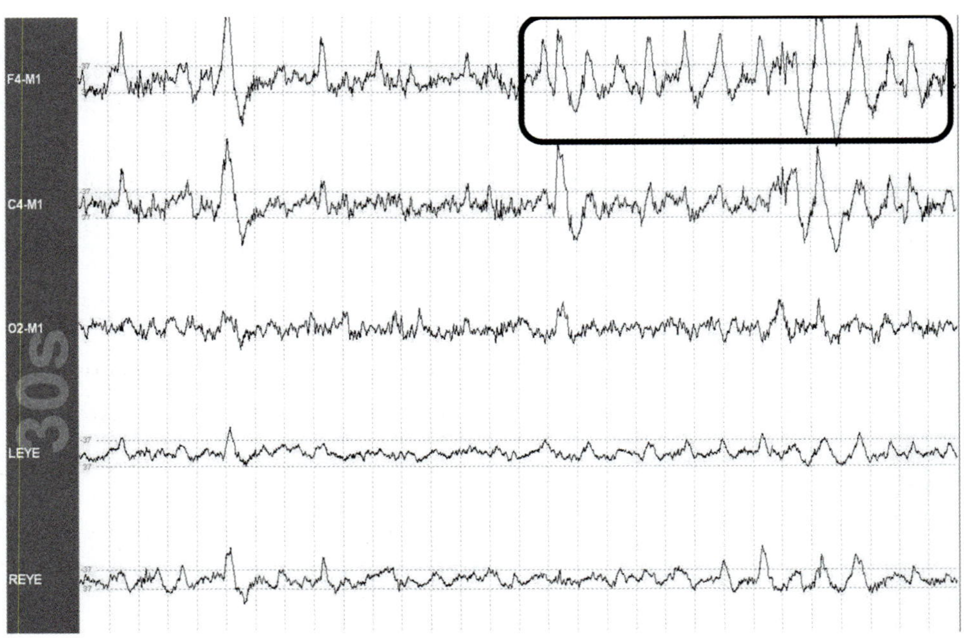

Figure 76-10 Slow-wave activity in a 19-year-old male; note the maximal amplitude in the frontal derivation.

replaced the human as the gold standard for detecting slow waves. The AASM Inter-Scorer Reliability (ISR) Committee has proposed a "zero-cross" method for measuring slow-wave activity.

Slow Eye Movements

The seventh waveform to recognize is slow eye movements (Figure 76-11). The AASM Scoring Manual defines slow eye movements as "conjugate, reasonably regular, sinusoidal eye movements with an initial deflection usually lasting >500 ms" (1).

Rapid Eye Movements

The eighth waveform to recognize is REMs (Figure 76-12). The AASM Scoring Manual defines REMs as "conjugate, irregular, sharply peaked eye movements with an initial deflection usually lasting <500 ms" (1).

SCORING SLEEP STAGES

Sleep staging is usually done on the first pass of the two-pass approach to sleep scoring. In the first pass, the scorer views the recording in 30-second epochs, using an epoch-by-epoch approach. One sleep stage (Stage wake [W], N1, N2, N3, R) is assigned to each 30-second epoch between lights out and lights on. In the event that two or more stages occur in a single 30-second epoch, the stage making up the greatest portion of the epoch is assigned to that epoch. In the event that three or more stages appear in a single 30-second epoch, observe the following:

I. Score the epoch as sleep if the majority of the epoch meets criteria for stage N1, N2, N3, or R.
II. Assign the sleep stage that occurs for the majority of sleep within the epoch (1).

Stage Wake

Stage W is scored when 50% or more of the epoch has alpha rhythm over the occipital region in people who produce the alpha rhythm (Figure 76-13). In people who do not produce alpha rhythm, stage W is scored when any of the following is present; eye blinks at a frequency of 0.5 to 2 Hz, reading eye movements, or REMs associated with high muscle tone (1).

Scoring Arousals

There is one rule for scoring arousals, but understanding it is important because arousals have implications for stage scoring (Figure 76-14). "Score an arousal during sleep stages N1, N2, N3, or R if there is an abrupt shift of EEG frequency including alpha, theta and/or frequencies greater than 16 Hz (but not spindles) that lasts at least 3 seconds, with at least 10 seconds of stable sleep preceding the change" (1). This is true for arousals scored in stages N1, N2, and N3 sleep. When scoring arousals in stage R, there must also be a simultaneous increase in submental EMG for at least 1 second (1).

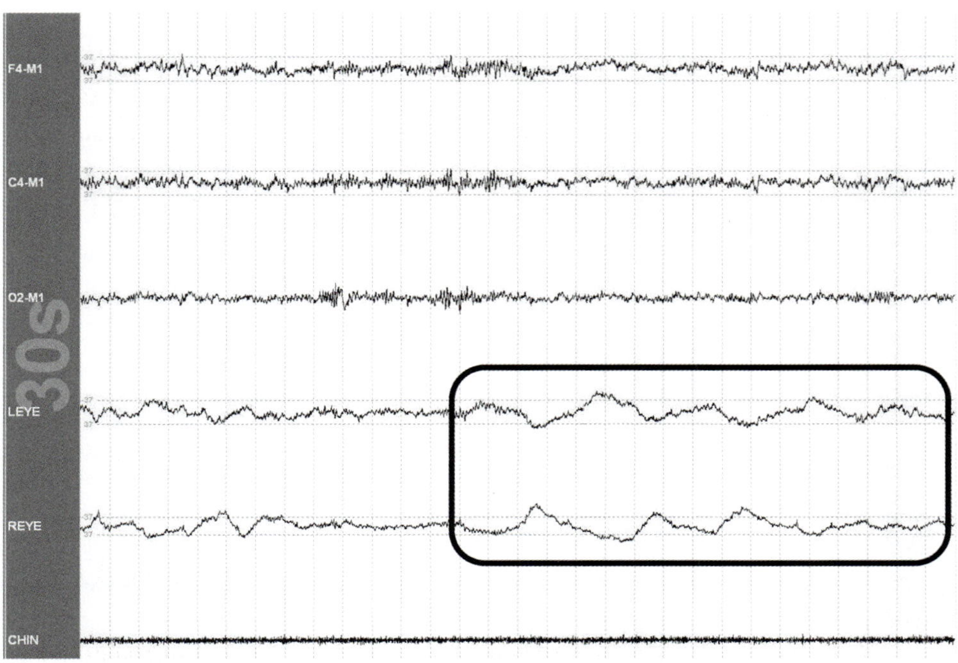

Figure 76-11 Slow-rolling eye movements in a 19-year-old male.

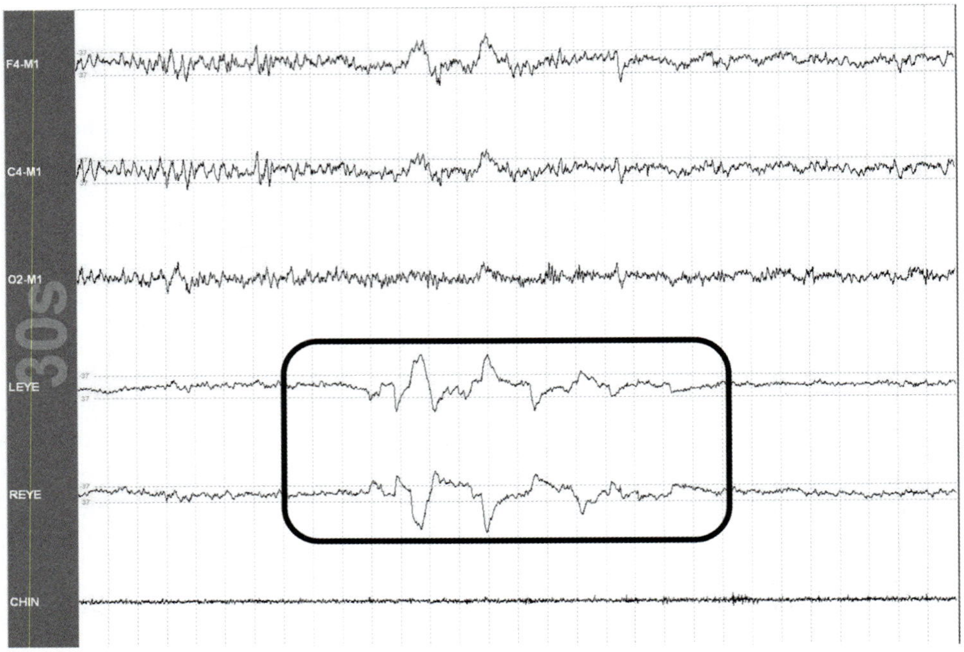

Figure 76-12 Rapid eye movements in a 27-year-old female.

Identifying Major Body Movements

The AASM Scoring Manual defines a major body movement as "movement and muscle artifact obscuring the EEG for more than half an epoch to the extent that the sleep stage cannot be determined" (1). There are three rules for what to do with epochs that contain major body movements:

1. If alpha rhythm is present for part of the epoch (even <15 seconds duration), score the epoch as stage W.
2. If no alpha rhythm is discernible, but an epoch scored as stage W either precedes or follows the epoch with a major body movement, score the epoch as stage W.
3. Otherwise, score the epoch as the same stage as the epoch that follows it (1).

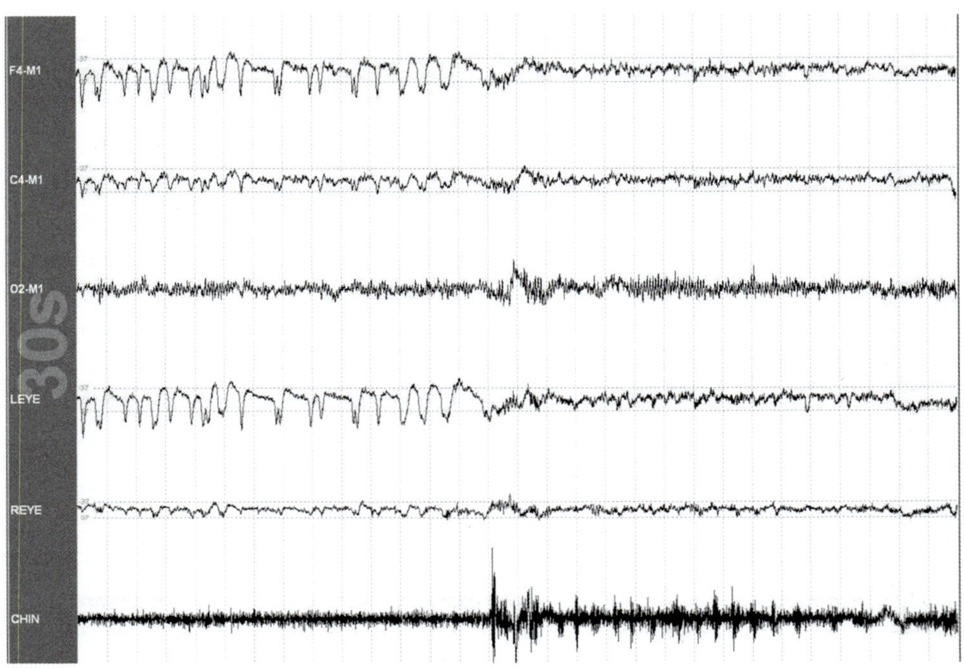

Figure 76-13 Wakefulness in a 31-year-old male. Note the eye blinks in the first 14 seconds and the alpha throughout.

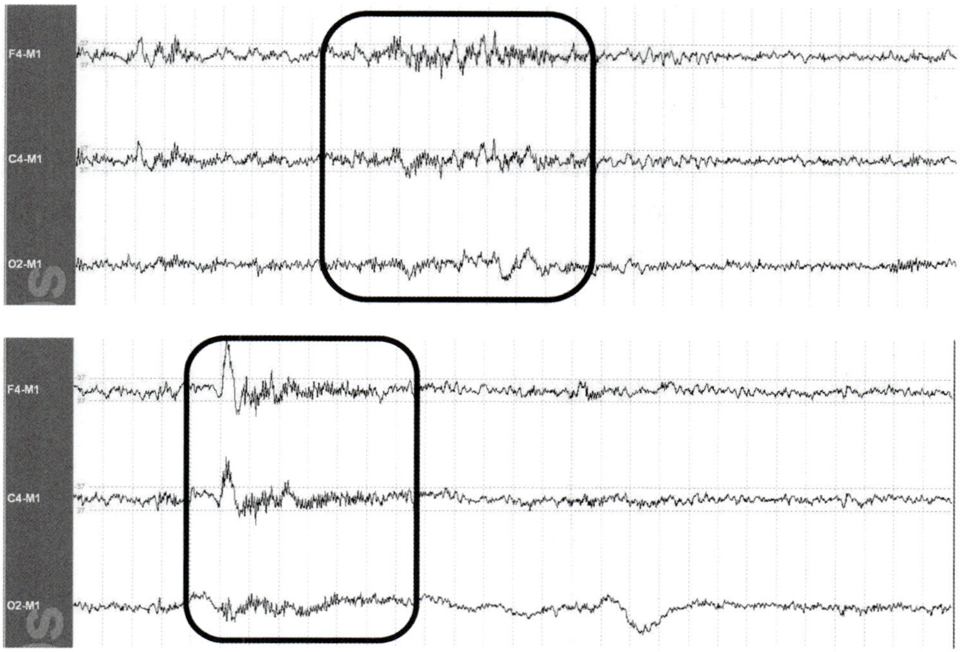

Figure 76-14 An example of an arousal without a K complex in a 22-year-old male at the top and an arousal with a K complex at the bottom in a 33-year-old male.

Major body movements are thus not scored as events themselves but are used to help the scorer decide how to score epochs with very little or no readable EEG activity due to movement or muscle artifact.

Stage N1 (NREM 1)

Stage N1 sleep (Figure 76-15) is scored when alpha rhythm drops out and 50% of the epoch comprises LAMF EEG in people who produce the alpha rhythm.

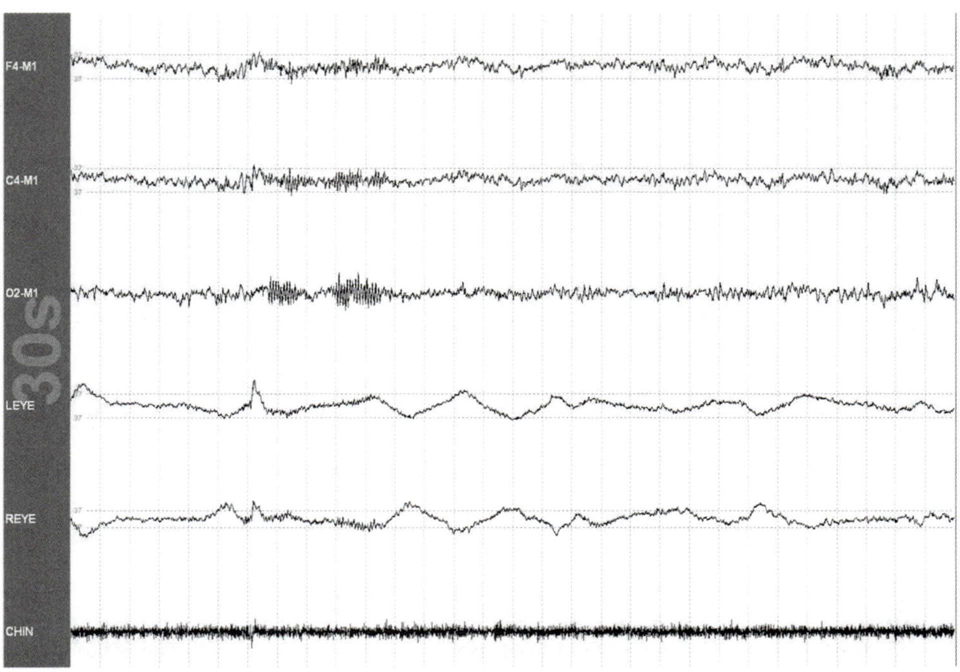

Figure 76-15 An N1 sleep in a 27-year-old female. Alpha activity is replaced by low-amplitude mixed-frequency electroencephalography activity. There are also slow-rolling eye movements present.

In people who do not produce the alpha rhythm, stage N1 is scored at the earliest appearance of any of the following: slowing of the background frequency by greater than or equal to 1 Hz and in the range of 4 to 7 Hz, the presence of vertex sharp waves, or the presence of slow eye movements. Further, an epoch is scored as stage N1 if the *majority* of the epoch meets the criteria for stage N1 and there is no evidence of another sleep stage. Continue to score stage N1 until there is evidence of another sleep stage (1).

There are two other situations when a score of stage N1 is recommended. When stage N2 is interrupted by an arousal, the following epochs are scored as stage N1 if LAMF EEG is present and K complexes and sleep spindles are absent, until there is evidence of another stage of sleep. When an arousal interrupts stage R and is followed by LAMF EEG and slow eye movements, score as stage N1, even with continued low chin EMG activity, until there is evidence of another stage of sleep (1).

Stage N2 (NREM 2)

Stage N2 sleep makes up the majority of total sleep time in most individuals (Figure 76-16). Stage N2 sleep is scored when there is a K complex or spindle in the first half of the epoch or the second half of the epoch that precedes it, with a background of LAMF activity. In the event that stage N2 sleep is interrupted by an arousal, score N1 sleep until the next K complex or sleep spindle appears (1). There are specific rules for the continuation and termination of stage N2 sleep, as well as a special set of rules for the transitions between N2 and REM sleep.

Continue to score stage N2 unless an arousal or stage change interrupts the EEG activity, even in epochs without K complexes or sleep spindles if preceding epochs contain either K complexes or sleep spindles. Transition from stage N3 to stage N2 when the EEG no longer meets criteria for scoring stage N3 as long as there is no arousal and criteria for stage W or stage R are not present.

Stage N2 ends when there is a transition to another stage (including stage W), an arousal results in a stage change, or a major body movement occurs. If a major body movement interrupts stage N2, score the epoch following the movement as stage N2 if there are no slow eye movements and as stage N1 if there are slow eye movements present (1). See the major body movement scoring rules for additional information.

Stage N3

Stage N3 (Figure 76-17) is scored when 20% or more of a 30-second epoch contains slow-wave activity. Thus, 6 seconds of activity in the frequency range of 0.5 to 2 Hz with an amplitude of greater than 75 μV measured in the frontal channels in a single epoch is sufficient to score N3 sleep. K complexes are scored as slow waves if they meet the definition of slow-wave activity. Pathologic slow-wave activity and artifact are not scored as stage N3 activity.

Stage R

Stage R (Figure 76-18) is scored when all of the following are present in the epoch: LAMF EEG, low chin EMG tone, and REMs. Sawtooth waves are a distinctive

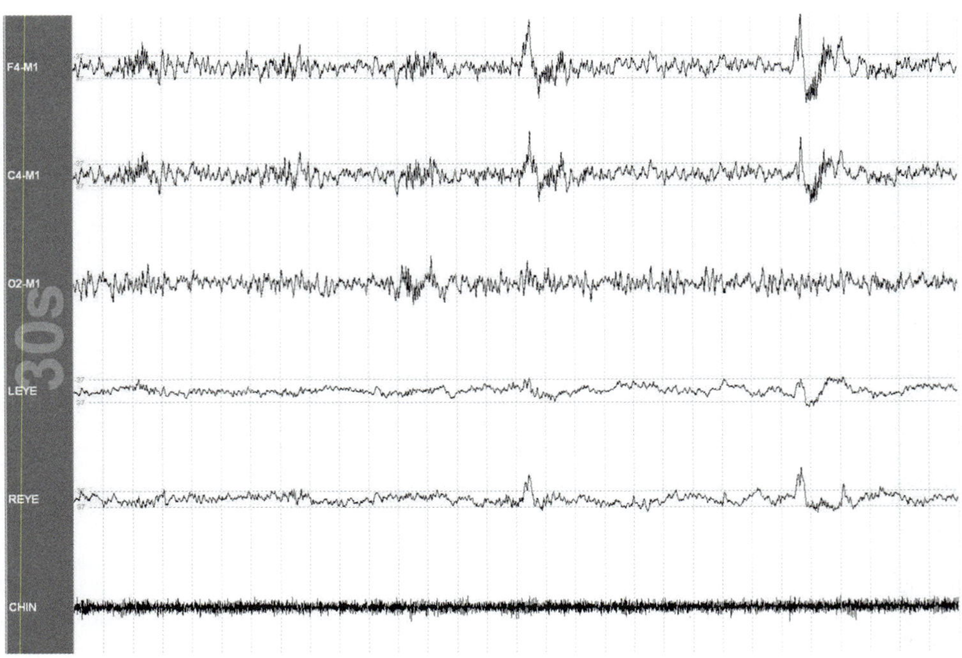

Figure 76-16 An N2 sleep in a 27-year-old female.

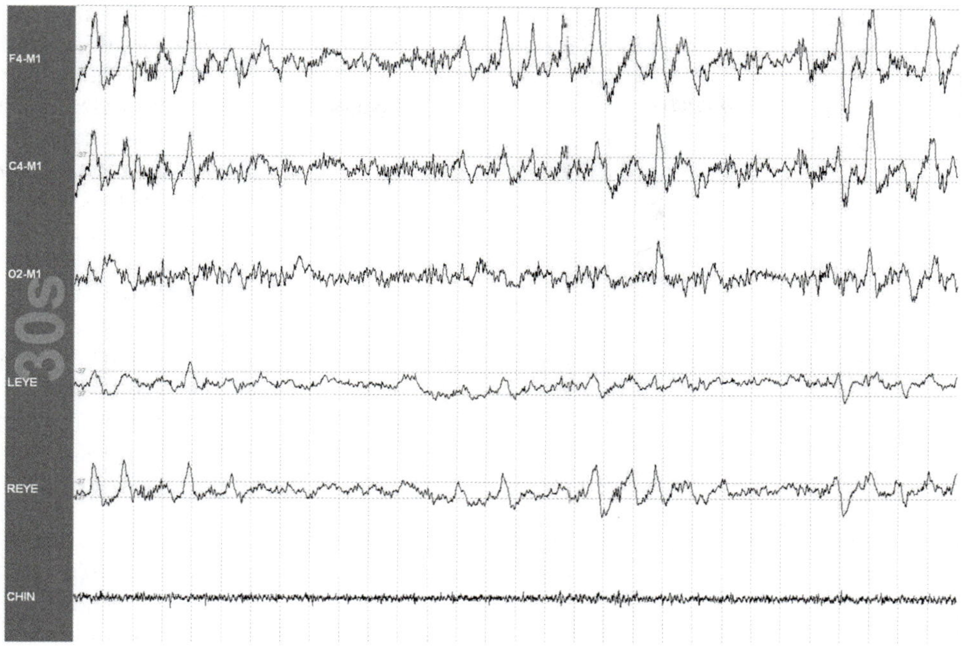

Figure 76-17 An N3 sleep in a 19-year-old male.

waveform observed during stage R but are not required to score the epoch as stage R. REMs are transient during stage R and are not required to be on each epoch to sustain scoring stage R. The continuation and termination rules address this. Stage R usually transitions from stage N2 or another NREM stage.

Definite stage R includes LAMF EEG activity without K complexes or sleep spindles, low EMG tone, and REMs. Score epochs that do not demonstrate REMs but precede or follow an epoch of definite stage R as stage R if chin EMG remains low, if EEG does not demonstrate K complexes or sleep spindles, and if there are no arousals or slow eye movements present. This is essentially the R&K lookback rule.

Note that stage R takes precedence over stage N2 rules. If the majority of an epoch meets stage R criteria,

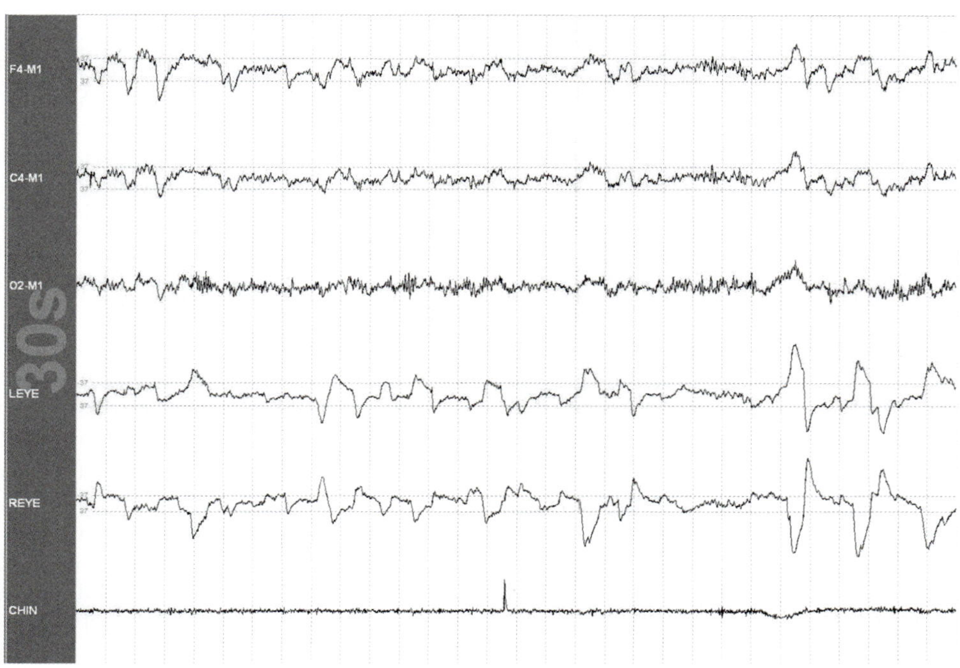

Figure 76-18 REM sleep in a 27-year-old female.

the epoch should be scored as stage R. Specific rules are outlined in the AASM Scoring Manual to address epochs that have a mixture of stage R and stage N2 features. In this instance, we need to determine which stage comprises the majority of the epoch. In an epoch that exhibits low chin EMG tone and a mixture of REMs, sleep spindles, and K complexes, score as follows:

- Segments of the epoch with no REMs that are between two K complexes, two sleep spindles, or between a K complex and a sleep spindle (regardless of which comes first) are stage N2.
- Segments with REMs and no intervening K complexes or sleep spindles are stage R.
- Score the epoch stage R or stage N2 on the basis of the segment that represents the majority of the epoch (1).

Stage R ends when there is a transition to stage W or N3. Following an arousal or major body movement, with slow rolling eye movements, score the following epoch on the basis of the features of the epoch.

- If increased chin EMG tone and slow eye movements are present, score the epoch as stage N1.
- If chin EMG tone remains low and no slow eye movements are seen, score the epoch as stage R.
- If K complexes and/or sleep spindles are present, even with low chin tone, score the epoch as stage N2 (1).

SCORING RESPIRATORY EVENTS

The AASM Scoring Manual provides technical considerations for scoring respiratory events. More specifically, it specifies channels to focus on for the scoring of different types of events as well as backup channels for times when the primary channels may fail or are not used due to the type of sleep study being done (positive airway pressure [PAP] titrations).

Identifying Apnea

During a diagnostic study, the recommended sensors for identification of apnea are the oronasal thermal airflow sensor for monitoring airflow and dual respiratory inductance plethysmography (RIP) belts (calibrated or uncalibrated) for monitoring respiratory effort. During a PAP titration study, the PAP device flow signal and dual RIP belts are recommended. Esophageal manometry is also a recommended technique for monitoring respiratory effort; however, it is rarely used today because it is an invasive measure.

Several alternate sensors are either recommended or acceptable if the primary sensors are not functioning properly. Recommended alternative flow measures for identification of apnea include a nasal pressure transducer (with or without square root transformation) or the RIP sum or RIP flow signal derived from calibrated or uncalibrated RIP belts. The polyvinylidene fluoride (PVDF) sum signal derived from PVDF belts is considered an acceptable alternative flow measure. An acceptable alternative respiratory effort measure is dual thoracoabdominal PVDF belts.

Identifying Hypopnea

During a diagnostic study, the nasal pressure transducer (with or without square root transformation of the signal) is the recommended sensor for monitoring airflow. Dual RIP belts (calibrated or uncalibrated) are recommended for monitoring respiratory effort. During a PAP titration study, the PAP device flow signal and dual RIP belts are recommended (1). The recommended alternative measures, if the nasal pressure transducer fails, are the oronasal thermal airflow sensor and the RIP sum or RIP flow signal from dual thoracoabdominal belts (calibrated or uncalibrated). An acceptable alternative for respiratory effort measurement is dual thoracoabdominal PVDF belts, and for monitoring airflow the PVDF sum (1).

Additional Respiratory Event Monitors

Oxygen saturation is an essential measure for determining oxygenation during sleep as well as for scoring hypopnea. Pulse oximetry with a signal averaging time of less than or equal to 3 seconds at a heart rate of 80 bpm is recommended. Monitoring snoring assists in the determination of respiratory event type and should be accomplished using an acoustic sensor (microphone), a piezoelectric sensor, or a nasal pressure transducer. A measure of carbon dioxide levels is essential for the detection of hypoventilation. During a diagnostic study end-tidal or transcutaneous Pco_2 may be used for this purpose. During a PAP titration, transcutaneous Pco_2 is recommended (1). Arterial Pco_2 measurement is a recommended alternative for use during a PAP titration study but is rarely used because this is an invasive measure.

There are four primary parameters to consider for scoring respiratory events, usually performed during the second pass of the diagnostic portion of a sleep study: the thermal channel, the nasal pressure transducer, the two respiratory effort channels (chest and abdomen), and the oximetry channel. There is a fifth channel that may be useful for scoring hypopneas and respiratory event-related arousals (RERAs): the EEG channel used for scoring arousals. The thermal channel and pressure transducer channel are replaced by the PAP machine-generated flow channel during PAP titrations. If hypoventilation is scored, a measure of Pco_2 must also be recorded. Of note, with subsequent versions of the scoring manual there has been an addition of PVDF belts as an acceptable alternative to esophageal manometry and RIP belts.

Currently, the AASM Scoring Manual indicates that event duration should be measured from the nadir preceding the first breath that is clearly reduced to the beginning of the first breath that approximates the baseline breathing amplitude (1). The AASM Scoring Manual indicates that when baseline breathing amplitude is difficult to determine, events can be determined to have ended when either there is a sustained increase in breathing amplitude or, with events associated with oxygen desaturation, the oximetry channel indicates a resaturation of at least 2% (1).

The recommended or alternate sensors for monitoring apnea must be used to determine event duration: preferably the oronasal thermal sensor signal for a diagnostic study or the PAP device flow signal for a PAP titration study. For hypopnea, the nasal pressure signal (diagnostic study) or PAP device flow signal (PAP titration study) should be used to determine event duration (1).

In adults, duration must be 10 seconds at minimum to score a respiratory event.

Scoring an Apnea

An apnea is scored when an almost complete absence of airflow (at least a 90% drop in amplitude pre-baseline) is seen on the thermal or PAP flow sensor. If the period of decreased amplitude lasts at least 10 seconds, then an apnea should be scored (1). Although a physiologic consequence such as a desaturation or arousal is often seen after an apnea, no such consequence is needed to score an apnea.

An apnea must be categorized in one of three ways: obstructive (Figures 76-19 and 76-20), mixed (Figure 76-21), or central (Figure 76-22). The AASM Scoring Manual describes the categories as given here:

- *Obstructive*—"meets apnea criteria and is associated with continued or increased inspiratory effort throughout the entire period of absent airflow" (1). Most apneas that we score are of the obstructive type.
- *Central*—"meets apnea criteria and is associated with absent inspiratory effort throughout the entire period of absent airflow" (1). Central apneas are seen less frequently than obstructive events.
- *Mixed*—"meets the apnea criteria and is associated with absent inspiratory effort in the initial portion of the event, followed by resumption of inspiratory effort in the second portion of the event" (1). Mixed apneas are generally considered to be obstructive events in terms of treatment decisions.

The apnea requires an almost complete cessation of airflow to be scoring. Events that have a smaller decrease in airflow are scored as hypopneas. The definition of hypopnea has undergone several changes from the 2007 version of the manual. These changes were primarily related to the definitions of the recommended and alternative hypopnea rules.

- The recommended rule allows scoring a hypopnea on the basis of a greater than 30% reduction in the

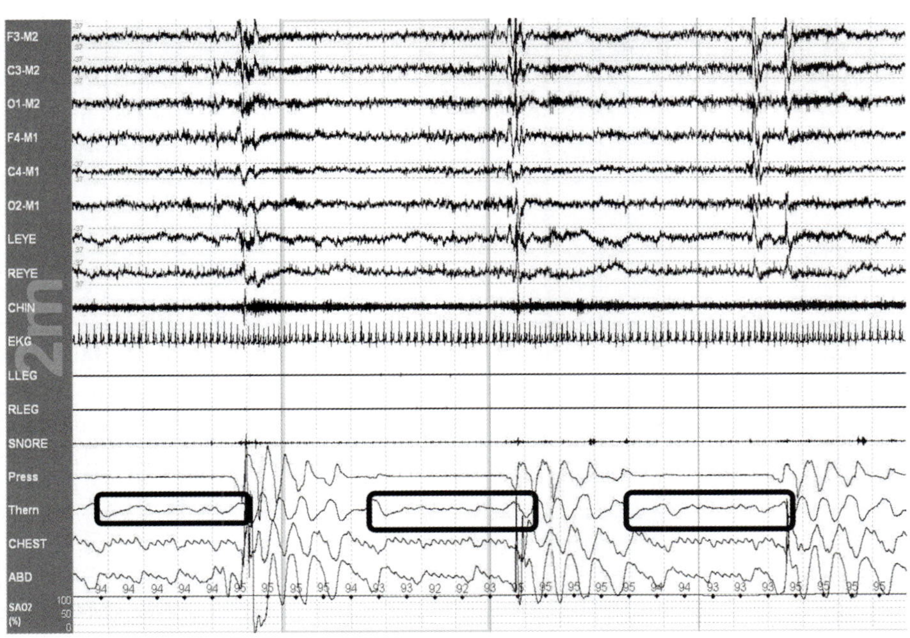

Figure 76-19 Three obstructive apneas in a 58-year-old female. Note the paradoxical breathing during the obstructive events.

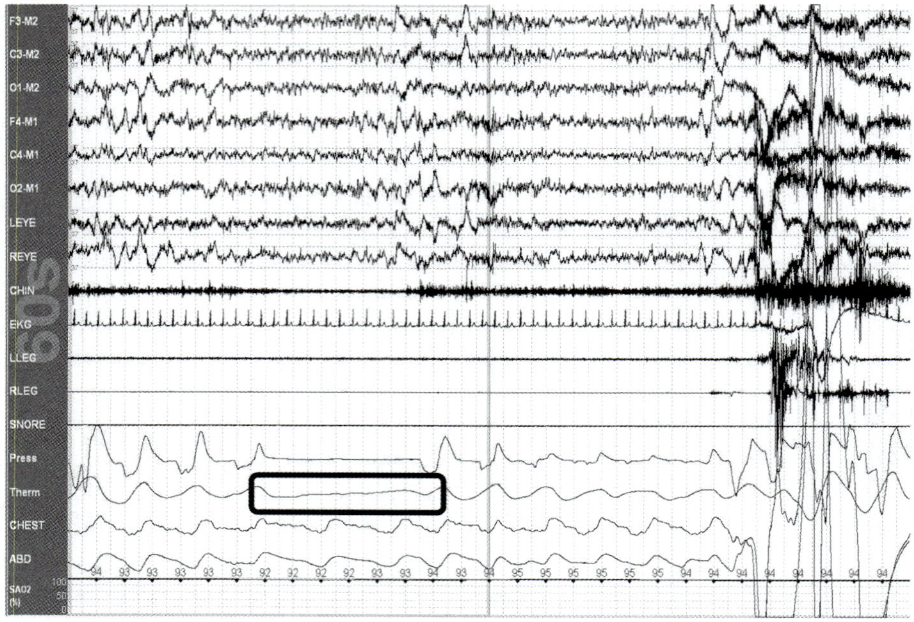

Figure 76-20 An obstructive apnea in a 59-year-old female.

flow signal lasting at least 10 seconds accompanied by either a 3% oxygen desaturation or an arousal.

- The alternative rule (required by Medicare and some insurers) requires a 4% oxygen desaturation and does not allow scoring a hypopnea on the basis of an arousal.

An additional change allows the clinician or investigator to further define hypopneas as either obstructive or central. The reader is encouraged to review the article by Berry and colleagues that explains these changes in detail (11).

Scoring a Hypopnea

Hypopneas are scored when at least a 30% reduction of airflow is seen in the nasal pressure signal (or PAP flow for a PAP titration) with a duration of at least 10 seconds.

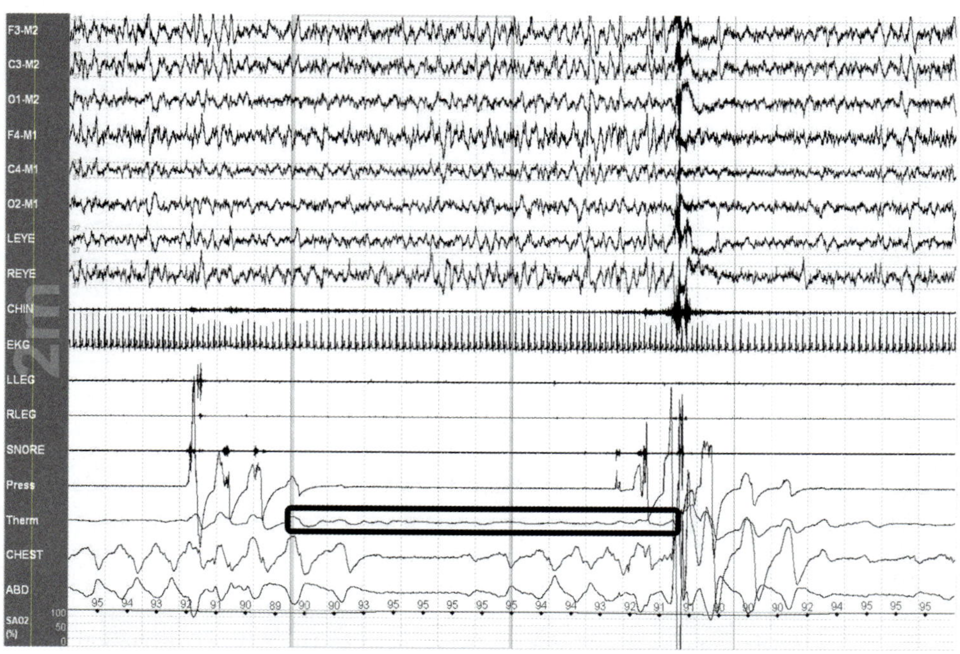

Figure 76-21 A mixed apnea in a 67-year-old male.

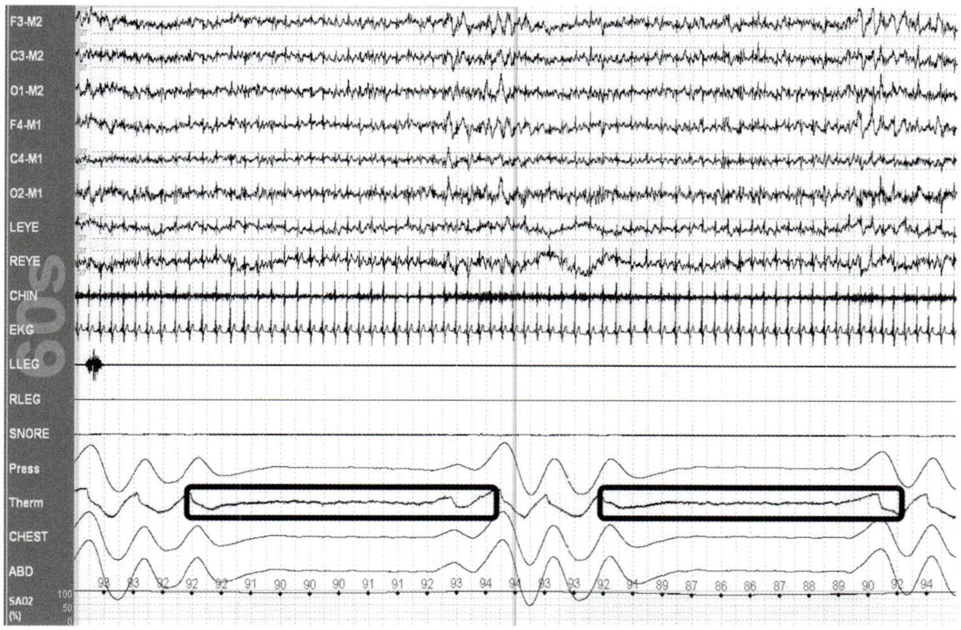

Figure 76-22 Two central apneas in a 60-second epoch in a 45-year-old male.

Unlike apnea, the scoring of hypopneas requires a physiologic consequence. Thus, scoring hypopneas requires a 3% desaturation or an arousal (Figure 76-23) or a 4% desaturation using the alternate scoring rule (Figure 76-24) (1).

Hypopneas may be further differentiated as either *obstructive* or *central* at the discretion of the medical director of the sleep center. If electing to categorize hypopneas as *obstructive* or *central*, the presence or absence of three features determines this categorization. *Obstructive* hypopneas may be scored if *any* of the following features are seen: snoring during the event, increased inspiratory flattening during the event, or thoracoabdominal paradoxical respiratory motion during the event. If one or more of these features are seen, then the event should be scored as *obstructive*. Only if *none* of these three features are seen may a *central* hypopnea be scored (1).

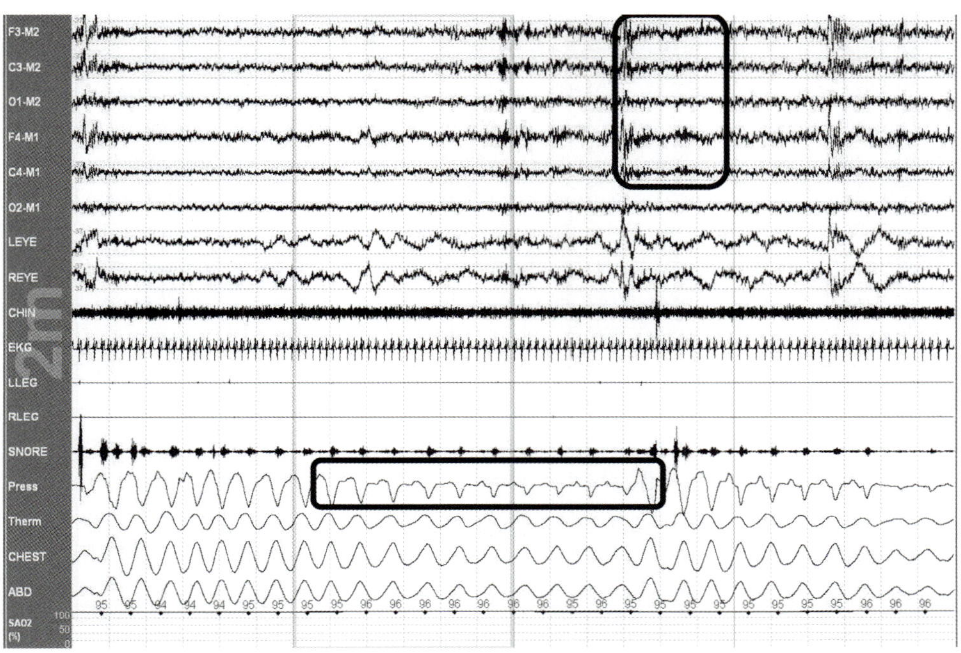

Figure 76-23 A 2-minute epoch displaying a hypopnea associated with an arousal in a 29-year-old male.

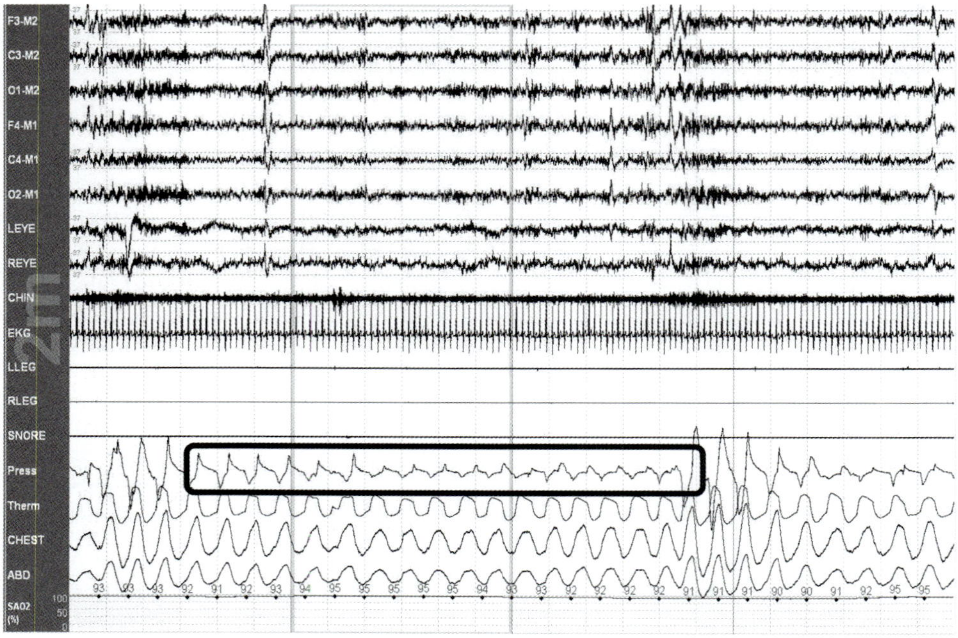

Figure 76-24 A 2-minute epoch displaying a hypopnea with 4% desaturation.

Scoring Respiratory Effort-Related Arousal

There are events that do not meet the criteria for either of the hypopnea rules or criteria to be scored as an apnea. These events are known as RERAs (Figure 76-25). The RERA always causes an arousal. The AASM Scoring Manual criteria for scoring a RERA requires a sequence of breaths showing increasing respiratory effort or flattening of the inspiratory portion of the nasal pressure (diagnostic study) or PAP flow (PAP titration) waveform that leads to an arousal (1).

Earlier versions of the manual specifically indicated that the preferred method for monitoring respiratory effort when scoring RERAs was esophageal pressure monitoring; however, RERAs are commonly scored on

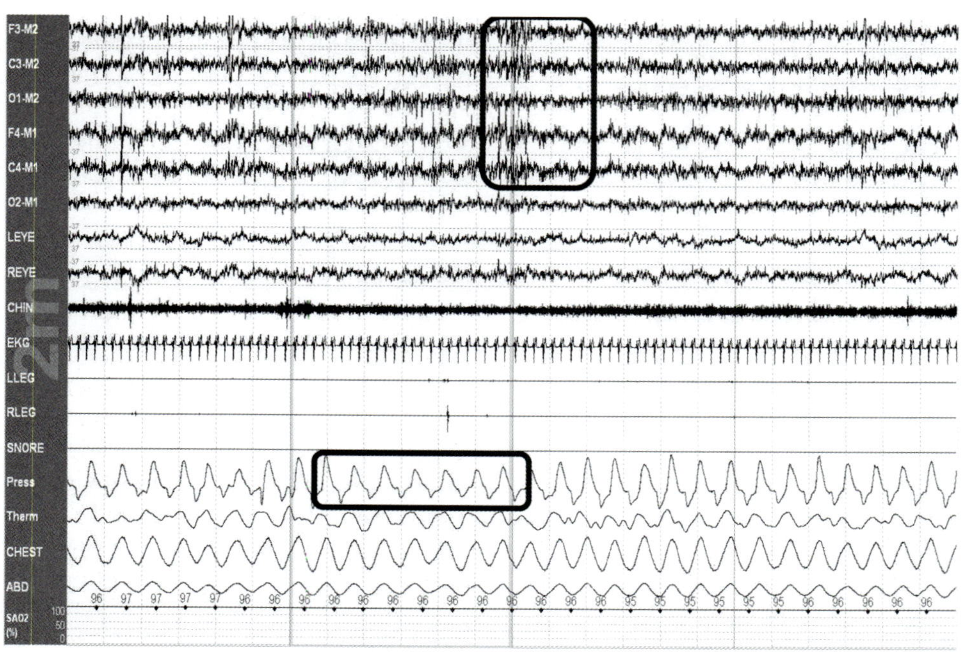

Figure 76-25 A 2-minute epoch displaying a respiratory event-related arousal in a 24-year-old male.

the basis of the pressure transducer signal in clinical practice, and thus, the current version of the manual mentions nasal pressure and PAP flow as adequate for scoring RERAs.

Scoring Hypoventilation

The AASM Scoring Manual also provides a rule for scoring hypoventilation during sleep if either of the following occurs:

a. Increase in the arterial P_{CO_2} (or surrogate) to a value greater than 55 mm Hg for greater than or equal to 10 minutes
b. Greater than or equal to 10 mm Hg increase in arterial P_{CO_2} (or surrogate) during sleep (in comparison to an awake supine value) to a value exceeding 50 mm Hg for greater than or equal to 10 minutes (1).

The reader is encouraged to review the article by Berry and colleagues that discusses monitoring hypoventilation in more detail (11).

Scoring Cheyne-Stokes Breathing

Scoring Cheyne-Stokes breathing requires meeting two specific criteria. This breathing pattern includes changes in breathing amplitude that follow a crescendo/decrescendo pattern and repetitive central apneas or hypopneas. Both of the following criteria are required to score Cheyne-Stokes breathing:

a. There are episodes of greater than or equal to three consecutive central apneas and/or central hypopneas separated by a crescendo and decrescendo change in breathing amplitude with a cycle length of greater than or equal to 40 seconds.
b. There are greater than or equal to five central apneas and/or central hypopneas per hour of sleep associated with the crescendo/decrescendo breathing pattern recorded over greater than or equal to 2 hours of monitoring (1).

Note that central apneas that meet duration criteria and occur during Cheyne-Stokes breathing must also be scored as independent events.

CARDIAC EVENTS

Scoring cardiac events is done on the basis of a single two-lead ECG signal. This signal is derived using a modified lead II placement of ECG electrodes, meaning that one electrode is placed on the right side of the patient's chest between the nipple and the clavicle bone and the second electrode on the left side of the patient near the bottom of the rib cage.

The *AASM Scoring Manual* outlines six rules of cardiac events that must be scored during sleep in adults:

1. Score sinus tachycardia with a sustained (greater than 30 seconds) sinus heart rate of greater than 90 bpm.
2. Score bradycardia with a sustained (greater than 30 seconds) heart rate of less than 40 bpm for ages 6 years through adult.
3. Score asystole for cardiac pauses greater than 3 seconds for ages 6 years through adult.
4. Score wide complex tachycardia for a rhythm lasting a minimum of three consecutive beats at a rate greater than 100 per minute with a QRS duration of greater than or equal to 120 ms.
5. Score narrow complex tachycardia for a rhythm lasting a minimum of three consecutive beats at a rate greater than 100 per minute with a QRS duration of less than 120 ms.
6. Score atrial fibrillation if there are irregularly irregular QRS complexes associated with replacement of consistent P waves by rapid oscillations that vary in size, shape, and timing (1).
7. Score second (identify Mobitz I or Mobitz II) or third degree atrioventricular (AV) heart block. Mobitz I (Wenckebach) is suggested by the PR interval that becomes longer until a nonconducted P wave occurs. Mobitz II is suggested by two fixed pr intervals prior to the nonconducted P wave. Third degree AV block (complete heart block) is suggested by complete AV dissociation with atrial (P waves) and ventricular (QRS complexes) activity being independent of each other (Figure 76-26 A-D).
8. Score cardiac pacemaker rhythm. The presence of cardiac paced rhythm will be manifested by sharp vertical spikes either immediately preceding the onset of P waves (atrial pacing) or QRS complex (ventricular pacing) or both on the ECG (Figure 76-26E).

SCORING MOVEMENTS

The movements most commonly scored in sleep are LMs (Figure 76-27). Limb movement EMG is monitored using surface electrodes on specific muscles. The technical guidelines for the recording of LMs outlined in the AASM Scoring Manual must be utilized to accurately score LMs. For LMs, the anterior tibialis muscle on both legs is always monitored. Additional upper extremity monitoring for LM activity is optional.

The AASM Scoring Manual has defined a significant LM event as an 8 μV increase in EMG voltage above resting EMG with a duration of 0.5 to 10 seconds. The onset of an LM is defined as the point at which there is an 8 μV

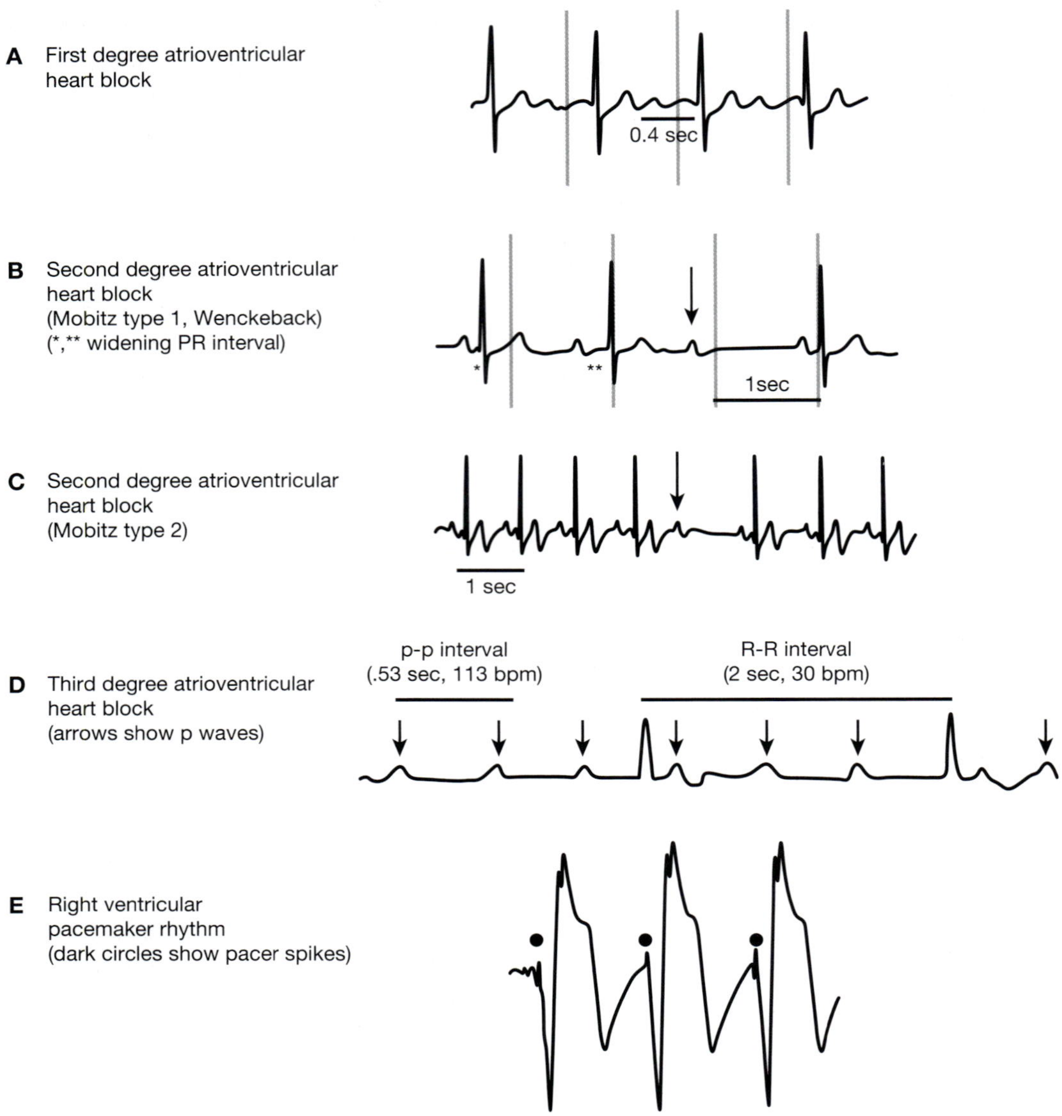

Figure 76-26 Scoring cardiac events from the *AASM Manual for the Scoring of Sleep and Associated Events.*

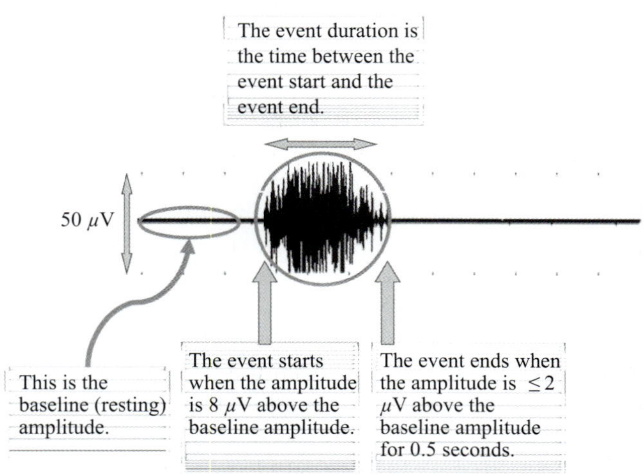

Figure 76-27 Duration criteria for the LMs from the *AASM Manual for the Scoring of Sleep and Associated Events.*

increase in EMG voltage above the resting EMG, and the end of the LM event is defined as the start of a period lasting at least 0.5 seconds during which the EMG does not exceed 2 μV above resting EMG (1).

LMs scored either as isolated (in which case they are simply marked) or as a part of a series. The rules that define a periodic limb movement (PLM; Figure 76-28) series indicate there must be at least four consecutive LM events with at least 5 seconds no more than 90 seconds between onset of the events. LMs on different limbs separated by less than 5 seconds between onsets are counted as a single LM (1). Note that PLMs that occur during an epoch of wake (stage W) are not counted as part of the series. However, it is also important to note that if the onset of the next scorable LM in the series occurs in an epoch staged as sleep and onset of the two events in sleep epochs on either side

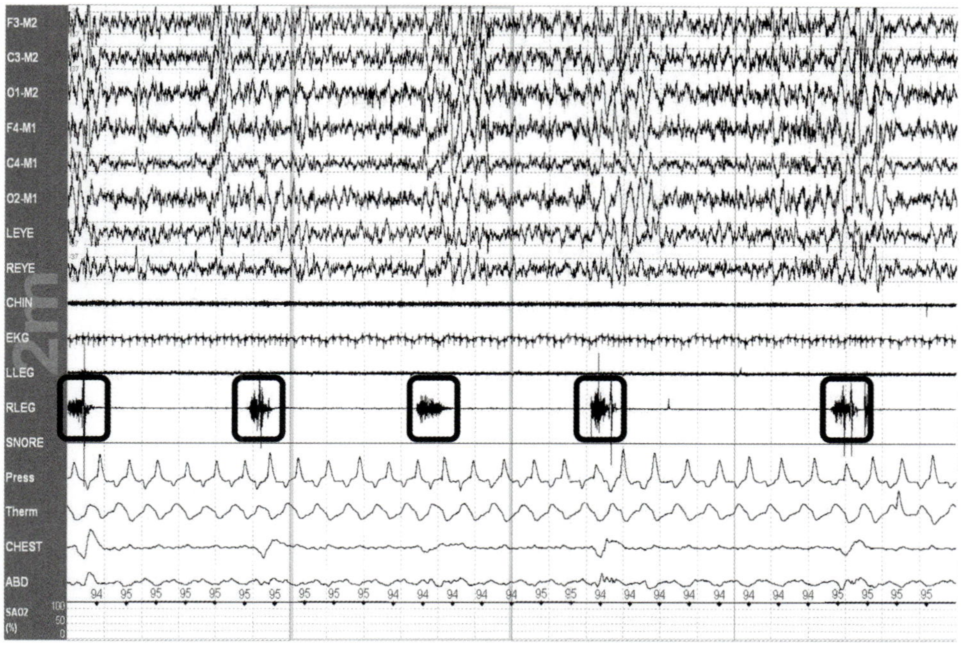

Figure 76-28 A periodic limb movement series in a 43-year-old female.

of the wake epoch is less than 90 seconds, the PLM series continues uninterrupted.

Arousals may be associated with LMs. When an arousal occurs simultaneously with or overlaps with the LM, or there is less than 0.5 seconds between the LM and the arousal, they are considered to be associated (1). LMs are typically scored with and without arousals. Scoring of LMs is also affected by the presence of respiratory events. For this reason, respiratory events should be scored before LM scoring.

An LM should not be scored if it occurs within 0.5 seconds preceding or following an apnea, hypopnea, or RERA.

There are several additional movement events that can be scored and reported. Alternating leg muscle activation (ALMA), hypnagogic foot tremor (HFT), and excessive fragmentary myoclonus (EMF).

- ALMA is defined as having a minimum frequency of 0.5 Hz and a maximum frequency of 3 Hz. To score an ALMA series, the minimum number of alternating EMG bursts on the right and left leg is four. The sequences occur during the transition of wake to sleep or are associated with arousals (1).
- HFT is defined as a minimum frequency of 0.3 Hz and a maximum frequency of 4 Hz. To score HFT, the minimum number of EMG bursts needed to make a train of burst in a train of bursts is four (1).
- EMF is defined as at least 20 minutes of NREM sleep, the maximum EMG burst duration seen is 150 ms. and at least 5 EMG potentials per minute must be recorded (1).

Bruxism

Bruxism is monitored using chin EMG and, if suspected, additional masseter muscle EMG. Bruxism in sleep (Figure 76-29) is scored when brief (phasic) or sustained (tonic) elevations of chin EMG activity at least twice the amplitude of background EMG are seen.

- Phasic chin EMG activity of 0.25 to 2 seconds in duration is scored as bruxism when at least three episodes occur in a regular sequence.
- Tonic (sustained) chin EMG activity of greater than 2 seconds is also scored.

To score a new episode of bruxism, either tonic or sustained, there must be at least 3 seconds of steady baseline chin EMG before scoring a new episode. It is important to note that bruxism can also be scored on the basis of audible tooth-grinding episodes. Specifically, there must be a minimum of two audible tooth-grinding episodes in the absence of epilepsy to audibly score bruxism (1).

Rapid Eye Movement Sleep Behavior Disorder

To score REM sleep behavior disorder (RBD), a time-locked video with recorded sound is essential to record dream enactment episodes occurring during REM sleep. Absent the occurrence of an episode during the polysomnography, demonstration of REM sleep without atonia (RWA) is required. Scoring rules for RBD require identification of sustained tonic muscle activity

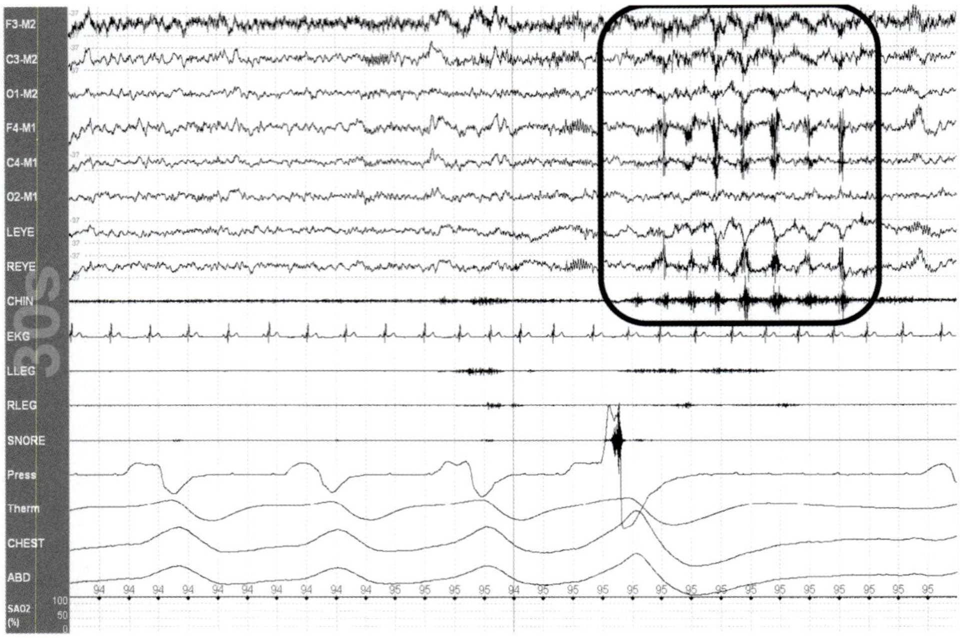

Figure 76-29 A 30-second epoch that displays bruxism.

and/or excessive transient muscle activity (phasic muscle activity) in REM sleep.

- To score tonic activity in REM sleep, 50% of the REM epoch must have chin EMG activity of an amplitude greater than that seen during NREM sleep.
- To score transient muscle activity, 30-second epochs of REM sleep are divided into 10 sequential 3-second mini epochs.
- To score RBD in an epoch of REM thus divided, at least five of the mini epochs (50% of the 30-second epoch) must contain transient muscle activity bursts 0.1 to 5 seconds in duration and at least 2 times as high in amplitude as the NREM if no stage R atonia is present.

In scoring RWA, you must have excessive sustained muscle activity in REM in the chin EMG or excessive transient muscle activity in REM in the chin or limb EMG, or at least 50% of the 3 second mini-epoch must contain chin or limb EMG activity bursts 0.1 to 5 seconds in duration and at least 2 times as high in amplitude as the stage R atonia level or the lowest amplitude in NREM, if no stage R atonia is present (1).

Rhythmic Movement Disorder

To record the movements associated with rhythmic movement disorder, a pair of electrodes are placed on the neck paraspinal muscles and referenced to each other in a bipolar montage. Scoring is based on evaluating movements recorded in this montage as follows:

Movements must have a minimum frequency of 0.5 Hz and a maximum frequency of 2 Hz. A cluster of rhythmic movements is identified as a minimum of four movements. The amplitude of the individual rhythmic bursts must be at least 2 times the background EMG activity to score rhythmic movements (1).

CONCLUSION

Scoring a PSG involves learning the rules outlined in the current version of the AASM Scoring Manual and reviewing as many PSGs as possible with an experienced scorer. It takes most people new to scoring about 2 weeks to become minimally proficient at scoring sleep stages and events. It takes frequent scoring practice to become an expert. The first time we score a record, we are tempted to try and get everything right, and this is a good instinct. There is, however, an old saying in sleep: "Don't take as much time to score a record as it did to record it." So make a decision about each epoch and move on, noting questionable epochs to be reviewed later with a more experienced scorer.

The AASM's ISR program is an online resource that allows scorers to score a common sample of PSG recording and compare their scores to a gold standard panel as well as other scorers who participate in the ISR program. In addition to participation in an ISR program being an AASM accreditation requirement, it is a convenient way to receive expert feedback on one's scoring. This is a valuable resource to the novice and expert scorer alike.

SUGGESTED READING

American Academy of Sleep Medicine. *A Technologist's Handbook for Understanding and Implementing the AASM Manual for the Scoring of Sleep and Associated Events: Rules, Terminology, and Technical Specifications.* American Academy of Sleep Medicine; 2009.

REFERENCES

1. Troester MM, Quan SF, Berry RB, et al; for the American Academy of Sleep Medicine. *The AASM Manual for the Scoring of Sleep and Associated Events: Rules, Terminology and Technical Specifications* (Version 3). American Academy of Sleep Medicine; 2023.
2. Silber MH, Ancoli-Israel S, Bonnet MH, et al. The visual scoring of sleep in adults. *J Clin Sleep Med.* 2007; 3(2):121-131.
3. Williams RL, Karacan I, Hirsch CJ, eds. *Electroencephalography (EEG) of Human Sleep: Clinical Applications.* John Wiley & Sons; 1974.
4. Himanen SL, Hasan J. Limitations of Rechtschaffen and Kales. *Sleep Med Rev.* 2000;4(2):149-167.
5. Webb WB. Recording methods and visual scoring criteria of sleep records: comments and recommendations. *Percept Mot Skills.* 1986;62:664-666.
6. American Sleep Disorders Association. EEG arousals: scoring rules and examples: a preliminary report from the Sleep Disorders Atlas Task Force of the American Sleep Disorders Association. *Sleep.* 1992;15(2):173-184.
7. American Academy of Sleep Medicine Task Force. Sleep-related breathing disorders in adults: recommendations for syndrome definition and measurement techniques in clinical research. *Sleep.* 1999;22(5):667-689.
8. Atlas Task Force. Recording and scoring leg movements. *Sleep.* 1993;16(8):748-759.
9. Anders T, Emde R, Parmelee A. *A Manual of Standardization Terminology, Techniques and Criteria for Scoring States of Sleep and Wakefulness in Newborn Infants.* UCLA Brain Information Service, NINDS Neurological information Network; 1971.
10. A glossary of terms most commonly used by clinical electroencephalographers. *Electroencephalogr Clin Neurophysiol.* 1974;37(5):538-548.
11. Berry RB, Budhiraja R, Gottlieb DJ, et al. Rules for scoring respiratory events in sleep update of the 2007 *AASM* manual for the scoring of sleep and associated events: Deliberations of the Sleep Apnea Definitions Task Force of the American Academy of Sleep Medicine. *J Clin Sleep Med.* 2012;8(5):597-619.

Chapter 77
Scoring Respiratory Events

LAREE J. FORDYCE

KEY CONCEPTS/LEARNING OBJECTIVES

The key concepts for this chapter include identifying sleep-related breathing events according to the American Academy of Sleep Medicine (AASM) adult respiratory scoring rules, defining the various types of sleep-related breathing events, and identifying common artifacts that occur in the respiratory channels.

KEY TERMS

Central apnea
Hypopnea
Hypoventilation
Mixed apnea
Obstructive apnea
Respiratory artifact
Respiratory event-related arousal (RERA)

Scoring respiratory events is an important part of our jobs as sleep technologists. The *AASM Manual for the Scoring of Sleep and Associated Events* has outlined the respiratory scoring rules for both adults and pediatrics. In this chapter, we review the respiratory scoring rules in adults as well as show examples to illustrate respiratory events and how these events should be scored.

The current parameters to be recorded as well as the technical specifications for respiratory rules for both adults and pediatrics are outlined in the *AASM Manual for the Scoring of Sleep and Associated Events* and should be reviewed to ensure collection of data meets these standards (1).

When scoring respiratory events, it is important to record the proper signals using the appropriate sensors (1). We should be recording airflow using an oronasal thermal sensor (this includes thermistors, thermocouples, or polyvinylidene fluoride airflow sensors) or a nasal pressure transducer. For respiratory effort channels, thoracic and abdominal respiratory inductance plethysmography (RIP) belts are recommended. The RIPsum and RIPflow channels can be a helpful tool for scoring respiratory events. See Figure 77-1 for an example of a normal respiratory pattern.

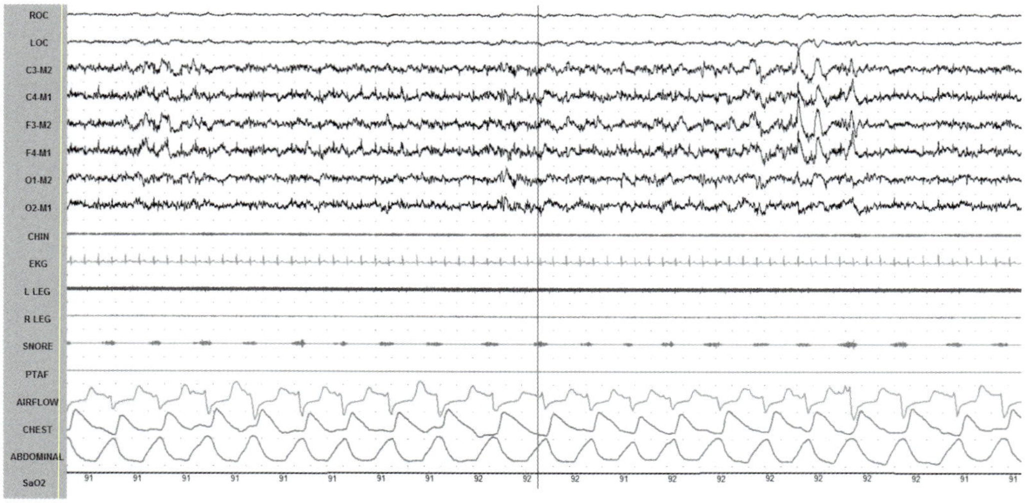

Figure 77-1 Normal respiratory pattern.

APNEA

An apnea should be scored using the oronasal thermal airflow sensor; however, alternatives such as a nasal transducer, RIPsum, or RIPflow may be used if this sensor is not functioning. When performing a positive airway pressure (PAP) titration study, use the PAP device flow signal to score apneas. There are three types of apneas: obstructive, central, and mixed.

Obstructive Apnea

1. An obstructive apnea (Figure 77-2A, B) is defined as cessation of airflow (drop in signal by ≥90% of the pre-event baseline using an oronasal thermal airflow sensor) with continued respiratory effort throughout the event.
2. The duration of the event is greater than or equal to 10 seconds.

Central Apnea

1. A central apnea (Figure 77-3A, B) is defined as cessation of airflow (drop in signal by ≥90% of the pre-event baseline using an oronasal thermal airflow sensor) with absent respiratory effort throughout the entire event.
2. The duration of the event is greater than or equal to 10 seconds.

Mixed Apnea

1. A mixed apnea (Figure 77-4A, B) is defined as cessation of airflow (drop in signal by ≥90% of the pre-event baseline using an oronasal thermal airflow sensor) for at least 10 seconds, with resumption of respiratory effort in the second part of the event.
2. The duration of the event is greater than or equal to 10 seconds.

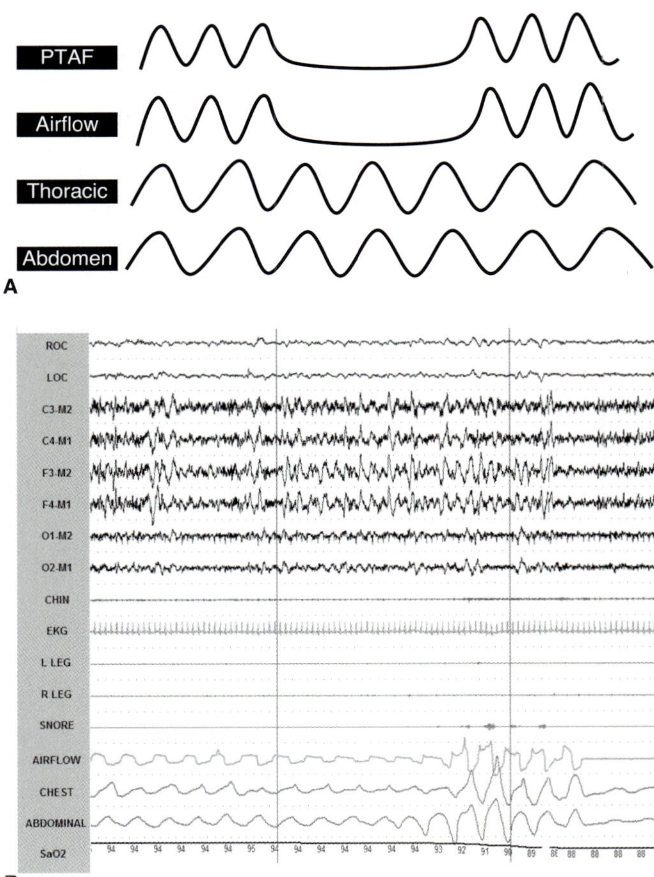

Figure 77-2 A, B: Obstructive apnea. PTAF, pressure transducer airflow.

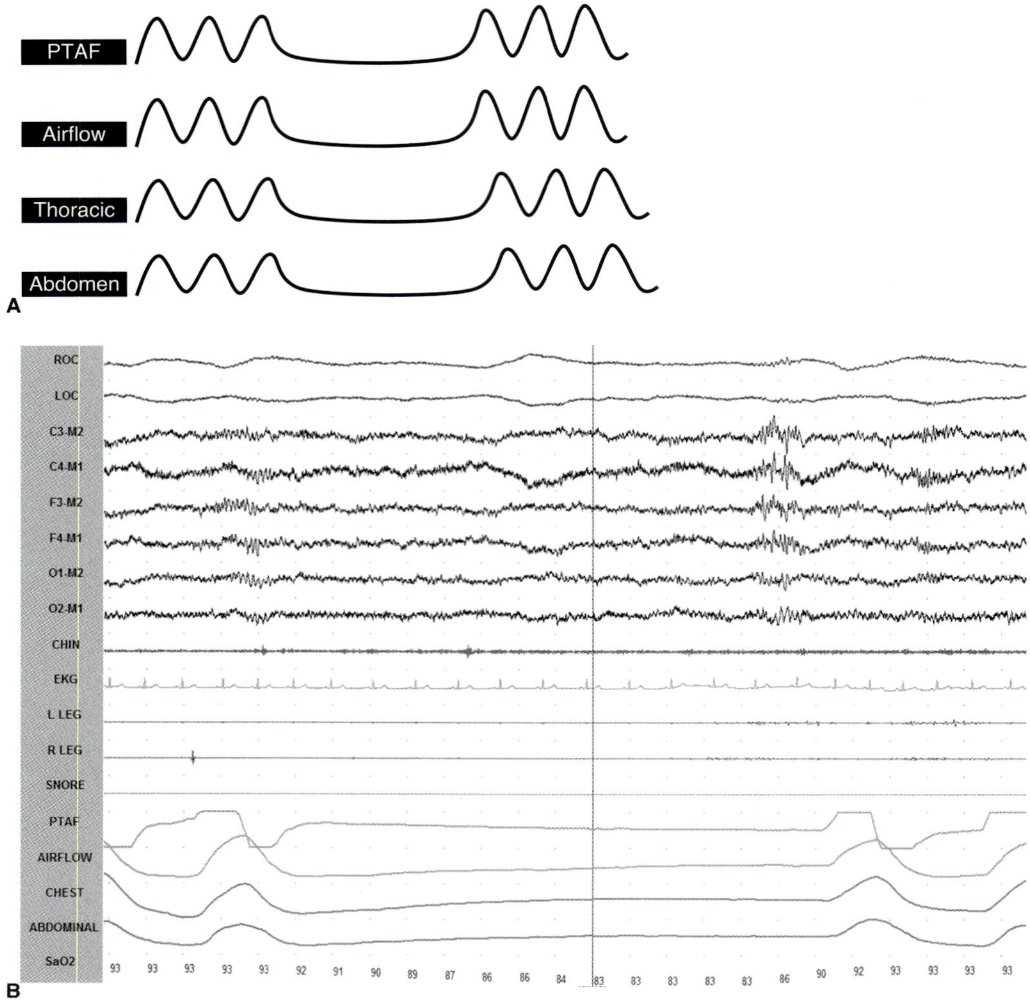

Figure 77-3 A, B: Central apnea. In this example, the airflow as well as the respiratory effort is completely absent. PTAF, pressure transducer airflow.

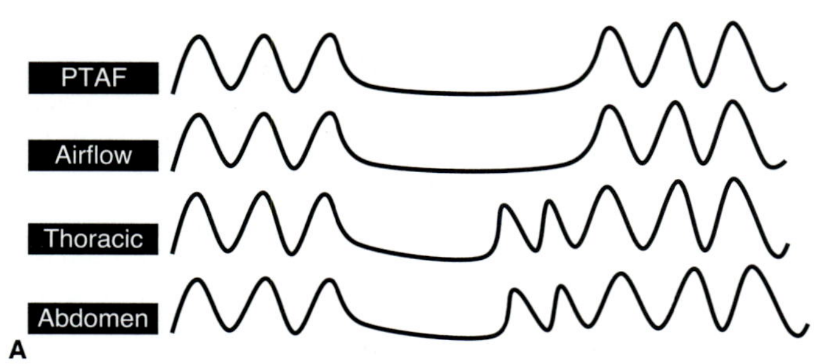

Figure 77-4 A, B: Mixed apnea. The airflow stops completely and does not resume until the end of the event. At the beginning of the event, there is no effort; then, effort resumes before the end of the event. Most often, a snore event is seen with resumption of airflow. PTAF, pressure transducer airflow.

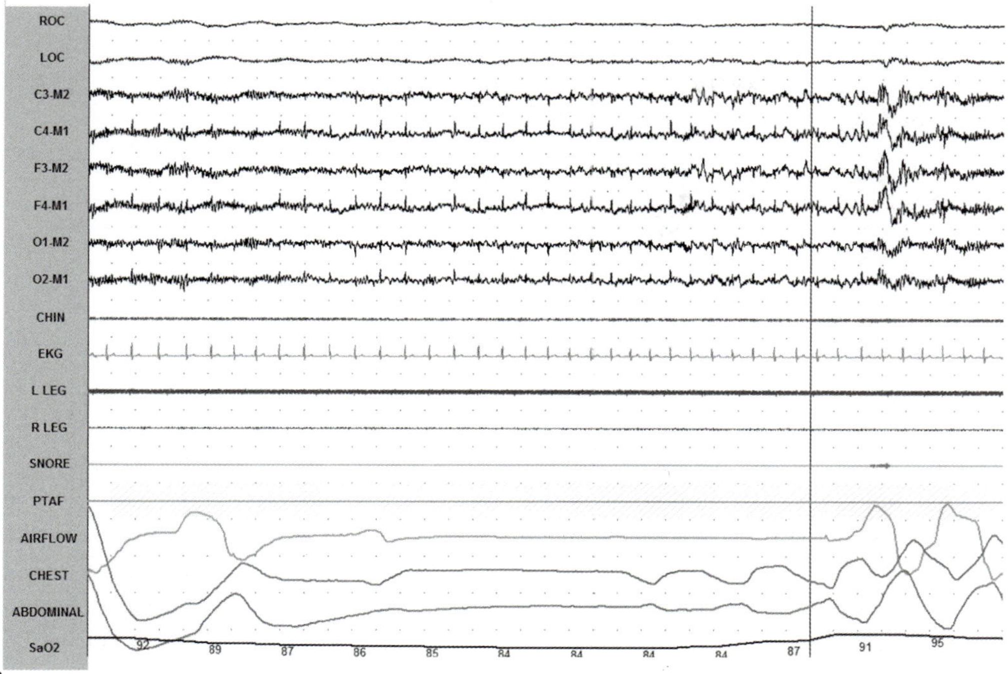

B

Figure 77-4 (*continued*)

HYPOPNEA

A hypopnea (Figure 77-5A, B) should be scored using a nasal pressure transducer; however, alternatives such as an oronasal thermal airflow sensor, RIPsum, or RIPflow may be used if this sensor is not functioning. When performing a PAP titration study, use the PAP device flow signal to score a hypopnea.

There are two rules that can be used to score hypopnea. It is important that your report specifies which scoring rule you have used to score hypopnea.

Hypopnea Rule 1A

1. A hypopnea is defined as a decrease in airflow (drop in signal by ≥30% of the pre-event baseline using a nasal pressure transducer) with continued respiratory effort throughout the event.
2. The duration of the event is greater than or equal to 10 seconds.
3. The event is associated with either a greater than or equal to 3% oxygen desaturation (from pre-event baseline) or an arousal. See Figure 77-6 for an example of a hypopnea with an arousal.

Hypopnea Rule 1B

1. A hypopnea is defined as a decrease in airflow (drop in signal by ≥30% of the pre-event baseline using a nasal pressure transducer) with continued respiratory effort throughout the event.
2. The duration of the event is greater than or equal to 10 seconds.
3. The event is associated with a greater than or equal to 4% oxygen desaturation (from pre-event baseline). An example of a hypopnea scored on the basis of an arousal is seen in Figure 77-7.

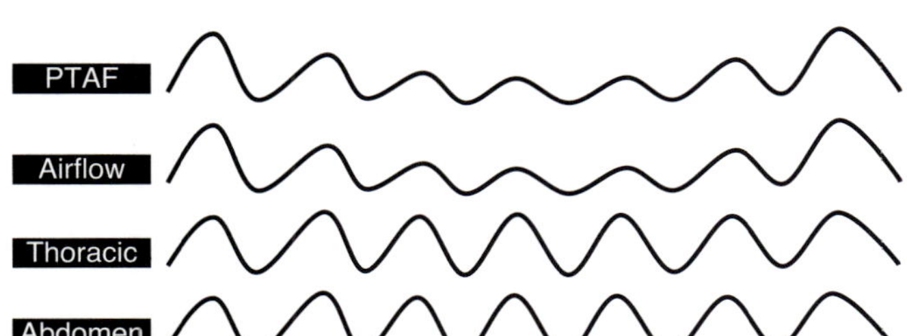

A

Figure 77-5 A: Hypopnea.

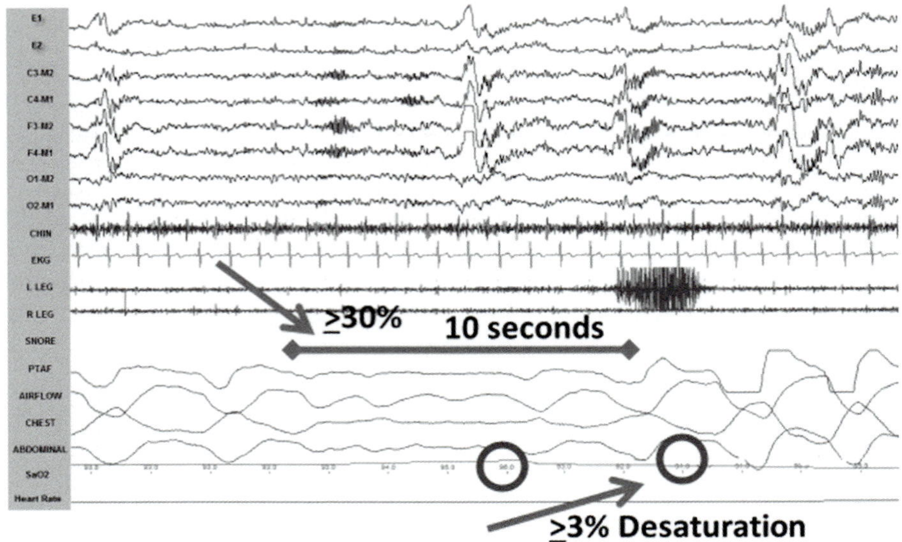

B

Figure 77-5 (*continued*) B: A hypopnea scored using rule 1A with greater than 3% desaturation. There is at least a 30% reduction in the flow channel. The event lasts a minimum of 10 seconds and is accompanied by at least a 3% decrease in oxygen saturation. PTAF, pressure transducer airflow.

RESPIRATORY EFFORT-RELATED AROUSAL

Scoring respiratory effort-related arousals (RERAs) is optional, as noted in the AASM scoring manual, Parameters to Be Reported.

A RERA is scored when an event that does not meet the criteria to be scored as an apnea or hypopnea occurs and yet leads to an arousal from sleep. A RERA should be scored if the event is greater than or equal to 10 seconds in duration. The event is characterized by increasing respiratory effort or by flattening of the inspiratory portion of the nasal pressure (diagnostic study) or PAP device flow (titration study) waveform followed by an arousal. An example of a RERA is seen in Figure 77-8.

HYPOVENTILATION

Monitoring hypoventilation in adults is optional, as noted in the AASM scoring manual, Parameters to Be Reported. To score hypoventilation in sleep requires

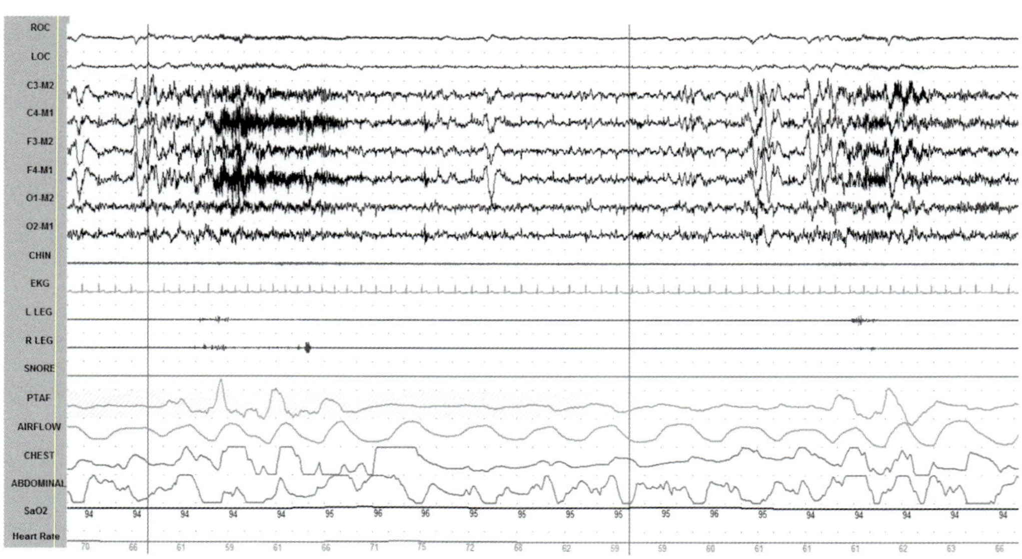

Figure 77-6 A hypopnea with arousal scored using rule 1A. There is at least a 30% reduction in the flow channel. The event lasts a minimum of 10 seconds. There is no oxygen desaturation, but there is an arousal associated with the event.

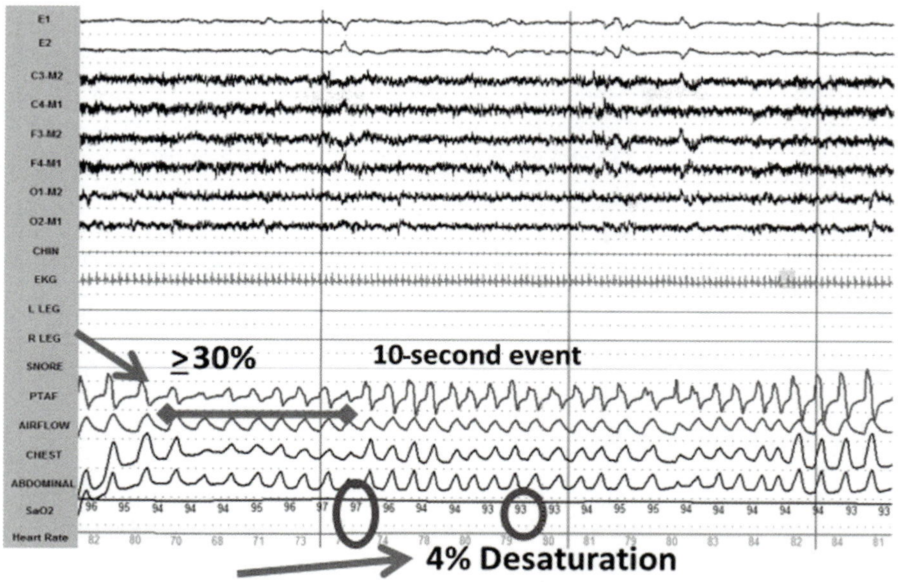

Figure 77-7 A hypopnea scored using rule 1B. There is at least a greater than or equal to 30% decrease in airflow using PTAF. The event lasts at least 10 seconds, and there is an associated 4% oxygen desaturation.

monitoring a measure of CO_2 (see Figure 77-9). Hypoventilation is scored when either of the following occurs:

1. There is an increase in the arterial Pco_2 (or surrogate) to a value greater than 55 mm Hg for more than or equal to 10 minutes.
2. There is greater than or equal to 10 mm Hg increase in arterial Pco_2 (or surrogate) during sleep (in comparison to an awake value) to a value exceeding 50 mm Hg for greater than or equal to 10 minutes (1).

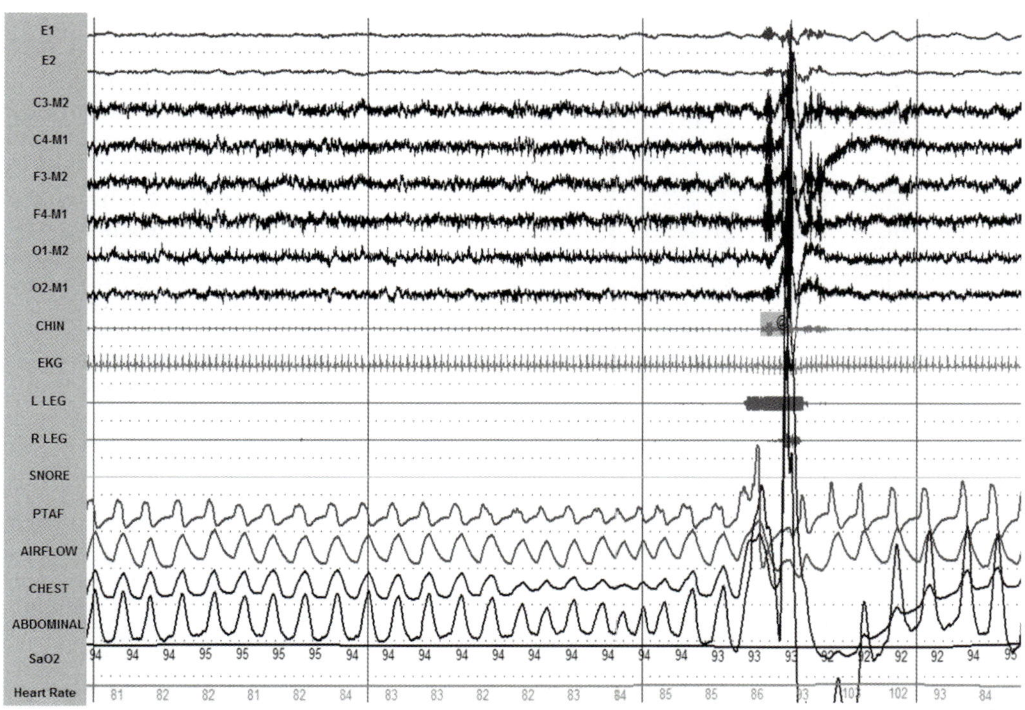

Figure 77-8 The airflow is reduced but does not meet the greater than or equal to 30% reduction required to score a hypopnea. There is no desaturation. The event does, however, lead to an arousal and can be scored as a respiratory event-related arousal.

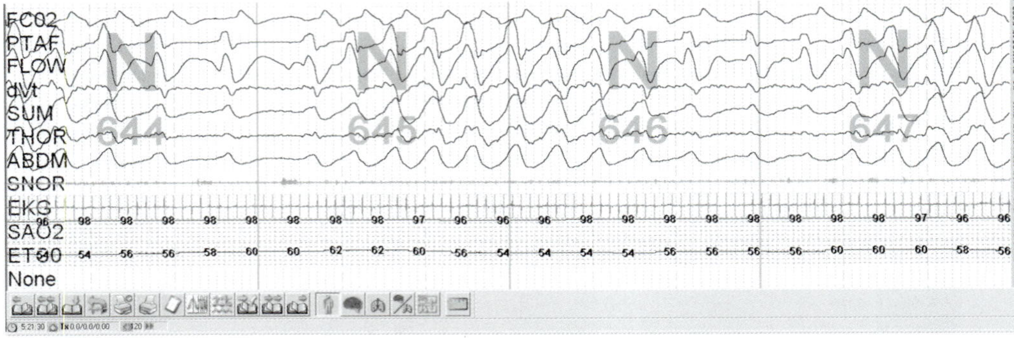

Figure 77-9 Hypoventilation identified in this recording by consistent high levels of CO_2 in the end-tidal CO_2 channel and the absence of discrete scorable events.

CHEYNE-STOKES RESPIRATION

We often see patients with Cheyne-Stokes respiration (CSR) who have other medical conditions such as heart failure, atrial fibrillation, or stroke. The pattern of CSR can be easily identified (Figure 77-10 for a classic example). Cheyne-Stokes breathing can be scored when there are episodes of greater than or equal to three consecutive central apneas and/or central hypopneas separated by a crescendo and decrescendo change in breathing amplitude with a cycle length of greater than or equal to 40 seconds. This looks like pearls on a string. Cheyne-Stokes breathing can also be scored when there are greater than or equal to five central apneas and/or central hypopneas per hour of sleep associated with a crescendo and decrescendo breathing pattern over greater than or equal to 2 hours of monitoring (1).

OTHER EVENTS

It is also important to document the presence, timing, frequency, intensity, duration, and pattern of events, as well as interventions if needed and other respiratory-related events that occur during the sleep study, including snoring, coughing, choking, stridor, wheezing, repetitive sneezing, or catathrenia.

RESPIRATORY ARTIFACTS

When recording and scoring respiratory events, it is important to ensure that the signals recorded are accurate and appropriate for scoring the type of event occurring in the recording. As mentioned earlier, thermal sensors, pressure transducer cannulas, and effort sensors are used to differentiate between apneas and hypopneas. If any of these signals are not working properly, other channels can be substituted to identify respiratory events. However, if there are few working signals or if there is artifact in the respiratory channels, it can be difficult to identify and score the correct respiratory events. See Figures 77-11 and 77-12 for examples of common respiratory artifacts.

SUMMARY

Scoring respiratory events can be challenging. Clinical examples of challenging events are not as clean as textbook examples. Figure 77-13 is another example of an obstructive apnea. Figure 77-14 shows a mixed apnea, and Figure 77-15 a hypopnea. It is essential to record the appropriate signals to identify the various defined respiratory events and score them according

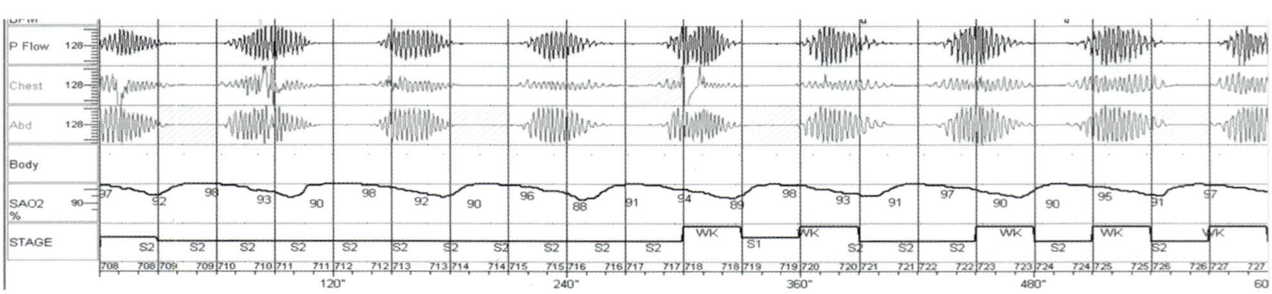

Figure 77-10 A sample of classic Cheyne-Stokes respiration over a period of 10 minutes.

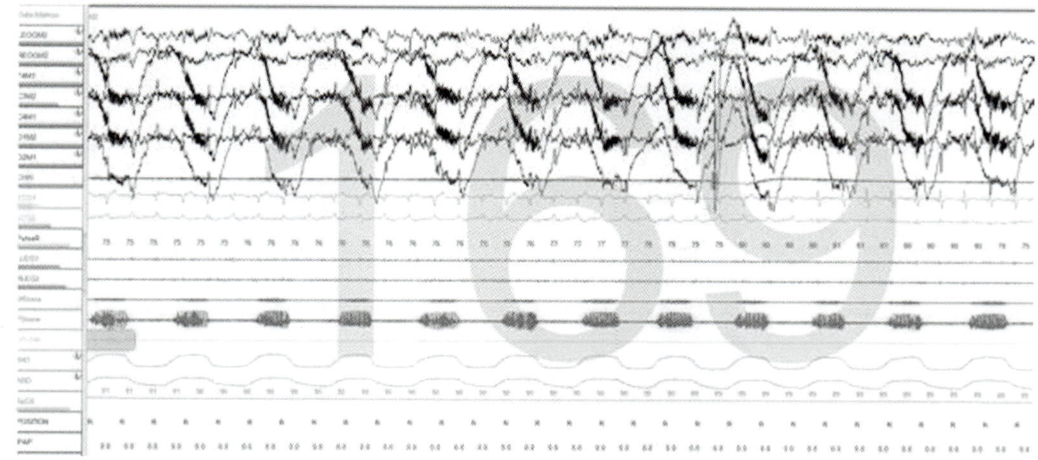

Figure 77-11 Respiratory artifact in the electroencephalogram can be mistaken for sweat artifact or a poor reference or ground electrode. Identifying the correct cause of artifact enables the technologist to fix the problem.

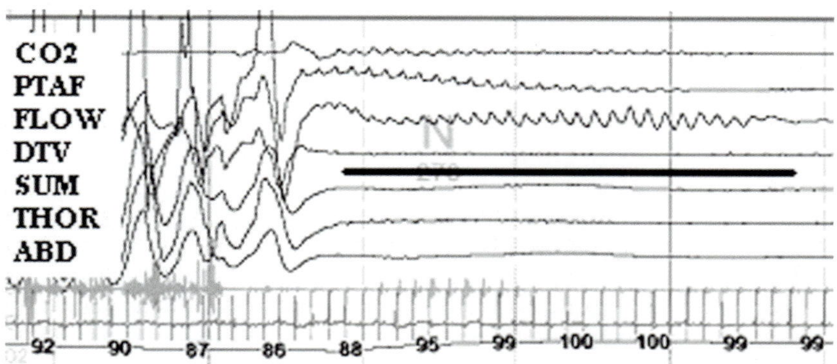

Figure 77-12 Cardioballistic artifact in the respiratory channels can be mistaken for respiratory effort or airflow. The ability to identify artifact in the respiratory channels enables correct scoring of the respiratory event—in this case, a central apnea.

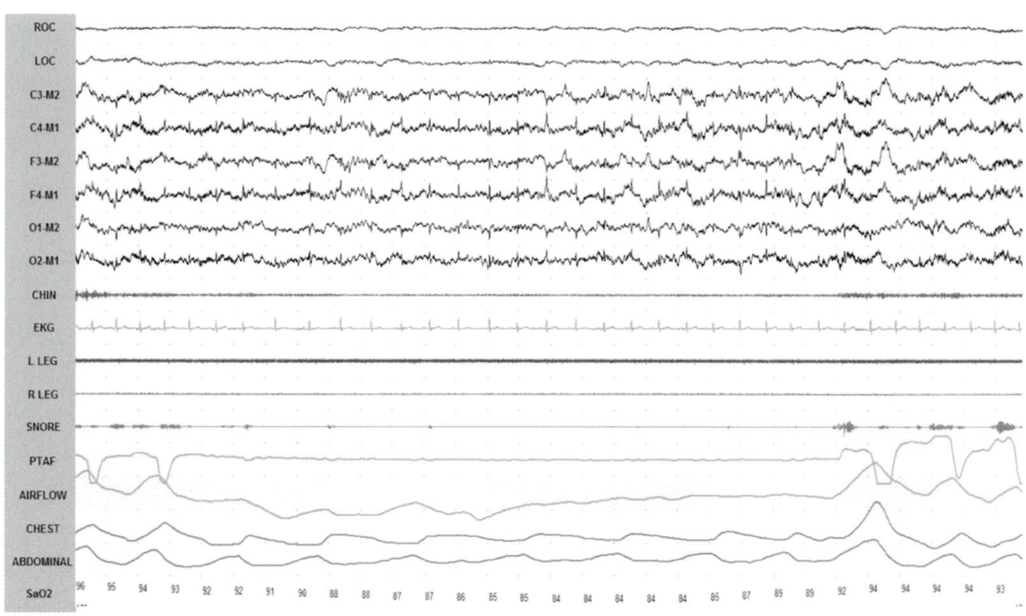

Figure 77-13 Obstructive apnea.

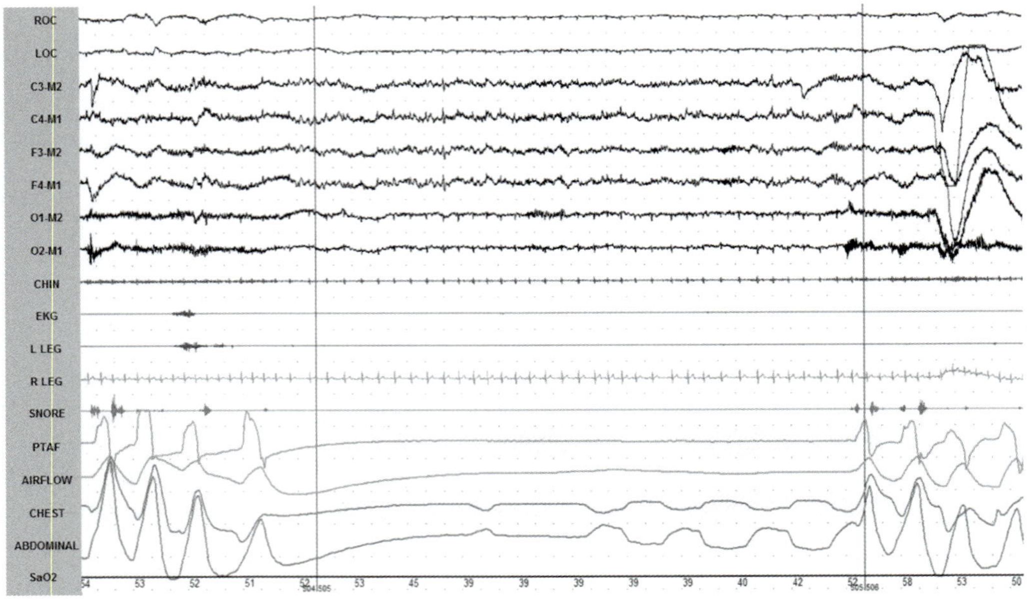

Figure 77-14 Mixed apnea.

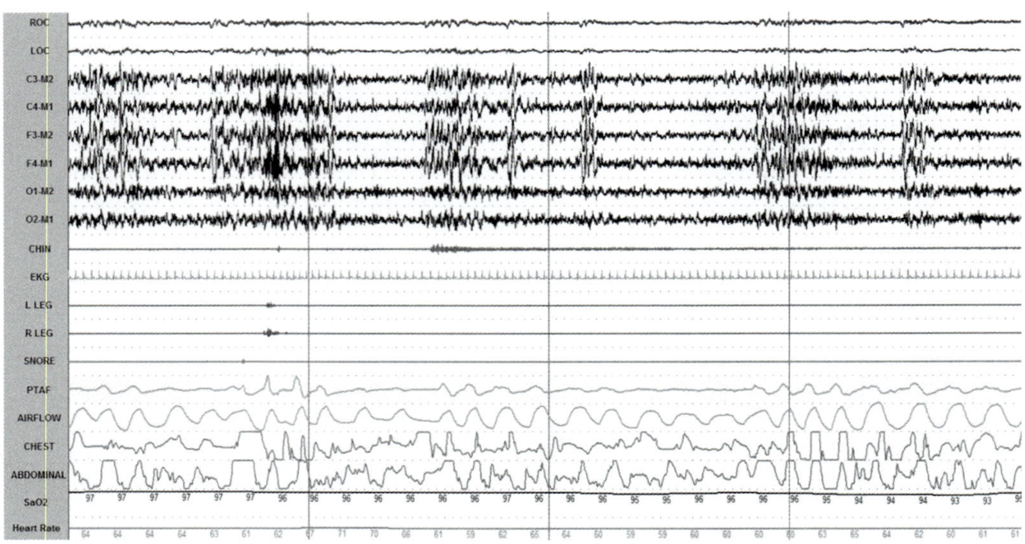

Figure 77-15 Hypopnea.

to accepted AASM scoring rules. The *AASM Manual for the Scoring of Sleep and Associated Events* outlines the appropriate parameters and sensors to utilize for collection of data as well as respiratory event scoring rules and examples that can assist in the scoring process (1). The wise technologist will keep a scoring manual handy!

REFERENCE

1. Troester MM, Quan SF, Berry, RB, et al; for the American Academy of Sleep Medicine. *The AASM Manual for the Scoring of Sleep and Associated Events: Rules, Terminology and Technical Specifications* [Version 3.0]. American Academy of Sleep Medicine; 2023.

Chapter 78
Scoring Movement Rules

LAREE J. FORDYCE

KEY CONCEPTS/LEARNING OBJECTIVES

The key concepts for this chapter include describing movement events and movement event scoring rules according to the standards of the American Academy of Sleep Medicine and identifying the common artifacts that occur in leg movement channels.

KEY TERMS

Bruxism
Excessive fragmentary myoclonus (EFM)
Hypnagogic foot tremor (HFT)
Periodic limb movements in sleep (PLMS)
REM sleep behavior disorder (RBD)
Rhythmic movement disorder (RMD)

In polysomnography (PSG), scoring movements is necessary but can be tricky. The *AASM Manual for the Scoring of Sleep and Associated Events* has outlined the scoring rules for scoring movements in both adults and pediatrics. Review the current sections' Parameters to Be Recorded as well as the Technical Specifications for Movement Rules in the *AASM Manual for the Scoring of Sleep and Associated Events* to verify you are using the most updated recording parameters for collection of data. In this chapter, we will review the movement scoring rules as well as provide examples to illustrate how these events should be scored.

When scoring movements, it is important to record the proper channels and use appropriate sensors. To assess movement activity in the lower limbs, both legs should be monitored. Surface electrodes are placed on the belly of the tibialis anterior muscle of each leg, about 2 to 3 cm apart (1). If upper limb movements are being assessed, both arms should be monitored. Surface electrodes should be placed on either the extensor digitorum communis or flexor digitorum superficialis muscles, or both (1).

Surface electrodes are placed on the neck over the paraspinal muscles (1) to record movement activity typical of rhythmic movement disorder (RMD). To record the electromyographic (EMG) activity seen with bruxism, surface electrodes are placed on the masseter muscle (1). For exact placements of the electrodes used for these EMG recordings, see the chapter on Movement Rules in the current version of the *AASM Manual for the Scoring of Sleep and Associated Events*.

PERIODIC LIMB MOVEMENTS IN SLEEP

1. Periodic limb movements in sleep (PLMS) are defined as leg movements with a duration of between 0.5 and 10 seconds.
2. The maximum amplitude of the event must be an 8 μV increase from the baseline limb EMG signal.
3. PLMS events may cause arousals. Arousals are scored as long as they occur within 0.5 seconds of the movement.

See Figure 78-1 for an example of a PLM that resulted in an arousal.

PERIODIC LIMB MOVEMENT SERIES

1. A PLM series is defined as four leg movements (Figure 78-2) with a duration of between 5 and 90 seconds.
2. The maximum amplitude of the event must be, at minimum, an 8 μV increase from the baseline limb EMG signal.
3. Events may cause arousals. Arousals are scored as long as they occur within 0.5 seconds of the movement.

RHYTHMIC MOVEMENT DISORDER

1. RMD will show a minimum of four individual clustered movements.
2. The amplitude of the activity will be twice that of the background EMG activity.
3. The frequency of RMD activity is 0.5 to 2.0 Hz.

See Figure 78-3 for an example of rhythmic movement activity.

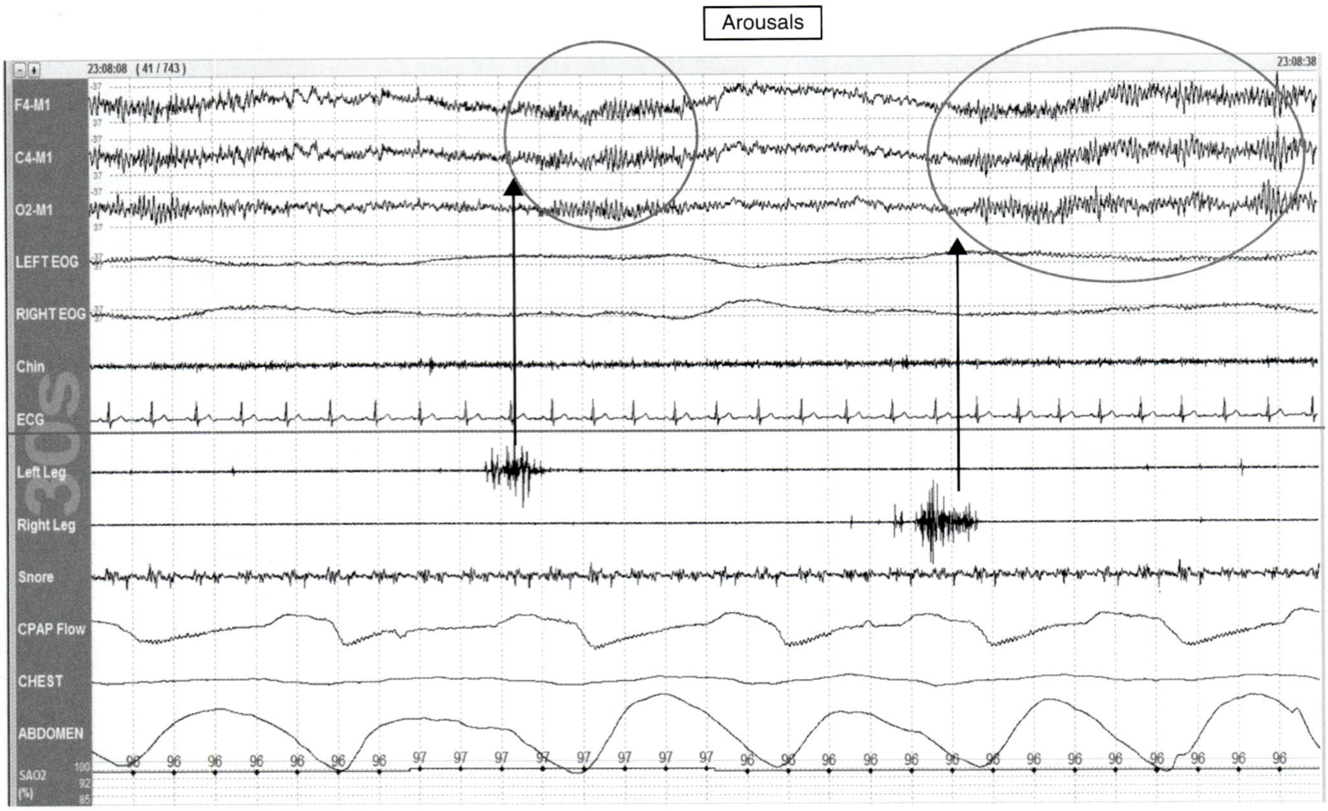

Figure 78-1 There is a greater than 8 μV increase in the leg electromyogram channels from baseline. The event duration is between 0.5 and 10 seconds. At the end of the movement event, there is an arousal.

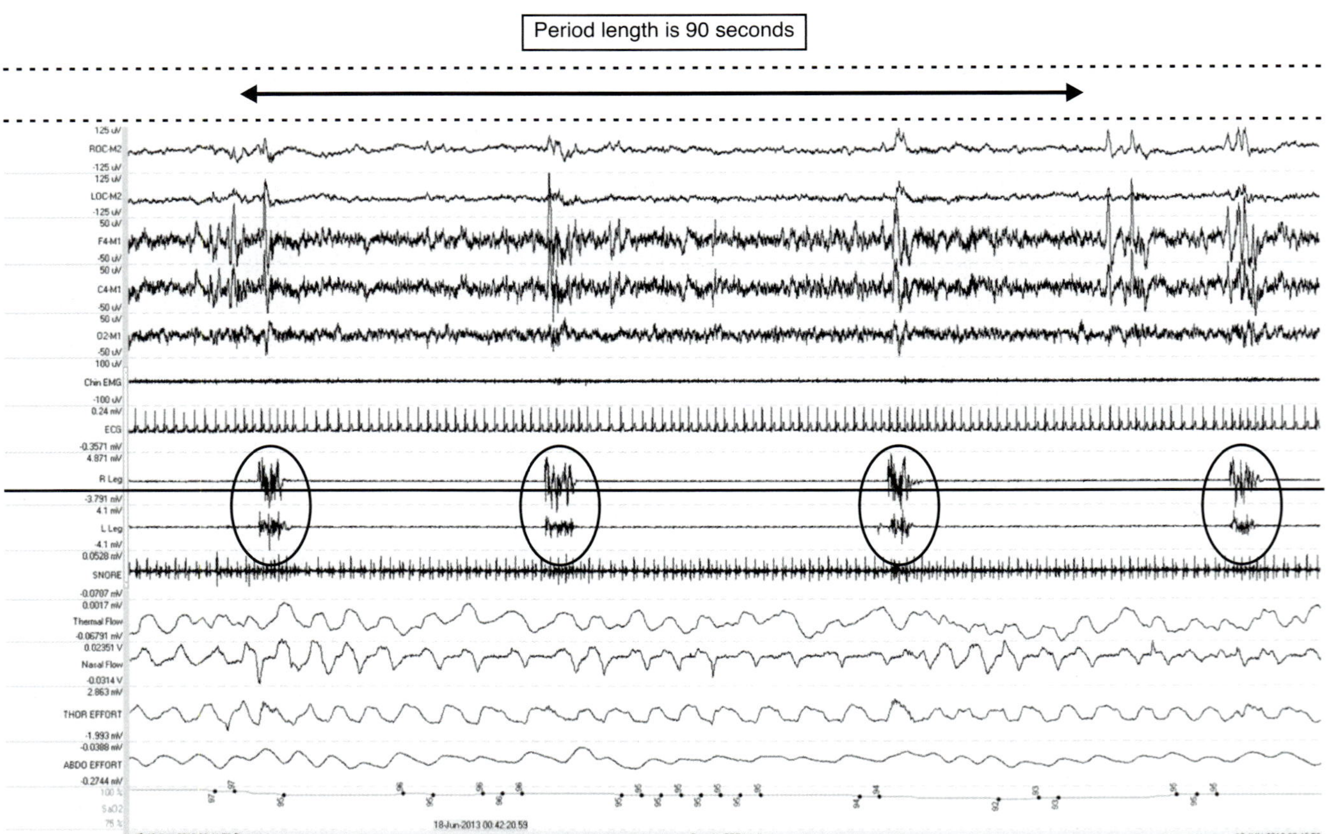

Figure 78-2 There is a greater than 8 μV increase from baseline. There are four leg movements. The period length is between 5 and 90 seconds. At the end of each movement event, there is an arousal.

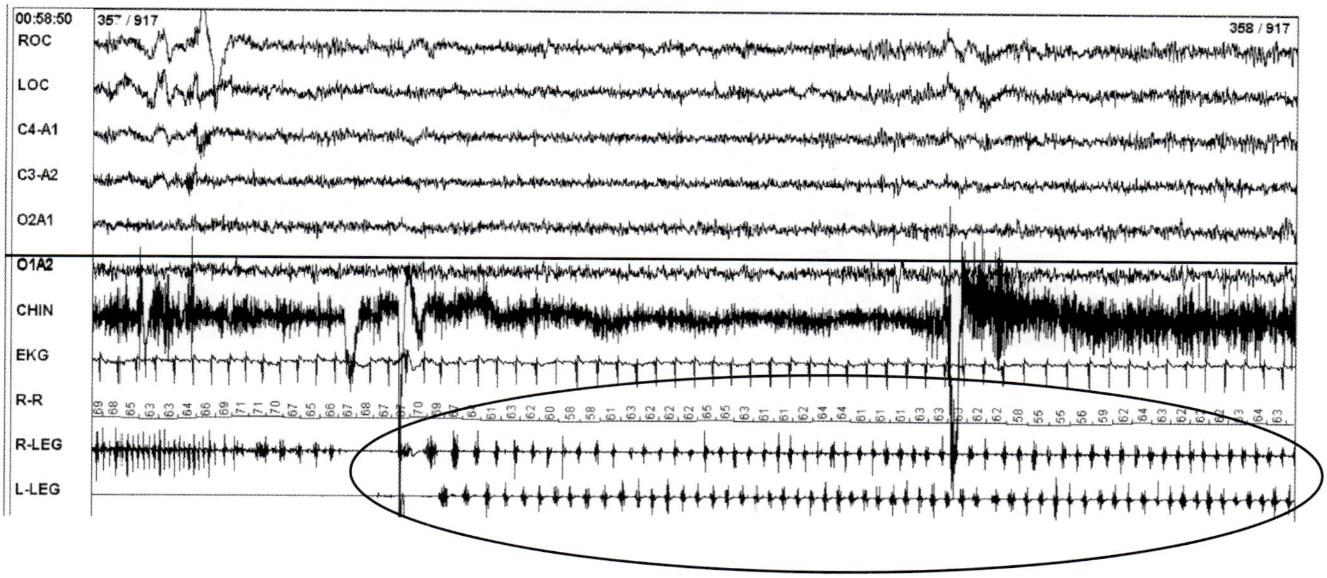

Figure 78-3 This epoch shows movements consistent with rhythmic movement disorder. There are more than four clustered movements. The activity is twice the amplitude of the baseline electromyogram activity.

LEG MOVEMENTS WITH RESPIRATORY EVENTS

1. Leg movements may occur in conjunction with respiratory events. It is important to know whether the leg movement or the respiratory event came first. Only one type of event is scored: either the limb movement or the respiratory event (Figure 78-4).
2. Leg movements should not be scored if they occur within 0.5 seconds before or after a respiratory event.

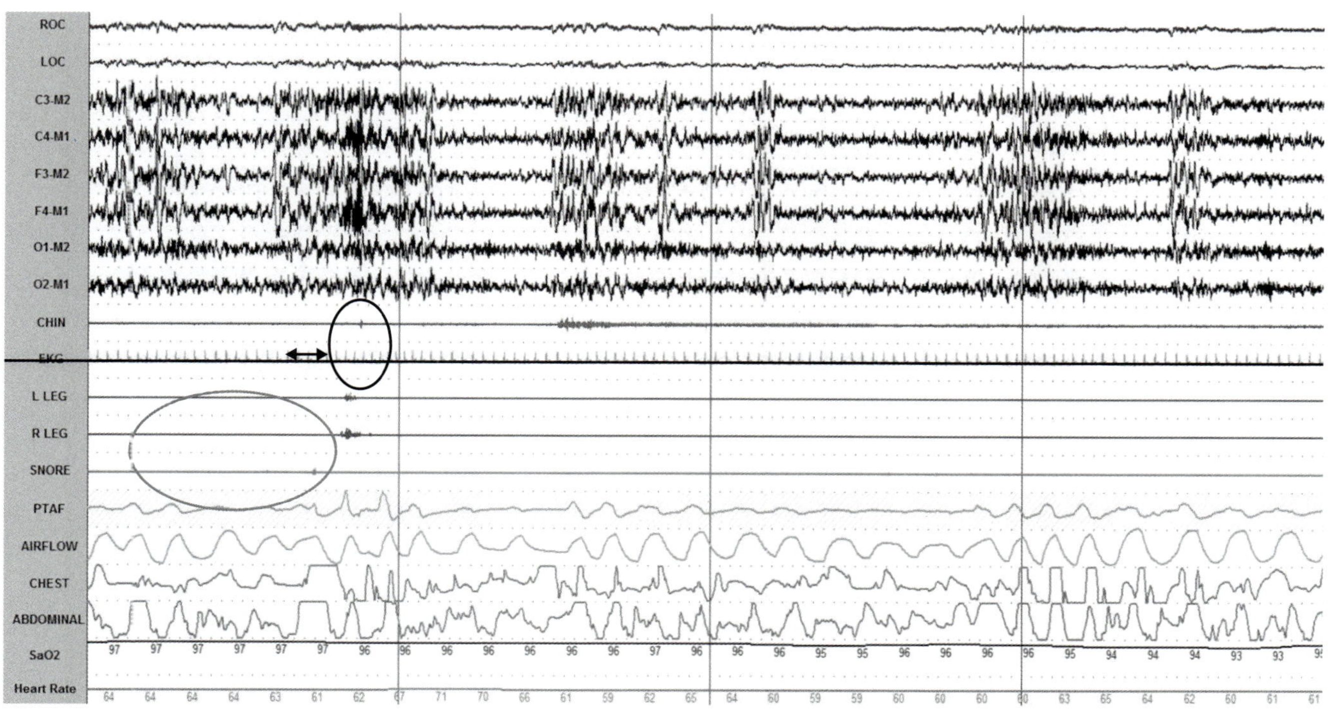

Figure 78-4 If a leg movement occurs within 0.5 seconds of a respiratory event, it is not scored. The respiratory event caused a leg movement at the end of this event.

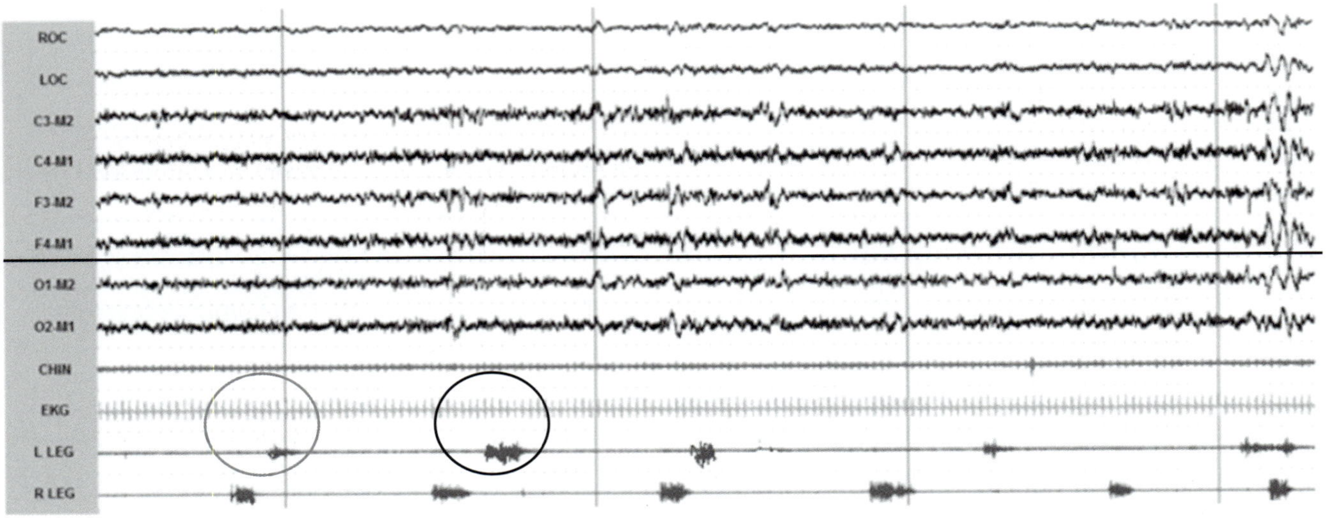

Figure 78-5 Alternating leg movement with a greater than 8 μV increase from baseline. There are four alternative leg muscle activations (ALMAs) circled in this figure. Each ALMA lasts between 100 and 500 ms.

ALTERNATIVE LEG MUSCLE ACTIVATION

1. Alternative leg muscle activation (ALMA) is defined as small bursts of muscle activity that alternate from one leg channel to the other.
2. For the activity to be considered ALMA, there must be a series of at least four alternating limb movements (Figure 78-5).
3. The frequency between ALMA events is 0.5 to 3.0 Hz, with a duration of 100 to 500 ms.
4. ALMA may also be a form of hypnagogic foot tremor (HFT).

HYPNAGOGIC FOOT TREMOR

1. HFT will show a series of at least four EMG bursts (Figure 78-6).
2. The frequency will be between 0.3 and 4.0 Hz.

BRUXISM

1. Bruxism is characterized by grinding or clenching of the teeth during sleep, usually associated with arousals from sleep.

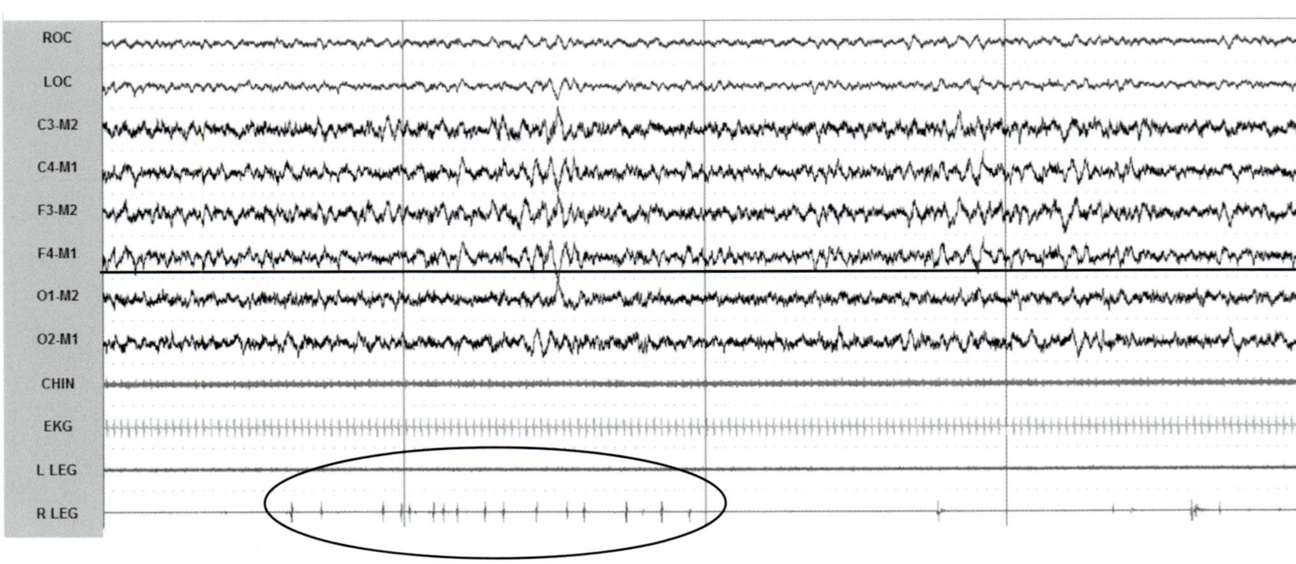

Figure 78-6 In this 120-second epoch, note the movements in the right leg channel. They meet the criteria to be scored as hypnagogic foot tremor.

2. The events consist of sustained (tonic) and phasic (brief) contractions of the jaw, usually 0.25 to 2 seconds in duration.
3. On the PSG, audio should be recorded to score bruxism more reliably.
4. A series of repetitive bruxism movements is called "rhythmic masticatory muscle activity."

See Figure 78-7 for an example of bruxism that was audible to the technologist and is reflected on the electroencephalogram (EEG) tracing as muscle activity in the EEG.

EXCESSIVE FRAGMENTARY MYOCLONUS

1. Excessive fragmentary myoclonus (EFM) is described as a benign movement. It is reported as not having any clinical consequences. See Figure 78-8 for an example of EFM activity.
2. The EMG burst duration is 150 ms.
3. A minimum of five EMG potentials per minute must be recorded.
4. During the PSG recording, 20 minutes of EFM activity must be seen during nonrapid eye movement (NREM) sleep in order to score EFM.

RAPID EYE MOVEMENT SLEEP BEHAVIOR DISORDER

Rapid eye movement sleep behavior disorder (RBD) is parasomnia that occurs in REM sleep where normal paralysis in REM is absent or incomplete. During REM sleep, RBD can be scored when the following criteria are present:

1. Sustained chin EMG muscle activity in REM sleep. The epoch will show at least 50% duration of chin EMG activity greater than the minimum amplitude seen in NREM sleep.
2. Excessive transient muscle activity occurring during REM sleep in the chin or limb EMG channels. The epoch will show bursts of EMG activity lasting 0.1 to 5.0 seconds with an amplitude that is 4 times greater than the background EMG activity.

Figures 78-9 and 78-10 are examples of scorable transient and sustained excessive EMG activity during REM sleep, respectively.

MOVEMENT ARTIFACTS

When recording and scoring movement events, it is important to evaluate the proper signals to determine what type of event is occurring. Physiologic signals such as electrocardiogram can obscure the desired activity and

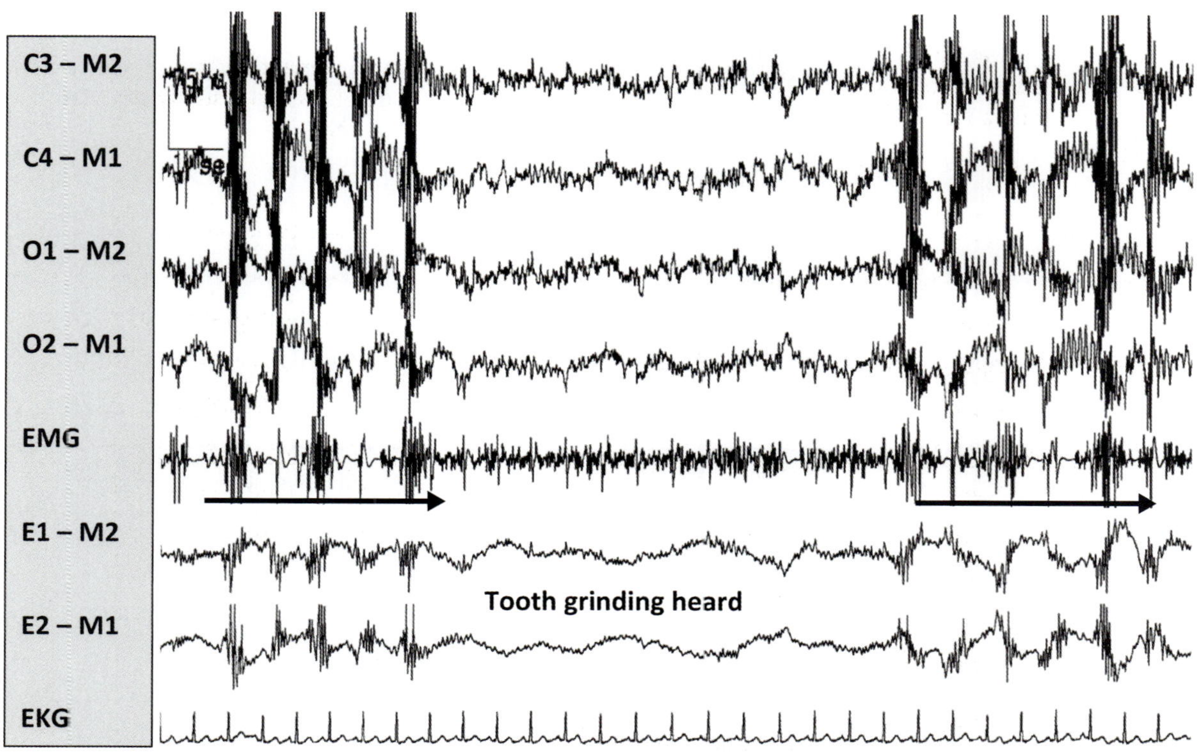

Figure 78-7 This is an example of bruxism reflected in the electroencephalogram channels. The technologist notes that audible tooth grinding was heard. EKG, electrocardiography; EMG, electromyograph.

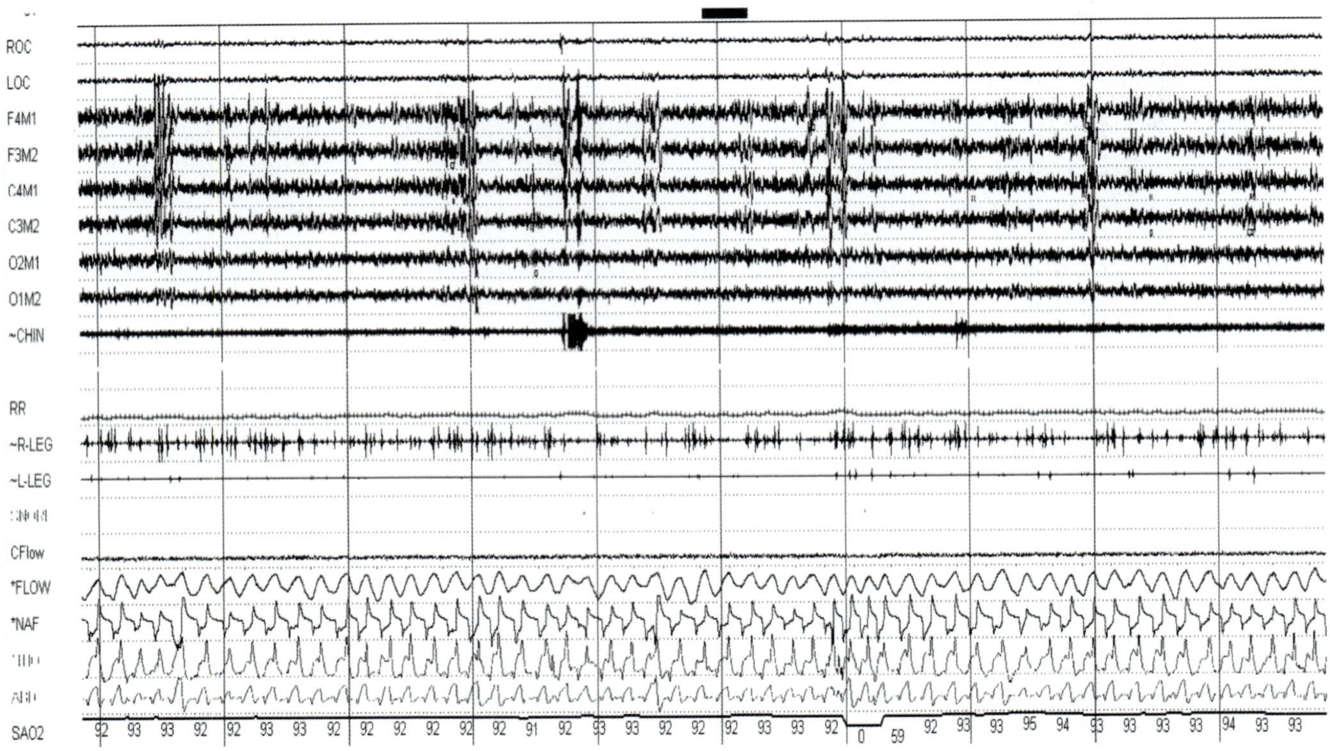

Figure 78-8 This is an example of excessive fragmentary myoclonus in the right leg electromyogram channel.

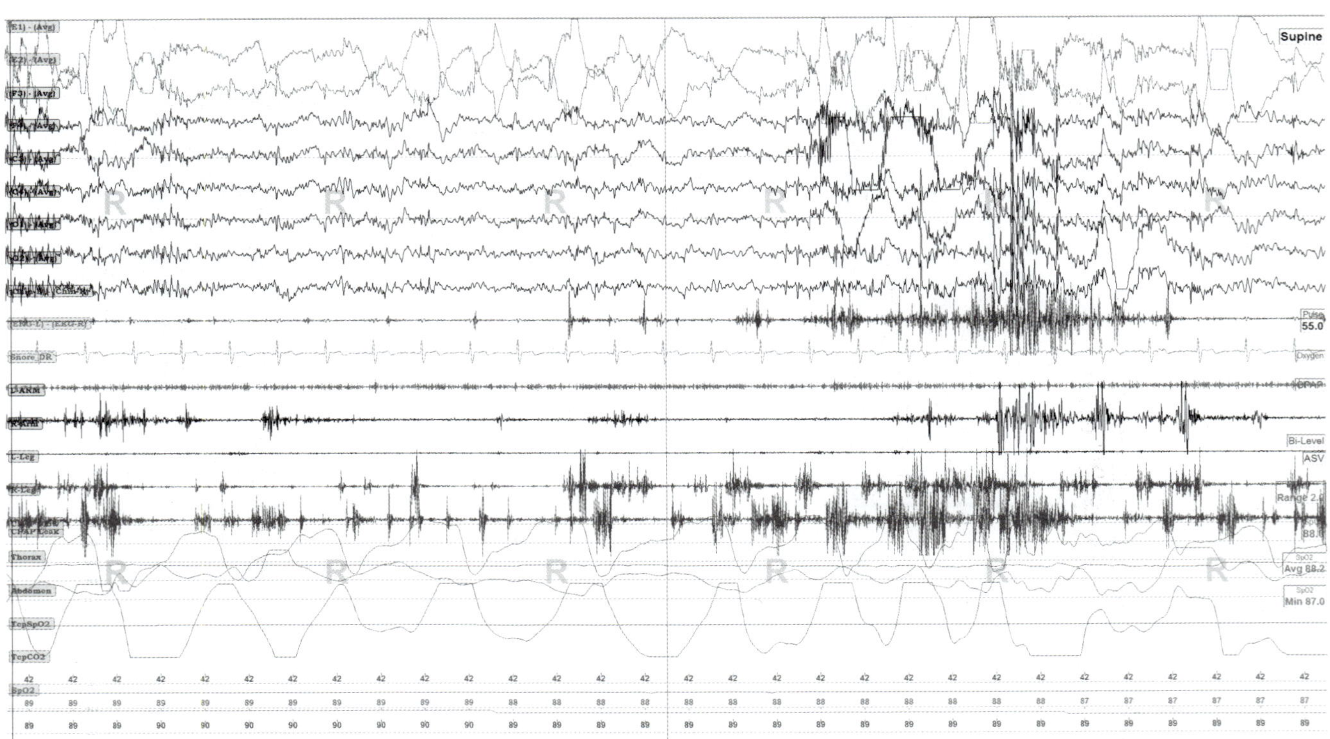

Figure 78-9 A 60-second sample of excessive chin and limb electromyogram activity during rapid eye movement (REM) sleep consistent with scorable transient muscle activity seen in REM behavior disorder.

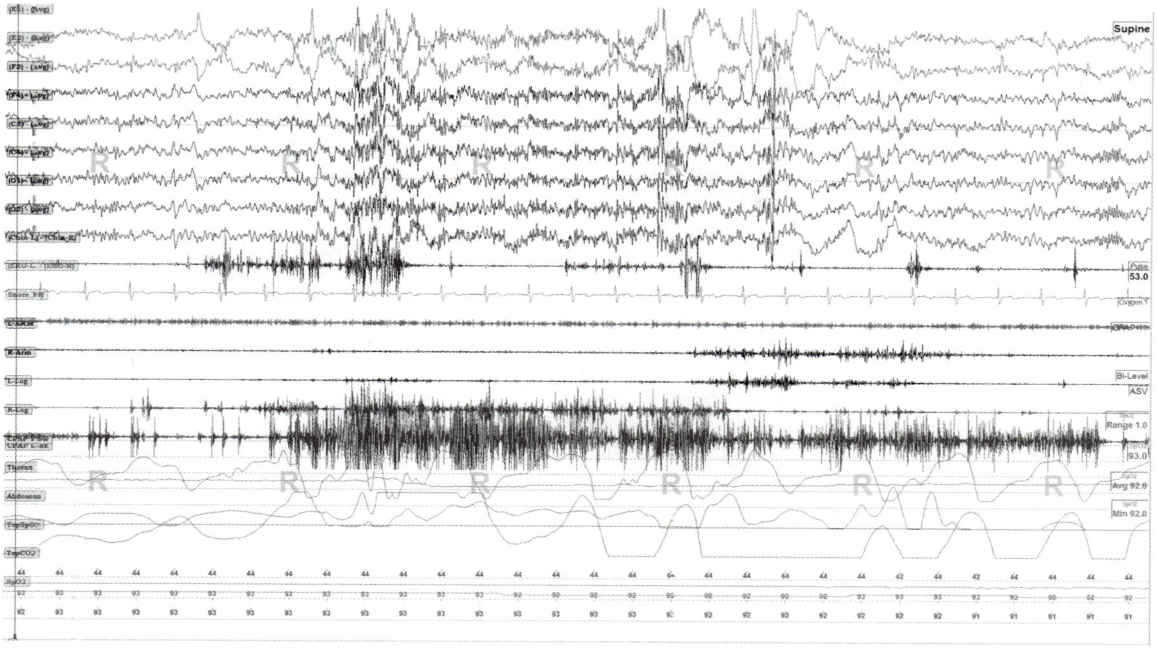

Figure 78-10 A 30-second epoch showing excessive chin and limb electromyogram activity during rapid eye movement (REM) sleep consistent with a scorable epoch of sustained muscle activity consistent with REM behavior disorder.

make it difficult or impossible to score limb movements (Figure 78-11). Patient movement itself can obscure activity in all of the channels, as seen in Figure 78-12.

If there are few working signals, poor signals, or artifact in the channels, this will prevent identifying or scoring significant movements occurring during sleep.

SUMMARY

Scoring movements in sleep can be challenging, even when the primary events being scored routinely are simple PLMS. Most importantly, the EMG signals recorded to assess movement disorders must be obtained using

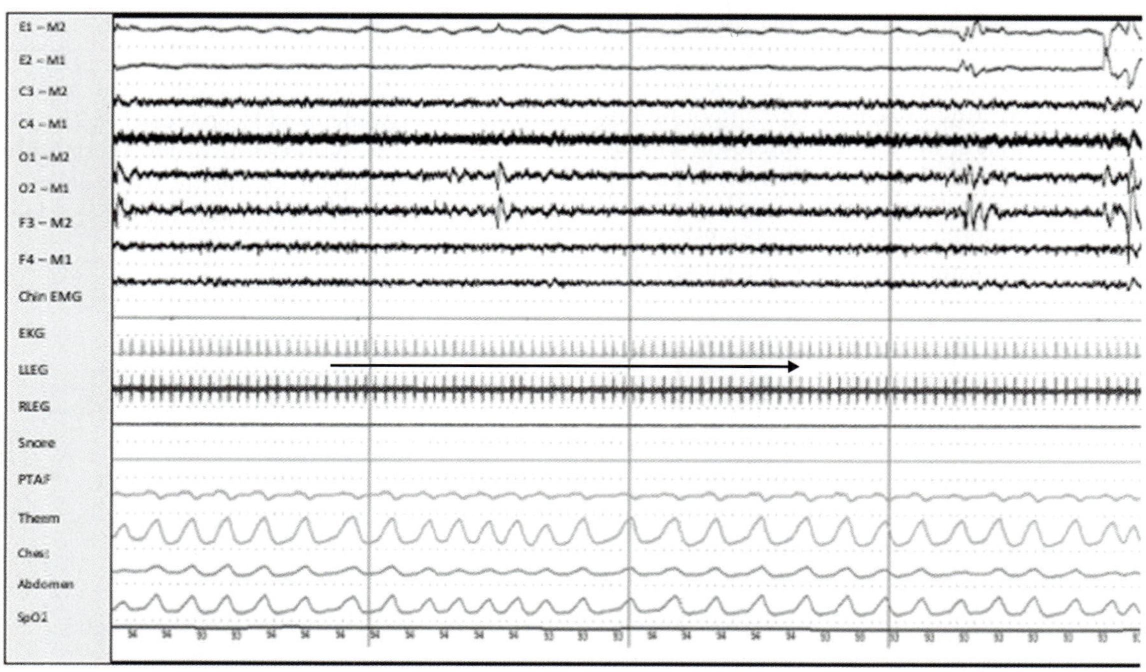

Figure 78-11 In this 120-second epoch, there is electrocardiogram artifact in the left leg channel. This artifact may mask any leg movements that might be occurring, such as REM sleep motor disorder. REM, rapid eye movement.

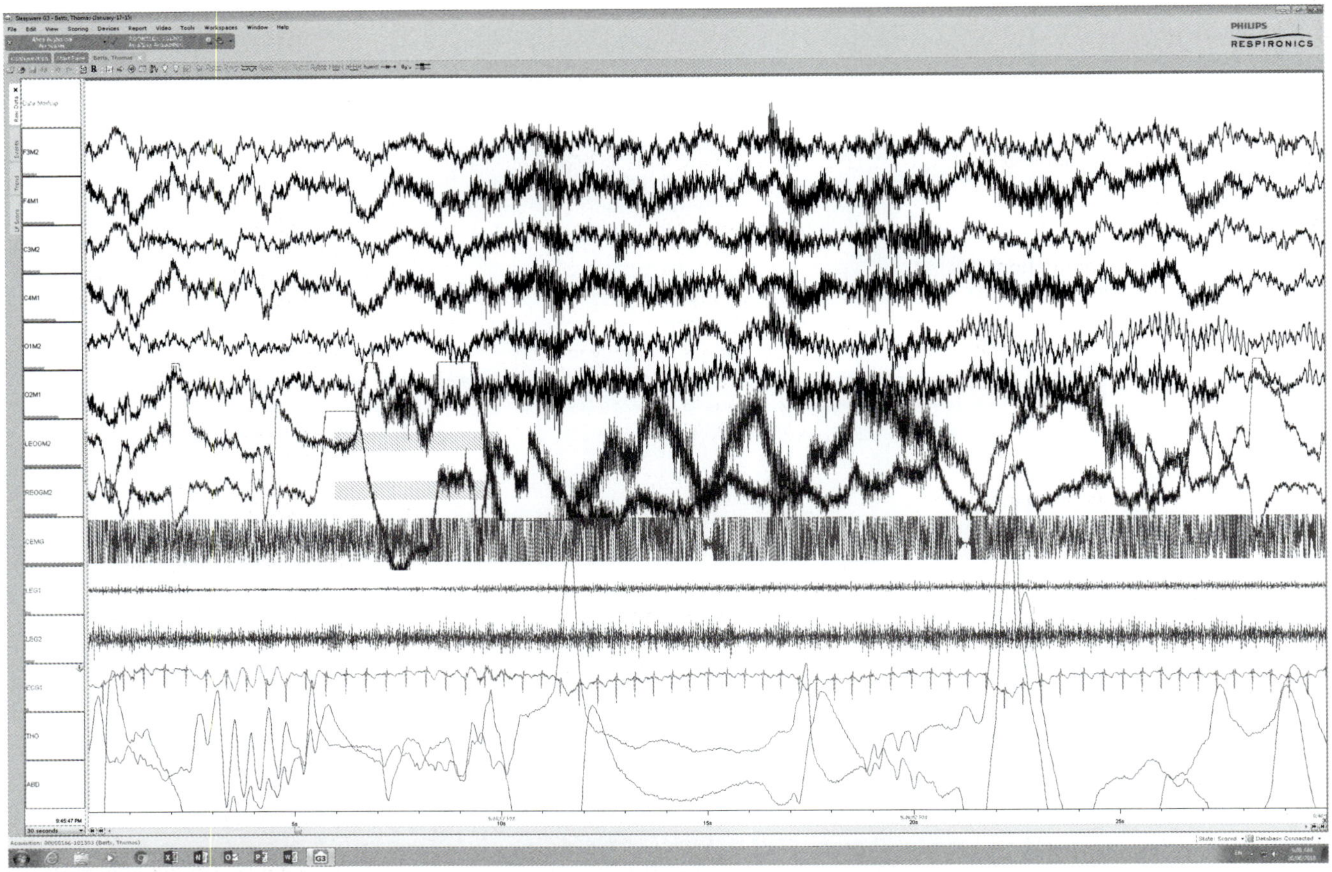

Figure 78-12 This is an example of a movement artifact that obscures the entire epoch.

appropriate electrodes and accurate placements. The scorer must be well versed in general sleep and arousal scoring as well as respiratory event scoring to accurately score PLMS. Scoring RBD, bruxism, and other unusual movements that are not so commonly seen may require a review of the scoring rules. Both the recording and the scoring technologist should always be aware of the patient history and the indication for the PSG in order to ensure that unusual events are not missed and that the patient receives an appropriate diagnosis.

REFERENCE

1. Troester MM, Quan SF, Berry, RB, et al; for the American Academy of Sleep Medicine. *The AASM Manual for the Scoring of Sleep and Associated Events: Rules, Terminology and Technical Specifications* [Version 3.0]. American Academy of Sleep Medicine; 2023.

Index

Note: Page numbers those followed by "*f*" denote figures and those followed by "*t*" denote tables

A

D

E

F

I

J

K

L

M

N

O

P

Q

R

S

T

QUADM0426